S0-BSF-367

PEDIATRIC TRANSPORT MEDICINE

PEDIATRIC TRANSPORT MEDICINE

KARIN A.L. MCCLOSKEY, MD
Associate Professor of Pediatrics
Division of Pediatric Emergency Medicine
The University of Texas
Southwestern Medical Center at Dallas
Children's Medical Center of Dallas
Dallas, Texas

RICHARD A. ORR, MD, FAAP
Associate Director, Pediatric Intensive Care
Medical Director, Pediatric Transport
Children's Hospital of Pittsburgh
Associate Professor, Anesthesiology/Critical Care Medicine and Pediatrics
University of Pittsburgh School of Medicine
Pittsburgh, Pennsylvania

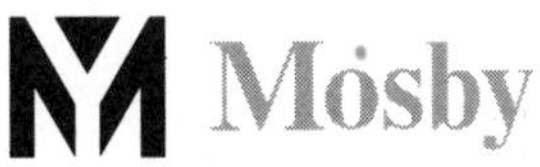

St. Louis Baltimore Boston Carlsbad Chicago Naples New York Philadelphia Portland
London Madrid Mexico City Singapore Sydney Tokyo Toronto Wiesbaden

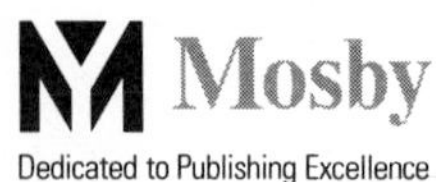

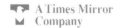

Editor: Laurel Craven
Developmental Editor: Dana Battaglia
Project Manager: Chris Baumle
Senior Production Editor: Shannon Canty
Manufacturing Supervisor: Betty Richmond
Design Manager: Sheilah Barrett

Printed in the United States of America
Composition by Progressive Information Technologies
Printing/binding by Maple-Vail

Mosby–Year Book, Inc.
11830 Westline Industrial Drive
St. Louis, MO 63146

Library of Congress Cataloging-in-Publication Data
Pediatric transport medicine / [edited by] Karin McCloskey, Richard Orr.
p. cm.
Includes bibliographical references and index.
ISBN 0-8016-7817-X
1. Interhospital transport of children—United States.
2. Pediatric emergency services—United States. I. McCloskey, Karin. II. Orr, Richard, 1951–
[DNLM: 1. Transportation of Patients—organization & administration—United States. 2. Emergency Medical Services—organization & administration—United States. 3. Patient Care Team—organization & administration—United States.
4. Emergencies—in infancy & childhood. WX 215 P371 1995]
RA995.5.A1P43 1995
362.1′9892—dc20
DNLM/DLC
for Library of Congress 94-41980
CIP

95 96 97 98 99 / 9 8 7 6 5 4 3 2 1

DEDICATION

To Mom, Da (who dedicated *his* last book to me), and "little brother" Wynn, whose love and support helped make this book possible.

Karin McCloskey, M.D.

To my God, the true author and sustainer of life, my wife, Margie, and my children, Jessica, Nathaniel, Rebekah, Hannah, and Joshua.

Richard Orr, M.D.

ACKNOWLEDGMENTS

This text has been produced through the efforts of many people who, unlike our contributors, go unrecognized. We would like to give thanks to our colleagues, friends and families who tolerated us with cheerful good humor and provided the needed supportive environment throughout the two years of this project. This includes, but is far from limited to: Dr. Carden Johnston, Linda Hambright, Jan Terry, David Patton, Dr. Michele Nichols, Dr. Lori Byron, Dr. Susan Day, Dr. Mary Pat Hemstreet, Andrea Rahl, and Marilyn Gilman.

Special thanks to those contributors and colleagues who assisted in review of chapters other than their own, or who offered their help with last minute challenges: Dr. Michele Nichols, Mary Gomez, and Dr. David Jaimovich.

Dr. Byron Aoki, who knows how many years later this book would have been written were it not for your intellectual stimulation and hard work on the transport manual whose publication directly led to development of this textbook project.

Thanks to our Editors, Dana Battaglia, Laurel Craven, and Stephanie Manning, for helping us maneuver through the maze of every step of this project, from proposal to publication.

Last, but definitely not least, great thanks to Sandra Shepherd who has read, typed, edited, and/or copied virtually every one of these 900 pages.

PREFACE

To the first edition of textbook entitled, "Pediatric Transport Medicine":

In 1969 an article on the topic of interhospital transport of children suggested that a tank of oxygen be taken on the trip and that the child's fever be reduced prior to transport. Since that time we have seen the advent of hospital-based medical helicopter services and mobile intensive care units with subspecialty teams in Neonatology, Pediatrics, and Adult Cardiac Care. Organizations have developed which are dedicated to the field of air transport (Association for Air Medical Services) and pediatric transport (American Academy of Pediatrics Section on Transport Medicine). Initially, most of the new transport systems were primarily designed for stabilization and immediate transport to a tertiary care center for victims of multiple trauma and myocardial infarction. In the past decade, Pediatric Intensive Care Units (PICUs) have become increasingly sophisticated and regionalized, and have been demonstrated to reduce morbidity and mortality for patients able to reach their services. Unfortunately, most critical childhood illnesses and injuries do not occur in proximity to a pediatric tertiary care center, and the child must spend minutes to hours in moving vehicles between hospitals. The quality of care received during transfer can make or break the ability of the PICU to provide an optimal outcome.

In the past five years, national educational conferences on the topic of neonatal and pediatric interhospital transport have proliferated, the AAP has appointed a Task Force on Interhospital Transport to review and revise existing guidelines for pediatric transport, more than a dozen articles on pediatric transport research have appeared in peer reviewed journals, the AAP Section on Transport Medicine has been established, a Critical Care Clinics issue has been devoted to pediatric transport, and Mosby–Year Book has published the first practical reference for caring for children before and during transport (*Evaluation, Stabilization and Transport of the Critically Ill Child,* Mosby–Year Book, February 1992). Fellowships in Pediatric Transport Medicine are being offered in conjunction with Pediatric Emergency Medicine Fellowships, dedicated pediatric transport physicians are being hired in some systems, and experience in transport has been added to the fellowship curriculum for Pediatric Critical Care and Pediatric Emergency Medicine. The tremendous interest in this new field of medicine has led to exponentially increasing research efforts and to a proliferation of teams wishing to transport children and to do it well.

Now this burgeoning field needs a definitive state-of-the-art textbook, designed as a reference for those starting a pediatric team, administering an existing pediatric team and planning medical management of children during transport, whether by a dedicated pediatric team or one with a more general focus.

The contributors to this text are physicians, nurses, paramedics and administrators currently involved in the practice of pediatric transport and in the direction of pediatric transport systems. Many of the physicians and all of the nurses participate in actual transports as well as practicing in pediatric subspecialty fields. This combination lends the unique perspective of indepth knowledge of a particular pediatric specialty (i.e., cardiology, pulmonary, etc.) combined with an understanding of the hands-on practicality of trying. to apply that knowledge to the outside-the-tertiary-care-center patient in a moving vehicle.

We hope that you find this text a useful tool in managing the transport of pediatric patients. Our goal is to provide information which will ultimately bring children to tertiary care in the most stable condition possible, ready to let all the forces of pediatric subspecialists have their best chance of providing an optimal ultimate outcome.

CONTRIBUTORS

NEEL ACKERMAN, JR., MD, FAAP
Medical Director, Neonatal Transport and North Texas Regional ECMO Center
Department of Pediatrics
Division of Neonatology
Presbyterian Hospital of Dallas
North Texas Neonatal Associates
Dallas, Texas

KENDRA BALAZS, RN, BSN, CCRN
Director, Medical Flight Services Administration
Samaritan AirEvac
Phoenix, Arizona

NICHOLAS BENSON, MD
Associate Professor and Vice Chair
Department of Emergency Medicine
East Carolina University School of Medicine
Greenville, North Carolina
Medical Director
Office of Emergency Medical Services
North Carolina Department of Human Resources
Raleigh, North Carolina

DEBRA M. BILLS, RN
Transport Nurse
Transport Team
Children's Hospital of Pittsburgh
Pittsburgh, Pennsylvania

ROBERT BOLTE, MD
Associate Professor of Pediatrics
University of Utah School of Medicine
Co-Director, Emergency Services
Primary Children's Medical Center
Salt Lake City, Utah

CHARLES W. BREAUX, JR., MD
Pediatric Surgery
The Children's Hospital of Alabama
Birmingham, Alabama

DENNIS BRIMHALL
President
University of Colorado Hospital Authority
Denver, Colorado

MARY BUSER-GILLS, RN, MS, NNP
Nursing Director
Children's Emergency Transport System
The Children's Hospital
Denver, Colorado

LORI G. BYRON, MD
Pediatrician, Indian Health Service
Crow Agency Public Health Service Hospital
Crow Agency, Montana

MICHAEL I. CINOMAN, MD
Fellow
Pediatric Critical Care Medicine
Children's Hospital of Pittsburgh
Pittsburgh, Pennsylvania

ROBERT S.B. CLARK, MD
Fellow
Pediatric Critical Care Medicine
Children's Hospital of Pittsburgh
Pittsburgh, Pennsylvania

ARTHUR COOPER, MD
Associate Professor of Clinical Surgery
College of Physicians & Surgeons of Columbia University
Chief of Pediatric Surgical Critical Care
Harlem Hospital Center
New York, New York

PAUL DAVIS, MD
Medical Rescue International
Braamfontein, Johannesburg
South Africa

SUSAN E. DAY, MD
Associate Professor of Pediatrics
Medical College of Wisconsin
Associate Medical Director, PICU
Co-Director, ECMO Program
Medical Director, Transport Program
Children's Hospital of Wisconsin
Milwaukee, Wisconsin

JOSEPH V. DOBSON, MD
Pediatric Emergency Physician
Maricopa County Medical Center
Phoenix, Arizona

DENNIS R. DURBIN, MD
Assistant Professor of Pediatrics
Senior Scholar, Center for Clinical Epidemiology and Biostatistics
University of Pennsylvania School of Medicine
Attending Physician Emergency Department
The Children's Hospital of Philadelphia
Philadelphia, Pennsylvania

DAVID N. FINEGOLD, MD
Associate Professor
Department of Pediatrics
University of Pittsburgh School of Medicine
Pittsburgh, Pennsylvania

GEORGE L. FOLTIN, MD, FAAP, FACEP
Director
Pediatric Emergency Medicine
Bellevue Hospital Center
New York City Medical Center
Assistant Professor of Clinical Pediatrics
Department of Pediatrics
New York University School of Medicine
New York, New York

ANGELO P. GIARDINO, MD, MSEd
Clinical Assistant Professor
Department of Pediatrics
Division of General Pediatrics
Children's Hospital of Philadelphia
Vice President for Ambulatory and Managed Care
Children's Seashore House
Philadelphia, Pennsylvania

BARBARA GOLZ, RNC, MS, NNP
Neonatal Nurse Practitioner
The Children's Hospital
Denver, Colorado

MARY GOMEZ, RN
Transport Nurse
Transport Team
Children's Memorial Hospital
Chicago, Illinois

ALVIN HACKEL, MD
Professor of Anesthesia and Pediatrics
Department of Anesthesia
Stanford University School of Medicine
Director
Northern California Perinatal Dispatch Center
Stanford, California

DANIEL M. HALL, MD
Associate Professor of Pediatrics
University of Colorado Health Sciences Center
Medical Director, Newborn Center
The Children's Hospital
Denver, Colorado

LINDA H. HAMBRIGHT, RN, EMT-P
Critical Care Transport Coordinator
Critical Care Transport
The Children's Hospital of Alabama
Birmingham, Alabama

KAREN N. (BATES) HAMILTON, RNC, CEN, CCRN, CFRN, MICN, NREMT-P
Chief Flight Nurse/Program Director
Aeromedical Transport Specialists, Inc.
Washington, DC
Los Angeles, California
Dallas, Texas

WILLIAM E. HARDWICK, JR., MD
Assistant Professor
Department of Pediatrics
The Children's Hospital of Alabama
The University of Alabama in Birmingham
Birmingham, Alabama

HARRIET HAWKINS, RN
Neonatal/Pediatric Transport Nurse
Transport Team
Children's Memorial Hospital
Chicago, Illinois

SUSAN M. HERRON, RN
Chief Executive Officer
AirEvac for Tulsa, Inc.
Tulsa, Oklahoma

DAVID JAIMOVICH, MD
Medical Director Transport Program
Section Head, Division Pediatric Critical Care
Department of Pediatrics
Christ Hospital and Medical Center
Oak Lawn, Illinois
Assistant Professor of Pediatrics
Rush Medical College
Chicago, Illinois

KAREN JOHNSON, RN
Adult/Pediatrics Flight Nurse—CN II
Samaritan Air Evac
Samaritan Health Services
Phoenix, Arizona

CARDEN JOHNSTON, MD
Professor of Pediatrics
Department of Pediatrics
University of Alabama at Birmingham
Children's Hospital of Alabama
Birmingham, Alabama

MADELINE M. JOSEPH, MD
Assistant Professor
Pediatric Emergency Medicine
University of Florida
Health Science Center in Jacksonville
Jacksonville, Florida

SUSAN L. KACZOROWSKI, MD
Fellow
Pediatric Critical Care Medicine
Children's Hospital of Pittsburgh
Pittsburgh, Pennsylvania

ROBERT K. KANTER, MD
Chapel Hill, North Carolina

VALERIE A. KARR

JOHN P. KINSELLA, MD
Assistant Professor
Division of Neonatology
Department of Pediatrics
University of Colorado School of Medicine
Assistant Director
Children's Emergency Transport Service
The Children's Hospital
Denver, Colorado

ELIZABETH KIRBY, RNC, NNP, MS
Neonatal Nurse Practitioner
Children's Emergency Transport System
The Children's Hospital
Denver, Colorado

KAREN KLEIN, RN, MSN
Staff Nurse
Emergency Department
Shadyside Hospital
Pittsburgh, Pennsylvania

PATRICK M. KOCHANEK, MD
Associate Professor
Anesthesiology/CCM and Pediatrics
University of Pittsburgh School of Medicine
Pittsburgh, Pennsylvania

STEVEN E. KRUG, MD
Director, Pediatric Emergency Medicine
Children's Hospital & Health Center
Associate Professor of Pediatrics
University of California, San Diego
San Diego, California

FORD N. KYES, RN, MPM
Director, Emergency/Trauma Services
St. Joseph's Hospital
Tampa, Florida

ROBERT B. LEMBERSKY, MD
Fellow, Pediatric Emergency Medicine
University of Alabama School of Medicine
Birmingham, Alabama

JAMES M. LYNCH, MD
Assistant Professor of Pediatric Surgery
Department of Surgery
University of Pittsburgh School of Medicine
Director, Benedum Pediatric Trauma Program
Department of Pediatric Surgery
Children's Hospital of Pittsburgh
Pittsburgh, Pennsylvania

ROBERT T. MANSFIELD, MD
Fellow
Pediatric Critical Care Medicine
Children's Hospital of Pittsburgh
Pittsburgh, Pennsylvania

DONALD W. MARION, MD
Assistant Professor
Neurological Surgery
University of Pittsburgh School of Medicine
Pittsburgh, Pennsylvania

CONSTANCE McANENEY, MD
Assistant Professor of Pediatrics
University of Cincinnati
College of Medicine
Attending Physician
Division of Emergency Medicine
Children's Hospital Medical Center
Cincinnati, Ohio

BENNIE McWILLIAMS, MD
Associate Professor of Pediatrics
University of New Mexico School of Medicine
Director, Pediatric Pulmonary Division
Department of Pediatrics
Albuquerque, New Mexico

SARAH NORWOOD MOORMAN, RN, MSN
Pedictric Consultant
Highsmith-Rainey
Memorial Hospital
Fayetteville, North Carolina

M. MICHELE MOSS, MD
Associate Professor of Pediatrics
Divisions of Critical Care and Cardiology
University of Arkansas for Medical Services
Medical Director of Pediatric Transport Service
Attending Physician, Pediatric and Cardiovascular Intensive Care Units
Arkansas Children's Hospital
Little Rock, Arkansas

DAVID V. MYERS, PhD
Clinical Psychologist
Pilot, Atlantic Southeast Airline
Tuscaloosa, Alabama

ZEHAVA NOAH, MD
Attending Physician, Division of Pediatric Critical Care
Department of Medicine
The Children's Memorial Hospital
Assistant Professor of Pediatrics and Anesthesia
Department of Pediatrics and Anesthesia
Northwestern University Medical School
Chicago, Illinois

DANIEL A. NOTTERMAN, MD
Director, Division of Pediatric Critical Care Medicine
Department of Pediatrics
The New York Hospital—Cornell Medical Center
New York, New York
Research Scientist
Department of Molecular Biology
Princeton, New Jersey

ANTHONY L. PEARSON-SHAVER, MD
Assistant Professor
Department of Pediatrics
Medical College of Georgia, School of Medicine
Augusta, Georgia

CATHERINE PETERSON, AS, RRT
Flight Respiratory Therapist
Respiratory Therapy
Samaritan AirEvac
Phoenix, Arizona

LAURA PHILLIPS, MD
Instructor, Department of Pediatrics
University of Arkansas for Medical Sciences
Arkansas Children's Hospital
Little Rock, Arkansas

IAN F. POLLACK, MD
Assistant Professor
Neurological Surgery
University of Pittsburgh School of Medicine
Pittsburgh, Pennsylvania

STEVEN PON, MD
Assistant Professor
Pediatric Critical Care Medicine
Cornell University Medical Center
New York, New York

KEVIN RAGOSTA, DO
Pediatric Critical Care Medicine
State University of New York
Health Science Center—Syracuse
Syracuse, New York

JAY S. RODEN, MD
Clinical Assistant Professor of Surgery
Southwestern Medical School
University of Texas
Dallas, Texas

MITCHELL R. ROSS
Assistant Professor of Pediatrics
Department of Pediatrics
University of Louisville
Louisville, Kentucky

ROBERT S. ROTH, MD
Associate Clinical Professor of Pediatrics
Medical Director of Pediatric Transport
Department of Pediatrics
University of California, San Francisco
San Francisco, California

JEFFREY S. RUBENSTEIN, MD
Associate Professor of Pediatrics
Chief, Division of Pediatric Critical Care
Department of Pediatrics
University of Rochester School of Medicine and Dentistry
Rochester, New York

FERNANDO STEIN, MD
Associate Professor of Clinical Pediatrics
Department of Pediatrics
Baylor College of Medicine
Medical Director of Progressive Care Unit
Deputy Director of Pediatric Intensive Care Unit
Department of Pediatrics
Texas Children's Hospital
Houston, Texas

DAVID TELLEZ, MD
Associate Medical Director
Critical Care
Phoenix Children's Hospital
Director, Pediatric Medicine
Samaritan AirEvac
Phoenix, Arizona

JANET L. TERRY, RN, MSW, EMT-P
Critical Care Transport and Emergency Department
The Children's Hospital of Alabama
Birmingham, Alabama

DEBORA TRALMER, RN, NNP
Transport Coordinator
Baylor University Medical Center
Dallas, Texas

SHEKHAR T. VENKATARAMAN, MD
Assistant Professor
Anesthesiology/CCM
University of Pittsburgh
Medical Director
Respiratory Care
Children's Hospital of Pittsburgh
Pittsburgh, Pennsylvania

DONALD D. VERNON, MD
Associate Professor of Pediatrics
University of Utah
Division of Pediatric Critical Care
Primary Children's Hospital
Salt Lake City, Utah

ELIZABETH A. WALLEN

JONATHAN M. WHITFIELD, MD
Director Pediatric and Neonatal Critical Care
Department of Pediatrics
Baylor University Medical Center
Dallas, Texas

MICHAEL S. WILLIAMS, MA, BS, AS, EMT
Director
Florida Emergency Medical Services
Florida Department of Health and Rehabilitative Services
Tallahassee, Florida

GEORGE A. WOODWARD, MD
Director of Transport Services
Department of Pediatrics
The Children's Hospital of Philadelphia
Philadelphia, Pennsylvania

PAUL WRIGHT, RRT, EMT-P
Flight Respiratory Therapist
Respiratory Therapy
Samaritan AirEvac
Phoenix, Arizona

LINDA YOUNG, RN, MNA
Manager, CQI/Research
Samaritan AirEvac
Phoenix, Arizona

BARBARA J. YOUNGBERG
Vice President
Insurance, Risk & Quality Management
University Hospital Consortium
Oak Brook, Illinois

ARNO L. ZARITSKY, MD
Co-Director, Pediatric ICU
Children's Hospital of the King's Daughters
Eastern Virginia Medical School
Norfolk, Virgina

CONTENTS

PART I

PRINCIPLES

1

PEDIATRIC TRANSPORT MEDICINE: AN EMERGENCY SPECIALTY

KARIN A. MCCLOSKEY
RICHARD A. ORR

Increasing knowledge and skills in pediatric emergency medicine, pediatric critical care, and neonatology have led to the steadily improving ability to decrease morbidity and mortality from critical illnesses and injuries. Optimal care during initial stabilization and the first few hours of treatment are needed to allow sophisticated intensive care units to provide the best possible outcome. Most pediatric critical illnesses and injuries do not occur in close proximity to a pediatric tertiary care center. The child will often first be treated by prehospital care providers, a community hospital emergency department, and/or an interhospital transport system. Medical personnel at these three stages of treatment need specific training in and understanding of the principles of pediatric transport medicine.

The words *pediatric* and *transport* represent separate concepts crucial to differentiate in the field of pediatric medicine. This text addresses issues in both areas of the specialty. Transport medicine, while sharing many similarities, is different from in-hospital emergency medicine and critical care. It is important to understand 1) how the practice of medicine differs in the transport environment, 2) the effects of transport on the patient and the team, 3) equipment specifications for moving vehicles, 4) the unique communication issues in transport, and 5) relevant local, state, and federal regulations as they relate to air and ground transport. These issues apply to the transport of patients of all ages. Teams that transport pediatric patients must also understand and prepare for circumstances unique to children. In addition to the need for training and experience in pediatric transport, consideration must also be given to differences in referring hospital capabilities with regard to children (as opposed to adults), differences in equipment and medications, ability to treat small patients in a helicopter differences in medical control, medical direction and protocols, possible differences in team composition, and the emotional differences and needs in children of varying ages.

Pediatric transport medicine is a very new field. In the development of transport systems in general, specific concerns about pediatric patients have often been neglected. Of all patients transported by both local prehospital care teams and critical care interhospital teams, less than 15% are young children. Training and transport equipment for this group generally consume a disproportionate amount of time and usually quite limited financial resources. In major urban areas this problem has been addressed by the development of dedicated pediatric and neonatal transport teams. In much of the country, however, low pediatric patient volume does not support the development of such specialty teams.

Recognition of deficiencies in the field of pediatric medicine transport has led to its rapid expansion in the past decade. Research and education are advancing quickly. In fact, the field has progressed to the point where there is sufficient information available to fill a comprehensive text. This book is divided into three broad sections. The first addresses administrative issues in the development and management of air and ground systems that transport children. The second section covers the medical management of infants and children during transport. Finally, "miscellaneous" issues are addressed including prehospital and intrahospital transport, psychosocial concerns, community outreach, perspectives of different parties involved in transport, equipment choices, and others.

2

HISTORY OF MEDICAL TRANSPORT SYSTEMS: AIR, GROUND, AND PEDIATRIC

ALVIN HACKEL

EARLY HISTORY

Medical transport had its early beginnings in association with warfare. A counterpart of Napoleon, Barron Larrey, arranged "for the speedy evacuation of battle casualties by dedicated horse-drawn vehicles."[58] In 1834 an elementary form of ambulance was used in England.[43] During the American Civil War, railroad cars were used for medical transport. In the Siege of Paris in 1870, civilians were airlifted to hospitals by hot-air balloon.[92]

The first known aeromedical transports using fixed-wing aircraft were conducted in 1915 during World War I by the Serbian army.[58] Later, in World War I, the French and American armies also performed aeromedical evacuations. During these transports, the patients were carried in litters on the outside of the aircraft.[35]

The first American air ambulance crash occurred in Maryland in 1921; seven lives were lost. Although the development of aeromedical evacuation did not cease as a result of the crash, progress was slowed. Emergency aeromedical transport continued to be used in connection with warfare. The German Air Force used aeromedical evacuation during the Spanish Civil War in 1936 and in Poland in 1940.[58] By 1941, 840 patients had been transported in fixed-wing aircraft by the American Army Air Force.[35]

The first American long-distance aeromedical evacuation occurred in 1943 when five patients were transferred in a DC-3 transport plane to a B-54 transport plane from the 159th Station Hospital in Karachi, India, to the Walter Reed Hospital by the Air Transport Command. The trip took seven days. Two of the patients required litters and were placed on army cots, which were strapped to the floor of the planes. The patients were accompanied by a nurse who had no previous medical transport or flight experience! She was so tired on her arrival at the Walter Reed Hospital that she could not remember her name.[7]

The present level of American military medical transport sophistication was reached during the Korean War. The concept of the "golden hour," the time period in which severely wounded trauma victims can be transported for emergency care while receiving fluid resuscitation and airway management, was popularized. Soldiers wounded in the battlefield received prehospital care from paramedics and then were triaged to Mobile Army Surgical Hospital (MASH) units by helicopter within a 20 to 30 minute transport radius for more extensive emergency care. From there, they were transferred to more traditional hospital trauma units. Frequently, the larger hospital trauma units were within 1 hour of the battlefield. If more definitive care was required, the soldiers were transferred to military hospitals hundreds or thousands of miles away from the battlefield. To do this, jet aircraft, specially outfitted for intensive care en route, were used. The relationship between time, distance, and the level of required emergency and definitive care was transformed.[99]

Hospital-based critical care transport systems, including aeromedical transport for adult civilian patients, were initiated in Europe in the 1950s when anesthesiologist-led intensive care teams transported polio patients requiring ventilatory support to regional care centers.[14,15] The same group initiated a system of intercontinental "repatriation" of medical teams specializing in the transport of critically ill patients.[57,102]

The term "Critical Care Transport" was coined in 1970 to describe a concept of medical transport that had been newly introduced onto the American medical scene. Medical transport teams, composed of health-care personnel from the intensive care units of regional medical centers, provided patient care as an extension of the critical care provided in their intensive care units. The goal of this concept was to extend the services of the intensive care units to patients in community hospitals.

The American military trauma prehospital transport program developed in the Korean theater had a tremendous impact on American civilian sector emergency and trauma care. Similar programs for trauma were developed in the United States.[8,18,20,83,95] The definition of critical care transport was thus extended to include critically ill patients requiring emergency transport from a prehospital area to a nearby hospital and then to a regional center. More than 200 hospital-based prehospital and interhospital transport programs exist in the United States today.

NEWBORN TRANSPORT: THE BEGINNING OF THE MODERN ERA

In the United States, newborn transport had its beginning at the turn of the twentieth century when premature and "weakly-born" infants were transferred to hospitals such as the Chicago Lying-In Hospital for care in "ambulance incubators."[24] The first dedicated neonatal transport vehicle in the United States dates back to 1934. Until the 1960s, there was no significant change in neonatal transport. Infants born at home who required hospitalization were transferred by ambulance in small hand-carried incubators.[49]

In the 1960s, new therapeutic modalities were introduced for the treatment of Infant Respiratory Distress Syndrome. These therapeutic modalities, such as cardioactive drugs, aggressive fluid management, supplemental oxygenation, and assisted ventilation, could be performed only in regional intensive care facilities by personnel specially trained in neonatal intensive care. Dr. Robert Usher reported on the value of a regional program for newborn infants that employed these therapeutic modalities.[97] He studied the outcome of 32,000 infants born in Quebec and found a twofold difference in the mortality rate between infants cared for solely in community hospitals as compared to a population whose critically ill neonates were transferred to regional centers. As a result regional neonatal intensive care networks were established centering around intensive care nurseries with hospital-based critical care transport programs as an important component.

The early belief that a newborn infant had to demonstrate "the will to live" before transport between a community hospital and a neonatal intensive care facility would occur was replaced by one in which the techniques of resuscitation and acute intensive care were begun with all critically ill infants in the community hospital and continued during interhospital transport.

The leader in the neonatal intensive care regionalization movement was Dr. Joseph Butterfield at the Children's Hospital in Denver.[12] His regionalization program included community hospitals in five western states—a geographic expanse greater than the size of Western Europe. The program emphasized close communication between physicians in outlying hospitals and the regional intensive care unit. "Hotline" telephones were placed in the nurseries of the community hospitals in the network. These regional networks, with their transport programs as the linkage mechanism, provided the latest in neonatal intensive care. They were successful in reducing the perinatal mortality rate. As a result of their success, they have become a standard part of modern neonatal intensive care and have fostered similar programs for high-risk maternity and critically ill children.

THE MOVEMENT SPREADS

In the 1970s, medical transport systems were developed to provide safe and effective interfacility transfer of critically ill neonates, which rapidly became a central component of regional neonatal intensive care networks.[21,30,59,77,90] The transport teams were staffed by teams of physicians, nurses, and respiratory therapists who used both traditional (surface ambulance) and aeromedical transport carriers (helicopters, chartered fixed-wing aircraft, commerical intercontinental airliners).

In 1970 the Stanford University Hospital reorganized its neonatal transport program and added an aeromedical component.[38] On the first flights, an attending pediatric anesthesiologist or neonatologist, accompanied by a pediatric resident, flew in a Bell Jet Ranger helicopter to community hospitals in the region. (The Department of Nursing would not permit nurses to go on aeromedical transports because it was "too dangerous.") A lightweight, compact, transport incubator was specifically designed for the provision of intensive care with the maintenance of a neutral thermal environment. For helicopter transport, this incubator could be placed on the lap of a member of the transport team. A 500-liter capacity oxygen tank connected to an infant manual ventilation system was placed on the cabin floor at their feet. Shortly thereafter, the Stanford program began to use small, fixed-winged aircraft. Other neonatal aeromedical transport programs operated similar programs. Critical care transport became the central point of the advance into regional care.

Ambulance carriers were studied to determine whether the use of a dedicated ambulance with a customized interior design was appropriate for neonatal transport.[3,32,46] Ultimately, this concept was abandoned because of the expense of maintenance, the lack of full-time use, and the simultaneous need for more than one carrier on an irregular, but frequent basis.

Because of the large number of referrals, newborn intensive care units frequently were filled to capacity. To ensure that all patients requiring transport could be accommodated, regional triage and communication networks between neighboring newborn intensive care centers were formed. With such a network, prompt referrals could be made from one intensive care unit to another. The importance of communication was stressed.[10,29,67,76,78] One example was the California Perinatal Dispatch Center system developed with the assistance of the National Foundation and funded continuously since 1976.[39]

Today, treatment of the critically ill infant begins in the delivery room and continues in the neonatal intensive care unit. Because many community hospitals do not have the personnel, space, or facilities for long-term newborn critical care, transfer of the infant to a regional care center is often necessary. The interhospital transport of critically ill infants can be accomplished safely without an increase in mortality.[11,17] If the neonatal transport is performed by an intensive care team that provides the needed therapy, the variables of transport, including transport time and transport distance, need not have an effect on mortality.[40] An example of the ability to transport neonates over long distances without a significant negative effect on outcome was the successful transport of a neonate with cyanotic congenital heart disease by a Stanford neonatal transport team in 1975 from the Queen Elizabeth Hospital in Hong Kong to the Stanford University Hospital in California in a commercial Boeing 747 airliner—a distance of 8700 miles.

The demonstration that regional neonatal intensive care programs are of value formed an environment in which similar programs for older children could be created. Regional critical care for children began to emerge in the 1980s and followed the same pattern of development. With their evolution, the need for hospital-based pediatric critical care transport systems became obvious.[25,93] Today, intensive care transport systems for older children are an integral part of pediatric intensive care.

STAFF RECRUITMENT AND TEAM COMPOSITION: DEVELOPMENT OF THE ICU TEAM CONCEPT

As the field of pediatric transport medicine evolved in the 1970s, there was considerable discussion as to the optimal team composition. The goal was to provide a level of care at the referring hospital and during transport as close as possible to the level of care provided in the receiving hospital. The issue under discussion was the make-up of the team that would be required to reach that goal. The debate continues to this day.

Initially, because there was no effective way to predict the type and level of care needed, team composition tended toward physician-led teams. It was apparent, however, that physician-led teams were expensive and difficult to assemble on a regular basis. Nevertheless, because there was no previous experience in the delivery of intensive care during neonatal and pediatric transport, it was essential that the response be at the maximum level even though resources might be wasted in doing so. With time, nurse-led transport teams have become more prevalent. In recent years, there has been considerable discussion regarding transport team composition but not enough to settle the issue.[19,66,69,93]

THE EMERGENCE OF PEDIATRIC INTERFACILITY TRANSPORT PROGRAMS AS SEPARATE HOSPITAL UNITS

As pediatic transport programs continued to evolve, the need for them to become separate organizational units within hospitals was identified. The volume of transports reached a level that required a significant percentage of the personnel, equipment, and outside expenditures of neonatal and pediatric intensive care units. The federal government recognized the need to study these issues at the regional level with the awarding of a Regional Medical Program grant to Stanford University. Hackel and Dobrin presented hospital-based models for such programs.[25,41] They viewed the pediatric transport program as a separate hospital unit whose personnel and equipment should have, as their first priority, transport. The personnel and their equipment need not be "borrowed" from a hospital intensive care unit, although transport team personnel frequently worked in such units on a part-time basis. They attempted to make the budget of the pediatric transport cost-center apply to charges covering operating expenses only, not for profit. Surprisingly, hospital administrators have not viewed these efforts as salutary. Administrators have continued to view transport as a means of attracting patients into their hospitals, irrespective of the cost of doing so. We know of only one major children's hospital in which the pediatric transport program can be viewed as a profitable cost-center.[85]

DEVELOPMENT OF GUIDELINES FOR PEDIATRIC INTERFACILITY TRANSPORT

The separate organizational concept has led to the development of guidelines for pediatric interfacility transport programs. There was a need to define the elements of a pediatric interfacility transport program that would deliver safe, high-quality care to its patients. There was also a need to address the problems associated with pediatric interfacility transport.*

The first attempt at establishing guidelines occurred in California in 1970. The Division of Maternal and Child Health and the Crippled Children's Service of the State Department of Health Services was concerned about the sudden increase in neonatal transports and their cost to the state. State officials called a meeting of neonatologists and neonatal transport carrier operators at which guidelines for the transfer of neonates from community hospitals to regional centers were established. Neonatal intensive care units were required to have a neonatal transport program to be licensed. To this end the program was defined in the State Health Code. Conferences were held, particularly in the western United States where the programs encompassed large geographic areas, at which the various elements of transport programs were discussed. In 1974 the Ross Symposium focused on the regionalization of perinatal care, including neonatal transport.[79]

As the field continued to develop, the movement toward establishment of national guidelines progressed. There was further discussion concerning the components of a pediatric interfacility transport program. Patient care had to be separated from the operational aspects of the transport programs. Other

* References 48, 60, 68, 70, 72, 88-89.

components had to be developed, including communications, data management, administration, equipment development and maintenance, and carrier operations. It was important to delineate functions performed by nonmedical personnel from those of caregivers so that health-care personnel could be used most effectively.

At a national meeting of pediatric interfacility transport held in Keystone, Colorado in 1980, national guidelines for pediatric interfacility transport were drafted at the request of Dr. Willis Wingert, a leader in pediatric emergency medicine. These national guidelines would be proposed to the Committee on Hospital Care of the American Academy of Pediatrics. The guidelines were based in part on work done earlier in California by the California Perinatal Dispatch Centers. Following submission to and approval by the Committee on Hospital Care, they were published by the American Academy of Pediatrics (AAP) in 1986.[1] These guidelines had little initial effect on the field of pediatric transport, mainly because they were not widely publicized. In 1991, however, an effort to revitalize the guidelines was proposed by a group of AAP members involved in pediatric interfacility transport. A task force created by the AAP revised and published the new edition of the guidelines in 1993.[2]

The focus on pediatric transport guidelines has now shifted to the state level in an attempt to put the national guidelines into practice. In California, the State Emergency Medical Services Agency recently approved a document entitled, "Guidelines for Pediatric Interfacility Transport Program Providers" that closely follows the national guidelines.

THE EMERGENCE OF A SECOND AEROMEDICAL TRANSPORT SYSTEM FOR PEDIATRIC TRANSPORT

The previously noted success during the Korean War with the use of helicopters for the emergency transport of wounded soldiers was transferred to the civilian arena in the United States in the 1970s.[8,18,20,83,95] Emergency transport programs, mainly hospital-based, were created throughout the United States to transport critically ill patients from the scene of injury to hospitals. The transport teams were composed of nurses, paramedics, and physicians experienced in emergency and trauma medicine. The focus of these programs that transported mainly adult trauma patients was on prehospital care ("scoop and run"). In such cases, time is of the essence. On the other hand, resuscitation and stabilization before transport are the focus of pediatric interfacility transport programs.

A rivalry developed between the new EMS-based programs that used emergency medicine-trained transport teams and the ICU-based programs that use neonatal and pediatric intensive care-trained transport teams. This rivalry continues to exist today. However, the most successful transport organizations have been able to bridge the gap of this rivalry by offering the type of transport team most qualified to transport specific classes of patients.

The cost of these transport programs in terms of dollars and time expended by health-care delivery personnel, as well as concerns about the most appropriate training and experience for transport personnel, mandates a solution to these complex problems. Proposals to regionalize pediatric transport would seem logical. It is not a simple matter to bring together the emergency medical, neonatal, and pediatric critical care groups. The rivalry between hospitals providing neonatal and pediatric intensive care has prevented regionalization from occurring in most areas.

EQUIPMENT DEVELOPMENT

The patient care equipment used in medical transport has evolved from equipment originally used for other purposes. Medical transport carriers were originally used in general passenger transport and then adapted for medical use. Thus, surface medical transport evolved from the horse-drawn carriage and the railroad train to the modern surface ambulance as automobile technology progressed. Aeromedical transport followed the same pattern, beginning with hot-air balloons and bi-wing aircraft, and progressing to the propeller, turbo-prop, and jet aircraft presently used. As each new carrier was put into service, its use in medical transport was evaluated. The special needs of medical transport such as safety, cost, space, accessibility, temperature control, temperature regulation, monitoring, pressurization, and lighting were considered. Ambulances were outfitted as mobile pediatric (neonatal) intensive care units and dedicated to pediatric transport, but the concept has not had continuing popularity due to the cost and unpredictability in the timing of transport requests.

In the first half of this century, neonatal transport primarily involved the transport of neonates from a home delivery to a pediatric hospital or ward for further care. The incubator equipment consisted of a closed box with a warming device such as a hot-water bottle,[49] a carrying handle, and a small window.

In the 1960s, with the advent of regional neonatal care, an effort was made to develop transport incubator systems that would allow care en route. Most of the transport incubators were based on the closed-box concept. They were a derivation of the isolettes being used in the newly outfitted neonatal intensive care units. For transport, these incubators were altered by adding a battery pack and individual monitoring and life support equipment. The result was a heavy unit that was difficult to use. Of particular note was the difficulty in maintaining a neutral thermal environment inside the transport incubator.[17,45]

During this time, radiant heat bassinets were coming into use in neonatal intensive care units. These bassinets facilitated intensive care in an "open" environment without the loss of heat. This type of environment, still in use, allows easy access to the infant for the multitude of therapies required. It was a more appropriate design for a transport incubator system than the closed box, which when opened to provide care, lost heat at a rapid rate.[63,65]

The author's initial experience was with a Taylor Incubator, which appeared to be identical to the "Acclibator."[13] The Taylor Incubator was powered through a plug that was inserted into the cigarette lighter of the ambulance. When care was given, the infant was removed from the unit and placed on the ambulance stretcher. Following is an account of a pediatric intern who assisted in retrieving a neonate who needed assisted ventilation.

> The pediatric intern indicated that during the transport the endotracheal tube had come out of the trachea. He had to remove the infant from the Taylor Incubator and reintubate him. The result was a chilled infant, pale and neurologically depressed on arrival. We decided rather quickly that, if we were going to provide intensive care during transport, the appropriate equipment to do so had to be available.

Professor Robert Moffat from the Thermosciences Division of the Department of Mechanical Engineering, Stanford University, whose area of interest was temperature measurement and regulation, was recruited to participate in developing a transport incubator that could provide a neutral, thermal, semiopen environment for the provision of intensive care. A modular approach was taken to the packaging of the monitoring and life support equipment. The system was lightweight, portable, and easy to use. Its capabilities included the following: 1) the provision of a battery-powered neutral thermal environment in external temperatures as low as −30°C for 2 hours; 2) easy access to the infant for intensive care, including assisted ventilation; 3) continuous on-line monitoring of heart rate, blood pressure, inspired oxygen, and core and skin temperatures; 4) a fail-safe humidified oxygen delivery system with a ventilator capable of delivering concentrations of oxygen between 21% and 100%; 5) adequate lighting under all conditions; and 6) portable, self-contained, lightweight rechargeable power for all electrical systems of the transport equipment. This unit was demonstrated to be superior to the closed type of transport incubator for the maintenance of a neutral thermal environment.[38,55,65] It was available for 16 years before being phased out by its commercial supplier.

Although it had been demonstrated to be superior for the care of the neonate during transport, it was phased out because of the merger and retrenchment of an interrelated group of medical equipment manufacturers. Today, the equipment used during transport is based on the closed-incubator concept. Although various approaches have been tried,[74,99] access to the patient during transport as well as weight, size, packaging, power capability, and simplicity of use in the transport environment remain significant problems.

The development of equipment for older infants and children has not been as dramatic as the history of neonatal transport incubator development. It has been underreported in the literature.[46] A transport incubator is not appropriate because of the larger size of the patient and the reduced need to provide a neutral thermal environment to maintain normal body temperature. The equipment currently in use is usually the same as that used to transport adult patients.

PEDIATRIC TRANSPORT IN OTHER COUNTRIES

Pediatric transport medicine is not only an American product. The contribution of European physicians must be mentioned in this recounting of pediatric transport history. The practice of showing premature infants at special exhibitions began in Europe and was brought to this country by Dr. Martin Couney, who sponsored exhibits at St. Louis, San Francisco, and other American cities beginning in the late 1800s.[13] Obviously, the infants had to be transferred to these fairs, although it is not clear how it occurred. In the 1970s, as neonatal interfacility transport became an important part of neonatal regional care in the United States, it attained the same position in Europe. Neonatal transport programs similar to those in the United States were developed.*

PEDIATRIC TRANSPORT MEDICINE EMERGES AS A RECOGNIZED AREA OF EXPERTISE

In the 1970s, with the development of regional pediatric intensive care, it became apparent that the models for neonatal interhospital transport should be applied to organize and maintain transport programs for older infants and children. As pediatric interhospital transport programs emerged and developed throughout the United States, the field of pediatric transport medicine achieved recognition at the national level.

Initially, the recognition came through requests for chapters in books on neonatal and pediatric intensive care,[41] requests for guidelines for pediatric interfacility transport from national organizations, and inclusion of the subject in published symposia on neonatal and pediatric intensive care. Conferences on pediatric interfacility transport were held in California, Utah, Colorado, and other states where 200 to 300 health-care providers involved in pediatric transport attended. It became apparent that a national forum for the discussion of many facets of pediatric interhospital transport was needed. The first national conference on pediatric interfacility transport was held in Keystone, Colorado, in 1980. It was co-sponsored by the Stanford University and the Denver Children's Hospitals, lasted two days, and was attended by 150 physicians, nurses, and other health-care providers involved in pediatric transport. There were calls for the development of a pediatric transport medicine society, but they were not followed up.

In 1989 a group of emergency medicine and critical care pediatricians who were interested in Transport Medicine convened at the annual meeting of the American Academy of Pediatrics in Chicago. The question posed was whether a more organized approach should be taken to this emerging field of pediatric medicine. The answer of the 50 individuals present was a resounding "yes". A leadership conference of medical directors of pediatric interfacility transport programs at Sun Valley, Idaho, followed in 1990. Issues facing the field were discussed.[22] Representatives of the American Academy of Pediatrics attended. A request to the Academy for the initiation of a new Section on Transport Medicine followed. This proposal was accepted the following year. Today, the Transport Medicine Section is active, with more than 150 members. In addition to the annual meeting of the Section at the Academy meetings each fall, a free-standing conference is held in the spring at which health-care providers working in pediatric transport medicine meet to discuss the latest advances in the field.

In this chapter the history of pediatric transport has been traced from its initiation as a needed service linked to neonatal and pediatric intensive care to its recognition as a separate field of pediatric medicine. To those of us who participated in part of its long history, it was an exciting time. The future holds as much if not more excitement as we reach out

* References 4-6, 16, 26, 28, 31, 33-34, 42, 48, 52-54, 56, 62, 71, 73, 80-81, 84, 91, 94, 96, 98.

to improve the quality of care for critically ill infants and children who require interfacility transport. Our world is in constant change. New methods and concepts are needed to cope with this change. Research, particularly outcome data, is needed to demonstrate the value, importance, and efficacy of pediatric critical care transport. The other chapters of this book discuss these issues and reflect the dynamic changes occurring in pediatric transport medicine.

REFERENCES

1. American Academy of Pediatrics Committee on Hospital Care: Guidelines for air and ground transportation of children, *Pediatrics* 78(5):943-50, 1986.
2. American Academy of Pediatrics Task Force on Interhospital Transport: *Guidelines for air and ground transport of neonatal and children*, Elk Grove Village, IL, 1993, The Association.
3. Baker GL: Design and operation of a van for the transport of sick infants, *Amer J Dis Ch* 118(5): 743-5, 1969.
4. Bakketeig LS, Bjerkedal T, Finne PH: Transfer of neonates to the pediatric department, *Tidsskrift for den Norske Laegeforening* 99 (13):626-8, 1979.
5. Balashova VG: Indicators and periods of transfer of sick newborn infants and premature infants from maternity homes into specialized wards of pediatric hospitals, *Feldsheri Akusherka* 41(9):5-6, 1976.
6. Barbier ML, Chabernaud JL, Lavaud J, and others: Emergency medical transport of children in the Ile-de-France area, *Archives Francaises de Pediatrie* 44(6):413-7, 1987.
7. Barger J: Strategic aeromedical evacuation: the inaugural flight, *Av Sp Envir Med* 57:613-6, 1986.
8. Baxt WG, Moody P: The impact of a rotorcraft aeromedical emergency care service on trauma mortality, *JAMA* 249:3047-51, 1983.
9. Beyer AJ, Land G, Zaritsky A: Nonphysician transport of incubated children: a system evaluation, *Crit Care Med* 20(7):961-6, 1992.
10. Bostick JS, Hsiao HS, Lawson EE: A minicomputer-based perinatal/neonatal telecommunications network, *Pediatrics* 71(2):272-6, 1983.
11. Brink LW, Chance GW, Matthew JD, and others: Neonatal transport: a controlled study of skilled assistance—mortality and morbidity of neonates less than 1.5 kg birth weight, *J Pediatr* 93(4):662-6, 1978.
12. Butterfield LJ: Regionalization for respiratory care, *Pediatr Clin North Am* 20:499-505, 1973.
13. Butterfield LJ: Historical perspectives of neonatal transport, *Pediatr Clin North Am* 40:221-38, 1993.
14. Cara M, Jolis P, Laborit G, and others: *Le transport d'urgence des insuffisants respiratoire anesthesie, analgesie, reanimation* no. 5, 1957.
15. Cara M, Poisvert M: *Premiers secours dans les detresses respiratoires*, Masson Ed, Paris, 1963.
16. Cara M, Hurtaud JP, Caille C, and others: Transport and liaison: evaluation in pediatrics, *Bull Inst Natl Sante Rech Med* 25(4):745-55, 1970.
17. Chance GW, O'Brien MJ, Swyer PR: Transportation of sick neonates 1972: an unsatisfactory aspect of medical care, *Can Assoc Med J* 109(9):847-51, 1973.
18. Cleveland HC, Bigelow DC, Dracon D, and others: A civilian air emergency service: a report of its development, technical aspects, and experience, *J Trauma* 16:452-63, 1976.
19. Cook LJ, Kattwinkel J: A prospective study of nurse-supervised versus physician-supervised neonatal transports, *Jogn Nursing* 12(6):371-6, 1983.
20. Cowley RA, Hudson F, Scanlan E, and others: An economical program and proved helicopter program for transporting the emergency critically ill and injured patient in Maryland, *J Trauma* 13:1029-38, 1973.
21. Cunningham MD, Smith FR: Stabilization and transport of severely ill infants, *Pediatr Clin North Am* 20(2):359-66, 1973.
22. Day S, McCloskey K, Orr R, and others: Pediatric interhospital cirtical care transport: consensus of a national leadership conference, *Pediatrics* 88(4):696-704, 1991.
23. DeBenedictis FM: Airline transport of premature and cardiopathic newborn infants, *Minerva Med* 71:3175-80, 1980.
24. DeLee JB: Infant incubation, with the presentation of a new incubator and a description of the system at the Chicago Lying-In Hospital, *The Chicago Medical Recorder* 22:22-4, 1902.
25. Dobrin RS, Block B, Gilman JI, and others: The development of a pediatric emergency transport system, *Pediatr Clin North Am* 27(3):633-40, 1980.
26. Droh R, Dortmann C: Transport of emergency patients by helicopter, *Der Anesthesist* 19(2):66-71, 1970.
27. Duncan AW, Mullins GC, Kent M, and others: A paediatric emergency transport service: one year's experience, *Med J Aust* 2(12-13):673-4, 1981.
28. Enocksson E: Transfer of newborn infants, *Lakartidningen* 70:1290-2, 1973.
29. Ehrenwerth J, Hackel A: Air-to-ground communications: a valuable aid in the transport of critically ill patients, *IEEE Transactions on Vehicular Technology* 28:303-6, 1979.
30. Ferrara A: Transportation of sick neonates, *Can Med Assoc J* 110:1233-4, 1974.
31. Fevrier YM, Cavadinin C, Gauthier JP, and others: Transport de nouveau-né pesant moins to 1500g, *La Revue de SAMU* 7:258-61, 1984.
32. Frank HD, Ballowitz L, Schachinger H: Ambulance with intensive care facilities for the transport of infants at risk, *J Perinat Med* 1(2):125-32, 1973.

33. Giroud M, Morlat C, Buffat JJ, and others: Value of helicopter evacuations in pediatric practice in the region of Lyons. Analysis of 40 cases in emergency and intensive care units of Desgenettes army instruction hospital, *Pediatrie* 27(7):783-8, 1972.
34. Goujard J, Saurel-Cubizolles MJ, Breat G and others: The transfer of babies in the neonatal period. Evaluation at the national level, *Arch Fr Pediatr* 36:827-35, 1979.
35. Grant DNW: Airplane ambulance evacuation, *Mil Surg* 88:238-43, 1941.
36. Green RG, Morgan DR: The effects of mild hypoxia on a logical reasoning task, *Aviation Space Environ Med* 56:1004-8, 1985.
37. Gunn T and others: Effectiveness of neonatal transport, *Can Med Assoc J* 118:646-9, 1978.
38. Hackel A: A medical transport system for the neonate, *Anesth* 43(2):258-67, 1975.
39. Hackel A: Regionalization and the Northern California Infant Medical Dispatch Center, Mead Johnson Conference on Newborn Air Transport, Denver, Colorado, 1978.
40. Hackel A, Wong R: The effect of interhospital transport variables on the survival of critically ill neonates with RDS, *Pediatr Res* 15:449, 1981.
41. Hackel A: Neonatal and pediatric transport. In Shoemaker W, Thompson WL, Holbrook P, editors: Textbook of critical care, Philadelphia, 1984 WB Saunders.
42. Hager-Malicka B, Grzymna W, Morsica-Boromka I, and others: Regional integration of intensive care and transport of severely ill newborn infants, *Pediatr Pol* 55:979-85, 1980.
43. Hart H: The conveyance of patients to and from the hospital 1720-1850, *Med History* 22:397-407, 1978.
44. Heluwaert A, Fournet J-P, Lapandry C, and others: Problemes thermiques poses par le transfer d'un nouveau-ne, *La Revue des SAMU* 2:288, 1979.
45. Heluwaert A, Lapandry C, Fournet P, and others: Une application du rechauffement par radiation au transfert des nouveaux-nés en difficultes. Banc d'essai de li'incubateur de transport cavitron IW 35 T, *Conv Med* 1,2:153-7, 1982.
46. Heluwaert A, Lapandry C, Fournet J-P, and others: L'adaption d'une ambulance de reanimation au transfert pediatrique, *La Revue des SAMU* 4:141-6, 1981.
47. Herve C, Gaillard M, Desfemmes C, and others: Neonatal distress. Interest of early medical care and medicalized transport, *Acta Anaesthesiologica Belgica* Suppl 35: 145-51, 1984.
48. Herve C, Gaillard M, Desfemmes C, and others: Etude analytique et critique des problemes immediats poses par la reanimation et le transport de l'enfant de moins de 1500g né a domicile, *La Revue des SAMU* 7:262-6, 1984.
49. Hess JH, Lundeen EC: *The premature infant,* Philadelphia, 1949, JB Lippincott.
50. Higgins EA, Chiles WD, McKenzie JM, and others: Effects of altitude and two decongestant anti-histamine preparations on physiological functions and performance, *Aviation Space Environ Med* 50(2):154-8, 1979.
51. Hitchcock FA: Paul Bert and the beginnings of aviation medicine, *Aerospace Med* 42:1101-7, 1971.
52. Hornchen H, Esser KJ, Marenberg J: The emergency transport of children, *Aneasth Intersivther Notfallmed* 15:69-71, 1980.
53. Huault G, Dehan M, Lejeune JA: Le transport du nouveau-né et du premature, *Gaz Med Franc* 79:6805-21, 1972.
54. Hurtaud JP, Caille C, Ivanoff S, and others: Transport medical des enfants en état grave, *Rev Prat* 19:150-8, 1969.
55. Indyk L: Evaluation of equipment in transport systems. In Sunshine P, editor *Regionalization of perinatal care: Report of the 66th Ross Conference on Pediatric Research,* Columbus, OH, 1974, Ross Lahs.
56. Irtel von Brenndorff A, Hook G, Hieronimi G: Transport of low birth weight infants. Experience with a new transport system, *Klin Paediatr* 190:168-74, 1978.
57. Ivanoff S, Hurtaud JP, de Courcy A: Les transports aeriens medicalises de longue durée, *Nouv Presse Medic* 8(16):1359-61, 1979.
58. Jones DR: Aeromedical transportation of psychiatric patients: historical review and present management, *Av Sp Envir Med* 51:709-16, 1980.
59. Jung AL, Smith K: Newborn intensive care in the intermountain west, *Rocky Mtn Med J* 68(1):16-21, 1971.
60. Kanter RK, Tompkins JM: Adverse events during interhospital transport: physiologic deterioration associated with pretransport severity of illness, *Pediatrics* 84(1):43-8, 1989.
61. Kanter RK, Boeing NM, Hannan WP, and others: Excess morbidity associated with interhospital transport, *Pediatrics* 90(6):893-8, 1992.
62. Koeven FW: Transfer of newborns with respiratory distress syndrome from obstetrical to pediatric wards for intensive care, *Z Prakt Anesth* 7:378-82, 1972.
63. LeBlanc MH: Evaluation of two devices for improving thermal control of premature infants in transport, *Crit Care Med* 12:593-5, 1984.
64. Levett J, Karras L: Effects of alcohol on human accommodation, *Aviation Space Environ Med* 47:867-71, 1977.
65. Levison H, Linsao L, Swyer PR: A comparison of infra-red and convective heating for newborn infants, *Lancet* 2(477):1346-8, 1966.
66. Macnab AJ: Optimal escort for interhospital transport of pediatric emergencies, *J Trauma* 31(2):205-9, 1991.
67. Martinez-Almoyna M: La communication et les contraintes de l'appel telephonique aux secours medicaux d'urgence, *La Revue des SAMU* 7:174-81, 1984.

68. Mayer TA, Walker ML: Severity of illness and injury in pediatric air transport, *Ann Emerg Med* 13(2):108-11, 1984.
69. McCloskey KA, King WD, Byron L: Pediatric critical care transport: is a physician always needed on the team, *Ann Emerg Med* 18(3):247-9, 1989.
70. Merenstein GB, Pettett G, Woodall J, and others: An analysis of air transport results in the sick newborn. II. Antenatal and neonatal referrals, *Am J Obstet Gynecol* 128:520-5, 1977.
71. Minoli I, Calciolari G, Cherubini P, and others: Transport of high-risk newborn infants to a neonatal intensive therapy unit, *Minerva Pediatr* 30:1131-6, 1978.
72. Morett L, Harin A, Ferrara A: Adverse effects of transportation on neonates as measured by PaO_2, *Ped Res* 12:530, 1978.
73. Nars PW: Fast and safe transport of newborns in an emergency, *Swiss Med* 2:69, 1980.
74. Nielsen HC, Jung AL, Atherton SO: Evaluation of the Porta-Warm mattress as a source of heat for neonatal transport, *Pediatrics* 58(4):500-4, 1976.
75. Opstad PK, Ehanger R, Nummestad M, and others: Performance, mood and clinical symptoms in medical personnel exposed to prolonged severe physical work and sleep deprivation, *Aviation Space Environ Med* 49:1065, 1978.
76. Perlstein PH, Edwards NK, Sutherland JM: Neonatal hotline telephone network, *Pediatrics* 64:419-24, 1979.
77. Pettett G, Merenstein GB, Battaglia FC, and others: An analysis of air transports: results in the sick newborn infant, *Pediatrics* 55(6):774-82, 1975.
78. Pinelli J, Ferguson MK: Transporting high-risk newborns: the importance of communication, *Neonatal Network* 3:23-6, 1985.
79. Sunshine P, editor, *Regionalization of perinatal care: Proceedings of the 66th Ross Conference on Pediatric Research,* Litchfield Park, Arizona, 1974, Ross Lahs.
80. Roget J, Beaudoing A, Gilber H: Helicopter transport of premature infants, *Med Infantile* 71:485, 1964.
81. Rosenkranz A: Reorganization of transportation of newborn infants, *Wien Med Wochen Schr* 124:180-2, 1973.
82. Roy RN, Kitchen WH: NETS: a new system for neonatal transport, *Med J Aust* 2(26-27):855-8, 1977.
83. Scheib BT, Foust J, Mueller W, and others: MAST: Military assistance to safety and traffic: a decade of service, *J Emerg Med Serv* 8:38-45, 1983.
84. Scheyer M, Iannascoli F, Brioude R, and others: Transport des nouveau-nés "a haut risque", *Ann Anesthesiol Fr* 130-4, 1975.
85. Schonfeld, N: *Personal communication,* June 10, 1992.
86. Segal S: *Manual for the transport of high-risk newborn infants,* Vancouver, 1972, Canacleau Pediatric Society.
87. Serre L, Tonellot JL, Blanc JF, and others: L'unite Mobile de Transport des nouveau-nés du SAMU de Montpelier, *Ann Anesth Franc* 15:780-9, 1974.
88. Shenai JP: Sound levels for neonates in transit, *J Pediatr* 90(5):811-12, 1977.
89. Shenai JP, Johnson GE, Varney RV: Mechanical vibration in neonatal transport, *Pediatrics* 68:55-7, 1981.
90. Shepard KS: Air transportation of high-risk infants utilizing a flying intensive care nursery, *J Pediatr* 77:148-9, 1970.
91. Srikasibhandha S and others: Transport of the newborn, *Z Geburtshilfe Perinatol* 181:460-4, 1977.
92. Shirley RE: Air evacuation prior to World War II. In Wright-Patteson AFB: Aviation Medicine Symposium on Civilian and Military Problems in Aeromedical Evacuation, OH, 1956.
93. Smith D, Hackel A: Staffing requirements for pediatric critical care transport teams *Crit Care Med* 9:277, 1981.
94. Storrs CN, Taylor MRH: Transport of sick newborn babies *Br Med J Aug* 3(718):328-32, 1970.
95. Thomas F: The development of the nation's oldest operating civilian hospital-based aeromedical service, *Aviation Space Environ Med* 59:567-70, 1988.
96. Unter CE, Cull A: Waikato Women's Hospital newborn transport service: the first year's experience, *NZ Med J* 13:95(717):683-5, 1982.
97. Usher RH: The role of the neonatologist, *Pediatric Clin North Amer* 17:199-202, 1970.
98. Vogel J: Transportation of ill neonates, *Cesk Pediatr* 35:563-6, 1980.
99. Wauer RR: Heat-protection foil for the prevention of heat loss in newborn infants, *Kinderaerztl Prax* 46:189-90, 1978.
100. White MS: Medical aspects of air evacuation of air casualties from Southeast Asia, *Aerosp Med* 39:1338-41, 1968.
101. Yadav J: Transportation of neonate with surgical disorders, *Indian J Pediatr* 46:96-9, 1979.
102. Ycard S, Perin M: Le transport de malades et le blesses a longue distance: l'experience d'Air France sur la ligne Ile de la Reunion-Metropole, *La Revue des SAMU* 3:323, 1980.

3

TRANSPORT REGULATIONS

General and Ground Regulations

MICHAEL S. WILLIAMS

Air Medical Transport Regulations

KAREN JOHNSON

General and Ground Regulations

This chapter will focus on regulations at the state, local, and federal levels that impact patient transport, transport personnel, and more specifically, pediatric air transport. Whether an individual system operates its own medical transport service or regularly relies on another organization, it must be familiar with the regulations that govern how that service operates. While regulations are often intimidating, remember that they are written with the best interest of the patient in mind.

First and perhaps most importantly, regulation of the medical transport system varies widely from one community to another. As a result the design and type of patient transport also vary greatly. No one text or reference can possibly address all the regulations that exist throughout the nation. Therefore it is imperative before beginning a new transport system or routinely calling on an established program to be familiar with the laws and regulations specific to the state and the local community. Each state's office of Emergency Medical Services (EMS) should be able to provide state laws and rules and referrals to appropriate county or municipal authorities who have further jurisdiction over local operations. For information on contacting individual state Emergency Medical Services offices, call the National Association of State Emergency Medical Services Directors at 619-431-7054.

EVOLUTION OF LAWS AND RULES

Federal laws are written by Congress, state laws by state legislatures, and local laws by county or city commissions (other terms may be used at this level of government) to protect the welfare of citizens. Federal laws always take precedence over state laws whenever the two are in conflict. However, state laws may exceed the minimum requirements of federal law and, likewise, local laws may exceed state law minimums. Therefore federal laws tend to be rather general in nature, outlining the intent of Congress for federal or state government operations. State law becomes more specific as to how the state is governed and local government law even more specific for how the local community will operate to protect its citizens.

A law written at any level will usually designate a department, agency, or office as having primary responsibility for enforcement. That entity then has the authority to write specific rules based on the law. For example, if the state law designates that a particular state agency is responsible for the licensure and certification of hospitals within the state, then that agency is responsible for writing rules to delineate the licensure and certification process.

The local community may exceed state laws and rules by writing ordinances (local laws) that are still in compliance with state law but which add further rules. For instance, the local community may require that before a hospital applies to the state for licensure or certification, they must first demonstrate the need for the hospital to even exist. To do so, the hospital may need to meet a series of tests established locally to demonstrate a need for service.

The intent of the process at each level of government is to ensure the public's welfare. When laws and rules are developed, they are always presented in a public forum to allow citizens an opportunity for input before enactment. Most citizens do not realize that these opportunities exist to have a significant impact on the final result. The time and location of these public hearings can be determined by contacting the organizational group primarily responsible for the law or rule. In addition, each agency is required to publish announcements. Once a law is passed by the legislative body and signed by the president, governor, county commission chair, or mayor, it becomes the "law of the land."

Laws can be changed or amended through the legislative process. Amendments can be introduced by citizens petitioning elected representatives in the legislative body that wrote the law. Rules can be similarly amended through petitioning the responsible agency. Once the amendment process begins, citizens can have significant influence on the results. The bottom line is, if the existing law or rule requires change, citizens can initiate that change. Familiarity with the system is essential to effective petitioning. It is imperative that anyone who operates a medical transport service be involved in relevant legislative processes and maintain awareness of any pending or recently implemented regulatory changes. Laws and rules have evolved over the years and have influenced the medical transportation of patients as mentioned in the following discussion.

PATIENT TRANSPORT REGULATION AT THE FEDERAL LEVEL

Two federal laws have had a significant impact on the transport of patients in need of medical care. They are the Emergency Medical Services (EMS) Act of 1973 and the Medical Treatment and Active Labor Act (commonly known as COBRA, since it was part of the Comprehensive OmniBus Reconciliation Act of 1985).[11] COBRA was subsequently amended in July and November 1990.

The EMS Act of 1973 essentially established the EMS system as we know it today. Responsibility was placed at the state level for the establishment and maintenance of EMS services. The Act recognized that an organized emergency response system is essential to the welfare of citizens who are struck by sudden injury or illness. Grant programs were established to encourage development of individual state EMS services. The Act further directed the National Highway Traffic Safety Administration (NHTSA) to establish an EMS office to design programs for training Emergency Medical Technicians, and later, paramedics and first responders. At that time, NHTSA seemed like the logical agency to oversee these programs because the major concern was traffic related injuries. Since the law did not specify that NHTSA or any other federal agency have regulatory authority, no regulations were ever written to accompany this law. The EMS Act remains the primary federal law without federal rules or a regulatory agency to oversee it.

Although not a regulatory agency, NHTSA, along with a number of other federal agencies, has established guidelines that are considered the national minimum standards for patient transport services. Although they are not mandatory, nationally accepted standards are generally employed in courts of law as the minimum standards that citizens should expect from their providers. NHTSA has established initial training and retraining curricula for paramedics, EMTs, flight medics, and first responders that serve as the minimum guidelines generally accepted throughout the country. The General Services Administration (GSA) has written the "KKK-A-1822-C Federal Specifications for Ambulances", which is better known as the "triple K" specs.[13] These specifications establish the minimum design and performance standards expected by the federal government when an ambulance is purchased. As a result, most ambulance manufacturers build their vehicles to meet triple K specs as the accepted minimum standard in the industry. In this somewhat haphazard way the federal government has influenced the EMS industry despite the lack of direct regulatory authority.

Providing citizens access to care is one

area in which the federal government *has* exercised significant regulatory authority. COBRA was drafted by Congress with an eye toward protecting indigent, uninsured patients from being denied access to emergency treatment by hospitals or from being inappropriately transferred between hospitals.[11] Most litigation and subsequent amendments have focused on misdiagnosis and subsequent complications rather than maintaining a focus on the patient's financial status. For the first time federal law defines terms such as *emergency medical condition, responsible physician, appropriate medical screening, transfer,* and *stabilize.* The federal law recognizes that all patients should have equal access to care and that it is incumbent upon the hospital, its employees, and physicians to ensure that proper care is provided.

Most relevant to this discussion are the sections of the law defining a medical emergency and referring to patient transfer. COBRA's definition of a medical emergency is as follows: "a medical condition manifesting itself by acute symptoms of sufficient severity (including severe pain) such that the absence of immediate medical attention could reasonably be expected to result in 1) placing the health of the individual (or, with respect to a pregnant woman, the health of the woman or her unborn child) in serious jeopardy; 2) serious impairment to bodily functions; 3) serious dysfunction of any bodily organ or part; 4) with respect to a pregnant woman who is having contractions, that there is inadequate time to effect a safe transfer to another hospital before delivery, or that transfer may pose a threat to the health or safety of the woman or the unborn child."

Under COBRA, the term *transfer* means "the movement (including the discharge) of an individual outside a hospital's facilities at the direction of any person employed by (or affiliated or associated, directly or indirectly, with) the hospital."[11] If transfer of the patient is necessary and the patient's condition is not yet stabilized, COBRA mandates that the following conditions be met: "1) the physician certifies in writing that in his/her professional opinion the benefits of the transfer outweigh the risks; 2) the transferring hospital treats the patient within its capacity to minimize patient risk; 3) the receiving facility agrees to accept the patient and provide appropriate medical treatment; 4) copies of all medical records, including treatment, certification, and consents, accompany the patient; and 5) the transfer is effected through qualified personnel and transportation equipment as required, including the use of necessary and medically appropriate life support measures during the transfer."[8]

Unlike the EMS law of 1973, enforcement of the COBRA law was assigned to the Department of Health and Human Services (HHS). HHS has been fairly aggressive in enforcing this law and has written a number of administrative directives on how they intend to enforce it. Unfortunately, the law can be confusing and has been given different interpretations in numerous (and sometimes inconsistent) court cases. Traditionally, once a court makes a decision on an issue, if one follows the direction that court gives, one should be confident of protection from legal action. But when different courts rule differently on the same issue, one can no longer have confidence that anything one does will not be subject to a successful law suit. In general, an attempt to act in consideration of the patient's best interest will be the most likely to be viewed positively.

COBRA has had a significant impact on hospitals and, of note to this discussion, how hospitals choose transport services to transfer patients. Medical transport services must be familiar with this law to determine appropriate responses to each request including vehicle staffing, equipment, and preparation for hospital personnel participating in such a transport.

NONREGULATORY NATIONAL STANDARDS

Despite the lack of direct legal mandates, national standards must be seriously considered when operating or choosing a patient transport system. Courts will often determine what standards will be followed when laws and rules do not exist. To do this they follow what is known as the "reasonable man" concept. The question addressed by the court is, "what would the reasonable man do in the same situation?"

To determine what is reasonable the courts will turn to professional organizations to review their minimum standards. The court willalso review any nonregulatory standards published by the federal government or by nationally recognized organizations. It is crucial to be aware that lack of specifically written laws and rules does not prevent a service being held to a local or national "reasonable guideline" or standard of care. Participation in recognized professional organizations and meeting their professional standards is an excellent way to meet the reasonable man concept and to demonstrate a commitment to education and quality service.

Two nationally recognized certifications that exist and are considered the "gold standard" for their respective industries are the Commission on Accreditation of Ambulance Services (CAAS)[8] and the Commission on Accreditation of Air Medical Services (CAAMS).[1] Should a service voluntarily comply with the requirements of these two accreditation processes and continue to provide service at that level after accreditation, it will probably meet the standards that exist at any level of government and should also meet the reasonable man test. These standards are high and the expectations of services that meet them are also high. These (currently elective) processes allow services that strive for excellence to have an objective evaluation by nationally recognized experts. Aside from the potential legal benefits, the accreditation process provides outside expertise and advice on potential areas of improvement.

Specific to pediatric transport, in 1993 the American Academy of Pediatrics published a manual entitled "Guidelines for Air and Ground Transportation of Neonatal and Pediatric Patients."[18] While there is no accreditation process associated with the guidelines, they are designed to recommend a minimum, reasonable goal for any service that transports pediatric and neonatal patients. Topics covered in the manual include the organization of a pediatric transport service, communication, administrative issues, transport personnel, team composition, selection and training, quality improvement, safety, vehicle choice, equipment and medications, outreach education, transport data base, and air-medical physiology. Suggestions are presented for practical ways to meet some of the recommendations offered in the document. In addition, more specific guidelines for neonatal transport are presented in "Guidelines for Perinatal Care" published by the American Academy of Pediatrics and the American College of Obstetrics and Gynecology.[12]

STATE AND LOCAL REGULATION

Since the EMS Act of 1973, the state has been viewed as the entity of primary responsibility for EMS oversight. Laws and rules are delineated and enforced at the state level. Should violations occur, the state will most often investigate and take appropriate action. Problems with a medical transport provider are likely addressed and resolved through state-developed processes.

EMS laws vary significantly between different states. Every state has established an office, bureau, division, or agency responsible for EMS oversight. That office is the focal point for enforcing the state's law(s) and writing the rules necessary to do so. It is essential to identify the state EMS director and his/her position in state government. The EMS director's office can provide copies of current laws and rules determining operation of patient transport services. Although regulatory in nature, the state office has a mission of ensuring the provision of quality care. Many state offices actively seek out advice from experts and have positive programs, such as Public Information, Education, and Relations (PIER), or grant awarding programs that can be very helpful. The service is intended to be helpful, not punitive.

The state EMS office may rely on a technical advisory group in which industry professionals help write the rules for the state. Further, many states have statewide advisory councils that assist the state EMS office in dealing with unforeseen issues that arise. Active participation with such groups have a significant influence on the operation of local services.

Like laws, EMS rules vary widely from state to state. The state EMS director and associated staff can provide the rules for individual states. Most state offices concentrate on the licensure of services, provision of vehicle permits, and certification of personnel. Some have very few rules in accomplishing these tasks, while others have extensive regulations to follow. Again, active participation is the key to ensuring that these rules serve the best interest of local citizens and allow reasonable operation of a medical transport system.

PATIENT TRANSPORT REGULATIONS AT THE LOCAL LEVEL

As with state governments, local forms of government vary from area to area. Traditionally, the terms county and city are the ones most frequently used, but individual communities may use different terminology. Most counties and cities across the country do not get involved in the regulation of medical transportation, instead relying on the state to address the issue. If they do get involved, it is usually in issuing some form of certificate of need (CON) for a service in the particular community.

The CON is a document that affirms that there is a need in that community for a particular service to exist. This is a way for the region to control local services. In some cases, it protects community-owned services from competition that threatens the optimal provision of care. For example, multiple services in a given area might not each have the patient volume to justify and maintain a high quality of equipment and of personnel training and experience. Usually the reason for more transport services than are justified by the patient referral population is competition to direct patients to a particular hospital. The program awarded the CON must be regulated to ensure patient access to any appropriate hospital. However, withholding of unnecessary CONs ultimately protects the patient. Additional CONs *may* be needed for services that provide a subspecialty role (especially pediatric and neonatal) if the existing service is inadequate in that area. Before beginning a service, it must be determined if a CON is needed before applying for state licensure. Few if any states will license a service before they receive a CON for the communities it intends to serve.

A few communities around the country actually have their own EMS oversight agencies armed with extensive ordinances to ensure the quality of service provided. These communities may go so far as to require special certification by ambulance personnel, special equipment to be carried on medical transport vehicles, and special procedures for operation within their community. All these requirements will exceed state requirements but are appropriate and allowed within the legal system. Again, it is incumbent upon any service, before commencing operation, to explore the requirements that the local community may have above and beyond state requirements.

In summary, before becoming involved in the business of medical transport, several steps should be followed:

1. Complying with all federal, state, and community laws, rules, standards, and regulations that impact the service;
2. Establishing a positive relationship with the state EMS office;
3. Becoming actively involved in the legislative process;
4. Gaining awareness of all nationally recognized standards;
5. Learning city and county requirements in other communities from which patients are referred;
6. Developing familiarity with all applicable Federal Aviation Regulations impacting the operation;
7. Understanding the requirements placed on each member of the transport team; and
8. Becoming familiar with all relevant safety requirements for air and ground operations.

Air Medical Transport Regulations

Transporting the critically ill or injured pediatric patient requires more than just ensuring optimal pediatric care and medical direction. Pediatric air transport programs must also actively participate in the daily aviation operations dictated by the Federal Aviation Administration (FAA) to provide safety for all patients and patient care providers in the air transport environment. Besides local, state, and federal laws, rules, and regulations, the pediatric air medical transport program/service must comply with Federal Aviation Regulations (FARs) imposed on the air taxi certificate holder. The FARs will apply to the program whether transporting in a fixed-wing or rotor-wing aircraft.

When establishing and implementing a pediatric air medical program, it is imperative that pediatric medical directors and program administrators develop a thorough understanding of aviation regulations and how they may influence the transport process, policies, operations of the service, safety, and ultimately patient care. This section will discuss the components of aviation regulations, such as the FAA's roles and responsibilities, definitions, and "general" FARs pertinent for a fixed-wing and/or rotor-wing pediatric transport program.

AVIATION OPERATION: FEDERAL AVIATION ADMINISTRATION

The Federal Aviation Administration regulates all civil aviation operations that involve air traffic control, airports, and aviation regulations for pilots, mechanics, and flight operations. The FAA is a branch of the US Department of Transportation (DOT).

FARs have been written and enforced by the FAA to regulate all components of aircraft operations including maintenance and certification of aircraft, pilots, and mechanics.[7] The majority of air medical transport and civil aviation programs must comply with the appropriate FARs (depending on who possesses the Air Taxi Certificate).

- FAR PART 91 — Pertains to general operating and flight rules for aircraft flying in US airspace.
- FAR PART 135 — Provides specific rules for air taxi operators and commercial operators.

The exceptions to these rules are the municipalities and government agencies that operate "public use" aircraft and are not bound by most portions of Parts 91 and 135.

Most air medical services are regulated under Part 135 of the FARs due to the nature of transporting "passengers" or "persons" for compensation or hire. Part 135 requires a program to comply with detailed regulations that are far more restrictive than when operating under Part 91. Part 135 stipulates not only the qualifications of the pilot in command, flight crewmembers, initial and recurrent testing, training, flight, and rest requirements, and maintenance and preventive maintenance, but also requirements for aviation management, record keeping, and visual/instrument flight rule operating limitations.[7] Future discussion of the FARs in this section will reference both Parts 91 and 135.

Currently, nearly half of the fixed-wing transport programs possess their own Part 135 Certificate.[9] On the other hand, the majority of rotor-wing air medical transport programs operate under an aircraft operator's 135 Air Carrier Certificate. These transport programs contract with a vendor or operator to provide the aircraft, pilots, and maintenance under the operator's certificate. This contract requires that the vendor meet the requirements of the Federal Aviation Act of 1958 to operate as a Part 135 Air Carrier under the terms and conditions approved in the operations specifications. Therefore the operator must comply with the regulations in their company's operations manual. There are approximately 15 aircraft operators who routinely advertise to assist or contract for aviation services.[13] Air medical programs have contracted for these services not only for financial reasons, but also for aviation expertise. If a program or hospital elects to obtain its own 135 Air Carrier Certificate from the FAA, which may take 6 months to 1 year to complete, the program must still comply with all FARs as outlined and approved in its own FAA approved operations manual. Failure to comply with the FARs is cause for suspending or revoking the operator's air carrier certificate by the FAA.

The FAA has district offices called Flight Standards District Offices (FSDOs) responsible for monitoring and inspecting operators, facilities, aircraft, and aviation personnel within their respective districts. The offices also interpret rules pertaining to aviation operations in their jurisdiction. Unfortunately, history has demonstrated that FSDOs interpret the FARs with very subtle differences from region to region, therefore the certificate holder should contact its FSDO for specific clarification on the FARs. These interpretations are "opinions" on the regulations and are not legally binding.

DEFINITIONS: PILOT IN COMMAND/ CREW/AIR MEDICAL PERSONNEL

The FAA outlines the responsibilities of pilots and flight crewmembers within the FAR Part 135. Specifically for pediatric air transport programs, it is important for the program administrators and medical directors to understand the appropriate titles and responsibilities necessary to comply with the FARs, and to avoid future confusion and conflict.

Pilot in command (PIC)

First, the program must have a thorough understanding of the responsibilities of the pilot in command (PIC), who is also a flight crewmember. According to FAR 91.3, the PIC is directly responsible for all aspects of safe operations in and around the aircraft (rotor-wing and fixed-wing).[7] The PIC has final authority for accepting or declining a flight based on weather and aircraft conditions. The pilot must also be responsible for overseeing the loading and unloading of patients, operating doors of the aircraft, briefing passengers, securing equipment, providing direction during aircraft emergency procedures, and aborting a medical mission due to a hazardous situation. Ultimately, all passengers are under the direction of the PIC.

Flight crewmember

Secondly, the FAA further defines the *flight crewmember* as a pilot, flight engineer, or flight navigator assigned to duty in an aircraft during flight time.[7] Furthermore, *flight attendant crewmembers* are also assigned to perform duties in the aircraft. All *crewmembers* are subject to specific qualifications, testing, training, duty, and rest requirements. If an air medical program designates medical personnel as *flight crew*, the above restrictions will pose additional time and financial responsibilities for the operator; therefore most transport programs prefer to avoid these liabilities for their personnel.

Air medical personnel (AMP)

After much discussion with the FAA, the Association of Air Medical Services (AAMS —formerly known as the American Society of Hospital-Based Emergency Aeromedical Services, or ASHBEAMS) was advised to avoid the use of the term *flight crewmember* when referring to medical staff. Air medical programs should approve a title for all RNs, MDs, RTs, and EMT-Ps to avoid confusion of crewmember requirements. *Air medical personnel* (AMP) has become a more frequently used title to refer to all patient care providers aboard aircraft. Pediatric medical directors and administrators should make a conscious effort to use such a title in job descriptions, policies and procedures, and patient care protocols and guidelines to avoid liabilities and provide consistency.

FEDERAL AVIATION REGULATIONS (FARs)

Introduction to federal aviation regulations

Since dedicated pediatric air medical transport programs continue to evolve, it is imperative that administrators and medical directors thoroughly understand the regulations that may influence the operation. Whether contracting with an operator or obtaining its own Part 135 Certificate, the pediatric transport program's key to success is to become knowledgeable regarding FARs. The program administrator, clinical supervisor, and medical director should be aware of the regulations that could affect transport policies and procedures, operations, safety, and pediatric patient care.

Many service and professional organizations in the air medical profession have published standards of patient care and safety for rotor-wing (RW) and fixed-wing (FW) operations. Besides referring to the various FARs, these standards of patient care typically can help a program comply with these regulations. For instance, the Association of Air Medical Services (AAMS) has been a driving force in developing standards for the air medical profession. AAMS has been involved in issues relating to reimbursement, research, continuous quality improvement, safety, and regulations.[6] Also, the Commission on Accreditation of Air Medical Services (CAAMs) has published Accreditation Standards and has been accrediting air medical programs since 1992.[1] The Commission provides a voluntary accreditation process to evaluate an air medical program's compliance with patient care and safety standards in the air medical profession.

In addition a pediatric transport program will have aviation resources available to educate the administration regarding the FARs. A program that contracts with an operator or vendor for a FW or RW service will have a pilot designated as the "lead pilot" or "base manager" by the operator. This pilot will be a resource when addressing the FAA and in referring to the appropriate FARs and operational policies. On the other hand, under Part 135.37, a program that possesses its own 135 Certificate must have qualified aviation personnel (pilots and mechanics) in the positions of the Director of Operations, Chief Pilot, and Director of Maintenance. These personnel will have the responsibility to ensure that the service is complying with the FARs and safety regulations.[7] These aviation experts will also educate the program director and medical director to the appropriate regulations.

A pediatric service must become aware of the issues and decisions necessary for the program to comply with regulations by reviewing the pertinent FARs for air transport operations. The service can then develop policies, procedures, and programs to ensure RW and FW compliance with the FARs. By briefly highlighting the areas of weight and balance, flight time limitations, rest requirements, passenger briefing requirements, weather minimums for RW versus FW (including visual and instrument flight rule limitations), maintenance issues, safety practices for flight operations, and aircraft emergency procedures, pediatric medical directors and program administrations can assist the program to comply with the FARs and ultimately with *SAFETY.*

PERTINENT FEDERAL AVIATION REGULATIONS: PIC RESPONSIBILITIES

Weight and balance requirements

Each RW or FW aircraft flown has specific weight and balance restrictions, as approved in the Airplane or Rotorcraft Flight Manual. The manual contains aircraft performance data on maximum certified gross weights, center of gravity limits, altitude limitations, runway lengths for takeoff (FW), and procedures for operating that specific aircraft. In the manual the gross weight of the aircraft is the maximum certified weight allowable for safe operations and optimal performance.

Furthermore, aircraft design specifications and performance data are based on "standard" conditions. Yet, ambient conditions such as air pressure, temperature, and humidity affect "air density" and can restrict gross weight. Lift and drag vary directly with the density of the air, so if air density increases, lift and drag also increase. However, air density also varies inversely to the altitude; therefore as air density decreases, the altitude increases.

High density altitude or conditions of high altitude, humidity, and temperature may cause the air to be thinner, thus reducing aircraft performance by reducing engine horsepower, thrust, and lift. On a hot, humid day, the rate of acceleration on ground roll and the rate of climb for a FW aircraft will be reduced, requiring a much longer distance for takeoff. For a RW aircraft, these factors will reduce the ability of the blades to produce the force and efficiency required for lift and hovering capabilities. It is particularly important for RW aircraft to be able to hover for takeoffs and landings at confined helipads and scene calls. The helicopter will also require a longer takeoff run to obtain the necessary forward speed and produce the required lift to climb.

High density altitude is most hazardous when combined with heavy loads, short runways, or obstructions near the end of the runway or surrounding a helipad. Airports and helipads located in geographic areas with high altitudes and warm weather will have conditions that modify the performance and limitations of each aircraft. Therefore the PIC will need to be aware of these conditions and the capabilities of the aircraft and will make decisions accordingly.

For instance, a FW aircraft taking off in Phoenix, at 1100 feet mean sea level (MSL) at 80°F will not perform the same when the ambient temperature is 122° F, which occurred in the summer of 1990. Taking temperature change into consideration, the aircraft that day in Phoenix "thought" it was at an altitude of 5500 feet MSL instead of the standard 1100 feet MSL. Also, even under normal circumstances, Denver is at 5000 feet MSL; therefore an aircraft would perform differ-

TABLE 3-1 BK-117 EQUIPMENT WEIGHT/CONFIGURATION LIST (212AE, 213AE, and 215AE)

On stretcher	*Wt [lbs]*	*Wt [kgs]*	*Arm*	*Moment*
1 Trauma Bag	25	11.3	4430	50236
1 LP—10	25	11.3	5300	60102
1 Ferno Stretcher	75	34.0	4800	163295
Medical wall				
1 Built-in Suction	4.1	1.9	4520	8406
2 Tubing & Yank.	0.5	0.2	4520	1066
2 Suction Liners	0.5	0.2	4520	1025
1 Minimed Pump	4.3	2.0	4520	8816
1 Minimed Charger	1.0	0.5	4520	2050
3 Minimed Tubing	0.04	0.1	4520	82
1 End-T. CO2 Det.	0.2	0.1	4520	410
4 4 × 4's	0.1	0.1	4520	246
1 PEEP Valve	0.1	0.1	4520	287
1 60cc LL Syringe	0.1	0.1	4520	256
1 Pulse Oximeter	2.0	0.9	4520	4101
Port pouch L/H AFT				
4 Hard Restraints	0.1	0.1	5350	291
1 Doppler W/Gel	1.0	0.5	5350	2427
1 Pulse Generator	2.0	0.9	5350	4853
Port pouch R/H AFT				
1 Extra BP Cuff	0.8	0.3	5350	1820
2 Pressure Infus.	2.0	0.9	5350	4853
Under L/H AFT seat				
2 Hot/Cold Packs	1.5	0.7	3650	2483
1 Peds Tubing	0.1	0.1	3650	215
1 D5W—250 cc	0.7	0.3	3650	1242
2 Blood Tubing	0.6	0.3	3650	1026
Under R/H AFT seat				
2 NS—1000 cc	5.0	2.3	3650	8278
4 LR—1000 cc	10.0	4.6	3650	1695

Courtesy of Samaritan AirEvac—Phoenix, Arizona.

ently than it would at 1100 feet MSL in Phoenix. Because of these temperature and altitude factors, an aircraft may not be able to perform with a full load of fuel, pilots, air medical personnel, patient, and family ride-alongs. Ultimately, the PIC will be required to limit the operational weight.

Since the gross weight is predetermined by the airplane or rotorcraft flight manual, the PIC must compute the daily operational weight, which is the weight of the aircraft, fuel, pilot(s), air medical personnel, and standard medical equipment. Part 91.605 requires the pilot to ensure that the aircraft is loaded within weight and balance limits at all times.[7] The PIC is responsible for the weight calculation before taking off on the medical flight.

It is imperative that the pediatric air transport program assist the vendor or operator by controlling weight factors for the flight operation. First, the program can develop policies to control the *total* weight of the medical equipment required for all pediatric transports, including a comprehensive list of items and their weights (Table 3-1).

"FIXED-WING CARRY-ON EQUIPMENT/AIR MEDICAL PERSONNEL WEIGHTS CHECKLIST"

Flight Log Sheet Number: ______

Adult/Ped:		
Adult/Ped Trauma Bag	(25 lbs.)	X ___ = ___ lbs.
Adult/Ped Drug Bag	(5½ lbs.)	X ___ = ___ lbs.
Maternal:		
Black Maternal Bag	(23½ lbs.)	X ___ = ___ lbs.
Teal Bag	(17 lbs.)	X ___ = ___ lbs.
Fetal Monitor	(23 lbs.)	X ___ = ___ lbs.
Maternal Drug Bag	(5 lbs.)	X ___ = ___ lbs.
Neonatal:		
Blue Neonate Bag	(5 lbs.)	X ___ = ___ lbs.
Red Bag	(20 lbs.)	X ___ = ___ lbs.
Neonatal Scene Bag	(11½ lbs.)	X ___ = ___ lbs.
Neonatal Drug Bag	(14½ lbs.)	X ___ = ___ lbs.
Other:		
Extra FW Black Bag	(19 lbs.)	X ___ = ___ lbs.
Infant Car Seat	(8½ lbs.)	X ___ = ___ lbs.
Doppler	(1 lb.)	X ___ = ___ lbs.
Ice Chest	(10 lbs.)	X ___ = ___ lbs.
UHF Radio	(2 lbs.)	X ___ = ___ lbs.

Fluids:		
Minimed Pump	(5½ lbs.)	X ___ = ___ lbs.
Syringe Pump	(2 lbs.)	X ___ = ___ lbs.
Pressure Infusers	(1 lb.)	X ___ = ___ lbs.
Trauma:		
Scoop	(20½ lbs.)	X ___ = ___ lbs.
MAST Suit		
Adult	(8½ lbs.)	X ___ = ___ lbs.
Peds	(6¾ lbs.)	X ___ = ___ lbs.
Splints:		
Sager	(3½ lbs.)	X ___ = ___ lbs.
Kleppel	(6¼ lbs.)	X ___ = ___ lbs.
Kendrick Traction Device	(1 lb.)	X ___ = ___ lbs.
Ventilator:		
6400 ST Vent.	(33 lbs.)	X ___ = ___ lbs.
IC2A Vent.	(15 lbs.)	X ___ = ___ lbs.
MVP 10 Vent.	(17 lbs.)	X ___ = ___ lbs.
M-1 Vent. Monitor	(2 lbs.)	X ___ = ___ lbs.
MIO Vent. Monitor	(3 lbs.)	X ___ = ___ lbs.

TOTAL WEIGHT: ______________

Fig. 3-1. Fixed-wing carry-on equipment/air medical personnel weights checklist.

This weight list should be limited to equipment only absolutely necessary to provide immediate pediatric care in-flight, for the time required during the longest anticipated patient flight. This list should not change, thus allowing the pilots to consistently count on a predetermined weight to calculate the operational weight of the aircraft. These medical equipment weight lists should only be approved and revised by administration and the chief or lead pilot.

Secondly, many air medical programs have policies in place for weight limits of air medical personnel. In October 1992, based on a survey distributed only to RW services, approximately 65% of the programs have an individual weight limit policy.[19] This kind of safety policy assists the program's operation, depending on the type and capability of the aircraft used. Many times the weight policy must also be guided or approved by an institution or hospital-wide policy, to comply with the Equal Employment Opportunity Commission (EEOC) and the Americans with Disabilities Act (ADA).[3]

Finally, air medical personnel should have a procedure for notifying the PIC before a flight when adding carry-on items, medical equipment, or an additional patient care provider (i.e. resident or fellow). The PIC must calculate the additional weight before takeoff. A program may develop a medical weight "worksheet" to assist the pilot as presented in Figure 3-1.

Once the operational weight of aircraft, fuel, equipment, and personnel is calculated, the pilot can determine the payload or weight available to carry a patient or second patient, physician, family ride-along, and patient belongings. Altitude and temperature conditions can further restrict the total payload from mission to mission as previously reviewed. The PIC is responsible for this calculation and has the final decision regarding weight limitations on any given flight.

Due to the "air density" factors, an aircraft may not be able to perform with a full load for each medical mission. Therefore the program must be aware of potential limitations and be responsive/flexible to complete the medical

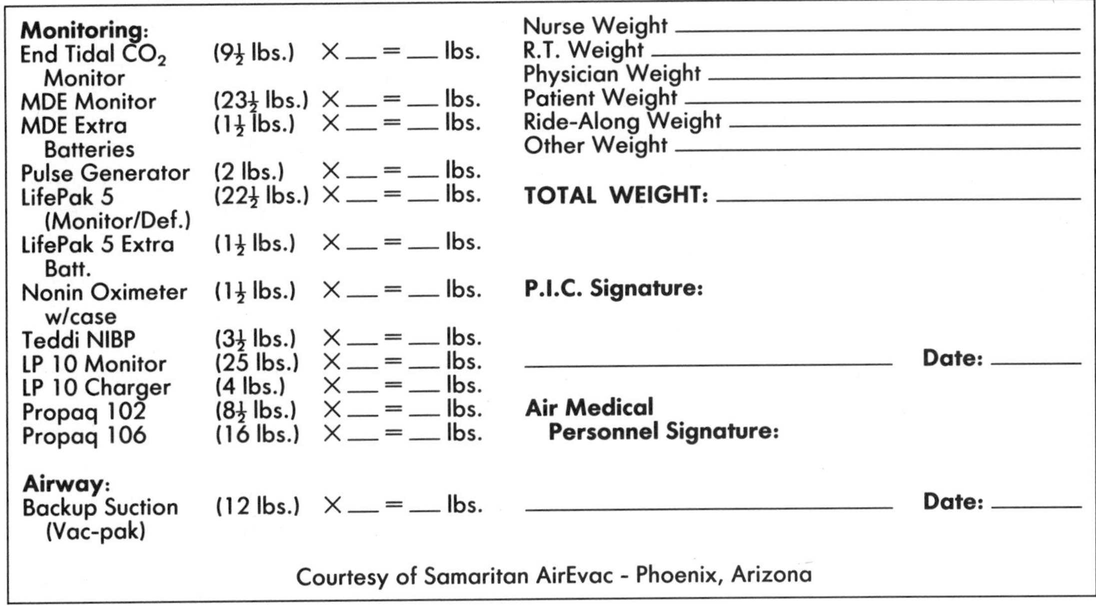

Monitoring:

Item	Weight	Quantity	Total
End Tidal CO_2 Monitor	(9½ lbs.)	× ___	= ___ lbs.
MDE Monitor	(23½ lbs.)	× ___	= ___ lbs.
MDE Extra Batteries	(1½ lbs.)	× ___	= ___ lbs.
Pulse Generator	(2 lbs.)	× ___	= ___ lbs.
LifePak 5 (Monitor/Def.)	(22½ lbs.)	× ___	= ___ lbs.
LifePak 5 Extra Batt.	(1½ lbs.)	× ___	= ___ lbs.
Nonin Oximeter w/case	(1½ lbs.)	× ___	= ___ lbs.
Teddi NIBP	(3½ lbs.)	× ___	= ___ lbs.
LP 10 Monitor	(25 lbs.)	× ___	= ___ lbs.
LP 10 Charger	(4 lbs.)	× ___	= ___ lbs.
Propaq 102	(8½ lbs.)	× ___	= ___ lbs.
Propaq 106	(16 lbs.)	× ___	= ___ lbs.

Airway:

Item	Weight	Quantity	Total
Backup Suction (Vac-pak)	(12 lbs.)	× ___	= ___ lbs.

Nurse Weight ___
R.T. Weight ___
Physician Weight ___
Patient Weight ___
Ride-Along Weight ___
Other Weight ___

TOTAL WEIGHT: ___

P.I.C. Signature:

___ **Date:** ___

Air Medical Personnel Signature:

___ **Date:** ___

Courtesy of Samaritan AirEvac - Phoenix, Arizona

Fig. 3-1, cont'd. For legend see opposite page.

mission. For instance, a service that transports with a pediatric nurse practitioner and pediatric ICU nurse may need to eliminate one caregiver to allow a pediatric fellow to fly on a specific mission. Also, if an air medical transport requires all three caregivers on a critical flight, the program should have guidelines in place not to allow a family ride-along due to weight limitations.

Center of gravity

Besides weight, it is essential that an aircraft is loaded within the Center of Gravity (CG) range or limitations.[4] Once the maximum weight has been determined, the weight distribution or where the weight is placed in an aircraft is critical for aerodynamic performance and safety in-flight. The weight must be properly loaded fore and aft, according to the manufacturer's Airplane or Rotorcraft Flight Manual, to meet the CG limitations especially along the longitudinal axis. If an aircraft is improperly loaded and out of CG, the aircraft could lose stability and control during flight manuevers and severe turbulence.

The pediatric transport program can assist with operations by developing not only a medical equipment weight list, but also an equipment configuration list and/or diagram. This list or diagram should be developed by the program director and lead or chief pilot to properly load the medical equipment to meet CG requirements. This list will clearly outline the location of all medical equipment, and it should not deviate without approval of the PIC. Table 3-1 provides an example of a configuration list.

Carriage of cargo

Once the weight and balance of medical equipment and personnel are completed, under FAR Part 91.525,[7] the pilot must ensure that all cargo is properly carried in a FAA approved cargo rack, bin, or compartment installed in the aircraft. Regulations also require that equipment be 1) properly secured by a FAA approved safety belt or other tie-down having enough strength to eliminate shifting; 2) packaged or covered to avoid possible injury to passengers; and 3) located in a position that will not restrict access to or use of required emergency or regular exits.

To comply with this Part, the transport program should attempt to permanently install the heavy medical equipment within the aircraft to ensure secure placement. As for other supplies and light portable equipment, the program should use various pouches, bins, drawers and FAA approved straps and belts to secure such items. All air medical personnel should properly secure ***all*** equipment during takeoff and landing and in-flight while providing patient care.

Flight time limitations and rest requirements

A request for an emergency pediatric transport is rarely "scheduled." Air medical transports are requested at all times of the day and night. Since the requests are unscheduled, FAR Part 135.267 places flight time limitations and rest requirements on all pilots.[7] The FAA regulates duty and rest time to ensure an alert, rested, and safe pilot is in command. The actual flight and rest times will vary depending on the number of pilots on board, the type of aircraft, the operations specifications (Op. Specs.) manual, and if flying a RW or FW aircraft.

For instance, RW aircraft have an additional FAR 135.271 that outlines specific requirements for Hospital Emergency Medical Evacuation Service (HEMES).[7] In the mid 1980s, helicopter EMS pilots were frequently assigned 24-hour shifts for a single pilot operation. This FAR 135.271 was developed to address pilot flight and rest time and to ensure at least 8 consecutive hours of rest during a 24-hour period. Fortunately, most air transport programs now only assign helicopter pilots to 12-hour shifts. The air medical profession ensured pilot rest by promoting a minimum of four pilots assigned to one RW aircraft as stated in the Accreditation Standards of CAAMS.[1] This 12-hour work schedule enables pilots to more clearly comply with the regulation for single pilot "unscheduled" flight time and rest requirements.

FAR Part 135.267 addresses various limitations of ***total flight time,*** such as 8 hours for a single pilot operation to 10 hours for a two pilot configuration.[7] Furthermore, this duty period must be preceded ***and*** followed by a rest period of 10 consecutive hours. The FARs do address circumstances beyond the control of the PIC where the ***flight time*** is exceeded due to adverse weather conditions. When flight time limitations are exceeded, the pilot must receive extended rest periods of at least 11, 12, or 16 hours depending on how long he or she flew. Finally, whether the pilot responds from the base operation, hospital, or from a pager at home, the duty time begins when the pilot is expected to respond. According to the FAA pager response is considered duty time, and this time is proactive in nature.[7]

Most pilots are assigned to work a 12-hour shift as their "assigned duty time." In addition, pilots have the latitude to legally complete their missions in up to a 14-hour period, even though they may exceed flight time limitations, provided this is caused by deteriorating weather or patient condition. For instance, if a flight request occurs within 1 hour of a pilot shift change, the day pilot may not be able to accept the medical flight, depending on the time involved. The day pilot may decline the flight due to the fact that *planned total completion* time will exceed either the legal duty time of 14 hours or flight time limitations. Yet if a program possesses its own 135 Certificate and the pilot's *planned completion* time was within the 14-hour duty time, but circumstances occurred beyond his/her control due to deteriorating weather or patient condition, the pilot may have another opportunity to complete the mission. The program, which operates its own 135 service, may be allowed to complete the flight as a FAR Part 91 flight because no patient is on-board this last leg of the flight. Even under Part 91, exceeding the standard Part 135 flight and duty time limitations should be permitted only under the rarest of circumstances.

All these limitations pose frustrating decisions for an air medical program, yet the program director/supervisor and medical director must understand these requirements. The transport program may need to develop procedures and guidelines with the chief or lead pilot to minimize the impact of these restrictions. For example, the program that operates more than one aircraft may use creative scheduling by staggering duty shifts by 1 to 2 hours to avoid having no pilot available for a mission at times of shift change.

TABLE 3-2 BASIC VFR WEATHER MINIMUMS

Altitude	*Flight visibility*	*Distance from clouds*
Class E: ≥ 10,000 feet MSL (Fixed-wing)	5 statute miles	1000 feet below 1000 feet above 1 statute mile horizontal
Class E: < 10,000 feet MSL	3 statute miles	500 feet below 1000 feet above 2000 feet horizontal
Class G: > 1200, but < 10,000 feet MSL (Rotor-wing)	Day: 1 statute mile Night: 3 statute miles	500 feet below 1000 feet above 2000 feet horizontal

Passenger briefings

According to FAR 135.117[7] the pilot in command should orally brief all passengers and air medical personnel before each takeoff. The briefing should include the following:

1. Prohibition of smoking as indicated by the illuminated "No Smoking" sign or placard;
2. Use of safety belts;
3. Placement of seat backs in an upright position before takeoff and landing;
4. Location and means for opening the passenger entry door and emergency exits;
5. Location of survival equipment;
6. Location and operation of fire extinguishers;
7. Ditching procedures and use of flotation equipment if flight involves extended overwater operations;
8. Normal and emergency use of oxygen if flight operates above 12,000 feet MSL.

Weather requirements/minimums

The FARs states explicit weather minimums and rules for the sole purpose of operating within consistent safety standards. Due to these rules, an air transport program will be faced with declining, aborting, and canceling flights, depending on the weather encountered in the geographical area.

Under Part 135, air medical transport programs operate within either Visual Flight Rules (VFR) and/or by Instrument Flight Rules (IFR). A service must comply with the appropriate rules, which define the limitations for flying in adverse weather conditions. VFR govern the procedures for conducting flight under visual conditions as interpreted by the pilot's judgment. Flight *visibility* is defined by the distance forward into the visible horizon, and *ceiling* (vertical boundary) is the height from ground/water to the base of the lowest (broken) *layer* of clouds. IFR govern the procedures for conducting instrument flight when weather conditions are below the minimum for flight under VFR.

FAR Part 91.155 addresses the basic VFR weather minimums that are maintained for "controlled" airspace for RW and FW as outlined in Table 3-2.[7]

In addition, according to Part 135.205, no person may operate an aircraft (other than a helicopter) in uncontrolled airspace or in a control zone below 1200 MSL under VFR unless flight visibility is 1/2 mile in daylight and 1 mile at night.[7] These rules are more restrictive for RW operations because the majority of RW air transport programs operate under VFR with aircraft only approved for VFR conditions. The majority of programs that operate FW aircraft have the capability to operate under IFR with other limitations, such as landing at approved airports with instrument approaches, complying with restrictions for takeoff, approach and landing minimums, and requiring plans for approved alternate airports.

These FAR requirements were developed over the years after a number of aviation accidents/incidents involving errors in pilot judgment due to adverse weather conditions. According to Adams and Taylor[2] in a study of 10 years of civilian helicopter accidents, 64% of the accidents were related to pilot error as the major factor. Dodd's Safety Study for the National Transportation and Safety Board also indicated that the majority of EMS accidents have been assigned as pilot error.[10] Many vendors and operators enforce RW weather minimums, which are more restrictive than the FAA requirements due to the increase of accidents/incidents in the air medical profession. AAMS played an integral role in assisting the air medical profession to come to a consensus with VFR/RW weather minimums. In addition these RW weather minimums are also presented in the Accreditation Standards of CAAMS.[1] RW minimums for day and night flights and local/cross country required visibility and ceiling limitations are listed in Table 3-3.

Under Part 135.213 IFR conditions, the pilot in command ultimately is responsible for accepting or declining a flight and may use weather information based on the pilot's observations for VFR conditions.[7] One must remember that even the pilot's observations for VFR flight at the base operation cannot fully predict the current weather briefings and forecasts enroute to and at the referring facility or accident scene. A pilot operating an aircraft under adverse weather conditions should use the US National Weather Service (NWS), a source approved by the NWS, or a source approved by the FAA, such as a Flight Service Station (FSS). Also, a pilot conducting a flight under IFR conditions is required to use the aforementioned sources of weather briefing information.[7] Unfortunately, many areas of the United States do not have round-the-clock aviation weather information from a local NWS or FSS. Also, pilots may not receive entirely accurate weather information, since some stations report "on the hour" and, therefore, the report may be up to 60 minutes past.

TABLE 3-3 VFR RW WEATHER MINIMUMS

Conditions	*Ceiling*	*Visibility*
Day/Local	500 feet	1 mile
Day/Country	1000 feet	1 mile
Night/Local	800 feet	2 miles
Night/Country	1000 feet	3 miles

Today, computers and modem/radar accessing systems provide more options to assist pilots in monitoring current weather briefings and forecasts.[5] The FAA currently sponsors a system called a Direct User Access Terminal Service (DUATS). This system provides not only hourly briefings, terminal forecasts, severe weather bulletins, but also notices to airmen (NOTAMS), significant meteorological information (SIGMETS), and radar briefings. There are other private companies that offer services similar to DUATS that provide color graphics and even real-time radar services by facsimilies of the actual NWS radar screen. These services have varying charges of per minute or per-item costs, monthly charges, or on-line rates.[5]

All these systems may assist the pilot in the decision making process to accept or decline a flight during marginal weather conditions. Over the past 10 years, 17 our of 64 (27%) of the helicopter accidents investigated by the NTSB relating to personnel error involved adverse weather.[12] Since many accidents have been related to weather, a pediatric transport program must understand the importance of pilots accessing the best weather system and must consider financial support of these options for the program's safety.

One disadvantage of using a weather accessing system is a delayed response time for the mission. Since the pilot will need to call either FSS or access another system, the response time may be delayed up to 10 to 15 minutes. However, safety must be the primary goal for an air medical program, and a delayed response time **should never be an** issue when marginal weather considerations are involved.

Finally, just because a mission has been accepted and the aircraft is enroute does not guarantee a completed mission. On RW or FW aircraft, the PIC can ultimately abort the mission based on deteriorating weather conditions below established minimums. Therefore protocols and procedures should be in place to address the weather limitations after takeoff. This should be clearly communicated to outlying referring facilities and physicians by outreach education providing public relations materials explaining the program's operation. The education should clearly explain how weather can affect the completion of an air medical transport and should offer alternatives for transport.

AVIATION MAINTENANCE ISSUES

One aviation issue that receives very little attention by air medical administration and medical directors is maintenance. Yet this very subject can cause a great deal of heartburn and frustration depending on the type and number of aircraft and the average number of flight requests the program receives in a week. The FARs relating to maintenance presents one issue for which administration and medical directors frequently require more education to understand. Use of "backup" aircraft may be needed if patient volume is high.

The purpose of maintenance is to ensure that the aircraft is kept at an acceptable standard of airworthiness while in operation. This includes the inspection, overhaul, and repair of an aircraft based on design, materials, workmanship, and performance. Once the FAA determines that an aircraft is in airworthy condition, they will issue an Airworthiness Certificate.[15] This is one of the most important activities in promoting safety in aviation. Issuance of the certificate means that the FAA, after inspection, found that the aircraft met the requirements of the FAR Part 43 and is in a condition for safe operation. A properly maintained aircraft is a safe aircraft.[15]

First, maintenance must include various inspections required by FAR Parts 43, 91, and 135 during specific intervals to determine the overall condition.[7] FAR Part 91 places primary responsibility on the owner or operator for maintaining an aircraft in an airworthy condition. These intervals are determined by the type of operation, so the aircraft may receive an annual inspection every 12 calendar months; after each 100, 250, or 500 hours of operation; or on another inspection cycle, such as progressive inspection requirements based on flight-time hours, calendar days, or engine starts/cycles, etc.

Typically, the annual inspections must be managed by a certified airframe and powerplant (A & P) mechanic holding an inspection authorization (IA). The 100- or 250-hour inspections can be approved by an A & P mechanic, an appropriately rated certified repair station, or by the manufacturer.

Second, maintenance encompasses not only the repair, but *scheduled* or *preventive maintenance* (PM). This maintenance consists of simple or minor preventive repairs or replacement of standard parts not involving complex assembly operations. The time intervals for PMs are based on the type and age of aircraft, operation, and climates. Maintenance regulations are found in FAR Parts 43 and 135 (maintenance, PM, and alteration) and must be followed and documented in the maintenance records.[7] All maintenance records must be available for inspection by the FAA or a representative of the National Transportation Safety Board.

The most commonly understood maintenance deals with *unscheduled* repairs and alterations, which are classified as major or minor. For major maintenance repairs or alterations, a certified A & P mechanic holding an IA or the FAA must approve the job. An A & P mechanic, a certified repair station, or the FAA must approve the minor maintenance before an aircraft can return into service.

If an air medical service contracts with an operator, the program will have dedicated mechanics assigned to the RW or FW aircraft. These mechanics will conduct the various inspections and complete the *scheduled* and *unscheduled* maintenance for the particular type of aircraft. Again, the program administrator and medical director need to understand the inspection requirements and FARs pertinent to that particular aircraft and operation. This understanding will reduce disputes and frustrations when an aircraft is out of service for maintenance at the time that a flight request is received.

Backup aircraft may be an option for some air medical programs during major maintenance to keep an aircraft in-service 24 hours a day. The program's contractual agreement should outline the type of aircraft, medical configuration requirements, guidelines for use, and financial liabilities for a backup aircraft.

IN-FLIGHT SAFETY OPERATIONS/ REGULATIONS

Numerous FARs refer to safety practices while in-flight. Although the flight crewmember or pilot must comply with the FARs, air medical personnel must be educated to the appropriate FARs to assist the pilot toward the goal of safety for *all* passengers. Ultimately, a pediatric air medical program must be safe or it will not benefit the community. In-flight safety regulations encompass not only the actual briefing of safety practices for FAR Part 135.117, but physical compliance with them. FARs should be reviewed for using safety belts, placing seat backs in an upright position, carrying fire extinguishers, prohibiting smoking, and securing equipment and cargo. AMP should be educated to these FARs during an initial education program and on an annual basis. For a more extensive review, see Chapter 49.

Safety belts

According to FAR 91.105, 135.171, and 135.128,[7] all flight crewmembers and passengers are required to wear safety belts for *all* takeoffs and landings. In addition, if the seat is equipped with a shoulder harness, then the air medical personnel must wear it. All air medical personnel should also attempt to wear safety belts during in-flight procedures when possible.

All patients should be secured to the litter or gurney during not only takeoffs and landings, but also during cruise flight. The patient should be secured to the litter with FAA approved straps, but due to the varying heights and weights of pediatric patients, other means may be needed for securing the smaller child, toddler, or infant. An infant or child car seat approved for aircraft will be more secure than the straps on the stretcher. This device is then secured to the stretcher. At no time should the child be held solely by the air medical personnel while in-flight.

Seat backs

FAA regulation 135.117 requires that all seat backs be in an upright position for all takeoffs and landings.[7] This may also affect various types of stretchers or gurneys. Some manufacturers require that the head of the stretcher be in the locked flat position during takeoffs and landings for the patient's safety, especially for fixed-wing operations.

Fire extinguishers

FAR Parts 91.513 and 135.155 note the requirements for fire extinguishers on board passenger carrying aircraft. All FW and RW aircraft must carry a minimum of one handheld fire extinguisher, conveniently located in the cockpit for use by the pilot.[7] In addition, flight crewmembers and air medical personnel should have annual education regarding fire safety and the use of the fire extinguisher against all types of fires. This education should include emergency procedures for fires within the aircraft while in-flight and while on the ground.

No smoking rule

FAR Part 135.127 states that smoking is prohibited and that all passengers must comply with the lighted "No Smoking" sign or posted placards. These signs should be posted visibly within the aircraft. In addition, there should be no smoking within 50 feet of the oxygen carrying system of the aircraft.

Securing equipment/cargo

All medical and patient equipment must be properly secured in an approved bin, cargo rack, or compartment installed in the aircraft according to FAR 135.87.[7] This is especially important while providing patient care. AMP must secure trauma and medication bags, cardiac monitors, O_2 cylinders, ventilators, and so on to prevent movement during air turbulence or aircraft emergency. Any loose medical equipment can become a missle within the cabin during air turbulence or if the pilot initiates an emergency aircraft maneuver due to rapid decompression in a FW aircraft or to avoid a midair collision.

AIRCRAFT EMERGENCY PROCEDURES

All AMP should receive initial and annual on-going education regarding *unscheduled* aircraft emergencies. The AMP should receive education appropriate for the type of aircraft.

According to FAR 91.505 and 135.331,[7] all flight crew should receive emergency training for each aircraft type, model, and configuration. In addition, at a minimum, an annual safety program should be conducted involving AMP to review all aviation emergency procedures so that crew members will be able to confidently perform the following tasks:

1. Anticipate the PIC's directives for emergency procedures and rapid egress during an aircraft emergency through the emergency exits.
2. Execute the emergency procedures as instructed by the PIC.
3. Execute emergency shut-off and rapid egress procedures in case of an incapaciated pilot in command.
4. Assist with post incident/accident procedures for location of the aircraft and initiation of techniques for personal survival.
5. Minimize personal stress to be able to perform emergency procedures calmly.

The pilots should review potential aircraft emergencies with AMP so that they can understand and assist the pilot with various procedures. Emergencies will depend on the make and model of the aircraft, but at a minimum should consist of training for the following emergencies:

- fire in-flight
- fire on the surface or ground
- electrical failure
- hydraulic failure
- engine failure in-flight
- autorotation (for RW aircraft)
- tail rotor failure (for RW aircraft)
- rapid decompression (for pressurized FW aircraft)
- water ditching, if appropriate for the geographic coverage area

First, the pilots should provide a didactic component to review the potential aircraft emergencies during the initial flight education program for all AMP. Secondly, the pilots should provide a "clinical" component or "hands-on" session to conduct the actual procedures. The didactic and clinical components should be continued on an annual basis. For further review of emergency procedures, see Chapter 49.

To transport the critically ill or injured pediatric patient, air medical transport requires more than just placing a patient in an aircraft. It requires a tremendous effort by both medical and aviation experts to work together towards the common goal of **SAFETY**. Therefore program directors and pediatric medical directors must understand the Federal Aviation Regulations that were developed for aviation safety. Only then can we provide quality pediatric patient care in the air transport environment.

REFERENCES

1. *Accreditation standards of the commission on accreditation of air medical services,* ed 2, Anderson, SC, 1993.
2. Adams R, Taylor F: *Investigation of hazards of helicopter operation and root causes of helicopter accidents, Technical Report DOT/FAA/PM-86/28,* Washington DC, 1986, Federal Aviation Administration.
3. Americans With Disabilities Act of 1990: *EEOC technical assistance manual, Equal Employment Opportunity Manual no. 124,* Chicago, 1992, Commerce Clearing House.
4. ASHBEAMS and Samaritan AirEvac: *Air medical crew national standard curriculum: Instructor manual,* Pasadena, CA, 1988, ASHBEAMS.
5. Berg KL: Is it time to upgrade your weather system, *J Air Med Transp* 11(3):11-3, 1992.
6. Brink LW and others: Air transport: transport medicine, *Pediatr Clin North Am* 40(2):439-56, 1993.
7. Code of federal regulations: *Title 14, Aeronautics and Space, Federal Aviation Administration,* Parts 43, 91 and 135, 1993, US Department of Transportation.
8. Commission on Accreditation of Ambulance Services: *Standards for the accreditation of ambulance services,* Dallas, 1991, Commission on Accreditation of Ambulance Services.
9. Directory of air medical services, *Air Med J* 12(5):151-67, 1993.

10. Dodd R: *Safety study-commercial emergency medical service helicopter operations, Technical Report NTSB/SS-88/01,* Washington, DC, 1988, National Transportation Safety Board.
11. *42 United States Code, Consolidation Omnibus Budget Reconciliation Act (COBRA) of 1985 (42USC1395dd),* as amended by the Omnibus Budget Reconciliation Acts (OBRA) of 1987, 1989 and 1999.
12. Interhospital care of the perinatal patient. In *Guidelines for perinatal care,* ed 3 1992, Elk Grove Village, IL, American Academy of Pediatrics, and Washington, DC, American College of Obstretrics and Gynecology.
13. *Federal Specifications for Ambulances KKK-A-1822C* Washington, DC, January 1, 1990 General Services Administration.
14. Lee G and others: *Flight nursing: principles and practice,* St Louis, 1991, Mosby-Year Book.
15. *Pilot's handbook of aeronautical knowledge,* Washington, DC, 1984, US Department of Transportation.
16. Preston N: 1991 Air medical helicopter accident rates, *J Air Med Transp* 11(2):14-6, 1992.
17. Product and service guide, *Air Med J* 12(5):125-32, 1993.
18. Task Force on Interhospital Transport: *Guidelines for air and ground transport of neonatal and pediatric patients,* Elk Grove Village, IL, 1993, American Academy of Pediatrics.
19. Wraa CE, O'Malley R: Flight nurse physical requirements, *J Air Med Transp* 11(10):17-20, 1992.

ADDITIONAL READINGS FOR GENERAL AND GROUND REGULATIONS

Dooley RE: Court upholds $20,000 fine in 'anti-dumping' case, *Emergency* 23(10):12-4, 1991.

Foster FE: Destination dilemmas, government opt the ante, *JEMS* 16(7):67-9, 1991.

Scarano RM: COBRA snakes its way around the system, *JEMS* 16(7):59-62, 1991.

Scarano RM: COBRA strikes again, *JEMS* 17(12):25-6, 1992.

Schanaberger CJ: Understanding COBRAs twists and turns, *JEMS* 14(4):101-4, 1991.

US Department of Transportation National Highway Traffic Safety Administration: *Air medical crew: national standard curriculum,* Phoenix, AZ, ASHBEAMS, 1988.

US Department of Transportation National Highway Traffic Safety Administration: *Emergency medical services dispatcher: national standard curriculum,* Washington DC, 1983, US Department of Transportation.

US Department of Transportation National Highway Traffic Safety Administration: *Emergency medical services first responder training course:* Washington, DC, 1979, US Department of Transportation.

US Department of Transportation National Highway Traffic Safety Administration: *Emergency medical services instructor training program: national standard curriculum,* Washington, DC, 1986, US Department of Transportation.

US Department of Transportation National Highway Traffic Safety Administration: *Emergency medical technician-ambulance: national standard curriculum,* Washington DC, 1984, US Department of Transportation.

US Department of Transportation National Highway Traffic Safety Administration: *Emergency medical technician-intermediate: national standard curriculum,* Washington DC, 1985, US Department of Transportation.

US Department of Transportation National Highway Traffic Safety Administration: *Emergency medical technician-paramedic: national standard curriculum,* Washington DC, 1985, US Department of Transportation.

US Department of Transportation National Highway Traffic Safety Administration: *EMT-ambulance refresher training program: national standard curriculum,* Washington DC, 1988, US Department of Transportation.

US Department of Transportation National Highway Traffic Safety Administration: *EMT-paramedic refresher training program: national standard curriculum,* Washington DC, 1988, US Department of Transportation.

US Department of Transportation National Highway Traffic Safety Administration: *First responder refresher training program: national standard curriculum,* Washington DC, 1988, US Department of Transportation.

US Department of Transportation National Highway Traffic Safety Administration: *National standard curriculum for bystander care,* Washington DC, 1992, US Department of Transportation.

US Department of Transportation National Highway Traffic Safety Administration: *Training program for operation of emergency vehicles,* Washington DC, 1978, US Department of Transportation.

4

RESPONSIBILITIES OF THE REFERRING PHYSICIAN AND REFERRING HOSPITAL

ROBERT BOLTE

"Not unlike the moment of birth, an emergency is pivotal to the chance for continued life and all that it offers, or the despair and the loss that accompanies the death of a child or the loss of his or her intactness" (Stephen Ludwig, 1992). For the child with a critical illness or injury, the difference between a successful outcome and a tragedy is usually determined by the care delivered before arrival at the tertiary referral (receiving) hospital. The referring physician, whether based in an office or clinic, urgent care center, or general emergency department is a vital link (perhaps *the* vital link) in the system of Emergency Medical Services for Children (EMS-C). The referring physician has major responsibilities both in the initial management of the child requiring transport and in the coordination of transport in conjunction with the medical control physician at the receiving hospital.

The referring physician has the responsibility to provide adequate stabilization and resuscitation for the acutely ill or injured child. The expectations for stabilization capability escalate from the office to the urgent care center and then to the general emergency department. However, all physicians involved in acute care for children should have the capability to provide emergency cardiorespiratory support. In addition, all physicians have both a professional and legal responsibility for appropriate arrangement of referral and transport. At its core appropriate referral involves timely communication with the receiving hospital. In the case of the critically ill or injured child, this generally implies communication with pediatric emergency or intensive care specialists at a tertiary care center.

STABILIZATION

Training

In the office or clinic setting, caring for a critically ill child is a relatively uncommon event. In the urgent care center or general emergency department, a life-threatening condition in a child is encountered less commonly than in the adult patient. This relative unfamiliarity leads to a great deal of anxiety in most physicians and increases the likelihood of management errors, both of commission and omission. A common theme in the successful management of the critically ill or injured child is the importance of planning and preparation.

When encountering a critically ill child outside of a pediatric tertiary center, one must overcome the instinctive "get this kid out of here" reaction. Certainly the referring physician should make arrangements for emergency transport, whether this be a call to 911 or the pediatric acute care specialists, however, the priorities of stabilization (airway, breathing, circulation) and initial management priorities must be addressed immediately.

If a local transport from an office setting is

needed, the responsibility of the referring physician would be to resuscitate and stabilize the child while awaiting the arrival of the ambulance team. This simple tenet, however, is often violated. A recent survey found that private practitioners generally opted to use the family car for transport of seriously ill children (49% for epiglottitis, 55% for meningitis, 63% for sepsis) despite an average driving time of 60 minutes to the tertiary center. The potential medical and legal consequences resulting from any adverse outcome in such a transport is obvious.

In the setting of the general emergency department, the pitfalls are more subtle. The child with a severe closed head injury may be inappropriately sent for a CT scan before endotracheal intubation and hyperventilation have been performed. Other potential errors may involve the choice of transport modality, particularly for the longer transport. In the case of a critically ill child, the use of local ambulance crews for transport to the tertiary pediatric center may be inappropriate even though ambulance transport may be faster. These personnel probably do not possess the expertise to manage the significant problems (airway compromise, circulatory insufficiency, neurologic deterioration, etc.) which may occur and may not have the appropriate equipment to optimally handle situations which may arise. In most cases it would be more appropriate to utilize a specialized pediatric transport team (air or ground) rather than transporting the child via an adult-oriented air transport team, even if initial response times may be faster with the adult team. These transport modality decisions need to be individualized and, ideally, should be jointly made with the pediatric acute care specialists at the receiving hospital. In all cases it is the responsibility of the referring physician to adequately stabilize the critically ill or injured child prior to the arrival of appropriate transport services.

Implicit in this responsibility is the need for all physicians providing acute care for children to be proficient at pediatric basic and advanced life support. Courses are available to assist the physician in maintaining and improving upon the knowledge base and technical skills which are important in the management of the critically ill or injured child. Pediatric Advanced Life Support (PALS) was developed conjointly by the American Academy of Pediatrics (AAP) and the American Heart Association (AHA). This course integrates current information (refer to AHA guidelines for pediatric resuscitation in JAMA, Volume 268, pages 2251-2281, October, 1992) and motor skills so the practitioner may accurately assess impending respiratory and circulatory failure and have the technical skills to effectively intervene. Advanced Pediatric Life Support (APLS) was developed conjointly by the American Academy of Pediatrics and the American College of Emergency Physicians (ACEP). The goal of this course is to provide the physician with the information necessary to assess and manage critically ill or injured children during their first 30 to 60 minutes in the emergency department.

A recent survey of pediatricians found that those who were PALS-certified were more comfortable with their resuscitation skills and, more specifically, the placement of intraosseous needles. For the physician in the general emergency department, proficiency in the simple but crucial skill of intraosseous needle placement cannot be overemphasized. Moreover, a recent study has emphasized the importance of rapid sequence intubation (with paralytic agents) in the emergency department management of the critically ill or injured child. Proficiency using this skill for emergency department-based physicians is vital. In the community hospital setting professional training standards for both physicians and nurses have been developed by the Emergency Departments Approved for Pediatrics (EDAP) program. This California program, developed by Dr. James Seidel and his colleagues, provides a national model. For additional information, refer to Chapter 6 in the American Academy of Pediatrics publication on *Emergency Medical Services for Children.*

Equipment/supplies

Trained personnel require appropriate resources to successfully manage the critically ill child. Again, organization and preparation should occur before the crisis event. Resources must be organized so that staff members can quickly access appropriate emergency equipment and medications. All medical personnel in the office or emergency department must know the location of emergency equipment and supplies and be trained in pediatric stabilization skills. "Mock pediatric resuscitation codes" with relevant scenario's utilize a facility's own staff, equipment, and supplies, are a useful tool in evaluating the true readiness of a system. It would be useful to designate a single interested physician in your group as the "Pediatric Emergency Coordinator." This coordinator is given the responsibility of assessing your facility's ability to respond to pediatric emergencies and should then develop a plan of action which addresses deficiencies or areas for improvement. This analysis would apply not only to equipment and supplies, but also to policies and procedures as well. Local pediatric emergency departments may also serve as a valuable resource in this evaluation.

There should be a designated treatment area for pediatric emergencies. This vastly simplifies the organization of emergency equipment and supplies. Equipment may be organized according to the Broselow® system, with color-coded equipment sizes and dosages based on the height of the child. Labeled, wall-mounted supply boards, providing easy access and visual cues for restocking, are also an option. Whatever system of organization is employed, equipment and medications should be available to treat infants and children of all ages. The Broselow® tapes, providing specific recommendations for total medication doses and equipment sizes, may be utilized in both office and emergency department settings. These tapes have been shown to be more accurate in estimating weight than age-based systems. Moreover, the potential for errors in calculation is eliminated with this system. Reference materials for pediatric resuscitation, such as drug/equipment information, age-based norms for vital signs, resuscitation algorithms, and phone numbers for consultation and transport, should be highly visible and mounted on a wall in the pediatric treatment area. The designated pediatric treatment area must have oxygen and suction capability. In the office, if built-in wall outlets are unavailable, portable oxygen tanks and suction units can be used. Personnel should be trained and regularly tested in the appropriate and efficient use of this equipment.

Equipping an office for pediatric emergencies should be relatively inexpensive. Many items are commonly stocked in most offices. The American Academy of Pediatrics has developed lists of suggested supplies, equipment, and medications for treating pediatric emergencies in the office setting (Table 4-1 and Box 4-1). In addition, the Broselow® tape should be considered "standard equipment." Note that expensive monitoring equipment, such as a defibrillator, is defined as optional and should not be necessary in most office settings. A pulse oximeter would be the most useful item of optional equipment. Inexpensive, disposable CO_2 detectors, useful in verifying appropriate endotracheal tube placement, may also be of value.

Guidelines for equipment and supplies necessary for managing pediatric emergencies in the general emergency department setting have also been developed (Table 4-2). The level of expectation for monitoring and invasive intervention capability in the emergency department setting is understandably higher than that of the private office. In general these recommendations would also apply to urgent care centers with the obvious exception of thoracotomy, tracheostomy, and peritoneal lavage capability. In addition to the items in Table 4-2, it is recommended that a pulse oximeter and disposable CO_2 detectors be considered standard equipment. Additional drugs to be considered include midazolam and flumazenil. 10% dextrose in water may be eliminated from "Pediatric IV supplies," and pre-filled syringes of 25% dextrose and 50% dextrose may be added as potentially safer alternatives.

REFERRAL/TRANSPORT

Communication

The essence of a successful transport involves effective communication between physicians at the referring and receiving (referral) hospital. A proactive referral strategy should be developed prior to the acute transport situation. A plan for pediatric referral

TABLE 4-1 SUGGESTED SUPPLY AND EQUIPMENT LIST FOR TREATING PEDIATRIC EMERGENCIES IN THE OFFICE*

Airway management
Oxygen source with flowmeter
Oxygen masks—preemie, infant, child, and adult sizes
Bag-valve-mask resuscitators, including reservoir for infant, child, and adult
Suction—wall unit or machine
Suction catheters—Yankauer, 8F, 10F, and 14F
Oral airways—0.5
Nasal cannulas—infant, child, and adult sizes 1-3
Optional for intubation
Laryngoscope handle with Miller blades—0, 1, 2, 3
Endotracheal tubes, uncuffed—3.0, 3.5, 4.0, 4.5, 5.0, 6.0, 7.0, 8.0
Stylets—small and large
Magill forceps

Fluid management
Intraosseous needles—15-gauge and 18-gauge
IV catheters, short, over the needle—20-gauge, 22-gauge, and 24-gauge
Butterfly needles—21-gauge, 23-gauge, and 25-gauge

Fluid management (cont.)
IV boards, tape, alcohol swabs, and tourniquet
Pediatric drip chambers and tubing
D5 one-half normal saline
Isotonic fluids (normal saline or lactated Ringer's solution)
Optional: over guidewire catheters 3F, 4F, and 5F

Miscellaneous equipment
Blood pressure cuffs—preemie infant, child, and adult sizes
Nasogastric tubes—10F and 14F
Feeding tubes—3F and 5F
Foley catheters—8F and 10F
Sphygmomanometer
Cardiac arrest board

Optional equipment
Portable monitor defibrillator
Doppler
Noninvasive blood pressure monitor
Pulse oximeter

* From Singer J and Ludwig S, editors: *Emergency medical services for children: the role of the primary provider,* Elk Grove Village, IL, 1992, The Committee on Pediatric Emergency Medicine, American Academy of Pediatrics.

BOX 4-1 SUGGESTED MEDICATIONS FOR TREATING PEDIATRIC EMERGENCIES IN THE OFFICE*

Aqueous adrenalin—1:1000 and 1:10,000 concentrations
Dextrose in water—25% and 50%
Atropine sulfate
Sodium bicarbonate—4.2% and 8.4%
Calcium chloride—10%
Lorazepam or diazepam
Phenobarbital
Antibiotics—parenteral
Diphenhydramine—parenteral
Methylprednisolone
Naloxone
Ipecac
Activated charcoal
Albuterol for inhalation
L-epinephrine for nebulizer

* From Singer J and Ludwig S, editors: *Emergency medical services for children:* the role of the primary provider, Elk Grove Village, IL, 1992, The Committee on Pediatric Emergency Medicine, American Academy of Pediatrics.

and transport should involve triaging the patient to the most appropriate facility by the most appropriate transport modality, thereby maximizing patient safety and utilization of resources. From the office setting many acute noncritical referrals can be directed to a general emergency department, whereas, the critically ill or injured child needs prompt referral to a tertiary center with pediatric critical care capability. A list of names and phone numbers of pediatric acute care consultants, transport systems, and receiving hospitals should be clearly posted in the pediatric treatment area of the referring facility. For interhospital transport the AAP has advocated the establishment of formal transfer agreements to facilitate appropriate and timely transports.

To optimize management of the critically ill child, early communication with the receiving facility is vital. This communication should occur between the referring physician and the pediatric acute care specialist (Emergency Medicine, Critical Care, Neonatology,

TABLE 4-2 EQUIPMENT, TRAYS, AND SUPPLIES FOR TREATING PEDIATRIC EMERGENCIES IN THE GENERAL EMERGENCY DEPARTMENT*

Standard requirements for equipment
Pediatric bag-valve resuscitation device
Transparent masks to use with bag-valve device in preemie, infant, child, and adult sizes
Laryngoscope with infant and child laryngoscope blades, curved and straight (sizes 0-3)
Pediatric Magill forceps
Cervical spine immobilization devices (sand bags, stiff neck headbed, etc); rigid four-post or plastic/Velcro collars in sizes for children and adults
Pediatric femur splint (pediatric antishock garments may be used to fulfill this requirement)
Blood warmer
An infant warming procedure/device
Infusion pumps—drip, or volumetric
Pediatric bone marrow needles for intraosseous infusion (15-gauge and 18-gauge)
Blood pressure cuffs—infant, child, adult and thigh sizes
Doppler-sensing device for blood pressure measurement
Monitor-defibrillator with 0-400 W/s capability
Pediatric scale
An appropriate procedure or device for ensuring pediatric restraint

Standard requirements for trays
Pediatric thoracotomy tray, including pediatric rib-spreader and aortic clamp
Pediatric tracheostomy tray with tracheostomy tubes (sizes 0-3)

Standard requirements for trays (cont.)
Setup for needle cricothyrotomy (3.5 Portex adapter and 14-gauge over-the-needle catheter acceptable)
Venesection tray appropriate for infants and children
Peritoneal lavage tray
Pediatric lumbar puncture trays with 22-gauge, 1.5-inch spinal needle

Standard requirements for supplies
Pediatric oral airways (sizes 0-5)
Endotracheal tubes (sizes 2.5-9.0)
Chest tubes (sizes 16-28 F; size 26 unavailable)
Pediatric IV supplies, including volumetric sets, butterflies, and over-the-needle catheters: 25-gauge through 14-gauge; 250 mL or 500 mL bags of NS, D5/0.25 NS, D5/0.5 NS, D5 NS, D10/W
Printed pediatric drug dosage reference material (calculated on dose-per-kilogram basis), readily available, preferably on a wall-mounted chart or the Broselow® tape system of drug dosing by length
Sodium bicarbonate, in 10 mEq/10 mL prefilled syringes
All drugs currently recommended for pediatric and adult resuscitation by the AHA
Pediatric nasogastric tubes, including sizes 3.0-F and 5.0-F infant feeding tubes
Pediatric Foley catheters (sizes 8-22F)

* From Singer J and Ludwig S, editors: *Emergency medical services for children: the role of the primary provider*, Elk Grove Village, IL, 1992, The Committee on Pediatric Emergency Medicine, American Academy of Pediatrics.

Pediatric Surgery) at the receiving tertiary center. It is important that the referring physician utilize the pediatric acute care specialist (medical control physician) not only as an agent to arrange the transport but also as a consultant. Immediate treatment can be reviewed, management options discussed, and the most appropriate mode of transport determined (ground, rotor wing, or fixed wing; general versus specialized team). The referring physician should have the patient's chart available at the time of the initial call in order to be able to provide specific details regarding vital signs, weight, medications, and fluids, as well as pertinent history and physical findings. Obviously, this type of interchange cannot meaningfully impact patient care if the call is placed after the patient is en route to the receiving hospital.

The importance of early physician-to-physician communication cannot be overemphasized. Significant changes in management may occur as a result of this conversation, often well before the arrival of the transport team. Decisions regarding the need for intubation (in general, aggressive recommendations will be made to ensure control of the airway prior to transport), use of paralytic agents, specifics of volume and vasopressor support, management of potential intracranial pressure elevations, and advisability of ancillary diagnostic studies at the referring hospital (e.g. CT scanning) are only a few of the topics which may be covered in the first few minutes of the consultation. The impact of these decisions has paramount importance for the child's ultimate outcome. These decisions need to be individualized utilizing the skills and experience of both the referring physician and pediatric medical control physician. Studies suggest that when this early communication is optimized, management errors are minimized and transport stabilization times (after team arrival at the referring facility) are reduced.

While the transport team is en route, it is the responsibility of the referring physician to attempt to implement the management plan agreed upon after consultation with the pediatric acute care specialist. Adaptation of the recommended management plan may be necessary based on changes in the patient's clinical condition and the technical expertise of the staff at the referring hospital. However, the referring physician should notify the medical control physician of any major changes in the patient's status. The referring physician should prepare a brief transfer note which highlights pertinent history, physical findings, and interventions. The parents should be briefed by the referring physician regarding the nature of the child's illness, potential outcome, and the reason for the upcoming transport. In addition, the staff at the referring hospital can greatly improve the safety and efficiency of the transport by completing several tasks prior to the arrival of the transport team. For the critically ill or injured child, two sites of stable intravascular access should be routinely obtained. The cervical spine and other potential fracture sites should be stabilized, if appropriate. Nasogastric and foley catheters are often indicated. All tubes and lines (most importantly, the endotracheal tube) must be secured. If the patient is at risk for hemorrhagic shock, blood products should be prepared for transport. In the emergent setting, uncrossmatched O negative blood is acceptable. However, type-specific (with 15 minute availability at most centers) or fully crossmatched blood is preferable provided the transport is not delayed. All records and radiographs should be copied. In addition, written consent for transfer and treatment should be obtained. Standardized "transport consent" forms may be available from the transport systems in your region. The parents should be present to briefly speak with the transport team prior to their departure from the referring facility. If emergent operative intervention is anticipated on return to the receiving hospital, a parent should remain at the referring hospital until an operative permit can be obtained via telephone by the responsible surgeon.

Depending on the clinical setting, the referring physician should remain at the patient's bedside and/or be available for immediate consultation, pending the arrival of the transport team. If requested, it may be necessary for the staff of the referring hospital to assist the transport team in ongoing stabilization of the patient after their arrival. Effective on-site communication between referring physician and the transport team is yet another important variable in a successful transport. Potential barriers to communication may arise as the referring physician encounters specialized expertise offered by younger, and often non-physician professionals. With the development of an ongoing professional relationship, these barriers inevitably fall. However, during the developmental phase, interactions must reflect mutual respect in an admittedly high stress environment, always keeping optimal patient care as the primary concern.

Legal issues

The medico-legal aspects of transport medicine, including the currently evolving implications of COBRA/OBRA legislation, are discussed in detail elsewhere in this textbook. This final section will briefly highlight some of these issues.

Legal responsibility for the transported patient represents a continuum. Increased involvement in the care of the patient implies an increased legal responsibility. At the time of initial consultation with the pediatric acute care specialist (medical control physician), a process of shared responsibility begins. The referring physician is obligated to attempt to implement the medical control physician's recommendations whenever feasible. It is obviously prudent to document any advice given or received in the context of a patient transport. When the transport team assumes care of the patient, primary responsibility shifts to the receiving hospital (assuming the transport team is based at the receiving hospital). Any significant conflict over patient management decisions occurring before the physical departure of the transport team from the referring facility should be resolved at the attending physician level.

In 1985 Congress enacted the Consolidated Omnibus Budget Reconciliation Act (COBRA) with the goal of assuring safe patient transfers between medical facilities and to prevent patient "dumping" between hospitals based on the patient's inability to pay. This legislation requires the referring hospital to assume liability for the adequacy of stabilization prior to transport. It also requires documentation that the receiving hospital has been contacted and that a receiving physician is willing to accept care of the patient before transfer. To transfer a patient before such arrangements are made is construed as medical abandonment. COBRA also places the referring hospital in the position of guaranteeing the adequacy of the receiving hospital. The referring hospital will ultimately be held accountable for choosing the most appropriate transport modality based on the medical condition of the patient. Degradation in the quality of care provided during the transport is also considered medical abandonment. The referring physician and hospital must ensure that the skills of the transport personnel and the equipment available during transport are adequate for the anticipated medical needs of the patient. The implications for both referring hospitals and transport services (particularly specialty transport services such as pediatrics) are obvious. Clearly COBRA, with its significant legal sanctions, focuses attention on the importance of effective communication. The Omnibus Budget Reconciliation Act (OBRA) amendment of 1989 requires referring hospitals to make an effort to obtain written consent from all patients involved in interhospital transfer. In addition, specialized units and hospitals are required to accept appropriate transfers if space is available without regard for ability to pay.

SUMMARY

The responsibilities of the referring physician and hospital in managing the critically ill or injured child include providing adequate stabilization and arranging appropriate referral and transport. Early effective communication between the referring physician and the pediatric acute care consultant (Emergency Medicine/Critical Care, etc.) is the key to a successful transport. Planning and preparation will facilitate an appropriate response to that pivotal moment, the pediatric emergency.

ADDITIONAL READINGS

1. Altieri M, Bellet J, Scott H: Preparedness for pediatric emergencies encountered in the practitioner's office, *Pediatrics* 85:710-14, 1990.
2. Aoki BY, McCloskey KA: *Evaluation, stabilization, and transport of the critically ill child,* St. Louis, 1992, Mosby-Year Book.
3. Baker MD, Ludwig S: Pediatric emergency transport and the private practitioner, *Pediatrics* 88:691-5, 1991.
4. Bourlier D, Pratt J: Pediatric office emergencies: a closer look (abstract), *Pediatr Emerg Care* 8:308-9, 1992.
5. Corneli HM: Evaluation, treatment, and transport of pediatric patients with shock, *Pediatr Clin North Am* 40(2):303-19, 1993.
6. Crippen D: Critical care transportation medicine: new concepts in pretransport stabilization of the critically ill patient, *Am J Emerg Med* 8(6):551-4.
7. Day S and others: Pediatric interhospital critical care transport: consensus of a national leadership conference, *Pediatrics* 88:696-704, 1991.
8. Dieckmann RA: *Pediatric emergency care systems,* Baltimore, 1992, Williams & Wilkins.
9. Emergency Cardiac Care Committee and Subcommittees, American Heart Association: Part V: Pediatric basic life support, *JAMA* 268:2251-61, 1992.
10. Emergency Cardiac Care Committee and Subcommittees, American Heart Association: Part VI: Pediatric advanced life support, *JAMA* 268:2262-75, 1992.
11. Emergency Cardiac Care Committee and Subcommittees, American Heart Association: Part VII: Neonatal resuscitation, *JAMA* 268:2276-81, 1992.
12. Frew SA, Roush WR, LaGreca K: COBRA: implications for emergency medicine, *Ann Emerg Med* 17(8):835-7, 1988.
13. Fuchs S, Jaffe DM, Christoffel KK: Pediatric emergencies in office practices: prevalence and office preparedness, *Pediatrics* 83:931-9, 1989.
14. Dean JM: Head trauma: management, intracranial-pressure control, and morbidity/mortality, *Emergency medical services for children, report of the ninety-seventh Ross conference on pediatric research,* Columbus, Ohio, 1989, Ross Laboratories.
15. Henning R: Emergency transport of critically ill children: stabilization before departure, *The Medical Journal of Australia* 156:117-124, 1992.
16. Hodge D III: Pediatric emergency office equipment, *Pediatr Emerg Care* 4:212-4, 1988.

17. Kanter RK: Evaluation and stabilization of the critically ill child, *Clinics in Chest Medicine* 8(4):573-81, 1987.
18. Krnoick JB, Kissoon N, Frewen TC: Guidelines for stabilizing the condition of the critically ill child before transfer to a tertiary care facility, *Current Review* 139:213-20, 1988.
19. Leicht MJ and others: Rural interhospital helicopter transport of motor vehicle trauma victims: causes for delays and recommendations, *Annals of Emerg Med* 15(4):450-3, 1986.
20. McCloskey KA, Orr RA: Interhospital transport. In Barkin RM, editor: *Pediatric Emergency Care*, St. Louis, 1992, Mosby-Year Book.
21. McCloskey KA, Orr RA: Pediatric transport issues in emergency medicine, *Emerg Med Clin North Am* 9:475-89, 1991.
22. McCloskey KA and others: *Guidelines for air and ground transport of neonatal and pediatric patients*, Elk Grove Village, 1993, American Academy of Pediatrics.
23. McDonald TB, Berkowitz RA: Airway management and sedation for pediatric transport, *Pediatr Clin North Am* 40(2):381-406, 1993.
24. Schoenfeld PS, Baker MD: Management of cardiopulmonary and trauma resuscitation in the pediatric emergency department, *Pediatrics* 91:726-9, 1993.
25. Schweich PJ, DeAngelis C, Duggan AK: Preparedness of practicing pediatricians to manage emergencies, *Pediatrics* 88:223-9, 1991.
26. Seider JS and others: Emergency medical services and the pediatric patient: are the needs being met? *Pediatrics* 73:769-72, 1984.
27. Seider JS: Emergency medical services and the pediatric patient: training and equipping emergency medical services providers for pediatric emergencies, *Pediatrics* 78:808-12, 1986.
28. Singer J, Ludwig S (editors): *Emergency medical services for children: the role of the primary care provider*, Elk Grove Village, Illinois, 1992, Committee on Pediatric Emergency Medicine, American Academy of Pediatrics.
29. Vernon DD, Woodward GA, Skjonsberg AK: Management of the patient with head injury during transport, *Critical Care Clinics* 8(3):619-31, 1992.

5

RESPONSIBILITIES OF THE RECEIVING HOSPITAL

GEORGE A. WOODWARD

The receiving hospital and control center for critical care transport are the backbone of a successful pediatric transport system. This chapter will assume that the receiving hospital is also in control of the transport, although much of the text will apply to other specialty hospitals to which transports are being arranged. A patient transport is a demonstration of the transport system in action and is not the time to discover deficiencies in organization, planning, training, or personnel. When involved with a transport system at a receiving tertiary care or specialty hospital, one must anticipate problems and organize plans of action before transports.

There are many patient and system needs which should be assessed prior to transport. These include the transport administrative structure along with the hospital or transport team administrator, the hierarchy of medical and nursing components, and the dispatch or phone operators at the receiving hospital. Breakdown at any level can result in a poorly organized transport system and potential adverse patient outcomes.

Inefficient entry into the transport system can be confusing and frustrating for the referring caretaker as well as potentially life threatening for the patient whose transport is delayed. A fool-proof system needs to be arranged for handling initial calls from referring hospitals. This can be done through a dispatch center with a centralized number, by direct calls to specific units such as the intensive care or emergency department, or with calls to a hospital operator.

Phone contact numbers for transport referrals should be widely disseminated and reviewed periodically with all potential referral sources. Toll-free numbers, phone index cards, phone stickers, brochures, calendars, and posters can all help easily identify the appropriate numbers for the transport system. All potential recipients of calls should understand where these calls should be directed, and this should be accomplished with a single transfer. Nonmedical persons receiving calls requesting transport, should immediately identify the nature of the requested transport (neonatal, pediatric, or adult) and direct it to the appropriate control physician while remaining on the line. There is no room in an effective transport system for multiple phone calls by the referring facility or endless transfers within the receiving hospital system. The medical control physician needs to be clearly identified and there must be a fail-safe system for locating this person at all times. Cellular phones add a dimension to initial phone contact which allows a control physician to be immediately available within the confines of the range and battery power of the equipment.

The types of patients that can be accepted by the transport team and the receiving hospital need to be established and continually reviewed. If a hospital or transport system is unable to accept certain types of patients, due to specific patient illness, injury, or severity or equipment or personnel problems; that information should be known by the control physician and be immediately relayed to the referring hospital. One can see how transporting a patient a long distance to a control or receiving hospital that has no intensive care capabilities or available ICU bed, may be detrimental to the patient. If a situation arises where the control hospital is temporarily unable to accept certain types of patients, the control physician should be aware of viable alternatives either at the control hospital or another center. The control physician has a responsibility to help arrange transport to an alternative center or at least to identify the steps to be taken by the referral center in order to obtain access to another center or transport system. It is unacceptable for the initial control physician to wash his or her hands of the transport request simply because there is currently no bed available at a particular institution. If the patient's financial status impacts the possibility or mode of transport, this should be clearly identified prior to transport initiation. Written transport agreements between referring and receiving institutions can be helpful in addressing these issues.

The referral hospital and control center should ideally have the capability to vary transport team composition to reflect the needs of the patient. While many transport teams function with a set group of personnel, regardless of the type or age of the transported patient, it is more beneficial for young patients to have pediatric specialty teams available. These specialty teams can respond effectively to the varied needs of children, such as a two-week-old with a hypoplasia, a four-year-old with epiglottitis, or an eight-year-old multiple trauma patient. The medical control physician is responsible for identifying the needs of the patient and establishing the appropriate team composition for that particular transport. The transport system should have the flexibility to amend team composition as needed to include specific physicians, nurses, respiratory therapists, and other specialty team members as indicated by the type and severity of patient to be transported. In addition to flexible team composition, one should also be able to choose between modes of transport (ground, fixed, or rotor wing), depending on the severity of the patient and the distance to be transported.

An ideal transport system would have ground, rotary wing, and fixed wing capability, with backup equipment immediately available. The transport hardware needs to be adequate, available, and functional. The receiving hospital should guarantee, to the best of its ability, that the hardware used for transport is safe, reliable, legal, and current. The medical equipment to be used on transport should be reliable, working, appropriate for the individual patient, and safe for the transport environment.

The receiving hospital and transport team should ensure that the transport team members are competent, well-educated, and current in all required certifications. Physicians are not qualified to transport an individual solely on the basis of their degree. Transport physicians, nurses, and respiratory therapists need to be specialists for whom transport is an integral part of their responsibility and who recognize the pitfalls that one may encounter during a transport. Transport protocols and guidelines can be very helpful for nonphysician teams to offer immediate response to compromised patients.

One must also ensure the psychological well-being of the transport team members. Realizing the stress these caretakers encounter and assuring adequate stress relief and psychological evaluations as necessary is critical in maintaining a functioning transport team.

The safety of the transport team and the transported patient should be ensured, as much as possible, prior to any transport. There should be no question of equipment familiarity or currency for any personnel. Weight can be an issue for rotary wing transports and, if so, current weights should be available for all transport personnel. Up-to-date safety briefings for each particular aircraft and ground ambulance should be documented. Weather-related decisions should be entirely at the discretion of the pilot or driver and should not be influenced by the patient's clinical status.

There should be instruction and routine reviews regarding emergency procedures that may vary depending on the mode of transport. For transport teams that routinely transport over long distances of barren, mountainous areas, wilderness and survival training should be an integral part of the safety training.

Once transports are initiated, it is critical that they be accomplished in a timely manner and that the referring hospital be aware of potential delays, so other arrangements can be made and the patient managed appropriately during the delay. Each receiving hospital should have guidelines regarding the dispatch of the transport team. Five minute rotary wing lift-off or 20 to 30 minute ground or fixed wing transport mobilization times are not unreasonable. Rapid mobilization and speed of transport do not ensure a successful transport, however. It may be more advisable to send a specialized pediatric team by ground than a nonpediatric team by air, because in effect the patient might receive and benefit from specialized pediatric care sooner. Decisions by the referring center to send potentially critically ill children by private vehicle so that they can arrive at the receiving hospital sooner should be discouraged. Decisions must be made which sometimes necessitate a compromise in speed or level of specialized service depending on the specifics of the individual transport. Alternative modes of transportation must also be available when weather or equipment problems necessitate a change in plans.

The control physicians should be emergency medicine or critical care physicians instead of specialists who may be more concerned with an individual organ system rather than the basics of cardiopulmonary resuscitation and stabilization. The control physician must, from the moment of contact, ensure adequate care of the patient. That includes reviewing the events leading to the transport decision, the medical care administered to date, and offering specific suggestions for further intervention. With a good control physician and an adequate referring hospital, unexpected contingencies regarding patient status on arrival to the referral hospital should be limited.

It is the responsibility of the control and the referring physicians together to determine the best receiving hospital for the particular patient. In some situations this decision may be very clear, while in others it may not be quite as obvious. Examples of patients which may be controlled by the tertiary care center, but directed to other facilities, include those with amputated limbs who need microvascular surgery which is available at another institution, patients who need dialysis, or patients with burns when a burn unit is not located in the control facility. These types of referrals may become more common as the medical system is redefined over the next several years. Prior to the arrival of the transport team, receiving physicians should be identified and the case discussed with them so that specific care can be suggested and enacted in anticipation of patient arrival at the receiving hospital.

The transport, once undertaken, should ensure that patient care does not deteriorate between the referring and the receiving hospital. The law demands that, at no time during the transport process, should the level of care be less than what was originally available at the referring institution. The transport team should, ideally, be capable of providing the same quality care that the patient will expect on arrival at the receiving or tertiary care hospital. Excluding rare mechanical limitations (x-ray equipment, blood gas analyzers) there is no excuse for a decrease in level of care during transport.

One must ensure that the referring hospitals are as knowledgeable as possible regarding the emergent stabilization of children as well as the limitations of the particular transport system. This can be accomplished by direct feedback concerning individual transports, but is probably more effectively achieved by means of outreach education by transport personnel as to the latest updates in resuscitative care and the capabilities of the transport system.

The transport team needs to develop an adequate billing system to arrange for reimbursement of transports. If possible this should be done through a separate billing center within the receiving hospital. Transport systems, especially those which involve aircraft, are very expensive to maintain, and few nonreimbursed transports can quickly undermine the solvency of the system.

The transport process brings with it a huge potential for medical and legal risk. All participants and hardware involved in the transport process should be insured to avoid financial instability secondary to medical or mechanical problems encountered during the transport. This should be arranged prior to the team embarking on transports and should be routinely reassessed for needs and adequacy.

ACTUAL TRANSPORT

Once the preceding basic arrangements have occurred, transports can take place. The transport is initiated by notifying the referring caregiver that a patient requires transport to a hospital with a different level or type of service available. A central contact phone number is preferable for entering the transport system. If this is not possible, however, all those who might potentially be on the receiving end of a transport call should know exactly how to locate a control physician immediately and efficiently. In cases involving hospital operators or nonmedical personnel, this should be in the form of written directives on immediately contacting the control physician and initiating the transport process. Initial questions should include the type of patient and transport desired (neonatal, pediatric, adult) and the name, location, and phone number of the referring hospital in case of inadvertent disconnection. The control physician should be identified to the referring hospital because this information will be required for their records.

Once the control physician has been contacted, it is imperative to review patient specifics including age, problem, pertinent medical history, interventions, and current status, including vital signs. A transport referral form can be invaluable in prompting the control physician to ask for specific information (Figure 5-1). It is imperative that the name and phone number of the referring physician, hospital, and the patient's location within the hospital be verified early in the initial contact so that the transport team is directed to the correct location. The transport referral form can help prevent an embarrassing misdirection of the transport team. The use of a similar form by the referring and receiving hospital can alert both centers to the expected information needed for an efficient transport. A control physician who neglects to review vital signs or type of fluids being administered and assumes that unstated care is appropriate care may be displeased when a patient arrives hyposensitive or comatose condition because of a D5/W bolus or similar mismanagement. The control physician should remember that he or she is becoming involved with the patient because he or she represents an increased level of expertise. This should be demonstrated by a complete pretransport review of the patient. Interventions should be suggested by the control physician as necessary. Interventions and suggestions should be discussed in detail with modifications made depending on the sophistication of the referring center. The control physician and the transport system accepts a legal responsibility to provide care for the patient once the transport call is initiated, although this responsibility is shared until the transport team has taken control of the patient and arrived at the receiving institution. One can appreciate the medical and legal importance of adequately documenting transport information and management suggestions as it is received. A summary of that interaction should be included in the patient's transport record.

The control physician should request that the referring hospital make copies of all pertinent medical material, including medical records, laboratory, and radiographic evaluations. It is not acceptable for the team to be delayed at a referring hospital while records are being copied because this should have been done beforehand. The control physician should also ensure that the parents or patient will give permission for transport. While emergency implied consent is available when a patient is at a location which cannot effectively manage the patient or when parents or guardians are not available, there will be instances when caretakers refuse transport. This situation should be identified early in the transport process, not upon arrival of the transport team. Written transport agreements between the referring and receiving hospitals, which as negotiated prior to transport, can be very helpful in obtaining permis-

☐ PCMC ☐ McKAY-DEE ☐ UTAH VALLEY ☐ DIXIE

DATE	TIME OF CALL	CALL RECEIVED VIA: ☐ DIRECT REFERRAL ☐ DISPATCH ☐ OTHER ______

PT NAME	AGE	DOB

REFERRING PHYSICIAN	PHONE

HOSPITAL/ CLINIC	CITY/STATE

ACCEPTING PHYSICIAN	☐ NOTIFIED	TIME
CONSULTANTS	☐ NOTIFIED	TIME

HISTORY, PHYSICAL EXAM & CURRENT MANAGEMENT

TEMP	PULSE	RESP ☐ INTUBATED	BP	WT	☐ IV ☐ NG ☐ FOLEY

LAB DATA

CBC CHEMISTRIES

BLOOD GAS (A/V/C) FiO_2

OTHER LABS

X-RAYS

RECOMMENDED MANAGEMENT

CALL BACK INFORMATION

TIME	ETA

ADMIT TO:
☐ NBICU ☐ ED
☐ PICU
☐ ______

TRANSPORTATION: ☐ ROTO ☐ FIXED ☐ GROUND ☐ PVT. VEHICLE

JUSTIFICATION FOR MODE OF TRANSPORT: ______

______

CONTROL M.D. ______

LIFE FLIGHT DISPATCH: **(801) 321-1234**

IHC NEONATAL/PEDIATRIC TRANSPORT INFORMATION

IHC TR-810/5-92

Fig. 5-1. Transport referral form

sion for transports. The transport team should also verify that there is a written order for transport by the referring physician. If it appears to the referring hospital or control physician that the patient may need operative intervention soon after arrival at the receiving hospital, a parent or guardian should be available by phone at all times until the child's condition is determined at the receiving hospital. Operative consents are needed prior to surgical intervention, and delays because parents are en route should be avoided. This should be anticipated by the control and referring physicians, discussed, and plans made for obtaining consent.

It is important for the control physician to understand the limitations of the referring hospital and personnel and to work within those confines. There is no room for a condescending control physician or one who humiliates or antagonizes referring caregivers. Unfortunately, it is often the young resident or attending physician who becomes angry with referring facilities whom he or she feels are not performing to his or her expectations, and in doing so, undermines the entire transport system. If the referring hospital has options for different transport arrangements, one can be sure these will be exercised in the future.

Once a transport request has been received, team composition must be evaluated. If the team composition cannot be altered, then this step involves merely identifying and notifying those transport team members who are currently on-call. If team composition is variable, however, then the control physician should make changes as necessary. Transport team composition may be dictated by the type of equipment used to transport the patient, (a large ambulance or fixed wing aircraft versus a smaller helicopter) as well as the severity of the patient's illness. Team composition can vary between physician teams, nurse-led teams, respiratory therapists, and paramedics or a mix of the above. The titles of the team members are not as important as the skills and training that those caretakers have received.

If time allows, communication between the control physician and transport team members should take place before transport. This initial contact can serve as an introduction to the patient's condition, a review of pathophysiology, discussion of priorities for that patient, and formulation of a treatment plan. Medication usage can also be discussed at this time, while dosages can be calculated en route. The time before arrival at the referring center can also be used to assign roles to each team member to help streamline care and avoid conflict while caring for the patient. Exception to the pretransport patient review may be made for helicopter-scene flights which, by character, necessitate immediate response. When possible, air-to-ground or ground-to-ground communication by on-scene medical personnel may serve to update the receiving institution regarding the patient's status. The control physician should have no questions as to the capabilities of individual transport team members including all necessary certifications and state licenses. These should be evaluated prior to any involvement in transport. The same should be said for insurance coverage of all those involved in a particular transport. There is no room for transport delay due to administrative or financial considerations that could have been attended to beforehand.

Along with team composition, the control physician must select the most prudent, safe, and cost-effective mode of transport depending on patient condition, available hardware, and weather. The control physician should be aware at all times of the availability of particular hardware and personnel. If the system has ground, fixed-wing and rotor-wing transports available, it is helpful to know if each is available prior to a call from a referring hospital. A system should be in place to notify control physicians if there are mechanical problems or transports in progress for which that control physician may not be intimately involved. Knowing this information can make transport management smoother from the initial call.

The control physician should anticipate what ancillary equipment, blood products, or medications might be needed for a particular transport and take steps to obtain those items. If a patient is being transported from a rural community clinic who has been hit by a truck, blood products may be needed during the transport, and O negative blood should accompany the transport team. The same can be said for specific equipment and medications which might be needed, such as central venous catheters for a septic child or prostaglandins for a 2-week-old infant with cyanosis.

Once the initial call has been received, the control physician and transport system have a responsibility to the patient being transported. The control physician should understand this responsibility and treat the patient to the best of his or her ability with phone advice to avoid any unexpected situations on arrival of the transport team. With the appropriate involvement of the control physician and a predictable medical or surgical process, the patient should be stabilized prior to transport to avoid delays in arriving at the tertiary care or receiving center. Specific tasks which generally should not wait for the arrival of a transport team (unless there are significant deficits in the capabilities of the referring institution) include making sure that an airway is available, adequately taping an endotracheal tube in place, IV placement, naso/orogastric tube and foley catheter placement, ensuring availability of blood products if necessary, obtaining patient medical history, having parents available for consent, speaking to the family about the plans, and copying all pertinent medical data. It is important to offer the referring hospital an estimated time of arrival and to update the hospital if there are delays which occur during the arranging of the transport.

The transport team is responsible for obtaining as much information as possible from the referring institution, because this will be the link that ensures continuity of care from the patient's arrival at the referring hospital through transport at the receiving hospital. Upon arrival at the referring hospital, the transport team should introduce themselves to establish a cooperative working relationship with the referring personnel. Care must be taken to avoid personality or turf battles while attending to the patient to be transported. The transport team needs to realize the stress which the referring team is undergoing concerning the care of the patient. Often, the referring hospital will have done their best with limited personnel, experience, and equipment, but still not have done the best possible for the patient. If a deficit in initial care is obvious to the transport team, it probably is also obvious to the referring team. As one can imagine, this stress can lead to less than ideal interactions. A nonphysician team is, unfortunately, especially vulnerable to personality confrontations as they suggest changes in therapy to the physician who is managing the case at the referral center. It is important for transport team members to realize that physicians and institutions may have modes of therapy that differ from routine transport care, but which may be appropriate nonetheless. If a conflict arises between personnel from the transport team and the referring hospital, the control physician should speak directly to the referring physician to negotiate a safe and effective solution for the patient. There is no excuse for leaving a hospital with a patient who is not completely stabilized because the referring physician refuses to allow interventions such as endotracheal intubation or chest tube placement. It is inexcusable to have patients removed from the referring institution to complete procedures in an ambulance or helicopter because the referring physician would not allow further intervention. Completing a transport checklist prior to leaving a referring center may be helpful in ensuring the completeness of prehospital stabilization (Box 5-1).

Patient disposition should be anticipated and arranged by the control physician. The control physician should have an idea whether a patient needs to go directly to an operating room, emergency department, intensive care unit, or to another specialty hospital. A receiving physician and location should be identified and a bedspace prepared so that the patient is not stranded in a hallway or elevator while waiting to be seen. If it appears that specific consultants may be needed, they should be identified and notified prior to the arrival of the transport so they can be immediately involved when the patient arrives. When these logistics are arranged before receiving a transported pa-

BOX 5-1 TRANSPORT PREPARATION CHECK LIST*

Patient status

- ( ) Acceptable respiratory status: PO_2†, pH, PCO_2†
- ( ) Chest radiograph for ETT† position in intubated airway
- ( ) Stable cardiovascular system: heart rate, rhythm, blood pressure, pulses, perfusion
- ( ) Adequate cerebral perfusion pressure
- ( ) Seizures controlled
- ( ) Reliable IV† access
- ( ) Appropriate IV fluids and rates
- ( ) Major metabolic concerns assessed, treated: glucose, Na^+, K^+, HCO_3^- and Ca^{2+}
- ( ) Urine output established
- ( ) Adequate Hgb,† Hct† values
- ( ) Bleeding controlled: mechanical, coagulation
- ( ) Antibiotics for presumed infection
- ( ) Antipyretics for fever
- ( ) Warmth for hypothermia
- ( ) NG† tube in all intubated airways
- ( ) Cervical spine precautions for potential spinal injury
- ( ) Appropriate restraints, analgesia, sedation
- ( ) Air transport considerations: air-filled cavities emptied: NG† (GI)†; chest tube (pneumothorax)

Equipment, supplies status

- ( ) Monitor(s) for patient evaluation: cardiorespiratory, pressure monitors; pulse oximeter
- ( ) Ventilator, IV pumps, suction
- ( ) Anticipated medications, supplies available

Records, communication

- ( ) Face sheet
- ( ) Copy of history, PE,† laboratory values, nursing notes
- ( ) Radiographs
- ( ) Laboratory specimens
- ( ) Signed consents
- ( ) Receiving facility notified before departure
- ( ) Exposure to communicable disease

* Aoki, BY, McCloskey, K: *Evaluation, Stabilization, and transport of the critically ill child,* St. Louis, 1992, Mosby-Year Book.

tient, it is amazing how smooth and effective the transfer of care can be as compared to when one struggles to arrange consults, labs, x-rays, CTs, and other procedures, after the arrival of a critically ill patient.

Once the patient arrives at the receiving hospital and is directed to definitive care, the acute transport is over. However, the transport system should still be in action. It is important to give follow-up information to the referring hospital concerning the patient's status. This knowledge can be communicated with a phone call to the referring hospital, other caretakers, and perhaps family, that the child arrived and in what condition. A more in-depth follow-up letter should be sent ot the referring hospital and caregivers, assuming permission is obtained from the parents, documenting the transport care and the patient's outcome. Perceived problems or positive feedback should be given directly to the referring physician or caretaker and, any significant system errors should be referred to the quality assurance (QA) departments at both the referring and the receiving hospital. It is not appropriate for the transport team to discuss the perceived quality of care with the referring hospital or the family during the transport if the care appears to have been substandard. There should be no negative feedback to the family or personnel of the referring hospital concerning the patient's pretransport care other than through direct physician contact or a QA process. Positive feedback can and should be given to the caregivers and family, if appropriate.

The quality assurance process should be undertaken in a positive manner by identifying needs and working on potential solutions. These solutions may include outreach programs, continuing medical education, case reviews, or other types of interventional discussions. Each transport allows physicians and team members to evaluate the function-

† For both referring hospital and transport team PO_2 = partial pressure of oxygen; PCO_2 = partial pressure of carbon dioxide; ETT = endotracheal tube; IV = intravenous; Hgb = hemoglobin; Hct = hematocrit; NG = nasogastric; GI = gastrointestinal; PE = physical examination

ing of the transport system as a whole and to evaluate specific transports and personnel. A continuous quality improvement and quality assurance program should be in place, therefore the transport system should improve with each transport. There should be routine transport review sessions with transport team members concerning individual transports, system-wide issues, perceived problems, and potential solutions.

In summary the transport responsibilities of the receiving hospital are much more involved than simply acting as a depository for an ill or injured patient. A substantial amount of planning and evaluation is required within a transport system prior to actual transports, and only after this has been accomplished can the transport be undertaken with the best potential outcome for the patient. Communication with a control physician, adequate planning and stabilization, and return to a center that is aware of the patient's condition and has appropriately planned for his/her arrival will help to assure optimal outcome for the patient. While problems will arise with specific transports regarding hardware, personnel, personality conflicts, and type of patient, these can be minimized by anticipating the above concepts. The level of care that the receiving hospital is capable of giving should be obtainable for the patient once the initial phone contact has been made. It is very rewarding to have a critically ill patient stabilized over the phone by a control phyiscian, transported by an appropriately trained team, and received in an improved condition.

ADDITIONAL READINGS

American Academy of Pediatrics, Task Force on Interhospital Transports: Guidelines for air and ground transport of neonatal and pediatric patients, 1993, Elk Grove Village, IL.

Aoki BY, McCloskey K: Transport process: referring and receiving hospital responsibilities. In *Evaluation, stabilization, and transport of the critically ill child.* St. Louis, 1992, Mosby-Year Book.

Day S and others: Pediatric interhospital critical transport: consensus of a national leadership conference, *Pediatrics* 88(4):696-704, 1991.

Dobrin RS and others: The development of a pediatric emergency transport system, *Ped Clin North Am* 27(3):633-646, 1980.

Frankel LR: The evaluation, stabilization, and transport of the critically ill child, *International Anesthesiaology Clinics* 25(2):77-103, 1987.

Hackel A and others: Guidelines for air and ground transportation of pediatric patients, *Pediatrics* 78(5):943-50, 1986.

Kanter RK and others: Excess morbidity associated with interhospital transport, *Pediatrics* 90(6):893-8, 1992.

McCloskey KA, Orr RA: Pediatric transport issues in emergency medicine, *Emerg Med Clin North Am* 9(3):475-89, 1991.

Reynolds M and others: The nuts and bolts of organizing and initiating a pediatric transport team, *Critical Care Clinics* 8(3):465-80, 1992.

Schneider C, Gomez M, Lee R: Evaluation of ground ambulance, rotor-wing, and fixed-wing aircraft services, *Critical Care Clinics* 8(3):533-64, 1992.

Smith DF, Hackel A: Selection criteria of pediatric critical care transport teams, *Critical Care Medicine* 11(1):10-12, 1983.

Youngberg BJ: Medical-legal considerations involved in the transport of critically ill patients, *Critical Care Clinics* 8(3):501-14, 1992.

6

INTERACTIONS BETWEEN THE REFERRING AND RECEIVING HOSPITALS AND THE TRANSPORT TEAM

LINDA H. HAMBRIGHT
KARIN A. McCLOSKEY

The decision to transfer a critically ill or injured child to a tertiary care facility is often a difficult and stressful one. The decision making process is easier if a relationship between the referring hospital, the receiving hospital, and the transport team has been established prior to the arrival of the critically ill or injured child at the referring hospital. When the need arises to transfer a critically ill child, the prevailing concern will be "crisis management."

Effective communication is the key to a successful transport. One of the most frustrating aspects of transporting a sick child occurs when there is miscommunication between any members of the referring and receiving teams. Everyone wants to do what is best for the child, but differing policies and protocols, information passed through several sources, attempts to maintain patient confidentiality, time constraints, and the underlying emotions of a group of people faced with the care of a sick child in a less than optimal environment create an atmosphere with great potential for conflict. Many situations are minor and quickly forgotten, but repeated problems with the transport team and with the referring hospital can, if left unresolved, result in unnecessary negative feelings. This can ultimately translate into poor morale and even be detrimental to the patient, for example, if the appropriate available team is not used because of communication or perception problems. The situation is worsened if referring hospital staff or transport team members complain amongst themselves about the other instead of openly discussing concerns with the transport director or the referring physician.

While most pediatric transports are completed with everyone satisfied that the child is safely in the care of those with the highest level of expertise, there are several recurring themes of conflict between the referring and receiving teams. This chapter addresses questions frequently asked by each group and answers which may help in mutual understanding. Community outreach programs which are initiated by transport systems should include up-front discussion of some of these frequent concerns before any negative incidents occur.

FREQUENTLY ASKED QUESTIONS

Referring hospital and transport team:

Why does it take you so long to get here? Most pediatric specialty teams are hospital-based and use air or ground Mobile Intensive Care Units (MICU). Typical mobilization times, the time the team receives the initial request for transport until the time of the departure to the referring hospital, are 15 to 30 minutes for ground transport, 5 to 15 minutes for helicopter transport, and 45 to 60 minutes for transport by fixed-wing aircraft. Helicopter teams specializing in adult medicine and trauma may arrive sooner but may not be the best choice for the transport of a critically ill or injured child. The receiving hospital is available by telephone to help with the stabilization and treatment of the child while the team is en route. The patient will generally receive better care in a stable environment with access to emergency department resources (lab, x-ray, consultants) than in the unstable environment of a helicopter. The extra minutes spent waiting for the specialized pediatric team can have a profound difference in a critically ill child's outcome. There is no evidence that the speed of transport is more important than the provision of pediatric critical care. A "swoop and scoop" philosophy may in fact not provide pediatric intensive care with a clinically significant time difference. For example, if the patient is 60 miles from the tertiary care center, and the available transport options are a helicopter with an adult-trained crew and a ground vehicle with a pediatric crew, the latter option may be better for the patient. If the helicopter mobilizes in 10 minutes, flies 20 minutes each way, and spends 15 minutes in stabilization, the patient reaches pediatric intensive care in 1 hour and 5 minutes, including a 20 minute flight time during which management is difficult. If the pediatric ground team mobilizes in 20 minutes and drives 60 minutes, the patient receives pediatric intensive care at 1 hour and 20 minutes but has remained in a stable environment with good telephone access and availability of subspecialty physicians, laboratory and x-ray facilities. While the referring hospital is being asked to provide care for a longer period of time, the best interest of the patient is served by maintenance in a stable environment. The exception is the patient with an immediate surgical emergency, such as an epidural hematoma, where time to the tertiary center might be the most important factor effecting outcome.

Why do you stay so long? (The other team only stayed 15 minutes.) Pediatric specialty teams performing interhospital transports operate under different guidelines than do most "scene response" teams. Helicopter teams historically utilize the "swoop and scoop" method of transportation, spending very little time stabilizing the patient at the referring hospital and preferring to defer intervention until arrival at the receiving hospital. Pediatric specialty teams utilize a different approach. These teams provide "bedside-to-bedside" mobile intensive care stabilization with only emergent intervention provided while in actual transport. As referring hospitals are often less experienced in the management of critically ill children (compared to adults), the team transporting a child may need to perform more assessment and stabilizing measures. Therefore, the pediatric team may need to spend more time at the referring hospital. The team should be independent and not require significant assistance of referring hospital personnel during stabilization. Choosing a team based primarily on speed of arrival or speed of stabilization, without regard to pediatric experience and expertise, is usually not in the best interest of the child.

Why did you change out our lines, tubes, etc.? The transport environment is not a stable or predictable one. The probability of losing IV tubing, endotracheal tubes, nasogastric tubes, etc. is very high even when the team is careful. Therefore, it is necessary to secure these as well as possible. Often this means moving tubing to a more secure location or a different taping method. Sometimes it is simply a matter of differences in equipment, in that what the referring hospital uses may not work with the transport team's monitors, pumps, etc. The team will also usually want more than one IV line due to the risk of losing one during transport. Certain types of equipment such as the "butterfly" or intraosseous lines) may be useful in the emergency department but not stable enough to be used alone during transport. Misunderstandings frequently occur when the team discovers that a perfectly appropriate tube or line has become dislodged, occluded, or otherwise nonfunctional. Without making a broad statement to everyone in the room that "the endotracheal tube is plugged" or "the IV is infiltrated," the team replaces whatever is needed. It may appear to others in the room that a perfectly good line or tube has been replaced. This is an area where communication is especially important. The team should be willing to explain any changes in treatment, if asked. The transport team is just as concerned with keeping the patient's tubes in place as the referring hospital and does not change anything that is not absolutely necessary. Routine changing of lines or tubes would not benefit anyone.

Why do we have trouble finding out what happened to the patient? Transport teams recognize that obtaining followup information can be difficult. The team transporting the patient may not care for the patient after the transport and, therefore, may not be aware of progress and plans. Most programs are attempting to eliminate this problem by instituting formal physician/nurse follow-up guidelines through quality assurance. Maintaining patient confidentiality precludes the routine communication of details of the patient's situation without written consent from the patient or parents. Teams which routinely give follow-up information to anyone but the patient's primary care physician may be incurring legal risks through breach of confidentiality.

Why do we need a "pediatric" team? There is a helicopter service closer to us which advertises for the transport of patients of all ages. Many "all-age" transport services have excellent training and ongoing experience with pediatric patients. A team transporting all ages may have different team compositions for different age patients, for example, adding a neonatal or pediatric critical care nurse or physician to the team when appropriate. A referring hospital should investigate the pediatric training and experience of the nearest transport service **in advance.** Problems arise when a service which reportedly transports patients of all age groups in fact transports only a small percentage of children and has minimal experience and training in pediatrics. Note that the percentage of pediatric patients transported should be examined based on patient age. If a service transports 30% pediatric patients, but three-fourths of those patients are adolescents, true pediatric experience may still be limited. When available within a reasonable time frame, a dedicated pediatric team offers extensive training and experience with children, excellent pediatric medical control, a full complement of pediatric equipment, and continuity of care with the tertiary care center.

How do we know which transport team to use for an individual child? There are no universally accepted guidelines in the area of transport service selection. The decision will depend on the severity of illness, distance to travel, available vehicles, and pediatric capabilities of individual teams. In general the most critically ill children, those who have to travel the farthest, and those who have required the most interventions need the highest level of pediatric capabilities. If the patient is transferred to a pediatric intensive care unit, that level of care should be used during transport if possible. The accepting tertiary care center physician can assist in decisions regarding transport service selection.

What can we do to prepare for the transport team before it arrives? Advance preparation is extremely important in making the actual transport process more efficient. Each transport service in the area should be evaluated in advance for pediatric capabilities, usual vehicles, usual response time, etc. Each team will have its own forms to complete and system to follow for access, parental consent, equipment preparation, etc. Asking in advance what the team will need can expedite the process of transferring the patient to the team.

What is the best way to get more experience with and information about stabilizing pediatric patients? It is very difficult to gain experience when there are small numbers of pediatric patients in a rural area or when staff members have multiple responsibilities and demands on their time. Ideally an individual could spend time working in a pediatric emergency department or pediatric intensive care unit. Also helpful is attendance at Pediatric Advanced Life Support (PALS) or other courses offered by children's hospitals or organizations with formal CME programs in pediatric emergency medicine. Practically speaking, it is difficult to find the time and resources for all of the emergency department staff to gain substantial pediatric experience. A small number of staff members could obtain additional expertise and then work different shifts or be on-call to provide coverage for pediatric emergencies. If that is not possible or opportunities are not available, or for staff members not undergoing extensive pediatric training, several options exist. The tertiary care center can be asked to provide community outreach programs in pediatric stabilization, a request can be made to the local American Heart Association affiliate to host a nearby PALS course, and reading materials can be obtained both for self-study and for use during crises. The transport team coordinator or director can provide suggestions for such material.

Why does the pediatric system make the parents stay here until the team arrives? The other teams let family members get a head start on the road to the tertiary care center. As part of the admission to a mobile pediatric intensive care unit, the team will want to obtain relevant pieces of information about the patient. This includes a detailed history of events preceding the current crisis and a complete medical history. Unlike adults, children are rarely able to provide such information about themselves. Parents also may incur a substantial delay in arriving at the tertiary care center because of the need to arrange for transportation, find caretakers for any other children, etc. As part of the critical care continuum, the team provides the opportunity for the parents to meet some of the tertiary care personnel, ask questions about the next steps in treatment, and obtain directions to the hospital and the unit within the hospital. True informed consent for transport can also be obtained. Teams which do not require the presence of the parents operate under "implied consent." The child can still receive care, but little benefit is derived from the parents trying to go on ahead and then wait "endlessly" outside the ICU or even risk not having the child arrive at all because of a terminal event prior to transport.

If we are comfortable stabilizing a child or are managing multiple victims, why do you insist on asking a lot of questions? Why can't the person answering the call just accept the patient and get the team on the way? Certain baseline information is needed in order to dispatch the team. For example, patient age and weight are needed in order to know whether to bring an isolette, car seat mechanism, or regular stretcher. It is also necessary to inform the pilots if there are any conditions requiring alterations in usual altitude. Additional information may be required if special equipment or large quantities of any medication are needed, or if any change in usual team composition (i.e., adding a fellow or attending for complex airway problems) is advisable. After obtaining the information needed for initial dispatch, there is a second level of details needed shortly after the initial call, if not originally provided. As part of the critical care continuum, the receiving physician is beginning to assume a level of responsibility for the patient. For this responsibility, and in the best interest of patient care, the receiving attending physician needs an in-depth understanding of the patient's status. Then, if there are any ideas or recommendations to improve patient care, they can be offered while the team is on the way. This allows earlier intervention and may aid in stabilizing the patient. The actual transport team will be mobilizing from the time of the initial call.

Why do you sometimes take so long to call us back about accepting a patient? Why can't you just get the team on the way? There are several potential problems, many of which are specific to individual transport systems, which can interfere with agreeing to transport a patient. The Pediatric Intensive Care Unit (PICU) or Neonatal Intensive Care Unit (NICU) may have no available beds (especially for special services like Extra-Corporeal Membrane Oxygenation (ECMO). Patients may have to be moved in order to free a bed. This may be time-consuming, since it may require consultation between multiple physicians and assurance of an appropriate bed for the patient being moved from the Intensive Care Unit (ICU). There may be multiple, simultaneous transport requests which have to be triaged. A team dispatched for another patient may have to be diverted. Vehicle availability may not be known if more than one hospital shares an aircraft or ambulance. Team availability may not be known if more than one unit shares the same transport staff. Also, if the transport team is not directed by the receiving hospital, administrative issues may cause delays. Many tertiary centers and transport teams will accept the patient immediately and then work out these details. This may result in a longer-than-hoped-for response time but allows early involvement by the tertiary center physicians.

Receiving hospital and transport team:

Why do you get so upset at how long it takes a pediatric team to get there? The referring hospital is often not equipped to deal with pediatric emergencies. The longer it takes the transport team to arrive, the longer referring hospital emergency staff have to care for a patient for whom they do not have the best facilities or specialists. Pediatric emergencies usually require more work and tie up more staff than adult emergencies. Aside from performing procedures which are more difficult in children, it is more emotionally stressful to deal with a critically ill or injured child. Once the child is stabilized and the parents have agreed to the transfer, the referring hospital would like the child to be on the way to tertiary care, rather than waiting, in the event that something goes wrong. Every minute seems longer when a patient is ready and the referring staff is forced to wait and watch the child while deferring other patients' care. Also, sometimes it seems as if the team does not care how long they take and does not even apologize or explain. One of the worst situations occurs when an estimated time of arrival is given to the referring staff and the patient's family, and then the team is significantly delayed (often for a perfectly reasonable cause). When they are not informed of the delay, problems are created and it makes staff appear callous or irresponsible to the family.

Why do you sometimes use a nonpediatric team who isn't comfortable with children? Non-pediatric teams are used because they arrive faster and do not stay as long. Many transport services, especially helicopter services, advertise the ability to transport patients of all ages. If they do not know the distinction, it makes sense to call the team that is nearest to our hospital. Sometimes, even if we know the dedicated pediatric team might be better, they are just too far away to provide the urgent tertiary care which the patient needs. The non-pediatric team often leaves the referring hospital sooner, freeing up staff and space for other sick patients. Also, (and this can happen with either type of team) sometimes one system gives us much better follow-up, both in terms of how the patient fared and in terms of any major things we did right or wrong. Usually nothing bad happens to the child with a non-pediatric team, especially if they are in a helicopter which makes the transit time much shorter.

Why do we have trouble getting all the information we need about the patient? Sometimes emergency department staff are overwhelmed with multiple trauma victims. There may be only one RN in the hospital and another coming in while someone asks about the birth date, capillary refill, total fluids, and insurance status of a patient to be transported. That case may be somewhat extreme, but the referring hospital does not always have the staff to quickly provide all patient information. In the interest of the patients, tasks are prioritized and some information is deferred. Tell the referring hospital in advance what is absolutely required to dispatch the team (i.e., patient age to decide between a neonatal or pediatric team/equipment pack). The staff usually contacts the family with more information as soon as possible. Also, sometimes the person who calls may not have all the information (i.e., the physician may not know exact vital signs and total fluids), and it may be necessary to call back to get the necessary information. It is helpful if copies of blank intake sheets are received in advance so that questions are anticipated and vital information is ready.

Why is the referring physician sometimes gone when we get there? If the referring physician is not full-time emergency medicine staff, then he or she probably has a practice with an office full of patients waiting to be seen. The ill or injured child has probably interfered with the physician's schedule of appointments. If the child is needing minute-to-minute changes in care, the doctor will usually stay (another reason for wanting the team to arrive quickly). However, if the patient is stabilized and the nurses are staying close, the physician can reasonably return to the office and stay in touch by telephone. If the team takes an hour or two to arrive, it is impossible to time exactly when to return to the emergency department, particularly in view of the aforementioned estimated time of arrival problems. If the patient is stabilized, the physician may feel that initial information and written transfer notes are sufficient. The physician may talk to the team by phone or may return to the emergency department if necessary.

Why didn't you do the things we suggested over the phone? There are several possible reasons for not following phone recommendations. Perhaps the suggestions were given to someone who did not pass them along or the patient's condition changed, making intervention unnecessary. Or perhaps hospital staff already had a plan to take care of the patient or were unable to perform the intervention, due to lack of equipment or experience. It is also possible that there was not enough time to follow recommendations prior to transport team arrival or that a specialist or consultant subsequently arrived to help.

Why don't you have the chart/x-rays/lab reports copied before we get there? Copies may not be ready due to limited staff resources & available equipment, especially after usual working hours. Also, if the chart is copied too soon, there may be additional nurses' notes or physician recommendations to copy regarding events which occur before and during the team's arrival or during their stabilization. There is usually enough time to perform copying once the team arrives for transport.

Why do we sometimes feel that you're trying to push us out the door before we're ready? Hospital staff need the space and want to get everything recorded, cleaned up, and completed. Of course, if the child is "crashing," there's no rush, but some teams seem to move out efficiently and others routinely take much longer talking to the patient's family, changing lines, making phone calls, getting lab work and x-rays, etc. Why can one team get their job done quickly and another take much longer to do essentially the same thing?

Why don't you call and tell us if you're upset about something that happened? There are a variety of possible reasons for not addressing concerns following a transport:

a. The staff is not sure exactly who to call.
b. The staff does not think much will change (for example, the attitude of residents towards "local medical doctors").
c. Staff members change shifts and keep missing each other (for example, if the night shift charge nurse has a concern and the contact person works a day shift).
d. The staff may not know the names of the people involved.
e. The staff becomes frustrated when placed on hold or transferred from place to place, only to wind up talking to an answering machine.
f. The problem may seem trivial (like changing an IV).

If you don't like something we do, why don't you just ask us why we did it? We don't want to sound patronizing by saying everything out loud we're doing. It is difficult to know what to ask. Staff members do not want to sound stupid or to hassle the transport team. Sometimes it is not clear who is in charge or who to ask. Occasionally, one of our staff members might be intimidated by the team, or if someone with a question has not been in the room all the time, they may not know if changing the line, for example, was already discussed. Sometimes the staff does not realize that there was a problem until after the transport team leaves.

As evidenced by the responses to the questions that were asked of each other, many perceptual problems between the referring hospital, the receiving hospital, and the transport team could be kept to a minimum through community outreach, communication, and a spirit of cooperation. The hospitals and the transport team must be able to freely discuss concerns and try to resolve misunderstandings in order to provide not only optimal continuity and excellence in care, but also the most effective and appropriate method of transfer to the receiving hospital.

It is unreasonable to expect that there will never be problems between the different individuals involved in the transfer process. The important thing to remember is that unless the patient is at risk, the problems should not be dealt with at the patient's bedside. Instead, concerns should be addressed to the appropriate supervisory personnel involved. Failure to report a problem will do nothing to prevent similar situations in the future. Often the problems are personality conflicts or differences in medical opinion where there are several "right" ways to approach a given situation. Communication is the key to solving conflicts involving referring hospitals, receiving hospitals, or transport team members.

7

DEVELOPING ADMINISTRATIVE SUPPORT FOR THE TRANSPORT SYSTEM

DENNIS BRIMHALL

Lack of institutional support for the transport system is a common frustration of transport clinicians and program directors. This real or perceived problem can many times be traced back to the clinician's dealing with non-clinicians (administrators) about clinical matters. The culmination of this frustration is represented by the transport program director's proverbial pilgrimage to the hospital administrator's office for the purpose of requesting or even pleading for the necessary resources. This exchange with the administrator is many times inconclusive. The administrator will ask questions for which the clinician is not prepared to answer. Sometimes these questions seem irrelevant, having significance only to a hospital administrator and not to a clinician. To be confronted with matters of insurance, indirect costs, political considerations, and competitive posturing seems somehow distant and obstructionist to the issues of delivering care to the 1500 gram neonate which should be on the way from a referring hospital.

Although many such encounters do result in appropriate support, almost all practitioners at one time or another have felt that "administration does not support or understand our program," or "we do not get the resource necessary to run our program for reasons unrelated to the care of the patient." In light of these frustrations, it is not uncommon for the program director to mentally, if not verbally, ask the question of how to develop administrative support for the transport system. Although there is no cookbook approach to obtaining administrative support, there are some important constants that will enhance communication with administration and improve the chances of appropriate support. At the risk of over-simplification, there are three keys for developing administrative support. First, understand the basic cost versus benefit analysis utilized by hospital administration in making decisions. Second, understand what questions administration will ask when confronted with the request for additional support; and third, understand those issues which administration will view as legitimate reasons to initiate or make changes to an existing program. When requests are made by practitioners or program directors to hospital administration, understanding these issues will assist in ensuring that communication with administration is accurate and effective, as well as making sure that the arguments presented are the most persuasive from the administrator's standpoint.

THE COST/BENEFIT ANALYSIS: IS IT WORTH IT?

The one question asked by virtually every business or corporation when confronted with a new opportunity is, "Will we benefit enough by the sale of the product or service to cover the costs associated with providing that service?" If an automobile manufacturer, through market research and product line review, determines that a new model should be developed, it usually comes after a very lengthy analytical process involving a technique commonly known in the corporate world as "the benefit minus cost analysis."[4] This simple process requires the automobile manufacturer to determine through every mechanism to the highest degree of accuracy possible, exactly what the cost will be to design, manufacture, market, sell, and warranty their new model. This determines the cost.

Next, through extensive market research and economic models trading off price with demand, the company will determine at what price the automobile will be sold and how many units will be sold at that price. This will be the benefit. If it turns out that the benefit exceeds the cost by a margin that satisfies the acceptable return on investment to the corporation with an appropriate factor for error, then the company will proceed with the project. If these projected revenues should not exceed their projected costs, then obviously the program will not proceed.

This example of an automobile manufacturer developing a new model is significantly simplified. The basic conceptual approach of benefit minus cost is the same, however, and is used repeatedly in American business, whether it is deciding to buy pencils by the gross or to develop a new model of automobile. In fact huge amounts of resources are expended on just the analysis itself, given reverence to the simple equation of benefit minus cost.

Although we are many times reluctant to compare a corporate methodology to the health care environment, the health care setting is also driven by exactly the same cost/benefit analysis. In the health care setting, however, there are variations on the cost/benefit theme that create problems.[1,4] These problems not only create difficulty in decision making, but also lead to poor communication between clinicians and administration. The most important and overwhelming variation to the cost/benefit equation comes from the fact that in health care, costs are usually measured quantitatively, and benefits are measured qualitatively. Compounding this difference is the fact that those who define and measure the costs are different from those who define and measure the benefit. Administration's training, expertise, orientation within the organization, and access to the cost (the dollars) information will naturally define the costs. The medical, nursing, and other professional staff who deal with patients will naturally define the benefits.

If the dichotomy of different people measuring different issues is not conflicting enough, additional stress is created by the fact that costs are by their very nature easier to measure than benefits. Most hospitals have good methods of cost accounting and can define through a relatively easy process the costs associated with any program. We also have a commonly accepted marker for measuring costs and that is dollars and cents. This, of course, makes the cost side of the equation simpler and very powerful in the sense that it can be measured and that there is a commonly accepted measurement. The benefits, on the other hand, are much more difficult to measure. They are measured qualitatively. Although it is true that one can measure the benefits by the question of whether or not it reduces cost, there are few examples of where new programs or changes in programs truly reduce cost while, at the same time, providing benefit to the patient. More usual is the question of whether or not the new program or program modification will reduce morbidity and/or mortality.

Generally, these are subjective evaluations. There are few, if any, objective and quantitative studies regarding the benefit of a transport system. Intuitively, we believe that faster is better, trained personnel provide better care than transport generalists, and that the right equipment is better than the wrong equipment. Although these assumptions are intuitively powerful, the enormous difficulties of running controlled studies make it difficult to isolate the benefits in such a way as to demonstrate that the impact on morbidity and mortality was a result of any element of the transport system alone.

It is simple to demonstrate how such an actual conflict with the cost/benefit analysis can occur. It may be intuitively very powerful to suggest that a transport system would benefit from the inclusion of a respiratory therapist on all transports. The arguments of having specifically trained individuals to handle the single most important issue associated with neonatal care during transport should be intuitive. In addition, there is the general benefit of having another set of hands, if not shoulders, to carry the load. Such a request made to administration would result in a very quick "costing out" of this program modification, hence, the cost side of the equation would be completed in a definitive way using a recognized unit of measure (dollars). When the program director was asked to quantify the benefit by indicating a reduction in morbidity or mortality, no quantitative marker is available to demonstrate this benefit. At best the program director is left with the frustrating, although not altogether ineffective, use of anecdotes to argue the case. Hospital administration will feel a certain amount of frustration in being asked to make a decision without all the facts (quantitative and documented costs but qualitative and undocumented benefits). The program director and practitioners are equally frustrated in that the benefit for them is defined through years of training, experience, and judgment regarding what is best for the patient. This judgment is now being challenged by someone unable by training and experience to make that judgment and who is also asking for a quantitative response about an issue for which such quantification is nearly impossible.

In summary, because of the different ways in which the costs and benefits are measured and the fact that different people measure benefits from those that measure costs, the cost/benefit question is complex and tortuous in the health care setting. In fact, given the different perspectives and challenges associated with using this analytical tool, one would wonder how any decisions are made at all. It is also not difficult to see why communication between clinicians and administration is difficult. The perspectives and responsibilities are profoundly different, and the tools utilized by each in carrying out the responsibility are different.

There is probably no way to make cost accounting less quantitative and benefit definition less qualitative. However, much can be done by simple recognition that both perspectives are legitimate and recognizing the respective views at both sides of this equation. Just as it is not possible for the clinician to set aside his or her concern for the patient, likewise, it is important to realize that administration, by nature of their responsibility and training, will not be able to set aside the cost/benefit analysis in making decisions about hospital resources. Almost every other consideration in developing administrative support for a transport program hinges on the understanding of the cost/benefit analysis and the respective roles played by each party in that process.

WHAT QUESTIONS DO ADMINISTRATORS ASK?

Administrators by nature should be inquisitive and curious beings. In their realm, answers do not come from basic or even clinical research but through asking people questions and then sifting through the answers. In some cases the answers will be accepted at face value and in other circumstances validated through an independent process. Even though the administrator will not weigh all the questions and answers the same, it is reasonably certain that at least most of the following questions will be asked. As with the answers to clinical questions, any question that has an incomplete answer or one that seems out of the norm then becomes the focus of attention, even on some occasions, to the point of distraction. These questions represent, however, a reasonable guideline for clinicians and program directors in preparing presentations or requests to administration.

How much will it cost?

For most administrators this is the first question that will be asked, and it should surprise no one. Such a question is inherent in the administrator's responsibility to the institution and some would suggest it is administratively pathological. Again, this question in most cases is not a difficult one to answer because of the availability of cost accounting techniques found in most hospitals.[6] The thing that will surprise most clinicians and program directors is the enormous number of elements that will make up the overall cost of a program or program modification. Many are of significant importance to the administrator but only of minor importance to the program director. The more comprehensive the analysis of costs, the more comfort the administrator will have in understanding the true nature of the issue. In the transport environment, costs associated with the program or changes in the program come from a variety of sources.

First, the cost of the **transport team**. Like everything else in health care, personnel costs usually make up the bulk of the expense. Costs associated with the team not only include salaries and benefits, but also training, insurance, special transport pay, the cost of replacing coverage within the unit if the transport team is pulled for transport, on-call, and over-time pay, and the cost of managing this select group of individuals. Even though there are a large variety of mechanisms to share the cost of the transport team with other functions within the institution, a significant portion of the cost associated with the transport team exists simply because of the decision to have a team. It is these stand-by costs which are the greatest. Ultimately, the total personnel costs must be spread out over the actual number of transports, because only when a transport has occurred is there an opportunity to recover costs either by billing for the transport or by admitting a patient to the hospital.

Although one of the many costs making up the expense of the transport team, it is appropriate to discuss the issue of transport team insurance. Insurance for the transport team falls into four categories: health insurance, accident and disability insurance, life insurance, and malpractice insurance.[5] Although the exact risk associated with transporting patients, whether it be in fixed wing, helicopters, or ground ambulance, is difficult to quantify, one thing is certain; there is more risk for the transport team while on transport than there is in the hospital caring for the patient in the unit. For this reason it is generally appropriate for the institution to consider assisting the transport team member in acquiring appropriate or additional insurance in consideration of this incremental risk. Most hospitals have insurance packages which either do include or can be adapted to include the transport team members while on transport. The risks associated with the transport usually are reflected in a higher premium to be paid for the insurance. Here the hospital can pay the higher premium, thus making sure that the insurance is available to the transport team member. Some transport team members feel that it is appropriate for additional insurance (usually life insurance) to be purchased as well. And here it may be appropriate for the institution to buy that additional insurance for the transport team member. Different approaches have been used by institutions in solving this problem. One includes blanket policies for all transport team members, while other institutions have provided flight pay which then can be used by the transport team member to purchase additional insurance or for other purposes.

It is true that the issue of insurance for transport team members usually carries with it more emotion than cost, and hence, most institutions have found that the incremental cost of additional insurance for the transport team member is marginal and certainly less of an issue than time-consuming and emotional debates over whether additional insurance should be provided and who should pay for it.

There is no credible argument that a transport team member should carry their own malpractice insurance as long as they are working within the course and scope of their assigned responsibilities as an employee of the institution. If, however, the transport team member is transporting in a situation where they are not an employee but rather billing a fee for their services directly to the patient, then the responsibility of obtaining malpractice insurance will rest with the individual team member. Ultimately, the responsibility to defend and indemnify a transport team member in a malpractice situation rests with the employer of that team member while on a specific transport. For a team member who bills for their own professional fee, they become the employer and are responsible for their own malpractice coverage.

The second very significant cost comes from the use of a **transport vehicle**. Just as the sophistication of transport personnel has grown significantly in recent years, so has the sophistication of the transport vehicle. Whether it is ground transportation, fixed wing, or rotor wing, and whether the vehicles are owned by the hospital or are leased by an outside vendor, the cost of the vehicle is a very important aspect of any transport system. Like the cost of the human resources, the transport vehicle cost must be spread out over a finite number of transport events, with each event sharing the enormous standby costs of having these vehicles available. Costs associated with the vehicle are those of acquisition, maintenance, insurance, normal operating costs, the human resources required to operate the vehicle (pilots and drivers), communication equipment, and items as mundane as specialized paint schemes and promotional material. Even though for many transport systems the human resource cost is the greatest, increasingly, the transport vehicle has become the dominant cost in the transport program.

The third cost area is that of **equipment**. Gone are the days of simple equipment and simple supplies. There are now vendors which specialize exclusively in transport equipment and who have come to realize that manufacturing equipment for the two most demanding and costly aspects of our society, aviation and medicine, can be combined to create a truly unique market with enormous returns. Equipment including incubators, monitors, ventilators, instruments, supplies, and equipment bags and the ever-present demand to create special modifications of this equipment for the transport team and vehicle can make the equipment component of the program costs seem insatiable to the accountant.

The fourth cost area deals with **supplies**. The very nature of a dedicated transport system and dedicated teams involve the treatment of severely ill or injured patients. These patients require a complex array of supplies including pharmaceuticals, blood products, disposable medical equipment and supplies, oxygen, and instruments, all of which make the few hours of a transport the most costly of the neonate's hospital experience. In addition to the clinical supplies, there are other expenses associated with the transport such as uniforms, paper products, and even meals. Not only are the costs of supplies high, it takes a significant amount of discipline on the part of the transport team to account for the use of the supplies and make sure the patient is appropriately charged. Predicting the cost of supplies for a transport program has always been risky. In this area, more than any other, a few months experience is overwhelmingly the best guide.

The fifth area of cost is associated with establishing the program. Given the lead time associated with starting or modifying the transport program, it is safe to assume that there will be significant costs incurred with people, training, equipment acquisition and modification, marketing, and promotion, all which will occur before the first patient is transported. In a cost accounting system that must ultimately account for all costs, to determine whether the cost/benefit analysis works, the start-up costs will be factored in.

Although there are many other costs associated with operating a transport system which have not been mentioned, there is one final area which is generally difficult for the program directors or clinicians to understand and is viewed many times as the hospital administrator simply looking for excuses not to support the program. These costs are the infamous indirect costs that exist in any hospital.[1,3,6] As with other revenue centers within the institution, the transport system must carry its share of the indirect costs; these are the costs generated in cost centers for which there was no opportunity to bill the patient. They include the human resource department, the billing office, medical records, the public relations office, foundation, and even administration. In many institutions indirect costs can run from 50 to 100 percent of the direct costs. Just when the program director believes that the program is economically viable, the program is hit with the indirect costs from other parts of the organization. Such an allocation of these costs seems grossly unfair because they represent expenses that appear to be completely unrelated to the provision of care to the patient. Although there are great debates about how these costs are allocated and whether or not the transport system should share these costs, they nonetheless exist within any organization and must be picked up through some type of allocation, by any programs in the hospital which have an opportunity to bill patients for services rendered.

Will it be reimbursed?

The next basic question increasingly asked by hospital administrators is the question of reimbursement.[6] In our current health care system, in which there is little linkage between what a hospital charges and what it gets paid, the hospital is faced with needing to determine whether or not those who reimburse the hospital (this is rarely the patient) will actually pay for the transport system or for any other modifications in the system. Most transport systems have been sobered by the reality that great care was rendered to a patient in an urgent situation only to find out that the transportation costs were excluded as a covered benefit for the patient. If the transport system is of value to the patient, will those who are responsible for paying the patient's medical bill recognize the value and be willing to reimburse the hospital for the cost of the system?

The analysis of the current reimbursement environment and the issues associated with that environment are extremely complex. This analysis begins with such basic questions as how much will be charged, identifying who is responsible for payment, and how to determine which part of the bill was paid and which part was not. Most successful programs have determined that enormous attention must be given to the education of insurance companies and other third party payers to maximize reimbursement. Increasingly, institutions are paid not for specific itemized units of service, but rather for lump sums associated with a day of service or a diagnosis associated with an admission. Increasingly, institutions will be involved in risk-taking associated with capitated patients where there, in fact, is no incremental reimbursement for any program such as a transport team. In these ever increasing scenarios, every program will be measured against its ability to reduce costs. This is a paradigm which is 180 degrees from the historical institutional approach of reimbursement being provided for services which generate charges. The new paradigm will be a reward for what is not done as opposed to a reward for what is done.

Once it is determined who will reimburse for services provided and what they will reimburse, the next question will surely involve the level of bad debt the system can tolerate or if the collections will cover the costs. If the program is important, even with a negative cost/benefit analysis, who will subsidize the transport team if, in fact, the transport system does not generate enough revenue to cover its own cost? The issues of reimbursement are becoming incomprehensible to many clinicians and, in truth, most administrators. It is now left to highly technical individuals who have the ability of analyzing contracts and insurance policies and predicting levels of reimbursement based upon volumes and types of patients.

Does it have medical staff support?

In most institutions where resources are limited, the administrator is forever faced with the dilemma of using limited resources in areas that will satisfy the greatest number of people. Medical staffs are historically the greatest demanders of resource and, understandably, the most parochial in their interest about resource allocation. The administrator will invariably want to know whether or not resources committed to the initiation or modification of a transport system will be viewed by the medical staff as appropriate or too narrow an expenditure of resource. If the medical staff of an institution generally does not view such a program as having broad enough institutional value, the administrator can be in the position of being a hero to a few members of the medical staff who want the transport system but a goat to many, many more who did not see its value. Hence, the question, "Does the proposed program modification have broad medical staff support?"

The development of support from the medical staff can rarely be managed or obtained by the administrator. It must, in all cases, be generated by the program's medical leadership. Support must spread from those directly associated with the transport system to the inpatient unit which might receive the patients as well as the ancillary and other clinical services that will be affected by the arrival of these patients to the hospital. If there is broad-based medical staff support for such a program, it might even overcome marginal cost/benefit analyses. Without strong, broad medical staff support, even the most optimistic cost/benefit analysis will be rejected because the internal political expense would be too high.

The transport system can actually be intimidating to medical staff. It is important to remember that the transport system is generally only valuable and effective if it brings patients back to the hospital. If the hospital does not have the resources to care for those patients when they arrive, then it will create problems within the hospital, particularly with the medical staff. If the transport system fills up the operating room with unscheduled cases, thus pushing out elective surgery, this will create problems amongst the surgeons. The same holds true for a transport system that fills the obstetrics unit with patients requiring antepartum care, thus restricting the overall capacity of the unit for normal deliveries. Careful planning with the medical staff will determine if the transport program will have institutional acceptance or whether it would become a threat to other practitioners within the hospital. An old saying goes about hospital administrators and medical staffs, "there are old administrators and there are bold administrators. When it comes to medical staff, there are no old, bold administrators." Issues of medical staff support for program initiation or change is paramount.

Who will provide the medical staff leadership in this endeavor?

There is a difference between medical staff support and medical staff leadership. For most institutions the hospital administrator is not in a position to champion the clinical program nor guarantee its success. The administration must rely heavily upon a specific leadership within the medical staff for the program. Wise administration will look for and evaluate the quality of the medical staff champion of the program.[5] If there is a passionate proponent of the program whose career and personal interest is at stake, it is almost certain that the program will be a success. If the medical staff leadership is lacking or comes by way of extra assignment or rotating responsibility, there is a high likelihood that the program will flounder, and the investment will be wasted. As previously mentioned, the ability to sell the program to other members of the medical staff, as well as members of the hospital board and other constituents, are dramatically enhanced if the administrator can rely on someone who is much more knowledgeable of the clinical benefits.

In reference to the cost/benefit equation, the benefits are best measured qualitatively by the clinician. This is based upon experience and judgment that places the burden of advocacy with the clinician. The hospital administrator is particularly suspect for promoting a benefit which cannot be quantified. If, as is generally the case, the transport system can be shown to enhance the hospital's financial situation by increasing the number of patients which come to the hospital and enhancing patient revenue, the combination of the hospital administrator's argument from a revenue standpoint with that of the clinician's argument for the patient benefit can be very powerful.

Will the system be used?

All of the previous questions may have been satisfied during the planning and analytical phase of the program development. It may satisfy the cost/benefit analysis. It may provide significant clinical benefit. It may be reimbursed, even adequately, and yet not be used. Just having a transport system or making a modification of a transport system in and of itself does not guarantee that the phone will ring and the request for service will come. It is very important to understand whether or not there is an external demand for the service, can that demand be created, and who are the current competitors for such a service. A careful analysis of the other transport systems within the service area, what impact the new system or modified system might have on the competition, and what the response of the competition will be needs to be conducted. It is important to remember that the simple presence of an additional transport system does not, in and of itself, create more demand. Most demand comes at the expense of other programs already in existence; it is an issue of competition. Competition in the existing healthcare market is not so much based on price, but on service, both quantity and quality. Yet quality and quantity of service almost always are associated with a higher price tag, which then can intimidate cost/benefit analysis.

It is also important to determine whether the program can be marketed successfully. This marketing must be done both internally and externally with the careful review and understanding of when the program will break even and how long a start-up phase can be tolerated.

What is the impact on the institution?

Mark Twain once commented, "there are two great tragedies in life; the first is not getting everything we want, and the second is getting everything we want." It is very important to analyze what impact a successful program will have on the institution. Will the transport system fill hospital beds? And, more importantly, are there beds available to be filled? Although it sounds like a great problem to have, many transport systems and clinical programs have been put under enormous stress by demands that cannot be realized. A successful program can create a demand for additional resources far beyond what was initially projected. This will usually mean recruiting additional staff which, in the case of professional staff, may or may not be available. Also, a demand for more equipment and for the precious commodity of space may be created.

A successful transport program obviously requires a round-the-clock response capability. Many institutions are not equipped to provide support for a transport system 24 hours a day. This is why it is also important to make sure that the clinical programs within the hospital exist to support the patients who are being transported. If the transport system were to retrieve a high-risk maternal patient who delivers a low birth weight infant but there is no newborn intensive care unit, then this becomes a disservice to the patient. Many institutions have initiated transport programs to enhance the movement of patients into the institution when inadequate clinical programs existed to properly care for the patient once they arrived. This is true not only for the hospital but for the medical staff as well. It is important for all to ask a sobering question as to whether or not the institution is the best one to provide such services and not become infatuated with transport capability beyond clinical program capability. There is also another even more fundamental question, and that is whether or not the transport program is consistent with the mission of the institution. A transport program by its very nature is highly visible and portrays a certain image throughout a referral area. It also creates expectations that ultimately the institution will need to meet. There are many institutions who have seen their balance of clinical programs within the institution changed by virtue of a transport system. Such change in image, focus, and balance may not be consistent with the stated mission of the institution and the institution's obligations to its various constituencies, including the community at large. Few institutions can afford to be known for or driven by a single, highly visible program.

What is the external impact to the institution?

Beyond the issue of competitive response and institutional image, it is important to analyze what the external response will be to a new program with the visibility and impact of a transport system. The response may not only come from competitors but from affiliated institutions as well. There may be a response from regulatory agencies who require review and oversight. There will also need to be a careful analysis of how aggressive the marketing should be and whether the marketing program might, in fact, compete with the very physicians or other programs that the institution relies upon for its own referrals. If, for example, the institution is heavily dependent upon referrals from community pediatricians for its pediatric programs, what might be the expected response from those pediatricians to an aggressively marketed neonatal transport program which might be taking patients away from those referring physicians? Although many times it is difficult to simply go into the community and solicit response prospective to starting a program, the more insight an institution has into those impacts, the more accurate the analysis will be concerning program initiation or modification and the less risk for program failure in the future.

What will it take to get the program going?

One of an administrator's worst nightmares is to go through all of the process and stress associated with making a major program commitment only to find out that the program never really got going. The administrator will want to know if he or she approves the program initiative, that there is a capability to actually make it work. These questions relate to such things as an organizational structure within the institution to support the system, dealing with all of the appropriate regulations, hiring and training the personnel, appropriate management of program personnel, adequate space, medical leadership, skilled marketing of the program, and a very important issue of timing. When is it right to initiate the program, to announce it, to market it, and dozens of other items that must be dealt with and worked on before anyone would dare hang out the "open for business" sign.

There are undoubtedly many other questions that can and will be asked by administrators concerning program initiation and change. Many of these will be unique to the given institution and to the relationship that exists between the administration and the program director. Although not always obvious at the outset, almost all of these questions will be used to help satisfy the cost/benefit analysis. On the part of the administrator, many of the questions will be asked in order to be comfortable with that qualitative, benefit side of the equation.

What are the basic reasons for program initiation or change?

Although it is often believed that programs are initiated solely from marketing and/or financial reasons, marketing/financial considerations are only part, and usually a lesser part, of the equation. Many institutions initiate transport systems because of programmatic needs. A review of these reasons is important. It is a fact that existing clinical programs of the institution may demand effective transport. An institution which considers itself a comprehensive medical center will have several tertiary programs. Usually these programs are so unique that there is not enough patient volume within the immediate area to support these programs. People from the outlying areas will refer patients to the medical center for care. This is true whether the programs are neonatal, high-risk maternal, transplants, trauma, burns, etc. Many transport programs have been initiated to facilitate the quick and safe transportation of patients who would be coming to the institution anyway, but would not arrive fast enough or safe enough using generic transport mechanisms.

The programmatic need is probably the soundest reason for developing a transport system. It guarantees that patients will be transported from an institution of less sophistication and capability to one of high capability, thus improving the potential outcome of the patient. With this programmatic logic, the transport system will be on the firmest foundation. The programmatic motivations, however, can be challenged if the cost/benefit is not satisfied, if institutional support is lacking, or if inpatient programs are not sophisticated enough or do not have high enough quality to serve the patients better than if they had been served at another institution.

The other compelling reason to develop a transport system is financial in nature. There are very few transport systems that can generate enough revenue from their own charges to meet the costs associated with the transport system. Consequently, most transport systems are financially justified based upon the fact that they bring additional patients into the hospital. Because a large portion of hospital costs are fixed, regardless of how many patients are in the hospital, any additional patients have large marginal revenues, thus making the transport program very attractive because of each additional patient brought to the institution.

Most institutions are capable of doing the type of analysis needed to determine whether or not the program ultimately is financially self-supporting. There are, however, several cautions associated with this type of analysis.

The first is that careful review must be made to determine whether or not the patients would have come to the hospital anyway. If this were the case, then there are no marginal revenues, only the marginal costs of the transport system. It is important to remember that the overall cost of health care within a community might be increased if patients are only redistributed between hospitals. That cost increase is associated with the new transport system. In this circumstance the overhead that is covered by the additional patients at the receiving hospital is generally equal to the overhead uncovered because the patient did not go to another hospital or did not stay in the referring hospital.

If there are not increased revenues from additional patients and the transport system is forced to stand alone, independent of other clinical programs or credits from associated revenue sources, there are several potential risks to the institution. They include an overemphasis on the number of transports as opposed to the movement of patients to support clinical programs and an overemphasis of the transport system as a means of marketing or advertising the institution. Next, they typically include a cost/benefit equation that will not be positive and insufficient overall institutional support. Finally, and probably the most serious, some proposals involve moving patients to an institution that is ill-equipped to deal with their ultimate clinical needs as opposed to moving patients to the appropriate clinical programs and appropriate facilities.

What about finances?

Economics have been and will forever be a crucial part of health care and, hence, a few summary comments about economics are appropriate. It is important to recognize that even though it is possible for a transport program to be initiated or changed against the current of negative financial analysis, it is almost impossible to imagine such initiation or change in the absence of economic analysis. It is also true that such overall review of a transport system will rarely be done solely in light of an economic analysis. It is very important to let the facts speak for themselves. Again, in reality, few transport systems can support themselves solely off the charges to the patient for the actual transport experience. Trying to force such economic justification, usually results in inappropriate assumptions and ultimate disappointment in the transport program's performance. A more pragmatic approach to what is possible economically and what is expected programmatically will create a much more healthy atmosphere when a program undergoes its annual review. Because of the training and unique purview that hospital administration has concerning dollars, it is generally best to let the institution's finance department and cost accountants do the number crunching. Program directors and clinicians arguing with cost accountants about dollars and cents is no more effective than administrators arguing with clinicians about the clinical efficacy of the program.

Next, by way of repeated emphasis, it is very important to recognize that for most transport systems, the cost/benefit equation will be satisfied by bringing additional patients into the hospital and by the overall support that the transport system provides to existing clinical programs. In many circumstances, once a clinical program has been committed to, a transport system is a natural consequence of such a programmatic decision. An institutional commitment to a high-risk perinatal program many times dictates the development of some type of transport capacity. A transport system development or modification in support of existing clinical programs and commitments will always have the strongest supporting logic and reasoning.

Finally, it is very important for everyone during a period of enormous national attention on health care and health care reform to ask the tough questions when initiating or modifying a transport system. A few of these tough questions might be as follows:[2]

- "Would these patients have come to the institution anyway through a transport system that already exists and is functioning well?"
- "What is the overall cost to the community of another transport system?"
- "Are the patients within the community being adequately cared for today by existing community resources?"

The answers to these questions might suggest that the development of the transport system is not primarily focused on enhancing the quality of patient care with its commensurate reduction in morbidity and mortality, but rather, simply attracting a large number of patients to one institution at the expense of another for competitive reasons. It is extremely difficult in today's environment for institutions to ask such tough questions and even more difficult to deal with the sobering answers. Such questions, however, help to keep the economic aspects of such a program in context and focus.

WILL ANY OF THIS WORK?

The reader might be initially tempted to look at the preceding material as a cookbook approach to dealing with hospital administration. In fact, every institution is different with different priorities, strengths, weaknesses, and expectations from its clinical programs. Program directors and clinicians would be well-advised to candidly discuss with administration the criteria that administration might use in evaluating requests for new programs or program modifications. The preceding material might be most valuable in enhancing a better understanding as to the respective positions and viewpoints of the unique combination of people who are involved in making decisions about health care. This material is not given as a secret formula for passing an administrative litmus test, but rather to enhance the quality of the communication between the various players so that the outcome of any decision is more objective and better understood by all players.

REFERENCES

1. Blum HL: *Planning for health, development and application of social change theory,* New York, 1974, Human Sciences Press.
2. Enthoven AC: The systems analysis approach In Hinrichs and Taylor, editors: *Program budgeting and benefit-cost analysis,* Pacific Palisades, CA, 1969, Goodyear Publishing Co, Inc.
3. Horngren CT: *Cost accounting, a managerial emphasis,* ed 5, Englewood Cliffs, NJ, 1982, Prentice-Hall, Inc.
4. Hyman HH: *Health planning, a systematic approach,* Germantown, MD, 1975, Aspen Systems Corp.
5. MacDonald MG and others: *Emergency transport of the perinatal patient,* Boston/Toronto, 1989, Little, Brown & Co.
6. Neumann BR and others: *Financial management, concepts and applications for health care providers,* ed 2, Baltimore, MD, 1988, National Health Publishing.
7. Price DP: Estimating the cost of illness, *U.S. Department of Health, Education and Welfare, Public Health Service, Health Economics,* Series No. 6, 1966.
8. Rado ER: Cost-benefit analysis, education and health, *United Nations, Research Institute for Social Development,* Report No. 7, 121-29, April 1966.
9. Wiseman J: Cost-benefit analysis and health service policy, *The Scottish Journal of Political Economy* 10:128-45, February 1963.

8

THE FINANCING OF AIR MEDICAL SERVICES

FORD N. KYES

Essential to an overall understanding of the financing of air medical services is an understanding of the component parts of this issue and their relationship to one another. In this chapter an overview of coverage policy, reimbursement policy, billing practices, and cost-effectiveness will be presented. Successful strategies for physicians and front line staff to assist the program in maximizing reimbursement will also be presented, and the author will speculate about how all of these issues might change as our health care system undergoes transformation in the 1990s.

COVERAGE ISSUES

The term coverage refers to the policies set by a health care insurance payor, public or private, which specifies the conditions that must be met for a health care service to be eligible for reimbursement. Before reimbursement can be considered, all insurance payors first seek to determine if a bill for services meets the payor's criteria for covered services.

Coverage requirements for air ambulance services vary widely between insurance plans, but most plans follow the principles set forth by the Health Care Financing Administration (HCFA) for Medicare recipients. HCFA regulations specify that air ambulance is a limited and specialized benefit under the Medicare program. The Medicare beneficiary's medical condition must require immediate and rapid ambulance transport that could not have been provided by land ambulance. Air ambulance transport is covered if the point of pickup is inaccessible by land vehicle or if great distances or other obstacles such as heavy traffic are involved in getting the patient to the nearest appropriate facility.

Most plans require documentation of medical appropriateness (medical necessity). Per HCFA regulations, "medical appropriateness is only established when the beneficiary's condition is such that the time needed to transport a beneficiary by land poses a threat to the beneficiary's survival or seriously endangers the beneficiary's health."[2] In general when it would take a land ambulance 30 to 60 minutes or more to transport an emergency patient, air ambulance is considered appropriate and therefore, covered. The term "emergency patient," as it pertains to air ambulance coverage requirements, is not specifically defined in the HCFA manuals.

If the full charges for an air ambulance transport are to be deemed "covered," the patient must also be transported to the nearest "appropriate facility." This provision can be of particular importance in determining coverage for pediatric patients, since, like trauma centers, children's hospitals are generally accepted as providing specialized services. Even if patients are transported long distances by air and other hospitals are bypassed, services are generally covered if a beneficiary's condition requires a specialized service available only at the more distance hospital.

Depending on the insurance provider, there may also be other special limitations to coverage. In some states, for example, it must be documented that neither land ambulances nor fixed wing air ambulances are sufficient to meet the patient's needs in order to justify coverage for helicopter air ambulance transport under Medicaid coverage provisions. Some insurance plans only cover emergent surface transportation services without preauthorization. Once again, preauthorization requirements generally follow Medicare (HCFA) requirements for determining medical necessity.

REIMBURSEMENT ISSUES

Once it has been determined that a particular air ambulance transport is a covered service under a particular insurance plan, the issue of how the reimbursement rate is determined becomes important. Again, there is variation among the policies used by different payor groups for determining reimbursement levels. Reimbursement for covered air ambulance services ranges from full payment of charges to partial payment at a prevailing rate schedule based on ground transport charges. Medicaid ground transport rates are usually the lowest level of reimbursement for ambulance services. When used as the basis for air ambulance reimbursement, Medicaid ground ambulance rates amount to approximately 10% of the cost of providing the service. As in most hospital and outpatient services, the key to attaining financial solvency is cost-shifting from payors reimbursing at less than cost to payors reimbursing at full charges or at negotiated discounts on charges. Pediatric and neonatal transport patients tend to have a high percentage of Medicaid payors. Unfortunately, in most states Medicaid has the lowest reimbursement rates. At the other extreme, auto insurance tends to be an excellent primary payor, particularly if air transport bills are authorized and paid prior to exhaustion of payment limits.

Reimbursement of an air ambulance transport charge for most managed care contracts is provided at a negotiated discount of full charges if coverage requirements are met. Strategic charge setting by air medical programs is an essential, yet often overlooked, action to improve financial success. If charges are set near or below cost, there is obviously no flexibility for either cost-shifting or for providing discounts on air medical charges during comprehensive negotiations for a managed care contract. Despite the obvious logic of that position, it is not uncommon for air medical transport programs to be priced at near or below cost due to a lack of understanding of costs and outmoded pricing strategies.

Because pediatric transport programs are frequently one component of a comprehensive adult and pediatric air medical transport service, it is important to understand the reimbursement principles at work under Medicare. Medicare is frequently the largest payor group in a comprehensive air medical transport program, and therefore, the applicable coverage and reimbursement issues are essential to the program's overall financial health.

Medicare reimbursement for air medical transportation services differs significantly if the service is provided directly by the provider hospital or "under arrangement." Where the service is provided directly, reimbursement is made on a "reasonable cost" basis. Where services are provided "under arrangement," reimbursement is made on a reasonable charge or prevailing charge basis. A service is deemed to have been provided directly if the provider (hospital) fully owns and operates the service. This principle also applies in a consortium program where all members of the consortium are provider hospitals. "Under arrangement" applies when the service is provided under contract with an entity not fully owned and operated by the provider.

Under most circumstances there are distinct advantages to providing the service directly and therefore receiving reimbursement on a reasonable cost basis. Under reasonable cost provisions, reimbursement is provided for all costs (both direct and indirect) applicable to the hospital's Medicare cost report. If the services provided to a qualified Medicare beneficiary are to be covered (based on the provisions noted above), the hospital receives an interim payment approximately equivalent to the reimbursement provided for ground transport services. At the end of the fiscal year, the hospital is also paid the percentage of their total allowable costs equivalent to the percentage of total covered transports provided that year to Medicare beneficiaries minus the interim payments already received. For example, if 30% of the hospital flight program's transports were authorized services for Medicare beneficiaries, then approximately 30% of the hospital's direct and indirect costs of operating the flight program would ultimately be reimbursed by Medicare.

Although reimbursement under the provisions of reasonable charges may seem desirable, total reimbursement is often substantially less than under the reasonable cost methodology. This is true because prevailing charges in the community are usually determined through a blending of ground and air charges. Therefore, reimbursable charges may be at or below direct cost, and there is no opportunity for additional payments to contribute to the hospital's overhead. A careful analysis must be completed in a program's geographic region to determine whether the program should be structured as a direct service or as a service provided under arrangement. The financial implications to these decisions are not always apparent in the casual analysis but are almost always significant if carefully reviewed and understood.

BILLING ISSUES

Since most air medical transport claims undergo full review by the payor's medical staff, proper documentation is essential to successful financial management. Internal review mechanisms should be in place at the program to ensure that submitted bills are timely and contain all necessary information to maximize the probability of acceptance without denial. If the payor has specific requirements to reach a determination that a claim is a covered service, one should be certain that information is submitted with the claim. If the payor allows certain elements to be bundled or unbundled from comprehensive charges, one should be certain that these charge coding conventions are followed accurately.

Medicare and many other payors specify that air ambulance services may be billed with two major components: a base fee and a per loaded mile fee. Some additional items such as oxygen and certain medical supplies can also usually be billed separately. ECG monitoring, pulse oximeter, and ventilator time are usually considered to be a part of the base fee and may not be reimbursed separately. A key strategy to successful billing is to know the payor's requirement in advance and comply by submitting accurate, substantiated bills for the first time and every time. A common oversight of hospital-based flight program managers is failure to track the billing process and success rate as submitted through the hospital's billing services. Air medical transport billing requires a certain level of complexity and attention which is often lost in a hospital billing structure oriented towards inpatient and/or physician billing.

Another key strategy for financial success is to appeal denials. If denials are consistently appealed, the program's management will gain a greater understanding of the payors interpretation of policy, and the payor's personnel will gain a greater understanding of the program's legitimate benefits to its beneficiaries. Failure to appeal denials will lead to more claim denials and set the precedence of a more narrow interpretation of payor's policies by the medical staff reviewing claims. Failure to appeal is frequently viewed by the payor as capitulation to the rationale for the denial. Failure to appeal a denial is a failure to take the opportunity to educate a regional payor about the benefits of air medical transport for the patient. Failure to appeal denials will result in declining reimbursement for the program's legitimate services.

COST-EFFECTIVENESS

In an environment where total reimbursement for all health care services is declining, the only opportunity to maintain positive margins is to decrease cost and/or improve efficiency. A number of opportunities exist for air medical transport programs to improve efficiency and decrease costs. The three most expensive components of an air medical program are aircraft costs, aviation management costs (including fuel, maintenance, insurance, and pilots), and the cost of medical and management personnel. Each of these components should be regularly evaluated for opportunities to reduce costs or improve efficiency.

It is incumbent upon the medical team and management personnel of an air medical program to carefully review the types of patients transported and their special needs in order to establish minimum requirements for aircraft capability. Some of the common reasons cited for needing to specify a larger helicopter for an air medical program include the need or desire to operate the aircraft under instrument flight rules (IFR), the need to complete neonatal transports with three medical team members, the need to transport two patients simultaneously, the need to complete intra-aortic balloon pump transfers, and the need to respond to requests for the transport of patients receiving ECMO. Each program's leadership team should carefully weigh the benefits and costs to their patients and the community of providing a comprehensive transport capability to respond to all potential requests. Are there other less expensive modes of transport available that would provide the same outcome potential for the vast majority of patients? If so, the cost savings of operating a smaller aircraft or transporting a greater percentage of the patients by ground ambulance could be very significant. It should be the goal of the entire flight team to use the most cost-effective aircraft that will meet the needs of the majority of the flight requests.

Once the optimal and minimum aircraft capability requirements have been specified, a thorough review of the aircraft options and financial advantages and disadvantages of different aircraft acquisition options should be considered. With the availability of low cost financing to non-profit and publicly affiliated institutions coupled with high residual values of most aircraft, the advantages to aircraft ownership can be tremendous. It is not uncommon for return on investment analysis of aircraft purchases to demonstrate a return of 15 to 20% at 5 to 7 years. The savings in gross operating costs over the entire life of the aircraft ownership can be substantial. In addition to purchase options or lease options with buy-out provisions, the prudent air medical program manager must also carefully evaluate aircraft on the basis of their direct operating costs. It is critically important to survey a number of credible sources to obtain meaningful estimates of direct operating costs for helicopters, since actual experience can vary substantially from manufacturer and profession published estimates. The differences in operating costs between a light, twin engine helicopter and medium, twin engine helicopter can be substantial when fuel, maintenance, and insurance costs are considered. Many programs have selected aircraft with capabilities in excess of their needs. Unless the aircraft selection criteria are regularly reevaluated for ongoing appropriateness, opportunities for improvement in cost-effectiveness will not be realized. As reimbursement shrinks it is quite possible that a shift toward smaller and fewer aircraft will occur in the air medical profession.

Since aviation management costs also make up a large percentage of a program's overall costs, it is important to evaluate that aspect of the program as well. One strategy used successfully by many programs is to hire an outside consultant with aviation management expertise to independently review the aviation management of the program and to offer suggestions for improving the contract or the execution of its provisions. For example, reducing unnecessary down time for maintenance through improved scheduling practices can improve overall efficiency significantly. Some programs have also decided to operate the aviation portion of the program directly without the assistance of a separate FAA certified Part 135 operator. There can be cost savings realized from this approach, but the risks can also be substantial and should be evaluated carefully. Another approach which is gaining acceptance by a number of large and small programs is to share in the risk of the aviation management of the program through a cost plus type contract with a Part 135 operator. In this scenario the hospital assumes some portion of the risk in financing the aviation portion of the program in exchange for a greater level of control and sharing of any cost savings.

ROLE OF PHYSICIANS AND FRONT LINE STAFF

In addition to participating in programmatic reviews to identify ongoing opportunities for cost savings, there are a number of steps that the physicians and front-line staff can take to assist the program in maximizing reimbursement. Documentation is key to minimizing denials based on coverage issues. Since most air medical transport claims undergo 100% review by the third-party administrator's medical review staff, it is important to provide the information they require to reach a positive determination. As mentioned previously, information should be gathered in advance about the requirements of all major payors for determinations that an air medical transport service is a covered device. The clinical record should contain the reasons for air medical transport and, if appropriate, the reasons for selecting the receiving hospital. The reasoning for destination hospital selection is particularly important if another potentially qualified hospital was closer than the actual destination hospital. All relevant information should be included at the time of the initial claim submission to assist the third-party administrator in promptly reviewing the claim and avoiding the need for them to request additional information.

The management and clinical team should develop and implement a timely chart review. In addition to seeking opportunities for improvement in clinical documentation, the reviewers should evaluate compliance with documentation requirements to maximize reimbursement. The staff should receive regular feedback and formal training regarding the types of documentation that are particular to the program's profile and reimbursement experience and has been successful in justifying transports. A process for the review of all flights to identify transports that may not meet medical appropriateness criteria should also be an important aspect of the program's comprehensive quality improvement program.

The need to gather accurate billing information at the time of the transport cannot be overemphasized. The front-line staff frequently has the best opportunity to obtain the patient's demographic and insurance information from the referring facility at the time of transport. If the patient is being transported from the scene, the flight crew can often assist with directing family members to the appropriate registration area or assist with timely follow-up with another receiving facility. The management staff should take an active role in monitoring the performance of the billing functions and take aggressive actions when opportunities for improvement become apparent.

FUTURE TRENDS IN REIMBURSEMENT

Health care system reform will clearly provide both significant opportunities and significant threats for the air medical profession. One strategy for cost savings in health care will be to limit the proliferation of advanced technologies. The only centers which will continue to deliver advanced technological services will be those that can offer competitive rates through volume and saturation of their high, fixed expenses. This will create an increased need for transportation of critical patients to these regionalized centers of excellence. Health care purchasers (corporation, HMOs, group purchasing alliances, managed care companies, etc.) will also have significant financial incentives to move their beneficiaries to health care systems with whom they have contracted for discounted rates. Since the American public is not likely to cease its appetite for travel, there will likely be increasing incentives to move patients back to their home systems for all but the most routine services. In an increasingly regionalized approach to health services delivery with large integrated provider networks, an infrastructure for the transport of patients to appropriate delivery sites will be essential. Air medical transport services will likely continue as a basic component of the public's expectation for a sophisticated delivery system.

The challenge for air medical transport services will be in developing processes that ensure the delivery of the most cost-effective means of transport available. Integrated transportation systems that provide access to helicopter, fixed wing, and ground transport services will be more common. These transport services will need to position themselves to either competitively bid for contracts to provide transportation services to multiple providers in a geographic region or absolutely minimize their cost impact on their sponsoring delivery network. If the transport service is a component of an integrated delivery network, their services will likely be provided as a part of the benefits package and will not be reimbursed separately from the capitated fee received by the network to provide all services to the covered lives in the plan. Under this scenario, where all services provided are an additional cost to the network, the incentive will clearly be to provide the least expensive means of transport appropriate to the patient's needs. The network will demand very rigid utilization criteria, and volumes for the more expensive modes of transport will decline. If the transportation service is competitively bidding to provide services independently in a region, the service will need to keep all of their direct and indirect costs as low as possible to remain competitive. Quality differentials are difficult to prove, and most purchasers assume a base level of quality and will make their decisions primarily based on cost. Under either scenario rigid guidelines will have to be applied to justify the use of the more expensive transport modes, and purchasers will demand to see documentation that air medical transport was cost-effective. The survival of air medical transport systems in the future will depend on its leadership's ability to control utilization and minimize the per unit cost. Per unit costs will be controlled by utilizing less expensive aircraft, minimizing direct operating expenses, and maximizing productivity on all aircraft.

SUGGESTED READINGS

Association of Air Medical Services: Position paper on the appropriate use of emergency air medical services, *J Air Medical Transport* 9:29-33, 1990.

Department of Health and Human Services, Health Care Financing Administration, Medicare intermediary manual: Part 3 claims processing, HCFA Publication 13-3, Section 3114C.11, June 1990, The Association.

Williams KA, Aghababian R, Shaughnessy M: Statewide helicopter utilization review: the Massachusetts experience, *J Air Medical Transport* 9:14-23, 1990.

9

ROLES OF THE MEDICAL AND PROGRAM DIRECTORS

STEVEN PON
DANIEL A. NOTTERMAN

The management of a pediatric critical care transport system, as with most medical units, consists of medical and nonmedical aspects of administration. Thus, a common model for the organization of transport systems includes a medical director who assumes the clinical responsibilities and a program director who bears the nonmedical administrative duties. Whether a transport organization is supervised by a single director or by a multidisciplinary team of professionals, the responsibilities are the same, though they may be apportioned differently.

The following exposition is a synthesis of numerous recommendations and guidelines but is not intended to be a regulatory document. Its goal is to stimulate the continuing improvement of pediatric critical care transport services.

THE MEDICAL DIRECTOR

Physicians play an integral part in the development and operation of all medical systems, including critical care transport systems. The major purpose of physician participation is to ensure the quality of patient care. To achieve this aim physicians must have the authority within the system to control its clinical aspects. It is this authority that defines the medical director.

There are many models which may apply to the medical directorship of a pediatric critical care transport system. Published guidelines and job descriptions exist for medical direction of prehospital emergency medical services,[15] air ambulance services,[19] critical care units,[17] pediatric intensive care units,[3] emergency departments,[5] and respiratory care departments.[8] Each of these guidelines and existing guidelines for pediatric critical care transport[2,4,11] stipulate precise qualifications for medical directors but are much less specific about the definitions of duties. Furthermore, there is no consensus regarding the specific functions and activities of the medical director among the many established transport programs that have well-defined directorships. However, the principal theme among all job descriptions is that the medical director is responsible for ensuring the quality, safety, and appropriateness of patient care. With these responsibilities, the medical director participates in many wide-ranging activities.

Qualifications

The medical director should have experience or training in transport medicine and medical control and should be familiar with the design and operation of transport systems. He or she should be knowledgeable about quality improvement processes and about the laws and regulations which pertain to transport systems. Familiarity with communications systems is also recommended.[13,15]

In accordance with the applicable guidelines, the medical director of pediatric transport systems should be a specialist in pediatric critical care, pediatric emergency medicine, or neonatology.[4] Systems which transport both adult and pediatric cases should have a pediatric medical director acting in collaboration with an adult specialist.[4]

Part of the medical director's duties, particularly aspects of off-line medical control, may be performed by a group or committee of physicians. A team approach is particularly useful when the transport system routinely serves diverse patient populations which require subspecialty expertise. Systems that transport neonatal patients should be advised by a neonatology codirector or medical advisor. The guidance of a pediatric surgeon is required for the transport of the pediatric trauma patient. In systems that serve a mix of adult and pediatric patients, respective specialties should participate in the medical direction of the program.

Some systems have multiple codirectors, whereas others have a single medical director with several medical advisors. The precise organization and relationships among the specialties vary among systems, but a formal, well-defined structure should be in place. Policies and procedures should be established to resolve or preempt potential conflicts among specialties, but most disagreements can be resolved with a team approach. The medical director may arbitrate irreconcilable differences by applying the stated priorities of quality, safety, and appropriateness of patient care.

Medical control

The principal duties of the medical director are related to medical control and can be divided into concurrent, prospective, and retrospective activities. The former constitutes on-line medical control, and the latter two comprise off-line medical control.

On-line medical control. On-line medical control consists of triage and patient management. These duties may be performed by the medical director or a designated medical control physician. The purpose of the on-line medical control physician is to ensure that the care of the patient conforms to acceptable standards and to serve as patient advocate during stabilization and transport. The medical control physician determines if the patient can be safely transported and may be responsible for deciding the mode of transport (e.g., air or ground) and team composition (e.g., physician or no physician) in programs which have such flexibility.

The patient care rendered by medical control is either in person or via direct communication. In transport systems which include physicians on the team, the transporting physician, certified by the medical director, may direct patient care.[11] However, the presence of a physician on transport does not obviate the need for a designated medical control physician.[13] Where the transport physician or other medical control physician lacks pediatric expertise, the receiving attending or pediatric medical director may serve as the on-line medical control physician.[11]

The qualifications for medical control physicians are similar to those required of medical directors.[11] The physician should have special expertise in pediatric critical care, pediatric emergency medicine, neonatology, or pediatric surgery, as appropriate.[4] This physician should be experienced and/or trained in receiving transport calls and in offering management suggestions. A thorough understanding of the transport environment, its potential impact on patient condition, and the limits it poses on therapeutic intervention is essential for any medical control physician. This may be especially important where patients are subjected to flight conditions.[13,19] The medical control physician must be aware of the capabilities and limitations of equipment, vehicles, and personnel and have practical knowledge of what can and cannot be accomplished in transit.[13] He or she must understand and apply all the policies, procedures, and protocols that address both medical and administrative issues (Box 9-1).

The medical control physician should be available at all times to respond promptly to transport requests or to transport management questions. He or she should be aware of bed and transport team availability and should have the authority to accept, refuse, or otherwise triage transports without further consultation.[4] The medical control physician should also have the authority to activate backup systems when necessary. Should dis-

BOX 9-1 DUTIES OF ON-LINE MEDICAL CONTROL

- Triage calls
- Ensure quality of patient care
- Determine patient transportability
- Select mode of transport
- Determine team composition
- Provide medical guidance for transport team
- Consult subspecialists when necessary
- Resolve conflicts & administrative problems
- Activate backup systems when necessary
- Communicate with transport team, referring physicians & receiving physicians
- Provide feedback to referring physician at transport completion

agreements arise between the transport team and the referring staff, the medical control physician should be available to intervene to resolve issues without confrontation.[12]

Subspecialty consultation may be sought once the transport mechanisms have been mobilized. A subspecialist or receiving attendant may serve as medical control for an individual transport if he or she has been appropriately trained.[4]

The transport team should always be able to communicate with the medical control physician to inform him or her of physiologic changes and adverse events and to elicit management suggestions. Medical control should also communicate with the referring physician to remain appraised of changes in clinical status, offer management suggestions prior to the arrival of the transport team, and provide timely feedback regarding the patient's condition at the completion of the transport. The medical control physician is obliged to inform the receiving physician of the status of the transport and of significant changes in the patient's condition in transit.

The medical control physician is assigned by the medical director to whom he or she reports.[4] The medical director or a designated physician must be available at all hours[4] to provide expert help and resolve problems not addressed by protocol.

Off-line medical control. The medical director conducts both prospective and retrospective off-line medical control activities. Prospective duties include participating in the design of the system, designating the on-line medical control physicians, developing and approving medical policies and procedures, promulgating standards of care, training, and testing, and certifying transport personnel.

The medical director must ensure that the protocols conform to the numerous guidelines established by various agencies. Guidelines regarding the proper selection of the mode of transport are examples.[2,9,10,11]

The curriculum for training programs, particularly those for nonphysicians and physicians-in-training, should be formulated or approved by the medical director. Determining staff cognitive and technical competency and documenting the completion of training requirements is imperative.[12] Mechanisms for continuing education and criteria for recertification should also be established. The training must satisfy regulations and guidelines where they exist, especially with regard to nonphysician personnel. Training requirements should be adjusted for the preexisting level of training and for the required level of function. The medical director should hold regular meetings of the transport staff, communications specialists, and medical control physicians for purposes of quality improvement, continuing education, introducing new technologies, and updating policies and procedures.

Retrospective medical control activities include continuing quality improvement programs directed at both patient care and the function of the entire system. Specific areas to be targeted for quality improvement efforts include safety, expediency, efficiency, triage, appropriateness, outcome of transport and hospitalization, and data collection.[4] Quality improvement activities include daily or periodic case review to address patient care or documentation issues and review of operational aspects, such as mobilization time or communications. Breaches in safety or medical protocol, equipment problems, and adverse events must be monitored. Appropriate protocols should be in place to provide timely and accurate documentation of adverse events, morbidities, and mortalities. Provi-

BOX 9-2 DUTIES OF THE MEDICAL DIRECTOR

- Train & certify on-line medical control physicians
- Assign on-line medical control physicians
- Provide expert help to medical control physicians
- Formulate clinical protocols
- Promulgate medical standards
- Design training curriculum
- Train & certify transport staff
- Provide continuing education for transport staff
- Conduct continuing quality improvement activities
- Perform case review
- Represent the transport system
- Establish and participate in outreach programs
- Provide continuing education for referring physicians
- Afford accessible consultation to referring physicians
- Approve transport agreements
- Serve as liaison to institutions & organizations
- Ensure compliance with guidelines/regulations of overseeing agencies/organizations
- Select/approve equipment & supplies
- Establish a database
- Promote research in transport medicine
- Maintain knowledge base
- Introduce new technologies and innovations

sions should be in place for remedial education or recertification when necessary (Box 9-1).

Although ensuring the quality of care is a responsibility of the medical director, some aspects may be delegated to associate directors, medical advisors, or nonphysician personnel, such as the program director or the transport coordinator.[12] Quality improvement activities are multidisciplinary and should include all aspects of the transport system. The program director (see above) may be responsible for the nonclinical aspects, but all quality improvement activities must be coordinated.

Outreach & liaison

The medical director has several responsibilities other than medical control. As an official of the transport organization, the medical director serves as a liaison to numerous groups and organizations.[13] He or she represents the transport program to the hospital, the critical care units, the emergency departments, and referring institutions.

The director often participates in outreach programs to referring institutions. Outreach education may include feedback to referring physicians regarding particular patient management issues. If the transport service originates from the receiving unit, status reports on the patient's progress also foster good relations that make future referrals more likely. Further outreach efforts should inform referring physicians of the specialized services available, educate referring physicians on the evaluation and the stabilization of critically ill or injured children, provide continuing education for receiving physicians, provide accessible consultation around the clock,[1] and formalize relationships with referring institutions.

Formalizing relationships with referring institutions by drafting transfer agreements has been suggested by some authorities.[6] These agreements outline the specific responsibilities of the referring, transporting, and receiving staff to preempt any confusion that would lead to unnecessary delay or a compromised level of care.[13,16] Furthermore, each member of the transport agreements as they must be for any other administrative protocol. The medical director must approve any transport agreements drafted with referring institutions and, where applicable, with receiving hospitals.

The medical director also interacts with local, state, regional, or national organizations and authorities. Compliance with the various standards and guidelines promulgated by these organizations should be ensured by the director. Agencies promulgating standards include the American Academy of Pediatrics,[1,2,4,11] the American College of Surgeons,[7] the American College of Obstetricians and Gynecologists,[1] the American Medical Association,[20] the Air Medical Physicians

Association (AMPA), the Association of Air Medical Services (AAMS),[9] the Commission on Accreditation of Air Medical Services (CAAMS), the Federal Aviation Administration (FAA), the Joint Commission on Accreditation of Healthcare Organizations (JCAHO),[14] the National EMS Pilots Association (NEMSPA),[12] the National Highway Traffic Safety Administration (NHTSA),[20] and the U.S. Department of Transportation.[20]

Other responsibilities

The medical director is responsible for ensuring that the transport team is suitably equipped to provide optimal care. With the suggestions and recommendations of transport program staff, biomedical engineers, and the program director, the medical director selects or approves the purchase and use of biomedical equipment.[12] Standards for patient care equipment and medications should be set or approved by the medical director.

Developing and maintaining a record-keeping system with meaningful data analysis is another responsibility of the medical director.[1] Data collection in a systematic fashion is important to study utilization and referral patterns, continuing quality improvement, and for billing purposes.[16] A number of data sets to be collected have been proposed.[1,4,7] Promoting research in the area of transport medicine and related fields should be another priority.

The medical director must maintain a knowledge level appropriate for the position,[15] since he or she is responsible for introducing medical innovations to the transport program and for developing or approving clinical protocols.[8,22]

THE PROGRAM DIRECTOR

Of the many models for the organization of transport systems[16] and other clinical units,[18,21] most include an individual assigned to deal with the nonmedical aspects of the system. In most transport organizations the program director is responsible for coordinating the activities of each of the system's components.

The program director can be a nurse, a paramedic, an administrator, or a physician. Where the medical director is also the program director, a nursing/paramedic administrator or coordinator may perform many of the nonclinical duties. Programs that use other nonphysician personnel could appoint an individual to coordinate the activities of those individuals.[12] The group of directors, administrators, and coordinators may serve as a management team that could facilitate interdisciplinary cooperation.[18]

The focus of the program director should be to ensure that the system conforms to all legal and safety regulations and operates within appropriate financial constraints. These responsibilities include: establishing administrative policies and procedures; developing system-wide continuing quality improvement programs; monitoring and recording licensure and certification of all personnel, vehicles and equipment; procuring equipment and supplies; ensuring the proper maintenance of transport vehicles; providing for appropriate communications systems; ensuring sufficient malpractice and disability insurance coverage; providing for adequate record-keeping and billing; preparing a budget; participating in marketing and strategic planning; and serving as liaison to other institutions, organizations, and agencies. Although the duties of the program director are somewhat different from the medical director, the overall priorities of quality, safety, and appropriateness of care should be shared. Significant overlap of duties should be divided to reduce duplication of effort.

Administrative protocols

The program director is responsible for setting policies and procedures for the nonclinical aspects of transport. Protocols regarding vehicular safety and communications are written or approved by the program director who ensures that they comply with the regulations and guidelines dictated by various overseeing agencies. Alternate medical, and communications equipment transportation, and transport personnel should also be identified in the program's policies and procedures.

One major function of the program director is to facilitate the safe and efficient operation of the transport system. Protocols should be in place to deal with problems that may arise during any phase of the transport. Problems may include loss of communication, equipment, or vehicular breakdown, inability to obtain consent for transport or procedures, and adverse events or incidents. Protocols should also be in place for routine procedures such as routing of referral calls, pretransport preparation, use of medications and supplies, and general safety precautions.[16]

Program evaluation

Continuing quality improvement requires the participation of the program director. The medical director may focus on the medical aspects, while the program director addresses the nonclinical aspects. All quality improvement activity should be coordinated among the professional disciplines, and provisions should be made for assessing the entire system as well as each individual component.[4] More specific objectives and requirements of quality improvement are outlined elsewhere[1,4] and later in this book. A systematic method of effectively evaluating and documenting the quality of patient care with appropriate response to the findings is the essential definition of a quality improvement program. The quality of care should be evaluated by standards of availability, accessibility, responsiveness, and effectiveness.[1]

Equipment & supplies

The program director is responsible for obtaining the appropriate equipment and supplies necessary for the safe transportation of patients. In collaboration with the medical director, new equipment should be evaluated, budgeted, and ordered. Equipment for use on aircrafts should be selected with extra care, given the potential for interference with navigational equipment. The U.S. Air Force School of Aerospace Medicine, the Aerospace Administration, the FAA, AAMS, and the Emergency Care Research Institute can provide some guidance.[1]

Supplies and equipment carried on transport should be standardized. The list of equipment and supplies should be formulated by the program and medical directors and should be in accordance with the standards and guidelines established by various regulatory agencies and supervisory organizations.[2,6,11,19] Separate supply packs for specific clinical circumstances such as burns, poisoning, or neonatal cases may be useful.[16,19]

The program director should establish procedures for restocking supplies and replacing damaged or malfunctioning equipment. Arrangements regarding medication acquisition and dispensing should also be made. Particular care regarding the administration and disposal of controlled substances is required by law (see Box 9-3).

Equipment and vehicles must be maintained assiduously for the safety of patients and staff. Pretransport inspections should be routine, and mechanisms for timely reporting and correction of malfunctions should be in place. Adequate backup systems should be readily available. The director should record and monitor licensure and certification of all vehicles, equipment, and personnel.

For transport programs which do not have their own vehicles, the administrator or program director must be responsible for con-

BOX 9-3 DUTIES OF THE PROGRAM DIRECTOR

- Formulate administrative procedures and protocols
- Develop and participate in continuing quality improvement programs
- Monitor licensure and certification of personnel & equipment
- Purchase and maintain vehicles or review transportation vendor qualifications
- Procure equipment and supplies
- Maintain communications system
- Ensure appropriate insurance coverage for the staff
- Provide for record-keeping/billing
- Prepare a budget
- Participate in marketing, outreach, and strategic planning
- Serve as liaison to institutions and agencies
- Comply with overseeing regulations and guidelines
- Arrange for backup personnel, vehicles, equipment, and communications

tracting specific items and services, such as properly equipped transport vehicles with drivers or pilots. The program director must ensure that such vehicles and personnel are properly maintained and certified by reviewing appropriate documentation. Furthermore, the organization, safety records, flight standards, personnel files, and financial reports of transport vendors should be scrutinized closely to avoid any compromise in the quality or safety of the transport program.[12]

A reliable communications system with appropriate backup is critical for any transport program, and the program director is responsible for providing and managing it. The director should also establish proper procedures and protocols for efficient communications. The system may entail a designated telephone line to receive referring calls and must include reliable communications between transport vehicles and the base station. Procedures should minimize both delays in responding to calls and risks of disconnection. Linking the communication system to other agencies, such as police, fire, emergency medical services, and landing facilities, should be arranged and agreed upon beforehand.[12] Coordination of vehicles and personnel can be accomplished via a communications center supervised by the program director. Adequate communications facilities are indispensable in the effort to coordinate the rendezvous of an aircraft with a ground ambulance at a landing site which is supervised by local fire and police departments.

Insurance

The program director must ensure that the members of the transport service have adequate insurance coverage or access to it. Transport personnel are typically exposed to greater risk to life and limb which may not be covered by an institutional policy. The program director should review new or existing disability and life insurance policies to ensure that all staff members are covered appropriately, particularly with regard to air transport for which there may be exclusions.[11] It should be noted that many disability benefits do not account for future potential earnings for individuals in training. Some systems provide "flight pay" so that individuals can purchase supplemental insurance.[4]

There is little precedence for malpractice by a transport organization.[13] Many programs operate under the auspices of the base hospital and should be covered as such if the transport is within the scope of employment and is recognized as such by the insurance carrier. The program director should determine if this is adequate or if further insurance is required.[11] Adequately covering the activities of the medical director and of the medical control physicians is another consideration of the directors.[4]

Budgeting & planning

The program director is responsible for formulating a budget and establishing and enforcing fiscal policies that enable the organization to operate within those bounds. Whether a separate entity unaffiliated with a hospital or completely owned and operated by a unit within the hospital, the transport program must reconcile costs and revenues if operations are to continue. Providing highly specialized services at a constant, high level of preparedness with wide fluctuations in demand is not an easy task.

One of the most important functions of the program director is to tabulate costs, project utilization, and arrange for sources of revenue. Several other activities are essential to this process. Accurate records documenting the utilization of the transport system will provide the historical data needed to formulate a budget. It may also elucidate seasonal or diurnal variations in utilization which could improve the efficiency of scheduling personnel coverage. Referral patterns could be identified to allow the formulation of specific marketing plans. Accurate data collection also facilitates billing patients or hospitals for service.

Outreach & liaison

As with the medical director, the program director represents the transport program and participates in outreach programs to maintain or expand the referral base. Outreach efforts include promoting the specialized services available and may involve formalizing relationships with referring institutions. Each of these activities must be coordinated with the medical director.

The justification of a transport system and a requirement for fiscal integrity is that the system is adequately used. Unused systems cannot survive. Marketing efforts are often needed to maintain or expand activity, particularly in regions with competing organizations. Methods of marketing include promotional visits, direct mailings, press releases, and displays at fairs. The most effective method, however, is to provide clinical follow-up to the referring institution or physician.[1,12] Mechanisms should be established for providing periodic updates of the patient's condition and discharge summaries to the original contact. When appropriate, transport back to the referring institution should be accomplished.

OBLIGATIONS OF THE SYSTEM

The pediatric critical care transport system has an obligation to provide both the medical director and the program director with appropriate authority and resources to fulfill their assigned duties. Appropriate liability insurance for the directors should be assumed by the transport system. The directors should also be adequately compensated for their time.[15]

The authority, responsibilities, and duties of both medical and program director should be agreed upon and documented. The medical director must have appropriate authority over all the clinical and patient care aspects of the system. Establishing and revising protocols, policies and procedures for triage, dispatch, treatment, and transport are within his or her purview. For effective quality improvement programs, the director must have access to all relevant records, including those from both referring and receiving institution, when relevant.

Hiring standards must be set or approved by both the medical director and program director. To ensure the competency of transporting personnel and of on-line medical control physicians, the medical director has the authority to certify, recertify, or decertify staff members. Certification and recertification include appropriate training and testing of personnel. Where problems arise, either director should have the authority to suspend providers given due cause. Appropriate mechanisms for review and appeal should be in place to ensure fairness with regard to disciplinary measures.

DISCUSSION

Medical administrative systems, including those of pediatric critical care transport organizations, must ensure the quality of care provided by each professional and integrate medical advances into their practice. They also must be consistent and reliable, yet responsive to their clients and adaptive to the requirements of regulatory agencies.[18]

A transport system requires a medical director who is responsible for the medical components and a program director who is responsible for coordinating the nonclinical, administrative activities. The complexity of the system determines the precise roles of the medical director and the program director. Interdisciplinary collaboration of physicians, nurses, respiratory therapists, paramedics, pilots/drivers, and dispatchers is essential for an effective transport service. The role of the directors is to ensure that the transport staff provides appropriate, safe, high quality medical care within a sound financial environment according to the applicable laws, regulations, and guidelines governing their practice.

REFERENCES

1. American Academy of Pediatrics, American College of Obstetricians and Gynecologists: *Guidelines for perinatal care,* Elk Grove Village, IL, 1992, AAP; and Washington, DC, 1992, ACOG.
2. American Academy of Pediatrics, Committee on Hospital Care: Guidelines for air and ground transportation of pediatric patients, *Pediatrics* 78(5):943-50, 1986.
3. American Academy of Pediatrics, Committee on Hospital Care and Pediatric Section of the Society of Critical Care Medicine: Guidelines and levels of care for pediatric intensive care units, *Pediatrics* 78(5):943-50, 1986.
4. American Academy of Pediatrics, Task Force on Interhospital Transport: *Guidelines for Air and Ground Transport of Neonatal and Pediatric Patients.* Elk Grove Village, IL, 1988, AAP.
5. American College of Emergency Physicians: Emergency care guidelines, *Ann Emerg Med* 20(12):1389-95, 1991.

6. American College of Surgeons, Committee on Trauma: Air ambulance operations, *Bull Am Coll Surg* 69(10):33-35, 1984.
7. American College of Surgeons, Committee on Trauma: Interhospital transfer of patients, *Bull Am Coll Surg* 69(10):29-32, 1984.
8. American Thoracic Society: Medical director of respiratory care, *Am Rev Respir Dis* 138(4):1082-3, 1988.
9. Association of Air Medical Services: Position paper on the appropriate use of emergency air medical services, *J Air Med Transport* 9(9):29-33, 1990.
10. Burney RE, Fischer RP: Ground versus air transport of trauma victims: medical and logistical considerations, *Ann Emerg Med* 15(12):1491-5, 1986.
11. Day S and others: Pediatric interhospital critical transport: consensus of a national leadership conference, *Pediatrics* 88(4):696-704, 1991.
12. MacDonald MG, Miller MK, editors: *Emergency transport of the perinatal patient,* Boston, MA, 1989, Little, Brown & Co.
13. Mookini RK: Medical-legal aspects of aeromedical transport of emergency patients, *Leg Med* 1-30, 1990.
14. Orr RA, McCloskey KA: Mobilizing critical care for interhospital and intrahospital transport. In Lumb PD, Shoemaker WC, editors: *Critical care: state of the art,* Fullerton, CA, 1990, Society of Critical Care Medicine.
15. Polsky S and others: Guidelines for medical direction of prehospital EMS, *Ann Emerg Med* 22(4):742-4, 1993.
16. Pon S, Notterman DA: The organization of a pediatric critical care transport program, *Pediatr Clin North Am* 40(2):241-61, 1993.
17. Society of Critical Care Medicine, Task Force on Guidelines: Guidelines for categorization of services for the critically ill patient, *Crit Care Med* 19(2):279-85, 1991.
18. Taft SH, Pelikan JA: Clinic management teams: integrators of professional service and environmental change, *Health Care Manage Rev* 15(2):67-79, 1990.
19. Thomas F, Gibbons H, Clemmer TP: Air ambulance regulations: a model, *Aviat Space Environ Med* 57:699-705, 1986.
20. United States Department of Transportation and National Highway Traffic Safety Administration/American Medical Association Commission on Emergency Medical Services: *Air Ambulance Guidelines,* DOT HS 806 703, Revised May 1986.
21. Zimmerman JE: Administrative structure of a critical care unit. In Parrillo JE, Ayres SM, editors: *Major Issues in Critical Care Medicine,* Baltimore, MD, 1984, William & Wilkins.
22. Zimmerman JJ, Coyne M, Logsdon M: Implementation of intraosseous infusion technique by aeromedical transport programs, *J Trauma* 29(5):687-9, 1989.

10

COMMUNICATIONS

SUSAN M. HERRON

A small paperback dictionary lists six short but distinct definitions of the word "communicate." Neither the size nor sophistication of this small dictionary should play a part in considering the size and sophistication of the word *"communicate."* To communicate is to make known, give or interchange thoughts or information, transmit to another, and be joined or connected. The communications center, like its root word, will follow these descriptive definitions.

In order to begin this discussion, terminology must be agreed upon. The area where incoming requests for service are received will be called the communication area or center. The personnel are communication specialists or coordinators. This area is not dispatch, and the specialist is not a dispatcher. If, for example, an air-medical transport program intends to charge patients for the service, and if either fixed wing or rotor wing aircraft are to be used as transport vehicles, the program will be operating under the Federal Aviation Regulation (FAR) Part 135. FAR Part 135 is "air taxi for hire," and the pilot in command of the aircraft is the dispatcher. Therefore, the pilot makes the final decision based on all the factors of flight, including if and when the aircraft will leave the ground. The communication specialist on the other hand "makes known" to the pilot a request for service. The pilot takes the information given, reaches a decision on the safety of flight, and then dispatches the aircraft.

The communications center is the designated area where the communication specialist is located. The communication specialist does much more than answer the phone and talk on the radio. This specialist should function as an integral part of the overall transport program and must ensure the existence of strong and regular operations to support the overall goal of optimal patient care and safety.

LOCATION

The communication center should be located in a place where cross-through traffic is limited, yet be visible and accessible to on-duty team members and administration. Visibility of the center will allow the communication specialists to request assistance when needed and enable their team members to observe when a transport is in progress and avoid interruption. Depending on the program's organization, it is advisable, and in many cases economical, for the communications center to be physically located separate from the transport vehicles and their personnel. The decision of where to locate the center should be made by taking into account the degree of physical and administrative support needed between the program's administration, transport personnel, and communication specialists. The area selected must have the physical layout and capabilities to provide adequate lighting, power supply, and ventilation to meet the needs of the equipment, power supply backup, and stor-

TABLE 10-1 RADIO SYSTEMS

Simplex	*Full duplex*	*Half duplex*	*Multiplex*
Transmit and/or send in one direction at a time using a single frequency, usually low band.	Transmit and receive at the same time, using two radio frequencies: one to transmit and the other to receive, usually Ultra High Frequency band.	Transmit or receive in one direction at a time using two frequencies, usually Very High Frequency band.	Transmit from two or more sources over the same frequency.

age. Additionally, since the center may be staffed 24 hours per day, frequently with only the communication specialist, other needs will include security and personal comfort items such as restroom and minimal kitchen facilities. Should the location not lend itself to including these personal needs, relief personnel must be available to maintain the center during the specialist's breaks.

EQUIPMENT

The equipment required for a program's radio communication will depend on the mission and scope of care.

Radio base station

The radio must be capable of transmitting information between the communication center, pilot or driver, and medical personnel on a designated radio frequency. This radio base station will be the one key element in the communication center. A detailed needs assessment must be completed by a technical radio advisor to assist in the final selection of the base station. A base station which has worked well in one agency may not always meet the needs of another.

The frequency used for the base station will be assigned by the Federal Communications Commission (FCC), based on the recommendation of a state public safety communication officer. The FCC will issue the radio license and call letters for the base station and radios. Several frequencies have been designated nationally to serve as EMS frequencies. These frequencies may be compatible with other EMS agencies in the region. A Continuous Tone Controlled Sub-Audible Squelch (CTCSS) or Private Line can be assigned to the national frequency for use during times when cross-over of radio transmissions between agencies is not desired. Listed in Tables 10-1 and 10-2 are the radio systems and frequency bands commonly used.

TABLE 10-2 RADIO FREQUENCIES

*Very high frequency (VHF) FM**	*Ultra high frequency (UHF) 450-850 MHz†*	*VHF AM 118-136 MHz†*
Simplex system used for a variety of communications, including base station, ambulance to hospital, hospital to hospital, and ambulance to ambulance.	Duplex system with limited range. A national set of medical channels are assigned to this system for use in EMS communications.	Primarily aircraft communication between aircraft and control towers. Included in this range is the national heliport advisory frequency 123.05.

* High Band 148-174 MHz† transmits by straight line. Low Band 30-50 MHz† has the greater range of VHF and follows the earth's curvature.

† A MHz is 1,000,000 cycles per second of electromagnetic wave.

Depending on the brand of radio base station selected, several options on the console will be available, such as paging from the console (either individual or group), radio to telephone patching capabilities, and additional radio frequencies which can be selected for use as a back-up frequency. Planning might include the option for agencies to program the main frequency of another agency into their base station and vice versa. In the event that one communication center experiences equipment failure or requires evacuation, another agency can take over the radio communications until the situation is corrected at the first agency.

Pagers

Any program will require the ability to page its on-duty personnel and administrative contacts. The system selected for use may be as simple as leasing pagers from a local paging service or paging from the radio console or as sophisticated as operating the program's own paging bridge which will allow alpha paging. Alpha paging is paging with the capability of sending messages which include both alphabetic and numeric data. The region of paging can be local, regional, or national, depending on the need of the program.

It is desirable for paging to be completed entirely from the communications center to avoid paging through a commercial system. Depending on the demand placed on the commercial system, a delay of up to several minutes may be experienced during peak times.

Telephone service

At least one dedicated telephone line must be available for service requests. Additional lines may be available by roll over capability or as separate numbers. Customers calling to request service should not reach a busy signal or wait extended periods of time for the telephone to be answered. Back-up telephone lines can be accessed by program personnel when requesting information which is not urgent but is related to a patient transport. These same lines may also serve as roll over emergency transport lines. More than one handset will be required, even if only one communication specialist is routinely scheduled. In many situations it is necessary for the specialist to be on more than one telephone line at a time or to have assistance in the center during a patient transport.

Logging recorder

A recorder should be in place to record all phone and radio transmissions regarding calls for service and communications regarding program patients.

The type of recorder selected might be a reel to reel logger or an audio cassette system. The reel to reel logger has the capacity to record more channels simultaneously than the audio cassette, but the reel to reel recorder and its tape is more expensive to purchase. In either case a dual logger should be purchased to provide redundancy in the recording system.

Many logging recorders have an instant playback option to allow the communication specialist the ability to replay the last phone or radio transmission quickly without physically going to the recorder. The playback option can be very valuable in avoiding the misdirection of a transport vehicle or misunderstanding a distress call.

Tapes or audio cassettes should be saved for a minimum of 30 days. Should a problem or concern be identified regarding a transmission recorded on a tape, either the original tape or a copy can be made for archive purposes.

Computers

As commercial software programs are developed specifically for EMS and critical care transport programs, it seems that the computer is less of an option and more an expected piece of communication center equipment. The hardware chosen for the communication center will vary depending on the level and demand the software will place on it. Standard software, such as a word processing package, spreadsheet, and database, should be installed immediately. Additional software may be purchased to provide real time recording of transports, pager messaging for access to the alphanumeric paging bridge, terminal access to a mainframe, modem access to other databases, and data communication direct with the transport vehicles by either Mobile Data Terminals or pager writing. If a computer is used an uninterrupted power source (UPS) should be attached to the system to prevent data loss due to power surges or blackouts. A UPS will maintain the computer without power interruption long enough to complete the current screen and allow for a controlled computer shut down. The extent to which a transport program involves computers is limited only by the creativity of the communication specialists and by the financial resources of the program.

Facsimile machine

A facsimile (fax) machine is also rapidly becoming essential equipment not only in the communication center but also in the transport vehicle. Fax transmissions allow good quality, rapid sharing of information regarding patient care, intervention, or treatment. The number of uses for this machine will quickly demonstrate its potential in any program.

Status board

For flight programs the FAA requires the communication center to have a large board with erasable marking ability to list on-duty personnel, on-call staff, such as maintenance and administrative, and specific information on the vehicle(s) being used that day. This board should be designed by the communication specialists who will be referring to the board during their duty shift. The board should list the pilot, physician, nurse, paramedic, mechanic and other staff who are on-call. The board should be updated at the beginning of the communication specialist's shift and as soon as any staff changes occur. The board will serve as a convenient reference for the communication specialist as well as a quick reference in the event of an emergency or a shift change during a transport. The status and location of all on-duty personnel must be maintained at all times to avoid delays in the departure of the transport vehicle.

Resource materials

The resource materials required will be very program-specific. Maps, whether aviation sectional, road, topographical, city, regional, state, or national will depend on the program's needs. In any case one should decide on the service area and transport method to locations within the service area and select maps which are appropriate. A good quality map which displays the program's service area and is covered with plexiglass must be located conveniently to the communication specialist. This map will be used to track the travel routes of the transport vehicle. By using an erasable marker, the communication specialist should highlight the intended route, follow the route by communication with the pilot or driver, and mark points along the line with the time the vehicle intersects with the marks. Transport following should occur at a minimum of once every 30 minutes for ground transports, once every 15 minutes by Visual Flight Rules (VFR) flight, and when possible during Instrument Flight Rules (IFR) flight. It may be necessary to share transport following with other agencies if the program vehicle travels out of radio or telephone range with the communication center. Other reference materials, such as the Program Policy and Procedure Manual, Communication Operations Manual, a listing of health care facilities and agencies with resources, phone numbers and landing zone information, Hazardous Materials Resource Guide, equipment manuals, state EMS agency manual, FCC part 90 rules and regulations, an airport directory, and the program's post incident/accident plan should also be readily available.

PERSONNEL SELECTION AND TRAINING

Communication specialists should be selected carefully and, as with all new employees, be offered a position only after multiple interviews with at least two different company employees. The communication specialist is the first and, in many cases, the only contact a customer or prospective customer will have with the company. Therefore, the communication specialist must exhibit positive human relations skills both in interdepartmental interactions and communication with customers. Additionally, the specialist must be able to work effectively under pressure on several simultaneous tasks to facilitate smooth operation procedures.

The specialist is responsible for all transport operations communication equipment. This will require the specialist to have expertise in radio communication systems and be proficient in the use of the radio console and recording equipment. The communication specialist must maintain and, whenever required, initiate appropriate equipment repairs.

Advanced knowledge of aviation safety, technology, and map reading, knowledge of the program's service area, medical terminology and/or Registered Emergency Medical Technician (EMT) training, self-motivation, assertiveness, and an aptitude for decision-making are also desirable skills for the position of communication specialist.

A newly hired communication specialist will require individualized training depending on the past experience of the individual and the scope of services provided by the transport program. In 1989 the Association of Air Medical Services (AAMS) produced a *Manual for Communications Operations*[1] which provides an exceptionally fine listing of aspects to be included in the training of communication specialists. This manual can be used as a course outline or as an aid to modify training specifically for their operation. The training section of this manual has been expanded in a publication prepared by the National Association of Air Medical Communication Specialists (NAACS). The *NAACS Air Medical Communication Specialist Training Manual*[5] is a comprehensive training manual with objectives and review questions for each unit. *Accreditation Standards,* published by the Commission of Accreditation of Air Medical Services[2] also outlines minimum training standards. All three of these references should be used in the development of a training program for communication specialists.

PATIENT TRANSPORTS

When a request for patient transport is received, the specialist should have pre-approved policies and procedures to address the request for service and a listing of authorized calling agencies. The initial request should be timed by either a time clock or computer time stamp. Stamping times are an important function of the communication specialist because questions frequently arise regarding the time lapses involved in a transport.

In the majority of programs the initial call received for transport is kept short with minimum information exchanged. Initial information would include patient name, patient location, working diagnosis, transferring and receiving physicians, and a number where the person requesting the transport can be reached. This basic information is adequate to initiate the standard operating procedures for notification of the on-duty personnel of the pending or approved transport request. Following notification of the on-duty personnel, the transport vehicle is either immediately released for transport or the appropriate persons are contacted to gain approval for the transport and the communication specialist should make a call back to the requesting agency. This call can be used to ensure the accuracy of the request and to obtain specific patient data. Some programs will gather this additional patient data prior to the departure of the transport vehicle, and others will supply this information to the on-board personnel after their departure while en route to the patient. In either case the communication specialist should be the primary coordinator of patient data. To receive and then transmit necessary data to the person who needs it is one of the prime reasons for having a communication center. Should another member of the transport team obtain additional information pertinent to the transport, they should share the information with the communication specialist. The communication specialist must be kept abreast of all pertinent data surrounding the transport to maintain the focal point of information within the communication center.

Federal legislation regarding transfer of patients between health care facilities, namely the Consolidated Omnibus Reconciliation Act (COBRA),[3] must be included in the program's development of standard operating procedures relating to intrahospital transfers. COBRA legislation places the burden of transfer on the transferring facility. Before a transfer can take place stabilization must be provided, and the transfer must be deemed appropriate. A transfer to a medical facility is defined as appropriate according to the following criteria:

(A) the transferring hospital provides the medical treatment within its capacity which minimizes the risks to the patient;
(B) the receiving facility
    (i) has available space and qualified personnel for the treatment of the patient, and
    (ii) has agreed to accept transfer of the patient and to provide appropriate medical treatment;
(C) the transferring hospital sends to the receiving facility all medical records (or copies) available at the time of transfer;
(D) the transfer is effected through qualified personnel and transportation equipment.

The communication specialist may be required to coordinate the landing zone for a helicopter or the use of ground ambulance transportation from the airport if the transport is by fixed wing. Information used to coordinate these situations should be easily accessible within the communication center.

A transport should be followed closely while in progress. The program should establish standard "on the ground" or "in the transferring facility" times, and if that standard time is extended for any reason, the medical personnel should communicate the reason for delay to the communications specialist and estimate a time of departure. The communication specialist will then relay the delay information to the receiving institution and physician.

All times associated with phases of the transport procedure, as with the time of the original call, should be stamped. It may be a vital element to know exactly what time the vehicle departed from the base en route to the patient, what time the vehicle arrived at the referring agency, what time the vehicle departed from the referring agency en route to the receiving institution, and what time the patient arrived at the receiving facility.

A request for patient transport from an area other than a health care facility is handled differently depending on the program and its mission. Standing protocols regarding the request from a prehospital care provider should be established. Information regarding the patient's medical condition when en route to a scene may be limited because the person requesting the transport may not actually be at the scene. In depth details of the patient's condition can be bypassed if the basic situation is communicated to the responding vehicle, for example, motor vehicle accident, gunshot wound, or cardiac arrest. Specific directional information must, however, be gained by the communication specialist, and this information must be relayed exactly to the pilot or driver. The communication specialist must realize that numerical addresses or small highway intersections will not be visible from a helicopter, therefore, other landmark data should be made available to the pilot. Air to ground communication with an agency on the scene, such as law enforcement or fire department, must be facilitated by the specialist, prior to the helicopter landing at the scene.

Patient data

Any information received by the communication specialist regarding the patient being transported must be considered confidential and therefore disseminated with caution. Most radio frequencies can be monitored with inexpensive radio frequency scanners. Each program should establish a policy regarding what confidential information can be transmitted over the radio and what information should be given only over more secure means of communication. Mobile data terminals or alpha paging may serve to meet the needs of the confidential information transmission and still be available to on-board personnel while en route. The communication specialist should not relay hearsay or unconfirmed information to the receiving institution. The decision whether to relay this type of information will be made by the senior medical team member during their report to the accepting medical personnel.

Medical control

Established and preapproved medical protocols must be in place before any patient transports are accepted by the program. These standing orders will address a broad spectrum of medical conditions and interventions. Should need arise for additional consultation with medical control, a standing medical control physician, or the receiving physician, the communication specialist may be asked to facilitate the communication and must be fully aware of the options for connecting the medical attendants to a physician. Radio to telephone patch capability, radio transmission directly to the medical control physician, cellular telephone contact, or a combination of these options may be necessary.

Missed transports

When a request for service is made and the program is unable to respond for whatever reason, the transport would be considered missed. Documentation of the time the service was requested and the reason the service was unable to respond should be clearly and completely recorded. Weather conditions, maintenance, another transport, lack of receiving physician or health care facility, or other situations may keep the program from providing service. Company policies should be in place which would allow referral to another service, if appropriate, or alternate means of providing service. Many critical care programs across the nation are now providing several vehicles within their program to match the appropriate vehicle to the patient. The vehicle may be selected depending on the distance of transport, acuity of the patient, weather conditions, medical equipment required during the transport, and cost-effectiveness.

TRANSPORT VEHICLE ACCIDENT/ INCIDENT PLAN

The program must be prepared for the worst possible case where an accident or incident occurs involving one of the transport vehicles. A well-planned policy must be in place in the event that the transport vehicle fails to report in a timely manner or if a situation is reported to the communication specialist by either the on-duty personnel or a witness. The plan must address who to notify, what information can be released and to whom, what to do to complete the transport of the patient on board, and who will make appropriate notifications.

Not only should this plan be in place in policy format, but it also should be tested on an annual basis to ensure that the content is complete, and the personnel of the program are familiar with the plan in its entirety.

DISCUSSION

The communications center of any organization is the heartbeat of that organization. Just as a heartbeat is vital to all of us, the heartbeat of the communications center is vital to the program's very existence. Without a strong and regular heartbeat, our health may falter and we may not survive. A transport program without a strong and consistent communications center will not be healthy and it too may not survive the test of time. Another important aspect of the heartbeat is the heart muscle, and in comparison to the communication center, the heart is the communication specialist. The muscle is the driving force between those with information and those who need the information.

REFERENCES

1. Association of Air Medical Services: *Manual for air medical communications operations,* Pasadena, 1989, The Association.
2. Commission on Accreditation of Air Medical Services: *Accreditation standards,* Anderson, SC, 1991.
3. Consolidated Omnibus Budget Reconciliation Act of 1985 (COBRA) amended by Omnibus Budget Reconciliation Act of 1989 (OBRA), 42 U.S.C. §1395dd
4. Lee G: *Flight nursing principles and practice,* St. Louis, 1991, Mosby-Year Book.
5. National Association of Air-Medical Communication Specialists: *NAACS air-medical communication specialist training manual,* Pasadena, 1993, The Association.
6. U.S. Department of Transportation: *Air medical crew national standard curriculum,* Pasadena, 1988, The Association.

11

HIRING, STAFFING, AND TEAM COMPOSITION

MARY GOMEZ

Ernest Hemingway's *Farewell to Arms* is a tale of a World War I ambulance driver. In one scene the young ambulance driver hastily loads a wounded soldier in the back of the ambulance and rushes him to the closest hospital. The severely injured man must try to stay alive until they reach the hospital. Today's scenarios are much different. Medical services are delivered to the patient, and medical care is rendered. Specialized teams are dispatched to referral hospitals or to the scene of an accident. Today, the transport team is brought to the patient to provide adequate stabilization before transport and proper monitoring during transport.[7,9,14]

Another trend is to organize specially trained transport teams rather than utilizing the unit-based staff in the neonatal intensive care unit (NICU), the pediatric intensive care unit (PICU), or the emergency department (ED). Indications such as referral center designation for specialty services, a level III nursery, or a level I emergency department highlight the need for coordinating transport services. This chapter will examine the issues associated with the type of transport team, hiring, staffing, and team composition that must be considered in developing a pediatric transport program.

TYPE OF TEAM

In the United States children are transported by various methods, vehicles, and teams. Regionally, many variables influence the type of team, team composition, and mode of transport available. Differences regarding team composition and the focus of training remain controversial. Factors such as distance, geography, availability of specialty services, and tertiary care dictate how a child is transferred. Thus, from state to state, hospitals implement a variety of team configurations.

Team structure can be a combination of the following:

Patient population:
- All-ages (general)
- Pediatric or neonatal
- Combination neonatal/pediatric

Team Base:
- Dedicated (designated or freestanding)
- Unit-based teams

Ideally, pediatric patients should be transported by experts in the field of transport medicine and in the care of children. This may not be feasible in certain areas, and many all-age teams have demonstrated the ability to adapt to and accommodate patients of different ages. It should be stressed that all teams which transport children need to consistently maintain education and practice in the medical care and transport of children. In the following sections dedicated (freestanding) and unit-based teams will be examined in detail.

Dedicated teams

Advantages. The dedicated team (all-age or pediatric) offers many advantages.[13] Usually, the team is composed of a small group of skilled practitioners. A designated group of specially trained nurses provides the core of the team. The team is supplemented by transport physicians, respiratory therapists, and/or paramedics as dictated by the circumstances. The nurses may have responsibilities that include endotracheal intubation, arterial catheterization, vascular access, and chest tube insertion. Depending on the hospital's policies and transport protocols, the team composition may vary. Transport physicians may be attendings or fellows in neonatology, critical care, and emergency medicine or PL-3 residents with transport incorporated as a part of the curriculum/PICU rotation. Moonlighting physicians can also be utilized for shifts that resident physicians may be unable to fill. Supplementing the team with respiratory therapists is prudent in situations which may require advanced airway management.

Expertise in the transport environment and its limitations is of paramount importance. The focus of clinical practice is in the impact of transport on the patient. Nurses concentrate on the anticipation of problems, reduction of possible risks, and stabilization for transport back to the base hospital. Consistency in care is maintained, since the same small group of nurses have extensive knowledge of transport stabilization and implementation of the treatment protocols developed to deliver specific care in the transport setting.

Training efforts are facilitated by the limited number of transport personnel that must be kept at advanced skill levels. In addition, team member responsibilities such as scheduling, protocol development and implementation, equipment maintenance, or restocking can be clearly delineated within the smaller group. Other advantages of a small group of transport staff is that the number of transports are rotated among the same staff. This maintains a high familiarity with transport protocols, vehicles, and equipment and even with referral hospitals. Transport vehicles necessitate consistent usage and familiarity of safety measures. Specialized transport equipment requires frequent use to implement proper monitoring and troubleshooting capabilities.[11]

The dedicated team can be mobilized rapidly, and its availability does not interfere with unit staffing or patient care. A rapid **response time** can be achieved by allowing the transport program to be separate from the critical care unit, since the nurses do not assume a patient assignment.

Lastly, the dedicated team serves a customer service function. It is able to immediately respond to transport requests by a direct access number or pager designated for emergency phone calls. They provide crucial stabilization advice on the phone when the transport is initiated. By rapidly communicating suggestions and recommendations, the referral hospital can implement measures to expedite the transfer process. As the team regularly interacts with referral hospitals, the opportunity for outreach education, data collection, and research opportunities may develop. As rapport develops the team may suggest educational offerings to the referral hospital which improves their ability to stabilize various pediatric conditions. Ongoing education and research may also result in reducing unnecessary transports and thus, cost containment. The team members can also send patient follow-up thank you letters that emphasize the public relations aspect of the dedicated team (see chapter on community outreach).

Disadvantages. Funding the dedicated team can be costly. The decision to establish a dedicated team requires examining many aspects of the hospital and its referral base. There is no magical number that determines when a dedicated team should be initiated, however, discussion with pediatric/neonatal teams demonstrates an industry trend of 500 transports per year as supportive of a dedicated team. Many hospitals seek alternatives for transport when potential expenses are closely examined. Transport reimbursement varies between states and third-party payors. Thus, the incentive to underwrite a dedicated team may be curtailed. Initial costs include equipment purchases, office allocation, possible construction of a helipad and an emergency access, as well as hiring and training team members. Continuing costs include office expenses, equipment replacement, salaries, aircraft, and ambulance expenses. Furthermore, dedicated teams require a separate cost center and clerical support. Specialized portable transport equipment is not purchased in large quantities, thus requiring payment of a premium price for such items. Transport nurses are usually higher on the pay scale than the average salaried nurse because of the level of expertise and seniority required for such positions. Space must also be allocated for an office area and equipment storage. Many institutions are hard pressed to part with precious office space.

Finally, dedicated teams incur downtime (non-patient care time). If hospital staffing is experiencing shortages or tight staffing patterns, dedicated transport nurses may be criticized for not assisting with patient care. Transport nurses can assist the units without assuming a patient assignment by starting intravenous lines or assisting with other procedures in the critical care units.

Financial resources must be fully examined. Careful analysis may show that bringing patients via a dedicated team proves beneficial for patient referrals and access to specialty services.

Unit-based (non-dedicated) teams

Advantages. Unit-based teams are composed of staff from a critical care unit that has received additional training in the stabilization and transport of their particular patient population. Many institutions utilize the unit-based team under various circumstances. This type of team is cost-effective for lower volume teams, since staff skills are maintained during patient care and downtime is not incurred. The unit can train a large pool of staff to assume transport responsibilities so when a transport request is received, any number of personnel can respond. Usually a physician is part of the team to assume direct visual medical control which does not necessitate advanced skill training for the transport nurse.

Non-dedicated teams may require less administrative attention, since training may be consolidated into the unit orientation. Administrative coordination may be incorporated into a clinical coordinator (unit manager) position or as an ancillary task of a unit member. It may also be advantageous for parents to meet unit-based staff immediately. During the transport process, parents may be able to begin developing a relationship with the nurse or physician who works on the unit. Non-dedicated teams may therefore add to the continuity of care in general.

Disadvantages. Numerous institutions implement a unit-based transport program. However, this approach is potentially disruptive to unit staffing if the designated transport nurse needs to relinquish a patient assignment. Other staff members must quickly absorb additional duties unless the transport nurse for the day does not take primary care of patients. The transport nurse may need more organizational time to set up the team, obtain a patient report, and gather equipment. This will often result in an increased response time.

Accommodating a larger pool of transport qualified nurses poses a challenge for the coordinator. Consistency in tasks, protocol implementation, assertiveness, and public relations may vary widely among the transport qualified staff. Training a large group is difficult unless the coordinator allows for numerous training opportunities and displays excellent communication skills. Also, individual team members may not perform the critical number of transports necessary to maintain adequate skills.

The referral hospital may encounter different team members each time they request transport services. Furthermore, transport nurses may not have time to devote to follow-up with the referral hospital. This may be due to time constraints with unit assignments and patient care unless the unit coordinator builds this time into non-patient care hours.

Finally, repeated vehicle orientation may be necessary for unit-based staff who transport patients infrequently. This orientation should consist of the use and location of pertinent equipment, oxygen hook-up, and accessory electrical power. A brief review of how to secure and release mounting systems, evacuation procedures, and location of fire extinguishers should also be included.[17]

Equipment and transport bags may not be carefully cared for from shift to shift unless restocking duties are clearly delineated.

JOB DESCRIPTIONS

Detailed job descriptions are essential to the developing transport team. If transport will be required or encouraged for staff working in a unit-based team situation, transport responsibilities should be clearly stated during the interviewing process. Please refer to other sections for detailed job descriptions.

ADMINISTRATIVE PLANNING

Clinical training must be a priority in the development of the new team. Initial training may include a variety of teaching modalities such as lectures, testing, skills labs, certification courses, and having a preceptor for transport. The team should establish an orientation program for future staff that will build on the new team's skills and experience. Continuing education minimums should be outlined. Activities such as attending conferences, recertification, case presentations, and transport review must be incorporated into the team's practice standards.

Methods should be available to reach team physicians twenty-four hours a day. Medical directors and other attending physicians should meet with the team regularly to advise and to review standards and protocols and their application to transport. Transport review allows the entire team to learn from an actual transport and to clarify circumstances that require independent judgement and interpretation.

Administrative and medical support are necessary to confront advanced practice issues. Some referral hospitals may not be accustomed to accepting stabilization advice from a transport nurse. Outreach education and team introduction may facilitate this process. However, efforts should always be made to accommodate the referral hospital's requests.

Another concern is the maintenance of advanced skills and procedures. The team must maintain records of current certifications, skills labs, lectures attended, and transport review with the medical director.

Secretarial support is integral to a well-functioning team. Ideally, this position can be part of the team and budgeted through the transport department. Responsibilities can include the following:

- Making preliminary transport arrangements
- Communicating information regarding the patient
- Sorting and distributing department mail
- Data entry
- Taking minutes at team meetings
- Processing ambulance, helicopter, or fixed wing paperwork charges to be posted on the patient bill
- Typing department memos
- Tracking and ordering department supplies
- Maintaining a customer oriented disposition
- Coordinating community outreach programs

If the developing team is unsure as to how workload and responsibilities will be distributed, a secretarial position could initially begin as part-time or be incorporated into a job-share with another department. It would be necessary to utilize this person at peak hours and reevaluate this arrangement at a later date. The dispatcher's job description may include additional clerical responsibilities during quiet periods.

Another option is to utilize resources available outside the department. If workload permits (if allowable within the job constraints), clerical personnel in the emergency department, neonatal intensive care unit, or pediatric intensive care unit may be able to incorporate additional responsibilities.

STAFFING

Several combinations of staffing are feasible for transport programs:

- Twenty-four hour in-house
- Twenty-four hour on-call
- Limited coverage in-house
- Limited coverage on-call
- Combination of in-house coverage for peak hours with on-call staff during non-peak hours

Two types of coverage can be utilized: twenty-four hour coverage or limited coverage. Full-time coverage provides the best service to the referral hospital. At any time of day or night referral physicians can obtain stabilization advice and transport services for critically ill infants and children. The team can be quickly mobilized if available on the premises. From the marketing point of view, a rapid response time is appealing to referral institutions. In addition, an on-site transport team is available to the base hospital for in-house emergencies. Expert transport staff can be readily utilized for intermittent situations such as a trauma code or difficult intravenous access as long as it does not compromise their ability to respond efficiently to a transport request.

However, twenty-four hour coverage is a costly proposition. Whether in-house or on-call, salary expenses may be prohibitive. If continuous in-house coverage is implemented, activities for nontransport time must be incorporated. Justification of such activities must also be documented for future reference of time appropriately utilized. Down-time activities should be defined and considered as a part of team responsibilities.

Limited coverage provides transport services for specific hours, primarily peak hours during the day. Newer teams may initially provide limited service until an assessment evaluates the needs of the referral base or until an analysis can be done to determine the amount of transport activity that will occur. This arrangement is difficult to implement for the following reasons. How will situations be handled if a call is received five minutes prior to end of service? Will on-call arrangements be utilized after hours? If on-call services are offered, how long will it take the team to be activated? These issues must be addressed in writing in the administrative plan of a developing team.

Another staffing consideration is whether to have in-house (on-site) or on-call (on or off-site) coverage for transport nurses and physicians. In-house staffing is more expensive. Furthermore, ancillary duties may be required to maintain productivity. Tasks may include starting intravenous therapy, assisting in the critical care unit (NICU or PICU), or other team responsibilities which will be reviewed later in the chapter.

Off-site, on-call staffing is the least expensive staffing option. However, the response time may be lengthy to allow for staff travel time to the base facility. On-site, on-call requires a staff rest area.

Staffing will vary for physicians, nurses, respiratory therapists, and emergency medical technicians. Possible options include the following:

- Physicians: —in-house resident physicians —moonlighting physicians on-call
- Nurses: —in-house with transport or unit responsibilities —on-call (on or off-site)
- Respiratory Therapist: —on-duty in critical care area with transport call responsibility
- Emergency Medical Technician (EMT): —on-duty in emergency department with transport call responsibility

SCHEDULING

Scheduling a twenty-four hour transport unit can be an intricate task. Because transport teams usually staff small numbers of personnel per shift, options for permanent shifts may not be feasible. Ideally, a team member can coordinate scheduling. The position of scheduling coordinator requires a diplomatic, objective, creative, and fair person! This person is usually revered by the team for doing the impossible. The job entails setting scheduling guidelines, tracking rotations, and plotting requests and team obligations.

The team must assess how many full-time equivalents (FTEs) it would require to properly cover the desired hours. If the team supports part-time staff, it must be decided how many of the FTEs can be split for part-time. The issue of the minimal number of hours to work in order to maintain adequate proficiency and experience must also be addressed.

Other scheduling concerns include peak hours, seniority, rotation expectations, weekend and holiday coverage, staffing for sick calls, leaves of absence, and vacation requests. Additional questions to confront are ideal vs. realistic schedule requests, daily minimal coverage needs, how long shifts will be and how many weeks are scheduled at a time.

The team that is able to respond to numerous transports at one time may want to consider flexible scheduling, such as staggering shifts, if patient assignments are not required. This cost-effective method would staff according to statistically peak hours. Previous transports can be carefully analyzed to determine overlap and hours of heaviest volume. Combinations of 8, 10, and 12 hour shifts are commonly utilized. The transport program at Children's Memorial Hospital in Chicago, Illinois, determined from past transport statistics that 11 am-9 pm had the most transport activity. Staggered shifts such as 7 am-3 pm, 9 am-5 pm, 1 pm-11 pm, and 9 pm-7 am are encouraged.

Transport programs that implement the one team/one vehicle concept can only respond to one transport at a time due to the sole availability of one vehicle, whether it is a ground ambulance, rotary wing or fixed wing aircraft. Scheduling under these circumstances is unique and must be coordinated with the pilots or ambulance personnel.

Scheduling practices are accomplished by assigned scheduling or self-scheduling. If self-scheduling is utilized, team members would enter their desired schedules as long as adequate coverage on all shifts was accomplished by the set guidelines. Guidelines might include a team member's expected off-shifts, weekends, and holidays for a specific period. The scheduling coordinator would oversee that all the requirements set by the team are honored. After the first draft of the schedule, team members would collaborate to cover the shifts that were not properly staffed and evenly distribute the hours. Advantages of this method are that team members have control of how the schedule is designed, how seniority is rewarded, and how holidays and weekends are distributed. Combinations of shifts and hours can be used as long as the shift is covered by the established guidelines. This flexibility may be appealing to a small group. However, disadvantages may outweigh the advantages if the team prefers assigned scheduling. Negative aspects of self-scheduling include the misinterpretation of guidelines by the various team members, which may lead to working only specific desirable days or shifts, too many hours in a row, and unwillingness of some team members to problem solve coverage for open shifts. Disagreements may occur if one team member is not flexible. Guidelines must be specific to avoid conflict.

If assigned scheduling is employed, rotations are determined, and work days are distributed according to the hiring agreement. Requests for vacations and days off are plotted by the scheduling coordinator.

Scheduling can be a source of on-going friction. It is prudent to devote significant time to thorough communication of staff expectations, deadlines for time off, and problem solving coverage for open shifts.

HIRING

Many criteria should be considered in the process of hiring a transport team member. Prerequisites such as psychological characteristics, physical capabilities, and clinical experience are important in selecting the best candidate.[1,10,17]

The transport nurse role requires several attributes specific to success in the transport environment. The position requires one to be independent and self-directed, flexible and diplomatic, and assertive and enthusiastic. Transport team members must be able to maintain a positive attitude even when circumstances are stressful. Since team members are working closely with referral facilities, these traits are important for establishing and maintaining a constructive relationship. Excellent oral and written communication skills are also vital. Commitment to the transport team should be substantial due to the time and expense involved in advanced skill training.

Physical capabilities are also pertinent to the transport role. Agility is necessary to manuever within the cabin area to deliver patient care in ambulances and aircraft. Stamina is essential to carry transport equipment, lift isolettes and stretchers, and perform patient care for extended periods of time in possibly adverse situations. Transport members should be tolerant of space constraints and a moving environment. Also, the team should address height and weight restrictions and compliance to fitness standards set by the program.[2]

Another requirement for hiring is clinical experience. Each transport program must decide the amount and type of previous experience necessary to succeed in the transport program. Prior pediatric or neonatal critical care experience or certifications such as Pediatric Advanced Life Support (PALS) are common prerequisites. Transport programs may also want to evaluate if the candidate has previous teaching or public speaking experience, if outreach education is a part of the department's mission. In today's computer-age, word processing skills may also be desirable.

Box 11-1 is a sample hiring process that stresses the importance of screening and selecting the best qualified candidate. Since training a transport nurse can be an expensive endeavor, it is essential to proceed with objectivity.

TEAM COMPOSITION

There are many influences that affect team composition. Many studies and transport programs have suggested the appropriate team configuration for various types of patients.* Further research and information sharing is crucial and necessary, since this complex issue continues to be a source of much debate.

It has long been supported that nurse-led neonatal teams have been able to provide expert and high quality care. Thompson[18] reported that neonatal intensive care nurses were able to effectively assess, manage, stabilize, and transport infants requiring advanced care. Since 1980 numerous institutions have developed such teams.[5] Some studies have suggested that team composition should be evaluated further. Additionally, indicators should be identified which would assist in sending the appropriate medical crew.[8,11-13,15,16] Studies on adult patient populations have reported that flight teams with a physician-nurse composition had a lower mortality rate than the nurse-paramedic team.[3,4]

The care of children is complex with diagnoses ranging from the 3 week old with sepsis to the 14 year old with status asthmaticus. Thus, it is essential to obtain accurate medical information prior to departure in order to mobilize the best possible team. Ongoing outreach education is fundamental. Practitioners not accustomed to decision-making in the care of a child can become increasingly skilled in the stabilization of various pediatric conditions. Hopefully this will lead to the appropriate use of transport resources.

Some of the variables that determine team composition include the distance or time to the patient, the diagnosis, status of the child's medical condition, age of the child, team size, and expertise provided by the team. Team composition can be designed by two basic methods: the variables noted above can determine which combination of team members are needed based on the available information or team composition can remain the same for all transports. If a program utilizes flexible team composition, emphasis should be placed on obtaining a thorough phone history. The cautious approach is to use the full team configuration if the information is incomplete, vague, or the patient has the potential for deterioration.

The task of predicting the ideal team is both a skill and an art. It requires sound judgment, consistency, knowledge of the referral population, and an ability to triage calls rapidly. Factors influencing team composition are illustrated in Table 11-1. This table is designed to be used as a decision checklist in order to take all pertinent variables into account. Guidelines on designing team composition should be decided in advance for objective evaluation, provision of a consistent standard of care, and to save time when actual transport requests are received. It is recommended that programs electing to use flexible team configurations should document specific circumstances that will dictate which team members respond to a particular transport and incorporate these team configura-

* References 3-6,8,11-13,15,16,18.

BOX 11-1 SAMPLE HIRING PROCESS

ANNOUNCING OPEN POSITIONS:

1. Posting Position (within institution)
   - Briefly describes position responsibilities and minimal educational and clinical experience desired and shift or schedule expectations.
2. Advertising (outside sources)
   - Select journals or newspapers that will attract potential candidates with desired skills.
3. Review legal "no-no's" or possible discriminatory questions in hiring practice (i.e., asking about family commitments, etc.).

SELECTING A TRANSPORT NURSE:

1. Application
   - Discuss applicant's potential with Human Resources recruiter.
   - Note previous clinical and management experiences, number of years in previous positions, level of responsibilities, number of persons supervised, educational level, expression of written content, and desired salary level.
   - If candidate meets initial criteria, request resume/vitae unless already included with application.
2. Resume/Vitae
   - Examine presentation of content via order of professional and educational history, neatness, and accuracy.
   - If applicant meets initial criteria, arrange phone interview.
3. Phone interview
   - Inquire as to how candidate(s) found out about position.
   - Describe position and qualities of desired candidate.
   - Review skills desired: transport, NICU, PICU, pediatric ER, flight experience, and physical requirements.
   - Describe team: include highlights of team history, types of transports, number of transports, size of team, mode of transport, and expectations.
   - Illicit in-depth description of current and previous positions, special certifications, advanced skills and experience, including computer familiarity, teaching, or public speaking experience.
   - Note confidence in candidate's voice, selection of vocabulary, expression of thought, and communication skills in completely answering questions.
   - If candidate meets initial criteria, arrange personal interview and describe the selection process.
   - If institution or team requires a prehire competency or critical care examination, arrange date and time.

2\. Personal Interviews (sample guidelines)

   A. Manager/Coordinator—
   - Describe expectations and responsibilities of transport nurse and stress of the transport environment.
   - Ask open-ended questions or describe scenarios that will require the candidate to explain their style of conflict resolution, judgment, problem-solving, teamwork, clinical expertise, and confidence.

   B. Medical Director—
   - Ask open-ended questions which will relate clinical judgment, medical knowledge of transport, and critical care.

   C. Team members (2-3 people)—
   - Illicit information regarding the candidate's ability to be a team player, resolve conflict within the team, handle crisis situations, enthusiasm, etc.

5\. Solicit input from interviewers
   - If there is more than one qualified candidate for a position, rank order of prospective candidates.

6\. References
   - If candidate(s) qualifies and meets desired criteria, arrange to check references.

BOX 11-1 SAMPLE HIRING PROCESS—cont'd

7. Follow-up
   - If references are favorable, arrange to offer position and salary via phone or letter. Confirm drug testing policy and medical exam with Human Resources.
   - If references are unfavorable, contact candidate(s).
8. Written contact
   - If offering position, confirm salary offer, hiring process, start date, and oritentation expectations.
   - If candidate was not selected, send thank you letter.

tions into their protocols. It should always be an option to upgrade the level of care based on actual patient information obtained.

Frew[8] highlights the legal expectations with regard to patient transport, stating that it is important to determine the highest level of training and skills required to manage a patient's anticipated condition during transport. If complications are anticipated the team must be able to manage the most serious

TABLE 11-1 CONSIDERATIONS INFLUENCING TEAM COMPOSITION (8,10)

	RN	*MD*	*RT/EMT*
DISTANCE/TIME TO PATIENTS*,*,*****			
• Under 10 miles or less than 20 minutes	______	______	______
• 10-25 miles or 20 minutes-1 hour	______	______	______
• Over 25 miles or over 1 hour	______	______	______
DIAGNOSIS/STATUS/AGE OF PATIENT+,++,+++			
• Neonate			
1. Stable	______	______	______
2. Unstable	______	______	______
• Infant (1 month-1 year)			
1. Stable	______	______	______
2. Unstable	______	______	______
• Child			
1. Stable airway status	______	______	______
2. Unstable airway status	______	______	______
• Trauma			
1. Stable airway status No head injury	______	______	______
2. Critical status Possible head injury	______	______	______
SIZE/EXPERTISE PROVIDED BY TEAM			
• Pediatric critical care experience	______	______	______
• Experience in transport medicine	______	______	______
• Size of transport vehicle/space constraints	______	______	______

RN—Registered Nurse; MD—Medical Doctor; RT—Respiratory Therapist; EMT—Emergency Medical Technician

* Depends on mode of transport (ground, helicopter, fixed wing)

** Urban vs. rural traffic

*** Weather

\+ Need for major procedures, resuscitation, endotracheal intubation, thoracostomy placement

++ Need for inotropic, vasoactive, anticonvulants, sedative, analgesic medications

+++ Circumstances when unable to determine status of child

BOX 11-2 TEAM ANCILLARY JOB ASSIGNMENTS

Outreach Coordinator
- Arranges educational presentations
- Maintains contact with referral hospitals

Training Coordinator
- Arranges orientation for new transport personnel
- Monitors educational needs of team members and implements measures to maintain skill level and protocol cognition and implementation

Statistics/Data Management
- Collects and inputs transport data
- Provides statistical analysis of pertinent data

Equipment
- Monitors restocking of storeroom and transport bags
- Initiates and communicates with vendors regarding equipment evaluation and purchase

Department Liaisons
- Maintains contact for problem solving with departments most affected by transport services such as NICU, PICU, Trauma, Emergency Department, Security

Development and Revisions
- Creates and revises team policies, transport forms, protocols, and standards

Vendor Contact
- Acts as liaison for aeroambulance and ground ambulance

Quality Management Coordinator
- Implements quality monitoring projects and reports information back to the team

Scheduling Coordinator
- Sets scheduling guidelines
- Monitors rotations and plots requests

Budget Planner
- Plans department operating and capital expenses
- Oversees annual spending activity

Safety Officer/Annual Review
- Arranges safety education for ground and aeroambulance vehicles and performs required hospital annual review such as fire, infection control, and disaster training

problems. McNab[15] summarized the importance of assessing the team's ability to provide optimal care for children, particularly on long transports, flights, or situations where the child is seriously ill or injured. Ultimately, team composition must be a collaborative decision between the medical control physician, the transport coordinator, and the referring physician.

Medical directors must be knowledgeable of team members' ability to make competent decisions and to perform necessary procedures. Nurses must be assertive and use restraint when a situation potentially requires skills and assessments beyond their capabilities or scope of practice. Respiratory therapists and paramedics should be included in annual safety training. Special transport skills can be identified and reviewed, such as oxygen hook-up in the various transport vehicles, how to use the transport ventilator, and anticipating airway needs during the transport. EMT training should include periodic training in pediatric anatomical differences, their stabilization priorities, implementation of pediatric sized equipment, and unique pediatric transport situations.

Lastly, expertise in the transport environment cannot be overemphasized. Priority setting in an ambulance or aeroambulance and implementing protocols approved by the medical control physician must be strictly adhered to.

TEAM ASSIGNMENTS

Delegating team assignments among the team members serves many purposes. The tasks can be completed during down-time.

These roles are essential for smooth team functioning and support a productive method for transport nurses to take "ownership" for their team. Box 11-3 illustrates possible team jobs that can be distributed. It is also important that jobs are evenly distributed, since some may entail more time than others. Renegotiation of jobs can be on-going as tasks are developed and redefined.

Communication with other team members is essential, since many of the tasks are interdependent. For instance, the budget planner should advise the equipment person of monies available for capital purchases or repairs. Similarly, the scheduling coordinator should consult with the outreach coordinator to confirm meeting dates and other team commitments. Utilizing a daily log and a monthly job summary can facilitate what has been accomplished and what still needs to be completed as well as keeping clear lines of communication open between team members.

DISCUSSION

Additional research and information sharing must be encouraged to improve pediatric transport services. This is especially notable in choosing an overall team structure and formulating an appropriate pediatric transport team for each patient.

Building a strong foundation is the key for the developing transport team. Upon this foundation long-term goals can be set to provide state of the art transport services for the pediatric patient. Structural decisions should include type of team, hiring prerequisites, staffing requirements, and team composition options necessary to provide expert services for the critically ill infant or child.

REFERENCES

1. American Academy of Pediatrics, Task Force on Interhospital Transport: Guidelines for air and ground transport of neonatal and pediatrics patients, Elk Grove Village, IL, 1993, The Association.
2. ASHBEAMS (currently Association of Air Medical Services) in cooperation with Samaritan Air Evac, Phoenix, AZ: *Air Medical Crew National Standard Curriculum*, St. Louis, MO, 1988, The Association.
3. Baxt WG, Moody P: The impact of a physician as part of the aeromedical prehospital team in patients with blunt trauma, *JAMA* 257:3246, 1987.
4. Burney RE, Fischer RP: Ground vs. air transport of trauma victims: medical and logistical considerations, *Annals of Emergency Medicine* 15:12, 1986.
5. Danzig D: Neonatal transport teams: a survey of functions and roles, *Neonatal Network*, October:41, 1984.
6. Dobrin RS and others: The development of a pediatric emergency transport system, *Pediatric Clinics of North America* 27:633, 1980.
7. Frankel LR: The evaluation, stabilization and transport of the critically-ill child, *Int. Anesthesiology Clinics* 25:77, 1987
8. Frew SA: Patient transfers: how to comply with the law, Dallas, 1991, American College of Emergency Physicians.
9. Kissoon N: The child requiring transport: lessons and implications for the pediatric emergency physician, *Pediatric Emergency Care* 4:1-4, 1988.
10. MacDonald MG, Miller MK: *Emergency transport of the perinatal patient*, Boston, 1989, Little, Brown and Company.
11. McCloskey KA, Johnston C: Pediatric critical care transport survey: team composition, mobilization time, and mode of transport, *Pediatric Emergency Care* 6:1-3, 1990.
12. McCloskey KA, King WD, Byron L: Pediatric critical care transport: is a physician always needed on the team, *Annals of Emergency Medicine* 18:247, 1988.
13. McCloskey KA, Orr RA: Pediatric transport issues in emergency medicine, *Emergency Medicine Clinics of North America* 9:475-89, 1991.
14. McCloskey KA and others: Variables predicting the need for a pediatric critical care transport team, *Pediatric Emergency Care* 8:1-3, 1992.
15. McNab AJ: Optimal escort for interhospital transport of pediatric emergencies, *The Journal of Trauma* 31:205, 1991.
16. Rubenstein JS and others: Can the need for a physician as part of the pediatric transport team be predicted? A prospective study, *Critical Care Medicine* 20:1657, 1992.
17. Schneider C, Gomez MA, Lee R: Evaluation of Ground Ambulance, Rotor-Wing, and Fixed-Wing Aircraft Services, *Critical Care Clinics* 8:533-64, 1992.
18. Thompson TR: Neonatal transport nurses: an analysis of their role in the transport of newborn infants, *Pediatrics* 65:887, 1980.

12

TRANSPORT TEAM TRAINING

KARIN A. McCLOSKEY

A wide variety of transport team training methods is currently in use, ranging from no training beyond that required for in-hospital practice to extensive, comprehensive courses involving multiple strategies and intense evaluations. The training program outlined in this chapter is substantially based on the American Academy of Pediatrics (AAP) manual entitled *Guidelines for Air and Ground Transport of Neonatal and Pediatric Patients*.[1]

Programs which transport children have a wide variety of challenges, including types of vehicles used, state laws concerning expanded practice nursing, availability of pediatric expertise for medical direction and control, availability of personnel with pediatric critical care experience, geography, size of territory covered, climate, percentage of patients in the pediatric age range, and referring hospital capabilities.[4] A tailored training program can be developed from the suggested options.

A team which is not appropriately trained or equipped for the individual pediatric patient's condition should not accept responsibility for the life and health of a child, especially if a better transport option is available. McNab and others,[13] have demonstrated significant benefits from intensive pediatric training for paramedics (as compared to routine paramedic training).

TEAM COMPOSITION

Team composition remains a controversial issue in transport of adult patients.[2,3,14,17] Many teams transporting adults do not use physicians as team members, and many neonatal transport teams successfully use neonatal nurse practitioners instead of physicians. No specific team composition for pediatric transport is recommended by the AAP or by any other organization.[1] Currently, dedicated pediatric teams tend to use physicians, largely based on lack of data to act otherwise.[5,7-13,15,16] The major difficulty in determining team composition for pediatric transport is the wide range of age, size, and illnesses encountered. Development of training and management protocols is thus more difficult than for the relatively narrower range of skills needed for adult or neonatal patients. One point often overlooked in transport systems is that if resident physicians are used, they require specific training in pediatric transport medicine. The fact of having obtained an MD degree does not in any way automatically infer that an individual is qualified to practice pediatrics or transport medicine. Intuitively, it would seem preferable to have the team led by a nurse who transports children every day than by a resident who occasionally "moonlights" by doing transports. McCloskey and others showed that, in 1989, 72% of dedicated pediatric teams used second year (PGY II) residents on transports.[10] Giardino and others then showed that only 39% of pediatric residency programs using residents on transport provided any significant education in transport issues.[6]

TRAINING GOALS: SKILL LEVELS

The AAP guidelines suggest that an individual's training and experience in pediatrics is more important than his or her educational degree. The document defines skill levels which should be achieved in order to perform pediatric transports. The basic skill levels are no different for dedicated pediatric transport teams than for teams transporting patients of all ages. The skill levels defined include cognitive skills, procedural skills, communication skills, and "other" skills.[1]

The cognitive skill level is the most important, the most difficult to achieve, and the most difficult to teach or evaluate. Skills include the ability to recognize and differentiate common pediatric symptoms (for example stridor vs wheezing) and to evaluate relevant laboratory and radiographic data (for example to differentiate croup vs epiglottitis). The team or a member of the team should be able to institute or continue definitive management, rather than delay treatment until arrival at the tertiary care center (surgical conditions excluded). Definitive diagnosis is not required, for example, for the child with apparent toxic ingestion or cyanotic congenital heart disease, but appropriate symptomatic treatment should be begun. In the ingestion example the team should determine the need for gastric decontamination, endotracheal intubation, and control of cardiac arrhythmias, hypotension, and seizures. In the case of presumed cyanotic congenital heart disease, the team should rule out the most common other causes of similar presentations and should determine the need for prostaglandins and endotracheal intubation. These decisions may be made with the assistance of the medical control physician.

Cognitive skills also include the ability to predict the most likely types of deterioration in the patient's condition, to recognize deterioration if it occurs, and to treat the condition appropriately. The team should be trained in the use of complex pharmacologic agents such as anticonvulsants, vasopressors, and paralyzing agents. They should recognize when such therapy is needed, institute treatment, and be familiar with and able to recognize and treat complications of medication use. The cognitive skill level is generally only achieved through significant training and experience in pediatric critical care.

Procedural skills emphasize airway management including facilitated intubation, vascular access including the central and intraosseous routes, chest tube placement, pericardiocentesis, and any other potentially life saving emergency procedures. It is in the realm of cognitive skills to determine the need for performance of procedures. Success at performance of procedures should be expected to approach 100%. A high level of training and experience with pediatric procedures is necessary because the transport environment is an adverse one compared with the base hospital's emergency department. There may not be a back-up person to attempt the needed intervention. In some states and hospitals, physicians are the only personnel permitted to perform certain necessary procedures. In these cases a physician should be available as a team member.

Procedural skills are often inappropriately considered the most important. In some cases it is erroneously assumed that teaching a team member to intubate and to achieve vascular access on children qualifies that individual for pediatric transport. It is not necessary for the same team member to possess both cognitive and procedural skills, but the team as an aggregate should possess both sets of skills. All team members should have the recommended communication and "other" skills.

The importance of communication skills is apparent if one considers the wide realm of individuals involved in the transport process, all of whom are under substantial stress. The referring physician and hospital staff are being forced to confront a situation which they are not equipped to handle, for whatever reason. The receiving physician is trying to help a patient he or she cannot see or examine. The transport team is working in an unfamiliar environment, often under adverse conditions. The patient's family is severely emotionally distressed, and the patient is often terrified and in pain. The transport team bears most of the burden of smooth communication between these groups while simultaneously trying to care for a critically ill child. The temptation to criticize prior management, the possible need to change current therapy, the need to explain interventions and expectations to an often uncomprehending family, and the need to give medications and perform procedures, without being able to write and sign off every order, are all potential communication minefields. In the particularly hazardous area of changing current therapy or replacing lines or tubes, the team must always operate under the premise that there is more than one right way to do things. The team must follow its own protocols, but conformance with protocols may be misinterpreted as being critical of prior care. Even innocent comments or questions may be interpreted as criticism, especially if the referring hospital has had prior negative encounters with any transport team. There should be absolutely no criticism of patient management in front of any member of the hospital staff, the patient's family, or a local ambulance crew driving the team to an airport. If significant mismanagement occurred the receiving attending physician or the transport medical director can take the issue up with the referring physician after the patient is safely transported.

Several other skills or personality traits are necessary for medical professionals who will be leaving their familiar home base and working with limited help under less than ideal conditions. Physicians or nurses who function very well in an emergency department or ICU may still lack certain characteristics which make for a good transport team member. The necessary traits include the ability to act independently (as no set of protocols will ever cover all possible events), physical stamina, emotional stability, flexibility, efficiency, ability to act as a team player, and, hopefully, a sense of humor. Lack of a tendency toward motion sickness is also quite helpful.

PRETRAINING CONSIDERATIONS

Prior to initiating a pediatric transport training program for an individual medical professional, the potential team member should be screened for existing qualities from the defined skill levels. If an individual is lacking in the communication and "other" skills, the transport team may not represent the best use of his or her expertise. Prior experience in the area of cognitive and procedural skills will be useful and may decrease the length of time needed for training.

A transport system may take one of two approaches for designing the transport training program. The first is to develop a basic set of requirements for anyone joining the team. For example, a nurse may be required to have at least two years of pediatric critical care experience, have taken certain courses such as Pediatric Advanced Life Support (PALS) or the Neonatal Resuscitation Program (NRP), and have supporting documentation from superiors of communication and "other" skills. A uniform training program is then designed using the methods described below. The second style of training is to develop a program tailored to each individual's background. In this case a highly experienced pediatric critical care nurse may need a program emphasizing physiology of the transport environment, use of transport-specific equipment, and several weeks of supervised initial transports. A nurse with extensive transport experience which is primarily with adult patients may need several months of pediatric emergency department or ICU experience. Nurses who are also paramedics often bring useful crossover experience to the team. Pediatric critical care nurses may need experience in a Neonatal Intensive Care Unit (NICU) if the team transports newborns as well as older pediatric patients. Similarly, NICU nurses may need PICU/Pediatric Emergency Department experience. Systems which use this selection and training style put more effort into individualizing programs but have a much larger pool of potential team members.

A final note on pretraining selection— whenever transport is to be a required part of an individual's job description, that fact should be made clear at the time of the job interview. This is especially true for residency programs which require air transport as part of the educational program. Enthusiasm for transport is another of the "other" skills required. There is no place on a transport team for an individual who feels extremely uncomfortable (some discomfort is normal and expected) practicing "alone" or who otherwise does not want to transport.

THE TRAINING PROGRAM

The goal of a training program should be to prepare individuals to meet the skill levels defined above. The accomplishment of that goal leads to fulfilling the overall program goal of safe, efficient, high quality initiation or continuation of pediatric critical care. The extent of the training program needed will depend on the background of the individuals being trained. Those with prior transport experience may need a program focused on developing pediatric cognitive and procedural skills, and those with pediatric critical care experience should focus on practice in the transport environment. All trainees will need an orientation to the particular program's operations, vehicles, and equipment.

The AAP guidelines outline three categories of training methods. Some strategies are specific to pediatrics, and some would apply to training for any transport system. Some of the strategies may already have been accomplished through prior job training. *Essential* training strategies are those considered to be the basic minimum needed to successfully transport pediatric patients. *Recommended* strategies include those that most programs transporting children regularly will want to use in order to extend the capabilities and competence of team members. *Helpful* training strategies will be most likely to benefit (and to be needed by) dedicated pediatric or neonatal transport team members.

Essential training strategies

The first part of any training program will be a formal orientation course for the particular system. Several components of that course are described, with the list not considered exhaustive. The goals of the transport system and its relationship to the mission of the hospital should be explained as a prelude to subsequent training. The paramount importance of public relations, especially maintaining a friendly demeanor and the importance of not criticizing referring hospital treatment, should be emphasized.

The role of each team member and the attendant responsibilities are discussed in detail and provided in a written job description. Specifics of this presentation include what paperwork is to be completed and by whom, expected interactions between team members (who is in charge of what), and channels for problem resolution. The steps involved in initiating a transport, the expected mobilization times, and individual responsibilities in mobilizing are explained. The basic administrative details of the system are presented, including consent for transport, existing contracts between referring and receiving hospitals, transport triage, handling of multiple simultaneous transport requests, conditions for diverting the team or transporting a different patient than the one originally planned, pathways for reporting, and resolving conflicts or concerns, etc.

Equipment availability and mechanics should be explained with hands-on experience provided. In addition, basic maintenance, troubleshooting, and channels for regular and emergency maintenance are discussed. The types of communication equipment available (radio, beepers, 800 numbers, cellular phones, etc.) and details of usage need discussion. Protocols for communication between the various individuals involved in transport for both routine and unusual situations should be explained.

A list of medications carried routinely on transport should be provided to new team members. The list should also include the total amounts of each medication carried. Infrequently carried or special situation medications should be noted along with how to obtain them expeditiously for transport. A checklist of potential conditions requiring medications not routinely carried should be provided for a brief review just prior to transport. The medication lists should be provided in an organized fashion, either alphabetically or by their location in the transport packs. Ideally, lists with each of those types of organizational arrangement should be provided.

Safety, first of the team and then of the patient, is of paramount importance on transport missions. A chapter of the AAP Guidelines is devoted to this topic.[1] Specifics of aircraft and ground vehicle safety should be discussed in detail, along with requirements for appropriate attire and protocols to be followed in emergency situations. Potential emergency situations should be decided on an individual basis for a given transport team. Helicopter safety issues are different from those for fixed wing aircraft, as air and ground transport issues are different. Some programs will need details of survival techniques in temperature extremes or in isolated regions. The team's responsibility to the patient when a safety concern arises should be addressed during the orientation. It should be emphasized that the safety of the team is of primary importance. If the team is not kept safe, they will be of no use to the patient. All reasonable efforts at patient safety and assistance with evacuation of the patient in an emergency situation should be discussed. Luckily, it is an extremely rare circumstance for the team to have to make a decision to abandon a patient in order to protect its own safety.

FAA regulations for air transport are standardized and are included in the general orientation for all transport members. Any changes in FAA regulations should be immediately reported in writing to members of the transport team. Other relevant regulations include those from the Department of Transportation (DOT) and those surrounding ground ambulance transport. Lack of understanding of specific ground ambulance regulations has caused deviations from required protocols at the time of a vehicular accident (personal communication).

Other regulations concerning air and ground transport exist at the federal, state, and hospital level (see Chapter 3). The transport team should be aware of these regulations, including the COBRA and OBRA regulations, state practice perimeters for nurses and paramedics, any restrictions an individual hospital might place on expanded nursing practice, conformance of transport protocols to in-hospital protocols, and required paperwork for patients admitted to or transported by the hospital's transport team.

The essential orientation should include a detailed discussion of the transport environment, specifically its differences from the hospital environment, and how patient management may differ from that in the hospital emergency department or ICU. An example of different management would be a patient who is intubated for transport, although he or she may not yet have met criteria for immediate intubation if already at the tertiary care center. The physical difficulty of patient assessment, performing procedures in a moving aircraft, and the effects of altitude on a patient's oxygenation (which may lead to deterioration in respiratory status) all potentially lead to the situation in which patient management differs from that in the hospital environment. It is better to anticipate potential problems and secure the airway prior to departure than to risk getting into trouble during the transport itself.

The physical comfort of both the team members and the patient should be included in a discussion of the transport environment. For example, the team should understand how altitude and pressurization changes will affect their own as well as the patient's oxygen saturation and pressure levels in closed spaces such as sinuses and the middle ear. The physical stress and often unexpected fatigue associated with working in a moving, vibrating environment should be addressed. Obviously, anyone prone to motion sickness should undergo a discussion of methods for anticipating or resolving that condition through nonsedating medications, home remedies which seem to work, and adjustment of meal schedules. The team should also understand up front that administrative personnel are aware of other physical stresses built into the system. These include enduring weather changes (especially on long distance transport), sleep deprivation, enhanced effects of alcohol, side effects of any medications, and the long-term effects of poor nutrition, as well as the short-term effects of hypoglycemia if meals are delayed through long or sequential transports.

The next essential training modality includes supervising transport team members on their initial transports. Lectures and discussions are necessary to begin the training process, however, nothing can replace the experience of hands-on treatment of critically ill children in the field. Team members, whether physicians, nurses, respiratory therapists, or paramedics, should perform their first transports accompanied by individuals with transport experience in the assigned role. The actual number of supervised transports is left up to the individual training program. Team members with prior skills and experience in pediatrics and pediatric transport may require only a few accompanied transports. Also, the acuity of illness in initial accompanied transports can play a role. If most of the patients happen to be critically ill and require a large amount of intervention, the team member is likely to be prepared to become independent sooner. Team members should not be expected to go out alone on transports until they are comfortable with operating in an unsupervised environment. If weight restrictions in helicopter transports preclude supervised transports, additional hands-on ground experience and case scenarios should be provided as well as specific protocols for additional communication during the orientation period. This is often less of a problem for pediatric transports because of low patient weight, allowing an additional team member to be carried on the helicopter.

Another essential training modality is didactic sessions in pediatric transport medicine. There should be initial sessions targeted to the group's experience followed by ongoing didactic sessions on a regular basis even after the team is experienced. For the team that primarily transports adults, sessions would cover the most common pediatric conditions likely to require transport. This includes respiratory distress, trauma, toxic ingestions, etc. For dedicated pediatric teams issues involving the transport environment and safety on transport will be more important as a lecture topic.

Follow-up case reviews of complicated or uncommonly encountered situations should be completed. These reviews should be done on a regular basis and should be presented to all team members, not just those involved in the individual case. For new team members, reviews of commonly encountered situations can be presented through cases which help integrate the educational process.

Maintenance of the transport team's skills and experiences are a critical part of the training process. If sufficient patient population exists for substantial on-going experience, current skill levels may be assessed through checklists of types of procedures performed, types of cases encountered, etc. Despite on-going experience, team members will need regular recertification in the Pediatric Advanced Life Support (PALS), Neonatal Resuscitation Program (NRP), Advanced Trauma Life Support (ATLS), Advanced Pediatric Life Support (APLS), and Advanced Cardiac Life Support (ACLS) courses, as appropriate. Maintenance of skills is more difficult if on-going experience in pediatrics is limited. This would be the case either for teams who infrequently transport children or for teams who transport children who are so thoroughly stabilized that interventions by the team are infrequently needed. In these situations a program of regular supplementation of experience should be designed. That program can include spending time in a pediatric intensive care unit, neonatal intensive care unit, or pediatric emergency department, spending time instructing pediatric resuscitation courses, rotating through anesthesiology, and animal labs or mannequin practice. *If ongoing experience is limited, ongoing training must include several of these modalities.* For example, simply practicing procedures in an animal lab does not ensure that staff possess an appropriate cognitive skill level to perform patient transports.

Recommended training strategies

Strategies in this category include an extended formal orientation course, increased frequency of didactic sessions, formal cases conferences on a regularly scheduled basis, participation in continuous quality improvement, and stress management lectures, courses, or seminars. The extension of the formal orientation course can include case scenarios, both administrative and medical, which deal with commonly encountered transport situations. Equipment scenarios are helpful, with personnel asked to physically find pieces of equipment in the transport packs within a limited time frame and to deal with simulated equipment failures. Expanded training in the public relations aspects of transport is also important. Role playing in communication scenarios can place team members "in each other's shoes" and provide insight into the emotions of referring hospital staff, family members, medical control staff, and the patient. Team members can also identify and discuss situations which may be causing anger, fear, or frustration.

Transport team members are exposed to many stresses outside of the usual realm of care for critically ill children. It is crucial that the transport team administration recognize these stresses and plan a program of diffusing them in any way possible. The stresses unique to the transport situation include.: 1) the potential for vehicular accidents; 2) having to practice medicine in an unfamiliar environment, often without access to many resources available in the usual hospital setting; 3) the sense of being isolated as possibly the only one who can make certain decisions or perform lifesaving procedures; 4) erratic work schedules involving being on-call and having to be prepared to leave rapidly or possibly staying on alert for the entire shift without going anywhere. In addition, the team member may end up on a long transport that goes well beyond the scheduled end of the shift, postponing planned activities after work; 5) pressure to work when off-duty because of personnel shortages and during periods of increased activity; 6) potential for having to work "alone" with other team members in whom one may not have total confidence; 7) for the not primarily pediatric team member, the additional emotions and fears involved in being responsible for a very sick child; and 8) the physical stress of working in a moving, vibrating, noisy environment. Transport team members can be helped by recognizing that the transport environment is particularly stressful, by taking opportunities to ventilate their fears and concerns, and by learning techniques for stress reduction. Techniques for recognizing excessive stress in other team members should be discussed. Team members who express higher than average anxiety or hostility, or those who routinely fail to attend stress management education opportunities should be identified and offered additional intervention. A formal critical incident stress debriefing program is crucial to the team's health and maintenance. Triggers for implementation of a critical incident debriefing should be sought, especially for night shift personnel who may have infrequent contact with the transport coordinator or medical director.

Participation in continuous quality improvement can serve to meet hospital standards and can assist transport team members in viewing the most effective areas of their system. It also provides the opportunity to identify areas for improvement.

Helpful training strategies

These strategies include regularly scheduled didactic sessions on the practice of pediatrics in the transport environment, participation in transport research, participation in community outreach programs, and attendance at national educational meetings with courses in the field of pediatric transport medicine. While not specifically addressed in the AAP Guidelines, joining organizations whose members transport children can be both educational for the individual and helpful in promoting the importance of pediatric issues in transport medicine.

Didactic sessions could include a monthly conference covering an individual medical topic. The general emergency management of the topic would be discussed, followed by consideration of differences in management during transport. Review of recent cases may be used for illustrative purposes. Involvement in transport research elevates the team members' understanding of how their system fits into a global process. The research can be local with basic data collection and evaluation of parameters for reporting to other members of the transport team, hospital staff, and administration. Formal studies can also be developed with the intent of evaluating unanswered questions and reporting findings outside the individual transport system, either in publications or at organized meetings. The organized meetings can be local, regional, national, or international.

Involvement in community outreach programs is an effective training tool both for the transport team members presenting the program and for the audience. The programs can improve pretransport care of sick children, improve the relationship between the transport team and referring hospital personnel, and contribute to good public relations for the team's base hospital (see Community Outreach chapter). A relatively easy form of community outreach is for transport team members to become instructors in nationally recognized pediatric stabilization courses such as Pediatric Advanced Life Support (PALS), Advanced Pediatric Life Support (APLS), and Neonatal Resuscitation Program (NRP). A transport system can also develop its own program to take to referring hospitals. Most of these programs include advice on pediatric stabilization, choice of a transport mode, and preparation for the transport team, as well as printed materials such as code cards and weight charts.

There is a rapidly increasing number of regional and national meetings devoted entirely to pediatric transport. Some courses emphasize hands-on medical management, while others also discuss administrative issues and present current transport research.

National organizations devoted to transport medicine but not necessarily to pediatrics include the Association for Air Medical Services (AAMS), National Flight Nurses Association (NFNA), National Flight Paramedics Association (NFPA), Air Medical Physicians Association (AMPA), and National Association of Emergency Medical Services Physicians (NAEMSP). Members of critical care and emergency medicine organizations will often consider issues in transport medicine. The AAP Section on Transport Medicine encompasses most providers and aspects of pediatric transport. National meetings can provide substantial education through informal discussion of policies of other transport programs.

In summary, all team members expected to transport children should have specific training and experience in pediatrics and in transport medicine. This training may be at a defined minimum level for teams rarely transporting children or may be substantially expanded for dedicated pediatric transport teams.[2] Individual training programs will vary depending on the goals and needs of each transport system, but many reasonable and varied modalities exist to develop a successful program.

REFERENCES

1. American Academy of Pediatrics, Task Force on Interhospital Transport: *Guidelines for air and ground transport of neonatal and pediatric patients,* Elk Grove Village, IL, 1993, The Association.
2. Baxt WG, Moody P: The impact of a physician as part of the aeromedical prehospital team in patients with blunt trauma. *JAMA* 257:3246-50, 1987.
3. Carraway RP and others: Why a physician? Aeromedical transport of the trauma victim, *J Trauma* 24:650 (abstr), 1984.
4. Day S and others: Pediatric interhospital critical care transport: consensus of a national leadership conference, *Pediatrics*; 88:4:696-704, Oct 1991.
5. Edge WE and others: Reduction of morbidity in interhospital transport by specialized pediatric staff, *Crit Care Med* S38, 1992.
6. Giardino AP, Burns KM, Giardino ER: The educational value of pediatric emergency transport: by design or by default, *Pediatr Emerg Care* 9(5):275-80, 1993.
7. Kanter RK, Tompkins JM: Adverse events during interhospital transport: physiologic deterioration associated with pretransport severity of illness, *Pediatrics* 84:43-8, 1989.
8. Kanter RK and others: Excess morbidity associated with interhospital transport, *Pediatrics* 90(6):893-8, 1992.
9. McCloskey KA, Johnston C: Critical care interhospital transports: predictability of the need for a pediatrician, *Pediatr Emerg Care* 6:89, 1990.
10. McCloskey KA, Johnston C: Pediatric critical care transport survey: team composition and training, mobilization time, and mode of transportation, *Pediatr Emerg Care* 6:1-3, 1990.
11. McCloskey KA, King WD, Byron L: Pediatric critical care transport: is a physician always needed on the team, *Ann Emerg Med* 18:247, 1989.
12. McCloskey KA and others: Variables predicting the need for a pediatric critical care transport team, *Pediatr Emerg Med* 8(1):1-3, Feb 1992.
13. McNab AJ: Optimal escort for interhospital transport of pediatric emergencies, *J Trauma* 31:205, 1991.
14. Rhee KJ and others: Is the flight physician needed in helicopter emergency medical services, *J Trauma* 24:680 (abstr), 1984.
15. Rubenstein JS and others: Can the need for a physician as part of the pediatric transport team be predicted? A prospective study, *Crit Care Med* 20:659, 1992.
16. Smith DF, Hackel A: Selection criteria for pediatric critical care transport teams, *Crit Care Med* 11(1):10-2, 1983.
17. Snow N, Hull C, Severns J: Physician presence on a helicopter emergency medical service: necessary or desirable, *Aviat, Space Environ Med* 57:1176, 1986.

13

QUALITY ASSURANCE AND CONTINUOUS QUALITY IMPROVEMENT

NICHOLAS BENSON

Everyone involved in health care today has had some interaction with quality assurance processes. However, many are left with the impression that quality assurance by definition is dull, repetitive, tedious, and results in punishment. Unfortunately, the process too often has allowed itself to be branded negatively, rather than being promoted as a way to improve patient care.

Many articles, books, and lectures have been produced on the performance of quality assurance, including several on quality assurance in emergency medical services and air medical transport.[2,3,5,7,9] This chapter will glean the essential points from these sources and offer a systematic approach for creating or renovating a quality assurance program.

In the early 1990s continuous quality improvement began to complement quality assurance. Continuous quality improvement is designed to constantly and consistently improve the process and the outcome of patient care (Box 13-1). The processes of quality assurance and continuous quality improvement are often confused as being the same, but actually complement each other instead.[6] Quality assurance is a specific review of patient care intended to ensure that the care delivered is both of a high quality and appropriate to the patient's needs. Typically, quality assurance is conducted after patient care is provided. Continuous quality improvement uses multidisciplinary teams to constantly review all aspects of a system, such as delivering care in the transport environment. Quality assurance seeks to maintain compliance with expected behaviors at a specific percentage, such as the maintenance of a normal core temperature in 80% of transported neonatal patients. Continuous quality improvement promotes constant striving to upgrade compliance with the expected behavior incrementally, such as reaching the goal of a normal core temperature in 100% of transports, rather than being satisfied with 80%.

In summary, the core concepts of quality assurance are to systematically and continuously monitor, evaluate, and ensure the caliber and appropriateness of the services offered. In continuous quality improvement the essential components are to measure, assess, and improve.

MEDICAL DIRECTION AND QUALITY ASSURANCE

Just as physicians have an integral and indispensable role in providing patient care in emergency departments and intensive care units, the physician's role in transport systems is inescapable. Although the physician may not be present in the transport vehicle, his or her experience, education, and judgment must be provided throughout the transport process. The physician should be actively involved as an advisor, educator, supervisor, patient care advocate, and reviewer. This is the role of medical direction.

While the specific job description of the

BOX 13-1 QUALITY ASSURANCE (QA) VERSUS CONTINUOUS QUALITY IMPROVEMENT (CQI)

- QA looks for people who are not performing at the expected level.
- CQI looks for system problems that do not allow people to perform.
- QA looks for methods to improve the level of performance.
- CQI looks for the root of the problem, to effect the optimal remedy.
- QA focuses on achieving the desired end.
- CQI decides what the consumer really needs and works to this end.
- QA works through the efforts of managers and specific staff members.
- CQI works through a philosophy of quality as a total management strategy from every level of the team.

medical director may vary from service to service, the success of the program will always depend on the medical director having a pivotal role. The physician chosen for this role must be enthusiastic and committed, providing leadership and creativity to all aspects of the transport service that directly or indirectly impact patient care. The role of the medical director is to maintain patient care at an optimal quality level: a goal shared by quality assurance and continuous quality improvement. Both medical direction and quality assurance have three general phases —prospective, concurrent, and retrospective.

Prospective quality assurance

Prospective quality assurance addresses the aspects of a transport service that are handled before serving patients. These include the interviewing, hiring, and education of personnel, as well as remedial education and potential disciplining of personnel who require it. Treatment protocols must be established to provide guidelines for the transport team to follow at the patient's bedside. The medical director must assist in the creation of the service's scope of care and mission statements, since these will describe the very nature of the service. In addition, the selection of mode of transportation and medical equipment, and the creation of dispatch and utilization criteria will involve the physician.

Concurrent quality assurance

Concurrent medical direction in a transport service includes oversight of patient care delivered by nonphysicians during patient stabilization and transport. This is also called online medical direction and is delivered by radio, telephone, or other means of direct voice communication. Physicians may also provide concurrent quality assurance by riding with the transport team members or meeting them in the field during the transport.

Retrospective quality assurance

Retrospective quality assurance entails an after-the-fact review of the process and outcome of patient care. A review is performed of written records, communication tapes, and other permanent records. This, as with prospective and concurrent methods, should lead to the development of a continuing education program for transport personnel that underscores the positive aspects of their performance and offers remediation for areas needing improvement.

All three phases have significant opportunities for effectively impacting the quality of the service, and transport programs should use all three. However, only the concurrent phase offers a chance to change the patient's care or the operation of the transport while it is happening. Therefore, concurrent quality assurance is especially important.

It is also important to remember that quality assurance is just a tool, albeit a useful problem-solving tool. It can make vague problems concrete and specific, and it can be used to gather data that uncover hidden problems. It can be used to identify resolutions and demonstrate their efficacy. If quality assurance and continuous quality improvement are always focused on assisting transport personnel in improving their process of patient care and the outcome of their transports, then the members of the team are more likely to understand the importance of the program and readily offer support. Using quality assurance and continuous quality improvement programs only to identify specific persons with problems and to punish them will lead to mistrust and to sabotage of these programs.

THE PLAN

A written plan is essential for the success of a quality assurance program. The plan must be used to map out each aspect of the program. A sample plan for a helicopter service is offered in Appendix 13-1.

The plan should begin with an explanation of the mission of the transport service and the purpose for the quality assurance and continuous quality improvement programs. The plan should delineate the lines of authority for performing quality activities and should list how that authority interfaces with the governing body for the transport service. It should specify the extent of involvement of individuals in the quality activities and the schedule of specific review and evaluation activities. Further, it should identify the importance of and methods for periodic reappraisal and revision of the quality assurance and continuous quality improvement programs. As the transport service evolves over time, so must its strategies for evaluating its impact on patients (Box 13-2).

Ten steps of quality assurance

In 1987 the Joint Commission on Accreditation of Health Care Organizations (JCAHCO) published the "Ten Step" approach to quality assurance for emergency departments.[8] This approach is also applicable to other areas of patient care, including the stabilization and transportation of patients. The ten steps provide a strong framework for organizing the overall approach to a quality assurance program (Box 13-3).

BOX 13-2 A PLAN FOR A QUALITY ASSURANCE PROGRAM

The plan for a quality assurance program should include all of the following:

- Statement of the purpose of the program,
- Lines of authority for the program within the transport service and its governing body,
- Scope of involvement of all key individuals in the program,
- Schedule for review and evaluation activities, and
- Strategy for periodic reappraisal and revision of the plan and the program.

BOX 13-3 JOINT COMMISSION ON ACCREDITATION OF HEALTH CARE ORGANIZATIONS[8]

1. Assign individual responsibility.
2. Write the scope of care.
3. Decide the important aspects of care.
4. Characterize the important aspects of care.
5. Establish thresholds for evaluation.
6. Gather data.
7. Evaluate the data.
8. Take action.
9. Reassess.
10. Report the results.

Step one: Assigning individual responsibility. Once the plan for the quality assurance program is created, the responsibilities of specific individuals in each aspect of the program should be made clear. Each individual must understand and be accountable for their designated responsibilities. With continuous quality improvement, a broader range of members of the transport team is typically involved in quality activities, since there are usually several task-oriented groups functioning simultaneously.

In classic quality assurance programs the range of individuals who take part may vary, usually including at least the following: the medical director, the manager of the transport service, the professional responsible for the transport team's education, selected representatives of the medical and nonmedical (drivers, pilots) personnel, and a representative of the governing body, such as a hospital administrator. Note that the quality assurance program should encompass all aspects of the transport service, not just the immediate patient care parameters. Therefore, the plan and the personnel should include drivers, pilots, mechanics, communication specialists, and other individuals as appropriate.

Step two: The scope of care. Defining the missions and goals of the transport service provide the quality assurance program with a focus to begin the review of its most essential elements. The entire breadth of care provided is specified, and an inventory is recorded of what the service provides. A sample is offered in Appendix 13-2.

Step three: Important aspects of care. Once the mission statement and scope of care are created, a listing of the important aspects of care and of system operation is easy to develop. The list should be simple and logical and should include the elements most important to the successful outcome of the patient's transport. It should include aspects which differentiate the transport service from other types of health care services. It must include the areas which are most crucial to enable the service to provide optimal patient outcome. Note that traditional, patient care-oriented quality assurance programs dealt only with quality of care issues, hence the term "important aspects of care." In transport medicine, however, operational issues are frequently just as important as patient care issues, therefore the term could be altered to "important aspects of care and operations."

The important aspects of care parallel the older quality assurance jargon of standards of care. These aspects establish the cornerstones of quality care and quality transport operations. They define the expectations of the service's management for the team's behavior and performance. They can be drawn from national programs such as Advanced Cardiac Life Support[1] or Advanced Pediatric Life Support,[4] or they may include requirements of the state regulatory agencies.

The service's medical director must be involved in creating the list of standards and important aspects, as should the rest of the transport team. The personnel actually performing the transports will know more about the operational requirements, obstacles, and keys to success in the transport environment than anyone else. The standards need to be set at a level high enough to motivate yet be achievable. The important aspects must be written in objective terms, so they are specific and amenable for measurable analysis. Finally, as with the quality assurance plan itself, the important aspects should be periodically revisited and updated to reflect the growth of the transport service.

Step four: Characterize important aspects. By creating a list of the most important patient care and operational aspects of the service the quality assurance program can focus on the highest priority areas for review. However, there are other components of the list that can be practically reviewed at any time.

The next step is to characterize those important aspects into three categories: *problem-prone, high-risk,* and *high-volume.* The relative importance of the aspects of patient care and operations are gauged using these descriptive terms.

Problem-prone areas include those that are typically difficult to perform or which frequently lead to complications. Examples include airway maintenance in a child with significant blunt trauma to the face, and patient care in a helicopter that has ventured into inadvertent meteorological conditions. When the very success of the patient's care or the transport's completion is involved, the aspect is said to be *high-risk* (this includes cardiopulmonary resuscitation during transport). The *high-volume* important aspects of care and operations are the vital practices that are done very frequently, such as maintaining intravenous access for fluid and medication administration, and properly managing the patient's airway with supplemental oxygenation and ventilation. A particular transport service may characterize an important aspect with two or three of the descriptors, such as management of circulatory failure (*high-risk* and *problem-prone*) (Box 13-4).

The next task is to rephrase the important aspects of care and operations into what JCAHO refers to as "clinical indicators."[8] This is a simple rewording of the important aspect into a description of the action or behavior that is appropriate for the setting. These clinical indicators must be stated in specific, objective, and measurable terms, and they must reflect current scientific or behavioral knowledge (Box 13-5). The clinical indicators should be reviewed with the staff of the transport service to verify that these are important aspects of their jobs. This increases the accountability of the personnel for the success of the quality assurance program and of the transport service.

BOX 13-4 POTENTIAL IMPORTANT ASPECTS OF CARE FOR A PEDIATRIC TRANSPORT SERVICE

Patient Care
- Patient's body temperature during transport (problem-prone; high-volume)
- Appropriate oxygenation and ventilation (high-risk)
- Infusion rates for intravenous medications (high-risk; high-volume)
- Accurate and complete patient assessments (high-volume; high-risk)

Operations
- Weather conditions during helicopter flights (for helicopters operating under Visual Flight Rules) (high-risk)
- Comprehensive vehicle preventive maintenance (high-risk; high-volume
- Flight following by communication specialists (high-risk; high-volume)
- Transport team response times (high-volume)

Step five: Thresholds for evaluation. Quality assurance strategies assume that people will rarely, if ever, be able to comply with an expected action or behavior 100% of the time. Thus, quality assurance allows for some margin of human error or mechanical malfunction; this is called the *threshold for evaluation.* When the compliance for the clinical indicator does not meet the threshold, then the quality assurance program must investigate the reason.

For example, the transport service may decide that trauma patient stabilization at the referring hospital is an important aspect of care. If the service transports many infants with major blunt trauma, this is both a *high-risk* and a *high-volume* operation. The clinical indicators written for this important phase of patient care may include the following: "Major blunt trauma patients with significant head/neck trauma or decreased mental status, neck pain, or acute upper extremity neurologic deficits will receive complete spinal immobilization. Major blunt trauma patients with respiratory distress, significant hypovolemia, head injuries, or major chest trauma will receive airway stabilization." Once these clinical indicators are written by the quality assurance program, they are reviewed with the general staff of the transport service. At that time the staff endorses the importance of the clinical indicators and agrees that their thresholds for evaluation should be 95% and 90%, respectively. A quarterly review of transports of major blunt trauma patients showed that the compliance with the first indicator for stabilization of the entire spine is 93%. Since the 95% threshold was not met, the 7% of instances not complying with the expected behavior are reviewed to determine where additional education, modification of protocols, change in equipment, or other interventions are necessary.

BOX 13-5 IMPORTANT ASPECTS OF CARE AND CLINICAL INDICATORS

Important Aspects:	Management of patients with circulatory failure (high-risk and problem-prone).
Clinical Indicators:	(1) All patients with poor peripheral perfusion will have two intravenous lines. (2) All patients with poor peripheral perfusion will receive intravenous crystalloid therapy (at least one bolus of 20 cc/kg) before vasopressors are attempted.
Important Aspect:	Prompt response times by transport team once they are notified (high-volume).
Operational Indicators:	(1) All helicopter transports (except neonatal) will lift off no more than fifteen minutes after the communication specialist accepts the flight. (2) All neonatal helicopter transports will lift off no more than forty minutes after the communication specialist accepts the flight.

Step six: Gathering data. Once the clinical indicators are written and the decision has been made about how often the staff will be expected to comply with those indicators, it is time to start gathering data. Some services attempt to evaluate all instances of a circumstance, such as every major blunt trauma patient transport. Others choose to review a representative sample. Reviewing every single instance of an event is usually not realistic, unless it happens infrequently, such as cardiopulmonary arrest in a pediatric patient with penetrating trauma to the torso. A good basic rule to follow is that the more often a circumstance or action occurs, the smaller a percentage of the instances must be reviewed. However, it is reasonable to suggest that a minimum of either 10% or 25% of all instances be reviewed for each listed situation.[8]

Sources of data for review are truly varied. The transport record, the patient's medical record at the referring facility, the assessments of the patient upon arrival at the receiving hospital, dispatch records, recorded voice communications, and other documentation reflecting the outcome of the patient and the transport are important. Additionally, questionnaires sent to the service's consumers can be very revealing. Consumers include patients, nurses, physicians, public safety officials, and others who come in contact with the transport service, transportation vehicle, and personnel. Criticisms, complaints, and incident reports are also meaningful sources of information.

Step seven: Evaluating the data. The next step is to review the data and compare the results to the threshold for evaluation. It is often tempting to review data gathered from just one aspect of the transport service, such as the actions of a specific individual or a specific crew. This, however, can be seen as a "witch hunt" and is not consistent with the goals of a quality assurance program. The purpose of the quality assurance program is to review the breadth and depth of the transport service for opportunities to improve the quality of patient care and quality of the transport environment for the patient. Isolating reviews of performance to a specific individual will typically lead to mistrust and will undermine the benefits of the quality assurance program.

Step eight: Taking action. Once the data have been reviewed and the results have been contrasted with the threshold for evaluation, it is time to decide whether action is necessary. Unless there are extenuating circumstances, the quality assurance system should be programmed to develop an action plan whenever an indicator's evaluation threshold is not met.

The action plan should include several elements: a description of the problem, identification of the person(s) or item(s) to change, a timetable for the expected change, an identification of the person(s) responsible for effecting the change, what the change in behavior specifically entails, and when this behavior or action will be evaluated again to determine the degree of success of the action plan (Box 13-6). If the evaluation reveals a problem beyond the service's direct sphere of influence, the action plan must detail how assistance from external resources will be rallied to affect the appropriate change in behavior or function. Action plans need to be considered in light of the transport service's continuing education calendar. Since the expected change in behavior or action will often require some reeducation of the personnel.

Step nine: Reassessment. As alluded to, compliance with a clinical indicator should

BOX 13-6 ELEMENTS OF AN ACTION PLAN

The action plan should include each of the following:

- Specification of the problem,
- What the change in behavior will specifically entail,
- Identification of the person(s) or behavior(s) to change,
- Timetable for the expected change,
- Identification of the person(s) responsible for effecting this change, and
- When this behavior will be evaluated again.

not be examined once and then discarded. The transport service should periodically evaluate the compliance of personnel with the expected action or behavior, at least until successive reviews have demonstrated consistent satisfactory compliance. Reassessment is especially important when a specific action plan has been instituted since the threshold for evaluation was not met during an earlier review.

The philosophies of quality assurance and continuous quality improvement programs differ. Quality assurance programs conduct periodic reviews of clinical indicators until satisfactory compliance with the threshold for evaluation is demonstrated. With continuous quality improvement, no threshold for evaluation exists, and the expected behavior is monitored over successive periods with the intent that each review will demonstrate incremental improvements in compliance with the expected behavior. In other words, continuous quality improvement typically does not include a threshold for evaluation; it continually strives toward 100% achievement of a desired outcome.

Step ten: Reporting results. For a quality assurance program to be successful, it must be conducted in a confidential manner with all records protected. Without this sense of confidentiality and protection, individuals cannot be expected to openly review another's efforts and outcomes. Nevertheless, the general results of the quality assurance work need to be periodically shared with the transport service staff and with the governing body of the transport service, even if it is only done verbally. Both the staff and the governing body must be aware of the successes of the transport service and of the plans developed to remedy problem areas. The peer review statutes of each state dictate methods for maintaining quality assurance information in a legally confidential manner and to minimize discovery by an attorney.

These ten steps are useful benchmarks in the development or renovation of a quality assurance program. They provide a structured strategy for building a program that will lead to meaningful data and to action plans that successfully impact the transport service.

CONTINUOUS QUALITY IMPROVEMENT

Based on the successful methods for researching problem areas used by experienced administrators for many years, continuous quality improvement offers a multifaceted structure for solving problems and improving quality. Experienced managers know that to accurately determine the extent and source of a problem, it is necessary to talk with many individuals to gain their perspectives and their suggested resolutions. With only one perspective on a situation, it is virtually impossible to develop a successful strategy for solving the problem. Continuous quality improvement formalizes this empirically successful approach.

The overall goal of continuous quality improvement is to infuse all aspects of the transport service with an unrelenting scrutiny toward providing the highest possible quality of service. The staff is therefore empowered to continuously improve the quality of their work. There is direct involvement by each staff member in the quality improvement process; they share a sense of individual and collective ownership to improve quality.

This is a consumer-oriented approach which is constantly seeking to meet the needs of consumers as they specify. The assumption that the service's management knows best what to provide and how to provide it is discarded. Instead, honest efforts are made to delineate and meet the needs of its customers.

The management team planning and implementing a continuous quality improvement program cannot be satisfied with the status quo. The continuous quality improvement program persistently dedicates resources to improve the quality or quantity of the final product. Specific, arbitrary goals of production are not relevant. The goal is to identify and utilize opportunities for improvement.

Another important contrast between quality assurance and continuous quality improvement involves the annual review or evaluation process. The annual review of the quality assurance program is a retrospective analysis of accomplishments. With continuous quality improvement the annual evaluation is a prospective process of setting the goals for the next year.

Multidisciplinary teams

Continuous quality improvement is built upon a team approach. Unlike quality assurance, continuous quality improvement is a program that envelops every member of the service to a greater or lesser degree. The responsibility for implementing and taking action is not relegated to a single person; rather it is a multidisciplinary process. The actual staff involved in the operation are vital to the success of the quality improvement effort, although managers should also be included. These multidisciplinary groups are created to monitor, analyze, and impact specific aspects of the service's operation. They may be called task groups, quality circles, task action groups or by another similar name.

The focus is on customer-oriented measures of performance that are developed after identifying customers' needs and expectations. The needs can be identified through a variety of approaches: surveys and interviews with customers, focus groups, careful observation and listening at referring and receiving facilities, complaints, and published articles.

Typically, the multidisciplinary team will begin the discussion by conducting a brainstorming session. This gives all members of the team a chance to share thoughts and expertise. No individual's perspective is discounted or rejected, and every idea or comment is heard and included. This promotes the review of all aspects of an operation and decreases the chances of overlooking a seemingly minor point that may prove important later.

The team should map out the process which is being reviewed. The specific operational issue is examined in minute detail. Examples include the refueling operation for a helicopter, the response times for preparing a neonatal team to embark on a transport, or the process of receiving and accepting a transport request. The team deliberately discusses each action that impacts this process. Every step whose success something or someone can impact is noted.

Once the detailed steps of the particular process are listed chronologically, the team can discuss the most likely sources of delay or confusion. Again, every potential should be appropriately examined.

Quality assurance methods may be needed to gather data and determine the exact extent of each step's impact on the outcome of the specific process. Data gathering and analysis, as well as developing of the action plan(s), follows the approach discussed previously in this chapter. These steps will lead to planning and implementation of effective strategies to resolve the problem(s). Of course the continuous quality improvement approach involves periodically and persistently reviewing the process to determine the effectiveness of the action plans that have been implemented and the areas where new strategies may be developed.

Seven steps of process improvement

The continuous quality improvement program consists of seven distinct steps which are designed to identify and improve a specific process. This is only a brief outline. Bringing a meaningful quality improvement program to life will require considerable education and background work, including learning statistical and analytical techniques which most health care professionals lack.

Step one: The problem statement. The team should begin by trying to state the problem as succinctly, objectively, and clearly as possible. This may or may not be the way the problem is finally identified and stated.

Step two: Information gathering. The team needs to turn to all available sources of information about the problem, including their own personal knowledge, to build a resource bank of information. The basic who, what, when, why, where, and how must be identified.

Step three: Revise the problem statement. Based on the information gathered in the second step, the problem should now be restated, if necessary.

Step four: List various solutions. Now that the problem is focused and adequate information is available, the team can strategize a variety of solutions for the problem. The solutions listed should be as broad and far-reaching as the team can generate. Initially, all solutions, no matter how unusual or impractical, should be listed. Then the list is streamlined as individual solutions are discarded or prioritized.

Step five: Analyze the solutions. Only after all the potential solutions are identified and catalogued can the team realistically review them and decide which ones stand the best chance of improving quality. Any risks and benefits of each solution should be reviewed, along with methods to minimize risks and maximize benefits. The issue of cost should also be considered.

Step six: Execute the solution. Now that the benefits and risks of the solutions are known, the team should proceed with the best available solution. A full action plan should be used, as is done with quality assurance.

Step seven: Analyze the results. Once the solution has been fully implemented, the team should step back and review the effect. The solution may have been fully effective, may have only partially resolved the problem, or may have created problems of its own.

Quality as a philosophy

Continuous quality improvement is deeply reliant on involvement and enthusiasm of personnel at all levels of a system. Senior administrative staff must receive an educational process that demonstrates the utility of continuous improvement. After appropriate education and planning at this level, the program expands to middle managers and staff. Many quality improvement programs have been doomed by inadequate planning and preparation, resulting in too little time for education. The result is personnel that do not sufficiently understand what the program has to offer and then fail to devote their interests and energies to its success.

Continuous quality improvement is not a quick fix. It may require anywhere from 1 year to 5 years, including educational programs, to be appropriately planned and implemented depending upon the sizes of the system and the problem involved. However, the team-oriented approach allows involvement from all personnel, helping to ensure responsibility and accountability in the program. Building slowly with careful groundwork will help to optimize the chances for success.

REFERENCES

1. American Heart Association: *Textbook of Advanced Cardiac Life Support*, Dallas, 1987, The Association.
2. Benson NH: Air medical transport. In Swor RA and others: *Quality management in prehospital care*, St. Louis, 1993, The CV Mosby Co.
3. Boyd CR: Ensuring quality, *Journal of Air Medical Transport* 10(8):5, 1991.
4. Bushore M and others: *Advanced Pediatric Life Support*, Elk Grove Village, Ill, 1989, American Academy of Pediatrics and American College of Emergency Physicians.
5. Eastes L: Implementing quality improvement for air medical services, *Journal of Air Medical Transport* 10(8):12-4, 1991.
6. Eastes L: Quality assurance v. quality improvement, *Journal of Air Medical Transport* 10(3):5-6, 1991.
7. Eastes L, Jacobson J: *Quality assurance in air medical transport*, Orem, Utah, 1990, WordPerfect Publishing Company.
8. Joint Commission on the Accreditation of Health Care Organization: *Agenda for Change Update* 1(1):3, 1987.
9. Stohler SA and others: Quality assurance in the Connecticut helicopter emergency medical service, *Journal of Air Medical Transport* 10(8):7-11, 1991.

APPENDIX 13-1

1993 LIFEFLIGHT XYZ
Quality assessment/improvement plan

Purpose:

The Quality Assessment and Improvement (QAI) Program for LifeFlight XYZ is designed in conjunction with the Hospital and Nursing Service Quality Assessment and Improvement (NSQAI) Programs. Its purpose is to provide:

1. A planned and systematic approach for monitoring and evaluating the quality and appropriateness of patient care/services provided,
2. A mechanism to resolve identified problems,
3. A forum to improve existing processes which will positively impact customer outcomes, and
4. A mechanism to assess improvements in services/effectiveness of action plans.

The program emphasizes the evaluation of nursing practice and working collaboratively with other members of the health care team to improve the quality of services delivered in our institution.

Authority:

Diagram A outlines the flow of authority and communication. The LifeFlight XYZ QAI Program receives direction and guidance from Nursing Leadership and the Nursing Service QAI Program. Bettie Smithfield, RN, MSN, the Nursing Manager, and Ronald Collins, RN, MSN, the Nursing Administrator of the Critical Care Division are responsible for

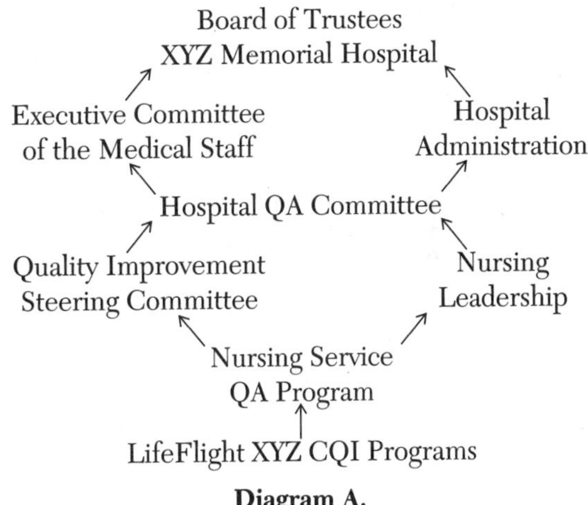

Diagram A.

setting expectations, developing plans, and implementing procedures/models to assess and improve the quality of the department's governance, management, clinical, and support process.

This is facilitated by:

1. Undertaking education concerning the approaches and methods of quality assessment and improvement,
2. Setting priorities for the review of activities that are designed to improve patient outcomes,
3. Allocation of adequate resources for assessment and improvement activities,
4. Ensuring that staff are trained in assessing and improving processes,

5. Using quality assessment and improvement data in the review of:
   a. Policy and procedures,
   b. The plan for providing nursing care to meet patient needs (budget),
   c. Education and training designed to maintain and improve knowledge and skills of all personnel,
   d. The effectiveness and appropriateness of the units orientation,
6. Including an orientation to the department quality assessment and improvement activities for new employees,
7. Fostering communication among individuals and among components of the organization and coordinating internal activities, and
8. Analyzing and evaluating the effectiveness of their contributions to improving quality.

All of the staff are expected to participate in QAI activities on the unit.

Scope of service:

As a regional air medical transport provider, the service offers emergency medical air transport services 24 hours a day to patients with all manner of critical illness or injury. Utilizing a helicopter ambulance allows the service to meet a broad range of needs. It also allows the service to transport patients up to a 120-mile radius of Our Town, New State. The service is prepared to perform interhospital transports, respond to trauma scenes, or in extreme situations, provide emergency transportation for medical or other modalities.

In its role as a regional service, although it is sponsored by XYZ Memorial Hospital, the service is closely integrated with all of the community hospitals in its rural referral area and the regional ground Emergency Medical Service (EMS) authority.

The air medical crew consists of: 1) one pilot and two flight nurses for adult/pediatric patients; 2) one pilot and one neonatal transport nurse, and one neonatal nurse practitioner for neonatal patients; and 3) one pilot, one flight nurse, and one neonatal transport nurse for small infant patients. (Small infant patients are defined as children over 30 days old and under 2 years old, and are nontrauma patients.)

Flight Nurses provide ALS care and may perform advanced nursing skills where indicated, under the direction (via Wulfsberg radio, EMS radio, or telephone) of medical control physician. The authorized advanced skills are as follows:

- Nasal and tracheal intubation
- Needle/surgical cricothyroidotomy
- Femoral vein and internal and external jugular vein cannulation
- Needle chest decompression
- Initiation of intraosseous infusion

Flight Nurses are well-versed in ACLS and PALS algorithms and in the use of other cardiac drugs such as nitroglycerine and thrombolytic agents. The nurses are expected to function proficiently with various types of equipment:

- Lifepak X cardiac monitor and defibrillator
- Lifestat 100
- MTP and syringe IV infusion pumps
- Doppler
- MAST garment
- CID, cervical collars, and long and short backboards
- Portable mechanical ventilator
- Transvenous and external cardiac pacemakers
- Oxygen tanks and equipment
- Laerdal portable suction and on-board in-wall suction equipment
- Pulse oximeter
- The Neonatal Airborne Unit

XYZ Memorial Hospital is a regional teaching medical center, fully integrated with the XYZ School of Medicine, and has over 700 beds. It has specialty critical care services in the following areas: cardiac intensive, cardiac surgery intensive, medical intensive, surgical intensive, neurosurgical intensive, pediatric intensive, and neonatal intensive. It is designated as a statewide Level I Trauma Center.

The service fulfills the following responsibilities:

1. Provides a fully trained and staffed critical care transport environment at all times for critically ill or injured patients.
2. Provides stabilization for patients at the referral site prior to loading the patient onto the aircraft for transport.
3. Maintains a comprehensive preventative maintenance program to ensure maximal availability of the aircraft.
4. Evaluates its operations and constantly reviews the safety of procedures and policies in order to provide the safest transport environment possible.

Common patient problems include the following:

Multiple trauma including closed head injury and spinal cord injury
Acute myocardial infarction
Acute respiratory failure
Septic shock
Pediatric respiratory emergencies
Premature neonates with respiratory insufficiency

Communication among all members of the air medical team is extremely essential. The communications center, located in the Emergency Department, is responsible for receiving requests for flights and referrals from other facilities, gathering and disseminating pertinent patient information, activation of the air medical team mission, flight following, and communication with receiving facilities.

The equipment on board the helicopter provides methods for treatment of almost any emergency from bleeding to anaphylaxis to pain control, etc. The helicopter is equipped with sophisticated radio systems to allow communication to take place between calling agencies and to allow reports to be called to the receiving hospital.

The program is marketed through intensive contact with surrounding hospitals in the service area.

All air transport requests are accepted without discrimination due to race, creed, sex, color, age, religion, national origin, ancestry, or handicap.

The helicopter provides a necessary link in the delivery of health care in Eastern New State. Flight Nurses with their equipment and health care expertise are able to augment existing prehospital personnel when needed. The Flight Nurse understands the pathophysiology of illness and provides emergency care and treatment for all critically ill patients.

Monitoring and review process:

The Nurse Manager, with the support of the QAI Department, reviews and revises the QAI Plan for the department annually. Revisions to the plan incorporate new JCAHO standards, feedback from the annual evaluation, and changes in the unit's scope of service and methods of delivering service.

As a part of this review, the Nurse Manager, the Unit QAI Representative, and the NSQAI Coordinator review the scope of service and identify high-risk, high-volume, and problem prone aspects of care which need to be evaluated during the year and areas they want to target for quality improvement activities. This list is shared with the staff to validate the priorities and get additional feedback. The list is then placed on an annual calendar indicating the quarterly intervals of review. The calendar is reviewed quarterly and adjusted based on issues which arise with patient care and results of the monitoring activities.

The Nursing Service QAI Program provides support to the Nurse Manager and Unit QAI Rep/Staff as they develop indicators to evaluate key components of structure, process and outcome related to each important aspect of care, establish thresholds for evaluation, and determine methods to collect and organize data. The information used to develop indicators and establish thresholds will be drawn from clinically valid sources. This information will be sent to key clinical experts to critique the indicators and review the methodology prior to implementing data collection.

All staff participate in the collection and organization of data as assigned. The cumulative data for each indicator will be continuously and periodically compared to its corresponding threshold. Based on this comparison a determination is made as to whether or not further evaluation (intense review) is necessary. The intense review will be used to evaluate if a problem or opportunity for improvement exists. If the evaluation concludes that a problem or opportunity for improvement exists, a corrective plan is developed with the input of the staff. The effectiveness of actions taken are assessed on a routine basis to determine whether there is a need for additional action.

The QAI office will assist the department with the use of CQI tools to analyze issues and display data.

Unit QAI program structure:

1. A LifeFlight XYZ QAI representative will be chosen to assist the nurse manager in establishing the monitoring and evaluation process. The selected staff nurse will serve a minimum of an eighteen month term of office. Responsibilities of the unit QAI representative will include the following tasks:
   a. Facilitating the periodic assessment of collected information in order to monitor the scope and effectiveness of practice,
   b. Communicating the monitor findings and opportunities to improve care on a quarterly basis to the Nursing Quality Assessment and Improvement Program,
   c. Communicating the responses and actions to the nurse manager and to his/her respective unit staff monthly,
   d. The unit representative will be expected to submit all reports in writing by the predetermined deadline and attend the scheduled quarterly meetings,
   e. Participation in the annual evaluation department and Nursing Service QAI Program,
   f. Attending the quarterly NSQAI Committee meetings,
   g. Participating in the Division QAI Committees.
2. The LifeFlight XYZ QAI representative and Program Manager will attend Divisional QAI Committee meetings. The Divisional QAI Committee will meet at least quarterly to provide support to the unit QAI representatives, identify issues across the division, and provide a forum for problem-solving.
3. The LifeFlight XYZ QAI Committee will consist of Robert Hurst, MD, Evelyn Copeland, MD, Bettie Smithfield, RN, Henry Vaughn, RN, Alice Miller, RN, Jack Hurley, RN, Suzanne Connolly, RN, Denice Spencer, Pilot, Jake Williams, Senior Secretary, and Nicole Warner, Communications Specialist. The committee will meet monthly to identify aspects of care which need evaluation, participate in identifying indicators, collection of data, identification and implementation of action plans, and evaluation of improvements.
4. Each committee is responsible for reporting activity quarterly, or more often as needed. The LifeFlight XYZ CQI Committee will then evaluate the activity report to identify high-risk, high volume, and problem prone aspects that may require monitor.

Annual appraisal:

The unit QAI Program will be evaluated annually to determine its effectiveness in evaluating the quality and appropriateness of patient care. This evaluation will include a comparison of the program to the Joint Commission Standards and the Commission on Accreditation of Air Medical Services. The results will be used to develop future goals and direct the department activities. The final report and goals will be forwarded to the following:

Nursing Service QAI Program
Hospital QAI
Nurse Manager
Nursing Administrator

Confidentiality:

All data, reports, and minutes are confidential and shall be respected as such by all participants in the QAI program. Names of patients, physicians, and other health care practitioners shall be coded so as not to identify the individual.

Data, reports, and minutes of the QAI program are the property of XYZ Memorial Hospital. This information is maintained in locked files in departmental or administrative offices as appropriate. QAI data, reports, and minutes shall be accessible only to those participating in the program. All other requests for information shall be in writing, stating the purpose and intent of the request and shall be addressed to the Nursing Administrator.

APPENDIX 13-2

TRANSPORT XYZ Scope of Care

As a regional pediatric transport provider, the service offers emergency medical air transport services 24 hours a day to patients under the age of 18 years with all manner of critical illness or injury. Utilizing a helicopter ambulance, a fixed wing ambulance, and a ground mobile intensive care vehicle allows the service to meet a broad range of needs and transport patients up to thousands of miles. The service is prepared to perform interhospital transports, respond to trauma scenes, or in extreme situations, provide emergency transportation for medications or other treatment modalities.

In its role as a regional service, although it is wholly sponsored by HOSPITAL XYZ, the service is closely integrated with all of the community hospitals in its rural referral area and the regional ground EMS authority.

The staff is composed of sixteen fully trained pediatric critical care flight nurses, six pilots, three drivers, two mechanics, a service administrator and a medical director. Each transport is staffed by two transport nurses and a pilot/driver. On-line medical control is provided by radio or telephone continuously for all transports. When the transport nurses are not actively engaged in transport duties, they are available to help in the sponsor hospital's pediatric units.

HOSPITAL XYZ is a regional teaching medical center which is fully integrated with XYZ University School of Medicine and has over 750 beds. It has specialty critical care services in the following areas: pediatric intensive, neonatal intensive, cardiac intensive, cardiac surgery intensive, medical intensive, surgical intensive, neurosurgical intensive, and pulmonary intensive. It is designated as a regional level I trauma center.

The service fulfills the following responsibilities:

1. Provides a fully trained and staffed critical care transport staff and environment at all times for critically ill or injured pediatric patients.
2. Provides stabilization for patients at the referral site prior to loading the patient onto the vehicle for transport.
3. Maintains a comprehensive preventive maintenance program to ensure maximal availability of the transport vehicles.
4. Evaluates its operations constantly to review the safety of procedures and policies in order to provide the safest transport environment possible.
5. Provides periodic refresher training for all staff members in their respective disciplines.

Common patient problems cared for include the following: sepsis, acute respiratory failure, complications of congenital anomalies, blunt trauma to the torso, closed head injury, spinal cord injury, cardiac surgical patients, and premature neonates with respiratory insufficiency.

Procedures frequently performed include the following: invasive airway maneuvers, establishing peripheral and central intravenous lines, maintenance of multiple intravenous medication infusions, mechanical ventilation, and intensive monitoring of vital signs of life.

14

ASSESSING SEVERITY OF ILLNESS BEFORE TRANSPORT

RICHARD A. ORR
VALERIE A. KARR

Health care reform is rapidly changing our approach to patient care. We are leaving an era in which more than 14% of our gross national product is spent on health care and entering one in which competition for the health care dollar is increasing. The health care profession is experiencing reductions in budgetary items, personnel, and services as a means of lowering costs. Therefore, health care workers are morally obliged to account for the costs of critical care transport services in which time, effort, and expense are major investments.

INDISCRIMINATE USE OF CRITICAL CARE TRANSPORT SERVICES

The indiscriminate use of transport vehicles and personnel can substantially increase the cost of medical care[10] and deplete the valuable resources available to patients who need them. Urdaneta and others.[58] evaluated helicopter transport in rural trauma situations and determined that the service was "not a factor" in the outcome for 57% of the patients. Rhee and others[48] looked at age differences in the patients transported according to physiologic scoring and determined that only 43% of patients transported by the participating air medical services were considered to be critically ill.

Within a 50 nautical mile radius of Pittsburgh, Pennsylvania, the use of air medical services has greatly increased over the past ten years. In 1984 only one hospital-based program leased two rotorcraft. By 1994 four competing services leased 10 rotorcraft despite no increase in the patient population. Referring hospitals, who have no financial accountability for patient transport, often demand the use of a rotorcraft to move patients quickly from their emergency departments to a receiving hospital, with threats of using a competing air medical service when response is not to their liking. Air transport is sometimes requested for distances as little as five miles away in instances where ground transfer would have been deemed more appropriate. Obviously, competition has played a major role in air transport proliferation, at the expense of the receiving hospitals (air medical services directly bill the receiving hospital) and, ultimately, the patient.

The golden hour: a knee-jerk response that is out of control

Emergency medical services (EMS) are essentially focused on the adult population and were developed to deal primarily with myocardial infarction and trauma, the major causes of morbidity in adults.[51] In 1973 Cowley and others[22] described the "golden hour" as being the period immediately after injury when intervention is critical. If the patient arrives at the definitive care facility within this "golden hour," survival is expected. One should note, however, that this study has never been validated and was performed during the era when prehospital personnel did little to manage the airway. Clearly, if the airway was not appropriately managed then travel time to the definitive care facility would be extremely important. The study was also performed on an adult patient population.

Later studies investigated the management of life-threatening injuries in the field and revealed that precious time is often wasted in attempts at securing vascular access, when the ultimate treatment for such injuries is prompt delivery of the patient to the surgical suite of the regional center.[24,45,46,54,59,61] The results of these studies have promoted the "scoop and run" approach often taken by EMS personnel. This philosophy might be appropriate for the 5% of patients who have severe, life-threatening injuries.[19] However, the use of precipitous haste in dealing with the remainder of the transport population often results in suboptimal stabilization,[29,30,40,54,55,62] particularly when the patients are children.[12,26,32]

For trauma calls originating at the scene or from a local emergency department, the air medical flight team launches before adequate information is known about the patient. The assumption is that *all* trauma is considered to be critical, and rarely is a trauma flight ever considered to be inappropriate. Could the patient have been safely transported by a ground unit? In our most recent set of 341 trauma patients (Level I and II) who were brought to the Children's Hospital of Pittsburgh by our air medical flight team, only 10 (3%) went to the operating room within the first 24 hours, whereas 68 (20%) had adverse events related to the airway during transport. One might ask whether the "golden hour" or "scoop and run" theory is a sufficient reason for minimizing scene and stabilization times to begin a race to the operating room when it was of questionable benefit to a small subset of patients. Unfortunately, flight teams in particular are often asked to document or offer a formal explanation to the medical director for *any* transport that exceeds the "trauma standard" of ten minutes at the scene or local referring emergency department. Team members may feel pressured to leave the scene before adequate resuscitation measures have been carried out. The goal of all transport teams, whether at the scene of an accident or in the emergency department of a referring hospital, should be to provide any treatment critical to the patient's survival. These issues underscore the need for effective triage and a better understanding of illness severity in the transport setting as it relates to outcome.

DETERMINING SEVERITY OF ILLNESS IN THE TRANSPORT SETTING

Only seeing is believing

The most obvious means of determining the severity of illness in the field is by getting an accurate description of the patient's condition from an experienced observer. The selection of an appropriate mode of transport and composition of the transport team should then follow. However, in the authors' experience, reporting mechanisms are, at best, erratic. The information may be accurate if the observer is a specialist in pediatric critical care or in emergency medicine with a strong background in pediatrics and if the person gathering the information asks the appropriate questions. Several studies have shown that severity of illness was significantly underestimated by the referring hospital when the Pediatric Risk of Mortality (PRISM) score[43] was used as a tool to compare information at the time of the referral request with that gathered by the transport team upon arrival at the referring hospital.[42,63] In the transport population at the Children's Hospital of Pittsburgh, a complete set of vital signs is available only 33% of the time for calls which are deemed "critical." "Stable" often means that a cardiac arrest is not imminent. We have seen a number of "stable" patients arrive in our emergency department in florid shock or respiratory failure that requires immediate intervention. The problem is that many prehospital providers have inadequate training in pediatric emergencies and are uncomfortable with their ability to assess a critically ill child's condition and perform any necessary interventions.[1,37,49,50]

Clinical scoring in the transport setting: does it work?

Because information at the time of transport request is often unreliable, it is no wonder that attempts to establish a severity of illness index for the purpose of triage in the transport setting have failed.[6,28,35,36] Severity of illness indices may be used either prospectively to predict individual outcomes on which treatment decisions might be made (triage), or retrospectively to characterize group trends in hospitals or therapeutic groups. However one decides to use these indices, one must take into account which outcome measure or endpoint is being considered, whether the information is available at the time it is requested, and how accurate the score is in predicting the endpoint.[47] This endpoint must be objective, clearly defined, measurable, and constant over time.

Severity of illness indices which have been validated for determination of in-hospital mortality, although objective, clearly defined, measurable, and constant over time, must be used cautiously in transport settings. Many of the physiologic variables required for scoring may be unavailable at the time of transport or may have been normalized by medical intervention; thus, the degree of physiologic instability and need for continuing intensive therapy may be underestimated. On the other hand, the more information that is available, assuming it is related to the outcome, and the longer the period of observation, the more accurate a severity score is likely to be. Also, mortality may not be the important event to measure since a number of other factors unrelated to transport may result in death. Variables within a score that influence a greater mortality risk may not necessarily indicate the need for a highly skilled transport team, if the score was used for the purpose of triage. The PRISM score[43] is a primary example of a severity of illness index that may prove to be unreliable in the field (Table 14-1). The PRISM score was validated in pediatric ICUs (PICUs) in order to predict mortality in children who were being monitored and treated by pediatric intensivists.[43] A child with a physiologic derangement indicative of respiratory failure, for example, is treated promptly in the PICU by a highly skilled physician and would be considered a low-risk item on a mortality scale. However, a child with the same physiologic derangement at a referring institution, where pediatric resources are limited, may be at high risk for morbidity or mortality. For example, a child in status asthmaticus with impending respiratory failure (gasping respirations at 40 breaths/min, PaO_2 of 60 torr in an FIO_2 of 1.0, and $PaCO_2$ of 55 torr), the highest PRISM score ever generated would be only 4 (risk of mortality <5%). This condition may seem to present a low mortality risk in a PICU; it becomes a potentially high-risk situation in a pretransport environment, especially if the health care providers are inexperienced with pediatric emergencies. On the other hand, a child with hepatic failure (total bilirubin >3.5 mg/dl with a prothrombin time or partial thromboplastin time of one-and-a-half times that of control value) and a stable cardiorespiratory system will generate a PRISM score of 8. Even though the child with hepatic failure has a greater predicted mortality than the child with asthma, the risk of morbidity during transport for the child with hepatic failure is considerably less. On this basis alone, one should question the validity of using the PRISM score as a measure of pretransport severity of illness.

Kanter and Tompkins[32] found a 10% rate of physiologic deterioration in their transport population; 20% of the patients who had PRISM scores of ≥10 deteriorated during transport, compared with only 4% of patients whose PRISM scores were <10. However, three (25%) of the 12 patients in their study who deteriorated during transport had pretransport PRISM scores of <10.

Amin and Ruddy[2] also used the PRISM score to determine the pretransport severity of illness. They examined the occurrence of physiologic deterioration and adverse events in patients during transport. Although neither physiologic deterioration nor adverse events were clearly defined, the most common adverse event noted was occlusion of the endotracheal tube. For children with a PRISM score of >11, 36% deteriorated physiologically, and 71% experienced an adverse event during transport. For patients with a PRISM score of <10, only 4% deteriorated physiologically, and 29% experienced an adverse event. The investigators concluded that patients with a PRISM score of >11 were at increased risk of physiologic deterioration and needed a specialized team. However, one

TABLE 14-1 PEDIATRIC RISK OF MORTALITY (PRISM) SCORE

Variable	*Age restrictions and ranges*			*Score*
	Infants	**All Ages**	**Children**	
Systolic BP (torr)	130-160		150-200	2
	55-65		65-75	
	>160		>200	6
	40-54		50-64	
	<40		<50	7
Diastolic BP (torr)		>110		6
HR (beat/min)	>160		>150	4
	<90		<80	
Respiratory rate (breath/min)	61-90		51-70	1
	>90		>70	5
	Apnea		Apnea	
PaO_2/FIO_2[a]		200-300		2
		<200		3
$PaCO_2$[b] (torr)		51-65		1
		>65		5
Glasgow Coma Score[c]		<8		6
Pupillary reactions		Unequal or dilated		4
		Fixed and dilated		10
PT/PTT		1.5 × control		2
		>1 mo		
Total bilirubin (mg/dl)		>3.5		6
Potassium (mEq/L)		3.0-3.5		1
		6.5-7.5		
		<3.0		5
		>7.5		
Calcium (mg/dl)		7.0-8.0		2
		12.0-15.0		
		<7.0		6
		>15.0		
Glucose (mg/dl)		40-60		4
		250-400		
		<40		8
		>400		
Bicarbonate[d] (mEq/L)		<16		3
		>32		

[a] Cannot be assessed in patients with intracardiac shunts or chronic respiratory insufficiency; requires arterial blood sampling.
[b] May be assessed with capillary blood gases.
[c] Assess only if CNS dysfunction is known or expected; cannot be assessed in patients during iatrogenic sedation, paralysis, anesthesia, and the like. Scores <8 correspond to coma or deep stupor.
[d] Use measured values.
From Pollack MM, Ruttimann UE, Getson PR: Pediatric risk of mortality (PRISM) score. *Crit Care Med* 16:1110-6, 1988.

TABLE 14-2 DISTRIBUTION OF PATIENTS WHO REQUIRED AT LEAST ONE MAJOR INTERVENTION BY THE REFERRING HOSPITAL OR TRANSPORT TEAM DURING TRANSPORT

	Referring hospital		*Transport team*	
PRISM Score	>10	≤10	>10	≤10
No. of children	20	136	20	136
No. of children requiring a major I intervention[a]	17 (85%)	42 (31%)	9(45%)	15(11%)
Fluids >20 mL/kg	5	5	6	5
Vasoactive drugs	7	7	4	4
Anticonvulsants for active seizures	8	16	3	3
Intubation	16	32	3	4
Chest tubes	2	2	2	3

[a] Some patients required more than one major intervention during the transport process.
Modified from Orr RA and others. Pretransport Pediatric Risk of Mortality (PRISM) score underestimates the requirement for intensive care or major interventions during interhospital transport, *Crit Care Med* 22:101-7, 1994.

should question whether a group with a 29% rate of adverse events was at "low risk."

Our own study[42] demonstrated that a pretransport PRISM score is often an insensitive indicator of physiologic instability and that some patients with low scores are so physiologically unstable that they require major life-saving interventions (Table 14-2). One must be careful in interpreting data implying a "low risk." On most transports, the risk of deterioration is reduced if the patient is well stabilized before departure. The transport team shall provide intervention if necessary. For example, a 5% rate of endotrancheal tube dislodgment may present a "low risk" situation in a PICU. However, if attendant personnel are not experienced in pediatric intubation, a 5% rate of dislodgment would be unacceptable.

Different physiologic or anatomic and mechanistic criteria have also been used to standardize and facilitate triage of trauma victims.[12,13,18] Attempts to validate the function of these systems have also emphasized their ability to predict only mortality rather than morbidity. Initially these scoring systems were thought to be predictive,[14-16] but recent reports have provided evidence to the contrary.[39,41] Baxt and others[4] reviewed trauma severity scores that might be used for triage and concluded that "each of the trauma prediction rules was able to accurately identify trauma victims who would die, but this was an obvious oversight since the majority of patients had profound physiologic abnormalities. The *rules* were incapable of accurately identifying those patients who appeared physiologically normal in the prehospital setting, but the patients were later determined by data obtained after hospitalization (Injury Severity Score and morbidity) to be major trauma victims."[4] In this particular study, the best simultaneous sensitivity and specificity that could be obtained in predicting major injury was 70% and 70%, respectively. Eichelberger and others[25] found similar results in a study of pediatric trauma. The use of prediction rules with low specificity leads to unwarranted evaluation of a large number of trauma center patients with minor injuries and burdens the trauma centers with higher costs of evaluation than are justified.[5]

Overall, one must be careful in using scores prospectively to predict outcomes of individual patients. The use of severity of illness scores for prehospital or interfacility triage suggests that individual outcomes can be predicted by an instrument that was intended to project the statistical outcome of groups. When carefully examined, severity of illness scores have not proved to be predictive enough to use in a prospective manner.[36]

Clinical scores used in children

Glasgow Coma Scale. The Glasgow Coma Scale (GCS)[56] (see Table 23-1) was derived from head-injured adults and focuses on three cortically-determined functions: eye opening, verbalization, and skeletal muscle movement. It has been modified in various ways to include age-appropriate behavior.[44,53] Scores range from 3 to 15 with higher scores indicating increased consciousness. This scale is widely used in prehospital and hospital phases, and has been correlated with both mortality and the level of ultimate brain function *(Glasgow Outcome Scale)*.[31]

Revised Trauma Score. The Revised Trauma Score (RTS) is based on the GCS, systolic blood pressure, and respiratory rate. These variables are assigned coded values from 4 (normal) to 0. A lower-than-normal coded value for any RTS variable suggests the need for trauma center care.[17] For outcome evaluation, these coded values are weighted and summed to yield the RTS, which ranges from 0 to 7.84; higher values indicate better prognoses.

Injury Severity Score. The Injury Severity Score (ISS)[3] is a summary of the Abbreviated Injury Scale (AIS). The latter is a list of several hundred injuries, each of which is assigned a score from 1 (minor injuries) to 6 (nearly always fatal) (Table 14-3). A summary score is needed to characterize the multiple injuries typically sustained by the trauma patient. The ISS scoring ranges from 1 to 75; a patient with an AIS of 6 corresponds to an ISS of 75. In other words, the ISS is calculated by summing the squares of the three highest AIS scores for injuries to different body regions. For example, a patient with a ruptured spleen, fractured ribs, a pulmonary contusion, and fractured femur would have the following AIS scores by region:

Abdomen: ruptured spleen—AIS 2
Chest: multiple fractured ribs—AIS 3
Extremities: fractured femur—AIS 3

The corresponding ISS is $2^2 + 3^2 + 3^2 = 22$, correlates with mortality.[8,20,21,52]

Pediatric Trauma Score. The Pediatric Trauma Score (PTS) (see Table 23-2) is a combined physiologic and anatomic scoring system for children.[57] One choice is made for each of the six variables, and the associated point values are summed to yield the PTS, whose values range from −6 to 12. It has been recommended that injured children with a PTS ≤ 8 be considered for transfer to a Level I pediatric trauma unit.[17] However, Kaufmann and others[33] concluded that the PTS offers no statistical advantage over the RTS, and the latter can be applied to patients of all ages.

TRISS methodology. The TRISS methodology is a combination index that is based on the RTS, ISS, and patient's age.[7,9,11] TRISS can be used to estimate the survival probability of an injured patient from a retrospective database using a logistic model:

$$Ps = 1/(1 + e - b),$$

where Ps is the probability of survival, e equals 2.7182 (base of Napierian logarithms), and

$$b = b0 = b1(RTS) + b2(ISS) + b3(A).$$

RTS is based on the patient's condition at the time of emergency department admission where A is 1 if the patient's age is > 54 years and 0 if ≤ 54 years, and b1 is the weight derived by applying the Walker-Duncan regression algorithm.[60] Pediatric patient (<15 years) outcomes are evaluated using the blunt injury norms for 15- to 55-year old patients. The TRISS methodology allows comparison of outcome between two patient populations while controlling for patient severity.

TABLE 14-3 THE ABBREVIATED INJURY SCALE (AIS) CODES FOR PATIENTS WITH CHEST INJURIES

AIS code	*Injury description*
1	Muscle ache or chest wall stiffness
2	Simple rib or sternal fractures
3	Multiple rib fractures without respiratory embarrassment
4	Flail chest
5	Aortic laceration

Modified from Baker SP and others: The Injury Severity Score: a method for describing patients with multiple injuries and evaluating emergency care, *J Trauma* 14:187-196, 1974.

Therapeutic Intervention Scoring System. The Therapeutic Intervention Scoring System (TISS)[23,34] quantifies ICU therapeutic interventions to characterize severity. The TISS is based on the premise that more interventions will be required for more critically ill patients.

Pediatric Risk of Mortality Score. The PRISM score (see Table 14-1) was developed from the Physiologic Stability Index[64] in order to reduce the number of physiologic variables required for PICU risk assessment.[43] The basis for these scoring systems suggests that physiologic instability directly reflects mortality risk. Mortality risk prediction in the PICU setting is obtained as follows:

$$r = a * \text{PRISM} + b * \text{age (months)} + c * \text{operative status} + d$$

where probability of death is:

$$p\ (\text{ICU death}) = \exp(r) / (1 + \exp[r])$$

and a, b, and c are the logistic regression coefficients for the PRISM score, age, and operative status (postoperative = 1, nonoperative = 0), respectively, and d is a constant.[43]

Neonatal scores. Several scoring systems have been published to evaluate the condition of transported neonates.[27,30] However, patient numbers in these studies are quite small.

Clinical scoring: Where do we go from here?

Obviously, the measuring of severity of illness for triage purposes poses a number of problems. Since scores derived from population data are not often predictive of individual patients, the authors agree with Rhee[47] and LeGall and Lemeshow[36] that severity scores should probably not be used for triage purposes, but may be retrospectively applied to stratify patient groups according to their severity of illness. This will allow administrators and clinical investigators to compare the performance of services or treatment strategies.[36] The only outcome variable that shares all the attributes of being objective, clearly defined, measurable, and constant over time is in-hospital mortality. However, as previously stated, in-hospital mortality may not necessarily be related to events that occurred during transport. McCloskey and others[38] examined the requirement for major interventions as performed by the transport team as an outcome variable. They reported an increased probability of needing a major procedure or pharmacologic intervention during the transport of patients who, at the time of the initial referral call, were intubated or were younger than one year of age with unstable vital signs. The conclusion was that such indications might allow one to make appropriate decisions regarding transport team composition. If a patient has a high probability of needing a major intervention, then a highly skilled pediatric team should be used. The obvious question one might ask in regard to this outcome variable is whether the patient actually needed the intervention. In this situation the outcome variable might not always be objective nor constant over time.

In the future the most effective method of triage might be found in the area of telecommunications. If the command or receiving physician was able to get a "real time" glimpse of the patient during referral, along with a report from the observer, he/she might be better able to make appropriate triage decisions; that is, does the patient need specialized transport services, or could he/she be safely brought in by an alternative mode?

In the meantime a transport severity of illness measure needs to be developed for children with nontraumatic diseases that would allow valid comparisons to be made between patient groups in different transport populations. Only then will we be able to determine what constitutes appropriate use of transport services, for example air versus ground, and in which groups of patients will specialized transport services really make a difference in outcome.

REFERENCES

1. Aijian P, Tsai A, Knopp R, Kallsen GW: Endotracheal intubation of pediatric patients by paramedics, *Ann Emerg Med* 18:489, 1989.
2. Amin N, Ruddy R: High risk interhospital pediatric transport, *Pediatr Emerg Care* 7:382, 1991 (Abstract).
3. Baker SP, and others: The Injury Severity Score: a method for describing patients with multiple injuries and evaluating emergency care, *J Trauma* 14:187, 1974.
4. Baxt WG and others: The failure of prehospital trauma prediction rules to classify trauma patients accurately, *Ann Emerg Med* 18:1, 1989.

5. Baxt WG, Jones G, Fortlage D: The trauma triage rule: a new, resource-based approach to the prehospital identification of major trauma victims, *Ann Emerg Med* 19:1401, 1990.
6. Bion JF and others: Validation of a prognostic score in critically ill patients undergoing transport, *Br Med J* 291:432, 1985.
7. Boyd CR, Tolson MA, Copes WS: Evaluating trauma care: the TRISS method, *J Trauma* 27:370, 1987.
8. Bull JP: The Injury Severity Score of road traffic casualties in relation to mortality, time of death, hospital treatment time and disability, *Accid Anal Prev* 7:249, 1975.
9. Champion HR, Sacco WJ, Hunt TK: Trauma severity scoring to predict mortality, *World J Surg* 7:4, 1983.
10. Champion HR: Helicopters in emergency trauma care, *JAMA* 249:3074, 1983 (editorial).
11. Champion HR and others: Trauma score, *Crit Care Med* 9:672, 1981.
12. Champion HR and others: An anatomic index of injury severity, *J Trauma* 20:197, 1980.
13. Champion HR and others: Assessment of injury severity: The Triage Index, *Crit Care Med* 8:201, 1980.
14. Clemmer TP and others: Outcome of critically injured patients treated at level I trauma centers vs. full-service community hospitals, *Crit Care Med* 13:861, 1985.
15. Clemmer TP and others: Prospective analysis of the CRAMS score for major trauma, *J Trauma* 25:188, 1985.
16. Clemmer TP and others: Comparison of the Trauma Score and CRAMS score for trauma triage, *Crit Care Med* 14:427, 1986 (abstract).
17. Commission on Emergency Medical Services: Air Ambulance Guidelines, Washington, DC, 1981, U.S. Department of Transportation.
18. Committee on Injury Scaling: The Abbreviated Injury Scale, 1980 Revision, Des Plaines, Illinois, 1980, American Association for Automotive Medicine.
19. Committee on Trauma of the American College of Surgeons: resources for optimal care of the injured patient, Chicago, 1990, American College of Surgeons.
20. Copes WS and others: The Injury Severity Score revisited, *J Trauma* 28:69, 1988.
21. Copes WS and others: A comparison of the Abbreviated Injury Scale 1980 and 1985 versions, *J Trauma* 28:78, 1988.
22. Cowley RS and others: An economical and proved helicopter program for transporting the emergency critically ill and injured patient in Maryland, *J Trauma* 13:1029, 1973.
23. Cullen DJ and others: Therapeutic Intervention Scoring System: a method for quantitative comparison of patient care, *Crit Care Med* 2:57, 1974.
24. Eggold R: Trauma care regionalization: a necessity, *J Trauma* 23:260, 1983.
25. Eichelberger MR and others: A comparison of the Trauma Score, the Revised Trauma Score, and the Pediatric Trauma score, *Ann Emerg Med* 18:1053, 1989.
26. Eisenberg MS, Berger L, Hallstrom A: Cardiac resuscitation in the community: importance of rapid provision and implications for program planning, *JAMA* 241:1905, 1979.
27. Ferrara A and Atakent Y: Neonatal stabilization score: a quantitative method of auditing medical care in transported newborns weighing less than 1,000 gm at birth, *Med Care* 24:179, 1986.
28. Fox J and others: An evaluation of potential prognostic indicators in cardiac patients, *J Air Med Transport* 10:18-30, 1991.
29. Greenburg DS: Health-care thrift spurs patient-dumping, Los Angeles Times, Part II:5, November 12, 1984.
30. Houtchens BA: Major trauma in the rural mountain West, *J Am Coll Emerg Phys* 6:343, 1977.
31. Jennett B and others: Predicting outcome in individual patients after head injury, *Lancet* 1:1031, 1976.
32. Kanter RK, Tompkins JM: Adverse events during interhospital transport: physiologic deterioration associated with pretransport severity of illness, *Pediatrics* 84:43, 1989.
33. Kaufmann CR and others: Evaluation of the Pediatric Trauma Score, *JAMA* 263:69, 1990.
34. Keene AR, Cullen DJ: Therapeutic Intervention Scoring System, Update 1983, *Crit Care Med* 11:1, 1983.
35. Kissoon N and others: The child requiring transport: lessons and implications for the pediatric emergency physician, *Pediatr Emerg Care* 4:1, 1988.
36. LeGall J, Lemeshow S: do we need a new severity score? *Crit Care Med* 19:857, 1991.
37. Macnab AJ: Optimal escort for interhospital transport of pediatric emergencies, *J Trauma* 31:205, 1991.
38. McCloskey KA and others: Variables predicting the need for a pediatric critical care transport team, *Pediatr Emerg Care* 8:1, 1992.
39. Morris JA and others: The Trauma Score as a triage tool in the prehospital setting, *JAMA* 256:1319, 1986.
40. Olson CM and others: Stabilization of patients prior to interhospital transfer, *Am J Emerg Med* 5:33, 1987.
41. Ornato J and others: Ineffectiveness of the Trauma Score and the CRAMS Scale for accurately triaging patients to trauma centers, *Ann Emerg Med* 14:1061, 1985.
42. Orr RA and others: Pretransport Pediatric Risk of Mortality (PRISM) Score underestimates the requirement for intensive care or major interventions during interhospital transport, *Crit Care Med* 22:101, 1994.
43. Pollack MM, Ruttimann UE, Getson PR: Pediatric Risk of Mortality (PRISM) Score, *Crit Care Med* 16:1110, 1988.
44. Raimondi AJ, Hirschauer J: Head injury in the infant and toddler, *Childs Brain* 11:12, 1984.
45. Ramenofsky ML and others: Maximum survival in pediatric trauma: the ideal system, *J Trauma* 24:818, 1984.

46. Ramenofsky ML and others: EMS for pediatrics: optimum treatment or unnecessary delay? *J Pediatr Surg* 18:498, 1983.
47. Rhee KJ: The use of severity scores in air medical transports, *Air Medical Transport* 10:5, 1991.
48. Rhee KJ and others: Differences in air ambulance patient mix demonstrated in physiologic scoring, *Ann Emerg Med* 19:552, 1990.
49. Seidel JS: Emergency medical services and the pediatric patient: are the needs being met? II. Training and equipping emergency medical services providers for pediatric emergencies, *Pediatrics* 78:808, 1986.
50. Seidel JS: A needs assessment of advanced life support and emergency medical services in pediatric patient: state of the art, *Circulation* 74:129, 1986.
51. Seidel JS and others: Emergency medical services and the pediatric patient: are the needs being met? *Pediatrics* 73:769, 1984.
52. Semmlow JL, Cone R: Application of the Injury Severity Score: an independent correlation, *Health Serv* Spring 1976.
53. Singounas EG, Volikas ZG: Epidural haematoma in a paediatric population, *Childs Brain* 11:250, 1984.
54. Smith JP and others: Prehospital stabilization of critically injured patients: a failed concept, *J Trauma* 25:65, 1985.
55. Stultz KR and others: Prehospital defibrillation performed by emergency medical technicians in rural communities, *N Engl J Med* 310:219, 1984.
56. Teasdale G, Jennett B: Assessment of coma and impaired consciousness: a practical scale, *Lancet* 2:81, 1974.
57. Tepas JJ and others: The Pediatric Trauma Score as a predictor of injury severity in the injured child, *J Pediatr Surg* 22:14, 1987.
58. Urdaneta LF and others: Evaluation of an emergency air transport service as a component of a rural EMS system, *Ann Surg* 50:183, 1984.
59. Von Wagoner FH: Died in-hospital: a three year study of deaths following trauma, *J Trauma* 1:401, 1961.
60. Walker SH, Duncan DB: Estimation of the probability of an event as a function of several independent variables, *Biometrika* 54:167, 1967.
61. West JG, Cales RH, Gazzangia AB: Impact of regionalization: the Orange County experience, *Arch Surg* 118:740, 1983.
62. West JG, Trunkey DD, Lim RC: Systems of trauma care: a study of two counties, *Arch Surg* 114:455, 1979.
63. Whitfield JM and others: The telephone evaluation of severity of illness of the neonatal/pediatric patient prior to interhospital transfer, *J Air Med Transport* 10:82, 1991 (abstract).
64. Yeh TS and others: Validation of a physiologic stability index for use in critically ill infants and children, *Pediatr Res* 18:445, 1984.

15

PRINCIPLES AND PHILOSOPHY OF TRANSPORT STABILIZATION

STEVEN E. KRUG

The mission of Pediatric Critical Care Transport (PCCT) is often misunderstood, even by its professional consumers. Historically, many interhospital transport systems have developed from prehospital precursors. It is therefore not surprising that PCCT is frequently lumped together with prehospital transport. Many interhospital transport services, particularly the aeromedical programs, provide patient transport from both prehospital and hospital environments, as well as transport for both adult and pediatric care. These situations have undoubtedly added to the significant confusion already present in emergency medicine regarding what constitutes optimal pediatric transport care. In many geographic communities, this confusion has led to a debate regarding what type of patient stabilization is necessary for the delivery of optimal pediatric transport care.

The purpose of this chapter is to illustrate how critical care transport systems differ from their prehospital counterparts, and the differences between adult and pediatric emergency care systems. The unique features and purpose of PCCT, as related to the needs of critically ill and injured children, will be identified. The chapter will also contrast the conflicting transport philosophies of "swoop, scoop and run" and "stay and resuscitate", explaining the relative merits and deficiencies of each approach. An analysis of the literature addressing the issue of pretransport stabilization will be presented. The perspective and expectations of the various consumers of transport services will be discussed, and suggestions will be offered on how PCCT programs can meet those needs. Finally, the chapter will provide insight into the issues pertaining to intrahospital transport of the critically ill child.

PREHOSPITAL VERSUS INTERHOSPITAL TRANSPORT

The differences between prehospital and interhospital transport services are summarized in Table 15-1. In general, prehospital transport serves as a mechanism for the initiation and transfer of emergency care for an acutely ill or injured patient. With the exception of certain rural communities, the distance traveled or transport time is typically less than 15-20 minutes. The skill of the prehospital care provider varies greatly among different Emergency Medical Service (EMS) systems, secondary to the level of training or certification of each EMS provider and the scope of practice permitted within the individual system. In general, the technical skill and level of care available ranges from basic to advanced life support, with or without specific pediatric focus.

While many interhospital transport systems provide a prehospital response, their typical role is to provide a critical care environment for patient transport between institutions. In theory these transport services are provided to patients for whom the initiation and main-

TABLE 15-1 PREHOSPITAL VERSUS INTERHOSPITAL TRANSPORT CARE

	Prehospital transport	*Interhospital transport*
Distance traveled	Generally short (minutes)	Generally long (minutes to hours)
Level of care	Basic and Advanced Life Support	Critical care
Personnel skill	Emergency Medical Technician and Paramedic	Nurse and/or Physician
Purpose	Initiation of and transfer for emergency care	Initiation and maintenance of critical care

tenance of emergency care has already occurred. These transported patients require interfacility transport for reasons ranging from the need for specialized or tertiary care not available at the referring hospital, to hospital preference of the patient or parent for a preferred primary or specialty care provider or a third-party payor. Of course, those patients requiring interfacility transfer due to preference rather than critical or specialized physiologic needs may be transported using a less sophisticated means of conveyance, such as the family car or a basic ambulance.

While the distance between hospitals can be short, the distances traveled by interhospital transport teams is usually greater than that traveled by prehospital transport teams. Additionally, while the team member configuration and associated skill level varies significantly between transport programs, the level of care and technical skill offered by interhospital critical care transport systems is typically more sophisticated than that found in prehospital transport systems.

Interhospital transport systems may therefore be viewed as extensions of hospital-based critical care units, moving severely ill patients to the hub of a regional critical or specialty care network.[41] It has been demonstrated repeatedly that these networks function to improve the outcome of the patients with special care needs, such as the critically injured* or neonatal patient.† The conveyance to a specialty care center is therefore an important contribution to the patient's overall medical treatment. Similar data have demonstrated that the outcome of critically ill children is improved when delivery by interhospital transport systems to a regional pediatric tertiary care center occurs,[55-58] creating an especially important point when examining the role of pediatric transport systems.

HISTORY AND STATUS OF EMERGENCY MEDICAL SERVICES

While the history of EMS can be traced back to the wars of Napoleon's era, it was the 1966 report of the National Academy of Sciences, "Accidental Death and Disability—The Neglected Disease of Modern Society," that served as the early catalyst for improvements in prehospital care.[68] The municipal EMS systems that followed were created with a primary focus on acute myocardial infarction. The Emergency Medical Services Act of 1973 provided the necessary funding for state and local governments to develop comprehensive EMS systems.[68,69]

As those EMS systems developed, it became clear that they were indeed successful in reducing the mortality and morbidity associated with certain sentinel illnesses. On closer examination, the reductions found for acute adult illness and injury were not paralleled in pediatric populations.[68,69] This apparent discrepancy in adult and pediatric emergency care served to stimulate the development of the federally legislated Emergency Medical Services for Children (EMS-C) program, which was designed to improve the quality of available emergency services for children. This program was funded in 1984, with a goal of integrating pediatric emergency care expertise into existing EMS systems through the development of equipment standards, patient care standards, education and training programs for prehospital and emergency care providers.[15,68,69]

In spite of the many improvements generated by numerous state and regional EMS-C

* References 8, 10, 14, 21, 71, 80, 81.
† References 13, 23, 24, 30, 73, 74.

programs, there remains a significant and widespread deficiency in the quality of pediatric emergency medical services in the United States.[15,66,68,69] These deficiencies have been well documented in both prehospital and hospital-based (e.g. emergency department) environments.* Most recently, the Institute of Medicine released its report "Emergency Medical Services for Children"; a comprehensive study on the status of pediatric emergency care in the United States.[35] The report, published in 1993, found the continued presence of significant problems in the delivery of emergency care to children, including inadequate equipment and personnel training in both prehospital and hospital based settings.

The findings of the Institute of Medicine demonstrate that the differences between pediatric tertiary specialty care centers and the institutions that refer children to them are not simply limited to critical care resources, but in general include deficiencies at more "basic" resuscitative care.[31,53,66] These pediatric emergency care (as well as critical care) deficiencies serve to illustrate an important distinction between adult critical care transport and PCCT. Adult critical care transport teams may rely more frequently upon an assumption that the acute and emergency care needs of the patient they are about to transport have been met by the referring team. Arguably, this same assumption cannot be made by PCCT teams. PCCT systems therefore serve as pathways in regional networks for the delivery of both pediatric emergency care and pediatric critical care.[41]

PHILOSOPHY OF PRETRANSPORT STABILIZATION

The question that logically follows is when and where should initiation and maintenance of the necessary emergency care, critical care, and definitive surgical care occur? Intellectually, as well as, physiologically it makes sense to provide the necessary intervention sooner rather than later. Considering the abysmal outcome of witnessed pediatric cardiopulmonary arrest in controlled hospital settings,† the early identification and intervention for pre-arrest states such as shock or respiratory failure will likely result in improved outcomes for acutely ill or injured children.[9,82]

In spite of the inherent benefits of early identification and intervention for life threatening illness and injury, there remain two prevalent, and somewhat different, approaches to transport care, "swoop, scoop and run" and "stay and resuscitate." The relative merits of these two different philosophies deserves closer examination.

"Swoop, scoop and run"

The philosophy of "swoop, scoop and run" is derived from the belief that the sooner a critically ill, and particularly a critically injured patient is delivered to a facility that can provide definitive medical or surgical intervention, the better the outcome of that patient. The assumption made here is that the patient's definitive care cannot be sufficiently met by either the referring facility and its health care team, or the transport team. If this is true, then it is in the patient's best interest to be transported as quickly as possible for a facility where those definitive care needs can be met. To accomplish this as little time as possible should be wasted at the scene or facility from which the patient is transported. Additionally, whenever possible, the means or method of transport should allow for the most rapid transfer that is physically possible (e.g. air transport versus ground transport).

Historically, this approach to transport care draws its greatest support from the American College of Surgeons ATLS (Advanced Trauma Life Support).[16] Mortality from trauma is known to have a trimodal distribution. The first group of deaths occur shortly after the injury and are due to lethal injuries (e.g. brain or brain stem injuries, aortic transection) that are essentially untreatable. The second peak occurs several minutes to a few hours after the injury. These deaths are usually due to surgically treatable injuries such as subdural or epidural hematomas, hemopneumothorax, or any injury which if left untreated might cause excessive blood loss (e.g.

* References 7, 29, 60, 66, 67, 70.

† References 42, 43, 52, 63, 76, 82.

laceration of the spleen, liver, or kidney, fractured pelvis and femur). The final group of patients who die are those who suffer sepsis or multisystem organ failure, usually several days after the injury occurrence.

The ATLS concept of the Golden Hour is best applied to those patients in the second mortality peak, namely those with potentially salvageable injuries. The golden hour represents a critical time window for medical and surgical intervention for the acutely injured patient that will limit the occurrence of preventable deaths. This mandates rapid patient assessment and stabilization, including rapid prehospital and interhospital transport times. In support there have been several studies on the management of life-threatening injuries in the field that have documented the wasting of valuable time in the pursuit of field-initiated life support.[61,72,77]

These published reports certainly support the perspective that the primary purpose of prehospital trauma care is the rapid delivery of the acutely injured patient to a trauma center. Unfortunately, the efficacy of this routine approach to trauma care has only been demonstrated in adult patients, specifically those with life threatening surgical lesions that require immediate definitive care.[27,36,41,61] There is in fact a growing literature base that identifies the advanced life support role of prehospital (and interhospital) care providers as a significant contributor towards improved patient outcome from life-threatening injuries.[6,51,61] Appropriate stabilization by a properly trained and experienced team should take precedence over speed of transport, especially for patients with illnesses or injuries not immediately requiring the physical facilities (i.e. operating room) of the trauma center.

"Stay and resuscitate"

In great contrast to "swoop, scoop and run" is the philosophy of "stay and resuscitate." This approach to transport care suggests that there are certain specific aspects of resuscitation that must be delivered as quickly as possible, either at the scene of an accident or at the referring hospital. In both settings it is imperative that these interventions take place prior to (or during) the patient's transport to the receiving specialty care center. The assumption here is that many definitive resuscitative care needs of the patient may be met by the transport team as a mobile intensive care unit. If this is true, the time taken to provide resuscitative care or stabilizing interventions prior to transport may contribute towards improved patient outcome.[41]

The adult transport literature contains several papers supporting the practice of pretransport stabilization. In 1990 Crippen published a fairly comprehensive and elegant review article on the controversy of optimal pretransport stabilization.[18] In this paper Crippen examines the transport literature for evidence supporting the philosophy of pretransport stabilization. The paper documents significant evidence in adult transport of a relationship between inadequate pretransport stabilization and poor patient outcome.[32,47,50,64] Moylan and others[49] compared trauma care delivery and the outcome from both air and ground transport systems. They identified that patients transported by air had significantly better survival rates (82% versus 53%) compared to those transported by ground. The patients transported by air had more therapeutic interventions (endotracheal intubation, fluid administration, blood transfusions) than did the ground patients. These therapeutic interventions were believed to be the primary contributor to the outcome difference. In a later review of aeromedical transportation, Moylan stated that the key factor in improving the survival of trauma victims was not the speed of patient delivery to a tertiary care center, but instead the time interval between the injury and the arrival of a team to the scene of the accident.[48] Baxt[5] examined the mortality rates of patients transferred to tertiary care centers by a basic EMS ambulance versus an interhospital helicopter program. The patients transported by helicopter were the only patients to experience a better than predicted survival outcome. This in spite of the fact that the patients transported by helicopter had on average a 23 minute longer transport time. More recently, Schmidt and others[65] published a comparison of the delivery of on-scene trauma care and outcome by a German and an American hospital-based helicopter transport service.

The transport services were somewhat different in that the team configuration in the American program was nurse/medic versus nurse/physician for the German team. The German program tended to provide more field intervention with a higher rate of intubation (37% vs. 13%), greater amounts of IV fluid administered (1800 cc vs. 825 cc), and more thoracic decompressions (9% vs. 0.5%). The comparison also found a significantly greater number of early deaths in the U.S. program. While the overall mortality in the two programs was similar, the German program had a better patient outcome using the TRISS *z* statistic (see Ch. 14).

Published support for maximal pretransport stabilization of critically ill children is greatest in the neonatal transport literature, with numerous papers demonstrating improved outcome with early and adequate stabilization of the critically ill newborn.[11,12,19,28,54] Chance, and others,[11,12] compared the care and outcome of neonates transported by experienced transport teams versus neonatal patients cared for by untrained personnel. Newborns transported by the experienced teams had longer scene stabilization times with superior maintenance of the neutral thermal environment, inspired oxygen concentration, blood pressure, and arterial PO^2 and PCO^2. These same infants also had lower mortality rates and shorter hospital stays compared to the infants transported by nonspecialized transport teams.[12] Gudavalli and others[28] examined the impact of physician's expertise on patient outcome in the transportation of sick neonates. In this study, care delivery by pediatric residents was compared to that provided by neonatology fellows. The comparison revealed that the presumably skilled fellows spent more time stabilizing patients at the referring hospital than the residents. The study found that patient mortality was lower for the fellow transports. One could infer that the additional pretransport/transport stabilization provided by the more experienced group of physicians was a primary determinant in the patient's outcome.

This approach to transport care is supported by the American Heart Association's PALS (Pediatric Advanced Life Support) concept for the recognition and intervention of prearrest states such as shock and or respiratory failure.[9] This approach has been echoed in a variety of publications on pediatric transport.* In their manual on pediatric transport care, Aoki and McCloskey[3] state: "The patient should be transported to the receiving hospital in as stable condition as is possible. For most patients stability and level of care during transport will be the major goal, superseding speed of departure from the referring hospital." These and other transport care experts have stated that the level of transport patient care provided should at least maintain if not exceed that provided by the referring hospital.†

Upon closer examination the transport care needs for most critically injured children may be optimized with in-field stabilization. For the majority of pediatric multiple trauma victims, the delivery of definitive resuscitative care most frequently occurs in a Pediatric Intensive Care Unit (PICU). Arguably, the "golden hour" for the pediatric trauma victim is not determined by the need to proceed to an operating suite, but instead by the initiation of emergency and critical care. The majority of injured children requiring surgical care need orthopedic and other procedures which, while important, are a secondary priority to resuscitative emergency and critical care.

In two studies of transport care delivery by nonpediatric transport teams, Kanter, and others[38,39] found excess patient morbidity associated with inadequate transport stabilization or the failure to recognize common critical care complications such as a plugged or dislodged endotracheal tube. The morbidity of these patients transported by the referring hospital was twice that of patients with a similar severity of illness cared for in a more controlled PICU setting.[39]

Macnab[44] published a retrospective evaluation of the incidence of preventable or secondary insults for transported children in relation to the level of transport team expertise. Compared to PCCT teams without a physician, PCCT teams with a senior pediatric resident or PICU fellow had longer transport

* References 1,3,20,41,46,75.
† References 1,3,15,20,41,46,75.

times, longer patient stabilization times, and fewer preventable insults (0.13 per transport versus 1.9 per transport). A third group of transports, performed by nonphysician teams with additional extensive pediatric training, demonstrated results closer to those of the physician-led teams. Inadequate stabilization, avoidable patient stress, and untreated changes in vital signs were the most common errors made by less experienced PCCT teams. While a statistically significant difference in the outcome of patients cared for by the different transport teams was not found, the patients cared for by the teams with physicians were significantly sicker initially compared to the patients cared for by the less experienced teams.

Clinical scenarios for "swoop, scoop and run"

Are there clinical scenarios where the "swoop, scoop and run" approach is preferable? Critically ill children with life threatening injuries requiring immediate surgical repair (e.g. an epidural or subdural hematoma requiring evacuation, unstable children with penetrating thoracic trauma) would be best served by this particular approach. While the efficiency or speed of the transport process is indeed critically important for the outcome of these children, it is also pertinent to point out that, in the advanced stages of these illnesses or injuries, certain resuscitative measures are necessary if outcome is to be favorable. As an example, for the child who has developed signs of early uncal herniation due to an expanding intracranial hematoma, aggressive management of that patient's airway along with hyperventilation and osmolar therapy may buy the time necessary to transport the child for definitive surgical evacuation.

POLITICS AND REALITY OF COMMUNITY NEEDS AND CONSUMER EXPECTATIONS IN INTERHOSPITAL TRANSPORT CARE

A call for medical assistance or the request to transport a sick child is generally accompanied by a sense of urgency. The magnitude of this urgency or anxiety is directly related to the perceived severity of the child's illness or injury. The message "baby sick, come quick!" conveys both that the patient is ill and that the referring team feels somehow unable to meet the needs of the patient. It is not at all surprising that, when asked to rank the most important characteristics of a transport system, many referring professionals will rank response time first.[40]

The ability to meet the expectation of a rapid response, as well as the definition of what constitutes an acceptable response time, varies from program to program, and is highly dependent upon available resources.[45] The time required for the transport team to arrive at the referring facility, or the response time, may be examined as follows:

$$\text{Response time} = \text{Mobilization time} + \text{Transit time.}$$

The dispatch or mobilization of the transport team relates to a number of factors including: the availability of the transport vehicle, team readiness, team specialization, the clinical data collected, and management advice provided prior to team departure. The presence of a dedicated transport team, one with no other responsibilities and poised to respond immediately, helps to limit mobilization time. It then follows that generic team composition, sending the same team for patients of all ages and illness severity, has a time-saving impact on response time. Conversely, taking the time to inquire in relative detail about the nature and severity of the patient's illness and specialized needs is time consuming, and if necessary should be done by someone not preparing to go on the transport.

Most adult-oriented transport programs have adopted a dedicated generic team composition for all transports, including those for children. While this translates to a brief mobilization time, it may result in little team preparation or specialization for the needs of a critically ill child.[41,46] Most standard transport teams consist of two health care providers. Patients that are critically ill may literally need a third or even a fourth pair of skilled hands.[22,41] Many transport programs electively utilize specialized personnel, such as respiratory therapists or senior level physicians for selected patients. Most programs cannot afford to support these specialized care providers in a transport dedicated mode.

Therefore including such personnel on transport when needed is time consuming and will lengthen mobilization time.

In addition to concerns regarding transport response time, there is the related considerations on the length of time a critically ill or injured child must remain in the referring unit once the decision to transport has been made. Extrication time may be defined as the time elapsed from the initial call for transport, until the transport team departs the referring facility with the patient, or:

Extrication time = Mobilization time + Transit time + Scene time

The amount of time the transport team spends at a referring facility or at the scene itself is another area of great concern for transport consumers.[40] The failure of some to differentiate interhospital care from prehospital care, combined with a general unfamiliarity with the literature advocating pretransport stabilization and an obvious preference to get a sick child out of one's emergency department or newborn nursery, have resulted in an expectation for brief scene times. The absence of universally accepted standards for the pretransport stabilization of children and the availability of interhospital transport systems have promoted an over-dependence at many health care facilities upon the transport system for provision of basic resuscitative care, rather than development of those skills in-house. Oddly, the development of PCCT systems has added to the deficiencies in the aforementioned quality of community-based emergency medical services for children.

The ability to transport patients with short response and scene times is an important feature of prehospital and some interhospital transport programs. While an efficient extrication time is certainly a reasonable goal for a critical care transport program, the identification of specialized needs and the provision of a sophisticated critical care response may require longer mobilization times. Additionally, the stabilization of the critically ill or injured child and the delivery of pediatric critical care may translate to longer scene times. Dobrin and others[22] suggest that there may be a narrow window of opportunity or an optimal time period in which to leave the referring hospital with a critically ill child. Leaving prior to this period might result in suboptimal pretransport stabilization. Conversely, leaving after the window has "closed" might risk the occurence of postresuscitation clinical deterioration (e.g. multisystem organ failure) prior to the patient's arrival to the receiving facility.

Part of the referring team's expressed urgency for rapid response and short scene times may be related to a perception of liability exposure as long as the patient physically remains in the referring unit. While professional liability exposure does exist during the patient's presence, that liability does not abruptly terminate upon the departure of the patient. The Consolidated Omnibus Budget Reduction Act (COBRA) of 1986 now requires the transferring hospital to assume liability for the adequacy of patient stabilization before any transport occurs and for the choice of an appropriate mode of transport.[26] However, it should be acknowledged that for many referring facilities, the presence of a critically ill or injured child poses a significant drain upon otherwise limited personnel and or equipment resources.

MEETING BOTH CONSUMER EXPECTATIONS AND PATIENT NEEDS IN SPEED AND CONTENT

The acknowledged deficiencies in the quality of pediatric emergency and critical care outside of pediatric tertiary care centers makes an especially strong argument for PCCT systems having rapid response times. It is undoubtedly in the best interest of a critically ill patient to limit the time spent in a potentially unstable environment (e.g. at the scene of an injury or enroute to the receiving hospital). As critically ill children pose a significant drain upon the resources of even the best equipped hospital, it is also in the best interest of the referring team to proceed efficiently with transport. Finally, in considering the potential transport needs of other patients, the sooner the team returns from a trip, the sooner they become available for the next patient needing transport.

One could therefore argue that the optimal PCCT system should meet the ideals of both philosophies, namely the provision of timely, efficient, yet comprehensive emergency and critical care. The balance between efficient and comprehensive care is indeed a delicate one, yet the resolution of this apparent conflict is frequently quite simple. Outreach education can be a most effective means towards that end. Pediatric transport care consumers should be made aware of the recently published standards for pediatric transport care, and the benefits offered by optimal pretransport stabilization and specialized pediatric transport services. This awareness may promote a greater appreciation of the efforts taken to provide critical transport care. Ultimately, the amount of transport care required by a patient is determined both by their illness or injury severity and the level of care provided by the referring team. If one goal of outreach education is to improve the ability of the referring team to recognize and meet the needs of acutely ill and injured children, then perhaps the need for extensive pretransport stabilization will be reduced.

INTRAHOSPITAL TRANSPORT ISSUES

Although intrahospital transport of the critically ill or injured occurs much more frequently than interhospital transport, the majority of the adult and pediatric transport care literature is focused on interhospital care in spite of the rather high complication rates found with intrahospital transport of the critically ill.[20]

In a study on intrahospital transfers of critically ill children from a PICU, Wallen, and others[79] found that nearly 60% suffered at least one adverse event associated with the transport, including hypothermia, significant heart rate, respiratory rate, and blood pressure changes, oxygen desaturation or blood gas deterioration, endotracheal tube mishaps, or significant changes in the level of ventilator or inotropic support required. Over half of these children suffered more than one adverse event. Similar studies on critically ill or injured adult populations of patients have found a similar occurrence of adverse events associated with transporting to or from an ICU setting.[2,33,34]

While conceptually similar to the issues faced in interhospital transport, the pretransport stabilization of critically ill children for the purpose of intrahospital transport, and the optimal timing for that transport, poses certain additional considerations. Generally, the population of children transported to and from tertiary care PICUs have a consistently greater illness severity than those transported from outside facilities. Children in PICU settings tend to require greater physiologic and technical support, and are also less tolerant of the stress and or adverse events associated with a physical transfer.

For critically ill children already in a PICU who require intrahospital transport for special diagnostic or therapeutic procedures, the risk benefit ratio of the procedure must be carefully examined. There are inherent hazards in moving an unstable patient and difficulties encountered in maintaining certain levels of care outside of a PICU (e.g. in the CT or MRI scanner). It may be in the best interests of a critically ill child to defer certain diagnostic procedures until the child's physiologic state is more tolerant of both the transport and the procedure itself.

For children in a tertiary care center emergency department who require transfer to a PICU for the continuation of definitive resuscitative care, the timing of that transfer should represent a careful consideration of the scope of care provided by that emergency department and whether the patient's needs have exceeded those capabilities. While there are inter-institutional variations, generally the scope of care provided by a tertiary center emergency department should include advanced physiologic support. Recognizing that such a department represents a relatively "stable" environment, the patient should not be transferred, and therefore subjected to an unstable environment (e.g. hallways, elevators, etc.), until definitive resuscitative care has been completed or the patient's condition has been stabilized to the point where they would be more tolerant of that transfer.

The timing of the transfer of a critically injured child from a PICU or a tertiary emergency department to an operating room for definitive surgical care represents a slightly different dilemma. A patient with a life threatening injury, such as an expanding epidural hematoma, or an unstable child with penetrating thoracic or abdominal trauma, should proceed rapidly for a definitive life saving procedure. While the mad dash down a hallway to an operating room with such a patient is inevitable, consideration must be given to doing so in a safe manner with the more basic resuscitative needs of the patient having already been met (e.g. placement of an airway and provision of assisted ventilation, and obtaining vascular access and the concurrent provision of fluids and medications). Additionally, the urgency to move such a patient quickly must be modulated by care taken so that harm, in the form of dislodged tubes, catheters, or monitoring devices, is prevented.

As should be the case for interhospital transports, the intrahospital transport of a critically ill patient should be conducted in a fashion so that there is no reduction in the level of care provided. This mandates the presence of a transport team with an adequate number of skilled health care professionals so that the many needs of these patients, such as airway, ventilation, and circulatory management, are met. The equipment and medications used in intrahospital transport should have the same portability features as that used for interhospital transport. Even for the most urgent transports, the patient should not be moved until the necessary personnel and equipment are present. Finally, the anticipation of the complex needs of critically ill children and the frequency of their intrahospital transport should prompt careful advanced planning. This planning should consider the development of necessary personnel and equipment resources to allow for the safest transport possible, and the development of institutional standards to guide the delivery of transport care.

REFERENCES

1. AAP Committee on Hospital Care: Guidelines for air and ground transportation of pediatric patients, *Pediatrics* 78:943-50, 1986.
2. Andrews PJD and others: Secondary insults during intrahospital transport of head-injured patients, *Lancet* 335:327-30, 1990.
3. Aoki BY, McCloskey K, editors: Evaluation, stabilization, and transport of the "critically ill" child, St. Louis, 1992, Mosby Yearbook Company.
4. Aprahamian CA and others: Traumatic cardiac arrest: scope of paramedic services, *Ann Emerg Med* 14:583-7, 1985.
5. Baxt WG: Impact of a rotocraft aeromedical emergency care service on trauma mortality, *JAMA* 249:3047-51, 1983.
6. Bowers SA, Marchall LF: Outcome of 200 consecutive cases of severe head injury treated in San Diego County: a prospective analysis, *Neurosurgery* 6:237-41, 1980.
7. Bushore M: Pediatric emergency care: where do we go from here? A pediatrician's view, *Pediatr Emerg Care* 2:258-63, 1986.
8. Cales RH: Trauma mortality in Orange County: the effect of implementation of a regional trauma system, *Ann Emerg Med* 13:1-10, 1984.
9. Chameides L, editor: *Textbook of Pediatric Advanced Life Support*, Dallas, Texas, 1988, American Heart Association.
10. Champion HR, Sacco WJ, Copes WS: Improvement in outcome from trauma center care, *Arch Surg* 127:333-5, 1992.
11. Chance GW, O'Brien MJ, Swyer PR: Transportation of sick neonates, 1972: an unsatisfactory aspect of medical care, *Can Med Assoc J* 109:847-52, 1973.
12. Chance GW and others: Neonatal transport: a controlled study of skilled assistance, *J Pediatr* 93:662-6, 1978.
13. Chou MM, MacDonald MG: Landmarks in the development of patient transport systems. In MacDonald MG, Miller MK, editors: *Emergency transport of the perinatal patient*, Boston, 1989, Little, Brown and Company.
14. Clemmer TP and others: Outcome of critically injured patients treated at Level I trauma centers versus full-service community hospitals, *Crit Care Med* 13:861-6, 1985.
15. Committee on Pediatric Emergency Medicine: *Emergency medical services for children*: the role of the primary care provider, Elk Grove Village, Illinois, 1992, American Academy of Pediatrics.
16. Committee on Trauma, American College of Surgeons: Advanced trauma life support course for physicians, Chicago, 1989, American College of Surgeons.
17. Copass MK and others: Prehospital cardiopulmonary resuscitation of the critically injured patient, *Am J Surg* 148:20-5, 1984.
18. Crippen D: Critical care transportation medicine: New concepts in pretransport stabilization of the critically ill patient, *Am J Emerg Med* 8:551-4, 1990.
19. Cunningham MD, Smith F: Stabilization and transport of severely ill infants, *Pediatr Clin North Am* 20:356-66, 1973.
20. Day S and others: Pediatric interhospital critical care transport: consensus of a national leadership conference, *Pediatrics* 88:696-704, 1991.
21. Detmer DC and others: Regional categorization and quality of care in major trauma, *J Trauma* 17:592-6, 1977.

22. Dobrin RS and others: The development of a pediatric emergency transport system, *Pediatr Clin North Am* 27:633-46, 1980.
23. Ferrara A: Evaluation of efficacy of regional perinatal programs, *Semin Perinat* 1:303-8, 1977.
24. Ferrara A and others: Effectiveness of neonatal transport in New York City in neonates less than 2500 gm: a population study, *J Comm Health* 13:303-8, 1988.
25. Fortner GS and others: The effects of prehospital care on the survival from a 50-meter fall, *J Trauma* 23:976-81, 1983.
26. Frew I, Roush WR, Lagreca K: COBRA: implications for emergency medicine, *Ann Emerg Med* 17:835-7, 1988.
27. Gervin AS, Fisher RP: The importance of prompt transport in salvage of patients with penetrating heart wounds, *J Trauma* 22:443-7, 1982.
28. Gudavalli M, Ferrara A, Harin A: The impact of physician's expertise on patient outcome in transportation of sick neonates, *Pediatr Res* 13:413, 1979 (abstract).
29. Haller JA: Towards a comprehensive emergency medical system for children, *Pediatrics* 86:120-2, 1990.
30. Harris TR, Isamen J, Giles HR: Improved neonatal survival through maternal transport, *Obstet Gynecol* 52:294-300, 1978.
31. Henning R, McNamara VL: Difficulties encountered in transport of the critically ill child, *Pediatr Emerg Care* 7:133-7, 1991.
32. Himmelstein DU and others: Patient transfers: medical practice as social triage, *Am J Pub Health* 74:494-7, 1984.
33. Indeck M and others: Risk, cost, and benefit of transporting ICU patients for special studies, *J Trauma* 28:1020-4, 1988.
34. Insel J and others: Cardiovascular changes during the transport of critically ill and postoperative patients, *Crit Care Med* 14:539-44, 1986.
35. Institute of Medicine Committee on Pediatric Emergency Medical Services: emergency medical services for children, Washington, DC, 1993, National Academy Press.
36. Ivatury RR, Nallathambi MN, Roberge RJ: Penetrating thoracic injuries: in-field stabilization vs. prompt transport, *J Trauma* 27:1068-71, 1987.
37. Jacobs LM and others: Prehospital advanced life support: benefits in trauma, *J Trauma* 24:8-13, 1984.
38. Kanter RK, Tompkins JM: Adverse events during interhospital transport: physiologic deterioration associated with pretransport severity of illness, *Pediatrics* 83:43-8, 1989.
39. Kanter RK and others: Excess morbidity associated with interhospital transport, *Pediatrics* 90:893-8, 1992.
40. Krug SE: Pediatric critical care transport: is time of the essence? Paper presented to Annual Meeting of the Ambulatory Pediatric Association, Anaheim, CA, May 1990.
41. Krug SE: Staff and equipment for pediatric critical care transport, *Curr Opin Pediatr* 4:445-50, 1992.
42. Lewis JK and others: Outcome of pediatric resuscitation, *Ann Emerg Med* 12:297-300, 1983.
43. Ludwig S, Kettrick RG, Parker M: Pediatric cardiopulmonary resuscitation, *Clin Pediatr* 23:71-6, 1984.
44. Macnab AJ: Optimal escort for interhospital transport of pediatric emergencies, *J Trauma* 31:205-9, 1991.
45. McCloskey KA, Johnston C: Pediatric critical care transport survey: team composition and training, mobilization time, and mode of transportation, *Pediatr Emerg Care* 6:1-5, 1990.
46. McCloskey KA, Orr RA: Pediatric transport issues in emergency medicine, *Emerg Med Clin of North Am* 9:475-89, 1991.
47. Mayer TA: Interhospital transfer of emergency patients, *Am J Emerg Med* 5:86-8, 1987.
48. Moylan J: Impact of helicopters on trauma care and clinical results, *Ann Surg* 208:673-8, 1988.
49. Moylan J and others: Factors improving survival in multisystem trauma patients, *Am Surg* 207:679-85, 1988.
50. Olson CM and others: Stabilization of patients prior to interhospital transfer, *Am J Emerg Med* 5:33-9, 1987.
51. Oreskovich M: Prehospital surgical care, Cited by Mayer TA: Transportation of the injured child, In Mayer TA, editor: Emergency management of pediatric trauma, Philadelphia, 1985, W.B. Saunders Company.
52. O'Rourke PP: Outcome of children who are apneic and pulseless in the emergency room, *Crit Care Med* 15:667-71, 1986.
53. Owen H, Duncan AW: Towards safer transport of sick and injured children, *Anaesth Intens Care* 11:113-7, 1983.
54. Pettett G, Merenstein GB: Stabilization of the high-risk neonate prior to transport. In MacDonald MG and Miller MK, editors: *Emergency transport of the perinatal patient,* Boston, 1989, Little, Brown, and Company.
55. Pollack MM and others: Accurate prediction of the outcome of pediatric intensive care: a new quantitative method, *N Eng J Med* 16:134-9, 1987.
56. Pollack MM and others: Efficiency of intensive care: a comparative analysis of eight pediatric intensive care units, *JAMA* 258:1481-5, 1987.
57. Pollack MM and others: Improving outcomes from tertiary pediatric intensive care: a statewide comparison of tertiary and non-tertiary care facilities, *Crit Care Med* 19:150-9, 1991.
58. Pollack MM and others: Improving the outcome and efficiency of intensive care: the impact of the intensivist, *Crit Care Med* 16:11-7, 1988.
59. Quan L and others: Outcomes and predictors for outcome in pediatric submersion victims receiving prehospital care in King County, Washington, *Pediatrics* 86:586-93, 1990.

60. Ramenofsky M and others: Maximum survival in pediatric trauma: the ideal system, *J Trauma* 24:808-12, 1984.
61. Ramsey CB, Holbrook PR: Pediatric Critical Care Transport. In Holbrook PR, editor: *Textbook of pediatric critical care,* Philadelphia, 1993, W.B. Saunders Company.
62. Rivara FP and others: Evaluation of potentially preventable deaths among pedestrian and bicycle fatalities, *JAMA* 261:566-70, 1989.
63. Rosenberg NM: Pediatric cardiopulmonary arrest in the emergency department, *Am J Emerg Med* 12:497-501, 1984.
64. Schiff RL and others: Transfers to a public hospital: a prospective study of 467 patients, *N Eng J Med* 314:552, 1986.
65. Schmidt U and others: On-scene helicopter transport of patients with multiple injuries: comparison of a German and an American system, *J Trauma* 33:548-53, 1992.
66. Seidel JS: Emergency medical services and the pediatric patient: are the needs being met? II. Training and equipping emergency medical services providers for pediatric emergencies, *Pediatrics* 78:808, 1986.
67. Seidel JS: History of EMS for children. In Dieckmann RA, editor: *Pediatric emergency care systems: planning and management,* Baltimore, 1992, Williams and Wilkins.
68. Seidel JS, Henderson DP, editors: *Emergency medical services for children: a report to the nation.* Washington, DC, 1991, National Center for Education in Maternal and Child Health.
69. Seidel JS and others: Emergency medical services and the pediatric patient: are the needs being met? *Pediatrics* 73:769-72, 1984.
70. Sloan EP, Callahan EP, Duda J: The effect of urban trauma system hospital bypass on prehospital transport times and Level I trauma patient survival, *Ann Emerg Med 18*:1146, 1989.
71. Simon JE: Current problems in the emergency management of severe pediatric illness. In Haller JA, editor: *Emergency medical services for children: Proceedings of the 97th Ross Conference on Pediatric Research,* Columbus, Ohio, 1989, Ross Laboratories.
72. Smith JP and others: Prehospital stabilization of critically injured patients: a failed concept, *J Trauma* 25:65-70, 1985.
73. Sumners J and others: Regional neonatal transport: impact of an integrated community/center system, *Pediatrics* 65:910, 1980.
74. Swyer PR: The regional organization of special care for the neonate, *Pediatr Clin North Am* 17:761, 1970.
75. Task Force on Interhospital Transport: Guidelines for air and ground transport of neonatal and pediatric patients, Elk Grove Village, Illinois, 1993, American Academy of Pediatrics.
76. Torphy DE, Minter MG, Thompson BM: Cardiorespiratory arrest and resuscitation of children, *Am J Dis Child* 138:1099-1112, 1984.
77. Trunkey DD: Is ALS necessary for pre-hospital trauma care? *J Trauma* 24:86-92, 1984.
78. Waisman Y and others: Management of children with epiglottitis during transport: analysis of a survey, *Pediatr Emerg Care* 9:191, 1993.
79. Wallen EA and others: Adverse events during intrahospital transport of critically ill children, *Crit Care Med* 19:S79, 1991 (abstract).
80. West JG, Cales RH, Gazzaniga AB: Impact of regionalization, *Arch Surg* 118:740, 1983.
81. West JG, Trunkey DD, Lim RC: Systems of trauma care: a study of two counties, *Arch Surg* 114:445, 1979.
82. Zaritsky A: Cardiopulmonary resuscitation in children, *Clin Chest Med* 8:561, 1987.

16

AEROMEDICAL PHYSIOLOGY

NEEL ACKERMAN

The aeromedical environment challenges medical transport personnel to understand and compensate for the dynamic and sometimes hostile conditions experienced during transport. A complete understanding of the physical laws related to altitude, the "stresses of flight," and the ability to understand and compensate for the physiological derangements inherent to the pathophysiology of the patient are the keys to a safe and successful aeromedical transport. This explains the important concepts and provides clinical examples which demonstrate the necessity of understanding the unique requirements of the aeromedical environment.

HISTORY

Many effects of altitude on humans have been known for hundreds of years. The Jesuit priest, Joseph de Acosta, made extensive observations of the natives of the Andes Mountains and published several speculations in his book *Natural y Moral de las Indias* in 1590. He noted ". . . I am convinced that the elements of the air in this place are so thin and so delicate that it is not proportionated to human breathing . . ."[10] It was, however, more than 200 years later, when balloons became fashionable, that the important effects of altitude became apparent.

In 1804 three Italians, Andreoli, Brasette, and Zambeccari, ascended in a balloon to an altitude in excess of 6,000 meters. They all experienced vomiting, lost consciousness, and suffered frostbite from the cold. Fortunately, the balloon crashed into the sea and they survived. Subsequently, Glasier and Coxwell in 1862 made flights in England and reported experiencing the classic signs of hypoxia and altitude sickness. Croce-Spinelli and Sivel in France in the early 1870s proved that supplemental oxygen abolished the symptoms related to altitude during simulated altitude chamber and balloon flights. Unfortunately, Croce-Spinelli and Sivel grossly miscalculated their oxygen requirements on a balloon flight in 1874 and died. Gaston Tissandier, the lone survivor of the ill-fated flight, subsequently wrote a classic description of the physiologic effects of hypoxia in Dr. Paul Bert's book *Barometric Pressure-Researches in Experimental Physiology*.[3,11,12]

By the early part of the twentieth century significant progress on altitude sickness had been made. A brave group of pioneering pilots, physicians, and physiologists strained to breech the lower levels of the atmosphere. The Wright Brothers' discovery of powered flight and the military advantages of the airplane in World War I further accelerated the efforts to go higher and faster. In 1919 Dr. Louis Bauer established the U.S. School for Flight Surgeons and in 1926 published *Aviation Medicine*, the first textbook of its kind in the United States. Advances made in many countries allowed the stratosphere to be breached. Auguste Piccard reached 51,795 feet in 1927 in a "space capsule" constructed by a beer barrel manufacturer.[12]

A significant group of "flying physicians" advanced the study of flight physiology during the 1930s and 1940s. In the U.S. Dr. Harry Armstrong was instrumental in establishing the Army Air Corp Aeromedical Laboratory. In Germany Dr. Hubertus Strughold accomplished major research efforts for the Aeromedical Institute of the German Air Ministry. The outbreak of World War II further accelerated the efforts and advances in aeromedical physiology. During WWII the first large scale, significant use of aircraft to move ill or injured patients was accomplished. Patient transport by fixed wing aircraft and by the more recently developed helicopter was further refined in both the Korean Conflict and Vietnam.[11,12]

The aircraft used for patient aeromedical transfers have changed little from a functional point of view since the time of the Vietnam War, but, advances in microprocessors, telemetry, and electronics (many from The National Aeronautics and Space Administration) have allowed the development of a thriving civilian aeromedical community. Critically ill or injured patients are routinely transferred by rotor or fixed wing aircraft to hospitals where they can receive definitive care. In addition, extraordinary support techniques such as Extra Corporeal Membrane Oxygenation, High Frequency Oscillation, and Aortic Balloon Pumps are routinely used as inflight support.[8,27] Indeed, while the military is still actively engaged in the research of problems and techniques for the aeromedical environment, many civilian medical centers and organizations are at the forefront of aeromedical physiology and patient care.

PHYSICAL LAWS

Boyle's law

Boyle's law describes the relationship between the volume and pressure of a gas. It states that the volume of a given mass of gas varies inversely to the pressure of the gas. So the same mass (number of gas molecules) has a smaller volume as pressure increases or a larger volume as pressure decreases.

$$P_aV_a = P_bV_b$$

where P_a = pressure at time a
V_a = volume at time a
P_b = pressure at time b
V_b = volume at time b

Real world problem. A calibrated ball and tube flow meter delivers 10 liters per minute flow of oxygen at sea level. How much flow will the flow meter deliver at 8,000 feet altitude?

The flow through a flow meter of this type is determined by an adjustable orifice with a high pressure source on one side and ambient pressure on the other. The size of the orifice determines the number of oxygen molecules that can exit per unit time. So if $P_a = 760$ torr and $V_a = 10$ liters at 8,000 feet, $P_b = 565$, and

$$V_b = (P_aV_a)/P_b$$
$$V_b = ((760)(10))/565$$
$$V_b = 13.45 \text{ liters}$$

Charles' law

Charles' Law describes the relationship between temperature and volume. As gas molecules are compressed, the temperature of the gas increases. Inversely as the temperature of a gas increases the volume increases since the gas molecules move faster and further apart.

$$V_a/V_b = T_a/T_b$$

where V_a = volume at time a
T_a = temperature at time a
V_b = volume at time b
T_b = temperature at time b

(temperature expressed as absolute = degrees C + 273)

Real world problem. A fixed wing aircraft flying at high altitudes pressurizes the ambient gas outside the aircraft to supply fresh air for the cabin. When the gas is compressed its temperature increases considerably. Therefore, even though the ambient temperature outside the aircraft may be below zero, the aircraft requires a cooling system after the pressurization system to deal with the temperature increase predicted by Charles's Law.

Dalton's law

Dalton's Law states that the total pressure of a gas is the sum of all the individual (partial) pressures of all the gases in a gas mixture. Thus, it can be seen that Dalton's Law describes the changes occurring within a gas mixture at different altitudes.

$$P_t = P_1 + P_2 + P_3 + P_4 + P_5 \ldots + P_n$$

where P_t = total pressure

and

$P_1 \ldots P_n$ = partial pressures of n gases

Real world example. During decompression of a previously pressurized aircraft cabin, the total pressure falls rapidly. This rapid fall in pressure (and the associated fall in temperature) suddenly reduces the capacity of the air to contain the water vapor previously present. Thus, an instantaneous fog occurs. It is interesting that interviews of survivors of several commercial aircraft crashes, in which explosive decompressions were a component of the emergency, describe the cabin rapidly filling with "smoke that didn't bother me." It is likely the passengers are describing the fogging phenomenon as the cabin rapidly depressurized.

Henry's law

Henry's Law describes the effect of soluble gases dissolved in liquids. The law states that the amount of gas dissolved in a liquid is proportional to the partial pressure of the gas over the liquid and the solubility of the gas in the particular liquid.

A problem in the real world. A recreational SCUBA diver spent several days investigating under-water shipwrecks in the Caribbean. He suffered a significant injury while exploring a wreck at a depth greater than 100 feet. His companions assisted him to the surface using appropriate decompression tables. Because of the seriousness of his injury, an aeromedical evacuation was ordered. Approximately 30 minutes after reaching cruising altitude (with a cabin pressure equal to 6,000 feet), the patient developed severe chest pain, dyspnea, cough, and a choking sensation. The symptoms were greatly reduced with the administration of 100% oxygen and pressurization of the aircraft cabin to sea level. A diagnosis of decompression sickness was made, and the diver was transported to a hyperbaric chamber where he made an uneventful recovery.

While the development of decompression sickness does not occur at typical cabin altitudes, Henry's Law easily explains this situation. Increased levels of gases are dissolved in the body tissues of the SCUBA diver due to the increased pressures encountered while diving. Every 30 feet of depth increases pressure by 1 atmosphere. Dive tables make allowances for gas egress from the tissues on return to sea level. However, if the patient is placed in the aeromedical environment and ambient pressure further decreases, there is a possibility that decompression sickness will result as the dissolved gases are no longer in solution. (For further information see section on Decompression Illness later in this book.)

STRESS OF FLIGHT

The stresses of flight are multiple and often interrelated (Table 16-1, Figure 16-1). They

TABLE 16-1 RELATIVE STRESSES DURING GROUND AND AIR PATIENT TRANSPORT

	Ground ambulance	*Rotor wing*	*Fixed wing unpressurized*	*Fixed wing pressurized*
Acceleration	–	–	+/–	+/–
Vibration	+	+	+/–	+/–
Noise	+/–	+	+	+/–
Thermal	–	+/–	–	+/–
Hypoxia	–	+/–	+	+/–
Gas expansion	–	+/–	+	+/–
Electromagnetic interference	+/–	+	+	+

Stresses of flight are compared to ground ambulance. A negative (–) indicates no significant problem in most situations. A sign of (+/–) indicates a potential for problems in some situations. A positive sign (+) indicates a significant problem which should be considered during every transport.

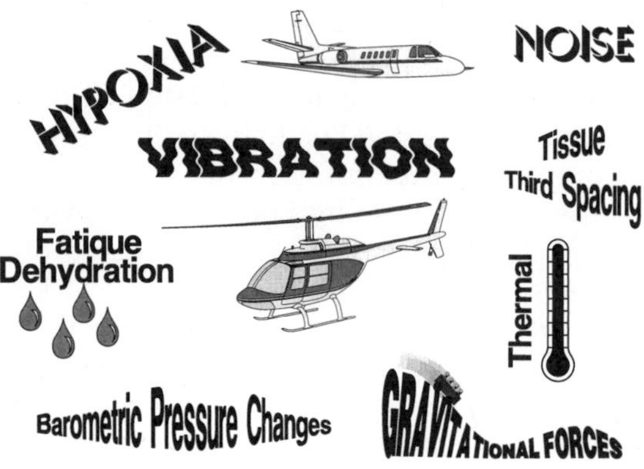

Fig.16-1. Stresses of Flight. The Aeromedical Environment is filled with stresses which must be routinely conquered by the pilots, medical crew, and patients.

include those factors that are pure manifestations of the physical laws as noted above. However, they also include many other factors related to the changes induced by man as we travel through the aeromedical environment. We will consider not only the impact of these stresses of flight on the patient but also on the crew and the medical equipment.

Barometric pressure changes

As we have noted, when considering the gas pressure laws, there can be dramatic and highly significant changes in both patients, crew, and equipment related to the physical alterations that occur with changes in altitude. There is a predictable change in gas volume at different barometric pressures and temperatures, as noted in the gas laws. Any gas-filled space in the human body or in the medical equipment is affected by the gas laws. We will consider these effects taking a systems approach (Figure 16-2).

Head, ears, nose, and throat. The sinuses and middle ear cavities are membrane-lined, air filled structures. Under optimal conditions these structures are vented to equilibrate with atmospheric pressure, therefore changes in barometric pressure have little or no effect. However, the presence of a cold, sinus infection, or allergies can be important during changes in the barometric pressure of the aeromedical environment.

Barotitis media, barometric pressure disturbance of the middle ear, is a common problem. The pressure in the middle ear is equilibrated via the eustachian tube that connects the middle ear with the nasopharynx. As external pressure changes occur, the air in the middle ear expands or contracts. Air then moves via the eustachian tube either into or out of the middle ear to allow equilibration. The situation is complicated somewhat since the eustachian tube functionally acts as a one-way valve which allows gas to escape from but not enter the middle ear. In most people equalization occurs spontaneously even during descent by normal breathing, swallowing, and jaw motion, provided the pressure changes do not occur very rapidly. In some individuals, equilibration of the middle ear requires active efforts such as opening the jaw widely, as in yawning or by exhaling slightly against a closed upper airway in order to create positive pressure in the nasopharynx (Valsalva maneuver).

A cold or allergies can result in problems with pressure equilibration. Barotitis media or ear block occurs most commonly on descent due to the unidirectional nature of the eustachian tube, but similar symptoms can occur with either increases or decreases in barometric pressure. Distortion of the tympanic membrane and over/under pressurization of the middle ear can cause tinnitus, mild to severe pain, bleeding, nausea, vertigo, and

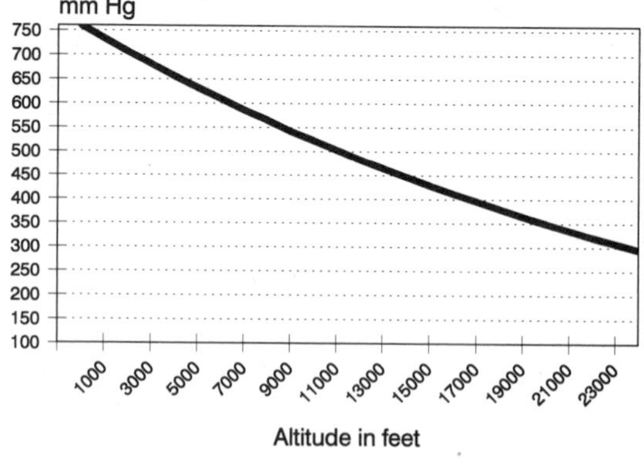

Fig. 16-2. Barometric Pressure Change as a function of Altitude. There is a predictable fall in total barometric pressure at increasing altitudes. The known change can be used to predict changes in gas expansion, patient/crew oxygenation, etc. using the Gas Equations, Alveolar Gas Equation, etc.

transient, conductive hearing loss. If the pressure differential is not relieved, a transudate will be formed in the middle ear that resolves when eustachian tube function normalizes. Perforation of the tympanic membrane occurs but is rare and usually heals without sequela.

The risks of allowing infants and children to fly with otitis media or serous otitis media are still debated.[38] In theory, if the middle ear is completely fluid filled, there should be minimal risk. Experienced ENT (ears, nose, and throat) specialists often allow children to take commercial flights within 36 hours of initiation of therapy for acute otitis media. Schwartz reports only two cases of ruptured tympanic membranes or intense otalgia in 36 years.[28] He suggests the administration of topical nasal decongestants 30 minutes before landing and drinking liquids during descent.

Treatment of in-flight barotitis media consists mainly of prevention and early recognition. Many flight organizations bar flight crew members with upper respiratory infections, sore throats, otitis media, or severe active upper respiratory allergic symptoms. There is an unresolved controversy regarding the risks of flying with otitis media. Medical personnel involved in air transport should be aware of early symptoms of barotitis media so that they can protect both themselves and their patients. The use of the Valsalva maneuver, frequent swallowing, yawning, etc. to open the eustachian tube at the earliest sign of problems is very important. The use of a vasoconstrictive nasal spray such as 0.25% phenylephrine is also frequently helpful. The Politzer procedure[29] may be helpful in that it forces air into the middle ear by means of a one ounce infant nasal bulb syringe inserted into one nostril while the other nostril is occluded.[29] The flight crew should be promptly notified of any illness to allow flight return to a slightly higher altitude which can relieve symptoms and allow easier equilibration.

A less well known, but equally painful, ear problem is external otic barotrama. This condition develops when airtight earplugs or other material completely seals the external auditory canal during descent. The negative pressure created behind the obstruction may damage the epithelial lining of the canal. Most commonly "blood blisters" are produced in the subepithelial areas. Air crews and aeromedical patients should not wear ear plugs or protectors that create an airtight seal, are unvented, or cannot be quickly and easily removed.[34]

The pathophysiology of barosinusitis is similar to that of barometrically induced ear problems. Barosinusitis can occur with ascent or descent but is most common during descent. Pus, mucous, blood, mucosal edema, or foreign bodies obstructing the openings to the sinus cavities may induce the condition. Treatment should begin at the first sign of symptoms and consist of clearing obstructing material if possible, using topical vasoconstrictive nasal sprays, and returning the cabin to the previous pressure, if possible. Obviously, crew members should not fly with acute sinus inflammation.

Patients with upper respiratory disease or injury are at high risk for developing sinus and middle ear problems. However, there are some patients with diseases that are less obvious. Sinus and middle ear problems in the infant or small child, who is unable to describe symptoms, will not likely be noticed until painful symptoms occur. Encouraging small children to chew gum, eat, or drink during ascent and descent will reduce the possibilities of air blockage. Older patients who sleep during flight, typically swallow less frequently and can experience painful symptoms. Symptoms can be magnified if patients are receiving poorly humidified oxygen, as this tends to dry the mucosa and potentiate the possibilities for obstruction of the eustachian tube or paranasal sinuses. Similarly, the intubated patient or patient with a large nasogastric tube may have enough edema of the nasopharynx to compromise eustachian tube function.

Air in structures which are not normally air filled can cause significant problems. Patients with recent neurosurgical procedures and residual intracranial air or patients who have had recent pneumoencephalograms should not be transported by air unless sea level altitudes can be maintained. Patients with gas within the globe of the eye from trauma or surgical procedures should not be transported in an unpressurized aircraft unless cleared by an ophthalmologist.

Respiratory system. Barometric pressure changes affect the respiratory system both by the physical effects of changes in gas density and volume and by the potential for creation of hypoxia due to decreased partial pressures of oxygen (Figure 16-3). We will discuss the influence of barometric pressure changes in producing hypoxia and its relationship to the respiratory system in the next section.

Expansion of extrapulmonary intrathoracic air is a major problem during aeromedical evacuation. A small pneumothorax that was assymptomatic at sea level expands approximately 30% at 7,000-8,000 feet altitude. This expansion, plus the decreased partial pressure of oxygen (also approximately 30% if the FiO_2 has not been increased), can create a situation where a patient with a small pneumothorax and normal arterial blood gases at ground level has significant respiratory distress at normal cabin altitudes. The use of a chest tube greatly reduces the possibility of respiratory deterioration. Other intrathoracic gas collections can also expand and compromise physiologic function.[4] Infants with severe cystic pulmonary interstitial emphysema and large intrapulmonary blebs will frequently have increased difficulties during transport.[1,4] This is quite likely due to expansion of the blebs with compression of functional pulmonary tissue. The gas in a pneumomediastinum expands according to Boyle's Law but rarely seems to cause physiologic compromise itself. It can however rupture into the pleural cavity as it expands and cause a new pneumothorax.

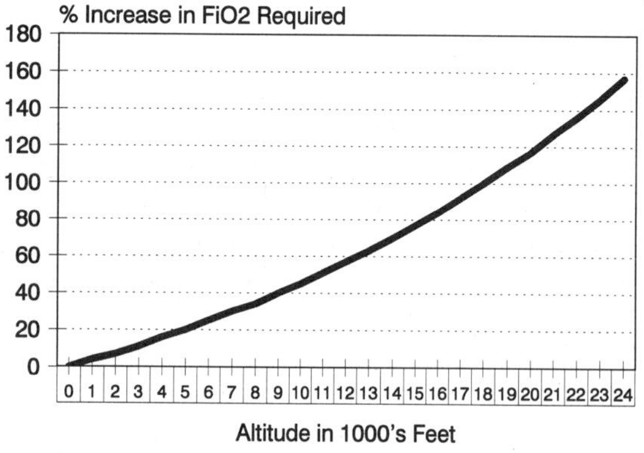

Fig. 16-3. Percentage Increase in Oxygen Required at Altitude. Predicted changes in FiO_2 requirement with increasing altitudes to maintain current alveolar PO_2 were calculated and graphically plotted. The plot accounts for only change in inspired PO_2 and not for changes in shunts, pulmonary vasoconstriction, etc.

Gastrointestinal system. There is usually no significant impact of altitude on the gastrointestinal system of healthy individuals. The gases in the stomach and intestine expand according to Boyle's Law. Thus, there will be approximately 30% expansion of the intestinal gas volume during ascent to normal cruising altitudes of 7,000-8,000 feet. Obviously, this could pose serious problems for certain patients with gastrointestinal problems.

Patients with a bowel obstruction or significantly distended stomach or intestines can experience severe pain with gas expansion. In addition, in patients who have had recent abdominal surgery, there is a risk of suture rupture. All patients with the possibility of experiencing gastric or intestinal distention require a vented nasogastric tube before transport.[24] Patients with recent abdominal surgery and a significant illeus should have transport delayed for approximatly 48 hours, if possible. Expansion of gas in the abdomen may splint the diaphragm and cause new or worsened respiratory distress. This is especially true in neonates with respiratory distress syndrome. Most neonates should have a nasogastric tube placed before transport to prevent gastric distension from causing or worsening respiratory distress.

Patients with hiatial hernias and gastroesophogeal reflux will occasionally experience increased symptoms, such as burping and pain during ascent, presumably related to gas expansion. Patients with health conditions that induce increased flatus may experience increased gas passage at higher altitudes. Probably due to similar mechanisms, patients with ileostomies and colostomies may require more frequent bag changes or venting of the bag apparatus. Unconscious patients will often have more frequent stools during air transports.[24]

Decompression sickness. Decompression sickness results from the formation of gas bubbles in various body tissues during periods of decreased ambient pressure exposure or following periods of increased ambient pressure exposure. Decompression sickness has been recognized for more than 250 years and has been responsible for significant morbidity with at least 18 cases of death in aviators. The development of pressurized cabins has greatly decreased morbidity from decompression.[3,12,20] The possibility of developing decompression sickness in the aeromedical environment is remote in typical situations. An incidence of 1.5% might be expected in situations where humans, previously at sea level, were exposed to altitudes of greater than 26,000 feet for longer than 30 minutes.[14] In fact, Davis and others reported that 79% of altitude decompression sickness cases occurred as a result of exposure to altitudes greater than 30,000 feet.[9] Thus, even in cases in which cabin decompressions occur, passengers would not be exposed to required altitudes for a long enough period of time to typically display symptoms.

There are profound dangers associated with flying following recreational SCUBA diving or aeromedical transport involving diving accident victims. Divers experience an increase in ambient pressure of approximately one atmosphere for every 30 feet of water. This can induce the dissolution of significant amounts of gas into tissues. If these individuals are then exposed to decreased ambient pressures during flight situations their chances of developing symptoms are greatly increased. Decompression sickness has occurred at altitudes commonly used by commercial and aeromedical transport aircraft (less than 5,000 feet cabin altitude) in patients who have very recently been SCUBA diving. Crew members should never fly within 24 hours of SCUBA diving. SCUBA accident victims should be transported by ground ambulance whenever possible. The use of low flying helicopters does not alleviate the risk.

Bubble formation in decompression sickness can induce a variety of symptoms. The bends accounts for approximately 70% of the cases. In the bends the patient experiences joint pain, which tends to be localized in the large joints but can also involve smaller joints. The pain occurs following exposure to decreased pressure and is relieved by return to increased ambient pressures. The chokes, another decompression sickness syndrome, is manifested as a choking sensation which includes chest pain, dyspnea, and cough. It appears to be related to the formation of multiple pulmonary gas emboli. Although rare, a number of other circulatory, peripheral, and central neurologic syndromes are associated with decompression sickness. Patients with known or suspected decompression sickness should be immediately returned to the highest ambient barometric pressure possible, placed on 100% oxygen, and be appropriately monitored and stabilized. All but the mildest cases, which are permanently and immediately relieved by returning to ground level, require transfer to a facility with hyperbaric capabilities.

Medical equipment. The effects of changes in barometric pressure on medical equipment are highly significant. Generally it is easy to anticipate and correct or compensate for many changes in barometric pressure. However, there are other alterations which are not as easy to anticipate, detect, or prevent.

The expansion of gas in closed containers, such as in the endotracheal tube cuff, can be anticipated. Gas in the cuff expands according to Boyle's Law. Obviously, a cuff inflated at ground level would expand with increasing altitude. The expansion could then rupture the cuff or compress the tracheal mucosa resulting in ischemic necrosis. This phenomenon can be prevented by partially deflating the cuff before takeoff or by inflating the cuff with saline instead of air. Alternately, one may use a large volume, low pressure cuff or a one of several designs of foam cuffs. An unvented sphygmomanometer cuff or pneumatic splint will also inflate as a result of the gas expansion which is seen at decreased barometric pressures, potentially causing vascular compromise to the extremity. Vacuum splints tend to soften with increasing altitude. Unvented glass IV bottles have shattered due to pressure build-up from gas expansion. The same mechanism can cause significant variation in IV flow rates as the air in the bottles and/or IV drip chambers expand and contract with altitude changes. The author experienced a near drowning of a dog during a simulated flight in an altitude chamber when the air in a sealed ventilator heated, resulting in the humidification system expanding and pushing approximately 500 cc of sterile water into the ventilator circuit.

The effect of altitude on flowmeters, ventilators, and other pneumatically-related equipment is difficult to anticipate. Most flowmeters appear to be delivering the same flow of gas at altitude as there were at ground level. Measurements at the United States Air Force (USAF) School of Aerospace Medicine have demonstrated that in fact gas flowmeters operated at high altitudes deliver the same mass of gas molecules but different volumes.[2] For example, an oxygen flowmeter set at 10 liters per minute on the ground would deliver approximately 13 liters per minute at a cabin altitude of 7,000-8,000 feet, due to gas expansion. However, the mass of gas (number of oxygen molecules) delivered per minute would not change. Ventilators may have behaved differently in response to changing barometric pressures. Because pneumatic ventilators are essentially flowmeters with exhalation valves, one might expect that the tidal volumes which are delivered would increase and, in many cases, they do. However, because peak inspiratory pressure, distending pressure, inspiratory time, expiratory time, etc., is typically determined by the bleed or pressurization time of pneumatic cartridges, the other ventilatory variables can increase, decrease, or stay the same. In fact, the ventilators often operate erratically until certain critical altitudes/pressures are reached. One widely used neonatal transport ventilator operates predictably until the aircraft reaches an altitude of approximately 22,000 feet, at which point it locks in an inspiration mode.[2] Electronically controlled ventilators usually do not experience significant variations in ventilatory parameters but may vary in flow rates and tidal volume delivery. Volume ventilators tend to deliver progressively smaller tidal volumes at increasing altitudes due to gas compression effects within the ventilator circuit.[2,26]

Evaluate the effects of changes in altitude on medical equipment before using this equipment in an aircraft. Airtight casings can produce shrapnel if they explode in a sudden decompression. An unvented mattress cover in an isolette blew up like an air bag during a sudden decompression from 7,000 to 50,000 feet. The memory of a baby doll being crushed between the mattress and the top of the isolette drove home the necessity of testing. Testing of equipment for use in the aeromedical environment is accomplished at the USAF School of Aerospace Medicine at Brooks Air Force Base in San Antonio, Texas. Information regarding the approval or disapproval of specific medical devices is available in technical reports published by the USAF.

Hypoxia

Hypoxia describes the situation in which body tissues do not receive or adequately utilize oxygen at the cellular level. Hypoxia in the aeromedical environment can occur within four (or various combinations of four) physiologic categories.

Hypoxic hypoxia. A failure to achieve adequate oxygen transfer at the alveolar level is called hypoxic hypoxia. Thus, the physical components impacting the development of hypoxic hypoxia are the inspired partial pressure of oxygen and the efficiency of gas exchange at the level of the alveolus. The role of altitude in Dalton's Law of Partial Pressures creates a situation of decreased partial oxygen pressures at increasing altitudes. Essentially, fewer oxygen molecules are available at the surface of the alveolar membrane (e.g. 30% less at 8,000 feet) for gas exchange. The partial pressure of oxygen at the alveolus is directly influenced by altitude and can be calculated from the alveolar gas equation.

$$PAO_2 = (PB\text{-}PH_2O)FiO_2 - PaCO_2[FiO_2 + (1\text{-}FiO_2/R)]$$

where PaO_2 = Mean alveolar oxygen pressure
PB = Ambient barometric pressure
PH_2O = Vapor pressure of water (body temp.)
FiO_2 = Inspired fraction of oxygen
$PaCO_2$ = Mean alveolar carbon dioxide
R = Respiratory exchange ratio

Patients with pulmonary problems and an increased alveolar-arterial O_2 gradient are at risk for developing hypoxic hypoxia even at normal cabin altitudes. It should be noted that in situations in which an increased $AaDO_2$ gradient is secondary to a fixed intracardiac or intrapulmonary shunt, altitude may have a minimal impact on the arterial PO_2. In practice it is often difficult to assess the relative importance of alveolar diffusion defects versus shunting. The safest approach is to assume that the diffusion defect is the primary component and then increase the inspired oxygen by an appropriate amount. However, since the reduction in cabin pressure may allow aircraft to fly further, faster, or higher (above bad weather), it is occasionally necessary to determine the relative importance of fixed shunting prior to transport or in a self-controlled trial and error experiment after takeoff.

Hyperemic hypoxia. If the oxygen carrying capacity of the blood is decreased, oxygen delivery to tissues may be limited. The vast majority of oxygen transport is done by hemoglobin. Thus, situations negatively impacting the amount or function of hemoglobin may produce hyperemic hypoxia.

Anemic patients or flight crew may encounter significant changes in tissue oxygen delivery. There are no absolute standards for determining hemoglobin concentrations and there are multiple factors to consider. The level of expected oxygen consumption is important. A stable chronically anemic immobile patient with no respiratory problems may do well with a hemoglobin of 7-8 milligrams per decliter. A child with respiratory distress and poorly compensated congestive heart failure or an infant with acute anemia and respiratory distress syndrome may deteriorate despite hemoglobin levels greater than 9 milligrams per deciliter. Similarly, a medical crew member with anemia who is actively involved in patient care may suffer significant performance deterioration at decreased barometric pressures. One must always remember that greater than 5 g of unsaturated hemoglobin is required to produce cyanosis. Thus, it is possible to have a significantly anemic patient with inadequate tissue oxygen delivery but no cyanosis.

Carboxyhemoglobin and methemoglobin are not effective in oxygen transport. Carbon monoxide is present in the exhaust of both conventional internal combustion and jet engines and can contaminate the aeromedical environment. Carbon monoxide (CO) is also present in smoke (from fires, cigarettes, etc.). Since CO combines tightly with hemoglobin, the hemoglobin is no longer available for gas transport. Methemoglobinemia occurs in response to many drugs in susceptible patients. The chocolately brown methemoglobin also does not carry oxygen well and can greatly reduce tissue oxygen delivery.

Stagnant hypoxia. Stagnant hypoxia results from inadequate blood flow to the body or to a particular area of the body. Patients with inadequate cardiac function may be unable to increase cardiac output to compensate for the "normal" decrease in oxygen tension that occurs with decreased barometric pressure. Any of the multiple factors producing shock act, in the end, by reducing oxygen delivery to the tissues. Localized tissues and organs can also be affected. Hyperventilation can reduce cerebral blood flow to potentially compromising levels. Pneumatic splint hyperinflation with decreased barometric pressures can compromise limb blood flow by compressing vessels. Vascular gas bubbles from malfunctioning intravenous equipment or decompression sickness can occlude vessels and compromise limbs and organs via stagnant hypoxia.

Histotoxic hypoxia. Many cellular poisons compromise the cytochrome oxidase enzyme system and impair the ability to use oxygen at the cellular level. Cyanide, carbon monoxide, hydrogen sulfide, and ethyl alcohol all can produce varying levels of histotoxic hypoxia. The effects of these agents (especially alcohol) may not be apparent at sea level but may produce serious tissue changes in reduced oxygen tension environments. It is especially important to note that the negative cellular cytochrome effects of ethyl alcohol can still be apparent many hours later, long after the CNS intoxicating effects have resolved.

Effects of hypoxia. Regardless of which of the four types of hypoxia occurs, there are several physiologic manifestations that range from minor to life-threatening. Many factors influence the individual response to hypoxia including heredity, fatigue, metabolic rate, alcohol intake, physical fitness, and emotion.

These interactions make predicting an individual's response to a specific degree of hypoxia unsure at best.

Cardiopulmonary response to hypoxia. Mild to moderate acute hypoxia may result in hyperpnea and an increased cardiac output. This effectively maximizes both gas exchange at the alveolar level and oxygen delivery by the circulatory system. Hypoxia also causes pulmonary vasospasm, on increase in pulmonary artery pressures, and right-sided cardiac work. The maximum cardiopulmonary compensation occurs at approximately 20,000 feet. Exposure to higher altitudes inevitably leads to cardiopulmonary failure with pulmonary edema, bradycardia, hypotension, and arrhythmia.

Hyperventilation. Hyperventilation may be a physiologic response to hypoxia but could just as well be a manifestation of a variety of other cardiorespiratory, neurologic, or metabolic abnormalities. The most common causes of hyperventilation in the aeromedical transport environment are pain, fear, anxiety, and the stresses of flight itself, such as heat and vibration. During hyperventilation the patient increases minute ventilation and decreases the alveolar CO_2 levels, producing a systemic alkalosis. An immediate effect of alkalosis is a shift of the oxyhemoglobin dissociation curve to the left and upward (the Bohr effect). The shift increases the ability of blood to carry oxygen but decreases its ability to release oxygen at the tissue level, potentially creating a situation of stagnant hypoxia. Extracellular/intracellular cation shifts, tachycardia, decreased cardiac output, decreased cerebral blood flow, muscular spasms, incoordination or tetany, and unconsciousness are all common symptoms of significant hyperventilation.

It is important to distinguish hypoxia with secondary hyperventilation and hyperventilation from other potential causes. Patients with hypoxia-induced hyperventilation tend to have a picture of a rapidly occurring cyanotic episode with decreased muscle tone and no signs of tetany. Those with hyperventilation from other causes usually have a gradual onset of symptoms. They commonly are pale with clammy skin and have muscle spasms and/or tetany.

Treatment of the hyperventilating patient must be aimed at the primary cause, if it can be determined. Although patients are commonly treated by breathing into a bag to increase CO_2 levels, this therapy should be carefully used and monitored frequently due to the possibility of harm if hypoxia is the primary cause. A safer approach may be to increase the inspired FiO_2 and quickly evaluate and treat the primary cause (e.g., alleviate anxiety, give analgesics, cool the patient, etc.).

Nervous system response. The CNS effects associated with hypoxia are especially dangerous as they are relatively insidious. Early signs include mild mental impairment, mild drowsiness, and decreased night vision. Mental impairment worsens progressively with increasing hypoxia. Individuals may not recognize the impairment, in fact many hypoxic patients experience a "buzz" similar to that experienced with alcohol intoxication. Often, poor judgement, decreased short-term memory, inability to perform calculations, and significantly delayed reaction times are also displayed. In some individuals there may be few intervening signs before the sudden loss of consciousness. This author was especially impressed while monitoring a simulated altitude exposure demonstration for twelve medical students. After less than 5 minutes, one student lost consciousness, while none of the other eleven had noticed the change in their colleague. During my first simulated exposure I remember thinking, "this is not a problem; I feel great; but, why can't I remember what four times seven is?" Each person's symptomatic response to hypoxia is different, yet neural function is always impaired. Effective performance time is the time a person can perform useful duties in an environment of inadequate oxygen.[30] This time can range from as long as 20 to 30 minutes at 18,000 feet altitude to 15 to 20 seconds at 40,000 feet. The brief time period available at high altitudes is the reason for commercial cabin crew reminding passengers to put on their own plastic cup mask first before attempting to help anyone else in an emergency decompression. Obviously, it is necessary for a medical flight crew to have an idea of the flight plan and cruising altitude to choose the correct sequence of actions in an emergency decompression.

Humidity

The absolute amount of moisture in the environment drops with increasing altitude. This decrease in relative humidity is due to a decrease in temperature and the lower absolute partial pressure of gases at higher altitudes. In addition, the methods used to pressurize the ambient air used in the aircraft tend to further dry air. In many large aircraft the cabin is pressurized by bleeding heated air from the engines. As this hot air is cooled for use in the cabin the small amount of humidity present is further depleted as it condenses during cooling.

Baseline fluid losses can increase several fold with altitude exposure. Both patients and crew commonly experience dry eyes and mouth, chapped lips, nasal drying, hoarseness, and sore throat. Dehydration can develop if adequate fluids are not provided by oral or intravenous routes.

A person breathing through the nose should experience no significant drying of the lower respiratory passages. However, patients breathing spontaneously through their mouth can experience significant airway drying. Patients receiving either medical or aircraft grade oxygen (which are essentially dry gases) are at even more risk of airway compromise from thickened secretions and airway damage from drying. Intubated patients are at special risk unless gases are well humidified.

Both patients and crew need to significantly increase fluid intake in the aeromedical environment. Patients with respiratory problems, especially those with endotracheal tubes or tracheostomies, are at special risk. Adequate humidification of the dry gases is important in flights of any significant duration.

Thermal

In the aeromedical environment it is likely that patients will be exposed to a variety of thermal variants. Besides those differences and stresses induced by the climatic changes from transport there are intratransport changes associated with altitude and aircraft design.

The availability of long-range jet aircraft makes moving patients long distances relatively common. Consequently, patients and crew may leave a warm climate and arrive several hours later in an area with subfreezing temperatures. Thus, careful planning to provide appropriate clothing for crew and patients is essential. The use of rotor wing aircraft for near door-to-door-interhospital transports occasionally leads flight crews to fail to dress appropriately for the outside weather. If the aircraft is forced to make an emergency landing, severe problems associated with outdoor exposure may be experienced.

A drop in ambient temperature of approximately 3.5°F is experienced for each 1,000 foot increase in altitude at altitudes in the flight range of commercial aircraft.[4] Therefore, at 10,000 feet the temperature will be approximately 30-35 degrees cooler than at sea level and more than 100 degrees cooler at 35,000 feet. An effective heating/cooling system is required in helicopters and nonpressurized fixed wing aircraft. In pressurized fixed wing aircraft an efficient thermal environmental control system is even more important because of the heat which is generated and added to the cabin atmosphere during pressurization.

Even in situations with a normal cabin air temperature, the crew must be aware of other thermal difficulties. Aircraft walls can be quite cold and, patients can loose significant heat via conductive mechanisms. Similarly, wet patients or patients in areas of increased ventilation flow can lose heat via convective and evaporative mechanisms. Covering and wrapping the patient with blankets can greatly reduce heat loss. On the other hand, direct sunlight can overheat patients, even if the surrounding air temperature is normal. In some older rotor aircraft, internal walls radiate heat from the engines and rotor mechanisms. Cooling with increased ventilation and fluids may be required, especially in older rotor and nonpressurized fixed wing aircraft.

Noise and vibration

Sound is produced by variations in air pressure within the frequency range that causes detectable vibrations of the tympanic membrane and inner ear structures. Vibrations and the disorganized sounds that we call noise are major problems in the aeromedical environment. Noise and vibration have been studied extensively in the workplace,[17] but few studies regarding the effects of noise in the transport environment are available.[31] There are significant variances in the levels of noise and vibration induced by different aircraft. In general, rotor wing aircraft produce greater noise and ongoing vibratory effects than pressurized fixed wing aircraft. However, peak vibratory and noise levels may be most intense during the takeoff of a fixed wing aircraft.

The effects of noise and vibrations on sick patients are well established. Campbell and others[5] reported on noise and vibration levels associated with the transport of neonates via ground, rotor, and fixed wing aircraft. They concluded, "When compared with adult tolerance levels, both sound and vibration exposures are high and potentially hazardous." He measured sound levels over 100 dB in all the aircraft. Since prolonged exposure to sound levels in excess of 80 dB is associated with sensorineural hearing loss[22] in adults, the effect of noise on immature systems with other simultaneous ototoxic exposures is disconcerting.[13]

The impact of vibration on patients is difficult to evaluate. The only specific vibration induced medical condition is the "white fingers" syndrome.[35] This is a syndrome caused by job exposure over years to certain vibrating construction tools and other tools such as chain saws. It appears to affect bones, joints, muscles, connective tissues, nerves, and the vascular system. Usual signs include impairment of either the peripheral nervous or circulatory systems. Raynaud's phenomenon, the most consistent presentation, states that vibration injury occurs through mechanisms related to tissue resonance.[32] Low compliance tissues have high resonant frequencies (e.g. skull = 500 Hz), while compliant tissues tend to have low resonant frequencies (e.g. brain = 20 Hz). The clinical significance of body tissue exposure to these potentially resonant frequencies during transport is unknown. Clark and others[7] demonstrated the development of pulmonary edema in adult humans and animals exposed to low frequency vibration. They also showed significant changes in mean blood pressure which seem to be related to exposure to vibration. Floyd and others[14] described changes in peripheral nerve conduction velocities in monkeys exposed to whole body vibration.

Noise and vibration clearly can affect the short term physiologic functions of the flight crew and also expose them to potentially auditory damaging levels over long-term exposures. Noise in aircraft typically are annoying, decrease flight crew performance levels, and hamper speech communications. Humans clearly perceive some sounds as noise, and in these situations, experience a clear decrease in tolerance to anxiety-producing or otherwise annoying situations. Tasks requiring vigilance are not performed as well in a noisy environment. Noise is said to increase the number of errors but does not reduce the speed at which work occurs. In addition, noise may contribute to general fatigue and irritability. Vibratory effects on the flight crew are real, including headache, visual fatigue, motion sickness, thermoregulatory problems, and chest or abdominal pain.[37]

Protection from noise can be obtained by using ear plugs, headsets, or helmets. Both patients and crew should be protected. To achieve this protection, however, the crew becomes unable to use a traditional medical tool, the stethoscope. This should not keep the crew from wearing protective devices in light of information provided by Hunt and others.[21] They demonstrated that flight nurses were unable to hear normal breath sounds with traditional or electronically amplified stethoscopes during helicopter flights. A new technological development uses a small computer to sense noise and then generate a mirror image sound that exactly cancels the noise. This technology potentially allows the wearer to filter out unwanted "noisy" portions of the auditory spectrum but still allow communication and patient evaluation including auscultatory findings.

Medical equipment can also be severely affected by vibration. Vibration in aircraft can occur along multiple axes simultaneously. Screws and bolts tend to "work out" over time, even with modest amounts of vibration.

Electrical connections to circuit boards, hinges, and joints secured with adhesives all tend to fail more frequently when exposed to vibrations. Many otherwise perfectly acceptable pieces of medical equipment have been reduced to nonfunctioning piles of plastic and metal within a few minutes following exposure to the vibratory phase of testing at the USAF School of Aerospace Medicine. Common sites of failure include metal and plastic connections, electrical connections, and circuit board cracks or securing failures. Medical equipment routinely used in high vibration environments should undergo routine preventive maintenance checks which includes tightening important structural screws and bolts and checking circuit boards of electronic devices to ensure stability.

Vibration can also interfere with the functioning of medical devices without harming the device itself. Cardiorespiratory monitors can give erroneous readings during periods of high vibration. Pulse oximeters frequently fail to "lock in" on the peripheral pulse and give questionable or clearly erroneous measurements. Gordon and others[18] and French and Tillman[15] have reported a pacemaker malfunction occurring during helicopter transport which is apparently related to vibratory interactions. The possibility of vibration-induced malfunctions in complex medical devices such as aortic balloon pumps and portable ECMO systems have been discussed at national medical meetings and cannot be ignored. Although no known complications have occurred, the complexity of the devices, associated sensors, and the critical nature of the patient makes vigilance an absolute necessity.

Acceleration and gravitational forces

Although patients and crew are routinely subjected to increased gravitational and accelerational forces, the current sentiment is that the changes are not so great as to be significant in the typical patient. The complex hemodynamic interactions of the cardiovascular system likely can compensate for the small changes in venous return, cardiac output, etc., during the ascent and descent of fixed wing aircraft.

In some patients there are theoretical reasons for patient positioning during takeoff and/or landings in fixed wing aircraft. With premature neonates at risk for intracranial bleeding or patients with head injury or fluid overload, there may be advantages to placing the patient's head toward the front of the aircraft in order to encourage fluid to pool in the lower extremities and to reduce the risk of a transient increase in intracranial pressure during takeoff. The arguments can be used to position patients exactly opposite during landings when the forces act in the opposite direction. Until controlled studies or other scientific data are accumulated, patient positioning within the aircraft should be more a function of the logistics of loading, unloading, and patient access than theoretical concerns regarding small accelerational changes.

Great care should be exercised, however, to adequately stabilize the patient, crew, and equipment to prevent shifting, falls, and other accidents during periods of acceleration, deceleration, or turbulence. The risks of unsecured medical equipment and monitors becoming dangerous projectiles should not be minimized. Whenever possible, equipment should be safely stowed away from the patient care area. Both patients and crew should be adequately restrained during the flight, except as required for patient care. Adequate restraints during takeoff and landings are a necessity.

Perceptual and spatial disorientation

The correct spatial and perceptual orientation of the pilot and other members of the flight crew is critical to success of any flight. Tremendous amounts of information have been written from the pilot's point of view.[16] Most of the problems are not directly relevant to the transport team except as spatial orientation and perceptions on impact motion sickness.

Motion sickness is a problem during all forms of transport. It is characterized by lethargy, headache, increased salivation, a warm sensation, nausea, pallor, cold sweats, and vomiting. It is said that as many as 40% of pilot trainees become airsick at least once during their training.[15] However, only about 1% are eliminated due to intractable airsickness.

Only about 1% of commercial passengers report airsickness.

Motion sickness seems to occur when motions and visual clues are unusual or unexpected or which produce sensory conflict. The simplest hypothesis states that conflicting information between several senses, including the vestibular system, produce the physiologic symptoms. This would explain why people can experience symptoms of motion sickness while sitting absolutely still and watching a movie with a chase scene. The visual findings conflict with the vestibular sensations. Treisman[36] proposes an extension of these observations which explains the problem from a teleologic point of view. He hypothesized that vestibular and other orientation systems serve as an emetic response to poisons. When an animal eats a toxic substance and consequently experiences the CNS effects it results in a reflex vomit response to rid the body of the poison. The theory has been validated in that labyrinthectomized animals are not only immune to motion sickness, but also show decreased emetic response to naturally occurring poisons.

The typical transport team member with airsickness will adapt successfully to the new environment within a few flights. Almost any member is at risk for developing the problem given the right set of circumstances. The Sopite syndrome is probably a subtle form of motion sickness which is very common.[19] Medications to treat motion sickness during adaptation periods or in unusual situations may be useful. The majority of oral medications, such as scopolamine, have enough side effects to make routine use by working medical crews inadvisable. The scopolamine transdermal patch system seems to have fewer side effects and may be used by medical crews. Unfortunately, their onset is relatively slow, making their use ineffective in acute situations.

Electromagnetic interference

Some electromagnetic interference is generated by the operation of almost all electronic devices. Electromagnetic interference includes any electromagnetic energy that interrupts, obstructs, or otherwise degrades or limits the effective operation or performance of another electronic device.[23] On modern aircraft the possibility of electromagnetic interference from a medical device adversely affecting the function of the aircraft or its navigation and communication systems is not an unjustified fear. One of the major reasons for medical equipment failing USAF testing procedures involves exceeding military standards for either radiated or conducted electromagnetic energy.[25] Although the FAA has not established standards for commercial aircraft, several airlines have banned the operation of certain electronic devices during all or parts of the flight. Pilots have reported significant malfunctions of the autothrottle, autopilot, navigational compass, and cockpit display instruments, apparently related to passenger use of computers, tape players, and electronic games.[33] NASA's confidential Aviation Safety Reporting System has logged 40 episodes of probable interference since 1986.[6] Certainly, members of flight crews should encourage medical equipment manufacturers to minimize design factors which lead to increased electromagnetic interference and should be extremely vigilant when using new or untested electronic devices for medical transport.

DISCUSSION

The aeromedical environment is dynamic and potentially hostile to the patient, flight crew, and medical equipment used for transport. The transport team is challenged to integrate and apply knowledge of the pathophysiology of disease with the physical laws and challenges of the transport environment to provide a safe, quick, & cost-effective means of emergency medical care.

REFERENCES

1. Ackerman N, Bell R, Yoder B: Personal observations, 1978-1984, Wilford Hall USAF Medical Center.
2. Ackerman NB and others: In house Studies USAF School of Aerospace Medicine, 1985-86, Crew Technology Division: Aeromedical Evacuation Group.
3. Bert P: Barometric pressure: researches in experimental physiology, Hitchcock M, and others, translators. Columbus, 1943, College Book Company.
4. Brink LW, Neuman B, Wynn J: Air transport, *Pediatric Clinics North Am* 40(2):439-56, 1993.
5. Campbell AN and others: Mechanical vibration and sound levels experienced in neonatal transport, *American Journal Diseases of Children* 138:967-70, 1984.

6. Chandler JG: Can your laptop reprogram your flight? *Travel & Leisure* 162, June 1993.
7. Clark JG, Williams JD, Hood WB: Initial cardiovascular response to low frequency whole body vibration in humans and animals, *Aerosp Med* 38:464-7, 1967.
8. Cornish JD and others: Inflight use of extracorporeal membrane oxygenation for severe neonatal respiratory failure, *Perfusion* 1:281-7, 1986.
9. Davis JC and others: Altitude decompression sickness, *Aviation Space Environmental Medicine* 48: 722, 1977.
10. de Acosta J: Natural y moral de las indias: Seville: 1590, English translation, London, 1604, Blount and Ashley.
11. DeHart RL: The historical perspective. DeHart RL, editor: Fundamentals of Aerospace Medicine, Philadelphia, 1985, Lea & Febiger.
12. Engle E, Lott AS: *Man in flight,* Annapolis, Maryland, 1979, Leeward Publications, Inc.
13. Falk SA: Combined effects of noise and ototoxic drugs, *Environ Health Perspect* 2:5-22, 1972.
14. Floyd WN, Brodeisen AB, Goodno JF: Effect of the whole body vibration on peripheral nerve conduction time in the rhesus monkey, *Aerosp Med* 44:281-5, 1973.
15. French RS, Tilman JG: Pacemaker function during helicopter transport, *Ann Emerg Med* 18:305-7, 1989.
16. Gillingham KK, Wolfe JW: Spatial orientation in flight. In fundamentals of aerospace medicine, DeHart RL, editor: Philadelphia, 1985, Lea and Febiger.
17. Goldman DE, Von Gierke HE: Effects of shock and vibration in man. In Harriss CM and Crede CE, editors: Shock and vibration handbook, New York, Vol 3, 1961, McGraw-Hill Book Company.
18. Gordon RS and others: Activity-sensing permanent internal pacemaker dysfunction during helicopter aeromedical transport, *Ann Emerg Med* 19:1260-3, 1990.
19. Graybiel A, Knepton J: Sopite syndrome: a sometimes sole manifestation of motion sickness, *Aviat Space Environ Med* 47:873-7, 1976.
20. Heimbach RD, Sheffield PJ: Decompression sickness and pulmonary overpressure accidents. In DeHart RL, editor: *Fundamentals of aerospace medicine,* Philadelphia, 1985, Lea & Febiger.
21. Hint RC and others: Inability to assess breath sounds during air medical transport by helicopter, *JAMA* 265(15):1982-4, 1991.
22. Kryter KD, Ward WD, Miller JD: Hazardous exposure to intermittent and steady-state noise, *J Accoust Soc Am* 39:451-64, 1966.
23. Military Standard, 463A, June 1977.
24. Moser R: Further significant medical and surgical conditions of aeromedical concern. In DeHart RL, editor: *Fundamentals of aerospace medicine,* Philadelphia, 1985, Lea & Febiger.
25. Nish WA and others: Effect of electromagnetic interference by neonatal transport equipment on aircraft operation, *Aviat Space Environ Med* 60:599-600, 1989.
26. Saltzman AR and others: Ventilatory criteria for aeromedical evacuation, *Aviation Space and Environmental Medicine* 58:958-62, 1987.
27. Saltzman AR and others: High frequency oscillation during simulated altitude exposure, *Critical Care Medicine* 18(11):1257-60, 1990.
28. Schwartz RH: Hazards of air travel for a child with otitis, *Pediatric Infec Disease Journal* 8(8):542-3, 1989.
29. Schwartz DM, Schwartz RH, Redfield NP: Treatment of negative middle ear pressure and serous otitis media with Politzer's technique: an old procedure revisited, *Arch Otolaryngol* 104:487-90, 1978.
30. Sheffield PJ, Heimbach RD: Respiratory physiology. In DeHart RL, editor: Fundamentals of aerospace medicine, Philadelphia, 1985, Lee & Febiger.
31. Shenai JP, Johnson GE, Varney RV: *Mechanical vibration in neonatal transport, Pediatrics* 68:55-9, 1981.
32. Silbergleit E and others: Forces acting during air and ground transport on patients stabilized by standard immobolization techniques, *Ann Emerg Med* 20: 875-7, 1991.
33. Stoller G: Is your laptop scaring the pilot? *Conde Nast Traveler,* June 32-34, 1993.
34. Stork RI, Gasaway DC: Evaluation of V-51R and EAR™ earplugs for use in flight, USAFSAM-TR-77-1: United States Air Force School of Aerospace Medicine, Texas, 1977, Brooks Air Force Base.
35. Taylor W, Pelmear PL, editors: Vibration white finger in industry, New York, 1975, Academic Press.
36. Treisman M: Motion sickness: an evolutionary hypothesis. *Science,* 197:493-5, 1977.
37. von Gierke HE, Goldman DE: Effects of shock and vibration in man. In Harris CM and Crede CE, editors: Shock and vibration handbook, New York, 1979, McGraw-Hill Book Co.
38. Weiss MH, Frost JO: May children with otis media safely fly? *Clinical Pediatrics* 26:567-8, 1987.

PART II
MEDICAL MANAGEMENT

17

ABC'S OF INITIAL STABILIZATION

CONSTANCE McANENEY

Previous chapters in this text have provided guidelines to set the stage for arrival to an emergency department of a critically ill or injured child who will ultimately require transport to a pediatric intensive care unit. Discussion of medical management of specific conditions requiring transport begins with the widely recognized ABC's of initial resuscitation and stabilization.

Stabilization is the shared responsibility of the referring facility, the receiving institution, and the transport team. The immediate resuscitation and assessment, as well as the decision to transport, is the burden of the referring facility. The receiving institution must provide consultation. The transport team faces the challenge of providing and maintaining both rapid and skilled pediatric intensive care at the patient's bedside throughout transport.[2]

Upon arrival a quick "once-over" visual assessment and a "barometer reading" of the comfort or tension level in the room should be done to determine whether immediate intervention is needed or a complete history with update can be obtained. A brief, polite introduction to staff and family in the room is essential. The team should immmediately perform its own assessment of the ABC's. From this evaluation of airway, breathing, and circulation one of three conclusions may be drawn: a) the system is stable — move on; b) the system is unstable — intervene as necessary, gauged by severity; c) the assessment is unclear — observe, reassess, intervene as necessary.[1] Assessment and intervention must occur almost simultaneously, a task which is difficult to convey in written text.

ASSESSMENT/INTERVENTION: CARDIORESPIRATORY ARREST

The worst possible scenario to walk into involves a child in cardiorespiratory arrest. It is easy to recognize; there is no question what the sequence of intervention should be, but it is a situation which causes high anxiety among health care personnel. The high anxiety is three-fold in etiology for an emergency department that normally only tends to critically ill adults: a) unfamiliarity with pediatric problems, b) lack of experience with and equipment for pediatric procedures, c) fear of the unknown and likely poor prognosis. Regardless of the reasons for anxiety, the sequence of events is the same as always with careful attention to the pediatric idiosyncrasies.

Determine responsiveness

In a nanosecond, through observation, the patient's color, amount of spontaneous movement, and level of consciousness can be determined.

Assess airway patency

Deliver oxygen (100%) via bag-mask ventilation. If the patient's own airway is not patent, suction the airway, reposition the head (using a jaw thrust, chin lift and/or head tilt if there is no cervical trauma) and re-attempt ventilation. An oral or nasopharyngeal airway may be helpful. Intubation may be required for airway patency (see below). If the patient is already intubated, check tube position visually and by assessment of breath sounds, and suction the tube. If ability to ventilate does not improve, remove and replace the tube.

Determine breathlessness

Spontaneous respiratory effort may be adequate or inadequate as determined by rate, chest rise, auscultated air movement, patient's skin color, signs of increased work of breathing, pulse oximetry and blood gases. If respiratory effort (with or without mechanical airway interventions) is inadequate or absent, bag-mask ventilation is needed. Consider a pneumothorax in the previously intubated or ventilated patient or in the patient with a related clinical history (asthma, chest trauma).

Access circulation

Listen for heart sounds, and feel for pulses. Begin chest compressions for profound bradycardia (infant's heart rate less than 80 or child's heart rate less than 60) without blood pressure, electrical activity of the heart without heart tones, or pulses (electromechanical dissociation) or absent heart rate or pulses. Place monitors on the patient (cardiorespiratory and pulse oximetry) if not already done, and begin intravenous line placement. Intraosseous lines are the easiest to insert in the infant and small child without a heart rate. If the child is school-age, then antecubital or (preferably) femoral line placement is the best.

Back to airway and breathing

The person in charge of airway should be preparing for intubation while the assessment and interventions are continuing. Gather equipment needed for intubation, such as suction (with tonsil suction catheter), oxygen and airway equipment (endotracheal tube, laryngoscope with blade, tape, benzoin). In selecting an endotracheal tube it is important to remember that uncuffed tubes are used in the child until the age of eight. When deciding on the appropriately sized tube it may be helpful to remember the following formula:

$$\frac{\text{Age (in years)} + 16}{4} = \begin{matrix}\text{endotracheal}\\ \text{tube size}\end{matrix}$$

Prior to the intubation attempt, a second person should place cricoid pressure (Sellick maneuver), as every person intubated emergently should be considered to have a full stomach. After the patient has been intubated, check placement by listening to breath sounds to ensure that they are bilaterally equal. Look for condensation in the endotracheal tube. The tube should be taped after benzoin is applied to the skin and allowed to dry. Taping the endotracheal tube is extremely important, as the patient will be moved in the ensuing hours. The tube must be secured in such a way that there is no movement in and out of the mouth when tension is applied. The placement of the endotracheal tube should be documented by noting the hash mark at the teeth (or gums). If the first attempt at endotracheal tube placement fails, do not get discouraged. Place the mask over the nose and mouth and continue to ventilate, preferably until the oxygen saturation is above 95%. Regroup, mentally review the problems that were encountered with the first attempt and, after oxygenating, try again. Order a chest x-ray to check endotracheal tube placement.

Back to circulation

If intravenous or intraosseous line placement are not obtained, remember that many of the resuscitation drugs, such as epinephrine, atropine, lidocaine, and naloxone, can be given via the endotracheal tube. However, do not give sodium bicarbonate via the endotracheal tube (Table 17-1). After intravenous access is accomplished, resuscitation drugs should be given (Box 17-1). To expand intravascular volume, fluids should be given, beginning with 20 cc/kg of normal saline. Normal saline boluses may be repeated based on cardiovascular status (see Chapter 20). Up to 80-100 cc/kg may be needed in the first hour for those in hypovolemic shock. If there is a return of heart rate, fluids have been given,

TABLE 17-1 COMMON DRUGS USED TO STABILIZE PEDIATRIC PATIENTS

Drug	*Dose*	*Volume*
Epinephrine 1 : 10,000	0.1 mg/kg IV or IO	0.1 cc/kg
Epinephrine 1 : 1,000	0.1 mg/kg ETT or, if no response to initial IV dose, may go as high as 0.2 mg/kg	0.1 cc/kg
Atropine	0.02 mg/kg min. 0.16 mg max. 1-2 mg	0.05 cc/kg min. = 0.4 cc max. = 2.5-5 cc
Na Bicarbonate	1-2 meq/kg	1-cc/kg
D_{25}	1 gm/kg	4 cc/kg
D_{10} (neonate)	200 mg/kg	2 cc/kg
Lidocaine	0.5-1.0 mg/kg	0.025-0.05 cc/kg
Thiopental	2-4 mg/kg	0.08-0.16 cc/kg
Succinylcholine	2 mg/kg	0.1 cc/kg
Vecuronium	0.08-0.15 mg/kg	0.08-0.15 cc/kg
Diazepam	0.1 mg/kg	0.02 cc/kg
Lorazepam	0.05-0.1 mg/kg	0.05-0.1 cc/kg
Racemic epinephrine	0.05 ml/kg	0.5 cc in 3 cc NS
Albuterol (0.5%)	2.5 mg in 3 cc NS	0.5 cc in 3 cc NS
Dopamine (infusion)	5-20 mcg/kg/min	
Dobutamine (infusion)	2–25 mcg/kg/min	

NS: Normal saline (0.9% saline solution)

and there are signs of poor perfusion or hypotension, inotropic support should be started. Dopamine is usually the first choice. After intravenous or intraosseous lines are obtained, then blood samples should be sent to the lab. The laboratory exam is somewhat dependent on the history of present illness but, in the arrest of unknown etiology, a complete blood count, blood culture, glucose (with bedside glucose check), electrolytes, type, and cross should be completed. If trauma is suspected (and it always should be), amylase and liver function tests are helpful. If sepsis is suspected, coagulation studies may be beneficial. Glucose (D25 2-4 cc/kg) should be given for hypoglycemia (<60). An arterial blood gas count can help in determining acid-base status and the effectiveness of therapy.

BOX 17-1 ASYSTOLE[1]

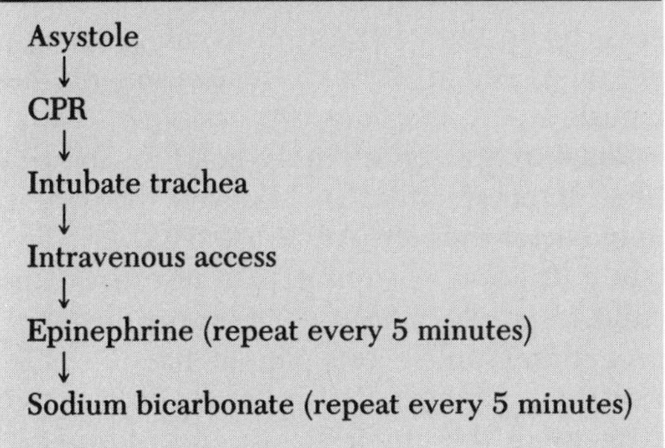

Asystole
↓
CPR
↓
Intubate trachea
↓
Intravenous access
↓
Epinephrine (repeat every 5 minutes)
↓
Sodium bicarbonate (repeat every 5 minutes)

POST-ARREST STABILIZATION

In the postarrest stabilization phase, careful assessment of the patient's cardiopulmonary status is essential. Cardiorespiratory monitoring and pulse oximetry monitoring should be continuous. If the patient begins to decompensate, go back to the beginning: airway, breathing, and circulation. Check the placement of all tubes and equipment. The following steps should be taken until the patient is safely delivered to definitive care:

- Vital signs should be obtained every five minutes until stable and every fifteen minutes thereafter.
- Frequent assessments of breath sounds and suctioning of endotracheal tube as needed are essential.
- Perfusion should be evaluated by capillary

refill, pulses, urine output, and level of consciousness.

- Place a Foley catheter for accurate urine output measurement and a nasogastric tube to relieve gastric distention and prevent emesis.
- Perform a full physical examination to determine the etiology of arrest. Appropriate treatment should be started (i.e., head trauma—hyperventilation to pCO_2 of 25-30; sepsis-antibiotics).
- Carefully assess neurologic factors including pupil size, pupil reactivity, and Glasgow Coma Score. Continuous assessments should be recorded with vital signs.
- Obtain the patient's temperature. Efforts should be made using an overhead warmer or warming pad to prevent hypothermia.
- Insert a second intravenous line in the patient, and if at all possible, two functioning lines should be obtained prior to transport (excluding intraosseous line, as it is difficult to secure and easily dislodged during transport).
- Check x-rays and laboratory data sent, making appropriate changes in therapy as needed. The endotracheal tube should be 1-2 cm above the carina.
- Make copies of all documents and x-rays.
- Secure all lines.
- Make all treatment decisions with the duration of the transport in mind.
- Have resuscitation medications drawn up and out for the ride back.
- Have extra fluids (normal saline) drawn up in syringes.
- Be prepared to increase inotropic support. Have enough dopamine infusion to be able to increase to the maximum amount. Have dobutamine ready for infusion.
- Carry extra airway equipment (especially the mask) should the patient extubate with movement.
- If a patient has ongoing blood loss, carry blood products for replacement infusion.
- Make a treatment plan for the way back and clarify roles should the worst happen.

ASSESSMENT/INTERVENTION: THE ILL CHILD

In many ways preventing uncompensated shock and cardiorespiratory arrest is a more difficult situation to handle. The ability to recognize a child in a state of compensated shock or impending respiratory failure requires astute observation skills and good judgment. The assessment sequence is the same (ABC's), but it is the decision-making, based on the degree and etiology of distress, that can be challenging in the pediatric patient (Refer to the appropriate chapter for in depth evaluation and treatment of specific system dysfunctions).

Assessment: airway and breathing

Ensuring the patency of airways and the adequacy of breathing should be the first priority. Listen to breath sounds, and pay attention to the amount of air entry. Note the respiratory rate, heart rate, temperature, presence of retractions, stridor, wheezing, rales, increased accessory muscle use, grunting, character of the voice or cry, presence and character of cough, presence of drooling, postural preference, color, toxicity, mental status, and level of anxiety. Determine oxygen saturation via pulse oximetry. With these observations the level of airway involvement and the severity of respiratory distress can be determined.

Stridor, increased accessory muscle use, hoarse cry, barky cough, drooling, tripod position, increased anxiety, and decreased mental status may all be indicative of upper airway obstruction. The differential diagnosis for upper airway obstruction is long but commonly includes: 1) infections (croup, bacterial tracheitis, epiglottitis, retropharyngeal abscess), 2) foreign body aspiration, and 3) congenital anomalies (hemangiomas, tumors, cysts, vocal cord paralysis). A number of approaches can be used in an effort not to agitate the child: a) do not separate from parents, b) do not restrain, c) examine from a distance, and d) defer visualization of the mouth.

Place oxygen (preferably mist) on the patient. If this agitates the child have the parent hold it near the face. Allow the child to maintain a position of comfort. Do not force the child to lay down. Do not perform invasive procedures unless the patient has unstable vital signs. Obtain a history to help discern the etiology of the upper airway obstruction. If the child is stable a portable lateral neck x-ray may be helpful in determining the etiology. It may be beneficial to begin empiric treatment with a racemic epinephrine nebulizer if the patient has stridor at rest, pallor or cyanosis, or altered mental status while the diagnosis is still unknown. If there are signs of supraglottic disease, foreign body impaction or angioedema, then preparations should be made for intubation. The most experienced person in the facility should handle the airway in these situations. The safest place for the intubation of a child with significant upper airway obstruction is the operating room. Generally paralytic agents are not used during intubation because these patients can be extremely difficult to intubate. Should intubation be unsuccessful, the patient will still have their own respiratory effort. The major errors made with children with an upper airway obstruction involve underestimating patient distress, examining the patient overzealously and performing lab work or other procedures.

Tachypnea, retractions, wheezing, rales, decreased breath sounds, increased accessory muscle use, grunting, cough, decreased mental status, and increased anxiety can be signs of lower airway disease. The differential diagnosis is long and includes infections (pneumonia, pleural effusion), asthma, bronchiolitis, pneumothorax, hemothorax, lower airway foreign body, congestive heart failure, and metabolic disorders. Immediately place the patient on oxygen and monitor cardiorespiratory and pulse oximetry status. Allow the patient to maintain a comfortable position. A nebulized treatment of albuterol may be administered empirically and repeated as needed. A chest x-ray should be obtained to rule out a pneumothorax, pneumonia, congestive heart failure, or foreign body. Chest thoracostomy tubes are to be placed for a pneumothorax or for a large pleural effusion causing moderate to severe respiratory distress. Arterial blood gas analysis is useful in those patients with moderate to severe distress in order to determine acid-base status and to track progress. Intravenous lines for fluids or resuscitation medications should be used. Laboratory studies should include the following: complete blood count, blood culture, and serum glucose. If a toxic ingestion is suspected, a patient urine sample for toxicology screening would be helpful.

The decision to intubate a patient is always a difficult one. The purpose of endotracheal intubation is to deliver high concentrations of oxygen to the patient, to protect the airway from gastric contents, and to keep the airway patent. Remember, the decision whether to intubate is one that should take into account the duration of the transport to the tertiary care center.

Assessment: circulation

After the airway and breathing has been assessed the circulatory status should be addressed. Careful attention should be paid to the vital signs. Tachycardia, although potentially derived from many different etiologies, is the first sign of hypovolemia. In children, blood pressure does not fall until very late in volume loss. Therefore, tachycardia with normal blood pressure can still be an ominous sign. The peripheral pulses and character (thready vs. full) are important. Skin perfusion may also provide a general idea of tissue perfusion. Check capillary refill, remembering that room temperature does adversely affect the results.[3] Level of consciousness, reaction to pain, reaction of pupils, and motor strength indicate the level of brain perfusion.

For any signs of hypovolemia, intravenous access should be obtained and fluids (normal saline) given in boluses of 20 cc/kg. Normal saline can be repeated as needed. Once 60-80 cc/kg of crystalloid is given, inotropic support should be considered. Blood samples for laboratory tests (complete blood count, blood culture, glucose, electrolytes) may be drawn during intravenous line placement. Antibiotics should be given when sepsis is suspected, and they should be treated empirically.

Sometimes there is a fine line between stabilization and too much intervention. The patient's vital signs should be acceptable, all foreseeable life-saving procedures completed, and all life-saving therapies initiated. The diagnostic work-up does not need to be completed or, in some instances, even begun (i.e., there is seldom an indication for a lumbar puncture on transport). Top priority includes stabilization and safe, expeditious transport to the tertiary care center.

REFERENCES

1. American Academy of Pediatrics and the American Heart Association: *Textbook of pediatric advanced life support,* 1990, The Associations.
2. American Academy of Pediatrics Committee on Hospital Care: Guidelines for air and ground transportation of pediatric patients, *Pediatrics* 78:943-50, 1986.
3. Gorelick MH, Shaw KN, Baker MD: Effect of ambient temperature on capillary refill in healthy children, *Pediatrics* 92:699-702, 1993.

SUGGESTED READINGS

Aoki BY, McCloskey K, editors: *Evaluation, stabilization, and transport of the critically ill child,* Philadelphia, 1992, Mosby-Year Book.

Corneli HM: Evaluation, treatment, and transport of pediatric patients with shock, *Pediatr Clin North Am* 40:303-19, 1993.

Day SE: Intra-transport stabilization and management of the pediatric patient, *Pediatr Clin North Am* 40:263-74, 1993.

Kanter RK and others: Excess morbidity associated with interhospital transport, *Pediatrics* 6:893-8, 1992.

Kanter RK, Thomkins JM: Adverse events during interhospital transport: Physiologic deterioration associated with pretransport severity of illness, *Pediatrics* 84:43-8, 1989.

Kissoon N: Triage and transport of the critically ill child, *Crit Care Clin* 8:37-57, 1992.

Pon S, Notterman DA: The organization of a pediatric critical care transport program, *Pediatr Clin North Am* 40:241-61, 1993.

18

AIRWAY MANAGEMENT

KEVIN RAGOSTA
ROBERT K. KANTER

The brain is the most vulnerable organ to injury after the disruption of oxygen supply. Four seconds of interrupted cerebral oxygen delivery results in unconsciousness, and four minutes may cause irreparable CNS damage. Respiratory insufficiency is the primary cause of most pediatric arrests, and is often responsible for physiologic deterioration and morbidity of transported children.[26,43] Respiratory function may deteriorate within seconds in a sick infant or child due to the obstruction of an airway apnea or aspiration. Yet, because of the inexperience of nonspecialized staff, children often do not receive the same degree of respiratory support as an adult.[1] Historically, failure to protect the airway was a major preventable cause of transport associated with morbidity and mortality in adults.[61] Thus, it is vital to ensure an intact respiratory mechanism during the transport of critically ill children. In most cases the likelihood of deterioration can be anticipated, and an endotracheal tube is placed prior to transport. However, some cases of unexpected deterioration, plugging of endotracheal tubes, and accidental dislodgment of endotracheal tubes during transport require that staff be capable of intubating the trachea. In this chapter the indications for endotracheal intubation are reviewed. In particular we emphasize high-risk situations for the transport setting. Anatomic considerations unique to the child are outlined. This is followed by a discussion of respiratory support equipment and the procedures involved in tracheal intubation and assisted ventilation during transport. This chapter concludes with an examination of some issues in training transport personnel and monitoring their proficiency in managing the pediatric airway

INDICATIONS FOR ENDOTRACHEAL INTUBATION

The transport vehicle is an unfavorable setting in which to provide intensive care and carry out emergency procedures such as endotracheal intubation. Except for the transport team and their equipment, personnel with other specialized skills and technology for diagnostic, monitoring, and therapeutic procedures are unavailable. Noise, vibration, dim lighting, and the need to cover the patient to reduce thermal stress make clinical monitoring difficult. Emergency procedures during transport are complicated by limited physical access to the patient and by the inability to control the environment. Therefore, every effort must be made to anticipate respiratory deterioration and gain control of the airway and ventilation prior to transporting the critically ill child from the referring hospital or scene. Some patients whose moderate respiratory problem might not require invasive support in an intensive care unit, would be safer if intubated before transport. The modest risks associated with placing an endotracheal tube in a severely ill patient are balanced by a substantial reduction of transport morbidity when the airway and ventilation are secure. Experienced pediatric transport specialists provide important assistance in making the decision to perform endotracheal intubation when indications are ambiguous. In the majority of cases the need for endotracheal intubation can be determined even before the arrival of the transport team, and personnel at the referring hospital should be able to place the endotracheal tube when necessary.[42] Delaying intubation until the arrival of the transport service may seriously compromise the patient's safety. The transport service physician must be prepared to provide guidance by telephone regarding intubation prior to arrival of the transport team. If a patient in a referring hospital has been intubated to stabilize a cardiorespiratory crisis, the endotracheal tube should usually be maintained in place for transport, even if it appears that the crisis is resolving. Elective extubation can be done under controlled circumstances after arrival at the critical care center.

In addition to cases involving a patient in cardiac or respiratory arrest, the usual indications for endotracheal intubation include the following pathophysiologic categories.

1) *Patency of the upper airway* may be impaired. Obstruction may result from mechanical or anatomical processes (infectious, foreign body, traumatic, or congenital malformations). In particular, the terminal event in children with epiglottitis may be a rapidly accelerating obstruction. Airway tone and protective reflexes also may be functionally depressed by central neurological or neuromuscular disorders, and the risk of aspiration is always present in comatose patients. Upper airway obstruction is recognized by inspiratory exacerbation with stridor or snoring and a prolonged inspiratory phase. Respiratory rate seldom exceeds 50-55 breaths/minute. Labored efforts to breathe are often fruitless and only increase the inspiratory collapse of the obstructed structure. Since airway obstruction or aspiration may evolve rapidly, endotracheal intubation is usually necessary before transporting any comatose patient or child with substantial obstruction of the airway.

2) *Controls of ventilation* are impaired in many critically ill infants and children, either as a result of underlying neurological illness (coma or seizures) or as the result of iatrogenic effects (especially sedatives, opiates, and anesthetics). Sustained hypoventilation and abrupt central apnea may occur. In the sick, stressed patient, normal compensatory mechanisms typically result in hyperventilation with increased respiratory frequency and use of accessory muscles. In the patient with irregular breathing, inappropriately comfortable respiratory effort, and $PaCO_2$ levels exceeding 40-45 mm Hg, respiratory drive is usually impaired, and immediate ventilatory support is usually indicated.

3) Abnormal respiratory mechanics with increased work of breathing often results in *respiratory insufficiency due to fatigue.* This may occur in patients with severe illness or injury involving the upper or lower respiratory tract. In an effort to compensate for illness, a patient may experience irritability, retractions, grunting, nasal flaring, head bobbing, and actively use expiratory abdominal muscles and may become fatigued unless a treatment is available to rapidly alleviate the underlying problem. In these patients, pallor is a sign of extreme stress. As fatigue develops, audible air entry diminishes. Less commonly, a patient with weakness due to a neuromuscular disorder may become fatigued by a minor respiratory illness, with similar clinical signs of labored respiratory effort. When the patient with impending respiratory fatigue must be transported, elective intubation is often warranted, even if blood gas analysis temporarily shows normal levels of gas exchange since hypoventilation, hypoxia, and CO_2 retention may worsen rapidly.

4) Patients with *severe lung disease and impaired gas exchange* often present with hypoxemia due to poor matching of ventilation to perfusion. They may also develop hypercapnia due to increased pulmonary dead space, even though air entry appears adequate. Hypoxia with a $PaO_2 < 60$ mm Hg while breathing supplemental oxygen at an $F_iO_2 > 60\%$, or acute hypercapnia with a $PaCO_2 > 50$ mm Hg often identifies the patient with lung disease who will benefit from endotracheal intubation, assisted ventilation, and sometimes positive end expiratory pres-

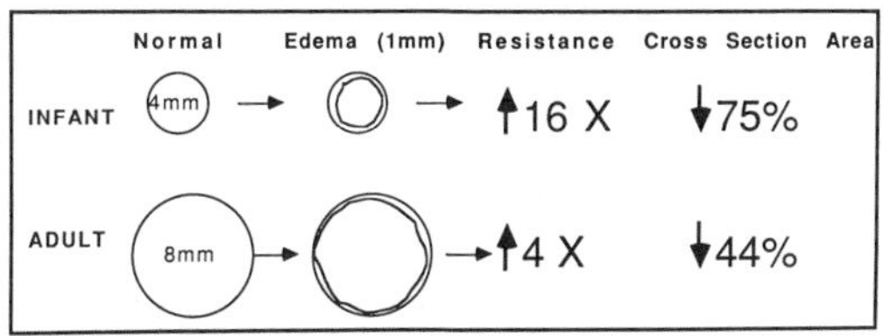

Fig. 18-1. Infant and adult airways.

sure support. While cyanosis provides clear evidence of hypoxemia, the anemic patient may not become cyanotic even when severely hypoxic. There are no specific clinical signs of hypercapnia. When time permits, analysis of blood gas tension adds to the objective evaluation of the patient. However, most cases of respiratory failure must be recognized clinically, and the distressed, fatiguing patient often must be intubated without measuring blood gases.

5) Finally, patients with severe *circulatory collapse* usually should be intubated and mechanically ventilated, even if respiratory function is temporarily compensating for their stressed state. Oxygen transport is often the limiting factor in such conditions. Metabolism in respiratory muscles diverts oxygen transport away from other compromised organs. Therefore, assisted ventilation improves physiologic reserve in shock.[5]

Many common pediatric disorders result in respiratory failure due to combinations of pathophysiologic mechanisms. Severe respiratory infections or asthma impair pulmonary gas exchange while imposing fatiguing work loads. Systemic infections may cause shock, encephalopathy, and pulmonary injury. Trauma and burns often compromise pulmonary function, upper airway patency, and neural controls of breathing simultaneously. Any insult to the child's airway may have significantly more physiologic effect than in the adult (Figure 18-1).

ANATOMIC CONSIDERATIONS

There are obvious size differences between adults and children. These differences are especially pronounced in the airway and its supporting structures. The physics of air flow in the respiratory system changes dramatically from infancy to adulthood (Fig 18-1). This chart assumes that the flow of air in the pediatric airway conforms to the Hagen-Poiseuille equation, $Q = \frac{P\pi r^4}{8nl}$, where Q is flow, P is driving pressure, r is radius, n is viscosity, and l is length of tubing.[79] This equation may only hold true for laminar air flow. The branching elastic airway of infancy may follow an equation that relates the airway resistance of the airway to the radius to the fifth power.[25] Physiologic demands differ in infancy as well (Table 18-1).

As in the adult, the neonatal and pediatric upper airways are made up of four different cartilages: hyoid, thyroid, cricoid, and arytenoid. The child's airway is made up of flexible cartilage that does not "mature" into the adult structure until the influence of hormones during adolescence.

Five major anatomic differences separate the young child's larynx from the adult. First, the infant tongue is large in comparison to the oral cavity. Especially if coupled with congenital anatomic abnormalities, ensuring control and instrumentation of the airway in infancy is more difficult than in the adult. Conditions found in infancy that may affect the tongue and oral cavity's relative size include: trisomy 21 (Down's Syndrome), Pierre Robin syndrome, Beckwich syndrome, and multiple bony, vascular, and lymphatic anomalies.[14]

The position of the larynx changes as the child grows and develops. The adult glottic opening is at the cervical level, C4-5. The infant's larynx is placed more anterior and more cephalad at C2-3. Positioning of the patient with excessive extension of the neck may

TABLE 18-1 PHYSIOLOGIC DEMANDS IN INFANTS AND ADULTS

	Infant	*Adult*
Tracheal diameter	4mm	8mm
Surface area (sq. meter)	4	70
Number of alveoli (million)	70	500
Size of alveoli (microns)	100	200
Respiration rate	25-35	13-18
Tidal volume cc/breath	6	6
Min vent cc/kg	200	100
Oxygen consumption (ml/kg/min)	8	4

exaggerate its anterior position. The combination of these anatomic differences and the soft cartilage make the child's airway more prone to obstruction by the tongue and other intrinsic and extrinsic insults.

The glottic opening is protected by the epiglottis. This structure is long, thin, and runs parallel to the larynx in the adult. In childhood this structure is more thickened, omega shaped, and tends to extend over the glottic opening more than in the older patient. There is also some concern that loose tissue may make the child's supraglottic tissues more susceptible to inflammation.

Vocal cords and folds are thinnest in the infant. The anterior vocal cords are attached lower in the airway than the posterior portion. This gives the vocal cords an angle with a prominent anterior commissure. It is not uncommon to feel an endotracheal tube "catch" in this space. When this occurs a slight twisting motion of the endotracheal tube usually resolves the problem.

The final anatomic difference of the larynx is the cricoid cartilage in the subglottic area. This rigid cartilage forms a ring with the trachea extending inferiorly, and its integrity prevents collapse of the infant's airway. It is also the narrowest portion of the child's larynx. Unlike the adult cylindrical larynx, the infant's is shaped like a funnel. Endotracheal tubes that pass easily through the vocal folds may fit snugly in the cricoid area. This may increase the risk of subglottic edema or stenosis due to pressure necrosis. Care should be taken to limit this risk.[23]

These five anatomic differences may add a level of difficulty in managing the pediatric airway. Techniques which are commonly used in adults may not work in a child. For example, blind nasotracheal intubation maneuvers in children often lead to esophageal intubation. Dentition patterns must also be kept in mind. Loose teeth are common in children ages 6-14 years.

Finally there are multiple congenital anomalies and conditions that may distort or obstruct the child's airway. These may be categorized into three areas: supralaryngeal, laryngeal, and tracheal. The most common are listed.

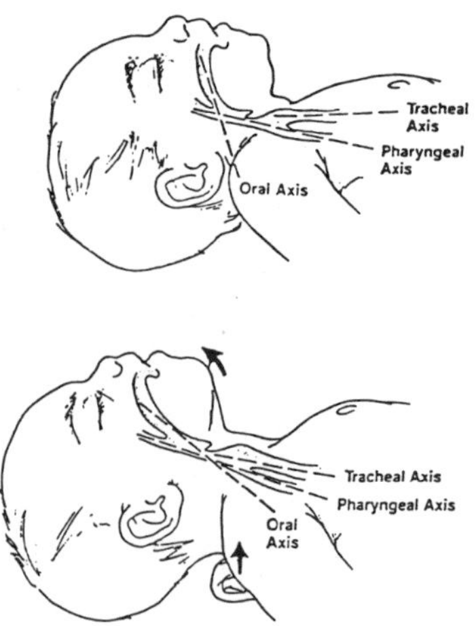

Fig. 18-2. Alignment of the mouth, pharynx, and trachea for intubation. (Reproduced with permission. Textbook of Pediatric Advanced Life Support, 1988. Copyright American Heart Association.)

Supralaryngeal—tonsils/adenoids, choanal atresia, teratoma, dermoid and other cysts, encephalocele

Laryngeal—laryngomalacia, congenital or acquired stenosis, vocal cord paralysis, webs, polyps, warts, hemangioma

Tracheal—tracheomalacia, tracheoesophageal fistula, tracheal stenosis, extrinsic mass, foreign body[59]

The airway is not the only anatomic structure that demands attention during the instrumentation of the pediatric airway. The large occiput of the infant causes flexion of the neck when the child lays in the supine position. This position may cause a posterior placement of the tongue in the oral cavity and accentuates the angles of the oral, pharyngeal, and tracheal axes. Positioning the child for airway management may include a towel roll under the shoulders and mild extension of the jaw and neck. These maneuvers will allow better alignment of the airway structures without undue anterior displacement of the larynx (Figure 18-2).

RESPIRATORY MONITORING

Transport monitoring devices has changed over the last 10-15 years. Pulse oximetry, capnography, and intravascular pressure measurement with electronic data storage and playback all have been added to conventional blood pressure cuffs, stethoscopes, and electrocardiogram monitors. These advances will grow in number as we attempt to better evaluate cardiopulmonary systems on a continual basis. Technology may extend the observations of experienced clinicians, but a skilled clinician is still necessary to integrate and interpret the multiplicity of data available in monitoring the unstable patient. Visual observation of the patient's thoracic respiratory movements during transport remains very important. When the clinician detects discrepancies between direct clinical observations and data obtained indirectly from monitors, the direct evaluation of the patient is likely to be more meaningful, and a source of artifact in the monitor should be suspected.

Pulse oximetry is reportedly accurate over a wide range of saturations. Several studies of infants with severe hypoxia secondary to congenital heart disease have shown that pulse oximetry is accurate at very low saturations.[12,49] It has helped predict beneficial efforts in the resuscitation of the newborn.[67] Its use in the operating room has eliminated many episodes of desaturation, and it has limited total hypoxic duration.[24,66] Battery operated units are now available, and many manufacturers of transport monitors have incorporated oximetry into their circuitry. Problems previously encountered with accuracy during motion and low flow states have been lessened with coupling of oximeter to QRS timing as the independent variable.[27,64,75] The presence of high levels of carboxyhemoglobin result in abnormally high measurements of saturation, while methemoglobin results in saturation percent measured in the mid 80s. Pulse oximetry is clearly of value in multiple clinical settings[33,73] and has become standard practice during most transports.

Capnography has not been used in the transport setting as widely as pulse oximetry. Reasons for this include poor accuracy of measurement, expense, and weight of machinery. Exhaled CO_2 monitoring, including disposable CO_2 indicators, have helped determine appropriate endotracheal tube placement in infants and children. These devices allow differentiation between tracheal and esophageal placement by the presence of CO_2 gas in exhaled alveolar air.*

EQUIPMENT FOR AIRWAY CONTROL

While one laryngoscope/blade and two or three endotracheal tubes may be adequate for most adult intubations, this is certainly not the case for children. Pediatric intubation trays need an array of face masks, oral/nasal airways, self inflatable resuscitation bags, endotracheal tubes, and suction catheters (see Box 18-1 and Table 18-2). This equipment must be immediately available at all times. These most important equipment items must be carefully checked before leaving on a transport mission.

Endotracheal tube size

There are three ways to estimate endotracheal tube sizes for children:

BOX 18-1 EQUIPMENT

Endotracheal tubes; 2.5-8 in ½ sizes, with / without cuffs if larger than 5
Suction catheters, suction tubing, saline, suction bulb, and Yankauer
Ambu bags and masks, infant, child, adult, PEEP system, manometer
Nonrebreather oxygen mask
Airways: oral; 70–100mm, and nasal; 14-26 Fr
Tape, benzoin, scissors, tongue blades
Oxygen source and tubing, nasal and mask systems, E cylinder with wrench
Laryngoscope handle and blades 0-3
Batteries, bulbs
NG tubes, Anderson and Replogle
Syringes, needles
Stylets, Magill forceps (two sizes)
Sterile jelly, viscous lidocaine, neosynephrine, anaesthesia spray, racemic epi
Monitoring devices and apparatuses; BP, pulsoximetery, ECG
Gloves, stethoscope
Nebulizer set-up

* References 9,10,17,22,30,31,54,55,63,76,77

TABLE 18-2 EQUIPMENT SIZES FOR AIRWAY CONTROL LISTED BY AGE/WT

Age	wt kg	Oral airway	blade	Endotrach tube	Mark at canine	Suction cath (Fr)	NG tube
Premature	2	00	0	2.5	8	5-6	5-6
Infant	3	0	1	3	9	5-6	5-6
6 months	7	1	1	3.5	12	8	8
1 year	10	2	1-2	4	12	10	10
2 years	12	2	2	4.5	14	10	10
4 years	14	2	2	5	16	10	10
6 years	20	3	2	5.5	16	12	12
8 years	25	4-5	2	6	18	14	14
10 years	>30	4-5	3	6.5	18	14	14
12 years	>40	4-5	3	7	20	14	14
Adult	>50	5	3	7-8	22	14	14

1. (Age in years + 16)/4
2. Diameter of the fifth digit of the hand
3. Diameter of naris

Small, premature infants usually require a 2.5 size endotracheal tube; small, term infants 3.0; and the larger, term infant 3.5 size ET tube. Endotracheal tubes may need to be down-sized when glottic or subglottic inflammation is suspected. A small, very debilitated older child may need a larger endotracheal tube than expected from body habitus. When the selected size is too small it may result in a large air leak and persistent impairment of gas exchange. In these instances the tube should be changed promptly to a larger size in order to gain better control of the airway.

Type of endotracheal tube

Children 8 years of age and younger are usually adequately ventilated with uncuffed endotracheal tubes. Cuffed tubes (low pressure/high volume) may be needed in the presence of high airway pressures or if caustic or hydrocarbon ingestion has occurred. In children older than 8 years cuffed tubes are desirable. One should inflate cuffs only to the point that eliminates excessive air leaks. The risk of pressure necrosis is less when cuff pressures are less than 20 cm/H_2O.[11,58]

Oral airway

Size can be estimated by placing the flange of the oral airway at the position of the incisors; the tip of the curvature should reach to the angle of the jaw. *Oral airways will not be tolerated in conscious patients.* Tongue blade insertion under direct visualization is preferred to decrease the risk of displacing teeth or lacerating the soft palate. After intubation these airways can be used as bite blocks.

Nasopharyngeal airway

The caliber of the nasopharyngeal airway is estimated by the diameter of the naris. Once placed, it should not blanch the skin around the external nares. Its length should approximate the distance from the nares to the tragus of the ear. These are better tolerated by conscious patients than oral airways, especially when insertion is accompanied with application of lidocaine jelly. The risk of nosebleeds is reduced by vasoconstricting the nasal mucosa using a cotton applicator soaked with 0.5 to 1% neosynephrine. Nasopharyngeal airways may be fashioned from endotracheal tubes.

Face mask

Masks, when used for bag-valve-mask ventilation, should fit easily over mouth and nose without extending over eyes or chin. Clear masks allow visualization of the mucosa and mouth. A tight seal should occur with minimal pressure from the caregiver's hand. When using a mask for ventilation the two-person technique may be useful. With this technique one caregiver ventilates with a self-inflating bag (Ambu), while the other holds the mask to the face insuring an adequate seal and good head position.

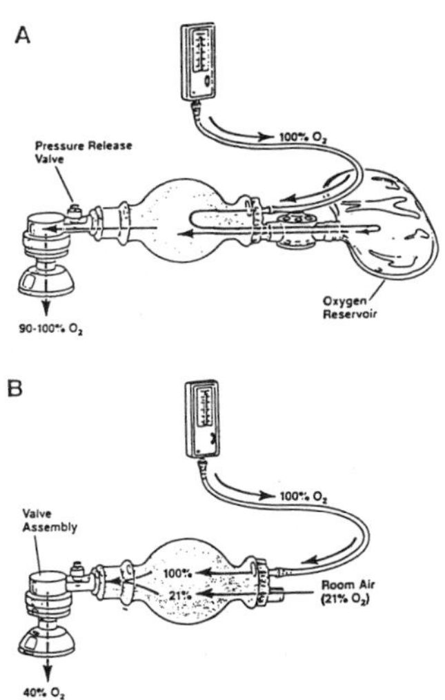

Fig. 18-3. Self-inflating bag-valve: A, with and B, without an oxygen reservoir. (Reproduced with permission. Textbook of Pediatric Advanced Life Support, 1988. Copyright American Heart Association.)

Resuscitation bag

Three sizes are available.

1. Infants—250-500cc with reservoir
2. Child—500-1000cc with reservoir
3. Adult—1500-2000cc with reservoir

The adult-sized bag can be used effectively in infants by titrating the tidal volume to visible chest excursion.[74] However, an infant-sized bag will be inadequate to deliver an effective breath to a child. Self-inflating bags are safer and more reliable than Mapleson anesthesia bags[41] which will not operate at all without a source of compressed gas. Delivery capabilities should be twice the expected tidal volume. An oxygen reservoir is essential to enable delivery of high F_iO_2. Manometers, an adjustable PEEP system, and controllable 35-45cm/H_2O "pop-off" valves are desirable[46] (Figure 18-3).

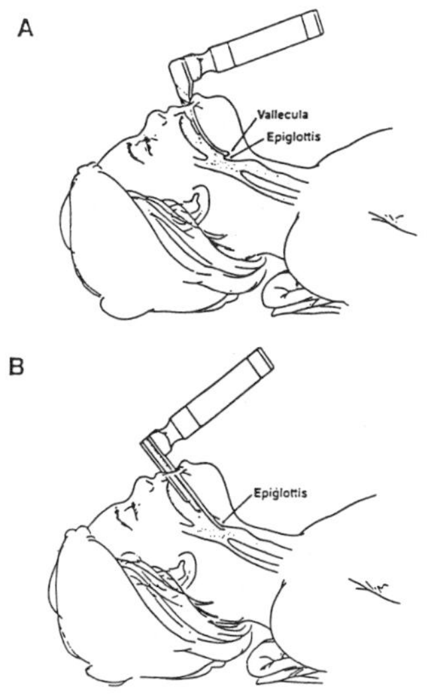

Fig. 18-4. Position of laryngoscope blade when using A, a curved blade versus B, a straight blade. (Reproduced with permission. Textbook of Pediatric Advanced Life Support, 1988. Copyright American Heart Association.)

Laryngoscope blades

The blade length should easily reach from the mouth to past the angle of the jaw. When in doubt a slightly larger blade will allow better visualization. Straight blades are usually used in a child. Curved or straight blades are used in the older patient. Oxyscopes with O_2 delivery are available in Miller 0 and 1 blades (Figure 18-4).

ADJUVANT MEDICATIONS

Except in the patient who is in an arrest, the use of sedation and muscle relaxants make the process of intubation easier. The use of medications to assist in airway management requires training and experience. Few medications could be listed as safe or as having negligible side effects. For patients who are profoundly hypoxic or in shock, sedation may have a more profound effect on blood pressure than expected. Knowledge of the actions, unique complications, and alternatives to drug therapy is necessary. The use of hypnotics, sedatives, and muscle relaxants is contraindicated unless a means exists to *guarantee* airway control.

Oxygen

Oxygen is the first drug of importance. Risk of short-term oxygen toxicity is minimal. Neonates with complex congenital heart disease who are dependant on a patent ductus arteriosus (for example, hypoplastic left heart syndrome) may have increases in cardiopulmonary symptoms with prolonged use of 100% oxygen. The best dictum is "oxygen is good." A nonrebreather mask that can deliver greater than 85% O_2 should be available.

Atropine

Atropine inhibits the action of acetylcholine at muscarinic receptors. With usual doses, atropine has little or no effects on the nicotinic receptor. Atropine differs from its quaternary ammonium analog in that atropine crosses the blood brain barrier, and may therefore stimulate the CNS, resulting in side effects.

Small doses (less than 0.01 mg/kg) may cause central stimulation rather than peripheral depression of the vagus nerve, causing bradycardia. Salivary, bronchial, and sweat gland secretions are depressed with low doses. Higher doses (0.02 mg/kg) dilate pupils, limit accommodation of the eye, and block the peripheral vagal effects on the heart. The highest doses (0.03 mg/kg) depress parasympathetic control of the GU and GI systems. Micturition and gut motility may be inhibited.

Atropine has a wide margin of safety. Only with large or repeated dosing should one expect to see undesired side effects. These might include restlessness, irritability, delirium, a persistently elevated heart rate, urinary retention, and fever.

The therapeutic effects of atropine have a rapid onset. Cardiac vagolytic action should begin to recede in 30 to 60 minutes. Salivary diminution and pupillary dilatation may persist longer but fixed pupils should not be expected. Use of ketamine and reversal of neuromuscular blockade agents is associated with bronchorrhea. Due to this risk their use should be coupled with atropine. Succinylcholine and intubation in the awake patient may elicit strong vagal stimulation which has been associated with bradycardia. The risk of bradycardia may be lessened with vagolytic doses of atropine. [Dose: 0.02 to 0.03 mg/kg intravenously, minimum single dose 0.1 mg]

Lidocaine

Lidocaine has been used to assist intubation in patients with elevated Intracranial Pressure (ICP). The topical use of lidocaine may be beneficial when placing nasotracheal tubes in the awake patient. Given parenterally, lidocaine will decrease the cough reflex and has been shown to decrease ICP in a manner similar to barbiturates.[41] Risk of lidocaine toxicity is limited with single and low doses. Symptoms of toxicity are usually seen in the elderly after repeated doses or when on a lidocaine drip. The toxic effects are usually CNS dysfunction, slurred speech, disorientation, paresthesia, and rarely, seizures. Hypotension has been reported after rapid administration. [Dose 1 to 1.5 mg/kg intravenously given 1 minute before the intubation attempt.[15]]

Sedation

Benzodiazepines. Benzodiazepines enhance the effect of gamma-aminobutyric acid (GABA) on the central nervous system. GABA is an inhibitory neurotransmitter, thus an increased effect results in CNS depression, amnesia, sleep, anxiolytic action, and sedation. These medications have a relatively large margin of safety, low incidence of secondary organ dysfunction, and a small but significant risk of addiction. By their pharmacologic action, one would expect the potential for CNS depression and apnea. This may be exaggerated in patients with hepatic failure, and in patients on barbiturates or opiates. Benzodiazepines and metabolites are eliminated by the liver. Hepatic dysfunction and use of other medications cleared by the liver may increase the drug's effect.[40] All benzodiazepines may cause hypotension.

Diazepam is commonly used in the child for sedation, its amnestic effect, and for anxiety and seizure control. It has a long distribution half-life and an extremely long elimination half-life, (20-50 hours). These pharmacokinetics may limit the usefulness of this medication in long-term patient care. The metabolites also are sedatives with very long elimination half-lives, which may be even longer in infancy. The dose is 0.1 to 0.2 mg/kg/IV. This dose may be repeated every 2-4 hours. Respiratory depression is common especially in young children or if used with barbiturates and narcotics. Intravenous administration may be associated with burning at the injection site. Intramuscular use of this medication has erratic absorption. Rectal use has been described, but onset of action is prolonged.[18,23,51]

Midazolam has several properties that may make it a good choice for acute airway care. It is water soluble, thus it can be given intravenously with little pain. It crosses the blood-brain barrier rapidly, and therefore, has a rapid onset, within 3 to 5 minutes with IV administration, and has marked amnestic effects. Its elimination half-life is 1.5 to 3 hours. Cardiorespiratory depression is most common with large doses, rapid administration, and with concurrent use of narcotics, barbiturates, and alcohol. Doses may vary greatly in different patients, and use of other medications may alter its effect. Patients given no medication may require a dose of 0.1 to 0.3 mg/kg IV for induction. Increments of 25 to 50% of the initial dose may be used every 2 minutes, if sedation for intubation is inadequate.[18,23,48,51]

Recently, a benzodiazepine receptor antagonist, flumazenil, has been developed. Given intravenously in 0.1 mg increments, this medication has been very effective in reversing the CNS depression of benzodiazepines. Risk of seizures may limit its use in the child.[18]

Narcotics. Morphine and fentanyl are the two most common opiates used in the ICU setting. When used in doses for intubation, respiratory depression is very likely, especially in the neonate. Onset of action is rapid, with fentanyl being greater than morphine. Duration of action is 2 to 7 hours for morphine, and 1 to 2 hours for fentanyl. Tolerance may develop with long-term use. Both medications may be reversed with naloxone. Special mention of morphine's effect on cardiovascular and pulmonary systems is warranted. Flushing, vasodilation, hypotension, and histamine release may complicate the care of an already unstable patient. Fentanyl has fewer cardiovascular effects, but it has been associated with bradycardia and chest wall rigidity, especially with high doses. Chest wall rigidity is amenable to muscle relaxants.[4,7,45,47,51] Morphine doses which may be used begin at 0.1 to 0.2 mg/kg/dose IV. Common dosages of fentanyl are 1-5 mcg/kg/dose IV. (Much higher doses are used in operative settings.)

Ketamine. Ketamine is a phencyclidine analogue, producing a dissociation anesthesia. Amnesia and anesthesia may be profound. Major advantages of this drug is its ability to stimulate release of catecholamine. This may make it the drug of choice for intubating the asthmatic person or patient with hypovolemia. Maintaining respiration and hypopharyngeal control are other advantages. Care is still needed with use of this medication. It may be associated with direct myocardial depression and may add demands to myocardial oxygen consumption. It is clearly associated with increasing intracranial pressure, hypersalivation, and laryngospasm. Pretreatment with atropine should be strongly considered. Hallucinations, more common in the older patient, may be lessened with concomitant use of benzodiazepines. The hypnotic effect is rapid, usually occurring with 1 minute, and the effect begins to dissipate in 3 to 5 minutes. The dose is 0.5-1.5 mg/kg/dose and should be given slowly intravenously to prevent apnea.[16,51]

Barbiturates. The ultra short-acting barbiturates continue to be popular for producing sedation and amnesia. Rapid onset of action with a very short duration of effect is attributable to their marked lipid solubility. Onset of the hypnotic effect occurs in seconds and lasts approximately 15 to 20 minutes. Repeated doses may cause accumulation in lipid stores with resulting prolonged sedation. A favorable effect of barbiturates is a reduction of intracranial pressure. Thiopental may be very useful in airway control of the patient with status epilepticus. The risks of thiopental (pentothal), and methohexital (brevital), are multiple. Both have a direct depressive effect on myocardial function, and both may cause the release of histamine. These concerns may eliminate the usefulness of these medications in patients with hypotension or bronchospasm. Methohexital may also lower seizure threshold.[16,18,19,50] Thiopental should be given in doses of 4-6 mg/kg IV and methohexital 1 to 1.5 mg/kg.

Muscle relaxing agents (paralytics)

Muscle relaxants have no sedative or amnestic effects. These medications are used in conjunction with a selected sedative agent. Moribund patients may not need muscle relaxants, while combative patients may benefit from sedation and paralysis. Multiple new and old medications are available, and each has benefits and limitations. It can be expected that new, rapid onset muscle relaxing agents, with very short duration times will be developed.

Succinylcholine, the only available depolarizing relaxant, continues to be useful because of its rapid onset and relative short duration of action. Onset of action is within 20 to 30 seconds, and duration is 4 to 5 minutes which may be longer in children. Compared with other muscle relaxants, use of succinylcholine is risky due to potential complications: muscle contraction (including trismus with masseter spasm), hyperkalemia, myoglobinuria, increased vagal effects, increased ocular & intracranial pressures, prolonged paralysis if there is a pseudocholinesterase deficiency, and malignant hyperthermia. Muscle contraction may increase gastric pressures, displace fractures, increase risk of eye injuries, and cause marked potassium release in patients with neuromuscular disease, crush injury, burn injury, chronic hypotonia, and spinal cord dysfunction. While this medication may be recommended by many anesthesiologists and critical care physicians, it is the authors' preference to use other muscle relaxing agents. This medication should be coupled with atropine. Typical dose is 1 to 2 mg/kg IV.

Pancuronium is commonly used for prolonged paralysis. The onset of action is long, although it can be shortened with a large (twice the ED_{95}) or a priming dose (one tenth the intubating dose given several minutes before time of intubation). Duration of action is also long. Cardiovascular effects include a vagolytic response, which commonly causes tachycardia. Histamine release is rare. While pancuronium is still used during emergent situations, its actions favor its use in long-term ventilator care. The paralytic dose is 0.1 to 0.2 mg/kg. The defasciculating (used before giving succinylcholine) and priming doses are each 0.01 mg/kg IV. High dose succinylcholine and pancuronium have been given intramuscularly in the rare situation where vascular access has not been established but paralysis is needed.

Vecuronium, a nondepolarizing agent of intermediate duration, has several advantages that have made it very useful in managing critically ill patients. Vecuronium has very little cardiovascular effect, little histamine release, both renal and hepatic clearance, and the onset of action may allow intubation within 1 to 2 minutes when using priming or higher doses. Duration of effect is between 30 and 40 minutes. Prolonged paralysis has been reported with extended use. The standard dose is 0.1 to 0.3 mg/kg given intravenously.

Although not usually necessary the paralytic effect of nondepolarizing agents may be reversed with the use of acetylcholinesterase inhibitors. Usual agents are neostigmine (0.06-0.08 mg/kg) or edrophonium (0.5-1 mg/kg). The use of these reversal agents *must* be accompanied by the use of atropine to avoid excessive muscarinic side effects, bradycardia, excessive secretions, and bronchoconstriction.[23,32,44,52,53,72] (Table 18-3).

TABLE 18-3 ADJUVANT MEDICATIONS FOR INTUBATION

Medication	*Dose (mg)*	*Indication*	*Concerns*
Atropine	0.2-0.3	Vagolytic effect	Tachycardia, dilated pupils
Lidocaine	1-1.5	Decrease cough and ICP	Occasional hypotension
Diazepam	0.1-0.2	Sedation	Resp. depressant, hypotension
Midazolam	0.1-0.3	Sedation	Resp. depressant, hypotension
Morphine	0.1-0.2	Pain/Sedation	Histamine release, resp. depress.
Fentanyl	0.001-0.005 (1-5 mcg/kg)	Pain/Sedation	Resp. Depress., Stiff chest wall
Ketamine	1-2	Sedation	Increase ICP, Bronchorrhea
Thiopental	4-6	Sedation, decrease ICP	Myocardial depressant
Methohexital	1-1.5	Sedation (ultra short)	Histamine release, Bronchospasm
Succinylcholine	1-2	Rapid sequence intubation	Hyperkalemia, MHT
Pancuronium	0.1-0.2	Muscle relaxant	Hypertension, Tachycardia
Vecuronium	0.1-0.3	Muscle relaxant	Prolonged paralysis (rare)
Naloxone	0.005-0.1	Narcotic reversal	Short action, arrythmias
Flumazenil	(see text)	Benzodiazepine reversal	Seizures

TABLE 18-4 LOW-FLOW OXYGEN DEVICES

100% Oxygen l/min	*Fraction insp. oxygen*
Nasal cannula	
1	24%
2	28%
3	32%
4	36%
5	40%
Oxygen mask	
5-6	40%
6-7	50%
7-8	60%
Mask with reservoir	
6	60%
7	70%
8	80%
9	>80%

Atracurium, mivacurium, and pipecuronium have advantages in patients paralyzed for treatment in the ICU or OR. Their onset of action and duration of effect limit their usefulness in rapid sequence intubation.

OXYGEN

Delivery devices

Nasal cannulas have been used to deliver oxygen to patients, but in conditions where determination of F_iO_2 is important, or when consistency of delivery is needed, these devices lose their usefulness. In adult patients the rule is that 1 l/min oxygen flow may increase F_iO_2 by 3 to 4%, but even high flow oxygen via nasal cannula probably does not increase tracheal oxygen above 50%. Attempts to increase O_2 concentration using both a nasal cannula and face mask have been met with varying degrees of success.

Nonrebreathing masks are designed with a series of one-way valves, so exhaled gases have minimal contact with inspired gas. This must be coupled with inspiratory flows which meet minute ventilation demands. This is accomplished by adding a reservoir that has additional gas available during the high flow phase of early inspiration. In a system where minute ventilation, flow rates, and reserve volumes are adequate to meet total ventilation needs, the system is called *fixed performance high flow*. When room air is entrained to meet ventilatory needs, the system is called *variable performance low-flow*, where precise determination of F_iO_2 is impossible.

High-flow systems deliver accurate oxygen concentrations, and all of the delivered gas may be warmed and humidified. However, oxygen flow rates of four times expected minute ventilation are needed. This may limit their usefulness during transport.

Low-flow systems are most commonly used because of convenience, economy, and availability. They are most accurate with even, slow tidal respiration. High respiratory rates with large, erratic tidal volumes may drop the expected F_iO_2[68] (Table 18-4).

OXYGEN TANKS

The oxygen tanks most commonly used in hospitals and in transport vehicles are the E and H/K cylinders. E cylinders are easily portable and are used for short trips. H or K cylinders are large and cumbersome but are needed for longer trips. When full, the pressure in these oxygen canisters is approximately 2200 PSI. Obviously, there is a difference in the amount of gas available for use in each cylinder. To approximate the time/flow capabilities of each tank, one may use the equations below:

E Cylinders:

$$(\text{PSI} \times 0.3)/\text{Flow in l/min} = \text{minutes of remaining oxygen}$$

H or K Cylinder:

$$(\text{PSI} \times 3)/\text{Flow in l/min} = \text{minutes of oxygen remaining}$$

Examples:

E Cylinder reads 900 PSI, and oxygen flow is set at 4 l/min.

$$(900 \times 0.3)/4 = 67 \text{ minutes}$$

H Cylinder reads 2000 PSI, and oxygen flow is set at 10 l/min.

$$(2000 \times 3)/10 = 600 \text{ minutes}$$

These equations are used for rough approximations. One should not depend on the gauge for accuracy when it reads less than 500 PSI. For safety one should plan for an oxygen volume to be two-fold over calculated needs.

TECHNIQUE OF INTUBATION

Once the need for intubation has been established the caregiver must evaluate the patient to determine the best approach (nasal versus oral), technique of instrumentation, and the choice of sedation and muscle relaxant.

A preintubation routine should be established in all nonemergent intubations, and every effort to follow the routine should occur with emergent situations (Fig. 18-5).

Preoxygenation with high concentration oxygen is always desirable. The patient will benefit from several minutes of spontaneous breathing from a mask delivering greater than 85% O_2. Normally, exhaled gases have oxygen tension of less than 80 torr; after preoxygenation the partial pressure of O_2 in the alveoli may be significantly greater than 100 torr for more than several minutes. This adds a margin of safety to any intubation.

Because of the increased risk of aspiration, a child who is experiencing respiratory difficulty should never be given anything by mouth. A child has a higher resting intragastric pressure, shorter esophagus, lower esophageal/gastric tone (especially in the neonate), and a longer gastric emptying time when compared with an adult. Studies have shown that gastric volumes may reach as high as 3 cc/kg after being NPO from 1 to 4 hours in children who are hospitalized for emergency surgery. Children hospitalized from 4 to 8 hours had residual volumes of approximately 1 cc/kg. NG emptying of stomach and medications that stimulate gastric emptying or increase gastric pH could be beneficial. Time and the clinical situation must be balanced when deciding on techniques that could limit risk of gastric aspiration.[20,21,65] Anesthesia techniques have been developed to decrease the risk of aspiration during intubation of the patient with a full stomach.[38,62]

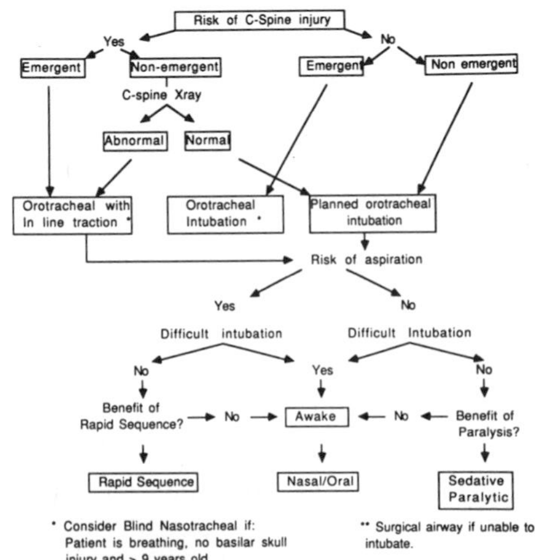

Fig. 18-5. Algorithm of intubation needed.

Rapid sequence intubation is a technique that has been developed to quickly take over control of a patient's airway. This technique using priming doses of muscle relaxants or high dose of muscle relaxants cause rapid onset of apnea. A priming dose of a muscle relaxant is a subtherapeutic dose of one of the nondepolarizing agents: pancuronium, atracurium, or vecuronium. This dose is usually given several minutes before planned intubation. The theory is that the subtherapeutic dose, which is usually one tenth of the intubating dose, will occupy approximately 70% of the neuromuscular receptors. This should allow very rapid onset of apnea when the intubating dose of the muscle relaxant is given.[53] This technique may be beneficial with patients who have a full stomach or elevated intracranial pressure.

The operator should quickly assess the patient, paying particular attention to mobility of neck, size and mobility of mandible, size of tongue, dental condition, and perfusion and volume status. The following sequence is then followed:

1. Start an IV infusion, ensure that there is free flow of fluid.
2. Check the equipment and clarify personnel's responsibility.
3. In a fully conscious patient, place a nasogastric tube, and empty the stomach of fluid and air. This tube may be left in place or removed.
4. Clean the mouth and pharynx with suction.
5. Preoxygenate the patient with either a nonrebreather mask or bag-valve-mask for at least 2 minutes with a high concentration of oxygen.
6. Prepare all medications.
7. Place the patient in a semierect position, approximately 30 degrees from supine.

8. Check to make sure that ECG, pulse-oximeter, and monitors are functioning.
9. Administer atropine and a priming dose of nondepolarizing muscle relaxant, if succinylcholine is to be used.
10. Give an IV sedative such as diazepam, midazolam, morphine, fentanyl, thiopental, or ketamine.
11. Position the patient for intubation. A roll placed beneath the shoulder in an infant or beneath the occiput in an older child may facilitate the alignment of the oral tracheal axis.
12. Give the IV muscle relaxant: succinylcholine, vecuronium, or pancuronium. Apply cricoid pressure and maintain until endotracheal tube is placed.
13. Allow the patient to become apneic. Apnea is a sign of complete muscle relaxation. *Do not allow hypoxia to develop.* Active intervention with bag-valve-mask should occur if saturations dip below 90%.
14. While maintaining cricoid pressure, expose larynx and intubate (Figures 18-6 and 18-7).
15. Confirm appropriate placement of endotracheal tube and secure and replace NG tube if previously removed. Restrain the patient's hands, and prepare for additional sedation.[35,70,81]

In patients with altered level of consciousness, one must maintain adequate oxygen delivery to the brain during manipulation of the airway. Many sedatives lower systemic blood pressure by vasodilatation or myocardial depression. This might compromise cerebral perfusion pressure. Thiopental is associated with depression of blood pressure, but it has the beneficial effects of lowering ICP and giving deep sedation. Ketamine may be contraindicated, since it is associated with elevation of ICP. Lidocaine will lower ICP, depress the cough reflex, and may add a measure of safety.[6,56] (Table 18-5)

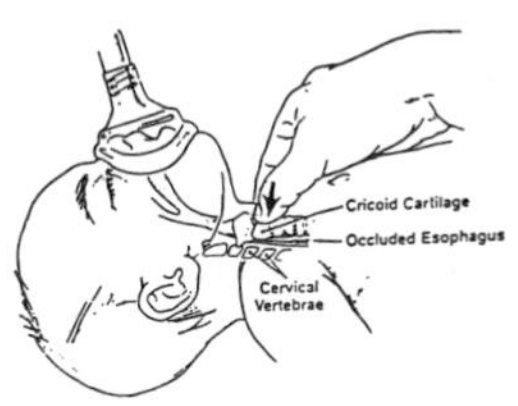

Fig. 18-6. Cricoid pressure (Sellick maneuver) with mask. (Reproduced with permission. Textbook of Pediatric Advanced Life Support, 1988. Copyright American Heart Association.)

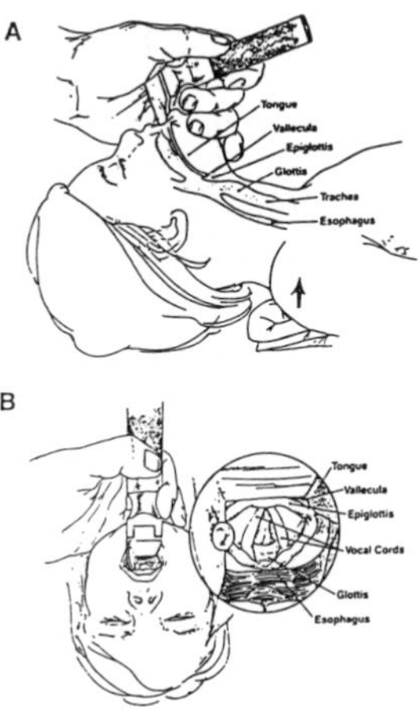

Fig. 18-7. A, Introduction of laryngoscope with anatomic landmarks. B, Operator's view of the internal anatomy. (Reproduced with permission. Textbook of Pediatric Advanced Life Support, 1988. Copyright American Heart Association.)

DIFFICULT INTUBATION

Even very experienced caregivers may face situations that demand special considerations with airway management. When difficult intubation is a possibility, several important points need to be mentioned. Use of muscle relaxants before intubation are contraindicated in certain circumstances: neck swelling, upper airway obstruction (epiglottitis), trauma to face with active nasopharyngeal bleeding or unstable mandible, and difficulty in ventilating patient using bag-valve-mask. In addition, succinylcholine should not be given in the following circumstances: hyperkalemia, penetrating eye injuries, or history of malignant hyperthermia. The loss of muscular tone may contribute to complete obstruction of the airway from an inflammatory process or a mass that is compressing the airway.

Fiberoptic intubation

Fiberoptic intubation is a newer technique in airway management. After placing an appropriately sized endotracheal tube over a

TABLE 18-5 MEDICATIONS FOR INTUBATION/SPECIFIC CONDITIONS

	Relaxant	*Sedative*	*Other*	*Rational*
Routine	Vecuronium/ succinylcho.	Narcotic/ben- zodiaz	Atropine	Vecuronium slower onset but less side effects than succi- nylcholine
Asthma	Vecuronium/ succinylcho.	Ketamine	Atropine	Ketamine is a bronchodilator
Obstruction	None	Ketamine/ben- zodiaz/nar- cotic	Atropine	Relaxants may worsen airway obstruction Awake intubation may be necessary
Elevated ICP	Vecuronium/ succinylcho.	Thiopental	Atropine and lidiocaine	If succinylcho used, a defas- ciculating med. (pancuro- nium) should be consid- ered. Thiopental and lidocaine lower ICP
Rapid sequence	Succinylcho./ high dose vecuronium	Thiopental or narcotic	Atropine	Succinylcholine has the most rapid onset high dose ve- curonium may be adequate thiopental causes rapid se- dation
Shock	Vecuronium	Ketamine/low dose nar- cotic	Atropine and fluids	Vecuronium has little hemo- dynamic effect ketamine may raise BP fluids will help prevent hypotension

bronchoscope, the operator inserts the bronchoscope via the mouth or nose through the larynx into the trachea. The endotracheal tube can then be passed over the bronchoscope into the airway. Appropriate position of the endotracheal tube can be determined immediately by observing the distance from the tip of the tube to the carina. However, this technique does require still and equipment that is not available to most transport teams. Instruments are now available with diameters smaller than 3.0 mm, allowing placement of a 3.5 to 4.0 endotracheal tube.

Tactile intubation

Tactile techniques for intubation have gained common acceptance in adult patients. This technique has also been described and used with great success in the neonate.[34] The approach to neonatal intubation is very similar to that of the adult.

While standing at the patients side, a gloved index finger of the nondominant hand is passed over and around the tongue until the epiglottis is passed, and the aryepiglottic folds are palpated. The thumb of that hand should apply gentle pressure at the cricoid cartilage. The endotracheal tube with stylet is passed like a curved pencil into the larynx, using the nondominant index finger as guide. The endotracheal tube is felt by the nondominant thumb as it passes into the trachea.

The advantages of this technique include no need for a light source, approach to the patient from any angle, and little concern for equipment failure. The risks are those that are inherent with any intubation, for example, vagal effects. Patients with teeth may also make this approach difficult and risky for the caregiver.[71]

Lightwand intubation is similar to tactile intubation. A lighted stylet is passed over and around the tongue. As the stylet is passed into the larynx the light can be seen as a red glow in the midline of the patient's neck. The endotracheal tube is then passed into the larynx over the stylet. Lightwand size is the factor that limits the use in children.[52]

Surgical airway intervention

Most surgical techniques for pediatric airway control, such as tracheostomy and cri-

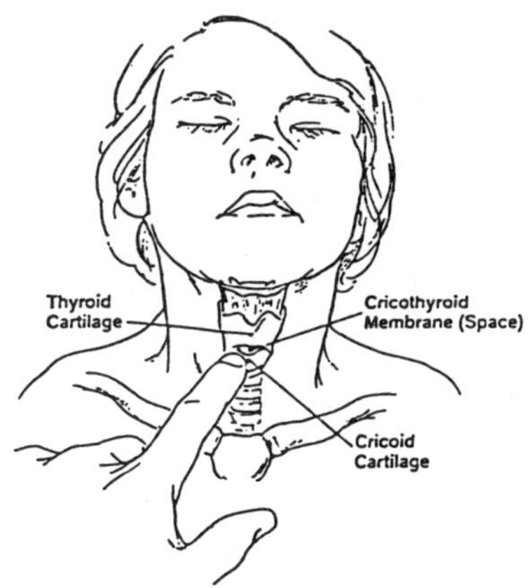

Fig. 18-8. Cricoid membrane anatomy. (Reproduced with permission. Textbook of Pediatric Advanced Life Support, 1988. Copyright American Heart Association.)

cothyroidotomy, require a high degree of surgical skill. These techniques are beyond the scope of this article; alternatives to these will be discussed below.[37,50]

Needle cricothyroidotomy is preferable to other surgical routes for emergency airway control in the child. A large, 12 to 16-gauge, caliber catheter over needle on a 10 cc syringe is passed through the cricothyroid membrane at midline (Figure 18-8). It is angled caudally at approximately 45 degrees. When air is freely aspirated the plastic catheter is advanced into the trachea. The hub of the catheter may then be attached to a 3.0 pediatric endotracheal tube adapter, or to a vascular Leur-lock apparatus that is modified for gas insufflation. The flow meter must be set at flush (>15 l/min), and the pressure source should be 45 to 50 PSI. Special connectors will be needed for the tubing in this high pressure system, since standard airway tubing and connectors will not maintain their integrity. Gas is delivered by jet insufflation not by a self-inflating bag. Y-connectors or a pressure button is needed to control gas delivery. One second on and 4 seconds off would be a reasonable starting rhythm. This form of jet insufflation assists with oxygenation, and assists little with ventilation. With this technique one may maintain oxygen saturation for 30 to 45 minutes. During this time other means of airway control can be attempted. This maneuver may have a unique benefit for airway obstruction secondary to a foreign body. Complications of this technique include asphyxia, infection, perforation of trachea, thyroid, esophagus or carotid, hematoma, and subcutaneous or mediastinal emphysema.[3,28,29,69,80]

Retrograde intubation is a technique which has been described in the spontaneously breathing patient who can not be intubated in the conventional manner. While angling cephalad the inferior cricothyroid membrane is punctured with a needle attached to a syringe. When air is aspirated, tracheal puncture is established. One to 2 cc of 1% lidocaine should be instilled at this time to help prevent laryngospasm. A guide wire is now passed through the needle. After the wire is located in the hypopharynx the endotracheal tube may be passed over it into the trachea. After the endotracheal tube is placed the wire is withdrawn. Distorted or very small airways would make this procedure more difficult to perform.[52] Complications of this technique include bleeding, infection, tracheal injury, and laryngospasm.

Stabilization and maintenance of endotracheal tube

There are a number of ways to stabilize an endotracheal tube. The authors prefer beginning by cleansing the perioral area with skin prep or benzoin. Tegaderm® is then applied over the cheek reaching to the angle of the lip. Two pieces of 1 inch elastic tape (Elastikon®) are measured to reach from the angle of the jaw to mid cheek on the opposite side. It is cut and split longitudinally for approximately half of its length. The base is applied to the Tegaderm®. One of the forks is applied over the lip, while the other is wrapped clockwise two times around the endotracheal tube. This is repeated with the second piece of tape, but now the first fork is applied beneath the lower lip while the other is wrapped counterclockwise around the tube. The endotracheal tube is measured from incisor to hub, and notation of the centimeter marking as the tube exits the mouth is made. Simple modification of this technique is possible for nasotracheal tubes.[60] Head harnesses have been used in patients who have facial burns or other problems that make facial taping difficult. When transferring the patient from a bed to a stretcher, one should disconnect the endotracheal tube from the resuscitation bag or ventilator to avoid dislodging the tube.

Some operators prefer to place oral endotracheal tubes, others prefer nasal. In either case it is the authors' experience that accidental extubations are more likely to occur in patients who are inadequately sedated or with tubes which are improperly secured. Therefore, chemical restraints (sedation) should be available for all intubated patients.

Once the endotracheal tube has been placed and stabilized, equipment is needed to maintain the patency of the endotracheal tube. The combination of small endotracheal tubes, dry gases, and airway secretions may cause the tube plugging and endotracheal tube occlusion. Instillation of 3 to 5 cc normal saline with suctioning of the airway every 15 minutes during transport is recommended. If thick secretions are a problem, more frequent suctioning and more aggressive use of saline may be indicated. If at any time the endotracheal tube were to become completely occluded, it should be removed and replaced.

TRANSPORT VENTILATION

Many intubated patients have been transported safely with ventilation by resuscitation bags. A bag valve device allows the caregiver to feel pulmonary compliance and intervene accordingly. PEEP valves and pressure manometers have added greatly to these systems. Limitations of hand ventilation include the following: 1) one person is needed continuously for ventilatory support, 2) fatigue, and 3) variation of rate and effort may change peak inspiratory pressure, mean airway pressure, and minute ventilation, placing a patient at increased risk for barotrauma or respiratory compromise.

Studies have shown that mechanical ventilation during transport may cause less variability of patient's blood gases when compared to manual ventilation.[13,39,78]

In order to use mechanical ventilators effectively, a basic understanding of their characteristics and nomenclature is necessary.

When a ventilator cycles independently of a patient's effort, it is referred to as controlled ventilation. Intermittent mandatory ventilation (IMV) refers to a pattern of controlled ventilation where spontaneous breathing is permitted. When this form of ventilation is synchronized to coincide with the patient's effort, it is termed synchronized IMV. In assisted ventilation, the ventilator cycles in response to each inspiratory effort. Assisted ventilation may have either volume or pressure modes.

Modes of ventilation are usually named by the physical factor that ends the inspiratory cycle, thus we most commonly use the terms volume, pressure, or time cycled. The most common modes of ventilation used for children are time cycled, volume-regulated, or time cycled and pressure-limited.

Time cycled volume ventilation is designed to deliver gas at a constant rate of flow over a given inspiratory time to yield a specific tidal volume. Thus, higher flows and longer inspiratory times yield larger tidal volumes. Peak inspiratory pressure is variable and dependant on flow rates, inspiratory times, resistance of the system, and compliance of the patient's lungs. The advantage of this mode of ventilation is that the volume delivered is reliably controlled and remains constant in the face of changes in patient's pulmonary compliance. Potential disadvantages are a loss of effective tidal volume when air leaks occur in the system, and high pressures can be unexpectedly generated.

Time cycled, pressure-limited ventilation delivers gas at some preset flow, usually 1-2 l/min/kg. Flow continues for a defined inspiratory time; the peak inspiratory pressure is limited to a preset value until the inspiratory time is terminated. The tidal volume is dependent on the pressure limit and the compliance of the system and lungs. The advantage of this system is simplicity, the ability to control peak airway pressure, and minimal change of effective tidal volume with air leaks around the endotracheal tube. This system is also very conducive to treatment of respiratory distress of the newborn where high rates, short inspiratory times, and higher mean airway pressures are needed. Important limitations include changing tidal ventilation with changes in pulmonary compliance or resistance in the circuit. This may result in decreased minute ventilation with worsening compliance or risk of pneumothorax with improvement of compliance.[68]

All ventilator systems should be designed with continuous or demand flow. Continuous flow circuits have gas flow through the tubing during all phases of the respiratory cycle. Demand flow is similar but requires a pressure-sensing device. With demand flow a spontaneous breath is sensed, and then a demand valve is opened which allows increased gas flow. This flow stops at end inspiration. Demand flow valves may lessen air trapping but may add slightly to work of breathing during the early phase of spontaneous inspiration. Ultrasensitive valves have been designed to lessen this effect. A mechanism to deliver positive end-expiratory pressure (PEEP) should be provided as well as a humidification and heating system. While transport ventilators allow ventilation to be more consistent during transport, they also add a level of complexity. They should be used only by personnel who are trained in their use and who understand the principles of gas consumption.

TRAINING AND SURVEILLANCE OF PERFORMANCE

Proficiency in respiratory support procedures is vital to safely transport the critically ill or injured child. Methods to train, maintain proficiency, and carry out surveillance of performance will vary among transport programs depending on type and experience of staff. General recommendations regarding qualifications of transport personnel should identify necessary procedures and abilities and are not dependent on their professional degree. A training process is required for both physicians and nonphysician transport staff which will develop cognitive abilities, judgment, and psychomotor skills in airway management. While some authors recommend the presence of a physician on pediatric transports,[2,82] recent experience indicates that nonphysician staff (nurses, paramedics, and respiratory therapists) can safely transport critically ill children.[8] It is likely that the transport performance of experienced nonphysician professional personnel will be superior to that of resident physicians, although no published data are available regarding this issue.

When training staff who lack previous experience in airway management procedures, the Pediatric Advanced Life Support course (PALS, American Heart Association/American Academy of Pediatrics) or its equivalent, will provide a satisfactory introduction in which endotracheal intubation is reviewed in written material and class discussions. Practice is achieved in the intubation of teaching models and anesthetized animals in the PALS course. Then, further experience is gained in supervised procedures in the well controlled environment of the operating room or intensive care unit. Judgment and experience with the unique factors involved in the transport setting are best attained by trainees working under the supervision of experienced staff during their first several transports. Specific protocols for intubation procedures will depend upon factors unique to each transport service. For example, experience in use of muscle relaxants by nonphysician staff to facilitate intubation has been published,[36] but risks and benefits of this approach in children by nonphysician staff have not been investigated.

A busy transport service may provide staff with enough practice in airway support procedures to maintain their proficiency. Surveillance of procedures and problems encountered by each staff member will allow the assignment of additional practice sessions on mannequins or supervised intubations on patients when necessary.

It must be emphasized that no data are available, which indicate the optimal educational curriculum or extent of practice necessary to become proficient in tracheal intubation. Nor have observations been made to indicate the amount of ongoing practice necessary to remain proficient in airway procedures. Since practice exercises may be carried out, in part, on mannequins, it is notable that no investigations have been published regarding the correlation between performance in actual resuscitation procedures and in simulations. As pediatric transport medicine becomes an active specialty, the highly structured training and surveillance processes involved provide an opportunity to evaluate the practical impact of specific educational methods in acute care procedures.

REFERENCES

1. Aijian P and others: Endotracheal intubation of pediatric patients by paramedics, *Annals of Emergency Medicine* 18:489-94, 1989.
2. American Academy of Pediatrics, Committee on Hospital Care: Guidelines for air and ground transportation of pediatric patients, *Pediatrics* 78:943-50, 1986.
3. American College of Surgeons, Advanced Trauma Life Support Instructor Manual, Chicago, 1989.
4. Arnold JH and others: Changes in the pharmacodynamic response to fentanyl in neonates during continuous infusion, *The Journal of Pediatrics* 119:639-43, 1991.
5. Aubier M, Trippenbach T, Roussos C: Respiratory muscle fatigue during cardiogenic shock, *J Appl Physiol* 51:499-508, 1981.
6. Bedford RF and others: Lidocaine or thiopental for rapid control of intracranial hypertension, *Anesthesia and Analgesia* 59:435-7, 1980.
7. Bergman I and others: Reversible neurologic abnormalities associated with prolonged intravenous midazolam and fentanyl administration, *The Journal of Pediatrics* 119:644-9, 1991.
8. Beyer J, Land G, Zaritsky A: Nonphysician transport of intubated pediatric patients, *Critical Care Medicine* 20:961-6, 1992.
9. Bhende MS, Thompson AE, Howland DF: Validity of a disposable end-tidal carbon dioxide detector in verifying endotracheal tube position in piglets, *Critical Care Medicine* 19:566-8, 1991.
10. Bhende MS, Thompson AE, Orr RA: Utility of an end-tidal carbon dioxide detector during stabilization and transport of critically ill children, *Pediatrics* 89:1042-4, 1992.
11. Bishop MJ: Mechanisms of laryngotracheal injury following prolonged tracheal intubation, *Chest* 96:185-6, 1989.
12. Boxer RA and others: Noninvasive pulse oximetry in children with congenital heart disease, *Critical Care Medicine* 15(11), 1062-4, 1987.
13. Braman SS and others: Complications of intrahospital transport in critically ill patients, *Ann Intern Med* 107:469-73, 1987.
14. Brink LW, Neuman B, Wynn J: Transport of the critically ill patient with upper airway obstruction, *Critical Care Clinics* 8:633-47, 1992.
15. Brucia JJ, Owen DC, Ruby EB: The effects of lidocaine on intracranial hypertension, *Journal of Neuroscience Nursing* 24:205-14, 1992.
16. Cada DJ and others, editors: *Drug facts and comparisons*, St. Louis, 1993, Wolters Kluwer Co.
17. Carlon GC and others: Capnography in mechanically ventilated patients, *Critical Care Medicine* 16:550-6, 1988.
18. Chernow B, editor: *The pharmacologic approach to the critically ill patient*, ed 2, Baltimore, 1988, Williams & Wilkins.
19. Cold GE, Holdgaard HO: Treatment of intracranial-hypertension in acute head injury with special reference to the role of hyperventilation and sedation with barbiturates: a review, *Intensive Care World* 9:172-6, 1992.
20. Coté CJ: NPO after midnight in children—a reappraisal, *Anesthesiology* 72:589-92, 1990.
21. Coté CJ and others: Assessment of risk factors related to the aspiration syndrome pediatric patients—gastric pH and residual volume, *Anesthesiology* 56:70-2, 1982.
22. Coté CJ and others: Intraoperative events diagnosed by expired carbon dioxide monitoring in children, *Canadian Anaesthetists' Society Journal* 33:315-20, 1986.
23. Coté CJ and others, editors: *A practice of anesthesia for infants and children*, ed 2, Philadelphia, 1993, W.B. Saunders Company.
24. Coté CJ and others: A single-blind study of pulse oximetry in children, *Anesthesiology* 68:184-88, 1988.
25. Cox PN: Current management of laryngotracheobronchitis, bacterial tracheitis and epiglottitis, *Intensive Care World* 10:8-12, 1993.
26. Edge WE and others: Reduction of morbidity in interhospital transport by specialized pediatric staff, *Crit Care Medicine* (In press).
27. Fanconi S: Reliability of pulse oximetry in hypoxic infants, *The Journal of Pediatrics* 112:424-7, 1988.
28. Fifield GC, Morton T, Ruiz E: Transtracheal catheter ventilation (TTCV) in a small animal model, *Annals of Emergency Medicine* 17:397-8, 1988.
29. Frame SB, Timberlake GA, Kerstein MD: Transtracheal needle catheter ventilation in complete airway obstruction: an animal model, *Annals of Emergency Medicine* 18:127-33, 1989.
30. Garnett AR and others: End-tidal carbon dioxide monitoring during cardiopulmonary resuscitation, *JAMA* 257:512-5, 1987.
31. Goldberg JS and others: Colorimetric end-tidal carbon dioxide monitoring for tracheal intubation, *Anesthesia and Analgesia* 70:191-4, 1990.
32. Goodman LS, Gilman A, editors: *The pharmacological basis of therapeutics*, ed 5, New York, 1975, Macmillan Publishing Co., Inc.
33. Gottrup F and others: Continuous monitoring of tissue oxygen tension during hyperoxia and hypoxia: relation of subcutaneous, transcutaneous, and conjunctival oxygen tension to hemodynamic variables, *Critical Care Medicine* 16:1229-34, 1988.
34. Hancock PJ, Peterson G: Finger intubation of the trachea in newborns, *Pediatrics* 89:325-6, 1992.
35. Hee MK, Plevak DJ, Peters SG: Intubation of critically ill patients, *Mayo Clinic Proc* 67:569-76, 1992.
36. Hedges JR and others: Succinylcholine-assisted intubations in prehospital care, *Ann Emerg Med* 17:469-72, 1988.
37. Heffner JE: Medical Indications for tracheotomy, *Chest* 96:186-90, 1989.
38. Hillemeier AC and others: Delayed gastric emptying in infants with gastroesophageal reflux, *The Journal of Pediatrics* 98:190-3, 1981.
39. Hurst JM and others: Comparison of blood gasses during transport using two methods of ventilatory support, *Journal of Trauma* 29:1637-40, 1989.

40. Jones EA and others: NIH Conference. The gamma-aminobutryric acid receptor complex and hepatic encephalopathy, *Ann Inter Med* 110(7), 532-46, 1989.
41. Kanter RK: Evaluation of mask bag ventilation in resuscitation of infants, *Am J Dis Child* 141:761-3, 1987.
42. Kanter RK, Tompkins JM: Adverse events during interhospital transport: physiological deterioration associated with pretransport severity of illness, *Pediatrics* 84:43-8, 1989.
43. Kanter RK and others: Excess morbidity associated with interhospital transport, *Pediatrics* 90:893-8, 1992.
44. Katz RL, editors: *Muscle relaxants,* Orlando, 1985, Grune and Stratton.
45. Kauffman RE: Fentanyl, fads, and folly: who will adopt the therapeutic orphans? *The Journal of Pediatrics* 119:588-9, 1991.
46. Kissoon N and others: Evaluation of performance characteristics of disposable bag-valve resuscitators, *Critical Care Medicine* 19:102-7, 1991.
47. Lane JC and others: Movement disorder after withdrawal of fentanyl infusion, *The Journal of Pediatrics* 119:649-51, 1991.
48. Lunn JJ, Larson JS: How best to provide sedation and analgesia for critically ill patients, *The Journal of Critical Illness* 7:1090-1104, 1992.
49. Lynn AM, Bosenberg A: Pulse oximetry during cardiac catheterization in children with congenital heart disease, *J Clin Monit* 2(4), 230-3, 1986.
50. Marsh HM, Gillespie DJ, Baumgartner AE: Timing of tracheostomy in the critically ill patient, *Chest* 96:190-3, 1989.
51. Marx CM and others: Pediatric intensive care sedation: survey of fellowship training programs, *Pediatrics* 91,2:369-76, 1993.
52. McDonald TB, Berkowitz RA: Airway management and sedation for pediatric transport, *Pediatric Clinics of North America* 40,381-406, 1993.
53. Motoyama EK, Davis PJ, editors: *Smith's anesthesia for infants and children,* ed 5, St. Louis, 1990, The CV Mosby Company.
54. O'Flaherty D, Adams AP: The end-tidal carbon dioxide detector, *Anesthesia* 45:653-5, 1990.
55. Paloheimo M, Valli M, Ahjopalo H: A guide to CO_2 monitoring, *Datex Instrumentarium Oy,* 1987 (pamphlet).
56. Paul RL and others: Intracranial pressure responses to alterations in arterial carbon dioxide pressure in patients with head injuries, *J Neurosurg* 36:714-20, 1972.
57. Propofol: A physician's guide to use in the intensive care unit, *Stuart Pharmaceuticals,* Wilmington, DE. (pamphlet).
58. Raphaely RC: Acute respiratory failure in infants and children, *Pediatric Annals* 15:315-8, 1986.
59. Richardson MA, Cotton RT: Anatomic abnormalities of the pediatric airway, *Pediatric Clinics of North America* 31:821-34, 1984.
60. Robson LK, Tompkins JM: Maintaining placement and skin integrity with endotracheal tubes in a pediatric ICU, *Critical Care Nurse* 29-32, 1984.
61. Rose J, Valtonen S, Jennett B. Avoidable factors contributing to death after head injury, *Br Med J* 2:853-5, 1977.
62. Salem MR, Wong AY, Collins VJ: The pediatric patient with a full stomach, *Anesthesiology* 19:435-9, 1973.
63. Sasse FJ: Can we trust end-tidal carbon dioxide measurements in infants, *Journal of Clinical Monitoring* 1:147-8, 1985.
64. Schnapp LM, Cohen NH: Pulse oximetry uses and abuses, *Chest* 98:1244-50, 1990.
65. Schurizek BAS and others: Gastric volume and pH in children for emergency surgery, *Acta Anaesthesiol Scand* 30:404-8, 1986.
66. Sellman GL, Patel RI, Hannallah RS: Changes in arterial oxygen saturation in the pediatric patient during postoperative transport, *Anesthesiology* 65:A447, 1986.
67. Sendak MJ, Harris AP, Donham RT: Use of pulse oximetry to assess arterial oxygen saturation during newborn resuscitation, *Critical Care Medicine* 14:739-40, 1986.
68. Shapiro BA and others: *Clinical application of respiratory care,* ed 3, Chicago, 1985, Year Book Medical Publishers.
69. Smith RB, Myers EN, Sherman H: Transtracheal ventilation in paediatric patients, *BJ Anaesth,* 46, 313-4, 1974.
70. Stept WJ, Safar P: Rapid induction/intubation for prevention of gastric-content aspiration, *Anesthesia and Analgesia* 49:633-6, 1970.
71. Stewart RD: Tactile orotracheal intubation, *Annals of Emergency Medicine* 13:175-8, 1984.
72. Stirt JA: Muscle relaxants in neurosurgical anesthesia: what should we do when the pressure's on, *Journal of Neurosurgical Anesthesiology* 2:1-3, 1990.
73. Swedlow DB: A primer on pulse oximetry, *Pediatric trauma and acute care* 1:25-6, 1988.
74. Terndrup TE, Kanter RK, Cherry RA: A comparison of infant ventilation methods performed by prehospital personnel, *Ann Emerg Med* 18:607-11, 1989.
75. Tremper KK, Barker SJ: Pulse oximetry, *Anesthesiology* 70:98-108, 1989.
76. Ward SA: The capnogram: scope and limitations, *Seminars in anesthesia* 6:216-28, 1987.
77. Weinger MB, Brimm JE: End-tidal carbon dioxide as a measure of arterial mandatory ventilation, *Journal of Clinical Monitoring* 3:73-9, 1987.
78. Weg JG, Haas CF: Safe intrahospital of critically ill ventilator-dependent patients, *Chest* 96:631-5, 1989.
79. West JB: *Respiratory Physiology,* ed 4, Baltimore, 1990, Williams & Wilkins.
80. Worthley L, Holt A: Percutaneous tracheostomy, *Intensive Care World* 9:187-92, 1992.
81. Yamamoto LG, Yim GK, Britten AG: Rapid sequence anesthesia induction for emergency intubation, *Pediatric Emergency Care* 6:200-13, 1990.
82. Zaritsky A, Beyer AJ, MD or not MD: is that the question, *Crit Care Med* 20:1633-5, 1992.

19

RESPIRATORY DISORDERS

BENNIE McWILLIAMS

Respiratory illnesses are very common life-threatening pediatric disorders that result in medical transports. The percentages of children transported with primary respiratory illnesses compared with all pediatric transports range from 19%[43] to 69%,[60] depending on the institution. Additionally, children of different ages have varying rates of primary respiratory illnesses. In a review by Beyer and others,[8] transported patients were divided by age into less than 1 month of age (including neonates), 1 month to 1 year of age, and greater than 1 year of age. The percentages of primary respiratory illnesses were 75%, 54%, and 28.4%, respectively.

Respiratory illnesses may be roughly divided into five major categories: upper airway diseases, lower airway diseases, parenchymal diseases, chest wall diseases, and disorders of the control of ventilation. The majority of children with primary respiratory disorders requiring transportation will have disorders of either the upper or lower airways. Upper airway disease comprises between 36%[43] and 65%,[60] while lower respiratory diseases comprise between 64%[43] and 38%[60] in transported children.

In addition to children with primary respiratory diseases, many other pediatric patients requiring transport undergo respiratory interventions. These include patients requiring intubation and ventilation because of poor central control of ventilation (trauma, meningitis, or other neurological disease), respiratory muscle weakness (sepsis or other type of shock), or other type of respiratory failure (flail chest secondary to trauma). The rate that pediatric patients being transported are intubated and ventilated ranges from 17%[64] to 69%.[8] Other pulmonary interventions occurring during transport include chest tube insertion (primarily for pneumothorax, but also for pleural effusions) and emergency reintubation.[43]

Pulmonary-related complications commonly occur during transport. Kanter and others[43] compared morbidity in transported pediatric patients with nontransported PICU patients with similar illnesses and severity of illness. Morbidity occurred in 21% of transported patients and 11% of nontransported patients (odds ratio of 1.85). The increased complication rate in transported children was primarily due to "intensive care-related adverse events," the majority of which were pulmonary related. Pulmonary adverse events accounted for 26% of the morbidity seen in transported patients and 9% of the morbidity in nontransported children. Fifty-nine percent of the transported children required intubation compared with 38% in nontransported children.

The above figures will vary widely between institutions, depending on the particular focus of the center, the patient population serviced by the center, and the experience of the transport team. They do, however, illustrate the significance of primary and secondary respiratory disease in pediatric transports. Thus, pulmonary disease and complications thereof are common and need to be considered in transported pediatric patients.

UNIQUENESS OF THE PEDIATRIC RESPIRATORY TRACT

There are unique aspects of the pediatric patient that put a child at risk for life-threatening pulmonary disorders. There are a number of review articles detailing lung growth and development.[46,56,58,74,80] A general knowledge of lung growth and development is necessary to understand the respiratory problems which are unique to children and the special considerations necessary for transporting children with respiratory disorders.

Lung development begins in utero and continues through the end of the adolescent growth spurt. The pattern of lung growth and structural features of the different components of the pediatric respiratory tract are important with regard to considerations in transporting pediatric patients. Lung growth may be considered in terms of upper airway development, lower airway development, and alveolar development.

Although the upper airways form very early in development, there are important differences between the infant upper airway and the older child or adult airway. In infants the airways are smaller than in adults, resulting in a significantly greater resistance to airflow in the larger airways compared with older children and adults. Thus, diseases causing airway narrowing have a much greater impact in small children than older children and adults. In addition to the differences in airway caliber, the mucosa is less adherent to the airways, resulting in easy edema formation. Additionally, the narrowest part of the infant airway is at the level of the cricoid cartilage rather than the level of the vocal cords as in older children and adults. Since the cricoid cartilage is a complete ring, any regional inflammation will decrease the airway diameter in an already narrowed area. Thus, diseases of the upper airways, such as viral laryngotracheobronchitis, may produce more severe symptoms in infants and small children than in older children and adults.

Likewise, the lower airways are relatively underdeveloped in infants. There is a decreased number of peripheral airways in infants compared with adults. The peripheral airways increase in number from the prenatal period until approximately 5 to 7 years of age and increase in size from the prenatal period until the end of adolescence. During the first 3 to 4 years (and especially during the first 2 years) the peripheral airways account for approximately half of the total airway resistance. As the number of small airways increase, the contribution of the peripheral airways to total airway resistance decreases to the normal value of approximately 20% by approximately 4 years of age.[40] Small children are therefore at a relatively higher risk of severe symptoms due to lower airway diseases than are older children and adults. Thus, diseases primarily affecting the small airways, such as viral bronchiolitis, are usually more severe in infants than in older children.

At birth the alveoli have only a single capillary bed (rather than two), and the alveolar-capillary barrier is thicker than in older children making gas exchange less effective. The alveoli develop into the typical adult architecture within the first year of life. Fully developed lungs have many connections between adjacent alveoli (Pores of Kohn) and adjacent alveoli and respiratory bronchioles (Lambert's channels). These connections aid the uniform distribution of air throughout the lungs. These connections develop over the first few years of life. As a result, infants have poor collateral ventilation and a greater tendency to develop atelectasis than older children and adults.

Other important differences in the lungs of infants and small children relate to the chest wall. The chest wall in infants is very compliant, and therefore retractions occur more readily in disorders causing decreased lung compliance. A very compliant chest wall results in inefficient breathing and greatly increases the work of breathing. Children often do not have large energy stores, therefore they are more likely to develop respiratory failure.

Thus, developmental factors of infant lungs place them at a greater risk for both upper and lower airway disorders, and these factors will affect the management of these children during transportation.

RECOGNITION OF RESPIRATORY DISTRESS AND FAILURE

Respiratory failure is defined as a state where there is inadequate oxygenation and/or inadequate elimination of CO_2 from the blood.[16] Respiratory failure may result from a number of diseases, ranging from decreased ventilatory drive to airway disease or parenchymal disease. In considering transporting children it is essential to quickly assess a child's respiratory status both before transport and at various times during transportation. A child in respiratory distress will display a number of signs indicative of impending respiratory failure. This "compensated respiratory failure" is analogous to compensated shock, and intervention may be required to prevent the progression to respiratory failure. The breathing pattern is assessed for rate and depth of the breath. The most efficient way for a patient to increase minute ventilation is to increase the depth of breathing more than the rate of breathing. This is seen in nonpulmonary causes for increased minute ventilation (diabetic ketoacidosis, exercise, etc.). In primary pulmonary diseases, however, there is usually a component of increased airway resistance and/or decreased lung compliance resulting in shallow breaths. The child responds by breathing in rapid, shallow breaths (tachypneic breathing). As respiratory distress progresses the breathing slows and may become irregular, indicating the development of respiratory failure. Measures to ensure adequate ventilation should be started immediately. As with continued respiratory distress, the respiratory muscles become fatigued and "see-saw" respirations may begin. In this type of respiration, the abdomen distends and the chest draws in during inspiration, and the chest wall extends and the abdomen withdraws during exhalation. This sign is also indicative of impending respiratory failure. Head bobbing, stridor, prolonged expiration, and grunting also indicate severe respiratory distress.[16]

When a child presenting with either stridor (indicative of upper airway obstruction) or wheezing (indicative of lower airway obstruction) fails to display either of these signs, it may either mean that the child is improving or that the child is worsening to the point that there is not enough air movement to produce the sound. Thus, the presence or absence of either stridor or wheezing must be interpreted in light of other clinical signs. Neurological findings such as hypotonia or lethargy also indicate impending respiratory failure. If a child in respiratory distress, who was previously very agitated, becomes quiet and "sleepy," the child's condition may be improving or it may indicate impending respiratory failure. Thus, the clinical signs of respiratory distress and failure must all be interpreted in light of the total clinical picture. This necessitates repeated assessment, especially during transport.

Oximetry is very useful in continually monitoring the respiratory status of transported children. Blood gases may be obtained prior to transport, and end-tidal CO_2 monitors may be used during transport.[9]

EMERGENCY TREATMENT AND STABILIZATION FOR TRANSPORT

Successful emergency treatment in preparation for the transport of children with impending or overt respiratory failure requires a very rapid systematic assessment before intervention. A convenient way of discovering the etiology and therefore treating a child in respiratory distress is to consider general principles of management and then examine specific disorders by dividing the respiratory system into the following components: upper airway disease, lower airway disease, disorders of the chest wall and respiratory muscles, parenchymal disease, and disorders of control of breathing.

General approach

As is true in all critically ill infants, addressing the basic "ABCs" is the most important factor in the emergency treatment of children with pulmonary diseases. The importance of stabilizing the airway and ventilation is emphasized by the fact that it is always the first system to address in any critically ill person. The general approach to managing respiratory distress and failure during transport includes the basics of advanced cardiac life

TABLE 19-1 INTUBATION EQUIPMENT GUIDELINES

Age	*Laryngoscope*	*Endotracheal* tube size (mm ID)*	*Distance from teeth to mid-trachea (cm)*
Preterm infant	Miller 0	2.5-3.0	8
Term infant	Miller 0-1	3.0-3.5	10
6 months	Miller 1	3.5-4.0	12
1 year	Miller 1	4.0-4.5	12
2 years	Miller 2	4.5	14
4 years	Miller 2	5.0	16
6 years	Miller 2	5.5	16
8 Years	Miller 2		
	McIntosh 2	6.0	18
10 years	Miller 2		
	McIntosh 2	6.5	18
12 years	McIntosh 3	7.0	20

* Generally, sizes below 5.5 are uncuffed and greater than 5.5 are cuffed.

support.[16] The major developmental considerations in managing pediatric airways have been outlined above. Specific guidelines for the general management of the pediatric airway during transport may be considered in terms of airway management, ventilation, and other considerations.

Airway management. Airway compromise is a common problem in children requiring transport[13,33] and is often the primary factor precipitating the request for transport. In a recent review of transported pediatric patients,[33] 97% had airway difficulties associated with their primary disease and 31% required further airway management by the transport team. Thus, airway management plays an important role in transported pediatric patients.

Pediatric airways are different from adult airways in that the larynx is more cephalad, the epiglottis is less stiff, and the vocal cords are shorter.[30] Thus, when positioning the head, excessive hyperextension may result in airway obstruction. Pediatric patients require different laryngoscope sizes, endotracheal tubes,[48] and distance from the teeth to the midtrachea (Table 19-1). As a rule, pediatric patients will have uncuffed endotracheal tubes, and a small endotracheal tube leak is usually present. Once an airway is obtained, it is important to adequately secure the airway. The distance from the teeth to the midcarina is very short in small infants (Table 19-1), and the tube may be easily dislodged (either accidental extubation or intubation of one of the mainstem bronchi). It is important to use tape that will not easily come off especially after it is soaked with oral secretions. Nasal intubation generally provides a more stable airway, but this should not be attempted unless the individual is skilled in this technique.

Ventilatory management. Once an airway is obtained, ventilation should be addressed. Numerous bags are available for pediatric transport which are either self-inflating[53] or flow-dependent.[27] As a rule, self-inflating bags are used during transport because they are not flow dependent. Care must be taken in selecting an appropriately sized bag and in not ventilating excessively. This is especially important during transport where there is often excessive noise and activity. Ideally, during transport a transport ventilator should be used rather than manual bagging. If manual bagging is necessary, a pressure-limited pop-off valve or an in-line manometer are useful. If a ventilator is used, basic settings are as follows:

- Tidal volume—10-15 ml/kg weight
- Ventilatory rate—15 to 30 breaths/minute
- Positive end expiratory pressure (PEEP)—+3 to 5 cm H_2O (or more, depending on the infant)
- FiO_2—1.0 (or less, depending on oximetry)

These settings are general guidelines and may need to be adjusted depending on the patient's disease and initial blood gases.

Other considerations. The neck should be stabilized using in-line traction if there is any indication of trauma.[3,16] Oropharyngeal and nasopharyngeal airways are usually unnecessary in small children, but care must be taken to use one of an appropriate size.[16,25] Oxygen should be administered at an FiO_2 of 1.0, or as high as possible, and weaned as appropriate using a pulse oximeter.

Upper airway disease

Upper airway obstruction is often a life-threatening emergency.[6] Concerns associated with the transport of children with upper airway obstruction has been reviewed.[13] Upper airway disease may be considered in terms of 1) neonatal patients and 2) older infants and children.

Upper airway obstruction in neonates. Neonatal upper airway obstruction is usually secondary to a congenital abnormality. One of the primary symptoms seen in upper airway obstruction in the *neonate* is apnea,[3] although stridor and, occasionally, wheezing may also be seen. Upper airway obstruction may be nasal and pharyngeal, such as in Pierre Robin Syndrome, Beckwith-Wideman Syndrome, or other abnormalities affecting the patency of the posterior pharynx.

Nasal obstruction. In cases of nasal obstruction the child may ventilate well when crying but, when crying stops, the child may turn cyanotic and apneic secondary to airway obstruction. Cyanosis and apnea result because infants are obligate nose-breathers, except when crying. Choanal atresia or stenosis are the most common causes of nasal obstruction in the neonate. If the obstruction is severe, placement of an oral endotracheal tube usually clears the obstruction and allows safe transport. Less severe patients may improve by suctioning the airway or by using a nasal decongestant (especially in children with upper respiratory tract infections in association with the congenital nasal stenosis).

Pharyngeal obstruction. Pharyngeal obstruction may be more difficult to manage during transport than nasal obstruction. The symptoms of pharyngeal obstruction are often more severe than with nasal obstruction, and crying and agitation may make the obstruction worse. The most common disorder causing pharyngeal obstruction is Pierre Robin Syndrome, but other congenital abnormalities may also cause pharyngeal obstruction.[19] Children with congenital pharyngeal obstruction often have abnormalities of the posterior pharynx making airway management very difficult. Placing an oropharyngeal airway may be effective in relieving the obstruction,[13] but if not, intubation may be difficult. Once an airway is secured, great care must be taken to stabilize the airway during transport. If the airway is lost during transport, it may be extremely difficult or impossible to replace the airway while in transit.

Upper airway obstruction in infants and children. Upper airway obstruction in infants and children results in exaggerated obstruction during inspiration compared with expiration. Thus, upper airway obstruction will result in a primarily inspiratory stridor. Disorders affecting upper airways in children are primarily infectious (croup, epiglottitis, and bacterial tracheitis)[31] foreign bodies, trauma, and other causes of extrinsic compression, such as vascular abnormalities and tumors.[13]

Croup. Croup, or laryngotracheobronchitis, is the most common cause of acute upper airway obstruction in children and will account for a number of transports. Croup is a viral process that typically affects the airways from the larynx to the bronchi in children 3 years of age and younger.[6,21] Because the cricoid area normally has the smallest diameter in the pediatric airway, severe symptoms are generally a result of swelling at this level. Croup follows a typical pattern consisting of a slow, progressive onset of symptoms over 2 to 3 days which slowly improves over the next 2 to 3 days. Croup is associated with a low-grade fever, a "barking" cough, and airway obstruction that is generally worse at night. These children are usually comforted by their mothers and prefer the supine position. Otitis media may also develop, resulting in a higher fever than is normally seen. When these children are calmed and supine, the symptoms usually are minimized. There is wide variability in the symptoms displayed by children with croup, but the most typical feature is a "barking" cough.

Management of croup initially involves calming the child as much as possible. Taking the child away from his or her mother and performing invasive procedures will agitate the child and may magnify the airway obstruction. Humidification and the administration of supplemental oxygen are the first recommended interventions.[4] The mechanism by which humidity improves the symptoms of croup is unclear, since the air reaching the larynx is normally fully saturated.[17,18] In fact, some studies have failed to demonstrate any therapeutic benefit of humidification.[11,39] If the obstruction is more severe, treatment with racemic epinephrine (0.25 to 0.5 ml of a 2.25% solution diluted with saline) via a nebulizer usually improves airflow past the obstruction by vasoconstriction.[21] For more severe obstructions, breathing a helium-oxygen mixture (75% to 80% helium and the rest oxygen) may significantly improve the symptoms[5] due to the decreased density of the gas mixture compared with air or oxygen alone. It is generally believed that corticosteroids shorten the course of viral croup,[21,44] however, they do not play a major role in the transport of these children. Severe patients will require intubation. Usually, when these children are intubated, an endotracheal tube 1/2 to one size smaller than the usual size is used. Concerns over possible complications that may result from intubating children with croup have been raised, but complications occur in less than 3% of cases.[52,63,66] Given the low percentage of complications, the highest priority remains establishing an adequate airway.

Children with croup requiring transport will usually have moderate to severe airway obstruction. If the child is intubated, care should be taken to maintain the airway (see section on Complications of Transport later in this chapter). If not intubated the child should be carefully monitored and given racemic epinephrine. One concern associated with the use of racemic epinephrine involves the drug's short duration of action. As a result, once the vasoconstrictive action of epinephrine has ended, the symptoms may return as bad or worse as before. Although it may not be a true rebound phenomenon, children who have received racemic epinephrine just prior to a 30 minute or one hour transport need to be carefully monitored.

Epiglottitis. Epiglottitis (or supraglottitis) is a bacterial infection of the supraglottic area occurring primarily in children 3 to 5 years of age.[21] The typical presentation is an explosive onset of symptoms that includes high fever, intense sore throat, hoarse muffled voice, drooling, and inspiratory stridor.[14] The "sniffing dog" position, characterized by neck extension, leaning forward, and an open mouth is the most comfortable position for the child. Historically, the most common etiology has been *H. Influenza* type B. With the advent of an effective vaccine against *H. Influenza* the overall incidence of epiglottitis has significantly declined. Gorelick and Baker[35] demonstrated a drop in incidence of epiglottitis from 10.9 per 10,000 admissions to 1.8 per 10,000 admissions. Likewise, the incidence of *H. Influenza* as the causative agent dropped from 76% to 25% of cases, with primarily Group A beta-hemolytic streptococcus being the main causative agent.

Children with acute epiglottitis are at high risk of acute, complete obstruction, and invasive procedures should be kept to a minimum. If a strong possibility exists that a child has epiglottitis, arrangements should be made to visualize the epiglottitis with direct laryngoscopy by the most experienced individual in the institution, generally the anesthesiologist. Usually the epiglottitis is visualized in the operating room with facilities to perform an emergency rigid bronchoscopy or tracheostomy in case the child develops complete obstruction and cannot be intubated. If a diagnosis of epiglottitis is made, the child should be intubated as part of his/her initial management,[66,81] preferably nasotracheal intubation. Unless there is a very unusual reason, such as the inaccessability of personnel trained in pediatric intubation, all children with epiglottitis or suspected epiglottitis should have a secure airway prior to transport.[13] Once a secure airway is established, attention should be focused on maintaining the airway during transport (see section on Complications of Transport later in this chapter).

Despite the potential morbidity and mortality associated with epiglottitis, there is relatively little consensus as to a protocol for transport.[76] Waisman and others[76] surveyed 43 transport teams and found a wide range of recommendations for airway management, sedation, muscle relaxation, and monitoring. Although there were significant variations in individual management, the general recommendations were to intubate the patient prior to transport, use sedation and muscle relaxation, and carefully monitor the patient via clinical, cardiac monitor, and pulse oximeter.

Foreign bodies. Foreign body aspiration may cause significant airway obstruction in children.[26,47] Children with suspected foreign body aspiration may be transported to a facility where rigid bronchoscopy and foreign body removal may be accomplished. An attempt at removal should not be attempted by inexperienced individuals unless the child has very severe symptoms and impending respiratory failure.[25] During transport the child should be placed in the position of comfort and given oxygen. A Heimlich maneuver may convert a partial obstruction to a complete obstruction[13] and should not be attempted.

Trauma. Facial trauma may result in airway obstruction associated with bleeding and soft tissue edema.[13] Hospital personnel should secure an adequate airway, if necessary, before transport. If there is a question about the airway, endotracheal intubation should be considered. These children may often have injuries so severe that endotracheal intubation is impossible and may, instead, need an emergency cricothyroidotomy.[5] Once an adequate airway is established, care must be taken not to lose the airway during transport.

Other causes of upper airway obstruction. Other causes of upper airway obstruction (vascular abnormalities such as rings and tumors) may be encountered in children requiring transport. Many of these children will be able to be transported without intubation, but some will require intubation.

Lower airway disease

Lower airway disease may be considered in terms of central (trachea and mainstem bronchi) and peripheral airways. If the airway obstruction is in the central airways, there is collapse with expiration. Central airway obstruction typically exhibit both inspiratory and expiratory obstruction, leading to both inspiratory stridor and expiratory wheezing. In small airway obstruction there is dynamic collapse during expiration leading to expiratory wheezing and air trapping in the lungs. The most common central airway disorders which frequently require transportation are tracheomalacia, aspirated foreign bodies, and vascular anomalies. The most common peripheral airway disorders requiring transportation are asthma, bronchiolitis, and bronchopulmonary dysplasia.

Central airway disease. Central airway disease may be confused with both upper and peripheral airway disease. The principles of management for foreign bodies and vascular anomalies have been previously discussed. Tracheomalacia is an important consideration in that it produces a more central "wheeze" that is often confused with lower airway disease. As a result, bronchodilators are often used in these children. Children with tracheomalacia, however, may worsen following the administration of a bronchodilator due to the decreased muscle tone and therefore, loss of integrity in the airway.[61] Children with tracheomalacia and an acute deterioration often respond to positive pressure from a mask.[32,42,55] Thus, during transport, acute wheezing in children with tracheomalacia may be more effectively treated with positive pressure from a mask than with bronchodilators.

Peripheral airway disease. Peripheral airway diseases that most commonly result in the need for transport are asthma, bronchiolitis, and bronchopulmonary dysplasia.

Asthma. Asthma is an inflammatory disease that affects approximately 5% of the population, and its incidence and severity have been worsening in recent years.[15] The reason for this increase is unclear. Asthma is characterized by intermittent bouts of airway obstruction caused by inflammation, edema, and bronchospasm. When a child experiences a severe asthma episode which requires transport, there is significant inflammation and bronchospasm as part of the pathophysiology of the episode. Oxygen is the first medication to administer during a severe asthma episode, since there is significant ventilation/perfusion mismatching. The next medication to administer is a bronchodilator, in particular, the beta-2-agonists. The most selective and rapidly acting beta-2-agonist which is available is albuterol.[12,41] There is much debate over the optimal method of administering albuterol in an acute asthma episode. The aerosol route is just as effective as the subcutaneous route, even in severe episodes. Most centers will administer albuterol by jet nebulizer at doses ranging from 2.5 to 5.0 mg diluted in saline. Albuterol, delivered via a metered-dose inhaler using a valved holding device (spacer), may be as effective as delivery using a jet nebulizer, but a large number of inhalations (10 to 20 puffs) may be needed in order to deliver the same dosage. Although there has been recent concern over the safety of long-term use of beta-2-agonists,[72,73] they should be liberally used in acute episodes. Albuterol is very highly beta-2-selective and is safe to use in very high doses. During severe acute episodes, albuterol may be administered by continuous nebulization at rates up to 20 mg/hr. The main side effects of albuterol administration are tachycardia and hypokalemia. Tachycardia may limit the use of albuterol, however, severe respiratory distress also produces tachycardia. For considerations of transport, the generous use of albuterol is the most important immediate intervention. A newer beta-2-agonist, salmeterol xinafoate (Serevent), has been recently released as a metered-dose inhaler for use in chronic asthma.[41,70] Salmeterol xinafoate is a very selective, long-acting beta-2-agonist and is very effective in chronic asthma management. It is, however, a partial agonist and what role, if any, it will play in the acute management of asthma is still unknown. Anticholinergic agents (ipatropium bromide by metered-dose inhaler or nebulizer solution) may cause additional bronchodilatation, but a beta-2-agonist is the first line medication.

Aminophylline (or theophylline) has been widely used in treating asthma for many years. Currently, there are numerous studies demonstrating no improvement in function in hospitalized patients (either in emergency room or hospitalized patients). Given the narrow therapeutic range and wide interpatient and intrapatient variability in metabolism, aminophylline or theophylline is not as widely used in the acute setting as it was previously. If theophylline is to be used (aminophylline is 80% theophylline), the loading dose is determined by the fact that 1 mg/kg theophylline will raise the serum theophylline concentration by 2 mcg/ml. The maintenance dose should then be 15 to 24 mg/kg/day, depending on the age of the child. Theophylline levels must be monitored frequently. Currently, levels of 5 to 15 mcg/ml (down from 10 to 20 mcg/ml) are recommended. If a child is receiving an oral sustained-release preparation of theophylline, has an adequate theophylline level, and is able to continue taking oral medications, there is no need to start aminophylline. The child may continue taking the theophylline orally. There are numerous adverse effects of theophylline (nausea, vomiting, arrhythmias, and seizures), and therefore, levels need to be monitored frequently. Since the additive effect of theophylline in the face of aggressive beta-2-agonist and anticholinergic therapy is marginal, many centers do not use theophylline (or aminophylline) in acutely hospitalized patients.

Antiinflammatory therapy is a fundamental aspect of asthma management, both acutely and chronically. Any child having an asthma episode severe enough for transport should be given corticosteroids. Prednisone (or methylprednisolone) at a dose of 1 mg/kg/dose should be administered as soon as possible. If a child is able to take oral medications and is not vomiting, there is no reason to administer intravenous corticosteroids. If the child already has an intravenous line or the child cannot or will not take the corticosteroid orally, hydrocortisone at a dose of 1 mg/kg/dose may be administered. The effects of corticosteroids are not seen for approximately 4 to 6 hours. Therefore, corticosteroids should be administered early in the course and aggressive beta-2-agonist therapy administered while waiting for the corticosteroid effects. Inhaled corticosteroids, cromolyn sodium, nedocromil sodium, and IV gammaglobulin all have very important roles in the chronic management of asthma but have minimal or no effect in an acute episode.

Thus, the primary treatments for acute asthma during stabilization and transport primarily include oxygen, high dose albuterol, ipatropium bromide aerosol, and IV or oral corticosteroids. The aggressive use of these modalities will treat the vast majority of acute severe asthmatic episodes in children.

Despite aggressive therapy, some children will require more intense therapy. If there is clinical and blood gas deterioration despite the above outlined therapy, intravenous terbutaline should be administered at a dose of 10 mcg/kg load over 10 minutes, followed by a 0.2 mcg/kg/min infusion. This may be increased by 0.1 mcg/kg/min increments every 15 minutes until there is a response.[10] If this is not effective, intubation may be necessary. Mechanical ventilation in asthmatic patients may carry a high incidence of morbidity in some[78] but not all studies.[29] All children requiring mechanical ventilation should be sedated and given muscle relaxing agents. The technique of "controlled hypoventilation" has been successfully used in some patients.[23,54] This technique involves allowing the $PaCO_2$ to rise. The respiratory acidosis is then corrected by administering bicarbonate.[69] Additionally, there are reports of other agents such as ketamine, halothane, helium-oxygen mixtures, general anesthesia, etc. being used in the treatment of severe, uncorrectable asthma,[20,34,59] but the use of these agents should be very rare and will not generally be used during transport.

Bronchiolitis. Bronchiolitis is a viral infection of the lower airways, usually caused by respiratory syncytial virus (but also caused by parainfluenza, influenza, and adenovirus) which severely affects primarily very young infants or children with underlying cardiac or pulmonary disease.[79] This infection produces significant inflammation, edema, and bronchospasm in the lower airways, and because infants have relatively underdeveloped lower airways, they tend to be the most severely affected group. These infants develop airway obstruction and wheezing similar to children with asthma, although the primary pathophysiology is different from asthma. Initial treatment is very similar to asthma in that aggressive bronchodilator therapy is indicated using primarily inhaled albuterol and also ipatropium bromide. Corticosteroids are occasionally used, but data on their efficacy is sparse. When infants begin to fatigue, nasal continuous positive airway pressure (CPAP) may be attempted.[71] This is often difficult to perform in children, especially those under 1 year of age, particularly during transport. If nasal CPAP fails, intubation and ventilation is necessary. As a rule, once children with bronchiolitis are intubated and ventilated, they are relatively easy to manage, and their respiratory symptoms dramatically improve. Infants with bronchiolitis produce copious secretions and are at a high risk for accidental extubation during transport. Thus, meticulous detail to airway stabilization is essential. Specific antiviral therapy (ribavirin) is sometimes used, but this plays no role in transport.

Bronchopulmonary dysplasia. With improved perinatal and neonatal intensive care, there is a growing number of children who have chronic lung disease or bronchopulmonary dysplasia (BPD). The overall pathophysiology and basics in management of BPD has been recently reviewed.[1] Children with BPD are primarily at high risk for severe symptoms during lower respiratory tract infections.[22,36,37] As part of their disease there is usually increased bronchial hyperreactivity, especially during an acute lower respiratory tract infection. The acute stabilization and management of these cases is similar to that described for bronchiolitis, with a few additions. First, many of these children will already be receiving supplemental oxygen, and the oxygen need may rise dramatically. These children may have other medical problems affecting transport. Often they are receiving diuretics, which may contribute to abnormalities in their electrolytes, and may have osteoporosis, making their bones fragile. These children have much less pulmonary reserve than normal infants and are at a much higher risk for rapid deterioration from respiratory illnesses. Lastly, these infants usually have been previously intubated and ventilated and may have difficult airways to manage.

Despite the many problems outlined above, the severity of BPD has taken a significant decline in recent years. This is probably due to three factors: improved perinatal care, surfactant administration, and high-frequency ventilation (jet and oscillator).

Disorders of the chest wall and respiratory muscles

This group of abnormalities is usually seen in the child developing paradoxical movements, such as with flail chest or other trauma. Additionally, children with underlying neuromuscular disease may develop respiratory failure very rapidly. The rapid deterioration is due to the relatively poor glycogen stores and the fact that infants and small children have more compliant chest walls which leads to ineffective ventilation.

Parenchymal lung disease

Diseases of the lung itself result in decreased compliance. Because the child's chest wall is more compliant than older children and adults, they tend to develop significant retractions. The most common diseases that result in parenchymal lung disease are pneumonia and the Adult Respiratory Distress Syndrome (ARDS). The management of pneumonia is similar to adults in that it involves antibiotics and supportive therapy. Small children may be at a higher risk of respiratory failure and should be monitored as outlined under "General Care".

ARDS also occurs in children and infants and has the same disease etiology. The background and management of ARDS in pediatric patients has been recently reviewed.[65] ARDS results in intrapulmonary shunting which is either minimally or completely unresponsive to oxygen administration.

The main aspects in the management of ARDS are treatment of the underlying disease and supportive therapy (oxygen, positive end expiratory pressure, mechanical ventilation, and cardiovascular support). If anything can be done to treat the underlying cause of ARDS (antibiotics, etc.), this should be instituted prior to transport. The primary intervention relevant to transport is intubation and positive end expiratory pressure (PEEP). As is the case in adults the mortality rate is high. Under the best circumstances children with ARDS should be intubated and ventilated with PEEP at levels of 5 to 15 cm H_2O pressure. Meticulous detail to airway patency and the maintenance of PEEP is essential for the best chance of survival. Maintaining adequate intravascular volume while minimizing the development of pulmonary edema is often challenging. These children may require pulmonary artery catheterization after transport to a tertiary care center. High frequency ventilation, nitric oxide, extracorporeal membrane oxygenation, and surfactant replacement are additional treatment modalities which have no impact on initial stabilization and transport.

Disorders of control of breathing

Abnormal control of breathing is manifested primarily by the apnea seen in infants who are premature and/or children with respiratory viral disease. It may also be seen in children with neurological abnormalities. In terms of transporting these children, the important aspects of management are to secure an adequate airway and ventilation. If there is a history suggestive of neurological disease, this needs to be evaluated after an airway is secured.

INDICATIONS/CONSIDERATIONS FOR TRANSFER TO TERTIARY CARE

Children should be considered for transport to a tertiary care center when the level of care exceeds the ability of the physicians, nurses, respiratory therapists, or other health care personnel caring for the child. Once the decision has been made to transport a child, preparations should be made to ensure that the child is as stable as possible. While transport arrangements are being made, it is very important for the referring institution to organize the records, including laboratory results and x-rays. This will facilitate a smooth transition of care from the referring institution to the transport team and then to the receiving institution.

COMPLICATIONS AND ADVERSE EVENTS RELATED TO TRANSPORT

One of the common and most feared complications during transport is extubation.[68] This is especially problematic when the transport team utilized is not dedicated to pediatric transports.[50,60] To minimize the incidence of accidental extubation during transport, stabilize the airway, monitor the airway during transport, sedate the child, and administer muscle relaxants.

The first consideration is appropriate airway stabilization. Different taping methods have been advocated during transport.[38,60] If any one thing deserves extra attention prior to transport, it is stabilization of the airway because of the ease in which small children may be accidentally extubated.

Monitoring the airway in the ambulance, helicopter, or airplane environment is difficult. Pulse oximetry has made a significant difference in the ability to monitor pediatric patients during transport. Unfortunately, oximetry may not immediately detect accidental extubation during transport. An end-tidal CO_2 monitor, however, has been successfully utilized in children greater than 2 kg.[9] Other recommended monitoring practices have been outlined.[28,38,49]

Sedation and muscle relaxation during transport greatly facilitates transport and minimizes the risk of accidental extubation.[51] Although there is concern regarding the use of muscle relaxants, the patients are at risk for greater complications in the event of accidental extubation. Using muscle relaxing agents has been shown to be safe when used by experienced nurse/paramedic teams.[57,76] The use of a short-acting narcotic (such as fentanyl) and a benzodiazepine (such as valium or versed) is very effective when used in conjunction with a muscle relaxing agent (such as vecuronium).

There are additional respiratory complications related to aeromedical transport.[62] Most airplanes are pressurized during flight to the pressure present at approximately 8,000 feet elevation. This results in a partial pressure of oxygen of 108 mm Hg (compared with 150 mm Hg at sea level) which may be significant in patients with intrinsic pulmonary disease. If a patient is unable to correct severe hypoxemia by supplemental oxygen, the patient should not be transported by air. Additionally, gas expands at higher altitudes. At an altitude of 8,000 feet, gas will expand by 30% compared with sea level. This may cause a small pneumothorax to expand and become a tension pneumothorax. Additionally, gas in the intestinal tract may greatly expand resulting in abdominal distention and occasionally, bowel rupture. Although cuffed endotracheal tubes are seldom used in pediatric patients, care must be taken when using cuffed endotracheal tubes during transport. The inflated cuff may expand and result in airway necrosis.

An additional, often unforeseen, complication during transport involves exhausting the oxygen supply.[24,62] The amount of time that a tank will supply oxygen is given by the following equation:

$$\text{Minutes of oxygen flow} = \frac{\text{Cylinder pressure} \times \text{Cylinder factor}^{*}}{\text{Liter per minute flow}}$$

It is important to keep this in mind when transporting a patient being administered oxygen, especially when a high liter flow rate is being used.

INTRAHOSPITAL TRANSPORT

Intrahospital transport is often given little attention. Considerations for intrahospital transports of critically ill pediatric patients have been made[77] and should be given the same considerations as interhospital transport in terms of preparation for emergencies and monitoring. Some procedures, such as magnetic resonance imaging, require special considerations,[75] therefore, arrangements should be made prior to transport.

SUMMARY

Respiratory disorders, either primary or secondary, are frequently seen in transported pediatric patients and, if improperly managed, can result in disastrous complications. Guidelines have been written for the stabilization and transport of the critically ill child, however,[2,45] there are many pulmonary complications which have not been adequately addressed. Additionally, many practicing pediatricians feel inadequate when faced with managing emergencies in their offices which may lead to transport[67] and therefore use private cars for transporting patients rather than professional transport services.[7] Reasons

* Cylinder size	Cylinder factor
D	0.16
E	0.28
H	3.14

cited for this were primarily related to cost and the difficulties associated with arranging transport.

Safe, effective transport of pediatric patients depends on a team of individuals who have an understanding of pediatric patients and who systematically monitor patients before and during transport.

REFERENCES

1. Abman SH, Groothius JR: Pathophysiology and treatment of bronchopulmonary dysplasia: current issues, *Pediatr Clin of North America* 41(2):277-315, 1994.
2. American Academy of Pediatrics Committee on Hospital Care, Guidelines for air and ground transport of pediatric patients, *Pediatrics* 78:943-9, 1986.
3. Ampel L and others: An approach to airway management in the acutely head-injured patient, *J Emerg Med* 6:1-7, 1988.
4. Anas NG, Goodman G: Croup. In Morriss LD editor: *Essentials of pediatric intensive care,* St. Louis, 1990, Quality Medical Publishing.
5. Backofen JE, Rogers MC: Emergency management of the airway. In Rogers MC editor: *Textbook of Pediatric Intensive Care,* Baltimore, 1987, Williams & Wilkins.
6. Backofen JE, Rogers MC: Upper airway disease. In Rogers MC editor: *Textbook of Pediatric Intensive Care,* Baltimore, 1987, Williams & Wilkins.
7. Baker MD, Ludwig S: Pediatric emergency transport and the private practitioner, *Pediatrics* 88(4):691-5, 1991.
8. Beyer AJ, Land G, Zaritsky A: Nonphysician transport of intubated pediatric patients: a system evaluation, *Crit Care Med* 20(7):961-6, 1992.
9. Bhende MS, Thompson AE, Orr RA: Utility of an end-tidal carbon dioxide detector during stabilization and transport of critically ill children, *Pediatrics* 89(6 Pt 1):1042-4, 1992.
10. Bohn D and others: Intravenous salbutamol in the treatment of status asthmaticus in children, *Crit Care Med* 12:392-396, 1984.
11. Bourchier D, Dawson KP, Fergusson DM: Humidification in viral croup: a controlled trial, *Aust Paediatr J* 20:289-91, 1984.
12. Boyd G, Anderson K, Carter R: Placebo controlled comparison of the bronchodilator performance of salmeterol and salbutamol over 12 hours, *Thorax* 45:340P, 1990.
13. Brink LW, Neuman B, Wynn J: Transport of the critically ill patient with upper airway obstruction, *Crit Care Clin* 8(3):633-47, 1992.
14. Butt W and others: Acute epiglottitis: a differential approach to management, *Crit Care Med* 16:43-8, 1988.
15. Centers for Disease Control: Asthma—United States, 1980-1987. *MMWR,* 39:493-7, 1990.
16. Chameides L, editor: *Textbook of Pediatric Advanced Life Support,* Dallas, Texas, 1988, American Heart Association/American Academy of Pediatrics.
17. Cole P: Some aspects of temperature, moisture and heat relationships in the upper respiratory tract, *J Laryngol Otol* 67:449-556, 1953.
18. Cole P: Further observations on the conditioning of respiratory air, *J Laryngol Otol* 67:669-81, 1953.
19. Corbet A: Respiratory disorders in the newborn. In Chernick V, editor: *Kendig's Disorders of the Respiratory Tract in Children,* ed 5, Philadelphia, 1990, W.B. Saunders Co.
20. Corssen G and others: Ketamine in the anesthetic management of asthmatic patients, *Anesth Analg (Cleve)* 51:588-96, 1972.
21. Cressman WR, Myer CM: Diagnosis and management of croup and epiglottitis, *Pediatr Clin of North America* 41(2):265-76, 1994.
22. Cunningham CK, McMillan JA, Gross SJ: Rehospitalization for respiratory illness in infants less than 32 weeks gestation, *Pediatrics* 88:527-32, 1991.
23. Darioli R, Perret C: Mechanical controlled hypoventilation in status asthmaticus, *Am Rev Respir Dis* 129:385-7, 1984.
24. Day SE: Intra-transport stabilization and management of the pediatric patient, *Pediatr Clin of North America* 40(2):263-74, 1993.
25. Dierking BH: Initial prehospital assessment of the pediatric patient, *J Emer Med Serv* 17:59-64, 1988.
26. Dierking BH: Managing the obstructed airway, *J Emer Med Serv* 7:89-92, 1990.
27. Dorsch JA, Dorsch SE: *Understanding Anesthesia Equipment,* ed 2, Baltimore, 1984, Williams and Wilkins.
28. Doyle E and others: Transport of the critically ill child, *Brit J Hosp Med* 48(6):314-9, 1992.
29. Dworkin G, Kattan M: Mechanical ventilation for status asthmaticus in children, *J Pediatr* 114:545-9, 1989.
30. Eckenhoff JE: Some anatomic considerations of the infant larynx influencing endotracheal anesthesia, *Anesthesiology* 12:401, 1951.
31. Ehrlich FE: Common pediatric emergencies. In Kravis TC and Warner CG, editors: *Emergency Medicine, A Comprehensive Review,* Rockville, MD, 1983, Aspen Publication.
32. Ferguson GT, Benoist J: Nasal continuous positive airway pressure in the treatment of tracheobronchomalacia, *Am Rev Respir Dis* 147:457-61, 1993.
33. Fuller J, Frewen T, Lee R: Acute airway management in the critically ill child requiring transport, *Can J Anaesth* 38(2):252-4, 1991.
34. Gluck EH, Onorato DJ, Castriotta R: Helium-oxygen mixtures in intubated patients with status asthmaticus and respiratory acidosis, *Chest* 98:693-8, 1990.
35. Gorelick MH, Baker MD: Epiglottitis in children, 1979 through 1992, Effects of haemophilus influenzae type b immunization, *Arch Pediatr Adolesc Med* 148(1):47-50, 1994.
36. Groothius JR, Gutierrez KM, Lauer BM: Respiratory syncytial virus infection in children with BPD, *Pediatrics* 82:199-203, 1988.
37. Groothius JR and others: Early ribavirin treatment of RSV infection in high-risk children, *J Pediatr* 117:792–8, 1990.

38. Henning R, McNamara V: Difficulties encountered in transport of the critically ill child, *Pediatr Emerg Care* 7(3):133-7, 1991.
39. Henry R: Moist air in the treatment of laryngotracheitis, *Arch Dis Child* 58:577, 1983.
40. Hogg J and others: Age as a factor in the distribution of lower-airway conductance and in the pathologic anatomy of obstructive lung disease, *N Engl J Med* 282:1283-7, 1970.
41. Johnson M and others: The pharmacology of salmeterol, *Life Sci* 52:2131-43, 1993.
42. Kanter RK and others: Treatment of severe tracheobronchomalacia with continuous positive airway pressure (CPAP), *Anesthesiology* 57:54-6, 1982.
43. Kanter RK and others: Excess morbidity associated with interhospital transport, *Pediatrics* 90(6):893-8, 1992.
44. Koren G and others: Corticosteroid treatment of laryngotracheitis vs. spasmodic croup in children, *Am J Dis Child* 137:941-4, 1983.
45. Kronick JB, Kissoon N, Frewen TC: Guidelines for stabilizing the condition of the critically ill child before transfer to a tertiary care facility, *CMAJ* 139:213-20, 1988.
46. Langston C and others: Human lung growth in late gestation and in the neonate, *Am Rev Respir Dis* 129:607-13, 1984.
47. Lee G: Maxillofacial, anterior neck, and eye trauma. In *Flight Nursing Principles and Practice,* St. Louis, 1991, Mosby Year Book.
48. Lee KW, Templeton JJ, Dougas R: Tracheal tube size and postoperative croup in children, *Anesthesiology* 53:S325, 1980.
49. MacNab AJ: Optimal escort for interhospital transport of pediatric emergencies, *J Trauma* 31(2):205-9, 1991.
50. McCloskey KA, Orr RA: Pediatric transport issues in emergency medicine, *Emerg Med Clin North Am* 9:475-89, 1991.
51. McDonald TB, Berkowitz RA: Airway management and sedation for pediatric transport, *Pediatr Clin of North America* 40(2):381-406, 1993.
52. McEniery J and others: Review of intubation in severe laryngotracheobronchitis, *Pediatrics* 87:847-53, 1991.
53. McPherson SP: *Respiratory therapy equipment,* ed 3, St. Louis, 1985, CV Mosby Co.
54. Menitove SM, Goldring RM: Combined ventilator and bicarbonate strategy in the management of status asthmaticus, *Am J Med* 74:898-901, 1983.
55. Miller RW and others: Effectiveness of continuous positive airway pressure in the treatment of bronchomalacia in infants: a bronchoscopic documentation, *Crit Care Med* 14:125-7, 1986.
56. Motoyama E: Pulmonary mechanics during early postnatal years, *Pediatr Res* 11:220-3, 1977.
57. Murphy-Macabobby M and others: Neuromuscular blockade in aeromedical airway management, *Ann Emerg Med* 21(6):664-8, 1992.
58. O'Brodovich HM, Haddad GG: The functional basis of respiratory pathology. In Chernick V, editor: *Kendig's Disorders of the Respiratory Tract in Children,* ed 5, Philadelphia, 1990, W.B. Saunders Co.
59. O'Rourke PP, Crone RK: Halothane in status asthmaticus, *Crit Care Med* 10:341-43, 1982.
60. Owen H, Duncan AW: Towards safer transport of sick and injured children, *Anaesth Intens Care* II(2):113-7, 1983.
61. Panitch HB and others: Effect of altering smooth muscle tone on maximal expiratory flows in patients with tracheomalacia, *Pediatr Pulm* 9:170-6, 1990.
62. Parsons CJ, Bobechko WP: Aeromedical transport: its hidden problems, *CMAJ* 126:237-43, 1982.
63. Postma DS, Jones RO, Pillsbury HC: Severe hospitalized croup: treatment trends and prognosis, *Laryngoscope* 94:1170-5, 1984.
64. Rubenstein JS and others: Can the need for a physician as part of the pediatric transport team be predicted? A prospective study, *Crit Care Med* 20(12):1657-61, 1992.
65. Sarnaik AP, Lieh-Lai M: Adult respiratory distress syndrome in children, *Pediatr Clin of North America* 41(2):337-63, 1994.
66. Schuller DE, Birckh G: The safety of intubation in croup and epiglottitis: an eight-year followup, *Laryngoscope* 85:33-46, 1975.
67. Schweich PJ, DeAngelis C, Duggan AK: Preparedness of practicing pediatricians to manage emergencies, *Pediatrics* 88(2):223-9, 1991.
68. Setzer N: Airway management during transport, *Crit Care Med* 21(9 Suppl):S365-6, 1993.
69. Shustack A, Noseworthy TW, Johnston RG: Combined ventilator and bicarbonate strategy in the management of status asthmaticus, (Letter to Editor) *Am J Med* 76(1):A88, 1984.
70. Simons FER and others: Bronchodilator and bronchoprotective effects of salmeterol in young patients with asthma, *J Allergy Clin Immunol* 90:840-6, 1992.
71. Soong WJ, Hwang B, Tang RB: Continuous positive airway pressure by nasal prongs in bronchiolitis, *Pediatr Pulm* 16:163-6, 1993.
72. Spitzer WO and others: The use of beta-agonists and the risk of death and near death from asthma, *N Engl J Med* 326:501-6, 1992.
73. Suissa S and others: A cohort analysis of excess mortality in asthma and the use of inhaled beta-agonists, *Am J Respir Crit Care Med* 149:604-10, 1994.
74. Thurlbeck WM: Postnatal human lung growth, *Thorax* 37:564-71, 1982.
75. Tobin JR, Spurrier EA, Wetzel RC: Anaesthesia for critically ill children during magnetic resonance imaging, *Br J Anaesth* 69(5):482-6, 1992.
76. Waisman Y and others: Management of children with epiglottitis during transport: analysis of a survey, *Pediatric Emerg Care* 9(4):191-4, 1993.
77. Weg JG, Haas CF: Safe intrahospital transport of critically ill ventilator-dependent patients, *Chest* 96:631-5, 1989.
78. Williams TJ and others: Risk factors for morbidity in mechanically ventilated patients with acute severe asthma, *Am Rev Respir Dis* 146:607-15, 1992.

79. Wohl MEB: Bronchiolitis. In Chernick V, editor: *Kendig's Disorders of the Respiratory Tract in Children,* ed 5, Philadelphia, 1990, W.B. Saunders Co.
80. Wohl MEB, Mead J: Age as a factor in respiratory disease. In Chernick V, editor: *Kendig's Disorders of the Respiratory Tract in Children,* ed 5, Philadelphia, 1990, W.B. Saunders Co.
81. Zulliger JJ and others: Assessment of intubation in croup and epiglottitis, *Ann Otol Rhinol Laryngol* 91:403-6, 1982.

20

SHOCK

ARNO L. ZARITSKY
SARAH NORWOOD MOORMAN

Shock is second only to respiratory failure as a cause of cardiopulmonary arrest in children. Thus, early recognition and effective therapy of shock are keys to the management of critically ill children undergoing transport. It is impossible, within this chapter, to cover all types of shock and their management. Our goal is to provide an overview of the pathophysiology, clinical classification, recognition, and therapy of shock in the child, with special emphasis on stabilization of the child undergoing transport. First, we will discuss the pathophysiology and compensatory mechanisms activated in shock and the physiologic determinants of cardiac output and tissue perfusion. With this understanding the therapeutic management techniques learned can be applied to the child with shock due to causes not specifically covered in this chapter.

DEFINITION

Shock is a clinical state characterized by inadequate delivery of oxygen and nutrients to meet tissue metabolic demands. Since shock represents a dynamic clinical state, its clinical recognition is not dependent on any specific set of vital sign abnormalities. Shock may occur with increased, normal, or decreased cardiac output, or with increased, decreased or normal blood pressure. For example, a child with sickle cell anemia in an aplastic crisis may have increased cardiac output, yet oxygen carrying capacity is inadequate to meet tissue metabolic demands due to profound anemia. Similarly, a child with coarctation of the aorta may be hypertensive but in shock secondary to inadequate blood flow beyond the aortic obstruction.

PATHOPHYSIOLOGY AND COMPENSATORY MECHANISMS OF SHOCK

The body's ability to control cardiac output and blood distribution ensures that tissue metabolic demand is met. During normal circulatory states, blood flow is matched to the local tissue metabolic demand by the release of local mediators, such as adenosine and endothelial-derived relaxing factor (EDRF).[5,25] Of note, the endothelial-derived relaxing factor appears to be nitric oxide.[30]

During steady-state conditions, neurohumoral control mechanisms, such as the sympathetic nervous system and renin-angiotensin system, generally do not play an important role in regulating local tissue perfusion. However, when circulating blood volume does not meet tissue metabolic demands, neurohumoral control mechanisms preferentially maintain perfusion pressure and blood flow to the brain and heart. These compensatory mechanisms are largely achieved by intense vasoconstriction of the splanchnic, skeletal muscle, and dermal vascular beds, which all redirect blood flow to the vital organs. Vasoconstriction is produced by increased sympathetic nervous system activity (release of epinephrine and norepinephrine) and renin-angiotensin system activity. Neurohumoral mechanisms also increase heart rate in an effort to maintain an adequate cardiac output. These changes characterize the *compensated* phase of shock in which vital organ perfusion and blood pressure are maintained by intrinsic compensatory mechanisms.

With prolonged or worsening compromise of organ perfusion, the child progresses to the *decompensated* phase of shock. Local autoregulatory mechanisms supersede the effects of neurohumoral activity, resulting in local vasodilation and pooling of blood. Anaerobic metabolism from inadequate tissue oxygenation reduces adenosine triphosphate (ATP) production and increases lactic acid production. Depletion of ATP, the major source of cellular energy, leads to further organ dysfunction. In addition, the elaboration of vasodilator peptides and the increased synthesis of EDRF in children with sepsis result in a loss of normal autoregulation of blood flow matched to tissue metabolic demand.[32,51] As the compensatory mechanisms fail, hypotension ensues. Factors at the cellular level also have important implications in the management of the child with shock. As seen in Figure 20-1, maintenance of normal cellular volume is dependent upon an energy requiring mechanism where sodium is pumped out of cells in exchange for potassium. When cells become ischemic, sodium moves down its concentration gradient into the cell, bringing water with it and sequestering extracellular fluid within the cellular compartment.[52] This intracellular movement of sodium and water

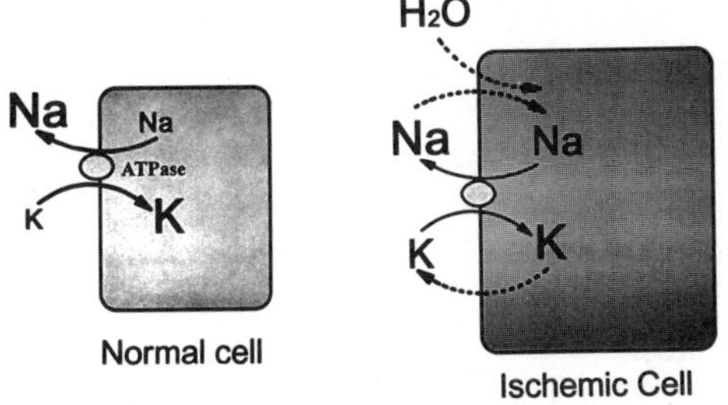

Fig. 20-1. Swelling of ischemic cells results from ATP depletion which prevents normal activity of the Na-K exchange pump. As sodium accumulates in the cell, water enters. ATPase is the sodium-potassium, ATP-requiring exchange pump.

further compromises the intravascular and extracellular compartments. Thus, the child in shock needs more fluid resuscitation than can be detected by the clinically observed fluid loss.

Furthermore, at the organism level it is important to recognize that about 70-80% of the blood volume is normally located in the venous system.[5] This distribution of blood volume helps maintain cardiac output as the intravascular volume is depleted. Increased venous tone moves blood from the venous capacitance system into the central circulation and subsequently out to the tissues. Conversely, with progressive acidosis and the production of vasodilator substances, venous tone may be diminished. This results in a pooling of blood and a drop in the venous return. When the venous tone decreases, large volumes of fluid are required to fill this increased capacity in order to restore an adequate blood volume.

DETERMINANTS OF CARDIOVASCULAR FUNCTION

Cardiac output is the total amount of blood pumped by the ventricle each minute; it is the product of stroke volume and heart rate. Stroke volume is the amount of blood ejected by the ventricle with each beat.

In the infant and child, stroke volume (ml/beat) is approximately equal to 1.5 times the child's weight in kg.[27] Thus, a 4 kg infant has a stroke volume of 6 ml/beat (4×1.5). Heart rate is an important determinant of cardiac output in the infant and young child, since they have limited ability to augment their stroke volume. Therefore, an increase in the child's heart rate is a common clinical manifestation of shock. An increase in heart rate provides one of the easiest mechanisms for maintaining adequate cardiac output when there is a decrease in circulating blood volume or stroke volume. Note that tachycardia is often the first sign of shock in children. Similarly, the heart rate may be elevated in children with an increase in metabolic demand requiring an increase in cardiac output. One common cause of increased metabolic demand is elevated body temperature. For every 1°C increase in core body temperature, the metabolic systems of the body increase oxygen consumption by 10-13%.[12] Thus, in a child with poor perfusion and a temperature of 40°C (104.0°F) basal metabolic demand is increased by 30-40%. Conversely, lowering the child's temperature to normal can often greatly improve their matching of cardiac output to tissue metabolic demand and, therefore, their clinical symptoms of shock.[11]

An inadequate heart rate is a very worrisome clinical manifestation in a child with shock. For reasons that remain unclear, hypoxic children often develop bradycardia rather than tachycardia. Thus, bradycardia in the child with poor perfusion is initially managed with attention to the airway by providing adequate oxygenation and ventilation.

Determinants of stroke volume include preload, afterload, and contractility. These terms have specific physiologic meanings that are often incorrectly estimated in the clinical setting. The interrelationships among these determinants are seen in Figure 20-2.

Preload

Preload is the degree or amount of stretch on the myocardial muscle fiber prior to the onset of contraction. Note, this definition does not relate preload to the pressure within the pumping chamber (i.e., right or left atrial pressures). As described by Frank and Starling and recently reviewed,[45] the amount of muscle fiber stretch determines the force of subsequent contraction. Thus, maintaining an adequate preload can sustain optimal myocardial contractility. In the working heart the degree of myocardial fiber stretch is related to the end-diastolic volume rather than the end-diastolic pressure within the ventricle. Since preload depends on ventricular volume, it is easy to understand how fluid administration augments preload.

When excessive, fluid administration may elevate the end-diastolic volume and pressure, compromising perfusion to the subendocardium. As a result, cardiac contractility falls rather than improves. This is much more common in the child with cardiogenic shock than in the child with hypovolemic or distributive shock.

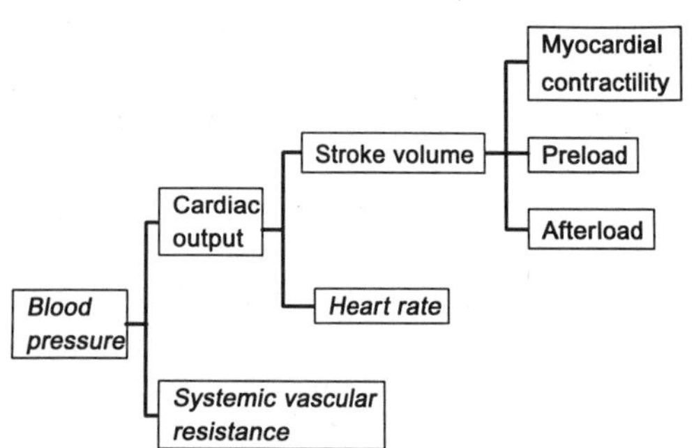

Fig. 20-2. Interrelationships between determinants of cardiovascular function. Clinically measurable or assessed functions are indicated in italics. Systemic vascular resistance is assessed by noting pulse volume, skin temperature, and capillary refill. Reproduced with permission from Chameides L, editor: *Textbook of Pediatric Advanced Life Support,* American Heart Association, 1990.

Afterload

Afterload refers to the sum of all the forces that resist ventricle emptying. Afterload is commonly estimated by calculating the systemic or pulmonary vascular resistance; however, this is only an approximation. Many factors influence the afterload of the ventricle including the caliber of the vessels, the viscosity of the blood, the presence of mechanical obstruction to ventricular emptying, the thickness of the ventricle, and the diameter of the ventricular chamber.

An increase in afterload (e.g., aortic obstruction or arterial hypertension) causes an increase in ventricular work and oxygen consumption and may result in decreased myocardial performance. With increased resistance, the ventricle cannot empty efficiently; fluid therefore backs up into the ventricles and pulmonary system, resulting in congestive heart failure with pulmonary edema. Afterload is manipulated by vasodilator or vasoconstrictor therapy. As cardiac output falls, increased afterload initially maintains blood pressure. The mathematic relationship between these factors is: $BP = CO \times SVR$ (BP is blood pressure, CO is cardiac output, and SVR is the systemic vascular resistance or afterload).

Note that a fall in stroke volume and cardiac output is not reflected in a change of blood pressure, since the rise in SVR maintains the product (i.e., BP). Thus, blood pressure often is a poor indicator of cardiac output. Vasodilator therapy is advantageous for observing the relationship between afterload and cardiac output in the child with myocardial dysfunction, as discussed in more detail below.

Contractility

Contractility refers to the force or strength of myocardial pumping. Contractility is the most difficult parameter to measure at the bedside. It is influenced by the metabolic state of the blood perfusing the myocardium and the intrinsic myocardial function, which may be altered by inflammation within the myocardium or congenital abnormalities in cellular pumping activity. Hypoxia, hypoglycemia, hypocalcemia, and acidosis all cause diminished cardiac contractility, while increased circulating catecholamines increase contractility.

Contractility is difficult to measure, yet it has an important effect on stroke volume. Inotropic drugs enhance contractility and thus increase stroke volume and cardiac output. In the child with an intraarterial pressure catheter, the contractility may be estimated by observing the upstroke of the arterial pressure wave. The upstroke graphically illustrates change in pressure over time. In the child with a nearly vertical upstroke of the arterial pressure wave, contractility is probably normal or enhanced. If the upstroke is more sloped, either the contractility is diminished or the pressure wave is poorly transmitted to the transducer. This poor transmission may occur from an obstruction to the vessel or monitoring system, from an air bubble in the pressure transducer system, or from the effects of intense vasoconstriction that diminish the transmission of the pressure wave to an arterial catheter placed in a distal artery.[16]

CLASSIFICATION OF SHOCK

Shock is produced by several clinical conditions, each causing different clinical manifestations. To help determine the approach toward a child with shock, the causes of shock may be classified into the following: hypovolemic, distributive, neurologic, and cardiogenic. Any classification system, however, represents an oversimplification, as many children manifest symptoms of more than one type of shock.

Hypovolemic shock

Hypovolemic shock is a state of inadequate intravascular volume. It is the most common type of shock seen in children. Hypovolemia may be caused by the loss of blood in the traumatized child or by the loss of fluids, which deplete the extracellular and intracellular spaces (e.g., diabetic ketoacidosis, diabetes insipidus, burns, diarrhea, and vomiting). Infants and children are predisposed to hypovolemic shock because their caretakers do not necessarily provide adequate fluid intake when they have increased fluid loss.

The pathophysiologic sequence of hypovolemia is seen in Figure 20-3. When the intravascular volume falls, inadequate volume remains to maintain the circulatory network. Venous return falls, and the ventricular chambers do not completely fill with blood. Decreased filling during diastole causes a decrease in the volume ejected during systole. As stroke volume decreases, so does cardiac output. As cardiac output falls, blood pressure is initially maintained by increased vascular resistance. With further compromise of tissue perfusion, local acidosis leads to vasodilation and pooling of blood in ischemic tissues. Blood pressure compensation then fails, and the child rapidly deteriorates.

The child's history often indicates the etiology of the child's hypovolemic shock. However, in infants and children with occult trauma secondary to child abuse, the history may be inconsistent. In these cases a careful, detailed examination usually suggests the diagnosis. Clinical manifestations of hypovolemic shock are discussed in the next section.

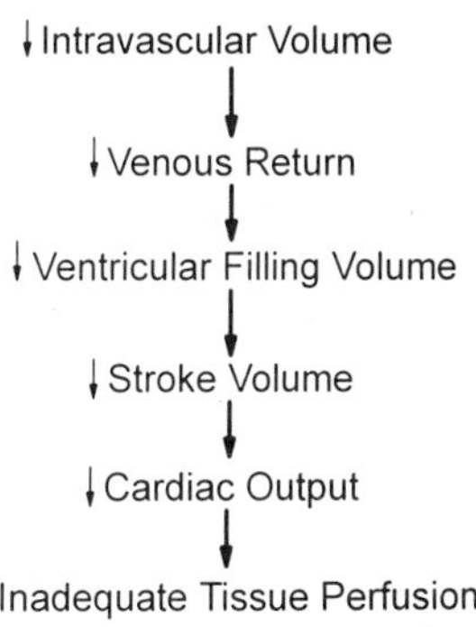

Fig. 20-3. Sequence of events leading from hypovolemia to inadequate tissue perfusion.

Distributive shock

This class of shock is characterized by a maldistribution of blood flow relative to tissue metabolic demand. Cardiac output, however, may be normal or increased. Typically, perfusion is maintained or enhanced in the skin and skeletal muscle vascular beds, but occult ischemia occurs in the splanchnic vascular bed.[50,54] The specific etiologies of distributive shock are sepsis, other causes of the systemic inflammatory response syndrome,[2] neurogenic shock, and anaphylactic shock.

Sepsis is the most common cause of distributive shock and is associated with high mortality rates in children. Because of the multiple factors involved, the clinical pattern and presentation of septic shock may vary depending on the dynamic interplay of the invading organisms, elapsing time, and host status.[46]

Septic shock is characterized by a loss of peripheral vascular resistance, initially producing a wide pulse pressure due to the fall in diastolic blood pressure. Hypotension usually occurs when the child develops excessive vasodilation and leakage of plasma through the capillary walls into the interstitial space. Hypotension also may result from poor cardiac contractility.

Neurogenic shock

Neurogenic shock refers to a clinical state of diminished or absent peripheral vascular tone caused by injury to the nervous system, most commonly to the upper cervical spinal cord. A loss of sympathetic nervous system tone in the peripheral vascular bed results, leading to a loss of normal systemic vascular resistance with intravascular pooling of blood. A neurogenic shock-like state may result from barbiturate or opiate overdoses as well as toxicity due to adrenergic blocking agents such as clonidine. Any of these drugs may cause sympathetic nervous system suppression leading to a loss of vascular tone and pooling of blood.

Anaphylactic shock

Anaphylaxis is an acute, life-threatening form of shock comprised of maldistribution of blood and increased capillary permeability[23] which is often complicated by an acute increase in afterload to the right ventricle.[43] Anaphylaxis results from the generation of inflammatory mediators in response to the activation of mast cells and basophil by an immunologic stimulus. Although uncommon in children, it may occur from exposure to medications or bee stings.

Some drugs also may degranulate mast cells or basophils independent of IgE-mediated activation and cause anaphylactic shock.[48] Commonly implicated agents include opiates, certain antibiotics, plasma expanders (e.g., dextran), muscle relaxants (e.g., atracurium), chemotherapeutic agents, and radiocontrast material. The management of children with nonimmunologic anaphylactoid reactions is the same as for anaphylaxis.

Cardiogenic shock

Cardiogenic shock results from a number of diseases, which either produce diminished contractility or pump failure secondary to the obstruction of blood return to the heart or blood flow from the heart. The causes of pump failure include (1) myocarditis, (2) drug toxicity (e.g., digoxin, propranolol or tricyclic antidepressant overdose), and (3) metabolic causes (e.g. hypoglycemia, hyperkalemia, and hypocalcemia). Acquired cardiogenic shock may occur after hypoxic ischemic episodes, such as ALTE (Apparent Life-Threatening Events, formerly called near-miss Sudden Infant Death Syndrome (SIDS) and near drowning.[36] In addition, infants experience cardiogenic shock, secondary to severe congenital outflow obstruction, within the first month of life.[4] The most common obstructions are aortic stenosis and coarctation of the aorta. Interruption to right ventricular outflow, such as from pulmonary valve atresia, also may present as neonatal cardiogenic shock.[27] Cardiogenic shock also may result from myocardial exhaustion secondary to increased metabolic demand exceeding coronary artery oxygen delivery. This condition most often is seen following supraventricular tachycardia.

As the heart's pumping ability decreases, a decrease in ventricle emptying results. Consequently, ventricular pressures rise, while stroke volume and cardiac output fall. Since the heart cannot pump blood effectively, tissue perfusion declines, with hypotension representing a late, decompensated state. In addition, pulmonary congestion develops from an increase in left atrial pressure and the resultant increase in pulmonary vascular pressure. Oxygenation of circulating blood decreases with lung congestion. Thus, in cardiogenic shock, the body not only receives less blood, but the blood it does receive is often less oxygenated.

All forms of shock, if not adequately treated, lead to at least some of the clinical manifestations of cardiogenic shock. This results from inadequate myocardial blood flow and secondary injury to the heart from the other forms of shock.

Compensated shock

Somewhat arbitrarily, shock also is classified as compensated or decompensated (hypotensive). This distinction is based on the maintenance of a normal systolic blood pressure for age. It is essential to recognize decompensated shock, since it represents a late state, which often rapidly progresses to cardiac arrest. As recommended in the Pediatric Advanced Life Support course (PALS),[17] compensated shock is distinguished from decompensated shock based upon the age-dependent systolic blood pressure (BP_{sys}). From newborn to 1 month of age, BP_{sys} should be >60 mm Hg; from 1 month to 1 year, BP_{sys} should be >70 mm Hg; and for children over 1 year of age, BP_{sys} should be $>70 + (2 \times \text{age in years})$ mm Hg. Note that the normal value for newborn blood pressure is only applicable for a full-term newborn. Also note that the upper limit for this equation works only until age 10. A systolic blood pressure of 90 mm Hg is acceptable as the lower limit for children >10 years of age.

RECOGNITION OF SHOCK

Since shock is a complex clinical state with varied physical signs, it is not always easily recognized. The clinical manifestations of shock depend on the underlying cause; typical clinical manifestations are summarized in Table 20-1. These clinical signs represent the components of a rapid cardiopulmonary assessment that can be completed in one minute. This cardiopulmonary assessment provides all of the necessary clinical information to both recognize and classify the child with shock.

Typically, the respiratory rate is elevated in all forms of shock, representing a compensation for the metabolic acidosis induced by the shock state. Besides respiratory rate, the work of breathing frequently provides very important information about the cause of the child's shock. In hypovolemic shock, children are typically tachypneic but do not have an increased work of breathing; this often is called "quiet tachypnea". In contrast, children with cardiogenic shock typically have an increased work of breathing due to pulmonary edema which results in diminished lung compliance. The child with septic shock may have a normal work of breathing. However, the child also may present with a significantly

TABLE 20-1 CLINICAL CHARACTERISTICS OF SHOCK*

Signs	*Hypovolemic*	*Cardiogenic*	*Distributive*
Heart rate	+++	++++	+++
Respiratory rate	++	+++	++
Work of breathing	normal	++ to ++++	0 to ++++
Pulse volume	0 to ++	0 to +	0 to ++++
Capillary refill	>2 secs.	>4 secs.	> or <2 secs.
Skin temperature	cool	cold	warm to cold
Skin color	pale	pale-ashen	pink-ashen
Mottling	+ to +++	++++	+ to ++++
Level of consciousness	normal to coma	depressed–coma	normal to coma
Liver size	normal	enlarged	normal
Acidosis	+ to +++	++ to ++++	+ to ++++
Urine output	<1 cc/kg/hr	≪1 cc/kg/hr	<1 cc/kg/hr

* The likelihood of a specific sign is indicated by the number of plus (+) signs.

increased work of breathing, due to pulmonary edema, which is more often caused by the adult respiratory distress syndrome (ARDS) rather than hydrostatic pulmonary edema.[14] Clearly, the child with grunting respirations who is using accessory muscles needs cautious fluid administration to augment intravascular volume and preload. Frequently, this child benefits more from intubation and ventilation along with vasoactive drug therapy.[6,29]

Determining pulse volume is also useful in the clinical evaluation of the child with shock. Assess pulse volume in both central and peripheral arteries. A bounding central pulse with a weak-to-absent distal pulse is consistent with early distributive shock. Note that the pulse volume is related to the difference between the systolic and diastolic blood pressure (i.e., the pulse pressure). Normal diastolic blood pressure should be two-thirds of systolic blood pressure; thus, for a systolic blood pressure of 90 mm Hg, the diastolic blood pressure should be 60 mm Hg. Diastolic blood pressure provides the best window on the child's systemic vascular resistance. Children with a low systemic vascular resistance have a wide pulse pressure and characteristically bounding pulses. The causes of a wide pulse pressure include distributive shock, fever, severe anemia (<8 gm %), acute or chronic liver failure, and hyperthyroidism. Children with intense vasoconstriction, as occurs in cardiogenic shock or hypovolemic shock, have thready pulses and a narrowed pulse pressure.

Capillary refill is related to the adequacy of distal perfusion. The technique used to assess capillary refill can influence the results. We recommend utilizing a consistent technique whereby the extremity is elevated above the level of the heart. This avoids capillary refill from retrograde venous refilling in the child exhibiting cardiogenic shock and high venous pressures. Apply pressure on the nailbed or digit until it blanches, then release the pressure. Color should return in 2-3 seconds. If the color does not return within that time, capillary refill is delayed. If the child is hypothermic or was exposed for a period of time, capillary refill becomes unreliable due to dermal vasoconstriction.

Skin temperature is influenced by environmental temperature, as well as the child's temperature and perfusion. Recognizing this limitation, determine the line of demarcation between warm and cool skin, since often this is a useful marker of restored perfusion in response to therapy. Skin color is produced by the hemoglobin concentration, the degree of vasoconstriction within the dermal capillaries and the oxygen saturation of the blood perfusing the skin. With vasoconstriction, the skin often appears pale; intense vasoconstriction often turns the skin gray or ashen. Note that cyanosis may be a late manifestation of hypoxemia in the child with anemia. In general, approximately 5 gm % desaturated oxyhemoglobin is required to clinically recognize cyanosis. In the child with a total hemoglobin of 10 gm %, the hemoglobin would have to be 50% saturated to achieve the threshold concentration of 5 gm %. For normal hemoglobin this level of hemoglobin saturation requires a $PaO_2 = 28$ mm Hg. Peripheral cyanosis may be seen at higher PaO_2 values, due to slow blood flow in poorly perfused distal extremities resulting in increased oxygen extraction in the tissues.

The level of consciousness provides very useful information in the child with shock. Often, one of the early manifestations of shock is a subtle alteration in the infant or child's interaction with their parents. The astute clinician recognizes that a child with open eyes who is not tracking the movement of individuals (especially parents) in the room is a child with significant impairment of consciousness. As hypoxia and/or perfusion to the brain is impaired the level of consciousness progressively declines. In septic shock, cerebral dysfunction is associated with a poor outcome.[57]

Laboratory studies are often performed, but only a few have specific utility in the child with shock. The most helpful laboratory study is a test to determine the level of arterial blood gas. Examine not only the absolute pH value but also the pCO_2 value and the calculated base deficit. In general, a child with altered perfusion and metabolic acidosis meets the criteria for shock. Metabolic acidosis results from the accumulation of protons (H^+) and lactate derived from inadequately perfused cells. There are other causes of metabolic acidosis, but the most common is the accumulation of lactic acid.

To further evaluate metabolic acidosis, examine the calculated anion gap (anion gap = [Na] − ([Cl] + [CO_2]),[47] which is readily available from standard electrolytes. The anion gap quantifies those anions (other than chloride and bicarbonate) that counterbalance sodium's positive charge. The normal anion gap is 8-12 mEq/L. The unmeasured anions constituting the normal anion gap are proteins, phosphate, sulphate, and various other anions. The largest portion of the anion gap is due to protein, particularly albumin.

When lactic acid accumulates the anion gap typically is greater than 12 mEq/L. In contrast, a normal anion gap acidosis usually results from the loss of bicarbonate in either the stool (most often caused by diarrhea) or urine. When normal anion gap acidosis is present, sodium bicarbonate is usually appropriate therapy. In contrast, treat wide anion gap acidosis by improving tissue oxygenation and perfusion. It is important to recognize the role of albumin in the normal anion gap. Since albumin is the major source of the normal anion gap, when the child is hypoalbuminemic, the anion gap may only be 4 mEq/L or less. Thus, when this child has a calculated gap of 10 mEq/L, it represents a wide anion gap acidosis, which otherwise may not be recognized.

Serum electrolytes are measured to ensure that the electrolyte balance is normal and to calculate the anion gap; however, other assessments such as an arterial blood gas are better indicators of shock. A complete blood count helps determine whether the oxygen-carrying capacity (i.e., hemoglobin concentration) is adequate. The white blood cell count is often elevated nonspecifically in children experiencing physiological stress and is not a reliable indicator of the presence of sepsis. Coagulation studies, including platelet count, PT, and PTT, are recommended in children with clinical evidence of bruising or bleeding. Other abnormalities that may occur in shock include hyperkalemia (resulting from the exchange of excess protons with intracellular potassium) and hyperglycemia (due to the neurohumoral stress response which may cause a misleading osmotic diuresis if not recognized).

A portable chest X-ray helps ensure proper endotracheal tube placement, and it also may provide valuable information about the etiology of shock. A child with poor perfusion, a small heart, and lucent lungs most likely has hypovolemic shock. Conversely, a child with an enlarged cardiac silhouette, congested lung fields, and poor perfusion most likely has cardiogenic shock.

Pulse oximetry, commonly available in referral emergency departments and during transports, provides very useful information about the adequacy of oxygenation and perfusion. Most pulse oximeters produce either a graphical illustration of the pulse wave or a quantitative illustration of the pulse magnitude using light-emitting diodes. When children have poor distal perfusion, the pulse wave appears small; thus, only a few diodes are illuminated during the arterial pulsation. Conversely, when pulse waves are large (with diodes illuminated from none to maximum), this suggests good distal perfusion, such as a low systemic vascular resistance state and wide pulse pressure in an infant with a large patent ductus arteriosus.

The pulse oximeter wave form can help guide therapy. For example, if the pulse oximeter waves are very small or the probe does not work on any extremity, inadequate distal perfusion is likely and fluid administration is indicated. Other causes of poor oximetry pulse waves include (1) applying the probe too tightly to the extremity, which compresses the vascular bed; (2) improperly placing the sensor so it is not directly across from the light-emitting diodes; (3) too much ambient light; (4) compromising the flow to the extremity due to a blood pressure cuff or because the extremity is taped too tightly to a broad; and (5) hypothermia. If these conditions are ruled out, it may be useful to follow the individual patient's pulse wave response to therapy.

MANAGEMENT OF SHOCK

Although management priorities are presented sequentially below, many therapies need to be provided almost simultaneously. The overall goals of shock therapy are to *in-*

crease tissue perfusion and oxygen delivery, and if possible, *decrease* metabolic demand to provide a better matching of perfusion to local tissue metabolism. Apply the following management principles based upon careful reevaluation of the child following each intervention. Recognizing that shock is an unstable, dynamic clinical state, it is critical to perform frequent rapid cardiopulmonary assessments to ensure that the child is maintaining adequate cardiac output.

Airway and ventilation

Even if the child's tissues are well oxygenated as shown by pulse oximetry, administer oxygen to all children with clinical signs of shock. Indeed, supplemental oxygen may be critical to a child with anemia, even when 100% saturated. For example, a leukemic child with a hemoglobin value of 3 gm % has an oxygen-carrying capacity (CaO_2) of 4.32 ml/100 ml of blood, assuming a PaO_2 of 100 mm Hg ($CaO_2 = 1.34 \times \text{Hgb} \times \%\ O_2$ saturation $+ PaO_2 \times 0.003$). If a nonrebreathing mask is used and the PaO_2 is increased to 600 mm Hg, the oxygen-carrying capacity increases to 5.82 ml/100 ml of blood, secondary to the increased quantity of dissolved oxygen in the plasma compartment. This represents a 35% increase in oxygen delivery to the tissues, which can make a critical difference in the child with shock secondary to anemia.

Since a diminished level of consciousness caused by shock may compromise airway reflexes, the airway must be evaluated to ensure that it is both open and stable. In the child with cardiogenic or distributive shock who has a substantial increase in the work of breathing, consider early intervention with intubation and ventilation. Normally, the respiratory muscles are responsible for only 2-5% of total body oxygen consumption. In the child with an increased work of breathing, however, respiratory muscle activity may comprise 25-30% of total oxygen consumption, leading to respiratory muscle fatigue and respiratory failure.[6] Therefore, reducing this metabolic demand by removing the work of breathing substantially benefits the child with shock and poor lung compliance.

Selection of the proper size endotracheal tube is guided by the child's size, utilizing a system such as the Broselow® Pediatric Emergency Tape.[35,37] The emergency tape is a tool that provides a simplified method rapidly estimating weight, based on length. Once the child's weight is known, the correct drug dosage, fluid boluses, endotracheal tube size, and other equipment needs are easily and quickly determined from the corresponding weight zone on the tape.

Once the child is intubated, they may relax and allow mechanical ventilation assistance. Some children, however, become more agitated and require sedation with or without neuromuscular blockade. Caution: sedative and analgesic agents must be used carefully in the child with shock. At particular risk is the child whose blood pressure is dependent upon enhanced sympathetic nervous system activity. Administering a narcotic or short-acting barbiturate to this child may cause the rapid onset of profound hypotension and cardiovascular collapse. Neuromuscular blockers either increase heart rate and blood pressure (e.g., pancuronium),[13] or maintain heart rate and blood pressure (e.g., vecuronium).[41] One of the other advantages of vecuronium is hepatic elimination, unlike the renal elimination of pancuronium. Since renal perfusion frequently is compromised in shock, pancuronium typically has a much longer duration of action than vecuronium.

Vascular access

Obtaining adequate vascular access in the child experiencing shock is often quite difficult. In the child less than 6 years old, placing an intraosseous (IO) needle provides a rapid method of obtaining vascular access. Once the child is fluid resuscitated through the IO needle it is often much easier to obtain venous access for transport. In children with shock, it is a good idea to obtain a second vascular access in case the first one is displaced or becomes nonfunctional during transport. However, do not spend too much time attempting a second IV line, particularly when the transport time is short.

Although determining central venous pressure might help guide the therapy of shock, central venous access is frequently difficult to obtain. The vast majority of children, including children with severe septic shock, are more than adequately managed initially with peripheral vascular lines. Regardless of the type of catheter placed, the transport team needs to ensure that all catheters are well secured and that the extremity is immobilized on an appropriate splint. If vasopressors are run through a peripheral venous site, careful observation of the site is necessary.

Fluid therapy

Fluid volume replacement is second in priority only to opening the airway and ensuring adequate oxygenation and ventilation in the child with shock. The quantity of fluid required to restore adequate perfusion often exceeds the calculated loss. This requirement reflects the fluid shift from the extracellular to the intracellular compartment of the ischemic cells[52] and the additive effects of the loss of vascular tone in both the microcirculation and the venous capacitance system.[5] Thus, the longer the child has been in shock, or the more severe the perfusion defect, the greater the amount of fluid required for effective resuscitation. Aggressive fluid resuscitation, however is not always appropriate. Children with prolonged shock, producing substantial myocardial dysfunction, may not tolerate large volumes of fluid. In these patients, give smaller rapid boluses of fluid (5-10 ml/kg) followed by careful reassessment, and then repeated bolus fluid administration.

Once IV/IO access is obtained, administer a bolus of 10-20 ml/kg. In the child with late compensated or decompensated shock, give the fluid bolus as rapidly as possible. This may require the use of a 20-60 ml syringe and a three-way stopcock to draw the fluid up into the syringe and push it through a small-bore IV catheter. Following each fluid bolus, reassess the child's perfusion. If systemic perfusion does not improve, repeat fluid boluses (10-20 ml/kg). Studies show that, in children with septic shock, survival is improved when more than 40 ml/kg is infused in the first hour of resuscitation.[14] The need for ongoing fluid requirements in sepsis is reflected by the six-hour mean fluid volume of almost 120 ml/kg in survivors.[14] The type of fluid used has been the subject of much controversy.[31] Fluid therapies are generally classified as colloid or crystalloid. Crystalloids are less expensive and more readily available. A one-liter bag of Ringer's lactate is approximately 1/100th the cost of a bottle of 5% albumin. Initially, either normal saline or Ringer's lactate is preferred. Do not use dextrose-containing fluid for bolus administration since hyperglycemia results. Five percent dextrose given in combination with salt solutions in a volume of 20 ml/kg delivers 1 gm/kg of glucose. This quantity represents the amount needed to correct hypoglycemia. Repeated administrations of 1 gm/kg of glucose can easily result in serum glucose concentrations >500 gm %. The resulting hyperosmolar state may worsen fluid loss by producing an osmotic diuresis as well as potentially injuring ischemic brain cells.

Colloid solutions contain either protein (5% albumin, plasmanate, or plasma protein fraction), or are comprised of an artificial colloid such as hetastarch. Colloids are substances that exert osmotic or oncotic pressure similar to plasma proteins. By increasing oncotic pressure in the vascular bed, fluid is pulled from the interstitial compartment, and the total blood volume is increased. Therefore, colloids are significantly better than crystalloids at selectively expanding the intravascular compartment.[31] Colloids may be preferable in the child with decompensated shock requiring rapid restoration of the circulating blood volume. Colloids must be considered in the child who fails to respond to 40-60 cc/kg of crystalloid. In general, administering a crystalloid adequately restores circulating blood volume and perfusion in most children, even if it is necessary to give 4-5 times the volume (compared with colloid). Blood products, such as fresh-frozen plasma and packed red blood cells, also act as colloids. Fresh-frozen plasma is overused and has limited acute utility in resuscitating the child with shock, unless a coagulopathy is present that requires replacement therapy.[20] Coagulopathy most commonly occurs in children with disseminated intravascular coagulation. Use of fresh-frozen plasma or packed red blood cells introduces the risk of allergic reactions and may transmit various viruses, such as non-A, non-B hepatitis and the HIV virus.

Packed red blood cells are specifically indicated in the management of the traumatized child who fails to restore adequate perfusion in response to two fluid boluses (i.e., 40 cc/kg) of crystalloid.[60] If needed, use O negative, uncrossmatched blood rather than permitting a state of shock to continue in the traumatized child. When available, substitute type-specific blood. Packed red blood cells are not indicated to maintain a hemoglobin concentration of 10 gm %. Unless the child is symptomatic, hemoglobin concentrations down to 7 gm % are usually tolerated well.[19]

In children with ongoing fluid loss, such as the child with traumatic shock, adjust fluid therapy in light of the ongoing losses. In addition, when large volumes of fluid therapy are required, ideally they are administered using a blood and fluid warming apparatus. Hypothermia often complicates the resuscitation of an infant or child receiving large volumes of room-temperature crystalloid and colloid combined with refrigerator temperature blood products.

During the fluid challenge, vital signs and clinical status should be followed closely. Children receiving fluid boluses are monitored closely for signs of volume overload: rales, increased work of breathing, cardiac gallop, hepatomegaly, and frothy respiratory secretions. If volume overload occurs, diuresis may be necessary. A dose of Furosemide® (1 mg/kg/dose) usually provides a prompt diuresis. An inadequate diuretic effect may indicate that renal perfusion is severely compromised. Frequent reassessment of the heart rate, quality of pulses, capillary refill, and color is imperative in the ongoing therapy for shock.

Determining the cause of shock

After attending to the basic needs of the patient, attempt to determine the cause of shock. This typically requires obtaining a history of the child's illness and evaluating the results of laboratory studies, as previously noted. Sometimes, even though the exact etiology of the child's shock is unknown, the child is successfully resuscitated. Early discovery of the cause of the child's shock, however, may be critical to successful therapy. Thus, a good history combined with the knowledge of age-specific causes of shock may suggest the diagnosis. For example, a one-week-old infant presenting with profound cardiogenic shock would be suspected of having a ductal-dependent congenital heart defect. If Prostaglandin E_1 (PGE_1) is given early, the infant often can be stabilized. Another example is a 3-year-old presenting with tachycardia and ventricular premature contractions. During the history it is discovered that the older sibling is receiving a tricyclic antidepressant. Therefore, therapy may be directed away from myocarditis and toward appropriate management of a tricyclic overdose using alkalization and phenytoin to manage the child's dysrhythmia.[24]

Cardiorespiratory monitoring

Careful monitoring of the child with shock is critical, both before and during transport. The goals of monitoring are to provide objective measures of vital organ function, response to therapy, and early identification of correctable problems. Monitoring methods include a continuous cardiorespiratory monitor to evaluate the heart rate and rhythm, invasive blood pressure monitoring, and pulse oximetry. Automated oscillometric blood pressure measurement (e.g., Dinemap®) may be inaccurate in the case of a child with shock.[16] A more accurate blood pressure can be determined using a manual blood pressure cuff and Doppler device. However, this system provides only the systolic blood pressure. Thus, the pulse pressure (systolic minus diastolic blood pressure), a significant evaluative tool, is not measured. Intraarterial blood pressure monitoring is ideal, but is often unavailable during interhospital transport.

Another additional useful monitoring modality is a bladder catheter to measure ongoing urine output, although the response time is not as rapid as some of the other monitoring modalities. Adequate splanchnic perfusion is suggested by a urine output ≥ 1 ml/kg/hr, provided that an osmotic diuresis (from mannitol or glucose), diabetes insipidus, or high output renal failure is not present.

Correct metabolic defects

Altered level of consciousness, poor perfusion, and diminished myocardial contractility all may be secondary to metabolic disorders which complicate the clinical state of a child with shock. When examining laboratory studies, always search for abnormalities in glucose and calcium, since these most often cause neurologic or cardiovascular complications. In addition, consider evaluating sodium, potassium, magnesium, and phosphorous levels. Hypoglycemia may be rapidly identified by a rapid bedside test, and the glucose concentration needs to be included in all early laboratory studies in a child with shock. Since the infant's myocardium is particularly dependent upon glucose as a metabolic substrate, hypoglycemia may present with all the clinical manifestations of cardiogenic shock. When hypoglycemia is present (<45 mg %), treatment consists of 2-4 ml/kg of $D_{25}W$.

Assess calcium concentration by measuring the ionized calcium concentration rather than the total calcium concentration.[15] Critically ill children often have reduced concentrations of albumin or the presence of drugs that may displace calcium from albumin binding sites. It is only the ionized (free) fraction of calcium that exerts a physiologic effect on the cardiovascular system.[22] Low-ionized calcium concentrations result in diminished cardiac contractility and peripheral vascular tone. Documented hypocalcemia is treated with the administration of 10-20 mg/kg of calcium chloride or 30-60 mg/kg of calcium gluconate; calcium chloride is preferred because of its greater bioavailability.[9]

Maintain temperature

Hypothermia commonly complicates the management of critically ill children in the emergency department. Typically, the children are disrobed and are not provided with an external source of heat. As previously noted, the clinical evaluation of the child with shock may be confounded by hypothermia, which causes cutaneous vasoconstriction and diminished distal pulse volume. A cold environment also adds a metabolic stress which may not be well tolerated in the child with shock.[1] Therefore, attempt to correct hypothermia using radiant heat in the emergency department or blankets and warming devices during transport. If hot packs are used to warm the child, they must not exceed a temperature of about 40°C (104°F). Children have been burned by the use of some commercially available chemical heating packs which achieve higher temperatures. Since a significant amount of radiant heat is lost through the head, cover the infant and child's head with a stockinette cap or a reflective cap.

Inotropic drug therapy

The need for inotropic drugs in the child with shock is limited and indeed contraindicated in children with hypovolemic shock. Their primary function in acute resuscitation is to rapidly restore perfusion pressure and blood flow to the vital organs. Since rapid resuscitation to normal or supranormal values of cardiac output and oxygen consumption are associated with improved survival,[14,53,59] it is important to avoid prolonged hypotensive shock. Therefore, it is usually most effective to use a potent agent initially. Once the child is stabilized, then change to a less potent, and hopefully less toxic, vasoactive agent. Complete discussion of all the available inotropic agents is beyond the scope of this chapter, but is available in other sources. The most commonly used vasoactive agents in the child with shock are epinephrine, dopamine, and dobutamine.[62] Other inotropic drugs, such as norepinephrine, amrinone, and isoproterenol, are less commonly required. The indications for all of these agents is included in Table 20-2.

Epinephrine is a potent, endogenous catecholamine that acts at β- and α-adrenergic receptors.[61,62] In the doses typically used to stabilize the child with shock, epinephrine increases heart rate, contractility, and myocardial conduction velocity. (Note that an increase in myocardial conductivity predisposes the child to arrhythmias). In the peripheral vasculature, epinephrine increases the systemic vascular resistance through its prominent effect on α-adrenergic receptors. At lower infusion doses, however, the action at peripheral β-adrenergic receptors results in a decrease in vascular tone. Epinephrine may be useful in all types of shock. Initial therapy for all forms of shock is directed at optimizing intravascular volume; therefore, if the child remains poorly perfused, and particularly, if the child is hypotensive, then an epinephrine infusion is the drug of choice to restore an adequate perfusion pressure.[17]

TABLE 20-2 SUGGESTED USES OF INOTROPES BY AGE. INOTROPES ARE LISTED IN ORDER OF PREFERENCE FOR INITIAL STABILIZATION

Condition	*Infant*	*Child*	*Adult*
Cardiogenic shock	EPI or Dobut DA[a] Amrinone	Dobut DA or EPI Amrinone	Dobut or DA EPI NE Amrinone
Septic shock (Distributive)	EPI or DA Dobut	EPI or DA Dobut	NE or Dobut or DA or EPI
Hypovolemic shock	Not Indicated	Not Indicated	Not Indicated
Shock from bradycardia	EPI or ISO	EPI or ISO	ISO or EPI
Anaphylactic shock	EPI	EPI	EPI
Decreased renal blood flow or urine output	DA[a]	DA	DA

DA = dopamine, Dobut = dobutamine, EPI = epinephrine, NE = norepinephrine, ISO = isoproterenol
[a] Dopamine is often combined with more potent vasoactive agents, such as epinephrine and norepinephrine. Dopamine infusions of 2-3 μg/kg/min may help maintain splanchnic perfusion when using these potent vasoconstrictors.

One of epinephrine's limitations is its potent action at α-adrenergic receptors with the potential for producing splanchnic and renal ischemia.[26] Studies show, however, that epinephrine (or norepinephrine) improves perfusion to these organs in hypotensive patients with cardiogenic or septic shock.[18,21,38]

Since epinephrine has potent vasoconstrictive effects, it must be administered through a secure vascular access. In emergency situations it may be given through an IO cannula. The usual starting infusion rate is 0.3-0.5 μg/kg/min; titrate to the rate necessary to restore an adequate blood pressure. When used in children with cardiogenic shock, careful monitoring of the cardiac rhythm is critical because epinephrine may produce either ventricular or supraventricular dysrhythmias. In addition, epinephrine has potent metabolic actions.[56] It typically elevates glucose concentration by both stimulating glucose production and inhibiting the action of insulin. Marked hyperglycemia results in an osmotic diuresis, which complicates the evaluation of splanchnic perfusion. Epinephrine also lowers serum potassium concentration by 0.3 to 0.8 mEq/L through a β_2-adrenergic receptor action.[10]

The preparation and dosage of epinephrine and other vasoactive drug infusions is outlined in Table 20-3. Since the half-life of all catecholamines is short, rapidly adjust the infusion to the level needed to maintain blood pressure and perfusion. As the child responds to therapy, reduce the infusion rate. Since this potent drug may produce profound hypertension if inadvertently run at a high rate, always use a carefully controlled infusion pump rather than a gravity drip.

Dobutamine is a synthetic catecholamine infused as a racemic mixture of the (+) and (−) isomers. The coinfusion of these isomers results in the β_1-adrenergic selective effect of dobutamine on the heart.[48] The (+) isomer is a β-agonist and an α-antagonist, whereas the (−) isomer is a potent selective α_1-agonist and a weak β-agonist. Since dobutamine possesses intrinsic α-adrenergic blocking activity, its use in children with septic shock may result in paradoxical hypotension, since sepsis is characterized by abnormal α-adrenergic vascular tone.[46,54] The primary indication for dobutamine use is to enhance cardiac contractility in children with diminished myocardial pumping function.[44] This may occur in children with primary cardiac diseases, as well as children with acquired cardiogenic dysfunction postarrest or following severe shock.[36] Since dobutamine lacks significant peripheral vasoconstrictive effects, it is a poor choice to initially increase the blood pressure in a child with decompensated shock. Dobutamine is largely reserved as a selective inotrope. Preparation of the infusion and the recommended infusion rate is outlined in Table 20-3.

TABLE 20-3 PREPARATION OF VASOACTIVE DRUGS USED BY CONTINUOUS INFUSION

Drug (how supplied)*	*Preparation for infusion*	*Dosage equivalents*	*Dose*
Dopamine hydrochloride (40 mg/mL)	6 times the body weight [kg] is the mg to add to the diluent to make a final volume of 100 ml.	Then, 1 ml/hr delivers 1 μg/kg/min.	Begin at 10 μg/kg/min; titrate to desired effect up to 20 μg/kg/min.
Dobutamine hydrochloride (12.5 mg/mL)			Begin at 5-10 μg/kg/min; titrate to desired effect up to 20 μg/kg/min.
Nitroprusside sodium (50 mg powdered vial)			Begin at 0.5 μg/kg/min; titrate to desired effect up to 8 μg/kg/min.
Epinephrine 1:1000 (1 mg/mL)	0.6 times the body weight [kg] is the mg to add to the diluent to make a final volume of 100 ml.	Then, 1 ml/hr delivers 0.1 μg/kg/min.	Begin at 0.1-0.3 μg/kg/min, and increase as needed to 1 μg/kg/min
Norepinephrine 1:1000 (1 mg/ml)			Begin at 0.1-0.3 μg/kg/min, and increase as needed to 1 μg/kg/min. Used in hypotensive septic shock.
Prostaglandin E_1 (0.5 mg/ml)			Begin at 0.05-0.1 μg/kg/min. Monitor for hypotension and apnea.
Isoproterenol hydrochloride (0.2 mg/mL)			Infuse like epinephrine; carefully monitor heart rate and blood pressure.
Lidocaine hydrochloride 2% (20 mg/mL)	60 times body weight [kg] is the mg to add to diluent to make a final volume of 100 ml.	Then, 1 ml/hr delivers 10 μg/kg/min.	Begin at 20 μg/kg/min (2 ml/hr), and increase to maximum of 50 μg/kg/min as needed.

* Concentration listed is either the form available in prefilled syringes or the most commonly used concentration.

Dopamine is an endogenous catecholamine with complex pharmacology.[40,62] When used in the child with shock, dopamine generally is infused at rates between 10 and 20 μg/kg/min. This results in peripheral vasoconstriction and increased cardiac contractility and heart rate. Dopamine is not as potent as epinephrine and, in our opinion, is not the first line agent to use in a child with decompensated shock. If the child responds to an epinephrine infusion, dopamine may be started. The transition from epinephrine to dopamine minimizes the potential for excess vasoconstriction and the metabolic abnormalities complicating the use of epinephrine (see Table 20-3). Like epinephrine and dobutamine, infuse dopamine through a central venous line or secure peripheral site. If an infiltration with any vasoconstrictor occurs, rapidly infiltrate the site with phentolamine (1-5 mg),[55] diluted with normal saline to a 1 mg/ml solution prior to subcutaneous administration.

Vasodilator therapy

In children with cardiogenic shock, vasodilators often improve cardiac output. When myocardial pumping function is diminished,

TABLE 20-4 CLASSIFICATION OF VASODILATORS BY THEIR SITE OF ACTION

Venous	*Balanced*	*Arterial*
Nitrates: nitroglycerin isosorbide dinitrate	Nitroprusside sodium	Hydralazine hydrochloride
	Phentolamine	Minoxidil
	Tolazoline hydrochloride	Dopamine hydrochloride
	Captopril and enalapril	Nifedipine
	Prazosin	
	Prostaglandin E_1	

increases in afterload produce proportional decreases in stroke volume.[39] A vasodilator often increases stroke volume while maintaining or increasing blood pressure, even though the systemic vascular resistance is reduced.[39,42] Furthermore, vasodilators may diminish myocardial oxygen demand even while they increase cardiac output. This is unlike inotropic agents, all of which increase myocardial oxygen requirements (except for amrinone which is a potent vasodilator as well). The commonly used vasodilators in the child with shock are nitroprusside,[3,7] and in selected infants, prostaglandin E_1 (PGE_1).[34] Less commonly used vasodilators are nitroglycerine[8] and amrinone.[33] Vasodilators may be classified by their site of action (Table 20-4) and mechanism of action (Table 20-5). The indications, dose, and route of these agents are outlined in Table 20-6. Dose information is included on agents not discussed in the text but used on occasion in children.

TABLE 20-5 CLASSIFICATION OF VASODILATORS BY THEIR MECHANISM OF ACTION

Mechanism of action	*Vasodilator agents*
Direct-acting	Hydralazine, minoxidil
Intracellular nitrate receptor	Nitrates, nitroglycerin, nitroprusside
Sympathetic nervous system blocker	Phentolamine, prazosin, trimethaphan
Calcium channel blocker	Nifedipine, diltiazem, verapamil
Renin-angiotensin system blocker	Captopril, Enalapril
Miscellaneous actions	Tolazoline, PGE_1

Sodium nitroprusside is a potent, rapidly acting systemic vasodilator that relaxes tone in both the arterial and venous systems. Also, sodium nitroprusside is a potent pulmonary vasodilator. The usual net actions of sodium nitroprusside are to increase cardiac output while decreasing the central venous and pulmonary artery wedge pressures. The latter occurs secondary to a change in ventricular compliance and a reduction in venous tone. Although the filling pressures go down, venous return increases if cardiac output increases.

If the child's intravascular volume is inadequate, sodium nitroprusside and other vasodilators pool blood in the venous system, decreasing venous return and thus cardiac output.[3,42] Hypotension results from an inadequate stroke volume combined with the decrease in systemic vascular resistance. Therefore, do not use vasodilators until the child's preload has been adequately augmented.

Sodium nitroprusside must be infused as a continuous drip since it has a short half-life. The usual infusion rate varies from 0.5 to 6.0 μg/kg/min. Sodium nitroprusside rapidly undergoes nonenzymatic degradation, releasing cyanide. Nonenzymatic degradation is rapidly metabolized by the liver to sodium thiocyanate.[58] Only in children with significant liver impairment does cyanide accumulate and potentially complicate the management of a child with shock. During transport of the child, significant thiocyanate accumulation is not a concern. Sodium nitroprusside must be prepared in D_5W, but it may be coinfused through the same IV access site with other vasoactive agents including any of the catecholamines prepared in other solutions.[28]

TABLE 20-6 INDICATIONS AND DOSES OF SELECTED VASODILATORS

Drug	*Actions and indications*	*Dose and route*
Sodium nitroprusside	Congestive heart failure or cardiogenic shock, aortic or mitral regurgitation, severe hypertension.	IV infusion at 0.5-8 μg/kg/min; adjust to desired effect
Nitroglycerine	Reduce high filling pressures, improve coronary blood flow, reduce pulmonary hypertension.	IV infusion at 0.5-10 μg/kg/min if special infusion set used
Hydralazine	Not used in shock, chronic therapy of congestive heart failure, and hypertension.	0.1-0.5 mg/kg IV every 6-8 hours 0.25-1 mg/kg orally every 6-8 hours; maximum of 7 mg/kg/day
Captopril	Very useful in children with congestive heart failure; no value in acute shock treatment; must be given orally.	*Neonates:* 0.03-0.15 mg/kg/day divided q 6-12 hours; maximum of 2 mg/kg/day *Children:* 0.5-1 mg/kg/day divided q 6-8 hours; maximum of 6 mg/kg/day up to 12.5 mg/dose q 8-12 hours in adolescents
Enalapril	Like Captopril, useful only for chronic therapy; major advantage is longer half-life, but limited pediatric data.	0.05-0.1 mg/kg/dose divided q 12h; little data in pediatrics
Prazosin	Limited pediatric use except occasionally in the hypertensive patient or in children with congestive heart failure.	0.01 to 0.05 mg/kg/dose orally q 6-8 h; maximum of 0.1 mg/kg/dose
Tolazoline	Complex pharmacology; used to treat pulmonary hypertensive crisis, although PGE_1 may be more useful and safer.	1-2 mg/kg load, then 1-2 mg/kg/hr
Phentolamine	Limited use; potent α-adrenergic blocking agent.	2.5-15 μg/kg/min for afterload reduction

SUMMARY

Optimal management of the child with shock requires careful attention to all the details of cardiorespiratory support outlined in this chapter and covered elsewhere in this book. As shock is a dynamic state, continuous monitoring and adjustments of therapy are critical during transport. The overall goals of shock therapy are to maintain vital organ perfusion, optimize oxygenation and ventilation, and prevent further injury to all organ systems. To minimize organ system injury, rapid correction of decompensated shock using aggressive fluid resuscitation and potent drug therapy is indicated.

Prior to transport, the child's cardiorespiratory condition must be stabilized. Secure the airway, as needed, and provide supplemental oxygen. Reliable vascular access is critical, since fluid therapy is the mainstay of shock treatment. During transport, maintain the hemodynamic and thermal stability by clinically assessing perfusion and maintenance of body temperature. Utilizing the treatments detailed above, most children with shock have an excellent outcome, especially if recognized in the compensated state.

REFERENCES

1. Adamson K Jr, Gandy G, James L: The influence of thermal factors upon oxygen consumption of the newborn human infant, *J Pediatr* 66:495-508, 1965.
2. American College of Chest Physicians/Society of Critical Care Medicine Consensus Conference: Definitions for sepsis and organ failure and guideliens for the use of innovative therapies in sepsis, *Crit Care Med* 20-864-74, 1992.
3. Artman M, Graham T: Guidelines for vasodilator therapy of congestive heart failure in infants and children, *Am Heart J* 113:994-1005, 1987.
4. Artman M, Graham TP: Congestive heart failure in infancy: recognition and management, *Am Heart J* 103:1040-55, 1982.

5. Astiz ME, Rackow EC, Weil MH: Pathophysiology and treatment of circulatory shock, *Crit Care Clin* 9:183-204, 1993.
6. Aubier M, Trippenbach T, Roussos C: Respiratory muscle fatigue during cardiogenic shock, *J Appl Physiol* 5:499-508, 1981.
7. Benitz WE and others: Use of sodium nitroprusside in neonates: efficacy and safety, *J Pediatr* 106:102-10, 1985.
8. Benson LN and others: Nitroglycerin therapy in children with low cardiac index after heart surgery, *Cardiovasc Med* 4:207-15, 1979.
9. Broner C and others: A prospective, randomized, double-blind comparison of calcium chloride and calcium gluconate therapies for hypocalcemia in critically ill children, *J Pediatr* 117:986-9, 1990.
10. Brown MJ: Hypokalemia from beta$_2$-receptor stimulation by circulating epinephrine, *Am J Cardiol* 56:3D-9D, 1985.
11. Buck SH, Zaritsky AL: Occult core hyperthermia complicating cardiogenic shock, *Pediatrics* 83:782-4, 1989.
12. Buran MJ: Oxygen consumption, In: Snyder JV, Pinsky MR, ed. *Oxygen Transport in the Critically Ill*, Chicago, 1987, Year Book Medical Publishers.
13. Cabal L and others: Cardiovascular and catecholamine changes after administration of pancuronium in distressed neonates, *Pediatrics* 75:284-7, 1985.
14. Carcillo J, Davis A, Zaritsky A: Role of early fluid resuscitation in pediatric septic shock, *JAMA* 266:1242-5, 1991.
15. Cardenas-Rivero N and others: Hypocalcemia in critically ill children, *J Pediatr* 114:946-51, 1989.
16. Carroll GC: Blood pressure monitoring, *Crit Care Clin* 4:411-34, 1988.
17. Chameides L, editor: *Textbook of Pediatric Advanced Life Support*, Dallas, 1990, American Heart Association.
18. Coffin LH Jr, Ankeney JL, Beheler EM: Experimental study and clinical use of epinephrine for treatment of low cardiac output syndrome, *Circulation* 33(Suppl 1):I78-I85, 1965.
19. Consensus conference: Perioperative red blood cell transfusion, *JAMA* 260-2700-3, 1988.
20. Consensus conference, National Institutes of Health: Fresh-frozen plasma: indications and risks, *JAMA* 253:551-3, 1985.
21. Desjars P and others: Norepinephrine therapy has no deleterious renal effects in human septic shock [see comments], *Crit Care Med* 17:426-9, 1989.
22. Drop L: Ionized calcium, the heart, and hemodynamic function, *Anesth Analg* 64:432-51, 1985.
23. Fisher MM: Clinical observations in the pathophysiology and treatment of anaphylactic cardiovascular collapse, *Anesth Intensive Care* 14:17-21, 1986.
24. Frommer DA and others: Tricyclic antidepressant overdose: a review, *JAMA* 257:521-6, 1987.
25. Fuhrman BP: Structure and function of the regional vasculature. In Furhman BP, Zimmerman JJ, editors: *Pediatric Critical Care*, St. Louis, 1992, Mosby-Year Book.
26. Gombos EA and others: Reactivity of renal and systemic circulations to vasoconstrictor agents in normotensive and hypertensive subjects, *J Clin Invest* 41:203-17, 1962.
27. Hazinski MF: Cardiovascular disorders. In Hazinski MF, editor: *Nursing Care of the Critically Ill Child*, ed 2, St. Louis, 1992, Mosby-Year Book.
28. Horrow JC and others: Intravenous infusions of nitroprusside, dobutamine, and nitroglycerin are compatible, *Crit Care Med* 18:858-61, 1990.
29. Hussain S, Simkus G, Roussos C: Respiratory muscle fatigue: a cause of ventilatory failure in septic shock, *J Appl Physiol* 58:2033-40, 1985.
30. Ignarro LJ and others: Endothelium derived relaxing factor from pulmonary artery and vein possess pharmacologic and chemical properties identical to those of nitric oxide radical, *Cric Res* 61:866-79, 1987.
31. Imm A, Carlson RW: Fluid resuscitation in circulatory shock, *Critical Care Clinics* 9:313-34, 1993.
32. Kilbourn RG and others: N^G-methyl-L-arginine inhibits tumor necrosis factor-induced hypotension: implications for the involvement of nitric oxide, *Proc Natl Acad Sci* 87:3629-32, 1990.
33. Lawless S and others: Amrinone in neonates and infants after cardiac surgery, *Crit Care Med* 17:751-4, 1989.
34. Lewis AB, Takahashi M, Lurie PR: Administration of prostaglandin E_1 in neonates with critical congenital cardiac defects, *J Pediatr* 93:481-5, 1978.
35. Lubitz D and others: A rapid method for estimating weight and resuscitation drug dosages from length in the pediatric age group, *Ann Emerg Med* 17:576-81, 1988.
36. Lucking SE, Pollack MM, Fields AI: Shock following generalized hypoxic-ischemic injury in previously healthy infants and children, *J Pediatr* 108:359-64, 1986.
37. Luten RC, and others: Length-based endotracheal tube and emergency equipment in pediatrics, *Ann Emerg Med* 21:900-4, 1992.
38. Marin C and others: Renal effects of norepinephrine used to treat septic shock patients, *Crit Care Med* 18:282-5, 1990.
39. Miller RR and others: Differential systemic arterial and venous actions and consequent cardiac effects of vasodilator drugs, *Prog Cardiovasc Dis* 24:353-73, 1982.
40. Notterman DA Inotropic agents. Catecholamines, digoxin, amrinone, *Crit Care Clin* 7:583-613, 1991.
41. O'Connor MF, Roizen MF: Use of muscle relaxants in the intensive care unit, *J Intensive Care Med* 8:34-46, 1993.
42. Packer M, Le Jemtel TH: Physiologic and pharmacologic determinants of vasodilator response: a conceptual framework for rational drug therapy for chronic heart failure, *Prog Cardiovasc Dis* 4:275-92, 1982.
43. Perkin RM, Anas NG: Mechanisms and management of anaphylactic shock not responding to traditional therapy, *Ann Allergy* 54:202-8, 1985.

44. Perkin RM and others: Dobutamine: a hemodynamic evaluation in children with shock, *J Pediatr* 100: 977-83, 1982.
45. Perloff WH: Physiology of the heart and circulation. In Swedlow DB, Raphaely RC, editors: *Cardiovascular Problems in Pediatric Critical Care,* New York, 1986, Churchill Livingstone.
46. Rackow EC, Astiz ME: Mechanisms and management of septic shock, *Crit Care Clin* 9:219-38, 1993.
47. Riley LJ, Ilson BE, Narins RG: Acute metabolic acid-base disorders, *Crit Care Clin* 5:699-724, 1987.
48. Ritter M, Lemanske RF Jr: Anaphylaxis. In Fuhrman BP, Zimmerman JJ, editors: *Pediatric Critical Care,* St. Louis, 1992, Mosby-Year Book.
49. Ruffolo RR Jr: Review: the pharmacology of dobutamine, *Am J Med Sci* 294:244-8, 1987.
50. Schneider AJ and others: Total body blood volume redistribution in porcine E. coli septic shock: effect of volume loading, dobutamine, and norepinephrine, *Circ Shock* 35:215-22, 1991.
51. Schumacker PT: Peripheral vascular responses to septic shock: direct or reflex effects?, *Chest* 99: 1057-9, 1991.
52. Shires GT and others: Alterations in cellular membrane function during hemorrhagic shock in patients, *Ann Surg* 176:288-95, 1972.
53. Shoemaker WC, Appel PL, Kram HB: Oxygen transport measurements to evaluate tissue perfusion and titrate therapy: Dobutamine and dopamine effects, *Crit Care Med* 19:672-88, 1991.
54. Sibbald WJ, Fox G, Martin C: Abnormalities of vascular reactivity in the sepsis syndrome, *Chest* 100 (Supplement):155S-159S, 1991.
55. Siwy BK, Sadove AM: Acute management of dopamine infiltration injury with regitine, *Plast Reconstr Surg* 80:610-2, 1987.
56. Soman VR, Shamoon H, Sherwin RS: Effects of physiologic infusion of epinephrine in normal humans: relationship between the metabolic response and β-adrenergic binding, *J Clin Endocrinol Metab* 50:294-7, 1980.
57. Sprung CL and others: Impact of encephalopathy on mortality in the sepsis syndrome, *Crit Care Med* 18:801-6, 1990.
58. Tinker JH, Michenfelder JD: Sodium nitroprusside: pharmacology, toxicology and therapeutics, *Anesthesiology* 45:340-53, 1976.
59. Tuchschmidt J and others: Elevation of cardiac output and oxygen delivery improves outcome in septic shock, *Chest* 102:216-20, 1992.
60. Young GM, Eichelberger MR: Evaluation, stabilization, and initial management after multiple trauma. In Fuhrman BP, Zimmerman JJ, editors: *Pediatric Critical Care,* St. Louis, 1992, Mosby-Year Book.
61. Zaloga GP and others: Pharmacologic cardiovascular support, *Crit Care Clin* 9:335-62, 1993.
62. Zaritsky A, Chernow B: Use of catecholamines in pediatrics, *J Pediatr* 105:341-50, 1984.

21
CARDIOVASCULAR SYSTEM

M. MICHELE MOSS

THE INFANT WITH SYMPTOMATIC CONGENITAL HEART DISEASE

Congenital cardiac defects constitute the majority of diagnoses in the pediatric patient with cardiovascular disease. Most of the defects needing acute intervention, medical or surgical, present in early infancy, often while the infant is still in the nursery. However, some infants with significant congenital cardiac diseases are discharged from the nursery before symptoms develop and the diagnosis is made, therefore, these infants present instead to clinics and emergency departments. Infants with congenital heart disease need to be evaluated in a tertiary center by a pediatric cardiologist with skills in echocardiography and cardiac catheterization. A pediatric cardiac surgeon also needs to be available for possible emergent surgical palliation. The timing of that evaluation depends upon the severity of symptoms. Frequently the symptoms are life-threatening and therefore require rapid transport to a pediatric cardiac care center. As a whole, infants with congenital heart disease can be transported safely by air or ground following adequate stabilization.

Cardiac defects can be divided into four categories of physiologic presentation: left-to-right shunt defects with symptoms of congestive heart failure; lesions producing obstruction to left heart outflow, resulting in dependence of the ductus arteriosus for systemic blood flow; defects including transposition of the great arteries and obstruction to right heart outflow producing cyanosis; and lesions where the systemic and pulmonary venous blood mixes at some level, resulting in symptoms of both congestive heart failure and cyanosis (see Box 21-1).

Most of the patients with significant defects will become symptomatic within the first three months of life. Left-to-right shunt defects usually manifest between 6 weeks and 3 months of age.[22] Defects causing obstruction to left heart outflow become suddenly symptomatic when the ductus arteriosus begins to close, usually from 24 hours to 12 days of age. Cyanotic defects generally become apparent in the immediate newborn period. However, some defects such as tetralogy of Fallot produce progressive cyanosis and may not become apparent for a few months.[8] Infants with the common, mixing lesions frequently will not be diagnosed until 2-4 weeks of age, older than infants with solely cyanotic disease and earlier than infants with isolated left-to-right shunts.

THE INFANT WITH CYANOSIS

The newborn infant with cyanosis can pose a diagnostic dilemma when presenting to a hospital not equipped with pediatric cardiac diagnostic capabilities. The differential diagnosis usually falls between cyanotic cardiac disease and pulmonary disease with or without pulmonary hypertension of the newborn. The history, physical examination, chest ra-

BOX 21-1 CONGENITAL CARDIAC DEFECTS AND THEIR PHYSIOLOGIC PRESENTATION

Cyanotic defects
- Transposition type physiology
  - Transposition of the great arteries
- Obstruction to right heart outflow
  - Tetralogy of Fallot
  - Pulmonary atresia with/without VSD
  - Tricuspid atresia with pulmonary atresia or severe stenosis
  - Critical pulmonary stenosis

Left-to-right shunts
- Ventricular septal defect
- Patent ductus arteriosus
- Atrial septal defects
- Atrioventricular canal defects

Obstruction to left heart outflow
- Coarctation of the aorta
- Interruption of the aortic arch
- Critical aortic stenosis
- Hypoplastic left heart syndrome

Common mixing lesions
- Single or common ventricle
- Common atrium
- Truncus arteriosus
- Tricuspid atresia without PS
- Total anomalous pulmonary venous return with or without obstruction

diograph, and blood gas and oximetry data can help determine whether the cause is pulmonary or cardiac and determine the severity of the process.

Cyanosis is a physical finding that relates to the amount of deoxygenated hemoglobin in arterial blood, not necessarily to the arterial oxygen tension.[30] Usually more than 5 grams of deoxygenated hemoglobin per deciliter of blood is necessary to clinically detect the presence of cyanosis. Arterial desaturation will be more difficult to diagnose if the patient is anemic because cyanosis will not be clinically detectable, even if the patient has low oxygen saturations. Also, a mildly desaturated infant will appear cyanotic with less deoxygenation when the total amount of deoxygenated hemoglobin is greater than five gm %. Cyanosis is best appreciated when examining the nailbeds and mucous membranes. It must be differentiated from the condition of acrocyanosis present in some newborns as blueness of the hands and feet and pink mucous membranes.

Information obtained from the history may be helpful to differentiate pulmonary from cardiac causes of cyanosis. A diabetic mother or a family history of congenital heart disease may suggest cyanotic heart disease. The presence of meconium at delivery, fetal distress during labor and delivery, and maternal fever may indicate pulmonary disease. The Apgar[2] scores at one and five minutes are also important, as they suggest the time the cyanosis appeared.

The physical examination should center around the infant's level of distress, work of breathing, and cardiac examination. The infant should be examined for signs suggesting distress such as agitation, irritability, tachycardia, and mild systemic hypertension. Respiratory symptoms such as tachypnea, grunting, flaring of the nasal alae, and intercostal and subcostal retractions point to pulmonary pathology as the cause of cyanosis. Despite low levels of oxygenation, infants with cyanotic congenital heart disease usually appear comfortable with no increase in the work of breathing. Their respiratory pattern is usually that of hyperpnea (deep, slow breaths).

Examination of the heart, although very important, may not be as specific as expected. The presence of a murmur may not always point to cardiac disease. The pansystolic murmur of tricuspid regurgitation is a frequent finding in infants with pulmonary disease. A continuous murmur might indicate a patent ductus arteriosus in tetralogy of Fallot with severe pulmonary stenosis or atresia. Infants with transposition of the great arteries often do not have murmurs. A split S_2 represents the presence of two semilunar valves which eliminates some cyanotic heart diseases, such as pulmonary atresia.

When an infant is believed to be cyanotic, continuous pulse oximetry should be performed to document the hypoxemia and to detect any rapid fluctuations in oxygenation. Further assessment of oxygenation should be done both on room air and under hyperoxic conditions as close to $FiO_2 = 1.0$ as possible.[12,30] Oxygenation can be measured during this test by both arterial blood gas and pulse oximetry. To perform the assessment, arterial blood gases should be obtained on room air and after 15 minutes breathing hyperoxic gas. The blood gases should be drawn preferentially from the preductal right radial artery. An infant with pulmonary disease will have an increase in arterial PO_2, usually greater than 200 mmHg, and a corresponding increase in arterial oxygen saturation as indicated by the pulse oximetry reading. An infant with significant cyanotic heart disease will not be able to increase arterial PO_2 greater than 150 mm/Hg and rarely will increase it greater than 100 mm/Hg. The arterial oxygen saturation also will not increase significantly, rarely greater than 95%. With significant cyanotic cardiac defects, often no increase in oxygenation is noted. Therefore, if the oxygenation improves dramatically with increased FiO_2, then pulmonary disease is most likely the cause; whereas if little change in oxygenation is seen, cardiac disease should be strongly suspected.

Infants with pulmonary hypertension of the newborn due to meconium aspiration, asphyxia, endotoxemia, or diaphragmatic hernia may show a pattern of rapid fluctuations in arterial PO_2 from very low levels to high levels when exposed to a high concentration of oxygen. This phenomenon is due to the pulmonary vascular response to oxygen which causes the pulmonary vascular resistance to fall and pulmonary blood flow to increase, thereby improving oxygenation. Pulmonary blood flow and the right-to-left shunt in these patients will change with the pulmonary vascular resistance, and therefore oxygenation fluctuates. In infants with severe pulmonary disease or pulmonary hypertension, the right-to-left shunt will appear fixed as in the infant with congenital heart disease.

The chest radiograph is examined for evidence of pulmonary pathology, presence or absence of pulmonary vascularity, and size and shape of the cardiac silhouette (Figure 21-1). Pulmonary infiltrates and atelectasis help identify pulmonary disease. Cardiomegaly, unusual cardiac silhouette (e.g., boot-shaped heart), and absence of pulmonary

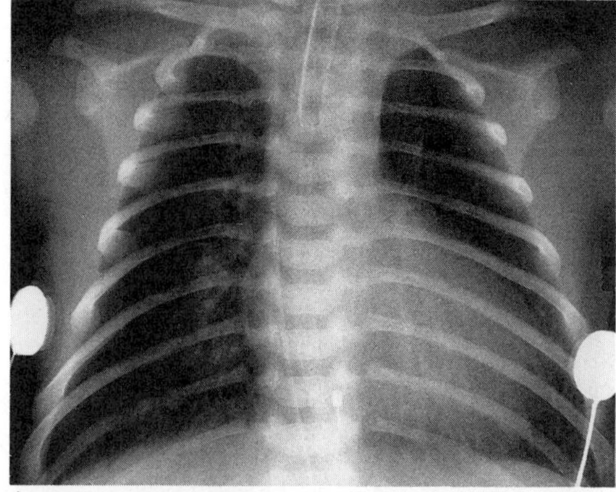

A

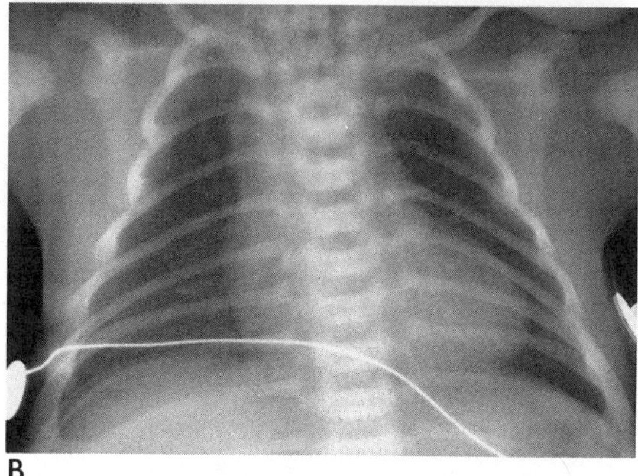

B

Fig. 21-1. a) Infant with transposition of the great arteries. Note the mild cardiomegaly but normal heart shape and pulmonary vasculature. b) Infant with tetralogy of Fallot with pulmonary atresia. Note the absence of a pulmonary artery segment causing the boot-shape of the heart. The pulmonary vasculature is diminished.

blood flow may indicate cyanotic cardiac disease. However, many infants with significant heart disease, such as transposition of the great vessels, can have unremarkable radiographic findings.

Once the cyanosis has been attributed to cardiac disease, arrangements should be made to transport the infant to a pediatric cardiac center. Transport should also be arranged for those infants whose diagnose is undetermined between pulmonary and cardiac disease. The severity of the cyanosis and the distress of the infant will determine the mode of transport and the skill of team members. Preferably, all infants with undiagnosed cyanotic congenital heart disease should be transported as rapidly as possible in the care of personnel trained specifically in neonatal or pediatric transport.

The management of the cyanotic infant before and during transport depends on the level of cyanosis. In the infant with severely low levels of oxygenation (O_2 saturations of less than 60%) the presence of metabolic acidosis and other evidence of tissue hypoxemia must be assessed. Such patients need to be treated aggressively to prevent tissue ischemia. Infants with mild hypoxemia (O_2 saturations above 80%) may need very little acute intervention.

Establishing the patency of the ductus arteriosus in severely cyanotic infants is crucial to their care.[10] Prostaglandin E_1 (alprostadil, Prostin VR Pediatric®) given as a continuous infusion can maintain or reopen the ductus arteriosus.[14] The starting dose is 0.1 mcg/kg/min until an improvement in oxygenation is noted. The dose can then be decreased to 0.05 mcg/kg/min. PGE_1 is a relatively safe drug, however, it does have notable side effects that are lessened at the lower dose. Infants, particularly those small for gestational age or premature, may develop apnea in the course of the PGE_1 infusion. Although the apnea usually occurs early after administration of the drug, it may be seen as late as 6-8 hours. Intubation prior to transport to control the airway and maintain ventilation is recommended, but is controversial. Although control of the airway is imperative, these infants do not always tolerate positive pressure ventilation. Positive pressure ventilation increases intrapulmonary pressure which decreases pulmonary blood flow. In infants who are dependent on the ductus arteriosus for pulmonary blood flow, this can dangerously restrict pulmonary blood flow. Therefore, if the airway needs to be secured because of periodic breathing, apnea, or inability to maintain the airway because of physical restraints during transport (i.e., small helicopter cabin), then low ventilator pressures and low rates should be used if possible.

Other complications of PGE_1 include systemic vasodilation with secondary hypotension.[20] This adverse effect can be managed with intravascular volume expansion. When PGE_1 is delivered through an umbilical artery catheter, the lower extremities may become dramatically red with bounding pulses secondary to this vasodilatory effect. Seizures, irritability, and fever may also be seen. Because the fever from PGE_1 can mask infection, these infants should have a sepsis evaluation performed if fever occurs.

Cyanotic infants, whether intubated or not, need to breathe higher concentrations of oxygen during air transport to overcome any decrease in inspired oxygen with altitude. Although helicopters rarely fly at altitudes high enough to decrease arterial PO_2 in normal patients, a cyanotic infant may show decreased oxygenation. This is also true for fixed wing aircraft with pressurized cabins, which are usually pressurized to an altitude that can maintain a comfortable inspired oxygen. However, altitudes above 5,000 ft may result in "uncomfortable" decreases in oxygenation in the cyanotic infant. Cyanotic infants also need to be kept hydrated, therefore total intravascular fluids should be delivered in maintenance amounts. A rate of 80-100 cc/kg/day of water plus age-appropriate amounts of glucose, sodium, and calcium should be given. Inotropic support with dopamine and dobutamine is occasionally warranted, especially in the severely cyanotic infant who may have diminished myocardial contractility due to hypoxemia.

THE INFANT WITH LOW CARDIAC OUTPUT AND SHOCK

Obstruction to systemic output from the left heart is the most common cause of cardiogenic shock in the infant less than one month of age. Severe sepsis with septic shock is the major differential diagnosis. Frequently, there are no symptoms or signs that can differentiate the two diagnoses, such as a bulging fontanelle or a pathologic heart murmur.[27] Therefore, the infant in shock under 3 weeks old must be treated for both conditions. Because these infants need tertiary care and diagnosis, a transport team is asked to transport them before the differentiation is made. The team must provide empiric therapy for both septic shock and obstruction to left heart outflow with antibiotics and PGE_1.

Patients with lesions causing obstruction to left heart outflow are dependent on the patency of the ductus arteriosus to provide blood flow to the body. The four major diagnoses in this category are coarctation, critical aortic stenosis, interruption of the aortic arch, and hypoplastic left heart syndrome (HLHS). The history usually is that of an infant who was doing well either still in the nursery or already discharged home. Some infants, in retrospect, will have a history of mild tachypnea. However, these infants "get sick" over the course of a few hours as the PDA closes and manifest with increasing respiratory distress, lethargy, poor feeding, and irritability.

The physical examination is that of shock: severely poor perfusion, diminished pulse rate, and low urine output. Patients will be lethargic and occasionally apneic. If the infant has a coarctation or interruption of the aorta, the pulses will vary in quality: stronger in the upper extremities and carotids and weaker or absent in the lower extremities. A measurement of blood pressure performed in all four extremities will reveal this difference. The BP will be higher in the arms (above the obstruction) and lower or nondetectable in the legs (below the obstruction). Infants with critical aortic stenosis and HLHS have weak pulses in all extremities. The cardiac examination reveals an S_3 gallop due to myocardial failure. A murmur of tricuspid regurgitation may be present with HLHS and right ventricular failure. A ventricular septal defect (VSD) murmur may be present with interruption of the aortic arch because of the high incidence of large VSDs. Infants with coarctation and critical aortic stenosis frequently do not have murmurs because the flow is too diminished across the coarctation or the abnormal aortic valve to cause a murmur.

The chest radiograph is useful because of the presence of massive cardiomegaly with pulmonary edema (Figure 21-2). Blood gas analysis shows a severe metabolic acidosis frequently with pH < 7.20 and low PCO_2. The arterial PO_2 is usually lowered to 50-70 mm/Hg because of pulmonary edema and right-to-left shunting across the patent ductus arteriosus (PDA).

Prostaglandin E_1 is crucial to the stabilization of these infants in order to open the PDA and provide blood flow to the body past the obstruction.[14] Following administration of PGE_1, blood flow improves with return of peripheral pulses, clearing of the metabolic acidosis, and improved urine output. Often the improvement can be appreciated clinically within minutes. Without patency of the ductus arteriosus, these infants will develop irreversible organ failure and death before surgical palliation or treatment can be performed.

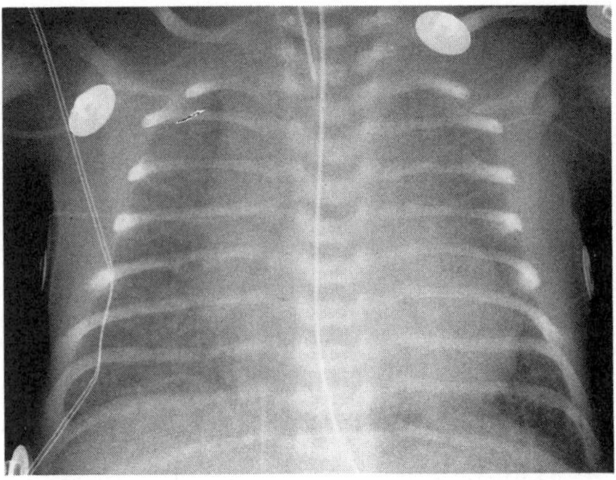

Fig. 21-2. Chest radiograph of infant with coarctation of the aorta who presented acutely after ductal closure. Note the cardiomegaly with pulmonary edema.

While the PGE_1 is improving perfusion, the infant must be stabilized conventionally. Intubation and mechanical ventilation are indicated because many of these infants are in profound shock at the time of presentation and need assistance overcoming the increased work of breathing due to pulmonary edema. Intravenous inotropic support with dopamine and/or dobutamine is also indicated because invariably the myocardium has poor contractility. The metabolic acidosis may also need to be buffered with sodium bicarbonate while the perfusion improves.

THE INFANT WITH CONGESTIVE HEART FAILURE

Infants with congestive heart failure generally present around one to three months of age. Although they do not usually have low cardiac output and shock, as in those with obstruction to left heart outflow, they may have respiratory instability or respiratory distress due to pulmonary edema or complicating infectious pneumonitis. Other causes of congestive heart failure (CHF) have to be considered in the diagnosis. Patients with obstruction to left heart outflow may present with symptoms of CHF before the PDA closes and shock ensues. Insufficiency of the aortic valve or the atrioventricular valves can cause CHF in infants. Other acquired causes are cardiomyopathy, especially endocardial fibroelastosis, infectious myocarditis, and incessant tachyarrhythmias. Most infants with congestive heart failure, however, have a left-to-right shunt defect, most commonly a ventricular septal defect as well as atrioventricular canal defects, patent ductus arteriosus, or a combination of defects.

The history of an infant with congestive heart failure is that of an infant who has exhibited a progressive increase in the work of breathing, often with wheezing symptoms. The infant gets tired while feeding, resulting in less oral intake over a longer feeding time. The mother often notes the infant becoming diaphoretic and stopping frequently to rest and breathe during feeding.

The general appearance of an infant with congestive heart failure is pale and thin but with normal length and head circumference. The pulmonary examination reveals tachypnea with intercostal and subcostal retractions. Auscultation of the lungs frequently will not demonstrate rales but may reveal wheezing or may be clear. With an intercurrent viral or bacterial pneumonitis, the lungs will have coarse rhonchi, rales, and wheezing. Examination of the heart shows the presence of an active precordium with a murmur typical of the cardiac defect: holosystolic murmur in cases of VSD, continuous machinery murmur in cases of PDA, or pulmonary flow murmur with a fixed split of the second heart sound in cases of ASD. The presence of a diastolic rumble at the apex of the heart indicates a significant increase in pulmonary blood flow from a large left-to-right shunt. This murmur represents relative mitral stenosis due to the large volume of pulmonary venous blood returning to the left atrium from the lungs. An S_3 gallop is also frequently heard. The liver will be congested and palpable below the right costal margin.

The chest radiograph of an infant with congestive heart failure will show an enlarged heart with increased pulmonary blood flow (Figure 21-3). The lungs may also be hyper-

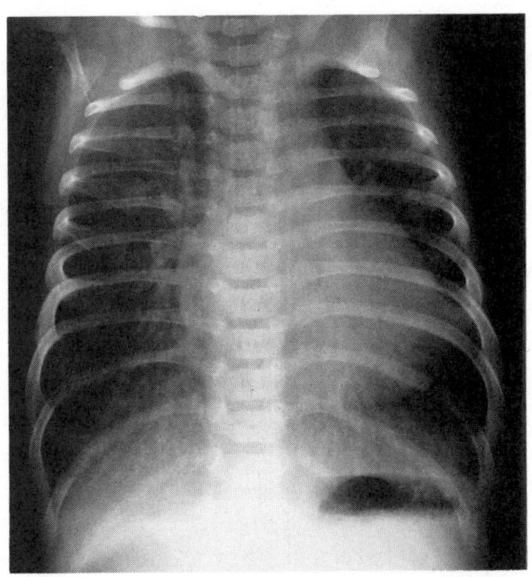

Fig. 21-3. Chest radiograph of a 3 month old infant with congestive heart failure from a complete atrioventricular canal defect. The heart is moderately enlarged. There are increased pulmonary vascular markings consistent with the left-to-right shunt. The lungs are hyperinflated due to wheezing from the pulmonary overcirculation.

inflated in infants with wheezing or may be atelectatic. There may be other, more subtle indications of cardiac pathology, such as an enlarged left atrium pushing the left mainstem bronchus upward and posteriorly while compressing its diameter. The electrocardiogram may be helpful in showing left ventricular hypertrophy and combined ventricular hypertrophy in patients with significant VSDs. In patients with ASDs the ECG reveals right ventricular hypertrophy, often with first degree heart blockage and atrial enlargement.

Initial emergency management of these infants focuses on improving the respiratory distress while maintaining perfusion. If the infant is in overt or impending respiratory failure, then intubation and mechanical ventilation is indicated. Infants who are working hard to breathe, but are still maintaining gas exchange, should be treated with an intravenous diuretic such as furosemide or bumetanide. Many patients will experience significant improvement in the work of breathing and tachypnea with diuretic therapy alone. Oxygen should be administered judiciously. Low concentrations of oxygen, around $FiO_2 = 0.30$, can result in relief of the dyspneic feeling. Because oxygen is a pulmonary vasodilator the left-to-right shunt may worsen with oxygen therapy, and therefore the respiratory distress may worsen. An infant with a left-to-right shunt and respiratory distress can be given oxygen but should be watched closely for improvement or deterioration in the respiratory effort.

Cardiac support is often not needed immediately and therefore can be started after the infant has been transported. If the infant is stable, digoxin is the drug of choice for support of cardiac function. Although the exact mechanism of action on the myocardium is controversial, longstanding clinical experience supports its use.[1] For an infant showing signs of poor cardiac output, a dobutamine infusion is effective, having mostly inotropic effects on the myocardium with mild peripheral vasodilation.[30] The effective dose range is usually 5-10 mcg/kg/min but may need to be as high as 20 mcg/kg/min. If the infant is requiring high doses of inotropic support to maintain perfusion, additional diagnoses such as sepsis need to be considered.

Of importance in the acute presentation of infants with left-to-right shunts is the determination if there is a coincidental pneumonitis which requires treatment. Bacterial antibiotics are often indicated empirically and can easily be administered while in transport. Antiviral therapy, such as ribavirin, may be indicated if the infant has respiratory syncytial viral disease, but this drug should not be given during transport because of the cumbersome delivery system, difficulty in delivering the drug to the ventilated patient, and the risk of exposing transport personnel to the drug. Studies indicate that ribavirin[1] may be useful when initiated within the first three days of the illness, so it should still be effective when given after arrival at the receiving institution.

THE OLDER INFANT AND CHILD WITH ACUTE HEART DISEASE

Rarely, an older infant or child with congenital heart disease will present acutely and need acute intervention and rapid transport. Both congenital heart defects, either preoperatively or postoperatively, and acquired heart disease can present in the older age groups. Many of these children will require postoperative surgical palliation or repair but some will not have yet received therapy. Arrhythmias, a common acute presentation for an older child with heart disease, are discussed below. Congestive heart failure and cyanosis may also present acutely outside the newborn period, although less commonly.

Congestive heart failure outside infancy is most often due to either decompensation of a preexisting congenital defect or acute infectious myocarditis. Occasionally, congestive cardiomyopathies may present with decompensated congestive heart failure. As in infants with left-to-right shunts and congestive heart failure, the symptoms are usually respiratory. Most patients will complain of shortness of breath and will experience respiratory distress due to pulmonary edema. On examination, perfusion will be poor with diminished pulses. The cardiac examination will reveal the presence of an S_3 gallop and a murmur of mitral insufficiency. Jugular venous distention and hepatomegaly are also present. Management is similar to the infant. The respiratory distress can be improved acutely by increasing the inspired oxygen and by giving a potent diuretic, usually a loop diuretic. Dobutamine is the drug of choice to improve cardiac contractility and improve tissue perfusion. During transport the patient may need to sit up or at least have the head elevated in order to breathe more easily. Lying flat may cause worsening dyspnea and respiratory distress.

Outside the newborn period, acute cardiac cyanosis occurs rarely. Congenital cyanotic defects that have not been palliated but have progressed in severity may present acutely with severe cyanosis. Patients with a cyanotic defect that has been palliated, usually with a systemic artery to pulmonary artery shunt, may have shunt failure and become acutely very cyanotic.

Hypercyanotic spells

Patients with uncorrected tetralogy of Fallot may experience progression of the obstruction to right ventricular outflow as they grow. At diagnosis many patients do not yet have right-to-left shunting and are therefore asymptomatic. However, when the pulmonary stenosis or subpulmonary stenosis worsens, the right-to-left shunt becomes clinically apparent. Patients with tetralogy of Fallot may have acute cyanotic spells called hypercyanotic spells, "Tet spells." These are episodes of acute cyanosis which may occur even in children who are not cyanotic at rest. The spells usually last from 10 to 15 minutes and are self-limited. A severe spell, however, may become life-threatening. They most often occur after waking in the morning and are triggered by eating, agitation, and exertion.[23]

The pathophysiologic cause of hypercyanotic spells is not completely understood but is theorized to be due to acute worsening of the subpulmonic stenosis due to increased tone in the infundibular muscle. Compounding the increased stenosis is a fall in the systemic vascular resistance. The blood then takes "the path of least resistance," and exits through the aorta instead of the pulmonary artery. The results are a dramatic decrease in pulmonary blood flow and an increase in right-to-left shunting. Frequently the murmur of pulmonic stenosis disappears in a patient having a spell because of the lack of blood flow across the pulmonary stenosis. Arterial oxygenation levels fall to extremely low levels, even to saturations of less then 20%. The infant becomes agitated and possibly syncopal from the severe hypoxemia.

Treatment of severe spells is emergent and focuses on calming the child, providing oxygen, and increasing systemic vascular resistance. Sedation, traditionally with morphine (0.1 mg/kg SQ, IM or IV), should be given to calm the infant. Oxygen should be provided by face mask with FiO_2 as high as possible. If the infant fights the mask, remove it and allow the oxygen to "blow by" its face. Placing the infant on its back with the knees held against the chest provides an increase in systemic vascular resistance and an increase in venous return to the heart. Systemic vascular resistance can also be increased by a continuous infusion of the vasoconstrictor phenylephrine in a dose of 0.1-0.5 mcg/kg/min. This increased systemic vascular resistance forces blood out the pulmonary arteries. Because of the severity of hypoxemia, the infant may develop metabolic acidosis. Acidosis also increases pulmonary vascular resistance and should therefore be treated empirically with sodium bicarbonate. Intravenous fluids should be given to maintain high ventricular filling pressures. When these standard measures do not result in oxygenation, general anesthesia with ketamine 1-6 mg/kg IM or IV may be given. Ketamine is an agent that also increases systemic vascular resistance. It can often break a hypercyanotic spell when no other measures can.

An infant or child in a hypercyanotic episode should have surgical palliation or repair performed as soon as possible after diagnostic evaluation. If there are extenuating circumstances to prevent surgery, then oral propranolol may be helpful in preventing subsequent episodes. The infant should not be allowed to become agitated; hence, minimize blood drawing and other noxious interventions like examination of the ears.

Cyanosis can also occur in patients who have been palliated, usually with aortopulmonary arterial shunts to increase pulmonary blood flow. With time the child usually gradually outgrows the shunt, and cyanosis will increase slowly with few symptoms. However, if the shunt suddenly becomes dysfunctional from clot, kinking, or infection, the patient will become severely cyanotic very suddenly. The patient must be transported to a pediatric cardiac surgical center as fast as possible in order to have pulmonary blood flow secured. If this cannot be done within minutes, then attempts to open the shunt by clot lysis may be effective. Using streptokinase (1000 units per kilogram bolus followed by 1000 units/kg/hr infusion) may lyse the clot and allow blood flow to return. This will not work if the shunt has kinked or become infected. The downside of clot lysis is that surgery may have to be delayed in order to improve clotting ability which was disrupted by the streptokinase.

EMERGENCIES IN THE POSTOPERATIVE CARDIOVASCULAR PATIENT

Surgery for congenital heart disease generally falls into two categories: reparative and palliative. Reparative indicates that the preexisting defect and abnormal physiology have been reversed and repaired by the surgery. Some examples of common defects that are completely repaired are ventricular septal defect, patent ductus arteriosus, atrial septal defect, and coarctation of the aorta.[31] Examples of more complex reparative surgeries are arterial switch operations for transposition of the great arteries, repair of tetralogy of Fallot with closure of the VSD and relief of the obstruction to right ventricular outflow,[18,19] and repair of complete atrioventricular canal defect with closure of the ASD and VSD and construction of two separate AV valves.[8] Although there may be minor residual abnormalities of anatomy or function after these surgeries, cardiovascular integrity is restored.

Palliative surgeries are designed to relieve the most significant symptoms in order to maintain the infant until more complex surgery can be done at an older age and larger size or to improve the quality of life for a patient whose defect will never be completely reparable. Most palliative surgeries can be performed without the use of cardiopulmonary bypass. An aorto-to-pulmonary artery shunt (e.g., Blalock-Taussig, Waterston, or central shunt) is performed in order to increase and secure pulmonary blood flow in patients with a severe restriction or absence of pulmonary flow, such as in pulmonary atresia patients.[7] The superior vena cava to pulmonary artery shunt (the bidirectional Glenn) also increases pulmonary blood flow but is usually performed in older infants and children and can maintain pulmonary blood flow for a longer period of time.[16] Restriction of pulmonary blood flow by banding the main pulmonary artery may also be done in patients with torrential pulmonary blood flow to relieve congestive heart failure.

Most of the serious complications of congenital cardiac surgery occur in the immediate postoperative period. These would include residual hemodynamically significant defects, cardiac tamponade from blood and fluid around the heart, hemorrhage either from isolated bleeding from suture lines or diffuse bleeding from postoperative coagulopathy, failure of the myocardium, or cardiac arrhythmias. However, complications which may be life-threatening can occur after the patient has been discharged from the hospital. These include arrhythmias, infection of the surgical wound or mediastinum, cardiac tamponade from blood or postpericardiotomy syndrome, or symptomatic pleural effusions.

Infection

The most common infections in the postoperative cardiac patient are surgical wound infections which usually are superficial. Most wound infections are caused by *Staphylococcus aureus* or *epidermidis*. Often these wounds require incision and drainage as well as exploration for foreign bodies aggravating the infection. Aggressive treatment is warranted to prevent deeper infection of the sternum or mediastinum.[11] These patients should be evaluated by their cardiovascular surgeon and may need transport to a tertiary facility even if relatively stable.

Patients who develop mediastinitis and sternal osteomyelitis are usually very ill. Although they may not develop overt septic shock, they typically exhibit toxicity with high fever, irritability, and often poor perfusion. Mediastinitis is usually caused by staphylococcal organisms but can be due to other organisms, especially if the patient had a prolonged postoperative ICU course. *Pseudomonas aeruginosa* and *Candida albicans* are also fairly common, particularly if the patient had delayed sternal closure for hemodynamic stability postoperatively. Mediastinitis must be treated quickly and aggressively with operative debridement and antibiotic therapy. Therefore, rapid transport to the cardiovascular surgical center is warranted.

Therapy in transport for both groups of patients is mainly supportive, including hemodynamic support if needed. The choice of antibiotics would include an antistaphylococcal drug with action against oxacillin-resistant staphylococcal species. Vancomycin (10 mg/kg/dose IV every 6 hours) is frequently used. Empiric treatment for pseudomonas species is also indicated with antibiotics such as ceftazidime, ticarcillin/clavulanate, or imipenem/cilastin. Treatment for candida usually is begun only after positive identification by staining of pus or by culture.

Postpericardiotomy syndrome

Postpericardiotomy syndrome is an autoimmune inflammatory process, occurring in about 30% of patients following heart surgery, in which the pericardium is disrupted.[11] Similar syndromes are seen following myocardial infarction (Dressler's syndrome) and trauma to the heart. Most surgeries causing this syndrome are open-heart but can be seen after closed heart procedures that involve the pericardium. Postpericardiotomy syndrome occurs about 1 to 3 weeks postoperatively. The patients develop fever, malaise, poor appetite, and serous effusions. The effusions may be pericardial and/or pleural. Generally, this is a benign problem easily treated with nonsteroidal antiinflammatory drugs or occasionally corticosteroids. Patients may, however, develop large collections of pleural or pericardial fluid in the chest, causing pain and shortness of breath.

Pleural effusions can cause dyspnea, pleuritic pain, and occasionally respiratory insufficiency and distress. Immediate drainage of the effusion by thoracentesis is indicated if the patient is acutely distressed. Thoracentesis may need to be performed prior to leaving the referring institution in order to adequately stabilize the patient during transport. The cause of the pleural effusions needs to be differentiated from other causes of postoperative pleural effusions such as chylous effusions, infectious effusions, and fluid overload from postoperative congestive heart failure.

Pericardial effusions usually are small and result in a pericardial friction rub on physical examination. However, the occasional patient will develop a large pericardial effusion without a friction rub. Cardiac tamponade can occur and must always be strongly suspected. The patient should be examined specifically for signs of tamponade including jugular venous distention, muffled heart sounds, pulsus paradoxus, tachycardia, and narrowing of the pulse pressure.[24] In infants whose jugular veins are difficult to examine, liver congestion and enlargement may be appreciated. Pulsus paradoxus is the accentuation of the usual variation in systolic blood pressure with respiration. A difference of greater than 20 mm/Hg with respiration is considered significant. Determination of the pulsus paradoxus must be determined by auscultory techniques, such as doppler or sphygmomanometer, or by continuous readout of the arterial wave form by pressure transducer. The noninvasive techniques for measuring blood pressure are unable to determine pulsus paradoxus. Occasionally, the presence of a significant pulsus paradoxus can be appreciated by simply palpating the peripheral pulses which vary in intensity with respiration.

Tamponade is treated by draining the pericardial fluid. As soon as tamponade is diagnosed, percutaneous pericardiocentesis should be performed.[29] A needle (steel lumbar puncture needle or a long 14- or 16-gauge intravenous catheter) is inserted below the xiphoid notch pointing at the left nipple and angled about 30-45° downward. Using a "slip-tip" syringe, constant negative pressure should be applied to the needle as it is inserted. As soon as fluid is obtained the stylet is removed and the fluid is aspirated. As much fluid should be drained as possible, although removing even a small volume may relieve the tamponade. During insertion of the needle the ECG monitor must be watched closely for ventricular arrhythmias which indicate that the needle is touching myocardium. The technique of using a steel needle and attaching alligator clamps and an electrocardiograph to the needle in order to detect an injury pattern to the myocardium is useful but cumbersome.

While pericardiocentesis is being performed the patient should be given intravascular fluid boluses which temporarily help cardiac output. If the patient were to deteriorate to cardiac arrest before the tamponade is relieved, the chest must be opened and open cardiac compression performed. Successful transthoracic CPR is unlikely in the presence of cardiac tamponade without drainage.

A patient with cardiac tamponade should never be transported without drainage of the fluid, although a patient with a pericardial effusion without tamponade can be transported safely prior to drainage. Once drainage has occurred the catheter can be left in place and aspirated repeatedly while the patient is transported. On arrival to the receiving institution an echocardiogram needs to be performed immediately to determine the presence of residual fluid which may need pericardial tube placement or surgical drainage.

ACUTE PEDIATRIC ARRHYTHMIAS

Although arrhythmias are infrequent in pediatrics, they are important in the mortality and morbidity of critically ill patients. Of course, the most frequent symptomatic arrhythmias in pediatric patients are bradycardia and asystole due to hypoxemia and hypoventilation. Of the arrhythmias primarily cardiac in origin, supraventricular tachycardia is the most frequent in all age groups. Other arrhythmias may be seen but with very low frequency. In the management of pediatric arrhythmias, carefully assessing the patient's symptoms is crucial. Many arrhythmias are asymptomatic; therefore, therapy can wait until the patient has arrived at the receiving hospital. An accurate diagnosis of the rhythm and specific therapy in a controlled environment can then be performed. Even in a patient having an asymptomatic arrhythmia, close observation should occur in order to note clinical deterioration. Symptomatic arrhythmias should be treated aggressively, preferably prior to transport if possible.

Supraventricular tachycardia

Supraventricular tachycardia (SVT) is the most common primary cardiac arrhythmia in children. In the pediatric population the most common age of onset is less than 4 months old, however SVT can be seen at all ages. Compared with patients older than 4 months, infants have faster rates of SVT, are more frequently symptomatic with congestive heart failure, and are less likely to have predisposing factors. Predisposing factors include aberrant conduction pathways like Wolff-Parkinson-White, drugs, myocarditis, preoperative or postoperative congenital heart disease, sepsis, or hyperthyroidism. Drugs that have been implicated in causing SVT include theophylline, beta-agonist drugs, caffeine, tricyclic antidepressants, methylphenidate, and phenylpropanolamine.

About 20% of all pediatric patients with SVT will have symptoms.[19] Those most likely to have symptoms will be younger (<1 year old), have faster heart rates, and have a longer duration of SVT. Young infants may be in SVT for more than 24 hours before the diagnosis is made. They often first experience symptoms of irritability and poor feeding but gradually develop the symptoms of congestive heart failure which include respiratory distress, pallor, diaphoresis, and cool, mottled extremities.

The diagnosis of SVT is made from the electrocardiogram. Although a single lead rhythm strip can frequently make the diagnosis, a complete 12 or 15 lead ECG is indicated for more specific diagnosis. There are multiple different electrophysiologic mechanisms that can result in SVT and have different electrocardiographic findings. The unusual mechanisms causing SVT are rare but difficult to treat so a complete ECG may be useful.

The ECG characteristics of most pediatric cases of SVT are listed as follows:[21]

- The QRS rate is most commonly around 280 beats per minute (bpm) in infants less than 4 months and 210 bpm in older patients. Tachycardia is defined as a rate greater than normal for age and patient situation.
- The QRS complex is of normal duration in 90% of patients with SVT. Occasionally, a right bundle branch block pattern may be seen but usually only in the patient with right bundle branch block or Wolff-Parkinson-White when in sinus rhythm.
- The P waves are visible in about 50% of patients. If present they may be retrograde (after the QRS) or have an abnormal axis. With normal sinus rhythm the P wave has an axis of 0-90°, positive in lead I and aVF. With SVT other P wave axes can be seen. There is almost always a 1 : 1 relationship between the P wave and the QRS complex when the P waves are visible. SVT with block is unusual in pediatrics except in patients with acute digoxin toxicity.

Supraventricular tachycardia must be differentiated from sinus tachycardia and ventricular tachycardia before therapy can be initiated. Table 21-1 summarizes the differential diagnosis. Sinus rhythm only rarely is greater than 230 bpm in infants and 210 bpm in older children. Sinus tachycardia also has the ability to change rates with various maneuvers like valsalva (decreases) or crying (increases), whereas the most common types of SVT are persistently regular. Ventricular tachycardia is always a wide complex tachycardia and P waves are rarely visible.

TABLE 21-1 DIFFERENTIATION BETWEEN SUPRAVENTRICULAR, SINUS AND VENTRICULAR TACHYCARDIA

EKG	*Sinus tachycardia*	*Supraventricular tachycardia*	*Ventricular tachycardia*
Rate	Rarely >240 bpm in infants and >210 bpm in children; varies with stimulation	Usually 280-300 bpm in infants; 220-260 bpm in children	>120 bpm in infants and children
QRS duration	Narrow complex; normal duration for age	90% narrow complex; 10% RBBB	Wide complex
P waves	Present and upright in lead II	Present in 50%; may be retrograde; usually not upright in lead II	Rarely seen; if present, retrograde
P:QRS relationship	1:1	1:1 conduction if P waves present even if retrograde	If P waves seen, P:QRS dissociation present
Predisposing factors	Anxiety, drugs, fever, dehydration	None in most; W-P-W, drugs, heart disease	Heart disease, metabolic abnormalities, drugs

Therapy of SVT is determined by the presence or absence of symptoms. In a symptomatic patient, conversion to sinus rhythm should be emergent. Prior to attempts at conversion, whether electrical, mechanical, or pharmacologic, airway equipment and resuscitation drugs, especially atropine and epinephrine, should be readily available. Often after conversion the patient returns to a slow sinus rhythm or even heart block with bradycardia for the first few beats. This bradycardia rarely needs treatment, but in the symptomatic infant, it may persist and need treatment.

The various methods of conversion include electrical techniques, vagal maneuvers, and drug therapy. Therapy is divided into initial "breaking" or conversion of the SVT and maintenance to prevent SVT. Synchronous cardioversion is the most effective means of conversion to sinus rhythm and therefore is the treatment of choice for patients with symptomatic SVT. The usual dose is one-quarter to two J/kg. For small infants the defibrillator may not go as low as needed, and therefore, the lowest amount of electricity (usually 2 or 5 joules) should be used. Other types of electrical conversion involve very rapid pacing, either transesophageally or transvenously, to overdrive the SVT. Both of these methods are very useful in the hospital setting but are not yet practical or safe for use during transport.

Other modes of therapy include vagal maneuvers like carotid massage and gagging. Retinal massage also stimulates a vagal response but is not recommended due to the risk of detached retina with permanent visual impairment. Stimulation of the diving reflex is particularly effective in infants and cooperative older children.[15] The reflex is triggered by applying ice quickly and firmly to the nose and mouth of the infant. The infant should be made to hold his breath briefly while the ice is in place. Sudden stimulation of the trigeminal nerve with cold as well as apnea are keys to the reflex. For convenience the ice can be placed in a rubber examination glove. While the defibrillator is being readied for cardioversion, the diving reflex and other vagal maneuvers should be attempted on the symptomatic patient.

Pharmacologic therapy to terminate the SVT is extensive,[26] but the drug of choice for most types of SVT is intravenous adenosine. Adenosine is an endogenous nucleoside which, when given intravenously, results in slowing of AV nodal conduction and interruption of reentry pathways causing paroxysmal forms of SVT.[25] The drug has a very short half-life of less than 10 seconds. The most common adverse effects are complete heart block, sinus bradycardia, bronchospasm, and vasodilation with flushing and headache. However, because of the short half-life these effects are also short-lived and rarely a contraindication to its use. Relative contraindications would include patients with sick sinus syndrome or advanced heart block, unless a pacemaker is present, and in patients with reactive airways diseases such as asthma or bronchopulmonary dysplasia. Methylxanthines (theophylline and caffeine) are the specific antidotes for adenosine.

The recommended starting dose for children is 0.1 mg/kg IV bolus up to a dose of 6 mg. If there is no response to this dose, the dose is doubled (0.2 mg/kg) and repeated. The usual starting dose for adults is 6 mg which is then doubled to 12 mg. If the drug is to be given by a central line with the tip in the heart then a lower starting dose of 50 mcg/kg can be used. The drug needs to be given rapidly as close to the heart as possible, preferably through a central line or a large bore IV in an upper extremity. The drug should be given rapid IV push followed immediately by a saline bolus. One technique for administering adenosine is as follows:

- Use a stopcock connected to a short (10-12 cm) IV tubing ("T-connector) attached to the IV catheter.
- Place the syringe containing the adenosine in the top port of the stopcock and a syringe containing 3-5 cc of saline in the end port.
- When ready, inject the adenosine into the stopcock, turn the phalange and rapidly flush all the saline behind the adenosine. This technique allows the adenosine to arrive at the heart as a "bolus," giving the best chance of effect.

Other drugs commonly used to convert SVT are listed in Table 21-2. Digoxin and oral propranolol are used in patients with asymptomatic SVT. Digoxin (intravenously) has been used safely for many years in infants to convert SVT, although the peak onset of action may be as long as 1 hour. This prevents its usefulness in the symptomatic patient. Verapamil is a useful agent to convert SVT in the older patient. Because of cases of irreversible asystole or hypotension in infants, this drug is not recommended for use in children less than 1 year old. The other drugs, phenylephrine and edrophonium, are used infrequently, due to the usefulness and effectiveness of adenosine.

Once sinus rhythm is established, medications to prevent recurrences should be given. The most commonly used drug is digoxin, but propranolol is also used. If the patient is known to have Wolff-Parkinson-White then propranolol is recommended. Often the infant who has been converted will have short recurrent runs of SVT. Giving digoxin or propranolol may be helpful to prevent this. Also be sure the infant is calm and comfortable. If not, benzodiazepines or morphine may be given to settle the infant, taking care to guard the airway. Occasionally, intravenous procainamide is needed to prevent the rapid recurrences.

Other atrial tachycardias

Atrial flutter and atrial fibrillation can also be seen in pediatric patients but much less frequently than in adults. Although both rhythms can occur in a paroxysmal manner, most of the time the patient has underlying heart disease. Both preoperative and postoperative congenital heart diseases may have associated atrial flutter or fibrillation. Any condition that results in high atrial pressures, such as mitral regurgitation or mitral stenosis or a large atrial septal defect, may develop these rhythms. Postoperatively, they may be seen in patients with atrial switch repairs for transposition of the great arteries (Mustard or Senning procedures) or with the Fontan procedure for complex single ventricular anatomy.[3]

The presence of symptoms with either rhythm depends mostly on the ventricular rate and the general health of the heart. Rates can be very rapid (in excess of 240 bpm), resulting in low cardiac output. If the patient has slowed conduction through the AV node, then the atrial beats are blocked to a higher degree and the ventricular rate is slower. This situation is usually tolerated well. Some patients with poor cardiac function, either due

TABLE 21-2 DRUGS FOR THE ACUTE THERAPY OF SUPRAVENTRICULAR TACHYCARDIA

Drug	*Dose*	*Adverse effects*
Adenosine	*Children* 100 mcg/kg IV for initial dose; repeat 200 mcg/kg if needed. *Adult* 6 mg IV initial; repeat 12 mg if needed.	Transient complete heart block or sinus bradycardia; bronchospasm; flushing, headache or dizziness.
Digoxin	*Infants and children* Load: Total digitalizing dose 30-40 mcg/kg IV; give 20 mcg/kg for initial dose followed by 2 doses of 10 mcg/kg; give doses 6-8 hours apart. Maintenance: 10 mcg/kg/day divided q 12 hours IV or po *Adolescents* Load: TDD 0.75-1.25 mg given ½ of TDD then ¼ of TDD for 2 doses every 6-8 hours. Maintenance: 0.125-0.375 mg IV or po as single daily dose.	Heart block including 1st, 2nd, or 3rd degree; nausea, vomiting.
Verapamil	0.1-0.3 mg/kg IV not to exceed 5 mg; may be repeated twice within 30 mins.	Not to be used in infants <1 yr; hypotension, bradycardia; have $CaCl_2$ readily available.
Phenylephrine	0.01 mg/kg IV bolus; double dose until systolic BP is twice baseline systolic BP; may be given as IV infusion of 0.01 mg/kg/min and double until desired BP reached.	Acute hypertension; poor perfusion; nausea and vomiting.
Edrophonium	Total dose is 0.2 mg/kg IV; give 0.04 mg/kg as initial test dose followed by 0.16 mg/kg.	Nausea and vomiting; severe bradycardia.
Procainamide	IV Load: up to 15 mg/kg given over 15 mins. IV Maintenance: 15-60 mcg/kg/min infusion.	Hypotension; intracardiac conduction delays; oral effects include lupus-like syndrome and thrombocytopenia.

to poor contractility, valve dysfunction, or complex anatomy, will not tolerate even slow rates.

In symptomatic patients as with SVT, synchronous cardioversion is the treatment of choice. Vagal maneuvers and adenosine are not useful in converting the rhythm back to sinus rhythm. Adenosine, however, may be useful in confirming the diagnosis of atrial flutter or fibrillation by transiently increasing block of the AV node. This can slow down the ventricular rate long enough to identify atrial flutter waves or atrial fibrillation more easily on the ECG. After cardioversion, digoxin should be given to slow AV nodal conduction, so if the arrhythmia recurs the rate will be slower. Other medications like procainamide and quinidine are useful in preventing recurrences of the flutter or fibrillation.

Ventricular tachycardia and fibrillation

Ventricular tachycardia is an unusual arrhythmia in pediatrics. The possible etiologies are listed in Box 21-2. The presence of a predisposing factor must be sought. There are patients with benign ventricular tachycardia who are perfectly asymptomatic from the ventricular tachycardia and do not require therapy.

As with most arrhythmias, assessing the

BOX 21-2 ETIOLOGIES OF VENTRICULAR TACHYCARDIA AND VENTRICULAR FIBRILLATION

Ventricular tachycardia
- Acquired heart disease
  - Myocarditis
  - Ischemia
  - Cardiac tumors
  - Hypertrophic cardiomyopathy
  - Dilated cardiomyopathy
- Postoperative congenital heart disease
  - Immediate postoperatively if ventricles were incised
  - Long term postoperatively especially tetralogy of Fallot
- Metabolic abnormalities
- Hypoventilation or hypoxemia
- Drugs (therapeutic or overdose)
  - Tricyclic antidepressants
  - Sympathomimetics
    - Albuterol
    - Isoproterenol
    - Oral decongestants
  - Amphetamines
  - Cocaine
  - Halothane
  - Antiarrhythmics
    - Quinidine

Ventricular fibrillation
- Normal heart
  - Hypothermia
  - Electric shock
  - Chest trauma
- Abnormal heart
  - Prolonged QT interval
    - Familial
    - Drug induced
  - Severe myocardial hypertrophy
  - Wolff-Parkinson-White with rapid conduction down pathway during atrial fibrillation
- Electrical injuries

presence and severity of symptoms is most important in determining the treatment of VT. If the patient is syncopal, shocky, or pulseless, cardioversion needs to be performed using 1-2 J/kg. Synchronous cardioversion is preferred, but if the VT is very chaotic, synchrony is not possible and defibrillation should be performed. Lidocaine may be given in a dose of 1 mg/kg prior to cardioversion if quickly available. Do not delay cardioversion to administer the drug; however, it should be given as soon as possible after conversion. An infusion of lidocaine (20-40 mcg/kg/min) should then be initiated. If there is no response to lidocaine, then procainamide or bretylium can be given. For asymptomatic patients, lidocaine may be given without using cardioversion. If the VT is self-limited then that may be the only acute therapy. Treatable etiologies must be sought and treated.

Ventricular fibrillation is a very rare cause of sudden cardiac death in children. Invariably there is a predisposing cause and usually underlying heart disease. (See Table IV). The treatment is emergency defibrillation *in a dose of 2 Joule/kg for children. For older children and adults the initial dose is 200 Joules. If no response then repeat a dose of 200-300 Joules followed by a maximum dose of 360 Joules.* Lidocaine should be given after defibrillation in order to raise the fibrillation threshold of the myocardium to prevent recurrences. Patients who have survived ventricular fibrillation need to be observed in an intensive care setting for evidence of organ hypoperfusion, especially the CNS. Also, underlying causes of the ventricular fibrillation should be diligently sought.

Bradycardic arrhythmias

Most bradycardias in children are due to hypoxemia with or without hypoventilation. As with the definition of tachycardia, bradycardia is relative to the condition of the patient. A sleeping infant may have a heart rate as low as 80 bpm, but an awake and active infant should not. Bradycardia may be a sinus mechanism, an escape rhythm, or a type of heart block. Escape rhythms occur when the sinus node does not fire after a pause, and another pacemaker takes over. This pacemaker may be atrial, junctional, or ventricular. Causes of bradycardia, other than hypoxemia and hypoventilation, include hypothermia, hypoglycemia, and hypothyroidism. Increased intracranial pressure, head trauma without increased ICP, and seizures may also cause sinus bradycardia or an escape rhythm. Placement or adjustment of nasogastric tubes or endotracheal tubes can cause vagal stimulation and bradycardia. Patients with cardiac transplants have denervated hearts that often develop bradycardia. Toxic ingestions, particularly with propranolol or organophosphates, can cause significant bradycardia.

Treating the underlying cause of the bradycardia is preferred. For most, airway management with oxygenation and ventilation will resolve the bradycardia. Patients who are symptomatic with bradycardia and are not improving may need treatment with atropine or a sympathomimetic agent. Atropine can be given (0.02 mg/kg) for up to four doses. Sympathomimetic drugs, particularly isoproterenol, are useful in increasing the sinus rate.

Symptomatic conduction blocks can rarely be seen in children. First degree heart block, PR interval longer than normal for age, does not produce symptoms and therefore is of little concern. Wenckebach block, or Mobitz Type 1 second degree block, is also rarely symptomatic. It is seen in the same clinical scenarios as described above, especially with vagal stimulation. Digoxin toxicity may also produce Wenckebach block.

Mobitz Type II second degree block and complete or third degree heart block indicate more serious cardiac pathology. Both can be seen in patients in the immediate postoperative period because of surgery or edema near the conduction system. However, they both can present later after surgery when scarring has infiltrated the conduction system. Inflammatory diseases, especially myocarditis, can produce these advanced heart blocks. Those patients are often quite ill both from the heart block and the myocarditis. Congenital complete heart block is seen in infants of mothers with collagen vascular diseases. In general, these children are either not symptomatic or they develop gradual symptoms of exercise intolerance or mild congestive heart failure. Ingestions of antiarrhythmic drugs can result in dangerous heart blocks with slow ventricular responses.

The rate of the ventricular response in Type II or complete heart block and the acuity of the development of the block determine the symptoms experienced by the patient. Most children will be symptomatic when the ventricular response is less than 50 bpm. Treatment of these advanced heart blocks involves increasing the sinus node rate and trying to improve AV conduction. Atropine is useful for both but can only be given for a short period of time. Isoproterenol can also increase the sinus node rate and improve AV nodal conduction.

Unfortunately, the response to these drugs is usually minimal. Temporary pacing is then necessary in the unstable patient. In pediatric patients, transvenous pacing is very difficult to accomplish safely and requires an experienced pediatric cardiologist. Transthoracic pacing has been used with limited experience in children but offers the only practical means of pacing a child during transport.[5,33] Some current defibrillators have the ability to perform transthoracic pacing. Smaller patches are made for use in children. This can be a painful procedure so sedation and analgesia may be necessary.

HYPERTENSIVE CRISES

Acute hypertension is not an uncommon finding in critically ill children. It may be secondary to an acute process, such as increased intracranial pressure, or to a more gradual process, such as chronic renal disease. Severe hypertension can be divided into three categories based on symptoms and acuity.[28] Malignant hypertension is a medical emergency. Neurologic symptoms are the common presenting complaints and are often associated with symptoms of congestive heart failure. Physical findings include papilledema, arteriolar retinal changes, and evidence of congestive heart failure. Accelerated hypertension usually occurs in patients with chronic hypertension who have rapid worsening of their hypertension. Accelerated hypertension is associated with retinal changes and often cardiac effects. Papilledema is not seen. Chronic hypertension usually has less severe symptoms but patients are more sensitive to rapid reduction in blood pressure.

Hypertensive encephalopathy is a common finding in children experiencing malignant hypertension. The symptoms may have a gradual onset over days with a persistent deterioration in neurologic function. Headache, lethargy, visual disturbances, and changes in mental status are seen. Level of consciousness may deteriorate to coma. Seizures are a very common finding and often are the cause of medical attention. Differentiating hypertensive encephalopathy from intracranial abnormalities with secondary hypertension may be very difficult. The history and physical findings outlined in Table 21-3 may be helpful. Urinalysis is useful if protein and red blood cells are present, suggesting renal pathology. Often a CT scan of the head is necessary to rule out intracranial pathology such as subarachnoid hemorrhage.

The management of hypertensive encephalopathy centers on gradually lowering the blood pressure, since the neurologic symptoms will not improve until the blood pressure is reduced. The reduction needs to be gradual and controlled in order to avoid hypotension. Lowering the blood pressure as low as normal is not always necessary to relieve symptoms. If seizures are present they need to be treated with valium or lorazepam to control them.

The etiologies of severe hypertension are numerous (Box 21-3) with renal disease being the most common.[6,28] Malignant hypertension with hypertensive encephalopathy often occurs in children with acute nephritis and chronic forms of glomerulonephritis. Patients with poststreptococcal glomerulonephritis, the most common nephritis in children, often present with a hypertensive crisis.[17] These

BOX 21-3 ETIOLOGIES OF HYPERTENSIVE CRISES IN CHILDREN

Renal
Acute glomerulonephritis
- Post-streptococcal
- Henoch-Schonlein purpura

Chronic glomerulonephritis
Hemolytic-uremic syndrome
Renovascular
Other chronic renal diseases
- Obstructive uropathy
- Renal dysplasia

Neurologic
Increased intracranial pressure
Seizures
Head trauma
Subarachnoid hemorrhages

Tumors
Pheochromocytoma
Wilm's tumor
Neurofibromatosis

Drugs (therapeutic and overdose)
Cyclosporine
Corticosteroids
Sympathomimetics
Cocaine

Other
Coarctation of the aorta

TABLE 21-3 DIFFERENTIATION OF HYPERTENSIVE ENCEPHALOPATHY FROM INTRACRANIAL PATHOLOGY

	Hypertensive encephalopathy	*Intracranial pathology*
Onset	Gradual over days	Sudden
Signs and symptoms	Prolonged headache; nausea and vomiting; seizures in 90%; diffuse pain; visual disturbances	Focal neurologic deficits; "worst headache in my life"; stiff neck
Level of consciousness	Progressive obtundation	May be alert; if comatose usually occurred suddenly
Fundoscopic examination	Papilledema; retinal hemorrhages; arterial fibrinoid necrosis; exudates	Normal or subhyaloid hemorrhage

Adapted from Stork JE: Hypertension. In Fuhrman BP, Zimmerman JJ, editors: *Pediatric critical care,* St. Louis, 1992, Mosby Year Book.

patients will have periorbital edema and abnormal urine findings, classically hematuria, red cell casts, and proteinuria. The history may reveal a previous infection with group A streptococcus such as impetigo. These patients are volume overloaded due to a decreased glomerular filtration rate which causes sodium and water retention. Renovascular hypertension and other forms of chronic renal disease, such as obstructive uropathy or renal dysplasia, also cause severe hypertension.

Managing patients with severe hypertension depends on the administration of antihypertensive medications with rapid onset of action. There are many medications available which can treat hypertension acutely. Close monitoring of the blood pressure response is crucial to the safety of antihypertensive therapy. During transport this may be a formidable problem because of the difficulty in accurately measuring blood pressure in a noisy, often turbulent environment. Direct measurement of arterial blood pressure by an intraarterial catheter with a visual readout of the pressure is the best technique available. Automated noninvasive blood pressure readings are useful in the hospital setting but may be inaccurate in transport. However, this technique is the most convenient and accessible for measuring blood pressure during transport.

The antihypertensive drugs most commonly used in pediatric hypertensive crises are listed in Table 21-4.[6,9,28] Most of the drugs are given intravenously, have a quick onset of action, and short duration of action. Overshooting blood pressure reduction can be a problem with many of the drugs, so blood pressure must be very closely and frequently monitored. Direct vasodilating drugs are the most commonly used. Sodium nitroprusside, a direct arterial and venous vasodilator, is given as a continuous infusion. The drug is started at a low dose (0.5 mcg/kg/min) and very gradually increased because of its potency and ability to lower blood pressure too far. Care must be taken to avoid increasing the dose until the drug has cleared the dead space of the IV tubing and entered the patient. No other medications can be given in the same IV, and flushes should be avoided. The drug is metabolized by the liver to thiocyanate which is then cleared by the kidney. Therefore use in renal or liver failure may result in toxicity at a low dose. This is not generally a problem in the acute setting such as transport.

Other direct vasodilators, such as intravenous diazoxide and hydralazine, are also commonly used. Diazoxide has an onset of action of less than 5 minutes and a duration of up to 12 hours. Overshoot hypotension and hyperglycemia are adverse effects of the drug. Hydralazine given IV has also been used with good safety in children. The onset of action is somewhat longer, 10-20 minutes, and duration of action is about 4 hours. Hypotension is rarely a problem, making this an attractive alternative in very sensitive patients. Reflex tachycardia is a bothersome effect.

The calcium channel blocker, nifedipine, is

TABLE 21-4 DRUGS USED FOR HYPERTENSIVE CRISES

Drug	*Dose*	*Onset of action*	*Adverse effects*
Sodium nitroprusside	0.5-10 mcg/kg/min IV continuous infusion	<30 secs	Hypotension; cyanide toxicity
Diazoxide	2-10 mg/kg IV bolus	1-5 mins	Hypotension; hyperglycemia
Hydralazine	0.1-0.2 mg/kg IV bolus	10-20 mins	Tachycardia; headache, nausea
Nifedipine	0.25-0.5 mg/kg up to maximum of 10 mg SL or PO	10-15 mins	Headache
Labetalol	0.5-3 mg/kg/min	1-5 mins	Hypotension; bronchospasm

also frequently used in hypertensive crises in conscious patients. This drug is given sublingual or p.o. so the patient should be cooperative with a competent airway. Dosing is difficult in small children because it comes as a viscous liquid in a capsule. The liquid has to be withdrawn by a small syringe in order to adjust the dose for the small child. The onset of action is about 10-20 minutes with a duration of 2-3 hours.

Labetalol is both an alpha- and beta-blocker that has had limited but effective use in pediatrics. The drug is given as an IV infusion but only until the desired effect is seen; then it is discontinued. Onset of action is within 1 minute but lasts as long as 6 hours once the goal blood pressure is reached. Complications include bronchospasm in asthmatic children and overshoot hypotension. The beta-blocking effects of labetalol do not affect cardiac output, as opposed to propranolol or esmolol.

There are many choices for acutely decreasing blood pressure during a hypertensive crisis. Experience with a certain drug is the best recommendation for its use. Control of the blood pressure and treatment of seizures are the focal points of therapy during transport. If the patient evidences congestive heart failure with pulmonary edema, then a diuretic may be beneficial. If, however, there is not evidence of pulmonary edema, the patient should not be diuresed until his volume status is established. In some cases of severe hypertension, intravascular volume depletion worsens the hypertension.

REFERENCES

1. Ackerman VL, Salva PS: Bronchiolitis. In Laughlin GM and Eigen H, editors: Respiratory disease in children: Diagnosis and management, Baltimore, 1994, Williams & Wilkins.
2. Apgar V: A proposal for a new method of evaluation of the newborn infant, *Anesthesia and Analgesia,* 32:260, 1953.
3. Artman M, Graham TP: Congestive heart failure in infancy: recognition and management, *American Heart Journal* 103:1040, 1982.
4. Beerman LB and others: Arrhythmias in transposition of the great arteries after the Mustard operation, *American Journal of Cardiology* 51:1530, 1983.
5. Beland MJ and others: Transcutaneous cardiac pacing in children, *Circulation* 74(suppl 2):176, 1986.
6. Berry PL: Nephrology for the pediatric cardiologist. In Garson A, Bricker JT, McNamara DG, editors: *The science and practice of pediatric cardiology,* Philadelphia, 1990, Lea and Febiger.
7. Blalock A, Taussig HB: The surgical treatment of malformation of the heart in which there is pulmonary stenosis or pulmonary atresia, *Journal of the American Medical Association* 128:189, 1945.
8. Bonchek LI and others: Natural history of Tetralogy of Fallot in infancy: clinical classification and therapeutic implications, *Circulation* 48:392, 1973.
9. Calhoun DA, Oparil S: Treatment of hypertensive crisis, *New England Journal of Medicine* 323(17):1177, 1990.
10. Chin AJ and others: Repair of complete common atrioventricular canal defect in infancy, *Journal of Cardiovascular and Thoracic Surgery* 84:437, 1982.
11. Culliford AT and others: Sternal and costochondral infections following open-heart surgery, *Journal of Thoracic and Cardiovascular Surgery* 72:714, 1976.
12. Driscoll DJ: Evaluation of the cyanotic newborn, *Pediatric Clinics of North America* 37(1):1, 1990.
13. Engle MA, Ito T: The postpericardiotomy syndrome, *American Journal of Cardiology* 7:73, 1961.
14. Freed MD and others: Prostaglandin E_1 in infants with ductus arteriosus dependent congenital heart disease, *Circulation* 64(5):899, 1981.
15. Hamilton J, Moodie D, Levy J: The use of the diving reflex to terminate supraventricular tachycardia in a 2-week-old infant, *American Heart Journal* 97:371, 1979.
16. Hopkins RA and others: Physiologic rationale for a bidirectional cavopulmonary shunt, *Journal of Thoracic and Cardiovascular Surgery* 90:391, 1985.
17. Hoyer JR and others: Acute poststreptococcal gomerulonephritis presenting as hypertensive encephalopathy with minimal urinary abnormalities, *Pediatrics* 39(3):412, 1967.
18. Kirklin JW and others: Surgical results and protocols in the spectrum of tetralogy of Fallot, *Annals of Surgery* 198:251, 1983.
19. Kirklin JW and others: Early primary correction of tetralogy of Fallot, *Annals of Thoracic Surgery* 45:231, 1988.
20. Lewis AB and others: Side effects of therapy with prostaglandin E_1 in infants with critical congenital heart disease, *Circulation* 64(5):893, 1981.
21. Ludomirsky A, Garson A: Supraventricular tachycardia. In Garson A, Gillette PC, editors: *Pediatric arrhythmias: electrophysiology and pacing,* Philadelphia, 1990, W.B. Saunders Company.
22. Mas MS, Bricker JT: Clinical physiology of left-to-right shunts. In Garson A, Bricker JT, McNamara DG, editors: *The science and practice of pediatric cardiology,* Philadelphia, 1990, Lea and Febiger.
23. Morgan BC and others: A clinical profile of paroxysmal hyperpnea in cyanotic congenital heart disease, *Circulation* 31:66, 1965.
24. Moss MM: Myocarditis, pericarditis, and pericardial effusions. In Blumer JL, editor: A practical guide to pediatric intensive care, St. Louis, 1990, Mosby Year Book.
25. Moak JP: Pharmacology and electrophysiology of antiarrhythmic drugs. In Garson A, Gillette PC, editors: *Pediatric arrhythmias: electrophysiology and pacing,* Philadelphia, 1990, W.B. Saunders Company.

26. Perry JC: Acute pharmacologic treatment of cardiac arrhythmias. In Garson A, Gillette PC, editors: *Pediatric arrhythmias: electrophysiology and pacing,* Philadelphia, 1990, W.B. Saunders Company.
27. Pickert CB, Moss MM, Fiser DH: Differentiation of critically ill infants presenting in the first month of life with sepsis or meningitis versus those with congenital obstructive left heart disease, Unpublished abstract.
28. Stork JE: Hypertension. In Fuhrman BP, Zimmerman JJ, editors: *Pediatric critical care,* St. Louis, 1992, Mosby Year Book.
29. Van Heeckeren DW, Moss MM: Pericardiocentesis and pericardial tube insertion. In Blumer JL, editor: *A practical guide to pediatric intensive care,* St. Louis, 1990, Mosby Year Book.
30. Victorica BE: Cyanotic newborns. In Gessner IH, Victorica BE, editors: *Pediatric cardiology: a problem oriented approach,* Philadelphia, 1993, W.B. Saunders Company.
31. Yeager SB, et al: Primary surgical closure of ventricular septal defect in the first year of life: results in 128 infants, *Journal of the American College of Cardiology* 3:1268, 1984.
32. Zaritsky A, Chernow B: Use of catecholamines in pediatrics, *Journal of Pediatrics* 105(3):341, 1984.
33. Zoll PM: Resuscitation of the heart in ventricular standstill by external electrical stimulation, *New England Journal of Medicine* 248:768, 1952.

22

TRANSPORT OF THE CHILD WITH NON-TRAUMATIC CENTRAL NERVOUS SYSTEM FAILURE

PATRICK M. KOCHANEK
SUSAN L. KACZOROWSKI
ROBERT S. B. CLARK
DAVID N. FINEGOLD
IAN F. POLLACK
MICHAEL I. CINOMAN

The relative sensitivity of the central nervous system (CNS) to physiologic instability (i.e., hypoxia, ischemia, trauma) makes it a prime target for secondary insults during stabilization and transport of the critically ill child. However, the complexity of the CNS, our limited monitoring capabilities, and the myriad of potential diagnoses, make it remarkably difficult to successfully intervene with a high level of confidence. Despite these problems, the prevention of secondary insults with interventions initiated during stabilization and transport may be more important for the CNS than any other organ system. Also, it is likely that emerging therapies targeting specific aspects of ischemic, traumatic, and other forms of CNS failure will need to be initiated during the stabilization and transport phase to produce a maximal beneficial effect. Finally, the vast majority of cases of CNS failure in children require highly specialized intervention and treatment in a pediatric emergency facility and intensive care unit supported by pediatric specialists in emergency medicine, critical care medicine, neurology, neurosurgery, nursing, and respiratory therapy. Based on the transport data base of the Children's Hospital of Pittsburgh, evaluating over 700 pediatric and neonatal transports between July 1992 and June 1993, in over 20% of cases a neurologic problem was listed as the primary indication for transfer (Table 22-1). Thus, the knowledge of procedures for optimal stabilization and transport of the child with CNS failure represents an important goal for any pediatric transport team.

In this chapter we review specific stabilization and transport issues for management of the child with "nontraumatic" CNS failure. Similar issues for the child CNS failure from head or spinal cord injury are reviewed elsewhere (see Chapter 25).

In distinct contrast to the traditional view of CNS failure, recent evidence suggests that specific aspects of the pathophysiology of each disease process involved should dictate therapy.[63,94,107,115] A single cookbook approach to CNS failure, even in the acute stabilization phase, may be suboptimal or even detrimental. We will partition the topic "nontraumatic" CNS failure in children into segments specifically dealing with these transport diagnoses (Table 22-1) with a particular focus on stabilization and transport issues.

SEIZURES AND STATUS EPILEPTICUS

Seizures are the most common neurologic problem in childhood, affecting about 7% of children less than five years of age. The presenting symptom of seizures or status epilepticus accounted for almost 12% of the transports between July 1992 and June 1993 in our referral area (Table 22-1) and was the second most common transport diagnosis (respiratory distress being the most common). The most severe form of seizures, status

TABLE 22-1 CNS-RELATED TRANSPORT DIAGNOSES AT CHILDREN'S HOSPITAL OF PITTSBURGH BETWEEN JULY 1992 AND JUNE 1993.*

Diagnosis	*Number (percent of transports)*
Seizures and status epilepticus	83 (11.5)
Cardiac arrest and asphyxia	22 (3.1)
Metabolic encephalopathy	15 (2.1)
Meningitis and encephalitis	7 (1.0)
Shunt malfunction	6 (0.8)
Brain tumor	4 (0.6)
Other CNS	15 (2.1)
Total	152 (21.1)

* Total number of transports for this period was 721.

epilepticus, is defined as "a condition characterized by an epileptic seizure that is sufficiently prolonged or repeated at sufficiently brief intervals so as to produce an unvarying and epileptic condition."[21,40,41] Any seizure or series of seizures lasting 10-60 minutes (average 30 minutes) is considered status epilepticus. The Commission for the Control of Epilepsy and Its Consequences estimates that between 60,000 and 160,000 people in the United States will have at least one convulsive seizure in a given year.[21,51] Twenty percent of children carrying a diagnosis of epilepsy will have at least one episode of status epilepticus in a given year.[21,51] Status epilepticus is more common in children less than three years of age.[3] Phillips found that 73% of patients in status epilepticus were less than five years of age, and 28% were less than one-year-old.[98] Of particular importance to the issue of stabilization and transport is the statistic that 20% of previously healthy children who experience an episode of status epilepticus will suffer permanent neurologic sequelae (ranging from mild to devastating) after their first episode.[102] Disability is inversely related to the age of the child.[15] Because of this potential for permanent brain damage, profound systemic effects, and even death, status epilepticus should be considered a medical emergency. Mortality rates as high as 3-18% are reported in the recent literature.[15,97,102] With early recognition and prompt management the neurologic sequelae and systemic effects may be minimized.

Though generalized tonic-clonic status epilepticus is the most common form, the term status epilepticus includes all forms of sufficiently prolonged seizure activity. Since children usually present with generalized tonic-clonic status epilepticus, the remainder of the discussion will focus on this entity.

Pathophysiology

Regardless of the underlying diagnosis, status epilepticus has a significant morbidity and mortality, especially when left untreated. The morbidity and mortality associated with status epilepticus are related to both the underlying diagnosis and the physiologic alterations that accompany prolonged seizure activity. Studies in experimental animal models of status epilepticus have clearly demonstrated that sustained status epilepticus (induced by the GABA-receptor antagonist bicuculline or the sodium channel agonist flurothyl) produces neuronal necrosis in the substantia nigra, neocortex, amygdala, thalamus, and hippocampus after periods of between 45 and 120 minutes.[75,88,95,131] This occurs despite rigorous control of extracerebral parameters including blood pressure, temperature, PaO_2, and pH. During bicuculline-induced status epilepticus lasting greater than one hour in rabbits, sustained cerebral energy failures occurs despite muscle relaxation, controlled ventilation, and controlled hemodynamics.[95] Cerebral energy failure develops despite tremendous increases in cerebral blood flow. Thus, uncontrolled status epilepticus should be approached as an ongoing, incomplete, hypoxic-ischemic cerebral insult even when extracerebral parameters are appropriately controlled.

In the clinical setting, early physiologic changes result from massive catecholamine release and autonomic discharge. Later effects and complications result from persistent hypoxia and acidosis. Blood pressure, heart rate, and respiratory rate increase as a result of sympathetic discharge.[26,43,67,71] Despite the increase in cerebral blood flow, cerebral oxygen delivery becomes inadequate to meet metabolic demands. Sustained status epilepticus may result in respiratory compromise and hypoxia from poor chest wall movement, accumulated secretions, aspirations, and airway obstruction. Metabolic acidosis, hypotension, pulmonary edema, hyperkalemia, myoglobinemia, hyperglycemia, hypoglycemia, hyperthermia, cardiac arrhythmias, cardiac arrest, and death can occur.

Diagnosis

Typically, status epilepticus is categorized as idiopathic or symptomatic (secondary to some underlying derangement). Aicardi and Chevrie reported that about half of children with status epilepticus had a defining precipitant.[3] Of the group with a precipitant, half of the episodes were associated with an acute event (i.e., meningitis, intoxication, trauma), and the other half with a chronic condition. About half of the idiopathic episodes of status were associated with fever. Phillips and Shananhan reported that episodes of status were more commonly associated with acute causes in younger children: 75% of children less than one year of age, but in only 28% of children older than three years of age.[97]

Though the differential diagnosis of status epilepticus remains similar throughout childhood, the relative frequency of the underlying derangement varies with age. In newborns, status epilepticus within the first 72 hours of life is most likely the result of hypoxia or birth trauma.[39,44,123,124,125] Seizures occurring on or after the third day of life are most likely the result of infection or metabolic disturbance, and all neonates should be evaluated and treated for sepsis (pending the results of the evaluation). Other common etiologies for seizures in the neonate include hypocalcemia, hypoglycemia, withdrawal from maternal drug use, developmental anomalies, and inborn errors of metabolism. Less common etiologies include pyridoxine deficiency and cerebral venous thrombosis. Trauma from abuse should be suspected in a child at any age presenting with afebrile seizures.

Beyond the neonatal period, fever is the most common etiology of seizures/status epilepticus in children less than five years of age, however, fever as a source of seizures is a diagnosis of exclusion.[3,31,37,39,97] Meningitis, encephalitis, and other endotoxic causes of seizures (Shigella, Cat Scratch disease) should be investigated. Hyponatremia is the most common cause of afebrile seizures/status epilepticus in this age group.[23,39,101,124] Hyponatremia results from the administration of dilute infant formula (water intoxication), or may be a marker of CNS or pulmonary disease producing the syndrome of inappropriate antidiuretic hormone secretion. Toxic ingestions, lead poisoning, trauma, and metabolic disorders should be considered in children less than five years of age.[23,101]

In children older than five years of age, infection, trauma, tumors, vascular malformations, ingestions, and degenerative CNS diseases are more likely causes of seizures than in younger children. The most common cause in this age group, however, is idiopathic, whether the episode represents a single event, the first manifestation of chronic epilepsy, or is the result of medication withdrawal in a patient known to be epileptic.[3,77,97]

Emergency treatment, stabilization, and transport

The goals of management of status epilepticus are to prevent the neurologic and systemic complications that stem from uncontrolled seizure activity (relative incomplete hypoxia-ischemia), and are exacerbated by secondary systemic derangements (i.e., hypoxia, hypotension, hyperthermia). Similar to other medical emergencies, the first steps in management include attention to airway, breathing, and circulation. First, the patient should be positioned, jaw maneuvered, and suctioned to provide airway patency. Respiratory effort and adequacy of gas exchange should be assessed and supplemental 100% oxygen provided. If ventilation and oxygenation are inadequate, or the patient becomes apneic, intubation is necessary. If intubation is needed, the patient should be considered to have a full stomach. A rapid sequence induction with vecuronium or pancuronium (0.2 mg/kg IV), or succinylcholine (1-2 mg/kg, IV) and cricoid pressure is preferred. In the absence of hypotension an intubating dose of thiopental (5-7 mg/kg) is the obvious choice for induction. If there is a suspicion of increased intracranial pressure, intubation should be done with appropriate additional precautions as indicated (i.e., lidocaine, mannitol). If the patient is paralyzed while experiencing a seizure, it is imperative to remember that while muscle contraction is inhibited, electrical seizure activity is not attenuated, and attempts at stopping seizure activity should continue. A full loading dose of a long-acting anticonvulsant (preferably phenobarbital, 20 mg/kg, IV) should be administered if paralytic agents are used on transport. While the patient is paralyzed, changes in heart rate, blood pressure, and pupillary size and reactivity may be the only indication of sustained or recurrent seizure activity. Additional anticonvulsant administration may be needed based on assessment of these clinical signs. Because of the risk of hypotension during prolonged seizure activity or as a result of anticonvulsant drugs, blood pressure should be measured repeatedly. Adequate blood pressure and peripheral perfusion can be maintained with volume administration and the judicious use of vasopressors.

Coincident with the initial stabilization the patient should be placed on a continuous cardiorespiratory monitor and vascular access established. While securing vascular access, blood may be drawn for laboratory evaluation (electrolytes, glucose, calcium, anticonvulsant levels, toxicology screen, complete blood count, and blood culture). A glucose containing crystalloid solution (D5-LR or D5-0.9NS) can be infused to avoid hypoglycemia. Toxic ingestions should be treated with the specific antidote, if available, as well as the appropriate supportive measures. A brief history and physical examination, aimed at determining the etiology of the seizure activity should be undertaken during this interval as well. Patient history should include any intercurrent illness and its therapy (dilute formula for an infant leading to hyponatremia), fever (meningitis, encephalitis, seizure with fever), prior seizure history, recent changes in anticonvulsant medications, possible ingestions, and trauma. Physical examination should include pupil size and reactivity and fundoscopic examination for retinal hemorrhages or papilledema. Specific note should be made of any rashes (petechiae, purpura) or other skin lesions (café-au-lait spots, ecchymoses).

After airway and breathing are stabilized, therapy should be directed at stopping seizure activity. Controversy exists over the preferred first-line drug of choice. Ideally, the drug should have a rapid onset of action, a sufficient half-life to avoid the need for frequent dosing, and minimal side effects. Obviously, no single drug fulfills all criteria. Diazepam is often suggested as the initial drug of choice for status epilepticus, primarily based on a relatively rapid onset of action in experimental animal studies. Recent clinical studies, however, suggest that diazepam affords no advantage over phenobarbital or phenytoin for rate of seizure control,[93,110] and diazepam, when used alone or in combination with phenobarbital or phenytoin, is associated with respiratory depression, apnea, and the need for intubation.[93] In addition, diazepam has a short duration of action, and the reemergence of seizure activity often results in the supplemental administration of phenobarbital or phenytoin.

Phenobarbital is a logical choice for the management of status epilepticus. Phenobarbital may be administered more rapidly than phenytoin (maximum rate of infusion of 100 mg/min vs 30 mg/min for phenobarbital vs phenytoin), is less likely to produce cardiac arrhythmias and hypotension in an already stressed system than phenytoin, and phenobarbital can be pushed to higher levels if usual loading doses are ineffective.[11,46,67,108,111] The initial loading dose of phenobarbital is 20 mg/kg IV. If the use of phenobarbital does not result in cessation of seizure activity, phenytoin can be added to the drug regimen. A full loading dose of phenytoin is also 20 mg/kg IV. If loading doses of phenobarbital and phenytoin are given and seizures persist, a benzodiazepine (diazepam, lorazepam), or short-acting barbiturate (i.e., thiopental, pentobarbital) should be administered. Intubation, by this point in time, may have already occurred. If not, the patient should be intubated and mechanically ventilated before or coincident with receiving these supplemental agents. Blood pressure should be monitored closely, and hypotension rigorously avoided using volume administration and vasopressor support if necessary. Table 22-2 lists commonly used anticonvulsants, dosages, and early side effects. Despite frequent use of paraldehyde in the past, and its common place among recommended anticonvulsants in many standard text books,[11,25,102,111] the intravenous form of paraldehyde has been removed from the market. Similarly, USP grade paraldehyde for rectal administration is not readily available.

During the initial stabilization and treatment period, continued thought must be given to both the underlying etiology of status epilepticus and the treatment required to correct the suspected derangement. Anticonvulsants may not be effective until correction of the underlying derangement is initiated. In some cases, treatment of the underlying derangement may stop the seizure activity. Antibiotics should be given if sepsis or meningitis is suspected (antibiotics should generally not be deferred pending lumbar puncture). Electrolyte abnormalities and hyperpyrexia should be corrected. Correction of hyponatremia in the face of ongoing seizures can be initiated by the administration of 4-6 cc/kg of 3% saline solution over 10 minutes (this should increase serum sodium by 3-5 mmol/L).[35] Hypocalcemia can be corrected with calcium gluconate (100 mg/kg IV) or calcium chloride (10 mg/kg IV, central access only). Glucose (25% dextrose) should be administered to correct hypoglycemia.

All patients should be stabilized and monitored as fully as possible before leaving the referring hospital to avoid any further decompensation while en route. This includes, but is not limited to, continuous cardiorespiratory and pulse oximeter monitoring and continued mechanical ventilation if appropriate. If possible it is optimal to avoid administration of muscle relaxants during the transport of patients with seizures/status epilepticus unless it is essential to maintain a patent airway or to ensure adequate ventilation and oxygenation. Recurrent seizure activity can generally be stopped with additional doses of phenobarbital, benzodiazepines, or thiopental in the intubated patient. Should a muscle relaxant be necessary, however, a short-acting nondepolarizing agent such as vecuronium (0.1 mg/kg, IV) or atricurium (0.5 mg/kg, IV) should be considered since these agents will allow for assessment of seizure activity every 15-20 minutes. Throughout the transport, continued attention must be paid to cardiorespiratory and neurologic status.

Transport equipment should allow the ability to monitor cardiorespiratory and pulse oximetry continuously, to measure blood pressure frequently, and to facilitate endotracheal

TABLE 22-2 DRUGS FOR USE IN SEIZURES

Drug	*Dosage*	*Early side effects*
Phenobarbital	10-20 mg/kg IV, IM up to 50 mg/kg (given as 5 mg/kg boluses)	Hypotension: CNS and respiratory depression with higher doses
Phenytoin	10-20 mg/kg IV	Arrhythmias, bradycardia, hypotension
Diazepam	0.1-0.2 mg/kg IV, IM 0.3 mg/kg PR Max. dose 10 mg	Respiratory depression apnea, bradycardia; effects potentiated when a second drug added
Lorazepam	0.05-0.1 mg/kg IV Max. dose 8 mg	Respiratory depression, apnea, hypotension
Thiopental	5 mg/kg IV bolus 1 mg/kg/hr infusion	Respiratory depression, hypotension, myocardial depression
Pentobarbital	5 mg/kg IV bolus 1 mg/kg/hr infusion	Same as above
Paralydehyde	300 mg (0.3 ml)/kg PR Mixed 1 : 1 with cottonseed or olive oil	Proctitis, pulmonary edema, pulmonary hemorrhage, hepatic and renal toxicity

intubation if necessary. Transport medications should include resuscitation medications, anticonvulsants, short-acting barbiturates, vasopressors, mannitol, standard crystalloid and colloid solutions, hypertonic saline, and muscle relaxants. Status epilepticus should be considered a medical emergency. Similar to other medical emergencies, prolonged seizures should be managed with meticulous attention to the "ABCs," aggressive attempts to control seizure activity, and attempts to define and treat an underlying cause.

CARDIORESPIRATORY ARREST

Despite the theoretical advantages associated with brain plasticity of infants and children, their outcome after cardiorespiratory arrest remains poorer than that reported for adults. Good outcome (defined as nonvegetative) from out-of-hospital cardiorespiratory arrest in children is less than 6%, while good outcome (defined as ability to function independently) is as high as 12% in adults.[62] These differences are explained by the different modes of arrest in children (generally asphyxia) versus adults (generally primary cardiac).[62] Most studies suggest that an episode of complete asphyxia lasting approximately 6-8 minutes produces cardiac arrest.[11,14,62,70] Thus, this period of hypoxic or anoxic perfusion precedes the actual cardiac arrest in children, resulting in a rather profound insult. Although the prognosis is generally grim for the child suffering an asphyxia-induced full cardiorespiratory arrest,[33,62,92,132] certain factors such as hypothermia during the insult (cold water submersion) or selected drug overdoses (barbiturates, calcium channel antagonists) can afford some protection.[69,112] In addition, as suggested above, children suffering isolated respiratory arrests often achieve a good outcome if managed appropriately. Recovery from respiratory arrest (without cardiac arrest) in children is markedly better, with good outcome ranging from 44%-75%.[33,62,92,112,119] A recent study by Frandsen and others in adults suggests that the application of advanced emergency medical services by a physician staffed ambulance team at the arrest scene and on transport can impact favorably on outcome.[35] If inroads are to be made in the area of cerebral resuscitation of children after respiratory or cardiorespiratory arrest, novel approaches initiated in the stabilization or transport setting will be essential.

Pathophysiology

The pathophysiology of the cardiorespiratory arrest is complex and poorly understood. Transient hypoxia-ischemia with reperfusion has profound detrimental effects which, in potentially resuscitatible patients, are maximal in the CNS. These effects are the result of transient energy failure which sets into motion a cascade of molecular events including excitatory amino acid release, calcium overload, intracellular acidosis, and oxygen-derived free radical injury.[62,106] In the CNS the physiologic derangements during the asphyxial event include a period of cerebral hyperemia and systemic hypertension. This is rapidly followed by progressive hypotension with cerebral hypoperfusion, and finally a no-flow state, if cardiac arrest occurs. During CPR, cerebral blood flow ranges from adequate (witnessed or short arrest) to none (prolonged arrest).[66] If restoration of spontaneous circulation (ROSC) is achieved and systemic perfusion is adequate a characteristic pattern of blood flow and metabolism is observed in the brain. Very transient (5-15 min) hyperemia is followed by a prolonged period (hours to days) of dynamic and heterogeneous hypoperfusion.[8,18,62,113] During this period, cerebral metabolic rate is generally reduced.[8]

Several features of the early postresuscitation period (stabilization and transport phases) are different from those observed in the more delayed (intensive care unit) phases. Cerebral acidosis, global cerebral energy failure, excitatory amino acid release, and transient cerebral hyperemia appear to be events which are very short-lived in patients with potentially resuscitatable insults.[106,113] Early postresuscitation myocardial stunning with dysfunction is also most important in the stabilization phase.[106] This suggests that relatively unique pathophysiologically-guided approaches may need to be applied specifically during the early postresuscitation phase, when stabilization and transport of the patient are occurring.

Emergency treatment, stabilization and transport

Starting basic and advanced cardiac life support maneuvers at the scene are fundamental and are discussed by Dr. Krug in Chapter 15. Restoration of spontaneous circulation unquestionably is the primary goal. Although it is currently unclear as to whether specific therapies administered after the arrest can be developed to ameliorate hypoxic-ischemic neuronal injury, it is well known that specific events can worsen outcome, and the major thrust of treatment during the stabilization and transport phases should focus on preventing these secondary insults.[48] Unfortunately, an optimal approach to specific clinical care issues in the child (or adult) in the early postresuscitation period has not been determined by controlled clinical trials. Remarkably, controlled clinical trials have focused on only novel, breakthrough therapies, while the optimal approach to standard care interventions has been less extensively studied.[1,2,48] It is necessary to select interventions based on the known pathophysiology of this process. This may be misleading because of wide variability of models and species used in resuscitation research. In addition, even studies in cardiac arrest models must be scrutinized to determine if "beneficial" effects increase the number of nonvegetative survivors, rather than just improved neurologic deficit score or survival. Despite these rather formidable limitations, general recommendations for emergency maintenance of key physiologic parameters are given in Table 22-3. These are discussed below.

The primary goal in the stabilization and transport phase is to avoid secondary arrest. Often, this can be achieved solely by continuing to provide optimal respiratory support, however, after prolonged arrests or arrests in the setting of other pathophysiologic derangements (i.e., sepsis, electrolyte disturbance, hypothermia, drug overdose) more complex interventions may be necessary. In particular, if an interhospital transport is undertaken shortly after a prolonged cardiorespiratory arrest, stability during transport may be facilitated by volume administration or the continuous infusion and titration of an inotropic/pressor agent (i.e., dopamine, epinephrine). In addition, correction of acidosis, electrolyte disturbances (hypocalcemia, hyperkalemia), or hypovolemia should occur before departing. It is imperative to avoid secondary hypoxemia or hypotension. Postarrest hypotension profoundly worsens outcome in primates.[48,81]

In general, based on the aforementioned pathophysiology, the postarrest brain is in a precarious position. Although studies have suggested that during the first few hours after global cerebral ischemia or cardiac arrest, cerebral blood flow and metabolism are coupled, and mild increases in cerebral metabolic rate are accompanied by adequate increases in flow,[79] cerebral blood flow is already low.[62,113] Further reductions in flow could produce a second ischemic insult. In addition, it is possible that major increases in metabolism (seizures, agitation, hyperthermia) are not compensated by appropriate increases in flow. Thus, these problems should be rapidly corrected, and interventions which could further adversely disturb flow/metabolism balance should be avoided. Specifically, hypotension and hypoxemia should be rigorously prevented. The use of hyperventilation in the early postarrest setting is a very controversial area which has been studied very little. In dogs, early after global cerebral ischemia or cardiac arrest, hyperventilation has been demonstrated to have either no effect or reduce cerebral blood flow.[80,117] In studies in which cardiac output is normal, intracellular pH in the brain normalizes or overshoots (resulting in alkalosis) quite rapidly after even prolonged global cerebral ischema.[72] Cerebral blood flow is generally low, and increased intracranial pressure is generally not a concern in the early postarrest setting, suggesting that hyperventilation would not be beneficial and would be potentially harmful.[48,62] However, a very recent study compared 8 hours of hyperventilation ($PaCO_2$) versus normoventilation in dogs subjected to a 15 minute arrest and demonstrated that histological injury (at 8 hours postarrest) was attenuated in the hyperventilated group.[121] Until definitive studies can be performed, normocarbia should be the therapeutic goal,

TABLE 22-3 EMERGENCY INTERVENTIONS FOR STABILIZATION AND TRANSPORT OF THE CHILD IN THE EARLY POSTARREST SETTING: RECOMMENDATIONS AND KEY REFERENCES FOR MANAGEMENT OF CRITICAL PHYSIOLOGIC VARIABLES

Blood pressure	*$PaCO_2$*	*PaO_2*
Key studies		
1) Hypotension produces devastating effects early postarrest in monkeys.[81]	1) Hyperventilation reduces postischemic CBF at a time when it is already low.[80]	1) Moderate hypoxia (PaO_2 = 40 torr) for 30 minutes produces devastating effects on previously injured brain but no damage in normal.[58]
2) Norepinephrine-induced hypertension (MAP of 200 mm Hg) beneficial in dogs at 1-5 min postarrest.[116]	2) Hyperventilation to $PaCO_2$ of 15 mm Hg produced no effect after 15 min arrest in dogs.[117]	2) Hyperoxia worsens outcome in brain ischemia models.[79]
3) Intermittent bouts of induced hypertension detrimental in dogs during the first 24 hours postarrest.[9]	3) Hyperventilation to a $PaCO_2$ of 10-15 torr for 8 hours reduced neuronal injury after a 10 minute arrest in dogs.[121]	
Recommendation for transport team		
Vigorously avoid hypotension. Early hypertension postarrest merits further study. Probably prudent to avoid aggressive treatment of transient hypertension during the first 5-10 min postarrest, unless it is severe or bradycardia occurs.	A very controversial area which needs further study. In the immediate postarrest setting (first 15 min) tradeoff intracellular acidosis reduction in brain/heart vs CBF reduction probably favors hyperventilation. Later (1-2 hours) intracellular acidosis usually has resolved, and hypoperfusion is seen, suggesting normocarbia may be optimal.	Avoid hypoxemia. Theoretical risk of increased oxidant injury by use of 100% O_2 deserves further investigation.
Key studies		
1) Bicarbonate administration (titrated to maintain base deficit <5 mmol/L improves neurologic outcome and markedly improves hemodynamic stability postarrest in dogs (including major reductions in pressor requirements).[126]	1) Induced hyperglycemia (GLU > 269 mg/dl) worsens outcome in global brain ischemia and cardiac arrest in adult models.[86] 2) Induced hyperglycemia (GLU 200-400 mg/dl) reduces damage in neonatal hypoxia-ischemia models.[122]	1) Mild (34°C brain hypothermia reduces brain injury in experimental animals, even when applied after the arrest.[42,49,115] 2) Moderate hypothermia (28-32°C) postarrest worsened outcome.[106] 3) Hyperthermia (39°C) markedly worsens ischemic neuronal injury.[42]

Continued.

TABLE 22-3 EMERGENCY INTERVENTIONS FOR STABILIZATION AND TRANSPORT OF THE CHILD IN THE EARLY POSTARREST SETTING: RECOMMENDATIONS AND KEY REFERENCES FOR MANAGEMENT OF CRITICAL PHYSIOLOGIC VARIABLES—cont'd

Blood pressure	*$PaCO_2$*	*PaO_2*
Recommendation for transport team		
Administration of bicarbonate to minimize base deficit during transport is a logical step to minimize instability. The optimal agent to treat acidosis in the arrest and postresuscitation setting is under investigation.	Avoid hypoglycemia in all patients. Avoid hyperglycemia in children. Study of therapeutic hyperglycemia is needed in asphyxial arrest models in neonatal animals. Further studies are needed.	Avoid and treat hyperthermia. Avoid active rewarming postarest if temperature is ≥34° C and patient is hemodynamically stable. Clinical trials of early transient (1-4 h) mild hypothermia after cardiorespiratory arrest are needed.

and if a significant metabolic acidosis is present, it should be treated with bicarbonate.[126] Seizures and agitation should be aggressively treated, and hyperthemia should be avoided. If anticonvulsant therapy produces hemodynamic instability, volume administration or pressor support should be initiated.

Strategies to improve early postarrest cerebral blood flow have not been thoroughly examined, and results are conflicting. For example, induced hypertension after cardiorespiratory arrest has produced beneficial and detrimental results in experimental models.[9,56,106,116] Postarrest blood pressure should be maintained in the normal range until such time that definitive studies prove otherwise. Similarly, studies attempting to reduce early postischemic metabolism have produced conflicting results. Administration of thiopental early postarrest did not improve outcome in adults.[2] However, novel strategies related to the inhibition of early postarrest cerebral metabolism are on the horizon (see Future Strategies).

The optimal PaO_2 after arrest has not been determined. Although future studies may demonstrate that oxygen radical induced injury may be minimized by careful attention to maintaining normoxia rather than hyperoxia,[79] currently, there is not enough data to suggest that transport should be on an FiO_2 of less than 1.0. This area deserves further study.

Optimal management of blood glucose level in the child after ischemic brain injury has been a point of confusion and debate. Hyperglycemia (a blood glucose level greater than 465 is associated with poor outcome in children after submersion accidents.[6] Similarly, induced hyperglycemia is associated with exacerbation of brain injury in adult models of global and focal cerebral ischemia.[12,27,86] This has been observed in cardiac arrest models with glucose levels as low as 269 mg/dl.[87] In contrast to these findings, induced hyperglycemia reduces infarct size in neonatal animal models of cerebral hypoxia-ischemia.[122] These differences relate largely to differences in glucose transport, utilization, and lactate accumulation between the neonatal and adult brain.[53] Induced hyperglycemia after the ischemic insult has not been examined in either neonatal models of cardiorespiratory arrest or the analogous clinical setting. In all cases, hypoglycemia should be treated, and hyperglycemia should be avoided. Controlled studies in the clinical setting are lacking.

Future strategies

Several novel therapeutic strategies have shown some promise in experimental models of cerebral ischemia or cardiorespiratory arrest. Notable among these studies and cogent to the issue of transport medicine, is the apparent brief time window for successful application of therapies in cerebral resuscitation.[42] The most promising strategies to watch for future development include transient mild brain hypothermia,[42,49,115] excitatory amino acid receptor blockade,[87] and inhibitors of oxidant injury.[84] Unfortunately, based on the severity of the insult, it is likely that a rather limited number of children suffering asphyxial cardiorespiratory arrest will attain good neurologic recovery even if new pathophysiologically-guided therapies are developed.

METABOLIC ENCEPHALOPATHY

There are many different etiologies of metabolic encephalopathy in children. When combined they are an important cause of central nervous system dysfunction. An underlying metabolic disturbance was the third most common CNS-related indication for transport to the Children's Hospital of Pittsburgh last year (see Table 22-1). Among these the most common diagnosis was diabetic ketoacidosis (DKA), which is the focus of this section.

Pathophysiology

Fluid, electrolyte, and metabolic disturbances are the genesis for all of the pathophysiology derangements observed in patients with DKA. The mechanisms for these disturbances are complex, but have been well described.[114,129] Essentially, patients experience a state of hyperosmolar dehydration. Along with hyperglycemia and ketoacidosis, there can be alterations in sodium, potassium, chloride, phosphate, calcium, and magnesium balance.[114,129] In advanced stages of dehydration, patients can progress to cardiovascular collapse and shock.

Among patients with DKA, cerebral edema and herniation remain significant causes of morbidity and mortality.[22,68,109] The mechanism of catastrophic cerebral edema associated with DKA has not been precisely defined and is probably multifactorial. Factors implicated in animal studies include fluid administration and the correction of hyperglycemia with insulin. In a canine model of hyperglycemia, rehydration, even without fluid overload or water intoxication, was associated with cerebral edema.[16] Arieff and others observed that in rabbits correction of hyperglycemia with insulin, but not with peritoneal dialysis, was associated with increased brain water, sodium, potassium, chloride, and "idiogenic" osmoles.[4] In a streptozotocin-diabetic rat model, brain edema developed during normalization of blood glucose with insulin and saline, but not with saline administration alone.[118] Clinical studies have documented elevated intracranial pressure and cerebral edema associated with "uncomplicated" DKA. In an adult study, Clements and others[17] continuously monitored lumbar CSF pressure in five patients. One patient had elevated CSF pressures initially, however the remaining four developed abnormally high CSF pressures within 6 hours following the start of treatment, and all patients displayed a rise in CSF pressure. When CT scans are done in patients with DKA, subclinical cerebral edema is the rule, rather than the exception.[54,65] In the study by Hoffman and others,[54] radiographic evidence of brain swelling (defined as a reduction in size of the lateral and third ventricles) was present before initiation of therapy, implying that cerebral edema and elevated intracranial pressures were as much as a complication of the disease itself, as they are a complication of therapy.

Emergency treatment, stabilization, and transport

Any child presenting with coma (Glasgow Coma Score <8) should be intubated with initial resuscitative efforts similar to those for any child with CNS failure. If the patient is hypocarbic, ventilatory rates should attempt to maintain the child's PCO_2 in a range close to that before intubation. This will prevent a rapid decrease in pH, as most patients have some degree of respiratory compensation for their metabolic acidosis.[85] The PCO_2 can be normalized at the receiving institution after treatment is initiated and acidosis begins to resolve.

Initial fluid resuscitation involves the correction of shock and hemodynamic instability. Dehydration is invariably present and is estimated to be in the range of 10-15%.[32] Isotonic fluid, such as normal saline, should be given in 10-20 ml/kg aliquots until hemodynamic stability is achieved. Once shock has been corrected the remainder of the fluid deficit is administered gradually over a 24-48 hour period. Several authors suggest that, in order to minimize the risk of brain herniation, rates of 4 L/m²/day should not be exceeded in a hemodynamically stable patient.[30,32,50] Herniation has been associated with rates in excess of 4 L/m²/day, and an inverse correlation has been found with the overall rate of fluid administration and the time of onset of herniation.[30] A recent review of 69 patients, however, failed to find an association between the rate of hydration or correction of hyperglycemia and CNS catastrophes associated with treatment of DKA.[103] Other authors suggest replacing fluid deficits over 24 hours, which could slightly exceed 4 L/m²/day depending on the estimated degree of dehydration.[82,114] In any case, fluid replacement should be undertaken carefully, and hypotonic fluids must be avoided.

Particular CNS issues unique to the transport of the patient with DKA involve the recognition and management of worsening cerebral edema. As mentioned above, radiographic evidence suggests that subclinical brain swelling is often present in patients with DKA. Because of this baseline swelling and the potential for significant fluid shifts even under optimal therapy, vigilant neurologic observation of the patient must be maintained during fluid resuscitation and correction of hyperglycemia. In the event of neurological collapse or clinical signs of herniation, fluids should be decreased, and the patient should be treated aggressively with mannitol[29,36] and hyperventilation.

The use of bicarbonate in patients with DKA is controversial. Theoretical risks involving the CNS, such as paradoxical worsening of intracellular acidosis and potential exacerbation of brain tissue hypoxia (through increased hemoglobin-oxygen affinity), have promoted avoiding the use of bicarbonate. Retrospective analysis and clinical studies, however, have failed to substantiate these theoretical risks.[68,85,103] As acidosis typically begins to improve after fluid resuscitation and usually corrects with continuation of fluid and insulin therapy, bicarbonate should be reserved for cases where acidosis is extreme and cardiac function is compromised. If required, bicarbonate can be added to the patients IV solution at concentrations of 25-50 mEq/liter. This will avoid rapid infusion which could potentially exacerbate hypokalemia and hypocalcemia.

In general, most patients can safely be transported once cardiorespiratory stabilization has been achieved before further correction of hyperglycemia with insulin. In the event of long or delayed transports a treatment protocol, such as that outlined in Table 22-4 or that used by the receiving institution, can be implemented.

MENINGITIS

Bacterial meningitis remains a significant cause of morbidity and mortality in infants and children and is a frequent indication for transport to a tertiary care center. An estimated 15,000 infants and children are affected by bacterial meningitis each year, with a 5-10% mortality rate and as many as 30% of survivors suffering long-term neurologic sequelae.[60] Approximately 7,000 children younger than 14 years of age develop aseptic meningitis each year as well,[13] although this is usually a self-limited disease.[104] The remainder of this discussion will focus on bacterial meningitis, since prehospital management of the patient with suspected meningitis is the same, regardless of bacterial or nonbacterial etiology.

Pathophysiology

Bacterial colonization of the CNS usually occurs during systemic bacteremia, but can also occur via direct extension from contiguous foci such as the sinuses or mastoids. The presence and release of various bacterial components into the subarachnoid space initiates an inflammatory cascade involving neutrophils, monocytes, macrophages, microglia, endothelial cells, and a host of inflammatory mediators.[60,105] Damage to the cerebrovascular endothelium (blood-brain barrier) occurs.[96] Hyperemia, vasogenic edema, loss of autoregulatory control of cerebral blood flow, and increased cerebrospinal fluid volume develop and contribute to intracranial hypertension.[5,57,59,96,120] Superimposed vasculitis, and thrombosis can also occur with accompanying neuronal injury and cytotoxic edema.[57,96] Uninterrupted, this cascade can progress to brain herniation, ischemia, infarction, and/or death.

TABLE 22-4 MANAGEMENT OF DKA (BASED ON PROTOCOL AND EXPERIENCE AT THE CHILDREN'S HOSPITAL OF PITTSBURGH)

Goal	*Hour*	*Specific management*
Initial assessment and management	0	1. Assess ABCs. a. If coma (GCS < 8) or respiratory, compromise intubate and secure airway. b. If patient is in shock, give 20 cc/kg NS boluses until adequate circulation established.
	0	2. Estimate degree of dehydration.
	0	3. Laboratory evaluation: draw glucose, electrolytes, serum osm, BUN, Creat, Ca^{++}, $PO_4^{=}$, blood gas, serum ketones. Obtain pertinent cultures (blood, urine, throat), urinalysis, and cardiac rhythm strip.
Fluid and electrolyte replacement	0-2	1. When hemodynamic stability achieved, continue volume resuscitation with NS at approximately 10 ml/kg/hr (assuming 10% dehydration).
	2-10	2. Give maintainance fluid rate + replace 50% of deficit over 8 hours. Include previous fluid resuscitation volume in the calculation of deficit. a. Change IVF to 0.45% NaCl. b. If patient is urinating and is not hyperkalemic, add 20-40 mEq potassium to IVF (consider giving $\frac{1}{2}$ as KCl and $\frac{1}{2}$ as KPhos if $PO_4^{=} < 2.0$). c. If pH < 7.1 consider adding 25-50 mEq $NaHCO_3$ to IVF.
	10-26	3. Give maintainance fluid rate and replace 50% of deficit over 16 hours. a. If KPhos added, replace with KCl. b. If $NaHCO_3$ added, remove it from IVF.
Correction of hyperglycemia	2	1. Begin continuous infusion of insulin at 0.1 units/kg/hr. Insulin should be delivered through a separate IV line or Y-shaped tubing via IV pump. 2. When patient's glucose approaches 250-300 mg/dl, or if glucose falls >100 mg/dl, then add 5% dextrose. If glucose continues to fall, increase dextrose to D7.5 or D10 or decrease rate of insulin infusion. 3. D/C insulin drip and change to subcutaneous insulin upon resolution of acidosis (pH > 7.34, HCO_3 > 18) and clearance of serum ketones.
Prevent sequelae	0-∞	1. Follow neurologic status, if any deterioration suggestive of elevated intracranial pressure: a. Secure airway and hyperventilate. b. Give mannitol 0.5-1 gm/kg IV. c. Decrease fluid rate. 2. Follow glucose q1h while on insulin infusion. 3. Follow electrolytes, osmolarity, pH, Ca^{++}, $PO_4^{=}$, q4h while receiving IVFs, and treat abnormalities as indicated.

Diagnosis

Infants and children with meningitis present with a constellation of symptoms including fever, lethargy or irritability, nausea, vomiting, and seizures.[6,60] Patients may appear toxic with altered mental status and signs of poor perfusion and septic shock. A bulging fontanelle can be observed in infants, and meningissmus is often but not always present.[60] Neurologic examination can reveal cranial nerve deficits and hyperreflexia. When significant intracranial hypertension develops, patients will be comatose and can display signs of cerebral herniation (i.e., Cushing's triad, decerebrate or decorticate posturing, pupillary changes, and abnormal oculocephalic and oculovestibular reflexes). Papilledema may be present, but its absence does not rule out intracranial hypertension.[6]

The gold standard for the diagnosis of bacterial meningitis is a positive culture from CSF obtained by lumbar puncture.[60] Rapid diagnosis can be made on clinical grounds and by initial examination of CSF. Pleocytosis, elevated CSF protein, and hypoglycorrhachia are observed in meningitis.[60] Gram's stain and bacterial antigen analyses can also provide etiologic information before culture results are available.

Computed tomography and magnetic resonance imaging often demonstrate a number of abnormal findings associated with meningitis in children, including cerebral edema, subdural effusion, infarction, and ventricular dilatation.[61] Normal scans are observed in between 4% and 89% of children, and cerebral edema can be observed in anywhere between 2% and 60% of patients imaged, depending on the severity of disease and the timing of the imaging study.[6,38,61]

BOX 22-1 INDICATIONS FOR INTUBATION IN PATIENTS WITH SUSPECTED MENINGITIS

Clinical

Signs of increased intracranial pressure
- Coma (Glasgow Coma Score < 8)
- Abnormal pupillary responses
- Abnormal oculocephalic or oculovestibular responses
- Decerebrate or decorticate posturing
- Cushings Triad (bradycardia, hypertension, bradypnea)
- Impaired or absent airway protective reflexes

Deteriorating level of consciousness
Seizures
Shock (hypotension, poor perfusion)
Hypoventilation

Laboratory

Hypoxemia
Hypercarbia
Metabolic acidosis

Emergency treatment, stabilization and transport

The goal of prehospital management is to recognize the disease and prevent sequelae. Once meningitis is suspected or confirmed, prehospital management is directed at treating the infection and stabilization of important physiologic parameters. If intracranial hypertension is suspected, it is imperative that hypotension, hypoventilation, and hypoxemia are avoided to minimize a superimposed secondary insult. Acute stabilization involves ensuring a stable airway, maintaining adequate ventilation and oxygenation, and correcting or preventing shock. Transport issues hinge upon the child's presentation and the progression of the disease. Endotracheal intubation should be performed whenever there are signs of CNS failure as listed in Box 22-1 or where respiratory or circulatory failure accompany meningitis. Intubation may also be appropriate if there has been an acute deterioration or if clinical signs suggest the likelihood of deterioration en route. A child with meningitis requiring intubation for the above reasons is undoubtedly at risk of having intracranial hypertension.[45,89] Adequate cerebral protection and muscle relaxation is essential to facilitate intubation and minimize iatrogenic increases in ICP. Thiopental is the drug of choice for intubation if the child is hemodynamically stable. If not, fentanyl and benzodiazapines can be used. Lidocaine and mannitol administration should be considered.

Cardiovascular stability is required to prevent inadequate cerebral perfusion. Hemodynamic compromise should be treated aggressively with colloid resuscitation and inotropes if necessary. Systemic hypotension carries a high likelihood of potentiating cerebral hypoperfusion in meningitis because of disturbances in cerebral autoregulation.[5,6,59,120] The risk of worsening cerebral edema with volume administration should be minimized by avoiding hypotonic fluids. As a practical matter a Foley catheter should be inserted if mannitol is administered or if intubation is required.

Intracranial hypertension occurs in the majority of children with meningitis,[46] and approximately 4-6% develop herniation syndromes.[55,100] If intracranial hypertension is present to a level where the Glasgow Coma Score has decreased to 8 or less, then meticulous attention is required in the event of neurologic deterioration and potential herniation. This is an especially difficult situation immediately before and during transport, when invasive monitoring of intracranial pressure is not available. Again, an adequate systemic blood pressure must be maintained to provide for cerebral perfusion.[24] Optimally, $PaCO_2$ is maintained between 30 and 35 torr. Aggressive hyperventilation ($PaCO_2 < 30$ torr) has fallen out of favor in the management of intracranial hypertension due to head injury, largely because of data suggesting the exacerbation of early post-traumatic hypoperfusion.[19,83] However, the application of hyperventilation to control intracranial hypertension in meningitis has not been specifically investigated. Theoretically, during the early phases of meningitis, some experimental models suggest that cerebral blood flow is excessive and hyperemia may contribute to increased cerebral blood volume.[6,96] Hyperventilation in this setting, particularly when clinical signs of intracranial hypertension are present, would be logical. However, clinical studies in children at more delayed times after presentation suggest that the early hyperemia may progress to hypoperfusion or ischemia.[6,7] Thus, cerebral blood flow studies are probably necessary to guide appropriate ventilatory therapy. During stabilization and transport, until a definitive study is performed, aggressive hyperventilation in children with meningitis should be reserved for the setting of impending herniation. Mannitol and possibly thiopental administration are therapies which should also be strongly considered in this setting. Muscle relaxation and alternative sedatives should also be considered, particularly if there are concurrent respiratory problems, or if agitation is present. Although these agents interfere with neurologic assessment, the primary source of monitoring the patient in the emergency department and during transport, judicious use of them may be necessary in order to safely transport the patient.

Seizures occur in 30-40% of children with meningitis,[6,60] and cause dramatic increases in cerebral blood flow, cerebral metabolic rate, and may produce intracranial hypertension.[26,43,67,71] Seizures should be aggressively treated with phenobarbital, phenytoin, or benzodiazepines. Often, refractory seizures in this setting require the use of a combination of anticonvulsants. Fever also increases cerebral blood flow, cerebral metabolic rate, and intracranial pressure and should be treated. The choice of antibiotics depends on the age of the child. For empiric therapy, ampicillin and gentamicin are appropriate for neonates, and a third generation cephalosporin, such as ceftriaxone or cefotaxime, for children beyond the neonatal period is recommended.[73] Antiinflammatory therapy with dexamethasone is currently recommended by the American Academy of Pediatrics.[73,98] In cases of known meningitis (lumbar puncture done before transport), it would be appropriate to administer dexamethasone (0.15 mg/kg IV) concurrent with antibiotics before or during transport.

Whether to perform a lumbar puncture before transport depends on the status of the patient. For diagnostic reasons, it is optimal to obtain cerebrospinal fluid before administration of antibiotics, however, antibiotic administration should not be delayed if the lumbar puncture cannot be done safely and quickly. Contraindications to lumbar puncture include hemodynamic instability, clinical manifestations of overtly high intracranial pressure, or coagulopathy. There have been reports suggesting an association between lumbar puncture and cerebral herniation,[52,100] though, there are others who argue that herniation was temporally but not causally related.[90] If there are concerns about hemodynamic instability, dangerously high intracranial pressure, or coagulopathy in a child with meningitis, it is appropriate to administer antibiotics and defer the decision to perform a lumbar puncture until after evaluation of the patient at the accepting institution.

ENCEPHALITIS

There were 350 cases of encephalitis in children less than 15 years of age reported to the Center for Disease Control in 1991.[13]

Etiologic agents, when recovered, are primarily viral and include herpes viruses, varicella-zoster, enteroviruses, arboviruses, and others.[64] Mycoplasma, parasites, chlamydia, and ricketsiae are less frequent pathogens.[64]

Presenting symptoms can include encephalopathy, altered level of consciousness, headache, fever, malaise, vomiting, and photophobia. Focal neurologic findings and seizures can also be observed, and meningeal involvement is often present.[104] Diagnosis before transport is presumptive and is made solely on clinical grounds, as laboratory diagnosis can only be made by identifying infecting agents in brain tissue or cerebrospinal fluid, or presumptively by measuring a rise in serum antibody titer over time.

Management and transport issues are similar to those discussed in patients with meningitis and are described above. Specific treatment involves consideration of antimicrobial therapy directed against the herpes or varicella-zoster virus, since these are the only viral agents for which specific therapy exists. Clinical trials using acyclovir reported a decrease in mortality from 70% to 28% for herpes encephalitis, and morbidity was also reduced with treatment.[130] Treatment before the onset of coma (Glasgow coma score < 7) correlated with better outcome.[130] If herpes or varicella encephalitis is suspected (or proven), and duration of transport is anticipated to be several hours, treatment with acyclovir should be considered before or during transport.

SHUNT FAILURE

When a child with a history of hydrocephalus and an intracranial shunt presents with severe headaches, nausea, vomiting, ataxia, mental status changes, hypertension, and/or fever, mechanical shunt malfunction and/or infection must be ruled out.[47,128] Diagnosis of shunt malfunction is made by clinical evaluation of the patient coupled with radiographic studies (computed tomography and plain films). Shunt revision in the operating room by a skilled pediatric neurosurgeon is the definitive treatment.

Since the manifestations of shunt obstruction may range from mild headache to profound neurological and cardiovascular compromise, the management of the patient must be appropriately tailored to the severity of the associated symptoms and signs. Communication with the neurological staff after receiving the initial transport call and upon arrival facilitates the choice of an optimal management plan.

If shunt failure is suspected, but the patient shows no signs of severe neurological compromise, such as somnelence, hypertension, bradycardia, posturing, or respiratory irregularity, urgent transport with careful monitoring of the patient's neurological condition is generally the treatment of choice. However, if the patient manifests signs of impending herniation, additional intervention is required at the scene. Patients who become severely symptomatic from progressive hydrocephalus have largely exhausted the buffering capacity of the intracranial cavity for additional cerebrospinal fluid; thus, further neurological deterioration, and, ultimately, cardiorespiratory arrest may occur precipitously. Accordingly, intubation with cerebral protective manuevers, hyperventilation, and mannitol and/or lasix administration, are useful temporizing measures, however, in selected cases, more definitive intervention is required. With appropriate neurosurgical consultation, whether by phone or on-site at the referring center, cerebrospinal fluid may be drained directly from the ventricular catheter reservoir or pumping chamber using a 23-gauge needle. In patients with distal shunt obstruction a brisk flow of cerebrospinal fluid will be obtained. In patients with proximal obstruction and in those without an accessible reservoir or valve, this technique will be ineffective and a 22-gauge needle may be directed through the ventricular catheter or, in young children, through the coronal suture into the ventricular system. After spinal fluid has been obtained, the needle hub is attached to a three-way stopcock and monometer; cerebrospinal fluid is then allowed to drip freely until the intracranial pressure is reduced to 10 to 15 cm of water. Excessive fluid removal or suction on the needle are to be avoided because of the risk of subdural hematoma formation.[28] Specimens of the spinal fluid should be retained for measurement of cell counts, protein and glucose,

BOX 22-2 ETIOLOGIES OF CENTRAL NERVOUS SYSTEM FAILURE

Trauma
- Head injury
- Spinal cord injury

Hypoxia/Ischemia
- Cardiorespiratory failure
- Asphyxia
- SIDS

CNS infection
- Meningitis
- Encephalitis
- Brain abscess

Seizures

CNS tumor

Hydrocephalus

Shunt failure

Cerebrovascular disease
- Intracranial hemorrhage
- Stroke
- Cavernous sinus or venous thrombosis
- Hypertensive encephalopathy

Shock

Sepsis

Endocrinopathies
- Adrenal crisis
- Thyrotoxicosis

Environmental
- Carbon monoxide
- Envenomation
- Heat stroke

Metabolic
- Hypoglycemia
- Hypo, hypernatremia
- Hypo, hypercalcemia
- Hypo, hypermagnasemia
- Hypophosphatemia
- Hyperammonemia
- Inborn errors of metabolism
- Diabetic ketoacidosis
- Renal tubular acidosis
- Hyperosmolar states
- Uremia
- Hepatic encephalopathy
- Reyes syndrome

Ingestion/toxin
- Alcohol
- Anticholinergics
- Sedative-hypnotics
- Narcotics
- Tricyclic antidepressents
- Salicylates
- Organophosphates
- Heavy metal poisoning

Nutritional deficiencies
- Nicotinic acid
- Pantothenic acid
- Thiamine
- Pyridoxime
- Vitamin B_{12}

and for culture and gram stain. Rarely, in patients with evidence of shunt obstruction on the basis of a cerebrospinal fluid infection in whom a lengthy transport time is anticipated, broad spectrum antibiotics (i.e., vancomycin and ceftazidine) may be initiated at the scene after a spinal fluid sample has been obtained.

CENTRAL NERVOUS SYSTEM TUMORS

Most patients requiring transport experience symptoms after tumor size and peritumor edema causes intracranial hypertension. Occasionally, children with central nervous system tumors present with specific neurologic deficits or seizures. Because of the ability of the intracranial contents to accommodate slow increases in tumor size, a large tumor volume must be reached before significant intracranial hypertension occurs.[91] Intracranial hypertension is produced via several different mechanisms. Hydrocephalus is the most important and occurs in approximately 80-90% of children with infratentorial tumors, and 60% of children with supratentorial tumors.[76,99] Hydrocephalus is most commonly noncommunicating with posterior fossa and midline tumors obstructing cerebrospinal fluid circulation.[99] Peritumor edema and tumor hemorrhage also contribute to intracranial hypertension. Peritumor edema is caused by structural and biochemical abnormalities in the tumor endothelium, and from local inflammation.[34] Spontaneous hemorrhage is a potentially devastating cause of intracranial hypertension associated with brain tumors. It occurs in 5% of children with brain tumors under 14 years of age and is associated with nearly 50% mortality.[127]

Diagnosis

Patients present with progressive headache, nausea, vomiting, and ataxia. When critical levels of intracranial hypertension are reached, an altered level of consciousness can develop and may often be a presenting sign in the emergency department. The basic principles regarding stabilization and transport of the child with an altered mental status apply. Indications for intubation are similar, with the exception that acute deterioration is less likely, for reasons described above. Medical treatment of intracranial hypertension in this setting involves the use of corticosteroids and diuretics. Corticosteroids decrease peritumor edema[74,127] and can decrease intracranial hypertension. Furosemide in combination with steroids also decreases edema.[74] However, in the presence of signs and symptoms of impending herniation, mannitol should be administered, and intubation should be performed using cerebral protective maneuvers (i.e., thiopental, vecuronium or pancuronium, and lidocaine) as described in the section on meningitis.

ESOTERIC

There are a large number of other causes of CNS failure that require stabilization and transport (see Box 22-2 on p 253). We have attempted to discuss the most common ones. Transport and early management issues are often etiology-specific, however, space limitations prevent a specific discussion of each of these disease processes. Prompt and meticulous attention to the acute stabilization of the infant or child with CNS failure is essential to providing optimal care before and during transport.

ACKNOWLEDGMENT

We thank Janet Santucci for preparation of this chapter and Dr. Richard Orr for access to the Children's Hospital of Pittsburgh Transport Database.

REFERENCES

1. Abramson NS: Effect of calcium entry blocker (lidoflazine) administration on comatose survivors of clinical cardiac arrest, *Crit Care Med* S132, 1989.
2. Abramson NS and others: Randomized clinical study of cardiopulmonary-cerebral resuscitation: thiopental loading of comatose cardiac arrest survivors, *N Engl J Med* 314:397, 1986.
3. Aicardi J, Chevrie JJ: Convulsive status epileptics in infants and children: a study of 239 cases, *Epilepsia* 11:187, 1970.
4. Arieff AI, Kleeman CR: Studies on mechanisms of cerebral edema in diabetic comas: effects of hyperglycemia and rapid lowering of plasma glucose in normal rabbits, *J Clin Inv* 52:571-83, 1973.
5. Ashwal S and others: Cerebral blood flow and carbon dioxide reactivity in children with bacterial meningitis, *J Pediatr* 117(4):523-30, 1990.
6. Ashwal S and others: Prognostic implications of hyperglycemia and reduced cerebral blood flow in childhood near-drowning, *Neurology* 40:820-3, 1990.
7. Ashwal S and others: Bacterial meningitis in children: current concepts of neurologic management, *Adv Pediatr* 40:185-215, 1993.
8. Beckstead JE and others: Cerebral blood flow and metabolism in man following cardiac arrest, *Stroke* 9:569, 1978.
9. Bleyaert A and others: Augmentation of postischemic brain damage by severe intermittent hypertension, *Crit Care Med* 8:41, 1980.
10. Brierley JB, Meldrum BS, Brown AW: The threshold and neuropathology of cerebral "anoxic-ischemic" cell change, *Arch Neurol* 29:367, 1973.
11. Browne J: The pharmacokinetics of agents used in the treatment of status epilepticus, *Neurol* 40(Suppl 2):28, 1990.
12. Calle PA and others: Glycemia in the post-resuscitation period, *Resuscitation* 17(suppl):S181-S188, 1989.
13. Centers For Disease Control: Summary of notifiable diseases 1991, *MMWR* 40(53):1-12, 1992.
14. Cerchiari EL and others: Protective effects of combined superoxide dismutase and deferoxamine on recovery of cerebral blood flow and function after cardiac arrest in dogs, *Stroke* 18:869, 1987.
15. Chevrie JJ, Aicardi J: Convulsive disorders in the first year of life: neurological and mental outcome and mortality, *Epilepsia* 19:67, 1978.
16. Clements RS, Prockup LD, Winegrad AI: Acute cerebral oedema during treatment of hyperglycemia: an experimental model, *Lancet* ii:384-6, 1968.
17. Clements RS and others: Increased cerebrospinal-fluid pressure during treatment of diabetic ketosis, *Lancet* 671-5, 1971.
18. Cohan SL and others: Cerebral blood flow in humans following resuscitation from cardiac arrest, *Stroke* 20:761, 1989.
19. Cold GE: Does acute hyperventilation provoke cerebral oligaemia in comatose patients after acute head injury, *Acta Neurochir* 96:100-6, 1989.
20. Commission on Classification and Terminology of the International League Against Epilepsy: Proposal for classification of the epilepsies and epileptic syndromes, *Epilepsia* 26:268, 1985.
21. Commission for the Control of Epilepsy and Its Consequences: *Plan for Nationwide Action on Epilepsy*, Bethesda, MD, U.S. Dept of Health, Education, and Welfare, 1977.

22. Connell FA, Louden JM: Diabetes mortality in persons under 45 years of age, *Am J Pub Health* 73:1174-7, 1983.
23. Corneli HM, Gormley CJ, Baker RC: Hyponatremia and seizures presenting in the first two years of life, *Pediatr Emer Care* 1:190, 1985.
24. Dean JM, Rogers MC, Traystman RJ: Pathophysiology and clinical management of the intracranial vault. In Rogers MC, editor: *Textbook of pediatric intensive care,* Vol. 1, 1987, Baltimore, Williams and Wilkins.
25. Dean JM, Singer HS: Status epilepticus. In Rogers MC, editor: *Textbook of pediatric intensive care,* Vol. 1, 1987, Baltimore, Williams and Wilkins.
26. Dehkharghani F: Status epilepticus. In *Handbook of Pediatric Epilepsy,* New York, 1993, Marcel Dekker, Inc.
27. D'Alecy LG and others: Dextrose containing intravenous fluid impairs outcome and increases death after eight minutes of cardiac arrest and resuscitation in dogs, *Surgery* 100:505, 1986.
28. DiRocco C, Iannelli A: Complications of cerebrospinal fluid shunting. In DiRocco C, editor: *The treatment of infantile hydrocephalus,* Vol 2, Boca Raton, 1987, CRC Press.
29. Duck SC and others: Cerebral edema complicating diabetic ketoacidosis, *Diabetes* 25:111-5, 1976.
30. Duck SC, Wyatt DT: Factors associated with brain herniation in the treatment of diabetic ketoacidosis, *J Pediat* 113:10-14, 1988.
31. Dunn DW: Status epilepticus in infancy and childhood, *Neurol Clin* 8:647, 1992.
32. Ellis EN: Concepts of fluid therapy in diabetic ketoacidosis and hyperosmolar hyperglycemic nonketotic coma, *Pediatr Clin North Am* 37:313-21, 1990.
33. Fisher DH, Wrape V: Outcome of cardiopulmonary resuscitation in children, *Pediatr Emerg Care* 3:325, 1987.
34. Fishman RA: Brain edema, *N Engl J Med* 293(14):706-11, 1975.
35. Frandsen F and others: Evaluation of intensified prehospital treatment in out-of-hospital cardiac arrest: survival and cerebral prognosis, *Cardiology* 79:256-64, 1991.
36. Franklin B, Liu J, Ginsberg-Fellner F: Cerebral edema and ophthalmoplegia reversed by mannitol in a new case of insulin-dependent diabetes mellitus, *Pediatrics* 69:87-90, 1982.
37. Freeman JM, Vining EPG: Decision making and the child with febrile seizures, *Pediatr Rev* 13:298, 1992.
38. Friedland IR and others: Cranial computed tomography scans have little impact on management of bacterial meningitis, *Am J Dis Child* 146:1484-7, 1992.
39. Fuchs S: Seizures. In Barker RM, editor: *Pediatric Emergency Medicine,* St. Louis, 1992, Mosby Year Book.
40. Gastaut H: Classification of status epilepticus, *Adv Neurol* 34:15, 1983.
41. Gastaut H: *Dictionary of epilepsy: part I, definitions,* Geneva, 1985, World Health Organization.
42. Ginsberg MD and others: Therapeutic modulation of brain temperature: relevance to ischemic brain injury, *Cerebrovasc Brain Metabol Rev* 4:189-225, 1992.
43. Glaser D: Medical complications of status epilepticus, *Adv Neurol* 34:396, 1983.
44. Glaze DG: Neonatal seizures. In Fishman MA, editor: *Pediatric Neurology,* Orlando, 1986, Grune and Stratton.
45. Goiten KJ, Amit Y, Mussaffi H: Intracranial pressure in central nervous system infections and cerebral ischemia of infancy, *Arch Dis Child* 58:184-6, 1983.
46. Goldberg MA, McIntyre HB: Barbiturates in the treatment of status epilepticus. In Delgado-Esqueta AV, Wasterlain CG, Triman DM, editors: *Adv Neurol,* Vol, 34: *Status Epilepticus,* New York, 1983, Raven Press.
47. Guertin SR: Cerebrospinal fluid shunts: evaluation, complications, and crisis management, *Pediatr Clin North Am* 34(1):203-17, 1983.
48. Gustafson I, Edgre E, Hulting J: Brain-oriented intensive care after resuscitation from cardiac arrest, *Resuscitation* 24:245-61, 1992.
49. Hall ED, Andrus PK, Pazara KE: Protective efficacy of a hypothermic pharmacological agent in gerbil forebrain ischemia, *Stroke* 24:711-15, 1993.
50. Harris GD, Fiordalisi I, Finberg L: Safe management of diabetic ketoacidemia, *J Pediatr* 113:65-8, 1988.
51. Hauser WA: Status epilepticus: epidemiologic considerations, *Neurology* 40(suppl 2):9, 1990.
52. Heldrich FJ, Walker SH, Crosby RMN: Risk of diagnostic lumbar puncture in acute bacterial meningitis, *Pediatr Emerg Care* 2:180-2, 1986.
53. Himwich HE, Fazekas JF: Comparative studies of the metabolism of the brain of infant and adult dogs, *Am J Physiol* 132:454, 1941.
54. Hoffman WH and others: Cranial CT in children and adolescents with diabetic ketoacidosis, *Am J Neuroradiology* 9:733-9, 1988.
55. Horwitz SJ, Boxerbaum B, O'Bell J: Cerebral herniation in bacterial meningitis in childhood, *Ann Neurol* 7:524-8, 1980.
56. Hossman KA: Treatment of experimental cerebral ischemia, *J Cereb Blood Flow Metab* 2:275, 1982.
57. Igarashi M and others: Cerebral arteritis and bacterial meningitis, *Arch Neurol* 41:531-5, 1984.
58. Ishige N and others: The effect of hypoxia on traumatic head injury in rats: alterations in neurologic function, brain edema, and cerebral blood flow, *J Cereb Blood Flow Metab* 7:759-67, 1987.
59. Kirkham FJ: Intracranial pressure and cerebral blood flow in nontraumatic coma in childhood. In Minns RA, editor: *Problems of intracranial pressure in childhood,* 1991, New York, Macbeth Press.
60. Klein JO, Feigin RD, McCracken GH Jr: Report of the task force on the diagnosis and management of meningitis, *Pediatrics* 78(suppl):959-82, 1986.
61. Kline MW, Kaplan SL: Computed tomography in bacterial meningitis of childhood, *Pediatr Infect Dis J* 7(12):855-7, 1988.

62. Kochanek PM, Uhl MW, Schoettle RJ: Hypoxic-ischemic encephalopathy: pathobiology and therapy of the postresuscitation syndrome in children. In Furhrman BP, Zimmerman JJ, editors: *Pediatric Critical Care* 1992, St. Louis, Mosby Year Book.
63. Kochanek PM: Ischemic and traumatic brain injury: pathobiology and cellular mechanisms, *Crit Care Med* 21(9):S333-4, 1993.
64. Koskiniemi M and others: Epidemiology of encephalitis in children: a 20-year survey, *Ann Neurol* 29:492-7, 1991.
65. Krane EJ and others: Subclinical brain swelling in children during treatment of diabetic ketoacidosis, *N Engl J Med* 312:1147-51, 1985.
66. Lee SK and others: Effect of cardiac arrest time on cortical cerebral blood flow during subsequent standard external cardiopulmonary resuscitation in rabbits, *Resuscitation* 17(2):105-17, 1989.
67. Leppik IE: Status epilepticus: the next decade, *Neurol* 40(suppl 2):4, 1990.
68. Lever E, Jaspan JB: Sodium bicarbonate therapy in severe diabetic ketoacidosis, *Am J Med* 75:263-8, 1983.
69. Lewis JK and others: Outcome of pediatric resuscitation, *Ann Emerg Med* 12:297, 1983.
70. Lougheed DW: Physiological studies in experimental asphyxia and drowning, *Can Med Assoc J* 40:424, 1939.
71. Lothman E: The biochemical basis and pathophysiology of status eplilepticus, *Neurol* 40:(suppl 2):13, 1990.
72. Mabe H, Blomquvist P, Seisjø BK: Intracellular pH in the brain following transient ischemia, *J Cereb Blood Flow Metabol* 3:109-14, 1983.
73. McCracken GH and others: Consensus report: antimicrobial therapy for bacterial meningitis in infants and children, *Pediatr Infect Dis J* 6(6):501-5, 1987.
74. Meinig G and others: Clinical, chemical, and CT elevation of short-term and long-term antiedema therapy with dexamethasone and diuretics, *Adv in Neurol* 28:471-89, 1980.
75. Meldrum BS and others: Systemic factors and epileptic brain damage, *Arch Neurol* 29:82-7, 1973.
76. Mercuri S, Russo A, Palma L: Hemispheric supratentorial astryocytomas in children, *J Neurosurg* 55:170-3, 1981.
77. Messing RO, Clossen RG, Simon RP: Drug-induced seizures: a 10 year experience, *Neurol* 34:1587, 1984.
78. Michenfelder JD, Milde JH, Katusic ZS: Postichemic canine cerebral blood flow is coupled to cerebral metabolic rate, *J Cereb Blood Flow Metab* 11:611-6, 1991.
79. Michel HS and others: Breathing 100% oxygen after global brain ischemia in monogolian gerbils results in increased lipid peroxidation and increased mortality, *Stroke* 18:426-30, 1987.
80. Miller C and others: Local cerebral ischemia. II. Effect of arterial PCO_2 on reperfusion following global ischemia, *Stroke* 11:542, 1980.
81. Miller JR, Myers RE: Neurological effects of systemic circulatory arrest in the monkey, *Neurology* 20:715-24, 1990.
82. Moon MR, Walker A: Emergency management: In Johnson KB, editor: *The Harriet Lane,* 1993, St. Louis, Mosby Year Book.
83. Muizelaar JP and others: Adverse effects of prolonged hyperventilation in patients with severe head injury: a randomized clinical trial, *J Neurosurg* 75:731-9, 1991.
84. Muizelaar JP and others: Improving the outcome of severe head injury with the oxygen radical scavenger polyethylene glycol-conjugated superoxide dismutase: a Phase II trial, *J Neurosurg* 78:375-83, 1993.
85. Munk P and others: Effect of bicarbonate on oxygen transport in juvenile diabetic ketoacidosis, *J Pediatr* 84:510-4, 1974.
86. Nakakimura K and others: Glucose administration before cardiac arrest worsens neurologic outcome in cats, *Anesthesiology* 72:1005, 1990.
87. Nellgard B, Wieloch T: Postischemic blockade of AMPA but not NDMA receptors mitigates neuronal damage in the rat brain following transient severe cerebral ischemia, *J Cereb Blood Flow Metabol* 12:2-11, 1992.
88. Nevander G and others: Status epilepticus in well-oxygenated rats causes neuronal necrosis, *Ann Neurol* 18:281-90, 1985.
89. Nugent SK and others: Raised intracranial pressure: its management in Neisseria meningitis meningoencephalitis, *Am J Dis Child* 133:260-2, 1979.
90. Obaro SK: Avoiding coning in childhood meningitis, *Br Med J* 306:1691-2, 1993.
91. Odom GI, Davis CH, Woodhall B: Brain tumors in children, *Pediatrics* 18:856-70, 1956.
92. O'Rourke PP: Outcome of children who are apneic and pulseless in the emergency room, *Crit Care Med* 14:466, 1986.
93. Orr RA and others: Diazepam and intubation in emergency treatment of seizures in children, *Ann Emerg Med* 20:1009, 1991.
94. Palmer AM and others: Therapeutic hypothermia is cytoprotective without attenuating the traumatic brain injury-induced elevations in interstitial concentrations of asparate and glutamate, *J Neurotrauma* 10:363-72, 1993.
95. Petroff OAC and others: Combined ^{1}H and ^{31}P nuclear magnetic resonance spectroscopic studies of bicuculline-induced seizures in vivo, *Ann Neurol* 20:185-93, 1986.
96. Pfister HW and others: Microvascular changes during the early phase of experimental bacterial meningitis, *J Cereb Blood Flow Metab* 10:914-22, 1990.
97. Phillips SA, Shanahan RJ: Etiology and mortality of status epilepticus in children: a recent update, *Arch Neurol* 46:74, 1989.
98. Plotkin SA and others: Dexamethasone therapy for bacterial meningitis in infants and children, *Pediatrics* 86:130-3, 1990.
99. Raimondi AJ, Tomita T: Hydrocephalus and infratentorial tumors, *J Neurosurg* 55:174-82, 1981.
100. Rennick G, Shann F, deCampo J: Cerebral herniation during bacterial meningitis in children, *British Medical Journal* 306:953-5, 1993.

101. Rosenberg D: Status Epilepticus. In *A Practical Guide to Pediatric Intensive Care,* 3rd edition, J Blumer editor, Mosby, St. Louis, 1990.
102. Rosenberg DI: Status epilepticus. In Holbrook P, editor: *Textbook of pediatric critical care,* St. Louis, 1993, WB Saunders.
103. Rosenbloom AL: Intracerebral crises during treatment of diabetic ketoacidosis, *Diabetes Care* 13:22-33, 1990.
104. Rubeiz H, Roos RP: Viral meningitis and encephalitis, *Seminars in Neurology* 12(3):165-77, 1992.
105. Saez-Llorens and others: Molecular pathophysiology of caterial meningitis: current concepts and therapeutic implications, *J Pediatr* 116(5):671-84, 1990.
106. Safar P: Cerebral resuscitation after cardiac arrest: research initiatives and future directions, *Ann Emer Med* 22:2(part 2):234-49, 1993.
107. Safar P and others: Systemic development of cerebral resuscitation after cardiac arrest. Three promising treatments: cardiopulmonary bypass, hypertensive hemodilution, and mild hypothermia, *Acta Neurochir* 57(suppl):110-21, 1993.
108. Sarniak AP, Lich-Lai MW: Transporting the neurologically compromised child, *Ped Clin NA* 40:337, 1993.
109. Scibilia J and others: Why do children with diabetes die? *Acta Endocrinol* 279:S326-33, 1986.
110. Shanahan DM and others: A prospective comparison of diazepam and phenytoin versus phenobarbital and optional phenytoin, *Neurology* 38:202, 1988.
111. Shields WD: Status epilepticus, *Ped Clin NA* 36:383, 1989.
112. Siebke H and others: Survival after 40 minutes submersion without cerebral sequelae, *Lancet* 1:1275-7, 1975.
113. Snyder JV and others: Global ischemia in dogs: intracranial pressures, brain blood flow and metabolism, *Stroke* 6:21, 1975.
114. Sperling MA: Diabetic ketoacidosis, *Ped Clin North Am* 31:591-610, 1984.
115. Sterz F and others: Mild hypothermic cardiopulmonary resuscitation improves outcome after prolonged cardiac arrest in dogs, *Crit Care Med* 19:379-89, 1991.
116. Sterz F and others: Hypertension with or without hemodilution after cardiac arrest in dogs, *Stroke* 21:1178-84, 1990.
117. Todd MM, Tommasion C, Shapiro HM: Cerebrovascular effects of prolonged hypocarbia and hypercarbia after experimental global ischemia in cats, *Crit Care Med* 13:720, 1985.
118. Tormheim PA: Regional localization of cerebral edema following fluid and insulin therapy in steptozotocin-diabetic rats, *Diabetes* 30:762-6, 1981.
119. Torphy DE, Minter MG, Thompson BM: Cardiorespiratory arrest and resuscitation of children, *Am J Dis Child* 138:1099, 1984.
120. Tureen JH and others: Loss of cerebrovascular autoregulation in experimental meningitis in rabbits, *J Clin Invest* 85:577-81, 1990.
121. Vanicky I and others: Prolonged postischemic hyperventilation reduces acute neuronal damage after 15 min of cardiac arrest in the dog, *Neurosci Lett* 135:167-70, 1992.
122. Vannucci RC, Vasta F, Vannucci SJ: Cerebral metabolic responses of hypoglycemic immature rats to hypopoxia-ischemia, *Pediatr Res* 21:524-9, 1987.
123. Vining EPG, Freeman JM: Introduction: epilepsy in children, *Pediatr Ann* 14:705, 1985.
124. Vining EPG, Freeman JM: Seizures which are not epilepsy, *Pediatr Ann* 14:711, 1985.
125. Volpe JJ: Neonatal seizures, *Clin Perinatol* 4:43, 1977.
126. Vukmir RB and others: Sodium bicarbonate improves hemodynamics and perfusion in canine cardiac arrest, *Crit Care Med* 21:S272, 1993.
127. Wakai S and others: Spontaneous intracranial hemorrhage caused by brain tumor: its incidence and clinical significance, *Neurosurgery* 10(4):437-44, 1982.
128. Walters BC and others: Cerebrospinal fluid shunt infection: influences on initial management and subsequent outcome, *J Neurosurg* 60:1014-21, 1984.
129. Weigle CM, Tobin SR: Metabolic and endocrine diseases in pediatric intensive care. In Rogers MC, editor: *Textbook of pediatric intensive care,* ed 2, 1992, Baltimore, Williams and Wilkins.
130. Whitley RJ and others: Vidarabine versus acyclovir therapy in herpes simplex encephalitis, *N Engl J Med* 314(3):144-9, 1986.
131. Winn HR and others: Changes in brain adenosine during bicuculline-induced seizures in rats: effects of hyposia and altered systemic blood pressure, *Circ Res* 47:481, 1980.
132. Zaritsky A and others: CPR in children, *Ann Emerg Med* 16:1107, 1987.

23

TRAUMA

JAMES M. LYNCH

Traumatic injury is the leading cause of death and disability in children after age one. In the United States, 8,000 to 10,000 traumatic deaths occur annually in children ages 1-15 years.[37] Five times that number suffer permanent physical or mental disability. Annual admissions to hospitals for traumatic injury of childhood number 340,000, while close to 9,000,000 visits to emergency departments occur because of lesser injuries.[21]

Since traumatic injury is usually an unforeseen event, the child with significant injury requires urgent transportation from the scene of the injury or from one hospital to another. Prior to transport, time should be effectively utilized attending to the basics of trauma resuscitation, the so-called ABCs. These include immobilization of the cervical spine and axial skeleton, clearing or establishing an airway, assessing respiratory dynamics, and attempts at correction of fluid volume deficit. In addition, control of hemorrhage by pressure dressings and immobilization by splints of limbs with obvious deformities are required interventions at the scene of the injury.

Further attempts at diagnosing exact injuries are not warranted. In the past, there have been numerous discussions of the relative values of deliberate stabilization and diagnosis at the scene ("stay and play")[5,24] versus rapid transport to a nearby hospital ("scoop and run").[17] While a more deliberate approach may be appropriate when transporting a patient from one hospital to another, extra time performing more than the required ABCs at the scene may have detrimental effects. The appropriate approach to managing the child suffering blunt trauma lies somewhere in the middle. Gaining control of the airway, evaluation of breathing, and initiation of fluid therapy are basic steps in the resuscitation of any trauma patient and are critical in the pediatric patient.

Because most pediatric traumatic injury occurs by a blunt mechanism, injury to more than one organ system often results. Combinations of brain, bone, chest, or abdominal injury are common. The approach to these injuries is resuscitation, followed by diagnosis and therapy. Resuscitation is directed at reconstitution of the circulating volume and optimization of oxygen delivery to the tissues. The investment of a small amount of time at the scene in establishing IVs, clearing the airway, and immobilizing the axial skeleton, thus initiating hemodynamic and cerebrovascular support and limiting the effects of any unrecognized spinal injury, pays considerable returns. In the state of Pennsylvania the on-scene time has been limited to 20 minutes when prolonged extrication is not a problem. Many crews accomplish these interventions in less than 10 minutes. The Pennsylvania Trauma Systems Foundation monitors this on-scene time as an indicator of quality care.[28] Other state and regional trauma system organizations need to establish their own criteria for the length of time that should be allowed preparing for transport. We have no information or knowledge of any adverse actions that have occurred because of these 20 minute on-scene times. However, literally taking the patient from the scene without attention to the ABCs and immobilization may have a profound negative effect on the seriously injured child, and may worsen preexisting fluid deficits, tissue oxygen delivery, and spinal cord lesions.

When faced with penetrating injury, particularly when the potential for involvement of major vessels of the trunk or neck is high, extremely rapid transport in the fashion of a "scoop and run" approach should occur. A few centers which see a high volume of penetrating adult-type injuries, feel that no time should be wasted in the field or even in the emergency department as only rapid definitive operating room resuscitation will result in survival.[17] In these systems the patient is placed on a backboard and loaded into the rescue vehicle. Attempts at aggressive fluid resuscitation are not encouraged for fear of raising the blood pressure and causing further bleeding. These patients do not require any preoperative work-up because the injuries will become evident during the operation, if the patient survives to that point.

Is this rapid approach worthwhile in children who are very seriously injured and have suffered a cardiopulmonary arrest at the scene? Studies have shown that resuscitation from cardiopulmonary arrest following blunt injury carries an extremely low survival rate. In this situation, attempts at resuscitation seem almost sophomoric.[4] Yet, the ABCs must be attempted as an occasional survivor has occurred.

TRANSPORT FROM SCENE

The often quoted study by Ramenofsky and others[30] implied that there was significant morbidity and mortality associated with transporting children with traumatic injury to the nearest hospital. This landmark paper was the impetus behind the establishment of a number of pediatric trauma centers across the country. Prior to this the establishment of regionalized adult trauma centers, most with air evacuation systems, was well underway and encountering success. A number of studies were done hoping to prove that it was better for a patient to be delivered directly to a trauma center than to go to a community hospital and then be transferred. Although these studies often showed contradictory or confusing statistics, Cowley and others[8] published a paper showing conclusively, that when definitive care was rendered in the first hour following traumatic injury in the adult, survival was markedly improved. This firmly established the phrase "the golden hour" in the trauma literature. This concept has never been studied critically in the pediatric trauma population but has been extrapolated to apply to children as well.

Cowley's paper established that trauma victims will do better when diagnosed and treated rapidly. In his study the only hospitals which could render such rapid evaluation and treatment were trauma centers where complete staffing was available on a 24 hour a day, seven day a week basis. The monetary outlay necessary to provide such intense staffing is beyond the means of most community hospitals. In addition, most community hospitals do not have complete pediatric medicine departments with specialists in pediatric surgery, neurosurgery, pediatric critical care, and to a lesser extent, pediatric orthopedics. Most facilities do not have the appropriate equipment including pediatric ventilators, monitoring devices, or other needed equipment in different sizes to fit the needs of each child. Therefore, it makes sense to transport injured children to regionalized centers to get the specialized treatment they deserve, especially if definitive care can be given within the "golden hour" following injury.

TRIAGE

Any number of factors may influence the decision to transport a patient to a recognized trauma center. These are usually based on anatomic and or physiologic factors, knowledge of the mechanism of injury, the preexistence of known disease, the judgment of the first response team, or at the direction of their medical command. A number of scoring systems have been devised and tested as indicators of who should be triaged to a trauma center. These include the Trauma Index,[15] the Injury Severity Index,[3] the Triage Index,[6] the Trauma Score,[7] the Hospital Trauma Index,[2] the Circulation, Respiration, Abdomen, Motor, Speech (CRAMS) scale,[13] the Glasgow Coma Scale (GCS),[35] and the Pediatric Trauma Score (PTS).[36] While the GCS is one of the most widely used of all these indices, it is pertinent only to head injury and must be modified to evaluate the infant and toddler (Table 23-1). The Pediatric Trauma Score is the most widely used triage score in pediatric trauma. It assigns relative value to six components of pediatric injury believed to be significant for morbidity and mortality. These are weight, airway status, blood pressure, level of consciousness, the presence of open wounds, and the presence of known fractures (Table 23-2). A score of less than nine indicates significant potential for morbidity and mortality. Children with scores of eight or less should be transported to a pediatric trauma center if one is available.[31]

In areas of the country where the PTS is not used, mechanism of injury, hemodynamic instability, and age may be prime determinants dictating whether a trauma center should directly receive the child.[38,39] In our trauma center at the Children's Hospital of Pittsburgh, we believe that all children with a mechanism of injury having the possibility of severe or multisystem injury should receive their initial evaluation by us (see Box 23-1 on p. 261). In addition, all children with respiratory or hemodynamic instability, major limb trauma, or any suspected neurologic, intrathoracic, or abdominal injury are transported directly to us.

TABLE 23-1 MODIFICATION OF THE GLASGOW COMA SCALE FOR INFANTS AND TODDLERS

	Infant / Toddler	*Child / Adult*
Eye opening		
4	Spontaneously	Spontaneously
3	To speech	To command
2	To pain	To pain
1	No response	No response
Best verbal		
5	Coos, babbles, smile	Oriented
4	Irritable, cries	Confused
3	Cry, screams with pain	Inappropriate words
2	Moans, grunts	Incomprehensible
1	No response	No response
Best motor		
6	Spontaneous	Obeys
5	Withdraws to touch	Localized pain
4	Withdraws to pain	Withdraws to pain
3	Flexion (decorticate)	Flexion (decorticate)
2	Extension (decerebrate)	Extension (decerebrate)
1	No response	No response

* From Benedum Pediatric Trauma Program, Children's Hospital of Pittsburgh: Trauma service guidelines, ed 6, 1992.

Additionally, specific injuries with a high chance of associated morbidity and mortality should be directed to a pediatric trauma center. Chest injury has a particularly high associated mortality when it occurs with

TABLE 23-2 PEDIATRIC TRAUMA SCORE*

Component	*+2*	*+1*	*−1*
Size	>20 Kg	10-20 Kg	<10 Kg
Airway	Normal	Maintainable	Unmaintainable
CNS	Awake	Obtunded	Comatose
Systolic BP	>90 mmHg	50-90 mmHg	<50 mmHg
Open wounds	None	Minor	Major or penetrating
Skeletal	None	Closed fracture	Open/multiple fractures

* If proper size BP cuff not available, BP can be assessed by assigning: +2 Pulse palpable at radial or brachial artery; +1 Pulse palpable at groin, but not radial or brachial artery; −1 No pulse palpable anywhere.
From Ramenofsky ML and others: The predictive validity of the pediatric trauma score, *J Trauma* 28(7):1038-42, 1988.

BOX 23-1 SIGNIFICANT MECHANISM OF INJURY

- Falls 15 feet or more
- Crash speed 20 mph or more: 30″ deformity of front end of automobile; rearward displacement of front axle
- Passenger compartment intrusion (8″ on patient side of car — 24″ on opposite side of car)
- Ejection of patient
- Rollover
- Death of same car occupant
- Motor vehicle-pedestrian accident victims

From Benedum Pediatric Trauma Program, Children's Hospital of Pittsburgh: Trauma service guidelines, ed 6, 1992.

other injuries.[27] Morbidity and mortality increases when fractured ribs are present.[27] The child's ribs are extremely pliable and deform to a marked degree without breaking. The force required to fracture the rib of a child is considerably more than that required to break one in an adult. Therefore, when a fractured rib is present, one must assume severe underlying lung injury as well serious injury to all organs in close proximity. When a fractured rib and severe brain injury occur simultaneously, mortality as high as 71% has been reported.[12]

Abdominal solid organ injury (liver, spleen, and kidney) may benefit from care at a pediatric trauma center.[23,26] The approach to these injuries is tending away from operation towards observation. However, the treating physician must have the medical expertise and experience to be able to decide when to treat nonoperatively and when to operate. A thorough understanding of the complications of nonoperative treatment is imperative.

Hollow organ abdominal injuries are becoming more common as the incidence of seat belt usage increases.[22] Unfortunately, adult seat belts are not designed for children. Commonly, when the grade schooler or preschooler uses an adult lap type belt, the belt does not lie across the hips as it should, but rather the lower abdomen. Sudden deceleration forces a loop of small intestine to become trapped momentarily between the belt and the spinal column. The sudden increase in pressure in the closed intestinal loop causes a small perforation of the bowel. Since the hole is usually very small, massive intestinal spillage does not occur early, and signs of peritonitis do not develop for three or more hours.

Another injury related to improper lap belt usage is the Chance fracture of the lower spine.[22] The child's lumbar column is violently flexed over the lap belt causing an unstable fracture. Often the abdominal injury causes more pain than the spinal fracture. However, many of these fractures are unstable and require repair. Lateral lumbar spine radiographs are usually diagnostic, but since this view is not routine, a high index of suspicion based on previous experience is needed to order this test.[33] Also, an orthopedic surgeon experienced in pediatric injuries is also required as repair must take into consideration the potential for spinal column growth.

THE PRIMARY SURVEY, EVALUATION AND STABILIZATION AT THE SCENE

The initial approach to the injured child should follow the basics of all trauma resuscitations. The evaluation of the ABCs of trauma care (Airway-Breathing-Circulation) as well as D (disability or neurologic injury) and E (exposure) should be accomplished within the initial 20 minutes of on-scene time.

Airway

Understanding airway management is based on recognizing the differences in anatomy between the child's and adult's lower face and upper airway. The child's mandible is smaller and not as protuberant. This allows the tongue to lie more posterior and predisposes to airway obstruction in the obtunded child. The tongue is relatively large, and the rescuer's fingers pressing in the submandibular region may push the tongue up and back, obstructing the airway when attempting to ventilate the child via bag-valve-mask. The child has more lymphoid tissue in the form of adenoids and tonsils which may infringe on the patency of the airway. The midface is smaller, and nasotracheal cannulation is more difficult, requiring a smaller tube than does orotracheal intubation. The glottis of a child lies more cephalad and anterior than in the adult. With the increased size of the soft tissues of the tongue and epiglottis, it is better to use a straight blade when attempting intubation. The vocal cords are not as well defined, approximating an omega shape in the very young and only assuming the characteristics of the adult cords in later childhood. Finally, the narrowest point of the airway in the child is the subglottic region. Because of this fact, uncuffed endotracheal tubes are used in children up to age 6 to 8 years of age. After this age, the vocal cords form the narrowest point, of the upper airway and cuffed endotracheal tubes are desirable.

Airway patency is first evaluated by asking the child his or her name. A clear and understandable name, or any word for that matter, is reassuring that the child's airway is indeed patent. If the child is unconscious the airway patency may be more difficult to evaluate. This evaluation can be confusing as a number of normal children have sonorous breathing when they are sleeping due to hypertrophied tonsillar and adenoidal tissues. These tissues may partially obstruct the sleeping child's airway. This commonly occurs in the supine rather than the prone position. These children normally find relief sleeping prone or on their sides. Because most trauma patients are transported supine due to spinal immobilization, airways may be inadvertently compromised as evidenced by sonorous respirations. It would be a mistake to intubate such children when stabilization may be obtained without invasive maneuvers. Gently opening the mouth to be sure no foreign material is present is the first maneuver. The second is to optimally position the child. The young child's posterior skull region is quite prominent. This prominence tends to slightly flex the neck when the child is supine. The resulting effect is to partially obstruct the airway due to the buckling of the posterior pharyngeal tissue on the already hypertrophied, partially obstructing tonsillar or adenoidal tissue. Reversal of this phenomena can be accomplished by placing a small pad beneath the occiput, thus slightly extending the neck. Immediately, the sonorous respirations should diminish or stop and the airway become clear. During this maneuver, great care must be taken not to manipulate the cervical spine. An appropriately fitted cervical collar should be in place, or, better yet, an assistant should hold the head in a midline, neutral position.

The chin lift and jaw thrust are the next maneuvers most often discussed in airway management. In our experience the chin lift has not been helpful in the child as there may be little to hold onto because of the small mandible, and the resuscitator's fingers may inadvertently force the tongue posterior causing further obstruction. The jaw thrust, on the other hand, is a commonly used maneuver even by pediatric anesthesiologists to maintain airways. The resuscitator's thumbs are placed behind the angles of the jaws and anterior pressure is applied to move the mandible, tongue, as well as the anterior soft tissues of the pharynx forward, thus clearing the airway.

If these maneuvers do not result in a clear airway, an oropharyngeal airway is the next intervention to try. Generally, these should only be inserted in the unconscious child. Some authorities advocate nasopharyngeal airways, others do not. We have not been impressed with any benefit from them, and when the possibility of a basilar skull fracture exists (e.g. blood from the ear or nose, hemotympanum, Raccoon's eyes), nasal insertion of any tube is contraindicated. The length of the oropharyngeal airway should be no longer than the distance from the corner of the mouth to the angle of the jaw. Ill fitting airways can force the tongue posteriorly, causing obstruction. Oropharyngeal airways that are too long can stimulate gagging, causing vomiting and potential aspiration of gastric contents. With an oropharyngeal airway in place the children can successfully ventilate themselves, or a bag-valve-mask can ventilate and oxygenate the apneic child for moderate periods of time. When bag-valve-mask ventilation is used, one should remember not to press on the soft tissues of the submandibular region, but rather on the mandible for control.

Endotracheal airways are required in a very small number of traumatized, usually brain injured, children. Apneic or comatose patients have lost the ability to protect their airways from vomitus and should always be intubated. Combative patients and any other patient showing the inability to protect their airway or signs of respiratory distress may require intubation. This procedure should be done by individuals trained and skilled in this technique. The importance of understanding the differences between pediatric and adult anatomy will be extremely helpful in performing a successful intubation.

Patients in arrest or comotose patients will not require drug therapy. In the field, some patients will require muscle relaxants. Rapid acting agents such as succinylcholine have been used with success by many systems. If the child requires endotracheal intubation in the more controlled situation of the emergency department, consideration should be given to using a combination of drugs designed to blunt the elevation of intracranial pressure (ICP) that generally occurs following tracheal stimulation. Lidocaine hydrochloride for control of airway irritability, fentanyl citrate for sedation, vecuronium bromide for paralysis, and thiopental for CNS protection have been very useful in the head injured, hemodynamically stable child in the emergency department setting.[20]

The use of drugs is not recommended for intubation in the unconscious, apneic, or hypotensive patient. Orotracheal intubation is the preferred technique with an assistant holding midline immobilization. Again, nasotracheal tubes are discouraged as they may cause laceration of the delicate tissues of the nasopharynx of the child. Nasotracheal tubes are also contraindicated when the presence of a basilar skull fracture exists and because the smaller diameter of the tube required by this route may be too small to effectively ventilate the child.

The two most common errors made during intubation is using a tube that is too small and inserting the tube too far into the trachea. Picking the correctly sized endotracheal tube requires some experience. However, a relatively accurate estimation can be made by selecting a tube of a similar diameter as the child's external nares or little finger. If possible, one should have the next larger and the next smaller size tube available in case the first tube has a poor fit. One formula for estimating an appropriately sized endotracheal tube is the child's age in years plus 16, divided by 4 ({Age in yrs + 16}/4) (Table 23-3).

The tip of the endotracheal tube should be visualized as it passes through the vocal cords. The tube should be secured and checked for accurate positioning in the trachea. One should avoid inserting the tip of the tube into the right main stem bronchus as this may cause either iatrogenic pneumothorax on that side from over distention of the right lung or atelectasis of the left lung with resultant hypoxia. Impaired oxygenation and/or iatrogenic respiratory acidosis for any period of time may aggravate any preexisting neurologic injury. Finally, a right main stem intubation may mimic a hemothorax or pneumothorax on the opposite side. Low oxygenation and signs consistent with a pneumothorax (i.e. decreased breath sounds) may cause the transport team to believe that the patient has a pneumothorax. In this scenario the team may insert a needle into the left chest to evacuate a nonexistent pneumothorax. Iatrogenic injury by the needle lacerating the lung tissue is an avoidable complication if accurate placement of the tip of the endotracheal tube is done prior to transport. Accurate insertion depth may be estimated by the mnemonics;

TABLE 23-3 DIAMETER AND INSERTION LENGTH OF PEDIATRIC ENDOTRACHEAL TUBE

Age	*I.D.*	*Length (cm)*
Newborn-6 months	3.0-3.5 uncuffed	10
6-18 months	3.5-4.0 uncuffed	12
18 months-3 years	4.0-4.5 uncuffed	13-14
3-5 years	4.5-5.0 uncuffed	16
5-6 years	5.0 uncuffed	16
6-8 years	5.5 cuffed	18
8-10 years	6.0 cuffed	18
10-12 years	6.5 cuffed	20
12-14 years	6.5 cuffed	20-22

From Smith RM: *Endotracheal intubation in anesthesia for infants and children,* ed 4, St. Louis, 1980, The CV Mosby Co.

ten plus the age in years or three times the internal diameter (ID) of the endotracheal tube. The resulting number is the depth of insertion in centimeters from the corner of the mouth (Table 23-3).

Prior to the final taping of the endotracheal tube into position, the chest should be examined for equal rise of the right and left sides of the chest wall. An observer from the head or the foot of the patient should be able to assess whether or not both chest cavities have equal excursions. This test may be extremely important when noise at the scene makes auscultation difficult.

Auscultation of both chest cavities should always follow. The smaller the patient, the more important it is to auscultate in the respective axillary areas rather than over the apical areas of the chest. In the small child, breath sounds are easily transmitted to the contralateral side especially during forceful bagging. Therefore, auscultation in both axillary areas during gentle ventilation may be very useful in evaluating the equality of ventilation of the right and left lung fields. Finally, auscultation over the stomach is indicated to be sure an esophageal intubation has not occurred.

Massive facial trauma is rarely seen in the child. The force necessary to injure the midface of a child to the point that immediate surgical airway is necessary usually will cause so much brain stem and cervical spine disruption that the child will expire immediately. However, in the rare event that a surgical airway is needed, a needle rather than surgical cricothyroidotomy should be attempted. Surgical cricothyroidotomies should be reserved for children over 12 years of age and adults. The structures in the neck of a young child are so small, mobile, and indistinct that lacerations of major vessels, vocal cords, and near complete transection of the trachea are very real possibilities with attempted surgical cricothyroidotomy. The needle cricothyroidotomy is a direct and quick approach providing for short-term ventilation and oxygenation and causes little damage if performed correctly. A 14-gauge needle catheter is inserted through the cricothyroid membrane. Feeling a single "pop" is indicative of being in the trachea. Aspiration of air through the catheter confirms successful placement. An adapter from a #3 endotracheal tube can be directly inserted onto the end of the #14 catheter, and either an Ambu bag or a 'Y' type connector can be attached for short-term ventilation using tracheal insufflation technique.

Following airway control, a nasogastric or orogastric tube is placed to prevent aspiration. This usually cures the child's abdominal distention. The abdomen often becomes markedly distended after injury due to fear, crying and the subsequent swallowing of air. Gastric distention has also been reported to cause obstruction of venous return from the inferior vena cava and intense vasovagal response resulting in a slowing of the heart rate with subsequent hypotension. Another common serious complication of a full stomach in a comatose or semi-comatose patient is aspiration. The early placement of a gastric tube may obviate these problems.

Breathing

Breathing is the involuntary act of bringing oxygen into the lungs for transport to the body cell mass and the removal of the major waste gas of metabolism, carbon dioxide. The former process is termed oxygenation while the latter is ventilation. Both are equally important to the trauma victim. Oxygen delivery is dependent on adequate amounts of oxygen being available for delivery, the amount of hemoglobin available to transport the oxygen, serum pH, intravascular fluid volume, and the adequate perfusion of metabolically active and injured tissues with oxygenated blood. Ventilation is dependent on the rate and depth of unobstructed air movement in and out of the lungs.

Oxygen saturation measurements can often be determined at the scene because of the miniaturization of pulse oximetry units. These devices transmit light of a specific wavelength through arterial blood. The refraction of the light by the saturated hemoglobin molecule is then measured by the receiving lens. These monitors give accurate measurements of oxygen saturation as well as pulse rate when the child is well perfused and the arterial flow is able to be found by the light probe.[18] However, the digital light beam may not be able to access the arterial blood in the patient who is hypovolemic, thus rendering the instrument inaccurate or useless.

While noninvasive oxygen saturation monitors have become reliable and relatively inexpensive, noninvasive CO_2 monitoring has not. End tidal CO_2 monitors do exist but need to be attached to endotracheal tubes. These monitors are expensive and, only now, are beginning to find their way out of the intensive care unit onto some rotorcraft rescue units. Therefore, the field evaluation of adequate patient ventilation is still based on clinical indicators.

The rate and depth of breathing efforts, along with the presence of full breath sounds over each hemithorax give the best indication of the adequacy of ventilation. Infants tend to have normal respiratory rates near 40 breaths per minute. Adult values range from 14 and 18 breaths per minute (Table 23-4). Adult values are attained by children between the ages of 12 to 14 years. Fear and pain may profoundly effect the rate of respiration and need to be taken into account when evaluating the respiratory rate and effort.

Significant defects in oxygen saturation may not be clinically evident without the use of pulse oximetry. Whether pulse oximetry is used or not, supplemental oxygen should be initially applied to all trauma victims. The resuscitation team should not be concerned that supplemental O_2 might harm the child, as most pediatric trauma victims have no preexisting pulmonary disease. Some awake children have a difficult time adapting to face masks, being fearful of suffocation. In such situations it may be better to switch to nasal prongs for the delivery of oxygen. So-called "blow by" oxygen-delivery systems generally deliver lower concentrations of oxygen as it mixes with air, and unless held very close to the nose of the child, are generally useless.

TABLE 23-4 VITAL SIGNS IN CHILDREN

Age	*Weight (kg)*	*Respirations (per min) (min-max)*	*Systolic BP (mmHg) (min-max)*
Newborn	3.5	30-60	50-80
6 months	7	30-60	65-106
1 year	10	24-40	72-110
3 years	15	20-40	78-114
6 years	20	18-25	80-116
8 years	25	18-25	84-122
12 years	40	14-20	94-136
15 years	50	12-20	100-142

From Benedum Pediatric Trauma Program, Children's Hospital of Pittsburgh: Trauma service guidelines, ed 6, 1992.

Adult respiratory mechanics differ from those of the child. The adult has a greater dependence on the accessory muscles of respiration including the shoulder girdle and intercostal muscles. The child has a greater dependence on the diaphragm and less on the thoracic muscles. Thus, the adult shows greater motion of the chest wall when breathing, while the child shows greater abdominal excursion and rather quiet chest movement during normal breathing in the supine position.

Because of the increased compliance of the chest in the young patient, partial or complete airway obstruction is evidenced by a paradoxical inward motion of the sternum and anterior ribs accompanied by the exaggerated thrusting out of the anterior abdominal wall. In this situation, attention to clearing the upper airway is initially made (positioning, jaw thrusts, oropharyngeal airway). If relief is not obtained, endotracheal intubation will be required for mechanical airway control.

Auscultation accompanied by careful observation of the major structures of the neck may give information about the presence of a hemothorax, pneumothorax, or cardiac tamponade. These abnormalities will generally evidence themselves by increased respiratory effort, distention of neck veins, shift of trachea to one side, or muffled heart sounds. If a patient does have evidence of any of these problems but is stable, and arrival at the receiving facility is imminent, it is best not to carry out any intervention. The information of a suspected problem should be conveyed to the receiving physicians. However, when symptoms, such as increased work of breathing, decreased mentation, hypoxia, or cyanosis, are present during transport which are consistent with the physical findings, and the patient is deteriorating, simple and rapid intervention should occur. The interventions are all designed, in one way or another, to increase oxygen delivery and/or facilitate ventilation.

A pneumothorax occurs when air enters the space between the parietal and visceral pleura of the lung. A simple pneumothorax is when air enters the pleural space and the leak is small or sealed. There is no evidence, in a simple pneumothorax, of a shift of the mediastinal structures. A tension pneumothorax occurs when air continues to enter the pleural space, causing a shift of the mediastinal structures to the opposite hemithorax. A tension pneumothorax is not tolerated as well in the child as the adult because of the mobility of the mediastinum. While the mediastinum in the adult is relatively fixed, the mediastinum in the child can shift so markedly that the venous return to the heart is impaired, and cardiac arrest may occur. An open pneumothorax is seen in penetrating trauma when the pleural space is open to the surrounding air. Thus, extrathoracic air is literally sucked into the pleural cavity during inspiration, giving rise to the term "sucking chest wound." An occlusive petroleum gauze pad will seal these chest wall rents.

In the adult trauma victim, a pneumothorax is most commonly associated with a fractured rib. The mechanism of injury is direct laceration of the pulmonary parenchyma by the bony fragments. However in the child, pneumothorax commonly occurs without evidence of fractured ribs. The mechanism is one of increased intrapulmonary pressure against a closed glottis causing rupture of alveoli and dissection of the air into the pleural space. External evidence of a rib fracture (e.g., point tenderness, contusion, rib instability) may be absent, even in the face of large accumulations of air.

The signs of a pneumothorax include decreased breath sounds on the side of the pneumothorax with deviation of the trachea to the opposite side. The neck veins may or may not be distended, and the cardiac sounds are usually shifted away from the side of the clinical pneumothorax. Thoracic pleural pain is often present in the awake child. The chest is hyperresonant, which is sometimes difficult to appreciate in the noise of the field.

The standard teaching for field treatment of a suspected pneumothorax is needle catheter decompression in the midclavicular line in the second intercostal space. This landmark is easily located and is safe in the adult and the large child but becomes more risky in the young victim. Missing the second intercostal space and entering higher up on the chest wall can, and has, resulted in laceration of the subclavian vessels. Entering lower may result in cannulation of the pulmonary vessels. Our preference for all children is to insert a needle catheter in the anterior axillary or midaxillary line at the level of the fifth intercostal space (level with the nipple). Though it may be difficult to identify the exact interspace, there are few major vascular structures that can be inadvertently cannulated or lacerated. Care should be taken to enter the pleural space by passing over the rib. Passing immediately under the rib may lacerate an intercostal vessel and lead to a hemothorax as well. After evacuating the air the catheter should be taped into position and attached to a one-way valve. A definitive chest tube should be placed shortly after arrival to the hospital. In the event of an open pneumothorax, a petroleum based bulky dressing is placed over the wound. Subsequent closure and insertion of a chest tube will occur at the hospital.

A hemothorax presents a different problem because the blood may not be able to be evacuated in the field. Fortunately, massive hemothorax is not as common as pneumothorax in the pediatric population. Laceration of the intercostal vessels is the most common cause of blunt trauma induced massive hemothorax. Because rib fractures are rare in children, the intercostal vessels are usually not lacerated. The signs of a hemothorax are similar to those of pneumothorax. There are decreased breath sounds and dullness to percussion on the side of the blood, some deviation of the trachea to the contralateral side, and usually, a lack of venous distention of the neck veins. The latter fact is related to a decreased circulating volume from blood loss into the chest. Therefore, the patient with a large hemothorax will often show signs of hemodynamic instability as large amounts of blood collect in the chest, while oxygen saturation decreases.

Since pneumothorax and hemothorax are often confused in the field, the insertion of a needle catheter is initially tried in both. Little or no air will be removed when a hemothorax is present, and the clinical situation will not improve as in the patient with a pneumothorax. Since evacuation of blood is not feasible through needle catheters, another approach to stabilization is used. Rapid intravenous infusion of physiologic fluid and/or blood in an attempt to correct the hypovolemic state and increase vital organ perfusion and oxygen delivery is appropriate. If respiratory failure occurs, the only alternative available in the field is intubation and mechanical ventilation. Immediate insertion of at least one large bore chest tube is required on arrival to the hospital.

Cardiac tamponade occurs when there has been direct injury to the myocardium or pericardium. Even small amounts of blood in the pericardial sac interfere with cardiac filling pressures resulting in hypotension and tachycardia. The patient appears to have air hunger and gasps during breathing. The heart sounds are muffled, and the neck veins are usually distended. (They may not be distended if there is marked blood loss from some other area of the body causing hypovolemia.) If the patient is attached to a cardiac monitor, the QRS complexes may appear small or diminished in size. The findings of muffled heart tones, distended neck veins, and hypotension constitutes Beck's Triad, the classic description of tamponade. However, all three signs may not be present even when tamponade is significant.

Since the basic pathophysiology of cardiac tamponade is a decreased filling pressure due to increased fluid in the nondistensible pericardial sac, therapy is aimed at either removing the fluid from the sac or increasing the filling pressures of the heart by increasing intravascular volume. Needle aspiration of the pericardial sac is described in every text on trauma and is potentially a life-saving maneuver. The problem with this procedure is that the needle may injure the myocardium or lacerate a major coronary vessel. Therefore aspiration should only be used in the face of true deterioration when other possibilities have been ruled out. Prior to that time, increasing the patient's intravascular volume will override, to some degree, the effects of the tamponade and is therefore an appropriate temporizing maneuver. Since the cause of most tamponades in pediatric trauma is blunt, simple aspiration of the pericardium, increasing the vascular volume stabilizes the child until reaching the hospital. Usually, bleeding into the pericardial sac stops. In tamponade due to penetrating trauma a catheter may be left in the pericardium for repeated aspiration as the injury to one of the chambers of the heart or coronary arteries continues to bleed.

Other thoracic injuries affecting breathing include pulmonary contusion, rib fracture, and flail chest. Pulmonary contusion is the most common lung injury in pediatric trauma. Yet, it is a diagnosis made by x-ray and not in the field. Rib fractures are rare, and by themselves, only indicate that massive forces were applied to the chest wall.[12] Flail chest segments occur when one or more ribs are each broken in at least two places. This results in unstable areas of the chest wall which show paradoxical motion on inspiration. It is extremely rare to see this lesion in young children. If one is seen, placing the patient on the side of the flail or applying sand bags around that area may stabilize the segment.

Circulation

The evaluation of a child's circulatory status consists of assessing peripheral pulses, blood pressure, skin perfusion, central pulses, and mentation. The evaluation of intravascular volume should be dependent on all these parameters, not just one. The ideal simple invasive measurement in children, urine output, is not available in the field and thus will not be discussed further in this section. Rather, clinical evaluation of intravascular volume depletion and its appropriate correction will be discussed.

Bleeding is a common problem in trauma. The control of bleeding and reestablishment of adequate circulating blood volume is basic to resuscitation. Not only should the volume of blood that has been lost be replaced, but losses of serum like fluid from the extravascular, extracellular fluid compartment must also be replenished.

Shortly after a bleeding episode the body attempts to preserve adequate circulating volume. A number of hormonal and vascular changes have been well described and will not be discussed in detail here.[9] However, basic to the process is the transfer of fluid from the extravascular, extracellular fluid compartment into the vascular space to help compensate for the volume lost. This has been called transcapillary refill. In appropriate fluid resuscitation, enough fluid is given to replace the shed blood as well as replace the fluid that has transferred from the extravascular, extracellular space. The amount of fluid that is required to replace these losses is roughly three times the amount of blood loss. Initial therapy consists of infusion of a physiologic fluid such as lactated Ringer's solution.

The child's total blood volume, between 80-85 ml/kg body weight is small when compared with adults. For example, a 3 year old weighing 15 kilograms (33 lb), has a blood volume of 1200 ml (80 ml/kg times 15 kg). A 25 percent blood loss would equal 300 ml (1200 ml times 0.25). This is 2 ounces less than an average can of soda (355 ml). Therefore, what appears to be relatively small amounts of blood to the uninitiated, may actually represent a major blood loss in small children. The accurate estimation of the amount of blood that a child has lost should be noted and reported at the hospital.

Large amounts of blood can be lost from lacerations of the face and scalp. These areas are extremely vascular, and all deep lacerations in this area must be adequately dressed in the field with pressure dressings. Children have become severely hypotensive from bleeding from the scalp. Brain injury, as in the adult, does not result in hypotension from bleeding, except in the infant. Massive blood loss can occur around the brain of the infant because of the presence of open fontanels and the expandability of suture lines. Fontanels usually close around the fourteenth month of life. Blood loss into the skull of the infant must be treated aggressively with fluid resuscitation as well as other means for brain resuscitation.

While intrathoracic, intraabdominal, and pelvic bleeding can lead to marked hypotension as in the adult, femur fractures do not. The muscles mass of the thigh is greatly decreased in the child, and the marked extravasation of blood seen in the adult from a femur fracture is much less in the child. If a patient appears to have an isolated femur fracture and is hypotensive, one must consider other causes for blood loss.

During discussions of pelvic, femur, and leg fractures and hypotension, the topic of the use of Pneumatic Anti-Shock Garments (PASGs) always surfaces. There is no credible evidence that PASGs trousers provide an "autotransfusion" or have any direct beneficial hemodynamic effect in the adult or child. Yet, PASGs may be beneficial when acting as a splint to immobilize fracture sites of the lower extremity, decreasing disruption of the clot and muscle. They can also be used to stabilize pelvic fractures if care is taken to prevent a marked increase in the patient's intraabdominal pressure, leading to impairment of diaphragmatic excursion and respiratory compromise. Care must also be taken to see that vomiting is not induced because of increased abdominal pressure on a full stomach. If, for some reason, the abdominal component of the PASG is inflated in the child, most authorities recommend that the child undergo endotracheal intubation to protect the airway.

Tachycardia and peripheral vasoconstriction are two early signs of the presence of hypovolemia. Blood pressure changes occur late in the hypovolemic child and indicate a significant blood loss (at least 30 to 40% of blood volume) and persistent deficit. Heart rate is an excellent indicator of intravascular volume and should be monitored carefully (Table 23-5). Changes in heart rate occur long before changes in blood pressure are seen. Cardiac output is equal to the product of stroke volume and heart rate. Changes in the heart rate is the only way the child can maintain cardiac output when intravascular volume falls. Heart rate is thus an early, sensitive indicator of intravascular fluid deficit and should be monitored closely for change and response to fluid therapy. Another mechanism the child has for maintaining blood pressure is the ability to markedly increase sys-

TABLE 23-5 AVERAGE PULSE RATE OF CHILDREN

Age	*Average*	*Range*
Newborn	140	170-80
0-12 months	120	160-80
2 years	110	130-80
4 years	100	120-80
6 years	100	115-75
8 years	90	110-70
10 years	90	110-70
12 years	85	110-65
14 years	80	110-60

From Kaplan S: The cardiovascular system. In Vaughn VC III, McKay RJ Jr, Behrman RE, editors: *Nelson's textbook of pediatrics,* ed 11, 1979, Philadelphia, W.B. Saunders Co.

temic vascular resistance in the face of hypovolemia. This is an attempt to maintain perfusion pressure to vital organs as well as increase filling of the heart.[34] A large outpouring of endogenous vasoactive catecholamines is responsible for this response. The peripheral signs of the presence of these catecholamines is intense vasoconstriction in the digits, decreased capillary refill times, and possibly peripheral cyanosis.

Unfortunately, fear can also elevate the cardiac rate and most alert children become fearful when put in the trauma situation. The child who is fearful but normovolemic may have tachycardia but also has normal distal capillary filling and bounding pulses. The child who is fearful and hypovolemic will have tachycardia with diminished capillary refill and weak peripheral pulses. In addition, vasoconstriction may be so marked that one may see cyanosis of the digits and around the lips. The child who is unconscious from a brain injury is much easier to evaluate, and the pulse may be used as an indicator of fluid volume, (unless brainstem herniation is imminent) in which case the patient becomes pathologically bradycardic.

Measurements of blood pressure in children are problematic. In order to get an accurate blood pressure the correct size cuff must be used, and it must be applied correctly. This automatically introduces a number of potential errors. In addition, there are a wide range of normal blood pressures in children (Table 23-4). Although a newborn generally has a systolic pressure of 80 mm Hg, a systolic pressure of 60 mm Hg may be normal for that patient. A useful mnemonic to remember the average systolic blood pressure in a child is 80 plus 2 times the age of the child in years.

Intravenous access must be established in all children who have suffered traumatic injury. In the field, only the percutaneous intravenous or intraosseous approaches should be used. Percutaneous vascular access should be attempted with the largest intravenous catheter possible. Sites for peripheral cannulation are at the elbow, back of the hand, and the saphenous vein at the ankle. With marked blood loss and subsequent vasoconstriction, percutaneous intravenous insertion attempts may be difficult at best.

The intraosseous infusion of fluids has regained popularity in situations where intravenous cannulation has failed and fluid infusion is necessary. It is most helpful in children less than 5 years of age where the marrow cavity has not filled with fat. It should only be used in the emergency situation and should be removed when venous access has been appropriately established. All intravenous fluids including blood and most medications can be given through intraosseous lines. Fluids can also be pushed through these lines, although some resistance will be met because of the bone's lack of distensibility. The site for insertion is the medial aspect of the tibia, one centimeter inferior and one centimeter medial to the tuberosity. A local anesthetic should be liberally infiltrated intradermally and subcutaneously prior to placement in the awake child. A bone marrow needle or one of a number of special needles manufactured as intraosseous devices can be used. A turkey thigh bone can be useful for practicing insertion techniques at home. The feeling of a "pop" indicates that the needle has passed through the cortex into the marrow cavity. Two "pops" indicate that the opposite side of the bone has been breached. Contraindications to intraosseous cannulation include fractures at or above the proposed insertion site, burns or abrasions at the insertion site. Interosseous infusion devices should not be left in place longer than 4 hours, as an increased incidence of osteomyelitis occurs.

The preferred initial intravenous solution in children, as in adults, is lactated Ringer's solution without dextrose. This solution contains physiologic amounts of sodium (135 milliequivalents) and chloride (110 milliequivalents). The lactate that is added to the solution (28 milliequivalents) is easily metabolized by the liver when normal perfusion returns and does not cause lactic acidosis. Glucose should not be added to the solution in the immediate post-injury period. Following injury, the normal endocrine response of the body in a child, as well as an adult, is to secrete a number of hormones including catecholamines, glucagon, growth hormone, and various steroids, all of which mobilize glucose from glycogen stores in the liver and muscles.[9,11,19] Added exogenous dextrose will not be utilized by the body and only serves to increase the serum glucose concentration to supernormal values.[10]

This elevation of serum glucose causes two problems. The first is an osmotic diuresis as the glucose concentration exceeds the ability of the kidneys to reabsorb it. The excessive glucose in the urine draws water into the urine and reduces the patient's vascular volume. This mechanism is similar to that seen in the dehydration in diabetic ketoacidosis. In the already hypovolemic patient, this diuresis will further decrease the effective circulating vascular volume, directly opposing what one is trying to accomplish in fluid resuscitation. The second undesirable effect has to do with incomplete utilization of the glucose molecule in injured brain tissue. There is evidence that when excessive glucose is presented to injured tissue, the glucose is not completely metabolized. This incomplete metabolism of sugar leads to a local build up of lactic acid, a drop in local pH, and results in a further decrease in vascular flow into that area, further hypoxia, and greater secondary injury.[16,32]

Therefore the ideal intravenous solution for children following traumatic injury is lactated Ringer's without glucose. This is given at maintenance rates with supplemental fluid boluses given for signs of hypovolemia. Two or three boluses of 20 ml/kg of body weight are given to restore volume. This fluid replaces both the intravascular and extravascular fluid losses that have occurred. If there is little or no response to three crystalloid fluid boluses, then 10 ml/kg of uncrossmatched type O, Rh-negative packed red blood cells are given. Further requirements for blood and fluid indicate ongoing hemorrhage and the necessity of surgical intervention.

EVALUATION OF DISABILITY AND IMMOBILIZATION

The presence of spinal column injury with an underlying spinal cord injury may not be immediately recognized but carries a high degree of morbidity and mortality. This may be due to the altered responsiveness of the child or distraction of the child's attention from the spinal injury to another area of the body where there is greater pain. Therefore, in all traumatized children great care should be taken in immobilizing the cervical vertebrae as well as the thoracic and lumbar axial skeleton.

This is accomplished by securing the child on a long board. Cervical spine immobilization should be a prime consideration while ensuring airway patency. The vast majority of cervical spine injuries in children occur at the levels of C-1, C-2, or C-3. Immobilization of the neck when significant trauma has occurred can prevent the disastrous results of completing a high cord lesion. Maintenance of midline position is the best way to immobilize the cervical spine. Otherwise, a well fitting cervical collar should be used.

Most children come in a variety of neck sizes, yet most cervical collars do not. Although rigid collars are preferred, sand bags or even bags of IV fluid wrapped in cloth will conform to the child's neck. Tape can be used to secure the head to the backboard. Following application of a collar, a cervical immobilizer device (CID) should be applied. The cervical collar serves to stop flexion and extension of the neck, while the CID stops rotational motion.

Further evaluation of the neurologic status should be limited to whether the child is normally awake, responds to verbal or painful stimuli, or is unresponsive. Evaluation of the movement of all limbs is made along with evaluation of pupillary response and size.

Further evaluation is useless and wastes precious time.

Extremity fractures should be immobilized in the position in which they lie using pneumatic splints or straight boards with towels. Although leg traction splints are used in adults, and their use is taught in all ATLS courses, our impression is that they are not very useful with children and often serve to further angulate a femur fracture. We prefer immobilization with pillows on a long board. Vascular injury in the pediatric trauma patient, particularly in the leg, is rare and most decreased pulses will return with reduction or pinning of the fracture. PASG trousers may be used to splint lower extremity fractures, but the leg should be wrapped in soft cloth if the PASG is to be on for any length of time. Skin burns have been described in the prolonged use of the PASG.

EXPOSURE

Children get cold very quickly. Although exposure of the patient is important in evaluating the child, every attempt must be made to limit the exposure for any length of time. The child rapidly loses heat to the surrounding environment by convection, conduction, evaporation, and radiation. Of these, conduction and convection cause the most rapid loss in the field. The child's skin is thinner than in the adult, fat is less abundant, blood flow to the skin and head is greater, and metabolic rate is much higher. Therefore, heat loss through the skin and the head is much greater than that of the adult, often three times as much. The metabolic requirements of a child for maintaining minimal bodily function is about 45 calories per kilogram per day. The adult requirement is on the order of 15 calories per kilogram per day for the same basic functions.

There are two major consequences of marked heat loss and lowering of body temperature. First, with cooling of the body, there is decreased perfusion of the skeletal mass in preference to the vital organs. This creates a state of hypoperfusion in the periphery and a change from aerobic metabolism to anaerobic metabolism, causing a build-up of excessive amounts of lactic acid. As the lactic acid builds the liver cannot further metabolize it and a state of generalized lactic acidosis develops. This leads to a reduced serum pH and detrimental effects on the myocardium with focal irritability and decreased contractility. This begins a downward spiral of increasing acidosis and decreasing cardiac function which may finally end in death.

The second effect of hypothermia has to do with the disruption of normal clotting mechanisms of the blood. As the body temperature is reduced, the coagulation system, as measured by prothrombin time (PT) and activated partial thromboplastin time (PTT) is markedly prolonged. Obviously, this is extremely detrimental to the patient if either solid organ laceration or brain injury with significant bleeding is present.

Every attempt should be made to warm the child. Aluminum lined blankets should be used to conserve heat loss. Radiant warmers should be turned on if available. IV solutions should be warmed. The rescue vehicle should also be warmed, even if it becomes uncomfortable for the crew to work.

SECONDARY SURVEY

The secondary survey is undertaken after the primary survey has been completed and the patient is hemodynamically stabilized. Each anatomic region of the body is examined for obvious injury such as laceration or abrasions, signs of injury such as hemotympanum in basilar skull fracture, or suggestion of other injury, such as tenderness over the spine or seatbelt marks on the abdomen. This survey directs the subsequent ordering of radiographs and laboratory studies and draws attention to potential surgical problems. Included in the secondary survey is a brief review of the child's medical history. These should include Allergies, Medications, Past illnesses, Last meal, and Events of the injury (AMPLE). Often parents are required for complete and accurate information on the younger child.

While a complete secondary survey should be done prior to transport from one hospital to another, the survey may have to be abbreviated due to weather conditions (e.g. cold) or the condition of the patient when transporting from the scene.

The head is examined by sight and feel. Palpation of the entire scalp may reveal unrecognized areas of injury evidenced by "bogginess" or crepitance. Occasionally, skull fractures may be identified, as will smaller, nonbleeding lacerations of the scalp. The eyes are next checked for pupillary response, symmetry, and size. Fundoscopic exam will identify abnormalities of the vitreous and fundus. Normal movement of the eyes: up, down, right, and left indicates intact cranial nerves III, IV, VI, and normal function of the muscles. The forehead, maxillary areas, and mandible are palpated for pain and instability. The mouth is checked for bleeding, laceration to the tongue or cheeks, missing or loose teeth, or malocclusion indicating midface fractures. Examination of the ears and nose for blood or CSF fluid is next. Otoscopic examination may reveal hemotympanum consistent with a basilar skull fracture. Other signs of basilar skull fracture include raccoon eyes (blood dissecting around the orbit) or Battle's sign (blood around the mastoid region of the skull).

The neck is then examined for evidence of trauma. If the patient is not intubated, they should be asked to talk in order to assess voice quality. Any hoarseness or gravel-like quality to there voice may indicate laryngeal injury. The skin over the larynx is carefully observed for signs of trauma. The trachea is assessed for abnormal position, indicating the possibility of a hemothorax or pneumothorax. Neck veins are assessed for distention, and the lateral soft tissues are palpated for any crepitance which might indicate air dissecting from a pneumothorax. The back of the neck is palpated for any "step-offs," indicating a possible fracture or dislocation. Pain and tenderness are signs of possible spinal column injury. If pain exists anywhere over the spinal column, one must assume underlying cord injury until proven otherwise, even in the face of normal radiographs. It is important to remember that a member of the resuscitation team should always hold the patient's head in a mid-line, neutral position until the cervical collar and CID are reapplied. Do not ever trust the child to hold still, as they inevitably will move to look at the activity going on around them.

Assessment of the thoracic cage begins with the observation of the chest wall movement during breathing. The motion should be symmetrical and full. In the older child, most motion will be in the chest and little of the abdomen. Younger children have greater abdominal motion and less chest motion during quiet respiration. Paradoxical motion with the chest moving inward and the abdominal wall moving outward may be the early sign of airway obstruction. The precordial area is auscultated for clarity as well as the proper location of heart tones. Lack of proper location or dullness of heart tones may indicate hemothorax, pneumothorax, or pericardial effusion. The bony thorax is palpated to find areas of tenderness (possible rib fractures) or crepitance (possible pneumothorax). Finally, auscultation of all lung fluids should occur, and the quality of air exchange on the right side is compared with the left.

The abdominal and flank region are next to be examined. The skin is noted for lacerations, abrasions, tire tracks, seat belt marks, and other signs of trauma. Auscultation is then performed in all quadrants of the abdomen. Since children may be frightened, palpation by hand may be inaccurate. Lightly palpating the abdomen while pretending to listen with the stethoscope is often distraction enough to the child for the examiner to get an accurate exam. The flanks should also be inspected and palpated for tenderness to the kidney region. Repeated exams may often be necessary in the frightened, uncooperative child, as the exam often changes depending on the degree of fright.

A common finding on abdominal examination is distention with tympany especially in the upper abdomen. This area may also be tender. The most common cause of this is gastric distention from swallowed air. The liberal use of a naso- or orogastric tube rectifies this finding.

The bony portion of the pelvis is next in line for palpation. While a larger number of pelvic fractures in children appear to be more stable than those in adults (unpublished personal communication), major ring disruption may be appreciated by this maneuver. Even if instability or tenderness is not appreciated, pelvic radiograph should be performed if the mechanism of injury puts the pelvic bones at risk for injury.

Visual inspection of the perineum for contusions, hematomas or bleeding is next. The urethral meatus is checked for blood. A urethrogram followed by cystogram may be necessary if evidence of trauma to the urethra or pelvis is present.

A rectal exam is performed to evaluate sphincter tone, the possibility of GI bleeding, and integrity of the rectal wall. The prostate gland of the young male, is not easily palpated, and the "absence" of one during palpation is not necessarily consistent with a disrupted urethra.

Each extremity is examined for obvious deformity, equality of pulses, and the presence of sensation. The child may be asked to move his or her toes, fingers, hands, feet, etc. to establish the intactness of neuromuscular function.

At this point in the examination, the patient should be rolled like a log to examine the back. One member of the team must maintain physical control of the patient's head and neck. Examination of the back is the most commonly forgotten portion of the exam. Yet, any tenderness over the spinal column may indicate the potential for spinal cord injury. In addition, significant bleeding lacerations may be missed if this half of the body is not examined.

It should be remembered that if at any time during the primary or secondary survey the patient's vital signs deteriorate, the examiner must immediately start anew with the ABCs. The logical progression of examination should then be repeated, even if it has already partially been done.

INTERFACILITY TRANSPORT

While increasing numbers of children are taken directly to a primary trauma hospital, a majority will still be taken to their local community hospital and are then transported either by ground or air to a tertiary facility. Studies confirm that the transfer of very ill children from community to tertiary institutions where pediatric facilities are available increases survival.[29] This usually occurs in areas of the country where rural communities are great distances from the trauma center. The physicians at these hospitals are generally not as comfortable treating children as are those at a children's hospital simply because the number of children is not large. When a traumatized child is brought to these facilities, there is a great deal of tension and fear. The physicians treat most things in a rote, almost mechanical way as is taught in the ATLS[1] course. The emergency department physicians, surgeons, and anesthesiologists at these hospitals are usually uncomfortable with the care of critically injured children and generally request transport early and often. Therefore, children who have not suffered significant injuries are none-the-less transported. There is no place for discussing the quality of care or intent of care in these situations. The child must be seen by someone who is going to be complete and thorough in their evaluation and understands the differences in diagnosis and treatment between pediatric and adult trauma.

The transport team's duty is to safely expedite the movement from one hospital situation to another with minimum morbidity and mortality. As such, it is the responsibility of the team to reevaluate the ABCs and secondary survey before and during transport. Additionally, paying meticulous attention to securing tubes and making sure all tubes are patent obviates problems during transport. Deliberate evaluation and stabilization should be done prior to transfer. Recent studies show that the sicker or more injured the child is, the greater the likelihood for deterioration during transport.[14]

One area of great concern that we have is the "clearing" of the cervical spine at the referring institution. Many times we have heard that "the cervical spines have been cleared by the lateral cervical spine x-ray." There is a misconception that this single x-ray view of the cervical spine, even if the alignment is correct, can rule out injury to the cervical cord. Nothing could be further from the truth. The cervical spine is only cleared when either a completely normal exam has been performed on a neurologically intact patient or a complete cervical spine series including lateral, AP, odontoid, and possibly flexion and extension views are obtained in someone who is not neurologically intact. Even when all films appear normal, there is a syndrome seen mostly in children called the SCIWORA syndrome[25]. In this syndrome, one may have totally normal x-rays but have an underlying injury to the spinal cord. SCIWORA stands for Spinal Cord Injury Without Radiologic Abnormality. This syndrome is very real and, in the comatose patient, may require Sensory Evoked Response Potential (SERP) exams to confirm the injury. Therefore, when there is the slightest doubt about the possibility of a spinal cord injury to the neck, one should leave the cervical collar in place or apply one for transport.

Oxygen should be administered to all trauma victims during transport. When air evacuation is performed, this is particularly important. All tubes in the patient should be checked for patency and made secure or retaped. Retaping an unsecured tube in the ambulance is difficult. In a helicopter it is dangerous for the patient and crew alike. Prior to transport, copies should be made of all x-rays, and the team should at the least review the latest chest film. If an endotracheal tube is present it should be checked for proper location and care should be taken to be sure it is not in one of the main stem bronchi. If it is, its position should be corrected prior to transport. Pneumothorax should be looked for. If one is present a chest tube should be inserted prior to transport, especially if the transport is to be by air. The stomach should be emptied with a nasogastric or an orogastric (if a basilar skull fracture is known or suspected) tube. Comatose patients, even if they have a patient airway, should have their stomachs emptied with a gastric tube.

All fractures should be completely immobilized and the patient secured to the transport bed. Warm blankets and radiant wraps should be secured around the patient to decrease heat loss.

If the patient is to be transported by air, appropriate monitoring devices need to be applied including automatic blood pressure monitoring, pulse oximetry, ECG monitoring, and end tidal CO_2 monitors if available. Doppler stethoscopes which transmit to the crew's helmets are also useful. All tubes that go into the patient must be checked for patency and need to be monitored during flight. If the endotracheal tube has a cuff, the volume of the cuff may have to be changed during ascent or descent. Everything should be taped securely so that the vibration of the aircraft does not dislodge anything.

REFERENCES

1. Ali, J and others: Advanced trauma life support instructor manual, Illinois, 1989, American College of Surgeons.
2. American College of Surgeons, Committee on Trauma: Field categorization of trauma patients and hospital trauma index, *Bull Am Coll Surg* 65:28, 1980
3. Bever DG, Veenker CH: An illness-injury severity index for non-physician emergency medical personnel, *EMT J* 3:45, 1979.
4. Bodai BI, Smith JP, Blaisdell FW: The role of emergency room thoracotomy in blunt trauma, *J Trauma* 22:487, 1982.
5. Bowers SA, Marshall LF: Outcome in two hundred consecutive cases of severe head injury treated in San Diego Country: a prospective analysis, *Neurosurgery* 6:237, 1980.
6. Champion HR and others: Assessment of injury severity: the triage index, *Crit Care Med* 8:201, 1980.
7. Champion HR and others: Trauma score, *Crit Care Med* 9:627, 1981.
8. Cowley RA and others: An economical and proven helicopter program for transporting the emergency critically ill and injured patient in Maryland, *J Trauma* 13:1029, 1973.
9. Drucker WR and others: Metabolic aspects of hemorrhagic shock: changes in intermediary metabolism during hemorrhage and repletion of blood, *Surg Forum* 9:49, 1958.
10. Elwyn DH and others: Influence of increasing carbohydrate intake on glucose kinetics in impaired patients, *Ann Surg* 190:117, 1979.
11. Gann DS, Dallmarr MF, Engelund WC: Reflux control and modulation of ACTH and corticosteroids, *Int Rev Physiology* 24:157, 1981.
12. Garcia VF and others: Rib fracture in children: a marker of severe trauma, *J Trauma* 30(6): 695-700, 1990.
13. Gormican SP: CRAMS scale: field triage of trauma victims, *Am Emerg Med* 11:132, 1982.
14. Kanter RK, Tompkins JM: Adverse events during interhospital transport: physiologic deterioration associated with pretransport severity of illness, *Pediatrics*, 84:43-8, 1989.
15. Kirkpatrick JR, Youmans RL: Trauma Index: an aide in the evaluation of injury victims, *J Trauma* 11:711, 1971.
16. LeBlanc MH and others: Glucose affects the severity of hypoxic-ischemic brain injury in newborn piglets, *Stroke* 24(7):1055-62, 1993.
17. Martin RR and others: Prospective evaluation of preoperative fluid resuscitation in hypotensive patients with penetrating truncal injury: a preliminary report, *J Trauma* 33(3):354-61, 1992.

18. Mihm FG, Halperin BD: Noninvasive detection of profound arterial desaturation using a pulse oximetry device, *Anesthesia* 62:85, 1986.
19. Moore FD: *Metabolic care of the surgical patient,* Philadelphia, 1959, W.B. Saunders.
20. Nakayama DK and others: The use of drugs in emergency airway management in pediatric trauma, *Ann Surg* 216(2):205-11, 1992.
21. National Center for Health Statistics: Vital statistics of the United States—1986, Vol 2, Department of Health and Human Services, Washington DC, 1988, U.S. Government Printing Office.
22. Newman KD and others: The lap belt complex: intestinal and lumbar spin injury in children, *J Trauma* 30(9):1133-8, 1990.
23. Oldham KT and others: Blunt liver injury in childhood: evolution of therapy and current perspective, *Surgery* 100(3):542-9, 1986.
24. Oreskovich M: Prehospital surgical care, Presented to the 67th Annual Clinical Congress, American College of Surgeons, San Francisco, 1981.
25. Pang D, Pollack IF: Spinal cord injury without radiographic abnormality in children—the SCIWORA syndrome, *J Trauma* 29(5):654-64, 1989.
26. Pearl RH and others: Splenic injury: a 5-year update with improved results and changing criteria for conservative management, *J Pediatr Surg* 24(5): 428-31, 1989.
27. Peclet MJ: Thoracic trauma in children: an indicator of increased mortality, *J Pediatr Surg* 25(9):961-5, 1990.
28. Pennsylvania Trauma Systems Foundation, 1991-95 Standards for Trauma Center Accreditation.
29. Pollack MM and others: Improved outcome from tertiary center pediatric intensive care: a statewide comparison of tertiary and nontertiary care facilities, *Crit Care Med* 19:150-9, 1991.
30. Ramenofsky ML and others: Maximum survival in pediatric trauma: the ideal system, *J Trauma* 24(9):818-23, 1984.
31. Ramenofsky ML and others: The predictive validity of the pediatric trauma score, *J Trauma* 28(7): 1038-42, 1988.
32. Robertson CS and others: The effect of glucose administration on carbohydrate metabolism after head injury, *J Neurosurgery* 74(1):43-50, 1991.
33. Savit CJ and others: Safety belt injuries in children with lap belt ecchymosis: CT findings in 61 patients, *Amer J Roentgenology* 157(1):111-4, 1991.
34. Simeone FA: Shock. In Davis L, editor, *Christopher's textbook of surgery,* Philadelphia, 1964, W.B. Saunders.
35. Teasdale G, Jennet B: Assessment of coma and impaired consciousness: a practical scale, *Lancet* 2:81, 1974.
36. Tepas JJ III and others: The pediatric trauma score as a predictor of injury severity: an objective assessment, *J Trauma* 82(4):424-9, 1988.
37. Waller AE, Baber SP, Szocha A: Childhood injury deaths: material analysis and geographic variation, *Am J Public Health* 79(3):310-4, 1989.
38. West JG, Cales RH, Gazzeniga AB: Impact of regionalization: Orange County experience, *Arch Surg* 118:740, 1983.
39. West JG and others: A method for evaluating field triage criteria, *J Trauma* 26:655, 1986.

24

TRANSPORT OF PEDIATRIC BURN PATIENTS

CHARLES W. BREAUX, JR.

The chances that a physician providing emergency care will encounter a burn patient are great, given that 2 to 2.5 million people seek medical attention for burn injuries annually in the United States. Most of these patients are treated as outpatients, but 60,000 to 100,000 require hospitalization with 10,000 deaths. Burn injuries are a major health problem in the pediatric population. Fires, burns, and deaths associated with fires are the third leading cause of accidental death in children aged 1 to 14 years (behind motor-vehicle accidents and drownings) and the leading cause of accidental death in the home in this age group.[11]

Burn injuries result from exposure to flames, scalding liquids, hot objects, caustic chemicals, or electricity. Younger children have more scald burns from kitchen (e.g., pulling cups of hot beverage, pots of boiling water, or skillets of hot grease off counters) and bathroom (e.g., bathtub immersion) incidents. Older children and adolescents are burned more often by flames from playing or working with fire.

The effects of the injury in burn patients can be wide-ranging. Local effects occur through the tissue destruction itself. Systemic effects can arise from circulatory derangements early on and hypermetabolism or infection later. If the circumstances of the burn are such that a smoke inhalation injury occurs, the respiratory insult may be of much more consequence than the cutaneous injury. In addition, burn patients may sustain other injuries (e.g., head trauma, fractures) from mechanisms of injury associated with the burn (e.g., falls, motor-vehicle accidents).

INITIAL MANAGEMENT

Immediate measures (life-saving steps)

The first priority is to stop the burn injury. At the scene, a victim on fire should be made to "stop, drop, and roll" or be wrapped in a blanket to extinguish the flames, and any smoldering clothing should be removed. With scald injuries, if clothing still holds the hot liquid, it should be quickly removed, and the wound can be briefly rinsed with cool water. Chemical burns should be copiously irrigated with water for 20 to 30 minutes to rinse off and dilute the chemical agent. Care should be taken to avoid spreading the caustic agent to unburned areas or to emergency personnel.

After the burning has been halted, airway patency and ventilation are of utmost concern. When these are clinical problems, they are usually associated with flame burns. If there is evidence of a smoke inhalation injury (e.g., history of burn in an enclosed space or physical evidence of facial burns, singed eyebrows and nasal hair, or carbonaceous sputum), oxygen should be administered via face mask. As facial and laryngeal edema develops following the burn, patency of the airway may become threatened. In this situation, early invasive airway control by endotracheal intubation should be performed. Airway concerns will be further discussed below.

Patients with significant burns will require intravenous (IV) fluids for circulatory support. This is especially true in infants and younger children who have higher fluid needs to begin with than do older pediatric patients and adults. One or two large-bore peripheral IV catheters should be inserted, and an infusion of lactated Ringer's (LR) solution should be started. Guidelines for fluid requirements will be discussed below.

Assessment of the burn injury (history and physical examination)

When taking the history, all pertinent details regarding the burn injury should be obtained, including when and under what circumstances it occurred and the nature of the burning agent. If the wounds are out of proportion to the story, or the report is unclear or changes, one must suspect child abuse or neglect and investigate appropriately, as a significant proportion of acute pediatric burn hospitalizations are due to inflicted injury. Important historical information includes any preexisting chronic or acute illness, current medications, and immunization status.

During the physical examination, the extent of the burn injury in terms of body surface area (BSA) must be determined accurately in order to guide fluid requirements during resuscitation and disposition beyond the emergency room. Errors in estimation of the extent of burn wounds are commonplace in community hospital emergency departments. Hammond and Ward found that, in 46% of referred cases, the pretransfer estimation of burn size was 25% higher than the charted size in their burn center; the estimated size was 100% higher than the actual size in 18% of cases.[8] Baack and others found that the outside emergency physician overestimated the extent of burn by more than 50% in 34% of patients helicopter transported to their center and underestimated the extent by more than 50% in 3% of patients.[2] The "Rule of Nines" gives a fair approximation of burn size in adults. However, in children, the proportionate surface area of the head is larger and that of the legs smaller in comparison to adults. A specialized pediatric BSA chart should be used to accurately calculate the burn size for a given age (Figure 24-1).[9]

The burn depth should also be determined because this parameter is an indicator of injury severity and influences patient disposition. *First-degree* burns involve the epidermis of the skin, are erythematous and painful, and are not blistered. They heal readily with minimal or no care and should not be used to calculate the BSA extent of the burn or determine patient admission or transfer. *Second-degree* burns extend variable distances into the dermis of the skin, are red or mottled in appearance, are covered with blisters or are open and wet, and are quite painful. These partial-thickness wounds will heal with good resuscitation, nutrition, and local wound care, and should be included in calculations of the extent of the burn. *Third-degree* burns extend all the way through the skin, are covered with dark or waxy white leathery eschar, and are anesthetic. These full-thickness wounds will ultimately require debridement and surgical coverage and are also included in burn extent calculations. Early on, especially with scald burns, it may be difficult to distinguish deep second-degree from third-degree wounds. During the early resuscitative phase of burn care, this distinction is not that important, as both depths of burn can be treated the same way.

Electrical injuries may result in more tissue destruction than is apparent on the surface. Deep muscle, nerve, and vascular damage may occur as the electrical current passes through the body. The ramifications of these injuries will be discussed below.

If present, other injuries must be picked up during the physical examination. The most life-threatening of these is an inhalation injury with or without carbon monoxide (CO) toxicity. Facial burns, singed nasal hairs and eyebrows, carbonaceous sputum, hoarseness, and/or wheezing suggest a smoke inhalation injury. CO toxicity manifests itself with increasingly severe neurologic symptoms as the carboxyhemoglobin (CO-Hgb) level rises. Patients are asymptomatic with CO-Hgb levels less than 15%; headaches, nausea, and fatigue occur at levels of 15% to 30%; visual impairment, ataxia, behavioral disturbances, and shock are seen with levels of 40% to 50%;

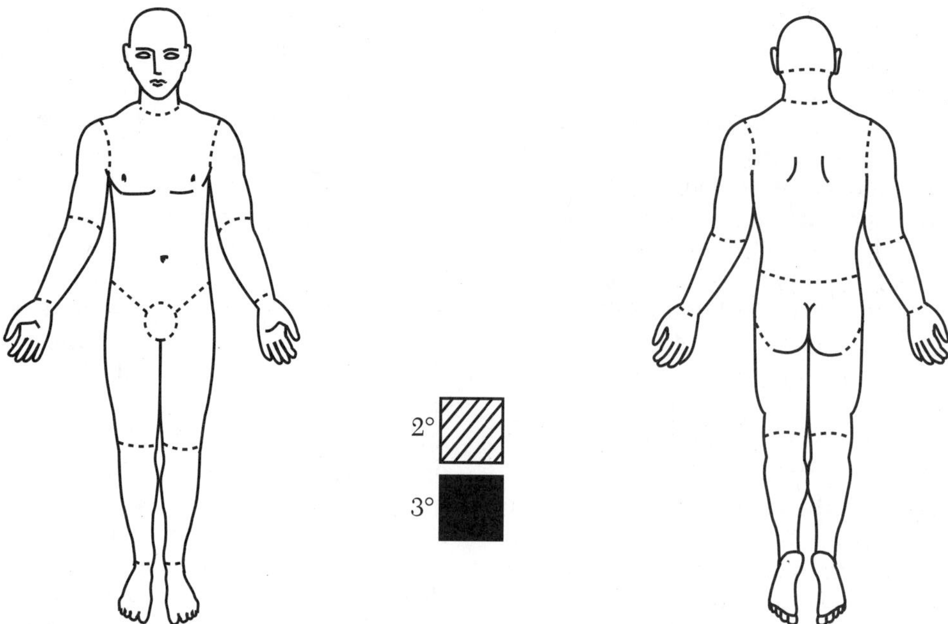

Area	Age in Years						% 2°	% 3°	Total
	0	1	5	10	15	Adult			
Head	19	17	13	11	9	7			
Neck	2								
Ant. Trunk	13								
Post. Trunk	13								
R. Buttock	$2\frac{1}{2}$								
L. Buttock	$2\frac{1}{2}$								
Genitalia	1								
R. U. Arm	4								
L. U. Arm	4								
R. L. Arm	3								
L. L. Arm	3								
R. Hand	$2\frac{1}{2}$								
L. Hand	$2\frac{1}{2}$								
R. Thigh	$5\frac{1}{2}$	$6\frac{1}{2}$	8	$8\frac{1}{2}$	9	$9\frac{1}{2}$			
L. Thigh	$5\frac{1}{2}$	$6\frac{1}{2}$	8	$8\frac{1}{2}$	9	$9\frac{1}{2}$			
R. Leg	5	5	$5\frac{1}{2}$	6	$6\frac{1}{2}$	7			
L. Leg	5	5	$5\frac{1}{2}$	6	$6\frac{1}{2}$	7			
R. Foot	$3\frac{1}{2}$								
L. Foot	$3\frac{1}{2}$								

______________________________, M.D.

Date: ______________________________

Fig. 24-1. Lund and Browder chart for estimation of burn size.

and levels greater than 50% can result in permanent damage to the central nervous system or death.[6] If another mechanism of injury occurs concurrently with the burn (e.g., fall, motor-vehicle accident), other injuries must be searched for, including head trauma, torso injuries, and fractures.

Finally, the patient should be accurately weighed early before the administration of much resuscitation fluid. This "dry" weight is important for calculation of fluid and nutritional requirements and drug dosages.

Stabilization

Patients with suspected smoke inhalation injury or CO toxicity should initially be placed on 100% oxygen by face mask or endotracheal tube. Although CO has a high affinity for the hemoglobin molecule, it can be displaced by high concentrations of oxygen. The half-life of CO-Hgb in room air is 250 minutes, and it is reduced to 40 to 50 minutes in 100% oxygen.[6] Once the CO-Hgb level is less than 7%, the inspired oxygen concentration can be weaned. The use of hyperbaric oxygen in the treatment of CO toxicity is controversial. This modality should only be considered in patients with high CO-Hgb levels (i.e., greater than 40%) and where there is a nearby facility with a hyperbaric chamber. Otherwise, ensuring adequate ventilation with 100% oxygen will suffice and should not be neglected while trying to set up transport for the patient.

Indications for endotracheal intubation in the burn patient are listed in Box 24-1. If intubation is necessary or may be necessary, it should be performed early before edema threatens the airway and makes intubation difficult. This is especially important in the pediatric patient with a relatively narrow airway diameter. As large an endotracheal tube as possible, taking into account the small, delicate pediatric airway, should be used to facilitate pulmonary toilet. The tube must be anchored securely. In patients with facial burns, taping the tube in place may be difficult. Umbilical tape or IV tubing can be tied tightly to the tube and then tied around the patient's head to secure the tube. Following intubation, a chest x-ray film is mandatory to ensure adequate placement.

The patient with smoke inhalation injury or CO toxicity must be monitored closely. Copious secretions may be produced in the airway requiring frequent suctioning. Pulse oximetry is helpful to document adequate or improving oxygen saturations in real-time, although high saturation measured by oximetry does not rule out carbon monoxide poisoning (see Chapter 30). Serial arterial blood gases, including CO-Hgb measurements, are helpful in determining need for intubation, ventilator adjustments, and improvement in CO toxicity.

Pediatric patients with greater than 15% BSA burns will require IV fluid resuscitation. Peripheral venous access is preferred, given that central venous catheterization is more difficult to perform and fraught with more complications in younger children and infants. However, a central venous catheter may be necessary early on in the patient with extensive extremity burns or later for hemodynamic monitoring, especially in patients on high ventilator settings. Ideally, the IV catheter should be placed through unburned tissue, although this becomes more difficult with extensive burns. The IV catheter should be dressed as securely and aseptically as possible.

Burned infants and children require more resuscitation fluids than do adults.[7,10] The volume needed in the first 24 hours is best approximated by the Parkland formula plus maintenance fluid requirements. The Parkland formula dictates 4 ml/kg/% BSA burn, half given in the first 8 hours from the time of injury and half given in the next 16 hours. Pediatric maintenance fluid requirements can be estimated at 100 ml/kg/d for the first 10 kg, 50 ml/kg/d for the second 10 kg, and

BOX 24-1 INDICATIONS FOR ENDOTRACHEAL INTUBATION IN BURN PATIENTS

1. Deep facial burns, especially of lips, mouth, neck, or oropharynx.
2. Significant smoke inhalation injury.
3. Significant CO toxicity (to truly deliver 100% oxygen).
4. Massive body burns, especially with circumferential chest burns.

20 ml/kg/d for any more kg. An example of a fluid resuscitation calculation is shown in Box 24-2. Note that maintenance fluids are given in addition to replacement fluids. The resuscitation fluid should be a balanced salt solution (e.g., lactated Ringer's), since calculated losses are based on the sodium deficit from the extracellular space. Administration of hypotonic fluids for burn resuscitation in the first day can result in significant hyponatremia. The initial fluids should be free of dextrose, since burn patients demonstrate glucose intolerance early on. Younger patients on IV fluids without dextrose, especially infants, should be monitored closely for hypoglycemia. After the first 24 hours postburn, the IV fluids are decreased to a maintenance rate, and a hypotonic solution containing dextrose and potassium is added (e.g., 5% dextrose in $\frac{1}{4}$ to $\frac{1}{2}$ normal saline plus 10 to 20 mEq potassium chloride/l). Colloid solutions (e.g., 5% albumin, dextran-40, dextran-70, hetastarch) are generally not administered until capillary permeability decreases 8 to 24 hours postburn.

The single best indicator of volume status over time is urine output, given normal renal function and nonglycosuric urine. Thus, major burn patients require urethral catheterization for accurate urine output measurement. The target urine output for pediatric burn patients is 1 to 1.5 ml/kg/hr (as opposed to 0.5 to 1 ml/kg/hr in adults). Other markers, including capillary refill, heart rate, mental status, blood pressure, hematocrit, venous PO_2, and venous oxygen saturation are helpful in the global evaluation of hemodynamic adequacy. However, each of these may be obscured by other factors such as pain, anxiety, or associated injuries. The calculation of resuscitation fluids is only an estimate of where to start. If signs of hypovolemia develop (especially decreased urine output), lactated Ringer's solution administered within the first 24 hours or colloid solution after 8 to 24 hours postburn can be given in boluses of 10 to 20 ml/kg.

If the urine is dark in patients with electrical burns, myoglobin from rhabdomyolysis should be assumed to be present. A urine sample can be sent for confirmation of myoglobinuria, but treatment should begin immediately. A brisk diuresis must be maintained (greater than 2 ml/kg/hr) to try to clear the pigment from the urine. Fluid administration can be increased, and mannitol in doses of 0.5 gm/kg can be given. In addition, sodium bicarbonate can be given to the patient to alkalinize the urine to increase myoglobin solubility.

Patients with circumferential third-degree burns of the extremities may develop inadequate distal arterial blood flow as subeschar edema develops. The adequacy of distal perfusion can be assessed by palpation or Doppler monitoring of the pulse and observation of capillary refill. In addition, a pulse oximeter placed on a digit of the involved extremity can give a constant readout of the pulse and oxygen saturation. If distal perfu-

BOX 24-2 EXAMPLE OF FLUID RESUSCITATION CALCULATIONS FOR A 14 KG PATIENT WITH 50% BSA BURNS

Parkland formula fluids:

4 ml/kg/% BSAB(14 kg)(50% BSAB) = 2800 ml over first 24 hr
1400 ml given over first 8 hr = 175 ml/hr
1400 ml given over next 16 hr = 87.5 ml/hr

Maintenance fluids:

100 ml/kg/d(10 kg) + 50 ml/kg/d(4 kg) = 1200 ml/d = 50 ml/hr

IV fluid rate:

First 8 hr: 175 ml/hr + 50 ml/hr = 225 ml/hr
Next 16 hr: 87.5 ml/hr + 50 ml/hr = 137.5 ml/hr

sion becomes threatened, escharotomies should be performed medially and laterally. No anesthesia is necessary as the third-degree eschar is anesthetic. The incisions must be deep enough to go completely through the eschar which pops apart because of the underlying pressure. There is usually little bleeding from the escharotomies due to coagulation of the superficial veins by the burn injury; small bleeding sites can be controlled with epinephrine-saline soaked sponges or suture ligatures. There should be immediate improvement in distal perfusion.

An ileus may develop in patients with burns greater than a 20% BSA. Vomiting with possible aspiration can result, and ventilation may be impaired due to limitation of diaphragmatic excursion from gastric dilatation. The stomach should be decompressed with a nasogastric tube. An orogastric tube is easier to place in infants and does not interfere with their obligate nasal breathing.

Thermoregulation can become a critical problem in pediatric burn patients. Compared to adults, infants and young children have a high BSA-to-mass ratio, resulting in increased conductive and convective heat loss. In addition, the burn injury damages the heat-retentive barrier function of the skin. Normothermia must be maintained with higher room temperatures, radiant warmers, heating blankets, and minimizing patient exposure.

Local wound care should be initiated in the primary hospital emergency room. Soot, dirt, gross debris, and loose skin should be gently removed with water and a dilute detergent soap. Excessive cooling of the patient must be avoided. The receiving burn team will want to perform its own assessment of the wounds, so one may be inclined not to dress the wounds for transfer. However, this tendency must be balanced against the length of time of transport and increasing microbial contamination of the wounds. How thoroughly the patient's wounds are dressed should thus depend on how soon he will arrive at the receiving burn center. For short transfers of less than 1 hour, the patient may be wrapped in sterile sheets/towels. With transfers of 1 to 4 hours, torso and extremity wounds should be wrapped occlusively with sterile gauze. For transfers exceeding 4 hours' duration, a topical antimicrobial agent (most commonly, silver sulfadiazine cream) should be applied to such wounds and then occlusive sterile gauze dressings. A petroleum-based antibiotic ointment (e.g., neosporin, polysporin) can be applied to facial burns which are then left open.

What drugs might be given to the burn patient? Generally, systemic antibiotics are not administered in early burn care but are reserved for later infectious complications. The patient's tetanus immunization history must be checked and prophylaxis given as needed.[4] Analgesics should be administered to patients in pain, especially before wound manipulation such as cleaning and dressing. For patients with minor burns (i.e., less than 15% BSA), oral (PO) analgesics (e.g. acetaminophen, codeine) can be given. Major burn patients with IV lines in place should receive parenteral analgesics (e.g., morphine, meperidine). The IM route should be avoided due to the possibility of altered circulation and erratic absorption.

INDICATIONS FOR TRANSFER TO A BURN CENTER

There are 138 burn centers in the United States with hospital beds designated specifically for burn patients.[3] It is estimated that 40% of all patients requiring inpatient care for burn injuries are admitted to designated burn centers.[5] Such facilities can provide optimal care for patients with significant burn injuries. The American Burn Association has devised guidelines for the development and operation of burn centers, including organizational structure, minimum census levels, personnel requirements, necessary facilities and equipment, and programs for rehabilitation, quality assurance, education, and research.[1] Patients admitted to a burn center are treated according to specific protocols by a dedicated multidisciplinary "burn team" including physicians, nurses, physical and occupational therapists, respiratory therapists, dieticians, pharmacists, and social workers.

Burn injuries usually requiring referral to a burn center as determined by the American Burn Association are listed in Box 24-3.[1] Since several transfer guidelines refer to the BSA involvement of the burn, an accurate

BOX 24-3 INDICATIONS FOR TRANSFER TO A BURN CENTER*

1. Second- and third-degree burns: greater than 10% BSA in patients less than 10 or greater than 50 years of age.
2. Second- and third-degree burns: greater than 20% BSA in patients in other age groups.
3. Second- and third-degree burns involving the face, hands, feet, genitalia, perineum, or major joints.
4. Third-degree burns: greater than 5% BSA in any age group.
5. Electrical burns, including lightning.
6. Chemical burns.
7. Burn injury with inhalation injury.
8. Burn injury in patients with significant preexisting medical disease.
9. Patients with burns and concomitant trauma.
10. Burn injury in patients who will require special social/emotional and/or long-term rehabilitation.
11. Hospitals without qualified personnel or equipment for the care of children should transfer pediatric burn patients to a burn center with these capabilities.

* (Adapted from the American Burn Association guidelines)[1]
J Burn Care Rehabil 11:100, 1990.

estimate of the extent of the injury must be made. There should be a lower threshold for transfer of pediatric patients, especially infants and toddlers, as many primary hospitals lack the specialized personnel and equipment to care for young children. If there is doubt about whether a patient would best be treated in a burn center, then a telephone consultation should be obtained with a burn center physician.

PREPARATION FOR TRANSFER

If necessary, transfer is ideally accomplished early before complications occur, making the move more difficult. Early telephone contact should thus be made with a burn center physician if transfer of a patient is desired, especially if the burn injury is moderate or severe. Sufficient information regarding the circumstances of the burn and an accurate description of the burn wounds and any associated injuries should be discussed to allow the receiving physician to make a decision regarding transfer. If accepted for transfer, matters of management such as airway control, resuscitation fluids, wound dressings, and need for escharotomies should be discussed with the receiving burn physician so that they can be initiated promptly and consistently. Many burn centers have developed a burn transfer form, usually in conjunction with a pediatric BSA chart, which is supplied to referring hospitals to expedite the transfer process and facilitate communication between physicians.[8,12] A burn transfer checklist can also be used to ensure that important details of assessment and treatment are not forgotten (Table 24-1).

Any patient who is endotracheally intubated or who is seriously enough injured to require frequent assessment and intervention should be accompanied by a highly skilled transport team with specific pediatric training and experience. The patient should be stabilized as thoroughly as possible (as outlined above) before leaving the referring hospital. A copy of the medical records and x-ray films should be sent with the patient.

Should the patient be sent by ground ambulance or air transport? Certainly, the transport distance and severity of injury of the patient should be taken into account. In a study of helicopter transport of acute burn patients, Baack and others found that 56% of the patients did not require a critical intervention within the first 24 hours postburn.[2] They felt that these patients did not benefit from helicopter transport, and therefore it was inappropriate in these cases. Based on their experience, they recommend that helicopter transport be reserved for patients requiring a formal IV fluid resuscitation, suspected of having a smoke inhalation injury, or needing an escharotomy.

TABLE 24-1 BURN TRANSFER CHECKLIST

Assessment	*Treatment (as needed)*	*Preparation for transfer*	*Potential complications*
History: When/Where/How? Child abuse? Current illnesses/ medications Immunizations up-to-date? Any allergies? Physical examination: Inhalation injury/CO toxicity Burn extent (% BSA) Burn depth Other injuries Weight Other data (as needed): Arterial blood gases (+ CO-Hgb) Chest x-ray film Other labs, x-ray films	Supplemental oxygen (+ pulse oximetry) Endotracheal tube Cardiac monitor IV fluids Foley catheter Escharotomies Nasogastric tube Thermoregulation Wound cleansing/ dressings Tetanus prophylaxis Analgesics	Call burn center physician early: Describe patient & injury Discuss management Discuss mode of transfer Insurance information Burn transfer form Patient accompanied by: Physician Nurse Copy medical records Copy x-ray films Choose mode of transfer: Ground ambulance Helicopter Airplane	Loss of airway Loss of IV access Hypovolemia Cardiac dysrhythmias

PRECAUTIONS TO TAKE AND COMPLICATIONS TO ANTICIPATE DURING TRANSPORT

Airway maintenance is of utmost concern during transport. A major burn patient whose airway is threatened by increasing edema should be intubated before, not during, transport. If uncertain whether to intubate the patient, go ahead and do it; the tube can always be removed later. An endotracheal tube that is in place needs to stay there during the trip. It must be securely taped or tied in place as described above and watched carefully. Any intubated patient should be accompanied by a physician or highly experienced team member capable of reintubating the patient.

Continued IV access is also important in burn patients requiring significant fluid resuscitation. It is prudent to place two IV catheters in case one is lost during transport. The IV lines must be taped or sutured securely. Adjustment of IV fluids is frequently necessary in burn patients undergoing resuscitation. Treat and others found this to be true in 42 (33%) of 129 acute burn patients during air evacuation to the United States Army Institute of Surgical Research.[13] In the majority of cases (38 of 42, 90%), fluid boluses were needed to treat hypovolemia. Fluid intake and output by the patient during transport must be accurately recorded and related to the receiving physician.

Patients with electrical injuries may have disturbances in cardiac rhythm. These abnormalities occur most often in the first 24 hours postinjury. Cardiac monitoring is thus necessary before and during transport, and one must be prepared to treat life-threatening dysrhythmias.

REFERENCES

1. American Burn Association: Hospital and prehospital resources for optimal care of patients with burn injury: guidelines for development and operation of burn centers, *J Burn Care Rehabil* 11:97-104, 1990.
2. Baack BR and others: Helicopter transport of the patient with acute burns, *J Burn Care Rehabil* 12:229-33, 1991.
3. Committee on the Organization and Delivery of Burn Care, American Burn Association: *Burn care resources in North America 1993-1994,* Cincinnati, 1993, American Burn Association.
4. Committee on Trauma, American College of Surgeons: *Advanced trauma life support course for physicians,* Chicago, 1989, American College of Surgeons.
5. Dimick AR, Brigham PA, Sheehy EM: The development of burn centers in North America, *J Burn Care Rehabil* 14:284-299, 1993.

6. Fein A, Leff A, Hopewell PC: Pathophysiology and management of the complications resulting from fire and the inhaled products of combustion: review of the literature, *Crit Care Med* 8:94-8, 1980.
7. Graves TA and others: Fluid resuscitation of infants and children with massive thermal injury, *J Trauma* 28:1656-9, 1988.
8. Hammond JS, Ward CG: Transfers from emergency room to burn center: errors in burn size estimate, *J Trauma* 27:1161-5, 1987.
9. Lund CC, Browder NC: The estimation of areas of burns, *Surg Gynecol Obstet* 79:352-8, 1944.
10. Merrell SW and others: Fluid resuscitation in thermally injured children, *Am J Surg* 152:664-9, 1986.
11. National Safety Council: *Accident Facts,* Chicago, 1991, National Safety Council.
12. Stein JM, Stein ED: Safe transfer of civilian burn casualties, *JAMA* 238:489-92, 1977.
13. Treat RC and others: Air evacuation of thermally injured patients: principles of treatment and results, *J Trauma* 20:275-9, 1980.

25

TRAUMATIC HEAD OR SPINAL INJURY

ROBERT T. MANSFIELD
DONALD W. MARION
PATRICK M. KOCHANEK

Trauma is the leading cause of death in children between the ages of 1 and 14.[61] Head injury is present in 80% of severely traumatized children and is the most severe injury in 60% of cases.[59] Mortality from severe head injury ranges from 6%[15] to 21.5%.[60] The mortality rate of trauma with head injury is almost triple that of trauma without head injury.[59] Morbidity is also high, with many children suffering permanent neurologic sequelae. These patients often require crucial, life-saving therapy immediately after the injury and during transport to a pediatric trauma center. A basic understanding of the pathophysiology and management of head injury is essential to optimize the chances of a good outcome.

Basic anatomy and physiology

Structure. The brain is encased in the rigid cranium and bathed in cerebrospinal fluid which acts as a cushion. Although the cranium is obviously an important protective feature, the sharp ridges along its base can cause physical damage when the brain moves within the cranium as in acceleration/deceleration types of injuries. The cerebral hemispheres are separated by the falx cerebri, and the cerebellum is similarly divided by the falx cerebelli. The tentorium cerebelli separates the cerebrum (anterior fossa) from the cerebellum (posterior fossa). These tough fibrous partitions restrict movement and expansion of the cranial contents and play a role in compression and herniation syndromes.

The main intracranial components are brain (about 87% of the volume), blood (about 4%), and cerebrospinal fluid (about 9%).[84] Because of very limited room for expansion within the rigid cranium, any increase in volume (e.g., subdural or epidural hematomas or brain swelling) requires a compensatory decrease in the volume of another component (e.g., egress of CSF or decreased blood in pial veins) or intracranial hypertension will result (the Monroe-Kellie doctrine). Small additions of volume may be tolerated with only a small increase in intracranial pressure (ICP), but ICP becomes exponentially greater with further volume increments (i.e., the compliance decreases). Intracranial hypertension compromises cerebral perfusion and may cause herniation of brain (see below).

Cerebral blood flow. The brain is very dependent on a stable blood flow because of its high metabolic needs and lack of metabolic stores.[9] Normal global cerebral blood flow (CBF) is about 50 ml of blood per 100 g brain tissue per minute in the adult[77] and slightly higher in children.[46,70] CBF is related to the cerebral perfusion pressure (CPP, which equals mean arterial pressure (MAP) minus ICP) and inversely related to cerebral vascular resistance (CVR). The CVR will vary with changes in CPP in order to maintain a constant blood flow.[49] This process is known as pressure autoregulation, and operates at a

CPP between 60 and 150 torr in normal adults.[98] Below this range, arterioles are already maximally dilated, and CBF falls passively as CPP falls. Above this range, arterioles are already maximally constricted, and excessive CBF may occur as CPP rises, causing vasogenic edema and intracranial hypertension.[49,97]

In order to maintain adequate oxygen delivery to the brain, CBF increases when arterial oxygen content decreases or when the cerebral metabolic rate increases (e.g., seizures).[9,50] The arterial PCO_2 also has a marked effect CBF, with flow linearly related to PCO_2 between 20 to 80 torr in the normal brain.[63,88] This CO_2-reactivity is mediated by alterations of the perivascular pH. Because it is nonionized, CO_2 readily crosses the blood brain barrier and therefore affects the perivascular pH.[50] On average, global cerebral blood flow changes by about 3% per torr change in PCO_2.[77] Therapeutic manipulation of CBF and cerebral blood volume may be achieved by altering the PCO_2, if CO_2-reactivity is intact (see below).

It is important to realize that blood flow and blood volume are related but are not the same. Blood volume is proportional to the diameter of the arteries (and veins) and directly affects ICP. Blood flow is related to arterial diameter (cerebral vascular resistance) but also to perfusion pressure. Thus, while an increased arterial diameter represents an increased blood volume and ICP, the effect on CBF depends on the concomitant changes in CPP.[9]

Pathophysiology

Primary injury. The mechanisms of injury in children involve motor vehicle accidents in 80 to 90% of cases with children as passengers, pedestrians, or bicyclists.[59,60] Falls, assaults and shaking injuries (often child abuse) also occur. Injury to the brain is traditionally thought of in terms of primary and secondary injury. Primary injury is the actual physical and mechanical destruction of tissue which occurs at the moment of impact. Acceleration and deceleration forces cause stretching and tearing of axons (diffuse axonal injury)[52,86] and blood vessels. Vessel injury may result in intracranial hemorrhage. Impact against the internal bony and fibrous structures of the skull can also occur, causing contusions.

Secondary injury. While some neurons are irreversibly damaged by the primary injury, others remain viable, but are vulnerable to necrosis in the ensuing cascade of inflammatory and ischemic damage known as secondary injury. Furthermore, traumatized brain tissue is extremely sensitive to ischemia, hypotension, and hypoxia[20,45,75,83,103] which also contribute to secondary injury.

Secondary injury is a very complex, incompletely understood cascade of self-destructive and self-perpetuating biochemical and cellular events. Ischemia, intracellular calcium influx, and oxygen-derived free radical damage are thought to be the prominent features.[96] Trauma to the brain causes spreading depolarizations and release of excitatory amino acids such as glutamate, aspartate, and dopamine.[29] These in turn trigger cellular receptors (NMDA and non-NMDA) resulting in calcium and sodium influx into the cell and potassium efflux.[96] Sodium influx causes cellular edema. Excess intracellular calcium activates proteases[21,96] and phospholipases, damaging cell membranes and providing free fatty acids and arachidonic acid, which are the substrate for eicosanoid production (prostaglandins, thromboxanes).[48] Eicosanoids cause microcirculatory disturbances (vasoconstriction) and platelet aggregation, causing further ischemia.[48] Important byproducts of arachidonic acid metabolism are oxygen-derived free radicals[36,42,47] which exert their pernicious effects via membrane lipid peroxidation, causing loss of neuronal and endothelial cell membrane integrity.[36,47] This causes further ionic disturbances, loss of an effective blood-brain barrier, vasogenic edema, microvascular obliteration, and ischemia. Thus the process perpetuates itself, engulfing adjacent neurons in the "penumbra" (surrounding tissue which may still be viable but is adversely affected by the inflammatory process).[94,95]

Cerebral blood flow. Disturbances of cerebral perfusion play a major role in brain injury. Both hypoperfusion and excessive flow (hyperemia) may be detrimental. Bouma[12] demonstrated low CBF (average 22ml/100g/min) early after head trauma (within 6 hours of injury) in adults using radioactive ^{133}Xe

and found an association between low flow and poor outcome. One-third of the patients had CBF in the ischemic range (defined as less than 18ml/100g/min)[6] when measured within 6 hours of injury, and this group also had the worst outcome and highest mortality. In a subsequent study using stable xenon-enhanced CT scanning, Bouma[12] found that 31% of severely head-injured adults had global or regional ischemia if measured early after trauma (average 3.1 hours). This was typically associated with early mortality. Other investigators have also described this phenomenon of low flow early after head injury.[43,57,78,79] These data are corroborated by the frequent occurrence of histopathologic ischemic changes in fatally-injured head trauma patients.[33,34] The etiology for this reduction in flow after trauma has not been elucidated. The significance of hypoperfusion is underscored by studies which demonstrate that the traumatized brain is sensitive to even mild ischemic insults.[45] As will be discussed later, hyperventilation applied early post-trauma may worsen hypoperfusion.

The above studies were performed on adults. Muizelaar[70] studied head-injured children with ^{133}Xe and also noted a relationship between low CBF and low Glasgow Coma Scale (GCS)[100] scores in the first 24 hours after trauma. Those children with favorable outcomes tended to have higher CBF (49ml/100g/min) in the first 24 hours than those with poor outcome (35ml/100g/min). This trend was reversed after 24 hours, with the more severely comatose children having higher flow (with the exception of those with a GCS of three, who had the lowest CBF). At any time point, the more extreme deviations from normal (high or low CBF) correlate with a more severe injury.

Though still at risk for low CBF, children with head injury have a higher incidence of hyperemia than adults. Muizelaar[70] found that 88% of severely head-injured children had hyperemia at some point during their course. This may be causally related to the higher occurrence of diffuse brain swelling found in children with head injury.[2,15] Hyperemia can be detrimental because it is associated with an increased ICP due to increased diameter of cerebral blood vessels (an increase in cerebral blood volume).[77,78] Hyperemia may exacerbate vasogenic edema[97] and is associated with a less compliant brain.[70]

Cerebral vasoreactivity. Global CBF usually changes by about 2 to 3% for each torr change in arterial PCO_2.[77,88] The CBF response to CO_2 is impaired after head trauma in about 50% of patients.[63,76,99] Furthermore, the CO_2-reactivity of injured brain is not uniform and varies between 1.3 and 8.5% within an injured hemisphere.[56] The importance of these findings is that hyperventilation can have paradoxical effects on different regions of the brain. For example, hyperventilation may reduce flow to normal or subnormal levels in a viable region of the brain with intact CO_2-reactivity, while exacerbating hyperemia in another region with impaired CO_2-reactivity (inverse steal).[25] It is therefore difficult to titrate hyperventilation without measurements of CBF and metabolism. In addition, the loss of CO_2-reactivity portends a worse outcome after traumatic or ischemic insults.[63]

Pressure autoregulation is defective in about one-third of adults and 41% of children after head trauma,[10,69,71] but unlike the loss of CO_2-reactivity this has not been found to be a negative prognostic sign. Regardless of whether pressure autoregulation is defective or intact, it is imperative to avoid hypotension. If pressure autoregulation is defective, a decrease of MAP will result in a direct decrease in CBF. Recall that early after head injury (the time when transport is usually occurring), CBF may already be low, and any further compromise could be catastrophic. If pressure autoregulation is intact, a decrease of MAP will produce compensatory vasodilatation (decreased CVR to maintain the same CBF) and thus an increase in the intracranial volume and intracranial hypertension.[10]

Intracranial pressure. After head trauma, intracranial hypertension may be caused by edema (vasogenic and cytotoxic), hyperemia, mass effect from unevacuated hematoma, and obstruction of CSF outflow. As one region swells it compresses adjacent regions and distorts blood vessels, thereby impeding perfusion, creating more ischemic tissue, and perpetuating the process. The duration and severity of intracranial hypertension are indicative of poor outcome.[65,66] Children have a relatively higher incidence of diffuse brain swelling as seen on initial CT scan.[2,15,70] Fortunately, from the standpoint of transport, posttraumatic elevations of ICP due to edema usually do not reach their peak until 24 to 72 hours after injury. However, intracranial hypertension can occur early after head trauma, due to intracranial hematoma formation or an extremely severe insult.

Herniation. Herniation of brain tissue is usually due to a clot or contusion causing a focal mass lesion. Cingulate (subfalcian) herniation occurs when a unilateral mass or asymmetric swelling forces the cerebral hemisphere laterally under the falx cerebri. Uncal herniation occurs when the medial portion of the temporal lobe (the uncus) is pushed over the edge of the tentorial notch, compressing adjacent brainstem structures. This process may also compress the third cranial nerve, causing the ipsilateral pupil to become fixed and dilated. Herniation is devastating because it damages the brainstem, compresses arteries, and obstructs venous drainage and CSF pathways.[84]

Diagnosis

Priorities. The physical examination begins with an assessment of the airway, breathing, and circulation. This takes precedence over all other activities of the transport personnel. Vital signs are checked to ensure adequate cardiopulmonary function (and clues to increased ICP). Initial assessment and management should proceed according to ATLS and PALS guidelines.[3,19] Only when hemodynamic stability has been achieved does the clinician directly address the neurologic problem. These issues are discussed in the management section.

Clinical. The diagnosis of head trauma usually does not pose a dilemma. Most often the event is witnessed, and there are obvious physical findings. If not, any child with altered mental status, seizures, or unconsciousness of unknown etiology should be suspected to have a head injury and managed as such until proven otherwise. Infants and toddlers who have been violently shaken may present with a vague history and no overt signs of trauma.

External signs of head trauma include lacerations, abrasions, contusions, and hematomas to the face and head. Fractures of the skull may be palpable. Raccoon eyes, Battle's sign, hemotympanum, CSF otorrhea, and rhinorrhea indicate a basilar skull fracture. Retinal hemorrhages are strongly suggestive of violent shaking as the mechanism of injury.[18]

The neurologic exam is extremely important is assessing the child with head trauma, and the transport personnel should make every effort to obtain at least an abbreviated exam before administering drugs that will prevent assessment. The level of consciousness can be described by the degree of stimulation necessary to arouse the patient (awake, arouses to voice, touch, or pain, or is unarousable). The motor exam should assess the patient's position, tone (normal, flexor or extensor posturing, hypertonic, flaccid, seizing) and symmetry. Flexor or extensor posturing suggests intracranial hypertension and may help to localize the lesion. The Glasgow Coma Scale[100] is a rapid and useful method to quantify the degree of neurologic impairment and should be calculated for all children with head injury (Table 25-1).[44] Generally, head injury with a GCS score of eight or less is considered severe. Children with very low GCS scores may still have a satisfactory outcome,[55] emphasizing the need for an aggressive initial approach in all cases. Pupillary size and reactivity can help to localize the lesion. In the case of uncal herniation, the patient may have a dilated and nonreactive pupil ipsilateral to the herniation, which should make one suspect a large clot or contusion. This brief CNS exam can be performed rapidly and provides important information on the nature and degree of injury and the need for any immediate life-sustaining interventions.

Computerized tomographic scan. The CT scan is the single most useful diagnostic test in the head-injured patient. It is never appropriate to delay transfer to a pediatric trauma center to obtain a scan, but if it has already been done then the transport command physician should make use of the information. Similarly, a CT scan should be obtained at the primary facility if there will be a delay in the arrival of the transport team and the patient can be appropriately stabilized. Although we

TABLE 25-1 COMA SCALES

Glasgow coma scale	Modified coma scale for infants	Point value
Eye opening		
Spontaneous	Spontaneous	4
To speech	To speech	3
To pain	To pain	2
None	None	1
Verbal		
Oriented	Coos, babbles	5
Confused	Irritable	4
Inappropriate words	Cries to pain	3
Grunting	Moans to pain	2
None	None	1
Motor		
Follows commands	Normal spontaneous movements	6
Localizes pain	Withdraws to touch	5
Withdraws to pain	Withdraws to pain	4
Abnormal flexion	Abnormal flexion	3
Abnormal extension	Abnormal extension	2
Flaccid	Flaccid	1

Data from Teasdale G, Jennett B: *Lancet* 2:81, 1974; and James HE: *Pediatric Annals* 15:16, 1986.

rely on the neurosurgeon and neuroradiologist to provide expert interpretation, clinicians involved in the care of head-injured patients should be familiar with the basic findings. The three major categories of pathologic findings on CT scan are hemorrhage, swelling, and shift. Large intracranial hemorrhage occurs in about 25% of children with severe head injuries[53] and can be extracerebral (epidural or subdural) or intracerebral (Figures 25-1 through 25-4). These are associated with a mortality rate of about 25%. Diffuse brain swelling, characterized by compression or obliteration of the perimesencephalic cisterns and ventricles, is seen in about 24% to 35% of initial CT scans of severely head-injured children.[2,53] Children with this finding have a three-fold higher mortality than those without it (53% vs. 16%).[2] Shift of the midline indicates asymmetric pressure due to brain swelling or a mass lesion which may cause herniation of the cingulate gyrus under the falx cerebri. This finding was noted in 16% of severely head-injured adults[28] and 10% of severely head-injured children[53] and is associated with poor outcome. The presence of these abnormalities indicates the severity of the head injury, the potential for rapid deterioration, and the need for immediate evaluation by a neurosurgeon. A copy of the CT scan (or the original) should accompany the patient on transport.

Management

Airway and breathing. The child with neurologic compromise may be in respiratory failure without any overt signs of respiratory distress. This must be avoided, since both hypercarbia and hypoxia produce cerebral vasodilatation which exacerbates intracranial hypertension.[50] Obviously, hypoxia is detrimental irrespective of its effects on CBF. The clinical exam (adequate respiratory rate, chest wall rise, air movement, color of skin and mucosa) as well as ancillary data (pulse oximetry, arterial blood gases) must be maintained in the normal range. Failure to achieve this mandates at the very least supplemental oxygen (which should already be in use) and possibly assisted ventilation via an endotracheal tube. In addition to the usual causes of respiratory failure, the respiratory system of the head-injured child may have been subjected to other insults, such as loss of protective airway reflexes, aspiration of blood or gastric contents, spinal cord trauma precluding effective muscle use, and direct trauma to the airway. These patients may require intu-

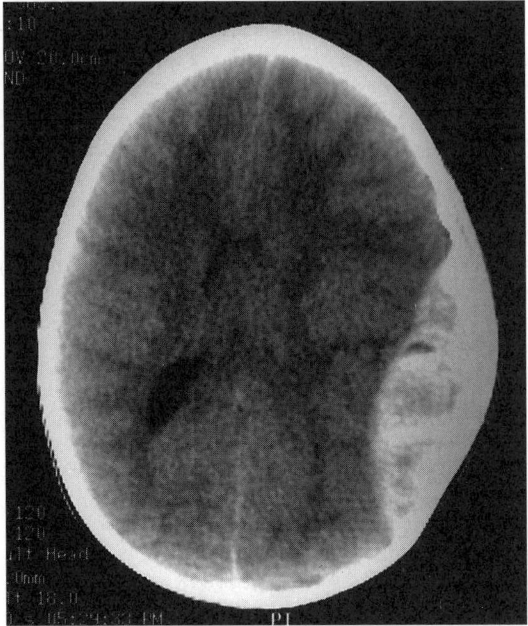

Fig. 25-1. Moderate-sized epidural hematoma with compression of ipsilateral lateral ventricle and minimal shift across the midline after falling from a grocery cart.

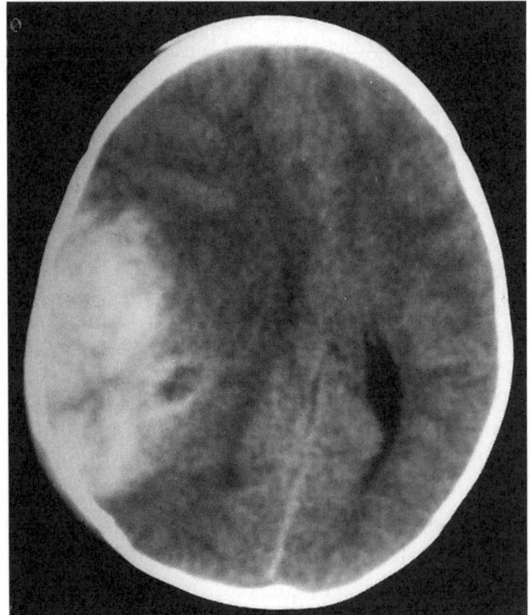

Fig. 25-2. Large epidural hematoma with compression of ipsilateral lateral ventricle and significant shift across the midline (consistent with herniation) after motor vehicle accident.

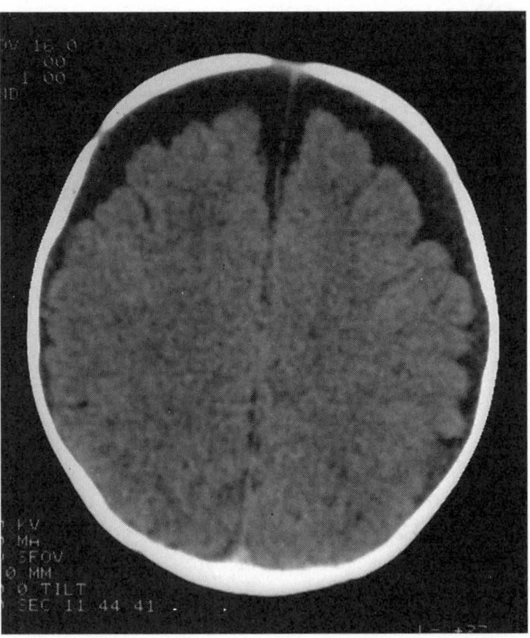

Fig. 25-3. Subacute bifrontal subdural hematomas after shaking injury in a toddler.

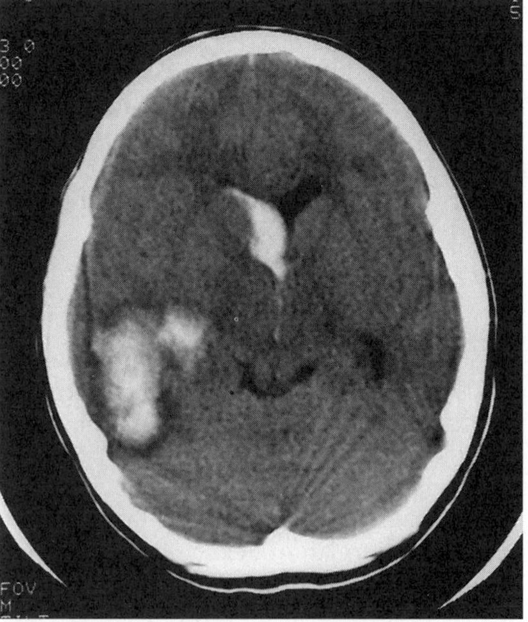

Fig. 25-4. Intracerebral hemorrhage in the right temporo-parietal region with blood in the lateral ventricle after motor vehicle accident.

bation for a variety of reasons (see Box 25-1). In preparation for transport, one should have a lower threshold for endotracheal intubation than if already at the tertiary care center. Deterioration may occur suddenly and it is more difficult to achieve airway control in a moving vehicle or aircraft.

When intubating a head-injured patient, a neuroprotective, rapid sequence technique should be used, if possible. This begins with preoxygenation with 100% oxygen. Ideally, one tries to avoid face-mask bagging, but if ventilation and oxygenation are inadequate or if there is evidence of herniation, the patient must be ventilated immediately. Apply gentle pressure to the cricoid to minimize the risk of aspiration (always assume a full stomach). The hemodynamic and neurologic status of the patient will determine the pharmacologic adjuncts used in securing the airway[74] (Table 25-2). If the patient is in cardiac arrest, CPR must be started immediately, and intubation should be performed without sedation or neuromuscular blockade. The patient who has sustained severe head trauma and is hemodynamically unstable should receive fentanyl, lidocaine, and vecuronium. If the patient is hemodynamically stable, a benzodiazepine (diazepam or midazolam) should also be used to provide better sedation. If there is clinical evidence of herniation, then fentanyl, lidocaine, thiopental (see below), and vecuronium are appropriate. The goals of this regimen are to avoid harmful alterations of MAP, ICP elevation, and aspiration.

BOX 25-1 INDICATIONS FOR INTUBATION OF THE CHILD WITH HEAD INJURY

Neurologic
- Coma (GCS 8 or less)
- Impending herniation
- C-spine injury compromising ventilation

Respiratory
- Cardiopulmonary arrest
- Apnea
- Arterial $PCO_2 > 45\text{-}50$ torr (relative)
- Arterial $PO_2 < 60$ torr ($SaO_2 < 90\%$)

TABLE 25-2 DRUGS FOR INTUBATION OF THE HEAD-INJURED CHILD

Situation	*Drugs*
Cardiopulmonary arrest	Resuscitation drugs
Hemodynamically unstable	Fentanyl, 2-4 mcg/kg Lidocaine, 1 mg/kg Vecuronium, 0.3 mg/kg
Hemodynamically stable	Fentanyl, 2-4 mcg/kg Lidocaine, 1 mg/kg Diazepam or Midazolam, 0.1-0.2 mg/kg Vecuronium, 0.3 mg/kg
Evidence of intracranial hypertension (and hemodynamically stable)	Fentanyl, 2-4 mcg/kg Lidocaine, 1 mg/kg Thiopental, 4-5 mg/kg Vecuronium, 0.3 mg/kg

Use with caution, see text.

Fentanyl blunts the dramatic elevations of systemic blood pressure, heart rate, and catecholamines[22,24,58,81] that occur during laryngoscopy and intubation, and lidocaine similarly blunts this sympathetic response.[1,40] More importantly, lidocaine mitigates the intracranial hypertension that occurs with ETT suctioning[27] or other noxious stimuli,[7] such as intubation.[8] Thiopental works by lowering the cerebral metabolic rate, and therefore blood flow, blood volume, and ICP.[82,93]

The issue of when to use thiopental during transport (and in preparation for transport) warrants discussion. Immediately after trauma, elevated ICP is uncommon, and there is the potential for hypotension when other injuries are present. Therefore, the use of thiopental is not recommended during the "scene run." However, tertiary pediatric centers are occasionally called to transport a patient with progressive neurologic deterioration 12 to 24 hours after the initial injury. An example of this situation is that of the shaken infant who is brought to medical attention after a latent period with a bulging fontanelle, blown pupil, and posturing. Another example is that of a child who is being observed at a nontertiary hospital after a head injury and begins to deteriorate. If the patient is manifesting signs of intracranial hypertension, then thiopental may be indicated prior to intubation and transport. Also, regarding intrahospital transport (typically for CT scan), once a patient has been hemodynamically stabilized and evaluated by the neurosurgeon, it is appropriate to use thiopental if intracranial hypertension is suspected. In summary, thiopental is not recommended for use by paramedics on a scene run in which intubation is needed. It is indicated prior to intubation of the hemodynamically stable head-injured patient with evidence of intracranial hypertension. It should be used only by personnel who are familiar with it. It is contraindicated when there is hypotension or significant bleeding, because it may cause severe and refractory hypotension.[106]

The choice of the neuromuscular blocker is controversial. Traditionally, succinyl choline has been favored because of its very rapid onset and short duration.[104] However, it causes undesirable side effects such as bradycardia in small children and fasciculations which can increase ICP and intragastric pressure. These side effects are diminished with prior doses of atropine and a priming dose of a nondepolarizing neuromuscular blocker, but this complicates the situation. A large dose of vecuronium (0.3 mg/kg) produces intubating conditions within 60 to 90 seconds, and maintains excellent cardiovascular stability.[51,102] The duration of this dose ranges from 83 to 111 minutes.[31,102] Although some would argue that this is too long, most of these children are transported and sent to CT scanner during this interval. Although one loses the ability to follow the neurologic exam for this time period, the neuromuscular blockade will decrease the risk of accidental extubation during transport and will allow for a high quality, motion-free CT scan. At this juncture, further management will often depend more on the CT scan than the clinical exam. Pupillary size and reactivity can still be monitored.[64] The sedatives used in this regimen will not last as long as the neuromuscular blockade, so administration of additional sedatives may be necessary.

The jaw thrust is used to maintain patency of the airway, not the head-tilt/chin-lift maneuver. Direct laryngoscopy with a designated person assigned to stabilizing the cervical spine (without traction) is the technique of choice for endotracheal intubation of the pediatric head trauma victim because it is the fastest and surest method of securing the airway.[39] Blind nasotracheal intubation is not advisable for children in this setting for numerous reasons. The anterior and cephalad position of the larynx makes this a difficult technique in small children. Flexion of the neck is often required, which is contraindicated in a child with a possible cervical spine injury. Multiple attempts are required 67 to 90% of the time,[32] and increases of arterial PCO_2 and ICP may occur. Furthermore, midfacial or basilar skull fractures are direct contraindications, and blind nasal intubation cannot be performed in the apneic patient.[3] Surgical methods of securing the airway, such as cricothyroidotomy and transtracheal ventilation, are associated with a high complication rate in children[73] and are generally methods of last resort.

Traditionally, head-injured patients have been routinely hyperventilated. However, this practice has come under serious scrutiny. As discussed earlier, hypoperfusion occurs commonly after head injury, particularly in the first few hours after trauma. Hyperventilation may exacerbate low CBF to produce hypoperfusion.[11,12,23,72,99] Obrist[77] noted a widening of the arterio-jugular venous oxygen content difference during hyperventilation in the first 24 hours after head injury, suggesting ischemia. During the initial management and transport this therapy should be used only when there is clinical or radiologic evidence of herniation. However, hypercarbia should be avoided and PCO_2 should be maintained in the low normal range (30 to 35 torr).

Circulation. It is imperative to support the circulation of all traumatized children, especially the child with head trauma. Hypotension after head injury is associated with a doubling of mortality.[20,103] In animal models, hypotension after traumatic brain injury causes a sustained reduction of cerebral oxygen delivery that persists even after restoration of systemic oxygen delivery.[90] With intact pressure autoregulation, a decreased perfusion pressure causes cerebral vasodilatation which may worsen ICP. Conversely, if autoregulation is defective, decreased perfusion pressure will directly decrease CBF. Isotonic fluids (0.9% sodium chloride), colloid, or blood products should be used as indicated in the resuscitation of the head-injured patient. Fluid overload should be avoided, once adequate perfusion is achieved. Recent data suggest that hypertonic crystalloid solutions may be superior to Ringer's lactate for improving cerebral blood flow and oxygen delivery and lowering ICP after focal brain injury.[91] Further studies are warranted in this area.

Herniation. The combination of a dilated, nonreactive pupil and asymmetric posturing is very strong evidence that the brain is herniating. Hypertension, bradycardia, and irregular respirations (Cushing's triad) may also be seen with herniation. If herniation occurs early after trauma, it is usually due to a large intracranial mass lesion (hemorrhage or contusion). Herniation is a life-threatening event. Neurosurgical intervention may be indicated, but this is not an option on transport. In the setting of herniation, it is appropriate to hyperventilate and administer thiopental[82,93] and mannitol.[62,68] As previously discussed, thiopental and mannitol should not be used routinely during transport of the child with head trauma. These agents are generally not recommended for use on a scene run, because thiopental may cause profound and refractory hypotension,[106] and mannitol may cause hypotension if given too rapidly.[26] These drugs should only be used by appropriately trained personnel in the setting of suspected brain herniation (and for intubation if indicated), and one must be prepared to treat hypotension with volume infusion and vasopressors as necessary.

Seizures. Posttraumatic seizures occur in 39% of severely head-injured children (GCS of 8 or less)[54] and are undesirable because they increase cerebral metabolic rate and blood flow, and therefore ICP. Dilantin is commonly employed to treat posttraumatic seizures, because it does not depress the level of consciousness. Studies in adults[101] and children[54] demonstrate the efficacy of prophylactic dilantin in preventing seizures early after severe head injuries.

Transport. Children with head injury can deteriorate rapidly, and continual reassessment during transport is mandatory. Although supportive care is extremely important to the child with a head injury, it is imperative that evaluation by a trauma surgeon and neurosurgeon take place as soon as possible. Thus, care should be efficient and the fastest mode of transport should be used for all moderately and severely head-injured children.

Future directions

Despite the best of supportive and neurosurgical care, head injury remains a formidable health problem. As the pathophysiology of brain injury is unraveled, multiple possibilities for therapeutic intervention are discovered. These include hypothermia, excitatory amino acid antagonists, free radical scavengers, and others. The optimal regimen may consist of several synergistic therapies applied early after the injury. This is currently an area of intense research. Treatment begun in the stabilization and transport phase will undoubtedly be important. Regardless of whatever advances are made, an aggressive and rigorous approach to ensure uncompromised cardiopulmonary stability will remain the foundation for optimal neurologic care.

SPINAL INJURY

Spinal injury in children is relatively uncommon compared with adults and accounts for only between 1 and 10% of all spinal injuries.[35,37,38,89] Cervical spine injuries occur in 1 to 3% of head-injured adults but only 0.5% of head-injured children.[39] However, the mortality rate associated with spinal injury is about 2.5 times higher in children than in adults.[38] Most spinal injuries in children result from motor vehicle accidents, falls, diving accidents, and other sports injuries.[35,37,38,41,89]

Anatomy

In contrast to adults, the vertebral column of the child is characterized by the following features: 1) increased mobility due to ligamentous laxity and more cartilage; 2) underdeveloped neck and paraspinal muscles; 3) incompletely ossified, wedge-shaped vertebral bodies; 4) horizontal facet joints between vertebrae; and 5) larger head size relative to torso.[30,37,89] Also, the fulcrum of neck motion is higher in the child than in the adult.[89] These features may offer some protection against bony injury, but predispose young children (less than 9 years) to high cervical injuries of greater severity.[5,35,37,41,80,89] The most severe high cervical spine injuries are sustained almost exclusively by children under eight years of age.[80] Children under four years of age demonstrate this trend even more,[89] underscoring the significance of developmental differences. Older children, like adults, suffer injuries that are more evenly distributed throughout the cervical and thoracic spine.

Pathophysiology

The pathophysiology of spinal cord injury is believed to be similar to that of head injury. Injury may be due to hyperflexion, hyperextension, compression, stretching, rotational forces, or penetrating trauma.[39] The cervical spine is the most mobile and least supported part of the spine and therefore the most prone to injury.[39] After the mechanical "primary" injury, the spinal cord becomes prey to the complex biochemical reactions of "secondary" injury, including excitotoxicity, ion fluxes, membrane lipid metabolism, eicosanoid and oxygen radical production, ischemia, edema, inflammatory cells, complement activation, etc.[4]

Diagnosis

In the awake and cooperative patient, pain or tenderness of the neck or back, decreased strength or sensation, and tingling of extremities are suggestive of spinal injury. In the patient with an impaired level of consciousness, one must have a high index of suspicion that the mechanism of injury is capable of producing spinal injury.

Some studies have reported the efficacy and safety of using plain x-rays and the clinical exam to rule out fractures of the spine.[67,92] A recent study of 216 adult patients with cervical spine injuries revealed that the standard "trauma series" (cross-table lateral, anteroposterior, and odontoid views) failed to identify 61% of fractures and 36% of subluxations and dislocations.[105] Most of the patients with spinal injury had signs or symptoms that prompted further evaluation, although 5% of the 216 were alert and cooperative but had no clinical evidence of spinal injury. Furthermore, spinal cord injury without radiologic abnormality (SCIWORA), accounts for up to 67% of spinal cord injuries in children,[80] making x-rays even less reliable in children. Given the uncertainty in this area, there is no reason for transport personnel to feel compelled to resolve the issue, and the most prudent course is to keep the spine immobilized if there is any suspicion of a spinal injury.

Management

Management of the child with possible spinal cord injury should proceed as for head-injured patients with the initial priority being support of the respiratory and cardiovascular systems. As discussed in the head trauma section, the safest and surest method for endotracheal intubation in this setting is direct laryngoscopy with manual in-line stabilization (not traction) of the cervical spine.[39] Spinal or neurogenic shock may occur with spinal cord transections above the T1 level due to interruption of the sympathetic nervous system. This results in hypotension accompanied by bradycardia. The treatment is volume infusion and a direct-acting vasoconstrictor such as norepinephrine.[87]

The cervical spine is most effectively immobilized with a Philadelphia collar and sandbags taped to each side of the head.[85] This combination maximally reduced the ability of conscious volunteers to move their necks. Sandbags and tape are nearly as effective without a collar as with one. Immobilization of the thoracic spine is best achieved with a long backboard.

Despite concerns that transporting a patient with an injured spine may be deleterious, Burney[17] reported the transport of 61 patients to a spine injury center (41% by ground, 54% by helicopter, 5% by fixed wing aircraft) without complication. Indeed, with the advent of an effective therapy that must be administered within 8 hours, it is in the patient's best interest to be transported to a spine injury center as soon as possible. Methylprednisolone has been shown in clinical studies to improve outcome after spinal cord injury in adults if the regimen is begun within 8 hours after the injury,[13,14] and this therapy now represents the standard of care.

Future directions

Novel antioxidant aminosteroids[36] may prove to be a more effective therapy than steroids. Clinical trials are currently underway to further evaluate these new therapies.

REFERENCES

1. Abou-Madi MN, Keszler H, Yacoub JM: Cardiovascular reactions to laryngoscopy and tracheal intubation following small and large intravenous doses of lidocaine, *Canad Anesth Soc J* 24:12-9, 1977.
2. Aldrich EF and others: Diffuse brain swelling in severely head-injured children, *Journal of Neurosurgery* 76:450-4, 1992.
3. American College of Surgeons: *Advanced trauma life support,* Student Manual, Chicago, 1989.
4. Anderson DK, Hall ED: Pathophysiology of spinal cord trauma. *Ann Emerg Med* 22:987-92, 1993.
5. Apple JS and others: Cervical spine fractures and dislocations in children, *Pediatric Radiology* 17:45-9, 1987.
6. Astrup J, Siesjo BK, Symon L: Thresholds in cerebral ischemia—the ischemic penumbra, *Stroke* 12:723-5, 1981.
7. Bedford RF and others: Lidocaine or thiopental for rapid control of intracranial hypertension? *Anesth Analg* 59:435-7, 1980.
8. Bedford RF and others: Lidocaine prevents increased ICP after endotracheal intubation. In *Intracranial pressure IV.* Publishers: Springer-Verlag, New York, 1979.
9. Bouma GJ, Muizelaar JP: Cerebral blood flow, cerebral blood volume, and cerebrovascular reactivity after severe head injury, *Journal of Neurotrauma* 9:S333-48, 1992.
10. Bouma GJ and others: Blood pressure and intracranial pressure-volume dynamics in severe head injury: relationship with cerebral blood flow, *Journal of Neurosurgery* 77:15-9, 1992.
11. Bouma GJ and others: Cerebral circulation and metabolism after severe traumatic brain injury: the elusive role of ischemia, *Journal of Neurosurgery* 75:685-93, 1991.
12. Bouma GJ and others: Ultra-early evaluation of regional cerebral blood flow in severely head-injured patients using xenon-enhanced computerized tomography, *Journal of Neurosurgery* 77:360-8, 1992.
13. Bracken MB and others: A randomzied controlled trial of methylprednisolone or naloxone in the treatment of acute spinal-cord injury, *N Engl J Med* 322:1405-11, 1990.
14. Bracken MB and others: Methylprednisolone or naloxone treatment after acute spinal cord treatment: 1-year follow-up data, *Journal of Neurosurgery* 76:23-31, 1992.
15. Bruce DA and others: Diffuse cerebral swelling following head injuries in children: the syndrome of "malignant brain edema," *Journal of Neurosurgery* 54:170-8, 1981.
16. Bruce DA and others: Outcome following severe head injuries in children, *Journal of Neurosurgery* 48:679-88, 1978.
17. Burney RE, Waggoner R, Maynard FM: Stabilization of spinal injury for early transfer, *J Trauma* 29:1497-9, 1989.
18. Buys YM and others: Retinal findings after head trauma in infants and young children, *Ophthalmology* 99:1718-23, 1992.
19. Chameides L, editor: *Textbook of pediatric advanced life support,* American Heart Association, 1988.
20. Chestnut RM and others: The role of secondary brain injury in determining outcome from severe head injury, *Journal of Trauma* 34:216-22, 1993.
21. Choi DW: Calcium-mediated neurotoxicity: relationship to specific channel types and role in ischemic damage, *Trends Neurosci* 11:465-9, 1988.
22. Chraemmer-Jorgensen B and others: Catecholamine response to laryngoscopy and intubation, *Anaesthesia* 47:750-6, 1992.
23. Cold GE: Does acute hyperventilation provoke cerebral oligaemia in comatose patients after acute head injury? *Acta Neurochirurgica* 96:100-6, 1989.
24. Cork RC and others: Fentanyl preloading for rapid-sequence induction of anesthesia, *Anesth Analg* 63:60-4, 1984.
25. Darby JM and others: Local "inverse steal" induced by hyperventilation in head injury, *Neurosurgery* 23:84-8, 1988.
26. Domaingue CM, Nye DH: Hypotensive effect of mannitol administered rapidly, *Anaesth Intens Care* 13:134-6, 1985.
27. Donegan M, Bedford RF, Dacey R: IV lidocaine for prevention of intracranial hypertension, *Anesthesiology* 51:S201, 1979.
28. Eisenberg HM and others: Initial CT findings in 753 patients with severe head injury, *Journal of Neurosurgery* 73:688-98, 1990.
29. Faden AI and others: The role of excitatory amino acids and NMDA receptors in traumatic brain injury, *Science* 244:798-800, 1989.
30. Fesmire FM, Luten RC: The pediatric cervical spine: developmental anatomy and clinical aspects, *J Emerg Med* 7:133-42, 1989.
31. Ginsberg B and others: Onset and duration of neuromuscular blockade following high-dose vecuronium administration, *Anesthesiology* 71:201-5, 1989.
32. Gold M, Buechel D: A method of blind nasal intubation for the conscious patient, *Anesth Analg* 39:257-63, 1960.

33. Graham DI, Adams JH: Ischaemic brain damage in fatal head injuries, *Lancet* 1:265-6, 1971.
34. Graham DI and others: Ischaemic brain damage is still common in fatal non-missile head injury, *Journal of Neurology, Neurosurgery, and Psychiatry* 52:346-50, 1989.
35. Hadley MN and others: Pediatric spinal trauma: review of 122 cases of spinal cord and vertebral column injuries, *Journal of Neurosurgery* 68:18-24, 1988.
36. Hall ED: Lipid antioxidants in acute central nervous system injury, *Ann Emerg Med* 22:1022-7, 1993.
37. Hamilton MG, Myles ST: Pediatric spinal injury: review of 174 hospital admissions, *Journal of Neurosurgery* 77:700-4, 1992.
38. Hamilton MG, Myles ST: Pediatric spinal injury: review of 61 deaths, *Journal of Neurosurgery* 77:705-8, 1992.
39. Hastings RH, Marks JD: Airway management for trauma patients with potential cervical spine injuries, *Anesth Analg* 73:471-82, 1991.
40. Helfman SM, Gold MI, DeLisser EA, Herrington CA: Which drug prevents tachycardia and hypertension associated with tracheal intubation: lidocaine, fentanyl or esmolol? *Anesth Analg* 72:482-6, 1991.
41. Hill SA and others: Pediatric neck injuries; a clinical study, *Journal of Neurosurgery* 60:700-6, 1984.
42. Ikeda Y, Long DM: The molecular basis of brain injury and brain edema: the role of oxygen free radicals, *Neurosurgery* 27:1-11, 1990.
43. Jaggi JL and others: Relationship of early cerebral blood flow and metabolism to outcome in acute head injury, *Journal of Neurosurgery* 72:176-82, 1990.
44. James HE: Neurologic evaluation and support in the child with an acute brain insult, *Pediatric Annals* 15:16-22, 1986.
45. Jenkins LW and others: Increased vulnerability of the mildly traumatized rat brain to cerebral ischemia, *Brain Research* 477:211-24, 1989.
46. Kennedy C, Sokoloff L: An adaptation of the nitrous oxide method to the study of the cerebral circulation in children, *Journal of Clinical Investigation* 36:1130-7, 1957.
47. Kontos H: Oxygen radicals in cerebral vascular injury, *Circ Research* 57:508-16, 1985.
48. Kontos HA and others: Prostaglandins in physiological and in certain pathological responses of the cerebral circulation, *Fereration Proc* 40:2326-30, 1981.
49. Kontos HA and others: Responses of cerebral arteries and arterioles to acute hypotension and hypertension, *Am J Phys* 234:H371-83, 1978.
50. Lassen NA, Christensen MS: Physiology of cerebral blood flow, *Br J Anaesth* 48:719-34, 1976.
51. Lennon RL, Olson RA, Gronert GA: Atracurium or vecuronium for rapid sequence endotracheal intubation, *Anesthesiology* 64:510-3, 1986.
52. Levi L and others: Diffuse axonal injury: analysis of 100 patients with radiological signs, *Neurosurgery* 27:429-32, 1990.
53. Levin HS and others: Severe head injury in children: experience of the Traumatic Coma Data Bank, *Neurosurgery* 31:435-44, 1992.
54. Lewis RJ and others: Clinical predictors of posttraumatic seizures in children with head trauma, *Ann Emerg Med* 22:1114-8, 1993.
55. Lieh-Lai MW and others: Limitations of the Glasgow Coma Scale in predicting outcome in children with traumatic brain injury, *Journal of Pediatrics* 120:195-9, 1992.
56. Marion DW, Bouma GJ: The use of stable xenon-enhanced computed tomographic studies of cerebral blood flow to define changes in cerebral carbon dioxide vasoresponsivity caused by a severe head injury, *Neurosurgery* 29:869-73, 1991.
57. Marion DW, Darby J, Yonas H: Acute regional cerebral blood flow changes caused by severe head injuries, *Journal of Neurosurgery* 74:407-14, 1991.
58. Martin DE and others: Low-dose fentanyl blunts circulatory responses to tracheal intubation, *Anesth Analg* 61:680-4, 1982.
59. Mayer T and others: Causes of morbidity and mortality in severe pediatric trauma, *JAMA* 245:719-21, 1981.
60. Mayer TA, Walker ML: Pediatric head injury: the critical role of the emergency physician, *Ann Emerg Med* 14:1178-84, 1985.
61. McKoy C, Bell MJ: Preventable traumatic deaths in children, *Journal of Pediatric Surgery* 18:505-8, 1983.
62. Mendelow AD and others: Effect of mannitol on cerebral blood flow and cerebral perfusion pressure in human head injury, *Journal of Neurosurgery* 63:43-8, 1985.
63. Messeter K and others: Cerebral hemodynamics in patients with acute severe head trauma, *Journal of Neurosurgery* 64:231-7, 1986.
64. Meyer S, Gibb T, Jurkovich GJ: Evaluation and significance of the pupillary light reflex in trauma patients, *Ann Emerg Med* 22:1052-7, 1993.
65. Miller JD and others: Significance of intracranial hypertension in severe head injury, *Journal of Neurosurgery* 47:503-16, 1977.
66. Miller JD and others: Further experience in the management of severe head injury, *Journal of Neurosurgery* 54:289-99, 1981.
67. Mirvis SE and others: Protocol-driven radiologic evaluation of suspected cervical spine injury: efficacy study, *Radiology* 170:831, 1989.
68. Muizelaar JP and others: Mannitol causes compensatory cerebral vasoconstriction and vasodilation in response to blood viscosity changes, *Journal of Neurosurgery* 59:822-8, 1983.
69. Muizelaar JP, Lutz HA, Becker DP: Effect of mannitol on ICP and CBF and correlation with pressure autoregulation in severely head-injured patients, *Journal of Neurosurgery* 61:700-6, 1984.

70. Muizelaar JP and others: Cerebral blood flow and metabolism in severely head-injured children: part 1, *Journal of Neurosurgery* 71:63-71, 1989.
71. Muizelaar JP and others: Adverse effects of prolonged hyperventilation in patients with severe head injury: a randomized clinical trial, *Journal of Neurosurgery* 75:731-9, 1991.
72. Muizelaar JP and others: Cerebral blood flow and metabolism in severely head-injured children: part 2, *Journal of Neurosurgery* 71:72-6, 1989.
73. Nakayama DK, Gardner MJ, Rowe MI: Emergency endotracheal intubation in pediatric trauma, *Annals of Surgery* 211:218-23, 1990.
74. Nakayama DK and others: The use of drugs in emergency airway management in pediatric trauma, *Annals of Surgery* 216:205-11, 1992.
75. Newfield P, Pitts L, Kaktis J, Hoff J: The influence of shock on mortality after head trauma, *Critical Care Medicine* 8:254, 1980.
76. Nordstrom CH and others: Cerebral blood flow, vasoreactivity, and oxygen consumption during barbiturate therapy in severe traumatic brain lesions, *Journal of Neurosurgery* 68:424-31, 1988.
77. Obrist WD and others: Cerebral blood flow and metabolism in comatose patients with acute head injury, *Journal of Neurosurgery* 61:241-53, 1984.
78. Obrist WD and others: Time course of cerebral blood flow and metabolism in comatose patients with acute head injury, *JCBFM* 13:S571, 1993.
79. Overgaard J, Mosdal C, Tweed WA: Cerebral circulation after head injury: part 3, *Journal of Neurosurgery* 55:63-74, 1981.
80. Pang D, Pollack IF: Spinal cord injury without radiographic abnormality in children: the SCIWORA Syndrome, *Journal of Trauma* 29:654-64, 1989.
81. Parker EO, Ross AL: Low dose fentanyl: effects on thiopental requirements and hemodynamic response during induction and intubation, *Anesthesiology* 57:A322, 1982.
82. Pierce EC Jr and others: Cerebral circulation and metabolism during thiopental anasthesia and hyperventilation in man, *J Clin Invest* 41:1664-71, 1962.
83. Pigula FA and others: The effect of hypotension on children with severe head injuries, *Journal of Pediatric Surgery* 28:310-6, 1993.
84. Plum F, Posner JB: *The diagnosis of stupor and coma*, ed 3. Philadelphia, 1980, FA Davis Co.
85. Podolsky S and others: Efficacy of cervical spine immobilization methods, *Journal of Trauma* 23:461-5, 1983.
86. Povlishock JT: Pathobiology of traumatically induced axonal injuries in animals and man, *Ann Emerg Med* 22:980-6, 1993.
87. Rawe SE, Perot PL, Jr: Pressor response resulting from experimental contusion injury to the spinal cord, *Journal of Neurosurgery* 50:58-63, 1979.
88. Reivich M: Arterial PCO_2 and cerebral hemodynamics, *Am J Phys* 206:25-35, 1964.
89. Ruge JR and others: Pediatric spinal injury: the very young, *Journal of Neurosurgery* 68:25-30, 1988.
90. Schmoker JD, Zhuang J, Shackford SR: Hemorrhagic hypotension after brain injury causes an early and sustained reduction in cerebral oxygen delivery despite normalization of systemic oxygen delivery, *Journal of Trauma* 32:714-22, 1992.
91. Shackford SR, Zhuang J, Schmoker J: Intravenous fluid tonicity: effect on intracranial pressure, cerebral blood flow, and cerebral oxygen delivery in focal brain injury, *Journal of Neurosurgery* 76:91-8, 1992.
92. Shaffer MA, Doris PE: Limitation of the cross-table lateral view in detecting cervical spine injuries: a retrospective analysis, *Ann Emerg Med* 10:508, 1981.
93. Shapiro HM and others: Rapid intraoperative reduction of intracranial pressure with thiopentone, *Brit J Anaesth* 45:1057-62, 1973.
94. Siesjo BK: Pathophysiology and treatment of focal cerebral ischemia: part 1: pathophysiology, *Journal of Neurosurgery* 77:169-84, 1992.
95. Siesjo BK: Pathophysiology and treatment of focal cerebral ischemia: part 2: mechanisms of damage and treatment, *Journal of Neurosurgery* 77:337-54, 1992.
96. Siesjo BK: Basic mechanisms of traumatic brain damage, *Ann Emerg Med* 22:959-69, 1993.
97. Simard JM, Bellefleur M: Systemic arterial hypertension in head trauma, *Am J Cardiol* 63:32C-35C, 1989.
98. Strandgaard S, Paulson OB: Cerebral autoregulation, *Stroke* 15:413-6, 1984.
99. Stringer WA and others: Hyperventilation-induced cerebral ischemia in patients with acute brain lesions: demonstration by xenon-enhanced CT, *American Journal of Neuroradiology* 14:475-84, 1993.
100. Teasdale G, Jennett B: Assessment of coma and impaired consciousness: a practical scale, *Lancet* 2:81-4, 1974.
101. Temkin NR and others: A randomized, double-blind study of phenytoin for the prevention of post-traumatic seizures, *N Engl J Med* 323:497-502, 1990.
102. Tullock WC and others: Neuromuscular and cardiovascular effects of high-dose vecuronium, *Anesth Analg* 70:86-90, 1990.
103. Wald SL, Shackford SR, Fenwick J: The effect of secondary insults on mortality and long-term disability after severe head injury in a rural region without a trauma system, *Journal of Trauma* 34:377-82, 1993.
104. Walls RM: Rapid-sequence intubation in head trauma, *Ann Emerg Med* 22:1008-13, 1993.
105. Woodring JH, Lee C: Limitations of cervical radiography in the evaluation of acute cervical trauma, *Journal of Trauma* 34:32-9, 1993.
106. Young WL, McCormick PC: Perioperative management of intracranial catastrophes, *Critical Care Clinics* 5:821-44, 1989.

26

RENAL DISORDERS

JOSEPH V. DOBSON
WILLIAM E. HARDWICK, JR.

Renal disorders are a common problem encountered in the transport of the critically ill child, and their prevalence has probably been underestimated in the existing literature. Of 2,124 patients transported to Children's Hospital of Wisconsin from 1989 to 1991, acute renal failure (ARF) or hemolytic uremic syndrome (HUS) was the primary diagnosis in 14 cases.[10] However, this does not include the many cases where renal insufficiency was a contributing factor, as in multisystem organ failure (MSOF), resulting from disseminated intravascular coagulation (DIC) or trauma, prerenal ARF from dehydration or shock, or the transport of neonates with congenital abnormalities (Potter's Syndrome, posterior urethral valves, or Prune Belly Syndrome). Thirteen of 125 pediatric patients transported to the Children's Hospital, Denver, from August 1979 to February 1980 were classified as having multiple organ/renal dysfunction (examples included acute renal failure and dialysis disequilibrium.[13] Accordingly, a thorough understanding of the evaluation and treatment of patients with renal failure is essential in pediatric transport.

RENAL PHYSIOLOGY

A basic understanding of renal physiology provides the cognitive framework necessary for the prediction of the metabolic derangements in renal disease and offers sensible methods of management.[20,44]

Through processes of glomerular filtration, tubular reabsorption, and secretion the kidneys are the major organs involved in maintaining electrolyte and volume balance. Metabolic end products (nitrogenous wastes), as well as many foreign chemicals and drugs, are eliminated by the kidney. The kidney also has important endocrine functions including the secretion of renin, erythropoietin, and the conversion of Vitamin D to its active metabolite (1,25 $[OH]_2D_3$).

The kidneys receive approximately 20 to 25% of cardiac output, and the nephron, the functional unit of the kidney, filters approximately 20% of the plasma delivered to it by way of the afferent arteriole. The efferent arteriole drains the unfiltered blood from the glomeruli and supplies blood to the peritubular capillaries or vasa recta. The glomerular filtration rate (GFR) is the product of single nephron GFR and the number of filtering glomeruli. In the adult male this is approximately 125 cc/min, but it is much less in the newborn (20-44 cc/min) or infant less than 1 year (60-80 cc/min).[6,24] The rate of filtration at the glomeruli is controlled by Starling's forces, the same forces that govern the movement of fluid across capillary membranes, and is proportional to the sum of the hydrostatic and osmotic forces favoring filtration minus the same forces opposing it. In general, hydrostatic forces favor filtration, and osmotic forces retard it. The kidneys can control or autoregulate GFR over a wide range of blood pressure by selectively dilating or constricting the afferent and efferent arterioles. The arteriolar resistance controls blood flow to the glomeruli by Ohm's Law (flow = pressure/resistance). Arteriolar resistance in the kidneys has several determinants: intrinsic mechanisms, neural innervation from sympathetic and parasympathetic activity, and hormonal influences. GFR can be estimated by measuring endogenously produced creatinine. Creatinine is largely a product of muscle metabolism, and unlike the BUN, it is produced in relatively constant amounts. It is not reabsorbed in the kidney but is secreted to a small extent leading to an overestimation of GFR in some instances (especially advanced renal failure).

Proximal tubule

The glomerular filtrate first enters the proximal convoluted tubule where approximately 60 to 70% of the water and solute is reabsorbed. Both active reabsorption and secretion occurs in the proximal tubule. Na^+ is actively reabsorbed by way of a Na-K ATPase in the basolateral membrane of the proximal tubular cell, and other solutes, such as glucose, amino acids, organic acids, and Cl^-, are reabsorbed by either secondary active transport with Na^+ or passive diffusion utilizing the electrochemical gradient established by the Na-K ATPase. K^+ is actively reabsorbed in the proximal tubule and secreted in exchange for Na^+ in the distal tubule. Water is reabsorbed by passive diffusion down the osmotic gradient created by the active reabsorption of Na^+ and other osmotically active solutes. Solute and water are reabsorbed in equal quantities in the proximal tubule, so the 30 to 40% of filtrate that leaves the proximal tubule is isotonic to plasma.[44]

Loop of Henle and distal tubule

The loop of Henle is responsible for establishing and maintaining an osmolar gradient in the medulla of the kidney by way of a process known as countercurrent multiplication. In the descending limb of the loop, where the epithelial cells are relatively impermeable to solute, water but not Na^+ is passively reabsorbed following the osmotic gradient between tubular fluid and interstitium. Approximately 15% of filtered water is reabsorbed in the descending limb. This creates tubular fluid with progressively increased osmolarity as it proceeds down the loop. In contrast, the ascending limb is impermeable to water but does cotransport Na^+, K^+, and Cl^- by Na-K ATPase powered active transport. The fluid leaving the loop of Henle is hyposmolar to plasma.[20] The osmolar gradient in the medulla of the kidney is critical for the final concentrating ability of the distal tubule and collecting ducts. In the presence of antidiuretic hormone (ADH), water is allowed to passively diffuse down an osmotic gradient as it passes through the progressively increasing osmolarity of the medulla creating concentrated urine (up to 1400 mOsm/l). Conversely, in the absence of ADH, hyposmotic or dilute urine (as low as 30 mOsm/l) is excreted. ADH is synthesized and released by the posterior pituitary. It is the hormone most responsible for maintenance of intravascular volume and osmolarity. As little as a 1% change in serum osmolarity can stimulate or inhibit ADH release. Hypovolemia through mediation of stretch receptors in the right atrium and baroreceptors in the carotid sinus also stimulates ADH release. Newborn infants do not have the concentrating capacity of older children and adults. The maximum urine concentration a newborn full-term infant can achieve is 700-800 mOsm/l (this is even less in premature infants). Similarly, neonates cannot maximally dilute their urine, which leads to problems handling both increased and decreased water load.[24]

Bicarbonate and hydrogen

Reabsorption of bicarbonate (HCO_3^-) and secretion of hydrogen (H^+) are coupled to sodium reabsorption. Under usual circumstances, approximately 85% of HCO_3^- is reabsorbed in the proximal tubule, while the remaining 15% is reabsorbed in the distal tubule. Premature and full-term infants have a lower capacity to reabsorb HCO_3^-. They excrete HCO_3^- when their capacity is exceeded (serum levels approaching 20-22).[24] Filtered HCO_3^- combines with H^+ secreted into the tubular fluid by H-Na countertransport to form carbonic acid (H_2CO_3) which is unstable and dissociates into H_2O and CO_2. The CO_2 passively diffuses into the tubule cell down its concentration gradient where it is rehydrated to carbonic acid by carbonic anhydrase in the cell. The H_2CO_3 breaks down into HCO_3^- and H^+. The HCO_3^- diffuses down its concentration gradient across the basolateral membrane into the interstitial fluid, and the H^+ is once again pumped into the tubular fluid in exchange for Na^+. In the proximal tubule, no net secretion of hydrogen is achieved, but HCO_3^- is reabsorbed. The energy is derived from a Na-K ATPase on the basolateral membrane which establishes the chemical gradient driving H-Na countertransport on the luminal membrane. After all the HCO_3^- is reabsorbed in the distal tubule, further secretion of H^+ combines with titratable phosphates or acidifies the urine through the production of ammonium (NH_4).[20]

Hormone effects

Aldosterone, a mineralocorticoid synthesized in the adrenal cortex, is the hormone responsible for Na^+ and K^+ balance. Aldosterone acts on the cells of the distal tubule to increase the reabsorption of Na^+ and the secretion of both H^+ and K^+ by coupled countertransport. K^+ and H^+ compete for the receptor responsible for their secretion. Increased Na^+ delivery to the distal tubule will thus increase secretion of H^+ or K^+ depending upon which is more readily available. Aldosterone secretion is regulated by the renin-angiotensin system. Renin, released from the juxtaglomerular cells of the afferent arterioles, stimulates the conversion of angiotensinogen to angiotensin I which is further metabolized to the biologically active angiotensin II in the pulmonary circulation by angiotensin converting enzyme. Angiotensin II is a potent arteriolar vasoconstrictor as well as being the major stimulator of aldosterone release from the adrenals. Accordingly, any process that stimulates renin release leads to aldosterone mediated Na^+ and water retention. Aldosterone secretion is also regulated by serum K^+ and serum Na^+ levels. Changes in K^+ concentration as small as 0.5 meq/L stimulate or inhibit aldosterone secretion where larger changes in Na^+ concentration must occur (as much as 10-20 meq/L) before aldosterone is affected.

Renin release is controlled by multiple inputs sympathetic innervation, hormones (angiotensin II, catecholamines, ADH), K^+, and Na^+ delivery to the distal tubules. Decreased renal perfusion pressure from any cause (hypoperfusion from hemorrhage or dehydration, CHF, renal artery stenosis) activates receptors in the walls of the afferent arteriole and stimulates renin release. Decreased Na^+ delivery to the distal tubule resulting from either decreased renal perfusion pressure (with resultant decreased GFR) or Na^+ depletion stimulates renin release, probably by way of the macula densa (specialized renal tubular cells at the junction of the loop of Henle and the distal convoluted tubule). Increased sympathetic activity through both circulating catecholamines and autonomic innervation also stimulates renin release. Renin release is inhibited by angiotensin II as well as by ADH and potassium.

RENAL INSUFFICIENCY

Renal failure is defined as a loss of renal function or glomerular filtration rate, leading to an inability to maintain metabolic and volume homeostasis.[4,6,34] While the transport physician will most often encounter children with acute renal failure (ARF), it is not infrequent that a neonatal patient or child with known chronic renal failure (CRF) should also require transport. For the purposes of transport, the principles of evaluation and management of both acute and chronic renal insufficiency will be discussed together with differences emphasized in the Special Circumstances section.

Etiology

The etiologies of acute renal failure are diverse and vary according to age. It is helpful to classify them pathophysiologically. One must remember that several mechanisms may be occurring simultaneously, and ARF may be superimposed on preexisting CRF[4] (see Box 26-1). Approximately 50% of ARF in children is secondary to hemolytic uremic syndrome and acute glomerulonephritis. In contrast, ARF in neonates is often due to perinatal insults (>60%) such as perinatal asphyxia, hypoxia, and sepsis.[34]

BOX 26-1 ETIOLOGIES OF ACUTE RENAL FAILURE

- Prerenal
  - Hypovolemia
    - Hemorrhagic shock
    - Dehydration (GI losses)
    - Insensible fluid loss (burns, prematurity)
    - Salt and water wasting (renal, adrenal, endocrine)
    - Hypoproteinemia
  - Hypotension
    - Congestive heart failure
    - Decompensated shock (cardiogenic, septic, hypovolemic)
    - Congenital heart disease
- Intrinsic
  - Primary parenchymal disease
    - Hemolytic uremic syndrome
    - Post-strep AGN
    - Lupus erythematosus
    - Henoch-Schonlein purpura
    - Pyelonephritis
    - Malignant hypertension
  - Acute tubular necrosis
    - Ischemia (prolonged prerenal ARF)
    - Nephrotoxins
      - Heavy metals
      - Uric acid
      - Drugs (aminoglycosides, vancomycin, indomethacin, sulfonamides)
      - Radiocontrast materials
      - Myoglobin or hemoglobin
  - Large vessel occlusion
    - Renal vein thrombosis
    - Renal artery stenosis
    - Thrombosis or emboles
  - Congenital anomalies
    - Renal agenesis
    - Infantile polycystic kidney disease
    - Bilateral multicystic kidneys
- Postrenal
  - Obstructive uropathy
    - Posterior urethral valves
    - Prune belly syndrome
    - Neurogenic bladder
    - UPJ obstruction
    - Tumor
    - Nephrolithiasi

Data from Anand SK: *Ped Clin N Am* 29:791-6, 1982; and Bergstein JM: *The urinary system.* In Behrman RE, editor: *Nelson Textbook of Pediatrics,* ed 14, Philadelphia, 1992, WB Saunders.

Prerenal. Prerenal ARF results from any process which leads to hypovolemia or hypotension, both of which result in a decrease in renal perfusion pressure. This affects GFR in several ways. Decreased arterial blood pressure under normal circumstances causes a reflex vasodilation of the afferent arteriole to maintain glomerular blood flow and GFR. This will maintain a relatively constant GFR to mean arterial pressures (MAP) as low as 80 mmHg. When MAP falls below the kidney's ability to autoregulate, a combination of neurohumoral and sympathetic stimulation results in afferent and efferent arteriolar vasoconstriction which decreases hydrostatic pressure at the glomeruli and decreases glomerular filtration by Starling's Law.[39] Sympathetic stimulation and decreased afferent arteriolar blood pressure also stimulates the release of renin from the juxtaglomerular cells, leading to angiotensin II mediated aldosterone secretion from the adrenal. Proximal tubular reabsorption of Na^+ and H_2O increases with decreasing proximal tubular flow and distal tubular reabsorption of Na^+ increases with aldosterone, resulting in near total (>99%) reabsorption of Na^+ (FeNa <1 and $U_{Na} < 20$). ADH release is also stimulated by hypovolemia leading to further concentration of urine ($U_{osm} > 500$ and $U_{SG} > 1.020$) in the distal tubule and collecting ducts (Table 26-1).[34]

With decreased GFR, less creatinine and urea are filtered, leading to their accumulation in serum. The urea which is filtered can be reabsorbed to a greater extent due to decreasing proximal tubular flow resulting in an elevated BUN/Cr ratio, since creatinine is not actively reabsorbed. If renal perfusion is restored promptly the process reverses itself, and renal function improves. However, if decreased perfusion is prolonged, intrinsic damage and acute tubular necrosis ensues.[2,6]

Intrinsic. The pathophysiology leading to intrinsic renal failure is diverse and depends upon the disease process, but all have a final common result of nephron damage and progressive, often irreversible, loss of glomerular function. In some cases, decreased glomerular function is a result of damage to the arterioles and glomerular capillaries from

TABLE 26-1 DIFFERENTIATION OF PRERENAL VS INTRINSIC RENAL FAILURE

	Prerenal		*Intrinsic*	
	Children	*Neonates*	*Children*	*Neonates*
FeNa*	<1	<2.5	>2	>3.0
Specific gravity	>1.020	>1.015	<1.010	<1.015
Urine osmolality	>500	>400	<350	<400
U_{osm}/P_{osm}	>1.5	>1.2	<1.2	
U_{Na}(meq/L)	<20	<40	>40	
BUN/Cr	>20		10-15	

* FeNa = $(U_{Na}/P_{Na})/(U_{Cr}/P_{Cr}) \times 100$

Data from Anand SK: *Kidney Intl* 43:1197-1209, 1993; Gaudio KM, Siegel NJ: *Ped Clin N Am* 34:771-85, 1987; and Schrier RW: *Hosp Pract* 16:93, 1981.

coagulation (HUS), inflammation (glomerulonephritis), or barotrauma (malignant hypertension). Acute tubular necrosis (ATN) from prolonged ischemia (prerenal ARF) or nephrotoxins is characterized by necrosis and sloughing of the cells of the proximal tubule and the ascending loop of Henle, resulting in obstruction of tubular flow and backleak of fluid into the peritubular space and plasma.[34] This is presumably due to the proximal tubular cells' inherent high metabolic demands and resultant vulnerability to ischemic insult. Occlusion of the renal arteries from thrombosis or emboli directly causes decreased renal blood flow and infarction. Renal vein thrombosis leads to vascular congestion and hemorrhagic necrosis. Angiotensin-converting enzyme inhibitors can lead to ARF in the patient with bilateral renal artery stenosis by inhibiting the angiotensin II induced efferent arteriolar vasoconstriction resulting from the high renin state.[6,39]

Postrenal. Decreased GFR and renal function in patients with postrenal ARF results from the alteration of Starling's forces favoring filtration at the glomerulus. Obstruction of urine outflow at any level (renal pelvis, bladder, urethra) results in transmitted increased hydrostatic pressure at the proximal tubule and glomerulus and decreased glomerular filtration. Prolonged unrelieved obstruction causes irreversible renal parenchymal damage by both increased prolonged hydrostatic pressure and ensuing infection.[38]

Diagnostic evaluation

The first step in the evaluation of a patient with renal failure is to obtain a complete history and physical. The transport physician must not let the signs and symptoms of the precipitating illness misdirect him/her from the consideration of renal insufficiency. The clinical manifestations are largely dependent upon the disease process that precipitates the renal insufficiency (fever and petechiae in DIC, thrombocytopenia and microangiopathic anemia in HUS, history of sore throat, hypertension and nephritic urine in post-strep AGN, shock or CHF in prerenal ARF). Most patients will have oliguria (<400 cc/m² or <1 cc/kg/hr) or anuria, symptoms related to nitrogenous waste retention (uremia) or salt and volume overload. However, not all patients have oliguria. In some patients, urine output is normal or increased (nonoliguric renal failure as in aminoglycoside nephrotoxicity and many instances of chronic renal insufficiency).[34,40] Symptoms of uremia include nausea, vomiting, diarrhea, pruritus, fatigue, peripheral neuropathy, seizures, and coma. Salt and water overload may present with edema, cardiomegaly, or hypertension.[6,22]

Laboratory and radiologic evaluation. Laboratory and radiologic evaluation on transport should be confined to either previously obtained or easily obtainable studies. Extensive laboratory evaluation and referral testing is usually not necessary. Essential evaluation includes electrolytes and calcium, urinalysis (and urine electrolytes if rapidly available), complete blood count and differential with platelet count, an ECG and a CXR[2] (see Box 26-2). Because of the kidney's role in maintaining volume and electrolyte status, abnormalities in electrolyte levels are common. Hyponatremia, while occasion-

BOX 26-2 LABORATORY AND RADIOLOGIC EVALUATION

Electrolytes
Calcium
CBC with differential and platelets
Urinalysis
Urine electrolytes
ECG
CXR

ally secondary to renal salt wasting in some forms of CRF, is usually dilutional secondary to water retention resulting from decreased GFR and ARF. Hyperkalemia (one of the most life-threatening complications of ARF) and metabolic acidosis result from decreased renal function and inability to secrete potassium and hydrogen in the distal tubules. Elevation of BUN and Cr often occur in renal insufficiency. It must be remembered that while serum creatinine crudely reflects GFR, up to 70% reduction in renal mass can occur prior to alterations in GFR or serum creatinine. Additionally, BUN and Cr may be normal early in the course of ARF, since creatinine rises only 0.5-1.0 mg/dl/day[2] in the presence of complete renal failure. The complete blood count is helpful in defining the etiology of the renal failure. Thrombocytopenia and evidence of microangiopathic hemolytic anemia should lead one to consider either HUS[18] or DIC as the precipitating cause. Examination of the WBC and differential, and consideration of the clinical course and physical findings, will usually allow differentiation of the two. Isolated anemia might suggest an underlying chronic renal insufficiency, especially with a history of polyuria, polydipsia, failure to thrive, or rickets.

Urinalysis and urine electrolytes are also quite helpful in determining the etiology of renal failure. In prerenal ARF the urine-specific gravity is usually high (~1.035). Acute poststreptococcal glomerulonephritis (APSGN) and other forms of acute glomerulonephritis show hematuria (often grossly bloody or "tea-colored"), proteinuria, as well as RBC, hyaline, and granular casts. A grossly positive urine dip for blood in the absence of microscopic hematuria suggests hemoglobinuria from hemolysis or myoglobinuria from rhabdomyolysis. A urine indicative of infection (WBC cells or casts, bacteria) suggests pyelonephritis or obstructive uropathy with coexistent infection. APSGN can also have marked leukocyte casts and should not be confused with pyelonephritis. The presence of renal tubular or bladder epithelial cells or casts may suggest nephrotoxic ARF or drug induced acute interstitial nephritis.[9] A urine with isolated proteinuria or an isosthenuric urinalysis should suggest a form of CRF.

Calculation of urinary indices, and especially the fractional excretion of sodium (FeNa),[14] can often differentiate prerenal ARF from intrinsic renal failure (Table 26-1). In prerenal ARF the kidneys are hypoperfused and respond by decreasing GFR and increasing Na^+ and water reabsorption. As previously discussed, this will result in almost total reabsorption of Na^+ and a highly concentrated urine. Conversely, tubular dysfunction in intrinsic renal failure generally leads to wasting of Na^+ (Table 26-1). These values are useful only if the patient has not received diuretics.[22] In many circumstances, obtaining urine electrolytes is not feasible in the transport setting. Examining the BUN/CR ratio, while less reliable than the FeNa, may help differentiate the etiology of the renal failure. It is often >20 in prerenal failure and normal (10-15) in intrinsic renal failure. However, it can be falsely elevated in the presence of significant GI bleeding (increased production of urea) or decreased in liver disease or starvation (decreased production of urea). A 12 lead ECG is of particular importance in evaluating the severity of hyperkalemia. The appearance of tall peaked T-waves is the first sign of hyperkalemia and correlates with serum potassium of 7.0-7.5. These may be followed by ST-segment depression and widening of the QRS interval (K^+ 7.5-8.0), prolongation of the PR segment (K^+ 8.0-8.5), loss of the P-wave (K^+ 8.5-9.0), and finally ventricular tachycardia, fibrillation (K^+ 9.0-9.5), and arrest ($K^+ > 10.0$). A chest x-ray is often helpful in aiding the clinical exam in differentiating volume overload and depletion, both of which may have oliguria in the presence of renal failure. More comprehensive radiologic studies such as renal ultrasound are rarely feasible in the transport setting.

Management

Basic treatment of the neonate or child with renal insufficiency can be focused on correction of volume status, metabolic abnormalities, and hypertension.

Fluids. Initially, determine whether the patient has prerenal ARF with volume depletion or other forms of renal failure with euvolemia or volume overload. If the patient appears to have prerenal ARF according to clinical evaluation and laboratory examination (Table 26-1), volume should be administered. An unnecessary delay in fluid resuscitation can convert potentially reversible renal failure into irreversible failure. Initially, 10-20 cc/kg of isotonic crystalloid or colloid should be infused, and this can be repeated hourly until urine output is established. If the patient is not in decompensated shock, this may be given over 20 to 30 minutes. Crystalloid (normal saline or lactated Ringer's solution) is usually an appropriate first choice except in obvious cases of hemorrhagic shock where colloid (5% albumin) or reconstituted PRBCs should be made available as soon as possible. If the patient's blood type is unknown, O-negative blood should be used. The one situation where providing fluid in prerenal ARF may be hazardous is in the case of cardiogenic shock (a relatively rare form of shock in pediatrics). Patients with cardiogenic shock require inotropic support with dobutamine to improve cardiac output and renal perfusion pressure and would probably benefit from CVP (central venous pressure) or PAP (pulmonary artery pressure) monitoring. Should the patient with apparent prerenal ARF not respond to volume as expected, clinical reevaluation and a chest x-ray should help differentiate this disorder. Placement of a Foley catheter early in the course of treatment is essential to closely monitor urine output and to diagnose urinary obstruction as a cause of renal failure. Once hypovolemia has been corrected, infusion of maintenance fluids must be carefully considered. The degree of fluid restriction should depend upon whether the patient is anuric, oliguric, or nonoliguric. Perhaps the easiest method of calculating fluid rate involves providing insensible losses (approximately 400 cc/m2/d or 30-50 cc/kg/d) plus replacement of UOP and other losses (GI losses or increased insensible losses secondary to fever or extensive burns).[16] Insensible fluids should contain minimal Na^+ (about 0.3 meq/kg/d) and no K^+, but UOP replacement may require highly variable amounts of Na^+. Measurement of urinary electrolytes can often tailor IVF choice, but in the absence of such studies, a sensible initial fluid might be $\frac{1}{4}$NS or $\frac{1}{2}$NS. High concentrations of dextrose are sometimes required to maintain serum glucose levels because of low IVF rates. Begin with D10 and monitor serum glucoses frequently. Central line access may be necessary to administer fluids containing greater than D12.5. In some patients with obvious volume overload, restriction to less than insensibles may be necessary utilizing high dextrose containing fluids. CVP monitoring may aid in managing volume status in critically ill patients.[6,34]

The use of diuretics in ARF is controversial except in the case of ARF secondary to myoglobinuria or hemoglobinuria. In such cases, lasix at a dose of 1-2 mg/kg IV, followed in 5 to 10 minutes by mannitol 0.25-0.5 g/kg IV, may be used to establish UOP. This can be followed with a solution of 5% mannitol in $\frac{1}{4}$ NS cc per cc of urine output until the myoglobin or hemoglobin has cleared.[9] The use of lasix in patients with renal failure with volume overload (acute glomerulonephritis) and symptoms of CHF, hyperkalemia, or hypertension may be therapeutic.[40] In other cases of euvolemic renal failure with oliguria, the administration of lasix may stimulate urine production, but improvement in renal function has not been proven.[16]

Electrolytes

Hyponatremia. Rapid correction of hyponatremia, unless symptomatic, is usually not necessary during transport. Hyponatremia in ARF is most often dilutional secondary to volume overload. Nonemergent treatment is with fluid restriction. Symptomatic hyponatremia causing seizures may be treated using hypertonic (3%) saline. A correction of serum

Na^+ by 1-2 meq/dl is often sufficient to stop seizure activity. The amount of NaCl to administer can be calculated using the following formula:

$$\text{meq NaCl required} = 0.6 \times \text{Wt(kg)} \times (\text{desired serum Na[meq/l]} - \text{actual serum Na[meq/l]})$$

Rapid correction of sodium beyond these limits carries the risk of exacerbating volume overload, causing shrinkage of the brain secondary to osmotic shifts and rupture of the bridging veins leading to intracranial hemorrhage.[6]

Hyperkalemia. Hyperkalemia is a potentially life-threatening complication of renal failure (see Box 26-3). Serum K^+ less than 5.5 in an asymptomatic patient (no ECG changes) requires only careful cardiac monitoring and the removal of and KCl in the IVF. Patients with a serum K^+ of 5.5-7.0 should receive kayexylate (sodium polystyrene sulfonate resin). Kayexylate exchanges equal milliequivalents of Na^+ and K^+, and each gram removes 0.5-1.0 mmol of K^+. Exchange occurs in the colon and ileum, so retention enema is the preferred route of administration. The onset of action for kayexylate is slow (approximately 1 to 2 hours). In patients with a serum K^+ greater than 7.0, or any patient with symptomatic hyperkalemia, additional measures are necessary. Infusion of calcium gluconate stabilizes myocardial membranes from the effects of hyperkalemia. Monitor the heart rate closely, and stop the infusion if the HR drops more than 20 BPM. Infusion of calcium has no effect on serum K^+, but can have immediate and impressive effects on stabilizing ventricular rhythm. Infusion of insulin with dextrose has a rapid effect on lowering serum K^+ (onset of action within 15 minutes with a decrease in serum K^+ by a mean of 0.6-1.0 mmol/l after 1 hour). When giving insulin, monitor serum glucose frequently to avoid hypoglycemia.

BOX 26-3 TREATMENT OF HYPERKALEMIA

$K^+ < 5.5$ and no ECG changes
- Careful monitoring and removal of KCl from IVF

$K^+ = 5.5\text{-}7.0$ and no ECG changes
- Measures above and in addition:
  - Kayexylate 1 g/kg in 70% sorbitol pr or 30% sorbitol po

$K^+ > 7.0$ or any level with ECG changes
- Calcium gluconate (10%) 0.5-1.0 cc/kg (50-100 mg/kg) IV over 10 min
- Dextrose and regular insulin IV
  - Children: $D_{25}W$ 2 cc/kg (0.5 gm/kg) IV + insulin 0.1 U/kg over 30 min-1 hr
  - Neonates: $D_{10}W$ 2 cc/kg IV + insulin 0.05 U/kg IV followed by a constant infusion of $D_{10}W$ at 2-4 cc/kg/hr and insulin 0.1 U/kg/hr[27]
- High dose nebulized albuterol(10-20 mg diluted in 4 cc NS over 10 min)
- $NaHCO_3$ 1-2 meq/kg IV over 30 min-1 hr

Data from Allon M: *Kidney Intl* 43:1197-1209, 1993; and Cronan KM, Norman ME: Acute Renal Failure and Acute Glomerulitis. In Fleisher GR, Ludwig S, editors: *Textbook of Pediatric Emergency Medicine*, ed 3, Baltimore, 1993, Williams and Wilkins.

Recent studies have shown a reproducible and rapid reduction in serum K^+ following administration of selective beta-2 agonists at high doses (four to eight-fold higher than the clinical dose prescribed in asthma) in patients with hyperkalemia from acute renal failure, end-stage renal failure, and normal subjects. The onset of action was rapid, occurring within 30 minutes, and action was sustained up to 6 hours with a decrease in serum K^+ comparable to insulin. Coadministration of nebulized albuterol and insulin with dextrose had both an additive effect on relieving hyperkalemia and helped protect against insulin-induced hypoglycemia.[1] Bicarbonate has long been advocated in the acute treatment of life-threatening hyperkalemia and does decrease serum K^+ during prolonged administration. However, the onset of action can be quite variable and may not be as reliable as the measures listed above. Lasix (1 mg/kg IV), in addition to inducing a saline diuresis, causes kaliuresis and may help to lower hyperkalemia in the presence of adequate renal function. The above measures are short-term and should be followed with immediate dialysis at a tertiary care center.[6,9,22]

Hypocalcemia. Hypocalcemia is usually a result of hyperphosphatemia and should not be treated unless symptomatic (tetany, seizures, or decreased cardiac contractility). Rapidly raising serum calcium in the face of hyperphosphatemia can result in deposition of calcium salts in body tissues. Nonemergent treatment is achieved by administering calcium carbonate by mouth. This serves to concurrently lower serum phosphate and increase serum calcium.[4] If symptomatic hypocalcemia is present, cautious infusion of calcium gluconate (10%) 0.5-1.0 cc/kg (50-100 mg/kg) IV over 15-30 minutes is recommended.

Metabolic acidosis. Metabolic acidosis is common but should not be treated unless severe and symptomatic. Rapid infusion of $NaHCO_3$ can cause cerebral acidosis, exposes the patient to a high osmotic load (known to precipitate intraventricular hemorrhage in neonates), and can worsen hypocalcemia.[22] If the patient has myocardial or respiratory depression secondary to acidosis (usually pH <7.15 or HCO_3 < 8), a slow infusion of $NaHCO_3$ can be given (if adequate ventilation is ensured) to raise the serum HCO_3^- to 12 or pH >7.20. The amount of HCO_3^- to give can be estimated using the formula:

$$\text{meq NaHCO}_3 \text{ required} = 0.3 \times \text{Wt (kg)} \times (12 - \text{serum HCO}_3^-(\text{meq/l})).^6$$

Miscellaneous

Hypertension. Hypertension associated with ARF is usually the result of salt and water retention. Emergency treatment of hypertension on transport should be confined to patients with evidence of end-organ damage: papilledema, retinal hemorrhage, retinal artery spasm, CHF, facial palsy, or hypertensive encephalopathy (hypertension, headache, visual changes, nausea and vomiting, altered mental status, and seizures).[6,9] An indepth discussion of evaluation and treatment of malignant hypertension is discussed under its own section.

Pressors. The use of inotropic agents (dopamine or dobutamine) are not often needed except in the circumstance of cardiogenic shock leading to prerenal ARF. In cardiogenic shock high doses of dobutamine, and occasionally other inotropic agents, are needed along with CVP monitoring. Low dose dopamine (2-5 mcg/kg/min) stimulates renal blood flow, increases GFR and socium excretion, and may maintain renal function.[16,26,37]

Anemia. Anemia from acute or chronic renal failure is often well compensated and mild except in cases of severe HUS or DIC. With severe symptomatic anemia in patients with nonoliguric renal failure, cautious infusion of PRBCs may be given with attention to the possibility of worsening volume overload. Infusing small amounts (5cc/kg) sequentially or in association with diuretics is often needed. Infusion of PRBCs in patients with oliguric or anuric renal failure carries a high risk of inducing hyperkalemia, hypervolemic hypertension, and CHF, unless done concurrently with hemodialysis.[6]

Dialysis. While not feasible on transport, the need for or complications of dialysis may be an indication for critical care transport. In general, indications for dialysis include neurologic symptoms secondary to uremia or electrolyte imbalance, rapidly rising serum creatinine, persistent hyperkalemia and metabolic acidosis refractory to medical management, and persistent volume overload with evidence of CHF or hypertension refractory to medical management.[9,16]

Complications of dialysis may result from the dialysis procedure itself, access devices used for dialysis, or may be related to the underlying uremic state. When dialysis is done in a dedicated experienced pediatric center, complications can be minimized. The major risks of hemodialysis which may require critical care include hypotension, the disequilibrium syndrome, associated electrolyte disorders, and the risk of infection of access devices. Hypotension during dialysis is more common in pediatric patients and is due to the rapid removal of intravascular volume by ultrafiltration. This leads to decreased venous return to the heart, with resultant decreased filling pressures and cardiac output. Due to their impaired ability to compensate by increasing peripheral vascular resistance or heart rate (perhaps secondary to medication, autonomic neuropathy, or the dialysis procedure itself), hypotension may result.[25] The disequilibrium syndrome results from the rapid fall in extracellular osmolarity during dialysis. Mild symptoms include headache, abdominal pain, nausea, vomiting, lethargy, and fatigue. More serious symptoms may include seizures or coma from cerebral edema. This is thought to result from unequal reduction in cerebral intracellular and extracellular osmolarity, leading to fluid shifts and cellular swelling.[32] The disequilibrium syndrome is more common during the first sessions of dialysis, particularly in dialysis for acute renal failure.[25] Shunts and fistulas used for dialysis access can become infected (usually with *Staphylococcus aureus*) if strict sterile technique is not used, resulting in thrombophlebitis or sepsis. Septic pulmonary embolus and DIC has been reported.[23]

Peritoneal dialysis, like hemodialysis, has the potential for inducing metabolic abnormalities (hypokalemia, hypoalbuminemia, hypophosphatemia, hyponatremia) and hypotension. Peritonitis is a common complication of peritoneal dialysis, but usually does not cause critical illness and can often be treated on an outpatient basis using intraperitoneal antibiotics with cover coagulase negative staphylococcus. However, if diagnosis is delayed, or infection with Gram-negative organisms occurs, more serious illness may ensue.[32]

Prognosis

Prognosis for recovery of renal function in patients with acute renal failure is largely dependent upon the underlying disorder. Prompt evaluation and appropriate treatment can improve outcome or facilitate complete recovery in many cases (ARF, HUS, APSGN, rhabdomyolysis, PUVs). With improvements in dialysis and transplant medicine, stabilization and transport of all critically ill patients with renal insufficiency offers potentially life-saving long-term therapy.

Special circumstances

Hemolytic uremic syndrome. The hemolytic uremic syndrome (HUS) is one of the most common causes of ARF in children and should always be considered in the differential of sudden onset of renal failure in a child.[41] It is characterized by a triad of microangiopathic hemolytic anemia, thrombocytopenia, and ARF.

Classically, the primary event in pathogenesis of the syndrome is thought to be endothelial cell injury in the renal cortex leading to localized coagulation and fibrin deposition.[36] The microangiopathic anemia results from damage to the red blood cells as they pass through the fibrin strands in the renal vasculature, and the thrombocytopenia results from consumption in the localized intravascular coagulation. Several infectious organisms have been implicated in the etiology of HUS, including several bacteria and viruses. In particular, verotoxin producing strains of *E. coli* have been associated with up to 75% of HUS in some studies.[30]

Clinically, HUS occurs primarily in infants and young children under 4 years of age. It is often preceded by a gastroenteritis type illness. Symptoms, including abdominal pain, vomiting, and often bloody diarrhea, can be confused with intussusception or an acute surgical abdomen. As the gastrointestinal symptoms abate, the child becomes suddenly ill with symptoms or irritability, restlessness, and pallor, signs of oliguria or anuria, fluid overload (peripheral or pulmonary edema and hypertension), and petechiae. Laboratory examination shows a Coomb's negative hemolytic anemia (Hematocrit values ranging from 15-30) with an elevated reticulocyte count, thrombocytopenia (20-100K), and evidence of ARF (elevated BUN and Cr, hyperkalemia, metabolic acidosis). The blood smear shows fragmented RBCs and a lack of platelets. Coagulation studies are usually normal, and there may be a leukocytosis up to 30,000 from bone marrow stimulation. Urinalysis, when the patient is not anuric, usually includes mild to severe proteinuria and microscopic hematuria.[41]

Treatment of HUS is supportive, but early recognition and aggressive management can result in low morbidity and mortality with recovery of renal function in about 85% of patients. Therapy focuses on control of fluid and metabolic balance, hypertension control, and early treatment of renal failure with hemodialysis or peritoneal dialysis.[35] The use of steroids, platelet inhibitors, anticoagulants, plasmapheresis, or plasma infusions show no clear benefit in HUS.[6]

While the prognosis in HUS is generally excellent with aggressive, early treatment, certain clinical features suggest a poorer outcome. These features include patients with an atypical nondiarrheal prodrome, a familial predisposition, recurrent episodes of HUS, severe central nervous system involvement, persistent thrombocytopenia, prolonged anuria, or adults with HUS.[36]

Acute glomerulonephritis

Acute glomerulonephritis (AGN) is a syndrome that is characterized by sudden onset of nephritis (gross hematuria, proteinuria, edema) and is often accompanied by hypertension, renal insufficiency, and symptoms of intravascular expansion. While a variety of organisms can induce an acute nephritic syndrome, by far the most common organism is Group A, beta hemolytic (type 12) streptococci. Acute poststreptococcal glomerulonephritis (APSGN) can occur following either pharyngeal or skin infections with Group A strepococci. This is in contrast to rheumatic fever which only follows pharyngeal infections with certain strains of streptococci.[7]

APSGN commonly occurs in school age children (average age 7 years), with more males affected than females. Most cases are sporadic, but epidemic disease does occur.[9] Clinical nephritis usually manifests 1-2 weeks after the infection; therefore, most patients are culture negative at the time of presentation. Thirty to 50% of patients have gross hematuria, often described as tea colored or coca-cola® colored.[7] Many cases of AGN are mild, asymptomatic, and do not require transport or hospitalization. Most patients requiring critical care transport have oliguria with symptoms of volume overload, including peripheral and pulmonary edema, CHF, and hypertension. The pathogenesis of AGN is thought to involve immune complex deposition in the basement membrane of the glomeruli with activation of the complement pathway leading to inflammation and glomerular damage.[9]

Laboratory analysis reveals a characteristic urinalysis with RBCs, RBC casts, proteinuria, WBCs, and WBC casts. The WBCs and WBC casts represent glomerular inflammation and not pyelonephritis. Evidence of renal insufficiency includes an elevated BUN and Cr, hyponatremia (dilutional), hyperkalemia, and acidosis (secondary to aldosterone suppression from volume expansion). The kidneys maintain their ability to conserve sodium, so the FeNa is usually low (<1%). Depressed C3 levels are important laboratory confirmation of AGN. Final confirmation of APSGN requires documentation of elevated antibody titers to streptococci (ASO, AHT, or anti-DNase B).[6]

Treatment of AGN is largely supportive. The severe manifestations of AGN which will most likely require transport involve volume overload from reduced GFR and oliguric renal failure. Hypertension from volume overload, if severe with symptoms of end-organ damage, requires immediate treatment as discussed elsewhere. Additional fluid in the form of IV fluids should not be administered, since this could only aggravate the patient's condition. Fluid and sodium restriction and the administration of loop diuretics (lasix 1-2 mg/kg/dose) are effective in relieving mild hypertension, edema, and circulatory congestion. If there is evidence of current streptococcal infection, a course of penicillin is appropriate, but this will not alter the course or prognosis of the nephritis. With appropriate management, full recovery with low morbidity is expected in >98% of children.[7]

Chronic renal insufficiency

Chronic renal failure (CRF) is rarely the sole presenting feature in a child requiring critical care transport. Most cases of CRF in children are diagnosed by pediatricians prior to development of end stage renal disease or metabolic derangements. This is because signs of growth failure, polyuria, or anemia may become manifest when renal function reaches 25-50%, but biochemical abnormalities do not develop until renal function decreases below 30%.[32] However, patients with undiagnosed chronic renal insufficiency (residual renal function of 25-50%) may present with complications when stressed. In particular, any precipitating cause of ARF can cause acute decompensation in a patient with decreased renal reserve. Additionally, patients with renal insufficiency have increased risk of infection secondary to defective granulocyte function and impaired cellular immune function.[6]

The etiologies of CRF are generally acquired, hereditary, or congenital (see Box 26-4). The most common cause of CRF in children is obstructive uropathy from reflux

BOX 26-4 ETIOLOGIES OF CRF

Acquired
- Glomerulonephritis
- Hemolytic uremic syndrome

Hereditary
- Hereditary nephritis (Alport syndrome)
- Cystic kidney disease

Congenital
- Hypoplasia
- Dysplasia
- Obstructive uropathy (posterior urethral valves, UPJ obstruction, reflux nephropathy)

nephropathy or congenital obstruction. Patients with CRF requiring transport present with many of the same metabolic derangements as patients with ARF (hyponatremia, hyperkalemia, metabolic acidosis, hypertension, anemia) and principles of diagnosis and management on transport are similar (See **Management** section above). Hyponatremia may be due to either salt wasting or water retention. Hyperkalemia and acidosis result from decreased excretion. Anemia occurs secondary to insufficient production of erythropoietin in response to reduced hemoglobin. Hypertension may result from salt and water retention or from the renin overproduction in the diseased kidney. An important difference between acute and chronic renal insufficiency is that most patients with early chronic renal insufficiency are not oliguric and can maintain water balance. Patients with congenital renal abnormalities may have salt and water wasting. Therefore, strict fluid restriction in these circumstances would not be appropriate. However, advanced CRF does generally have salt and water retention similar to ARF and may require use of fluid restriction or diuretics. A thorough clinical evaluation of the individual patient's fluid status is essential to management.

Cardiac complications of CRF, in particular CHF from hypertension or volume overload or uremic pericarditis, may be important indications for transport.[17] In neonates, cases of severe Potter's syndrome (renal agenesis, PUVs, or polycystic kidneys leading to pulmonary hypoplasia from oliguria) can present particularly difficult transport situations primarily because of the severe pulmonary compromise.

No definitive treatment exists for CRF, but with improvements in renal replacement therapy (dialysis and renal transplantation), patients with CRF can lead increasingly normal and productive lives. Because of this potential, stabilization, management and transport of patients with renal insufficiency has had growing importance for minimization of morbidity and mortality.

Drug dosing in renal failure. Drug dosing in patients with acute or chronic renal failure is an important consideration, since many drugs utilized widely on transport are primarily excreted through the kidney. In order to minimize toxicity, dose and interval need to be adjusted according to the patient's renal function.[39] When possible, substitute a medi-

BOX 26-5 DRUGS IN RENAL FAILURE

Drugs requiring adjustment in renal failure:
- Muscle relaxants
  - pancuronium (pavulon)
- Antibiotics
  - vancomycin
  - aminoglycosides
  - most penicillins and cephalosporins
- Anticonvulsants
  - phenobarbital
  - carbamazepime (tegretol)
- Miscellaneous
  - insulin
  - digoxin

Drugs **not** requiring adjustment in renal failure:
- Muscle relaxants
  - vecuronium (norcuron)
  - succinylcholine
- Antibiotics
  - nafcillin
- Vasoactive agents
  - dopamine
  - dobutamine
  - nipride
- Anticonvulsants
  - phenytoin (dilantin)
  - valproic acid
- Benzodiazepimes
  - midazolam (versed)
  - lorazepam (ativan)
  - diazepam (valium)
- Miscellaneous
  - lidocaine

cation which does not require adjustment (i.e., vecuronium for pancuronium). Box 26-5 lists drugs which are commonly used on transports and which do and do not require adjustment in renal failure. Antibiotics like vancomycin and the aminoglycosides have greatly prolonged half-lives. A single loading dose will generally be sufficient to maintain therapeutic drug levels through the duration of transport.

HYPERTENSIVE EMERGENCIES

In the past a numerical value for blood pressure has been used to define a hypertensive emergency.[31] But an isolated blood pressure measurement is probably a poor determinant of the seriousness of the clinical situation or of the need for emergency treatment, transportation, or hospitalization. For example, adults with chronic hypertension may have great elevations of blood pressure (greater than 150 mm Hg diastolic) without complaints or outward evidence of end-organ dysfunction; however, a child with poststreptococcal acute glomerulonephritis may be seen in a truly life-threatening state from an acute but more modest elevation of blood pressure. Therefore, the definition of a true hypertensive emergency should not be based on any absolute level of blood pressure, but should consider multiple factors, including rate of rise of blood pressure, duration of hypertension, and clinical indications of immediate threat to the patient. The Joint National Committee on Detection, Evaluation, and Treatment of High Blood Pressure suggests a more functional classification system using two categories: emergencies and urgencies. Emergencies are defined as situations in which elevated blood pressure must be lowered immediately (within 1 hour) to prevent progression of end-organ damage, whereas urgencies are situations where severe elevations in blood pressure are not causing immediate threat, but should be controlled within 24 hours to reduce potential patient risk.[15,28] For the purpose of transport, we will concern ourselves only with the emergency situations (see Box 26-6).

Pathophysiology

In order to safely treat hypertensive emergencies, the transport physician must be aware of some basic regulatory mechanisms affecting blood pressure. If arterial blood pressure rises too high or falls too low, the cerebral arteries respond with constriction or dilatation, respectively, to maintain uniform cerebral blood flow. This phenomenon is referred to as autoregulation. Although cerebral blood flow is maintained uniformly over a wide range of blood pressures, there is a lower as well as an upper limit to autoregulation.[19] In normotensive adults, cerebral blood flow is decreased when mean arterial pressure (MAP) falls below 60 mm Hg. However, in chronically hypertensive adults, this lower limit of autoregulation appears to be set higher with symptoms suggesting cerebral ischemia developing in patients with MAP as high as 120 mm Hg.[33,42,43] Coronary artery perfusion and renal perfusion are similarly maintained by autoregulation. Clinical manifestations of cerebral and coronary hypoperfusion includes seizures, transient ischemic attacks, blindness, myocardial infarction or dysrhythmias. Renal ischemia, in contrast to cerebral or myocardial ischemia, is generally more reversible, but if hypoperfusion is excessive or prolonged, renal ischemia may cause acute tubular necrosis. Thus, there are risks associated with too rapid or excessive reductions of elevated blood pressure.

In a hypertensive emergency setting, however, these risks of rapid reduction of blood pressure are less than the risk of continued vascular damage and should not delay treatment. The need to lower blood pressure rap-

BOX 26-6 HYPERTENSIVE EMERGENCIES

Emergencies
- Hypertensive encephalopathy
- Severe malignant hypertension accompanied by
  - Acute left ventricular failure
  - Acute myocardial infarction or unstable angina pectoris
  - Dissecting aortic aneurysm
  - Stroke or head trauma
  - Progressing renal insufficiency
  - Eclampsia with convulsions or fetal distress
  - Postoperative bleeding
  - Extensive burns

idly, however, does not imply the need to achieve normotension. The goal is to reduce blood pressure to a level that avoids hypertensive complications, but at the same time, maintain it at a level above the lower limits of autoregulation and ensure adequate perfusion to the brain and other organs. A review of hypertensive adults suffering neurologic injury in association with antihypertensive therapy found that, in the majority, the MAP was reduced by more than 50%, and the diastolic blood pressure was reduced to less than 90 mm Hg. These low pressures were maintained for hours to days.[19] Suggested guidelines to avoid these complications include decreasing the blood pressure in the first 6 hours by not more than one-third of the total reduction planned and then by the final two-thirds over the following 2 to 4 days.[12] A simpler guideline is to acutely lower the MAP by no more than 20 to 25% of the original value.[3] To avoid cerebral hypoperfusion, any sign of neurologic deterioration during therapy should prompt upward adjustment of these guidelines.

Emergency treatment

Unlike other disease processes, if blood pressure is indeed deemed a threat to life or organs, treatment must be begun immediately, even before the cause is known. History and physical, investigative procedures (laboratory, x-ray) should be performed simultaneously with treatment (see Box 26-7). The ideal drug for treating hypertensive emergencies should have several characteristics:

BOX 26-7 INITIAL DIAGNOSTIC STUDIES

Urinalysis, bun, creatinine, electrolytes
CBC and PLT count
Chest x-ray
ECG

1. It should be easily titratable with a rapid onset and offset of action permitting smooth, precise control of blood pressure.
2. It should be easily administered and monitored.
3. It should be effective in a variety of scenarios.
4. It should have minimal side effects.

Such an ideal medication does not exist. A number of drugs do possess some but not all of the above characteristics and should be considered during the transportation of a hypertensive emergency. Sublingual nifedipine, intravenous labetalol, and intravenous sodium nitroprusside presently are the drugs of choice in hypertensive emergencies (Table 26-2).

Nifedipine, a calcium channel antagonist, is listed by virtue of its oral/sublingual administration with its major advantage being administration in the emergency setting before IV access or intensive care monitoring is available. When puncturing the capsule and expressing the contents sublingually, nifedipine has a relatively rapid onset of action. Drawbacks of nifedipine use include less control

TABLE 26-2 DRUGS OF CHOICE IN HYPERTENSIVE EMERGENCIES

Drug	*Dose*	*Onset*	*Comments*
Nifedipine (Procardia)	0.25-0.5 mg/kg SL (Max = 10 mg)	20-30 min.	Sublingual administration
Labetalol (Normodyne, Trandate)	1-3 mg/kg/hr IV (Max = 3 mg/kg/hr 300 mg total daily dose	1-5 min.	Contraindications: Congestive heart failure Heart block Asthma
Sodium Nitroprusside (Nipride)	0.5-8.0 μgm/kg/min	1-5 min.	Intensive care monitoring Cyanide toxicity
Diazoxide (Hyperstat)	1-2 mg/kg IV (Max = 150 mg/dose)	3-30 min.	Unpredictable BP control—Long duration of effect

Data from Jung FF, Ingelfinger JR: *Pediatr Rev* 14:169-79, 1993.

over the rate of blood pressure reduction as well as a longer duration of action, thus making it less useful than other drugs in the titration of blood pressure in a true hypertensive emergency.[5,21]

Labetalol is an antihypertensive drug possessing both alpha and beta adrenergic blocking properties. With continuous intravenous infusion, there is a prompt and controlled reduction in blood pressure. Because of its dominant beta adrenergic blocking effects, labetalol should not be used in patients with congestive heart failure or asthma. However, it may be useful in the management of hypertension associated with catecholamine excess states (thyrotoxic disorders or pheochromocytoma).[12,15]

Sodium nitroprusside acts as a direct vasodilator with a balanced effect on both arterioles and venules, decreasing preload, afterload, and myocardial oxygen demand. When given intravenously, effects of nitroprusside are seen almost immediately, and when therapy is discontinued, blood pressure rises rapidly to previous levels within five minutes.[19] Because of this precise control of blood pressure, as well as the sparing of sympathetic reflexes, nitroprusside has been used widely and successfully to treat acute hypertensive emergencies in pediatric patients. Disadvantages of the drug include the need for intensive care monitoring during its use, inactivation of the drug by light, and the possibility of cyanide intoxication.[21]

Diazoxide, another direct acting vasodilator, historically has been recommended for hypertensive emergencies but now is considered a second-line drug.[12] Disadvantages of diazoxide include a reflex increase in sympathetic activity, a less predictable reduction of blood pressure (particularly with bolus administration), and a duration of action anywhere from 2 to 12 hours, thereby preventing rapid return of blood pressure to baseline, should hypotension occur. To avoid such complications, use of diazoxide should be limited to repeated intravenous mini-boluses of 100-150 mm or to continuous infusion.[19,45]

In general, when treating hypertensive emergencies it is probably best to use a single antihypertensive agent and avoid the unpredictable responses associated with multiple drugs. The majority of children who present with hypertensive emergencies will have an ECF volume which is normal or reduced; the administration of diuretics at this time is contraindicated and may actually potentiate the action of another antihypertensive medication, causing profound hypotension. Unless fluid overload is obvious, it is appropriate to reserve diuretics until the hypertensive emergency is stabilized.[11] Sedatives are also contraindicated in this situation because they can only serve to confuse the evaluation of neurological symptoms.[8]

Complications and adverse events

As discussed previously, there are risks associated with overaggressive reduction of elevated blood pressure. All patients being transported for hypertensive emergencies should be closely monitored and observed for signs of complications, including shock, seizures, transient ischemic attacks and blindness. Any evidence of shock or hypoperfusion in these patients should be treated aggressively with volume resuscitation. If a child in hypertensive crises is having a coexisting seizure, an appropriate anticonvulsant can be administered as long as steps are also being taken to reduce blood pressure.[12]

REFERENCES

1. Allon M: Treatment and prevention of hyperkalemia in end-stage renal disease, *Kidney International* 43:1197-1209, 1993.
2. Anand SK: Acute renal failure in the neonate, *Pediatr Clin North Am* 29:791-96, 1982.
3. Aoki B, McCloskey K: Hypertensive emergencies. In Aoki B, McCloskey K, editors: *Evaluation, stabilization and transport of the critically ill child,* St. Louis, 1992, Mosby Year Book.
4. Barratt TM: Acute renal failure. In Holliday MA, Barratt TM, Vernier RL, editors: *Pediatric nephrology,* Baltimore, MD, 1987, Williams & Wilkins.
5. Bauer JH, Reams JP: The role of calcium entry blockers in hypertensive emergencies, *Circ* 75:174-9, 1987.
6. Bergstein JM: The urinary system. In Behrman RE, editor: *Nelson textbook of pediatrics,* ed 14, Philadelphia, PA, 1992, W.B. Saunders Co.
7. Berry PL, Brewer ED: Acute poststreptococcal glomerulonephritis. In Oski FA, editor: *Principles and practice of pediatrics,* 1990, J.B. Lippincott Co.
8. Burris JF: Hypertensive emergencies, *Cardiovasc Clin* 16:3:163-79, 1986.

9. Cronan KM, Norman ME: Acute renal failure and acute glomerulitis. In Fleisher GR, Ludwig S, editors: *Textbook of pediatric emergency medicine,* ed 3, 1993, Williams & Wilkins.
10. Day SE: Intra-transport stabilization and management of the pediatric patient, *Pediatr Clin North Am,* 40:265, 1993.
11. Dillon MJ: Modern management of hypertension. In Meadows R, editor: *Recent advances in pediatrics,* Edinburgh, 1984, Churchill Livingstone.
12. Dillon MJ: Drug treatment of hypertension. In Holliday, editor: *Pediatric nephrology,* ed 2, Baltimore, 1987, Williams & Wilkins.
13. Dobrin RS and others: The development of a pediatric emergency transport system, *Pediatr Clin North Am* 27:633, 1980.
14. Espinel CH: The FeNa test, *JAMA* 236:576, 1970.
15. Ferguson R, Vlasses P: Hypertensive emergencies and urgencies, *JAMA* 255:1607-13, 1986.
16. Fildes RD, Springale JE, Feid LG: Acute renal failure: II. management of suspected and established disease, *J Pediatr* 109:4:567-71, 1986.
17. Fine RN: Recent advances in the management of the infant, child, and adolescent with chronic renal failure, *Pediatr Review* 11:9:277-82, 1990.
18. Fong JSC, de Chadarevian JP, Kaplan BS: Hemolytic uremic syndrome, current concepts and management, *Pediatr Clin North Am* 29:835, 1982.
19. Franklin SS: The case for more rapid lowering of blood pressure. In Narins, editor: *Controversies in nephrology and hypertension,* ed 1, New York, 1984, Churchill Livingstone.
20. Ganong WF: Renal function. In Ganong WF, editor: *Review of medical physiology,* ed 12, Los Altos, CA, 1985, Lange Medical Publications.
21. Garcia JY, Vidt DG: Current management of hypertensive emergencies, *Drugs* 34:263-78, 1987.
22. Gaudio KM, Siegel NJ: Pathogenesis and treatment of acute renal failure, *Pediatr Clin North Am* 34:3:771-85, 1987.
23. Grushkin CM, Fine RN: Management of the child on chronic dialysis. In Lieberman E, editor: *Clinical pediatric nephrology,* Philadelphia, PA, 1976, J.B. Lippincott Co.
24. Guignard JP: Renal function in the neonate, *Pediatr Clin North Am* 29:777-9, 1982.
25. Hakim RM, Lazarus JM: Complications during hemodialysis. In Nissenson AR and others, editors: *Clinical dialysis,* Norwalk, CT, 1984, Appleton-Century-Crofts.
26. Henderson IS, Beattie TJ, Kennedy AC: Dopamine hydrochloride in oliguric states, *Lancet* 2:827, 1980.
27. Ingelfinger JR: Renal conditions in the newborn period. In Cloherty JP, editor: *Manual of neonatal care,* Boston, MA, 1991, Little, Brown and Co.
28. Joint National Committee on Detection, Evaluation, and Treatment of High Blood Pressure: The 1984 report of the joint national committee, *Arch Intern Med* 144:1045-57, 1984.
29. Jung FF, Ingelfinger JR: Hypertension in childhood and adolesence, *Pediatr Rev* 14:5:169-79, 1993.
30. Karmali MA and others: The association between idiopathic hemolytic uremic syndrome and infection by verotoxin-producing E. coli, *J Infect Dis* 151:775-82, 1985.
31. Koch WJ: Current concepts: hypertensive emergencies, *Med Clin North Am* 63:127-40, 1979.
32. Kohaut EC: Chronic renal failure and end-stage renal disease. In Oski FA, editor: *Principles and practice of pediatrics,* Philadelphia, PA, 1990, J.B. Lippincott Co.
33. Lassen NA: Cerebral blood flow and oxygen consumption, *Physiol Rev* 39:183-238, 1959.
34. Marisculco MM: Acute renal failure. In Oski FA, editor: *Principles and practice of pediatrics,* Philadelphia, PA, 1990, J.B. Lippincott Co.
35. Mayes TC, Terhune PE: Hemolytic uremic syndrome. In Oski FA, editor: *Principles and practice of pediatrics,* 1990, J.B. Lippincott Co.
36. Miller K, Kim Y: Hemolytic uremic syndrome. In Holliday MA, Barratt TM, Vernier RL, editors: *Pediatric nephrology,* ed 2, Baltimore MD, 1987, Williams & Wilkins.
37. Parker SP and others: Dopamine administration in oliguric and oliguric renal failure, *Crit Care Med* 9:630, 1981.
38. Porth CM: *Pathophysiology, concepts of altered health states,* ed 3, Philadelphia, PA, 1990, J.B. Lippincott Co.
39. Ramon JC, Ongkingo MD, Bock GH: Diagnosis and management of acute renal failure in the critical care unit. In Holbrook PR, editor: *Textbook of pediatric critical care,* Philadelphia, PA, 1993, WB Saunders.
40. Schrier RW: Acute renal failure, pathogenesis, diagnosis and management, *Hosp Prac* 16:93, 1981.
41. Stewart CL, Tina LU: Hemolytic uremic syndrome, *Pediatr Review* 16:6:218-24, 1993.
42. Strandgaard S: Autoregulation of cerebral blood flow in hypertensive patients, *Circulation* 53:720-6, 1976.
43. Strandgaard S and others: Autoregulation of brain circulation in severe arterial hypertension, *Br Med J* 1:507, 1973.
44. Thies R, Person RJ, editors: *Physiology,* 1987, Stringer-Verlog.
45. Wilson DJ, Vidt DG: Control of severe hypertension with pulse doses of diazoxide, *Clin Pharmacol Ther* 23:135-40, 1978.

27

ENDOCRINE AND METABOLIC DISORDERS

DAVID JAIMOVICH

Patients presenting with metabolic derangements due to primary metabolic disorders and illnesses of nonmetabolic etiology which may lead to secondary metabolic imbalance may be frequently encountered by medical personnel caring for critically ill children. This chapter is intended to provide personnel who care for critically ill children in the pretransport and the intertransport periods with the necessary information to comprehend the important principles, pathophysiology, differential diagnosis, and effective therapy for the most common endocrine and metabolic disorders encountered in an emergency setting.

INBORN ERRORS OF METABOLISM

Altogether, these diseases belong to a large group, but singularly, a transport team may only see a few of these patients per year (see Box 27-1). These patients generally present during the neonatal period or early infancy, since their critical illness presents after the initiation of feedings and the introduction of protein in the diet. Patients who present later in life usually have a more insidious course of onset and are often initially misdiagnosed.

These patients will frequently present with vomiting, lethargy, central nervous system depression, failure to thrive, hyperventilation, seizures, and respiratory depression. Jaundice, hepatomegaly, hyperpigmentation, and sometimes dysmorphic features may indicate one of these disorders. Should the infant present with a fever and one or more of the above signs and symptoms, sepsis should be considered, but one must keep in mind that many disorders may be indicated by these symptoms.

There are three major groups into which these disorders are commonly divided. The first is based on biochemical findings including acidosis, hyperammonemia, high anion gap, and ketosis.[61] The other group includes metabolic intoxicants, including ammonia, amino acids, galactose, fructose, and/or organic acids. The third group is based on the failure of energy in organs such as the brain, heart, liver, and muscle. This may be due to fatty oxidation defects, congenital lactic acidemias, gluconeogenesis defects, dysfunctional peroxisomes, or defective mitochondrial function.[130]

The most common disorders which the transport team may be faced with include urea cycle defects, organic acidemias, amino acid metabolism disorders, and defects associated with carbohydrate metabolism.

After a patient's medical history and physical examination have been conducted and the severity of illness and stability have been established, a minimum set of laboratory data should have been obtained or recommended. When the transport team arrives, these results should be available. Necessary laboratory results include an arterial blood gas, an arterial sample of blood for ammonia (placed

BOX 27-1 EXAMPLES OF INBORN ERRORS OF METABOLISM

Defects of Amino Acids Metabolism
- Tyrosinemia
- Phenylketonuria
- Maple syrup urine disease

Defects of Carbohydrate Metabolism
- Lactose intolerance
- Glycogen storage diseases
- Mucopolysaccharidoses

Defects of Lipid Metabolism
- Hyperlipoproteinemias
- Congenital adrenal dyperplasia
- Metachromatic leukodystrophies

Defects on Erythrocyte Metabolism
- Methemoglobinemia
- Glucose-6-Phosphate dehydrogenase (G-6-PD)

Defects of Vitamin and Mineral Metabolism
- Vitamin D—dependent rickets

Primary Defects of Renal Tubular Transport Mechanism
- Fanconi syndrome
- Nephrogenic diabetes insipidus

in ice), calcium, electrolytes, glucose, BUN, creatinine, liver enzymes, bilirubin, prothrombin time (PT), partial thromboplastin time (PTT), a complete blood cell count, and if the patient is febrile, a blood culture. A complete urinalysis, including microscopic analysis and culture, Clinitest and Phenistix testing should be included. Urine pH results and microscopic examination results will be as important as the serum determination to establish renal function, since many of these patients may present with renal tubular acidosis.[145]

Differential diagnosis

It is not the intent for the transport team to perform a complete and detailed differential diagnosis during the interhospital transfer of a critically ill infant, but the team must consider other possible life-threatening illnesses.

Patients may be hypoalbuminemic due to recurrent or chronic illnesses. This will significantly change the anion gap and thereby mask the biochemical imbalance of a lactic acidemia. Renal failure, toxins, and other organic acids may cause an elevated anion gap with normal lactate and albumin. Anion acidemia should be suspected if the patient presents with elevated ammonia levels and a high anion gap acidosis, since a secondary urea cycle defect is often produced. A urea cycle defect should be suspected if the patient has significantly elevated ammonia levels without other anion deficiencies and without acidosis.

Carnitine deficiency,[17,59] congenital lactic acidosis, transient hyperammonemia of the newborn, valproate toxicity, and salicylate toxicity are among some of the other potential causes of pediatric hyperammonemia.

Principles of management and initial therapy

As with any critical emergency, initial assessment of the patient must begin with airway, breathing, and circulatory status (ABCs). Airway compromise from depressed mental status, seizure activity, or depressed respiratory drive will be an indication that endotracheal intubation should be strongly considered prior to transporting the patient. Respirations should be supported throughout the transport until the patient has arrived safely at the tertiary care facility and is in a more controlled environment.

Blood glucose by rapid bedside determination method should be assessed and kept within normal range. If hypoglycemic the patient should be treated accordingly with 0.5 to 1 g/kg of a dextrose solution. A repeat bedside glucose determination should be performed within 30 minutes after the administration of dextrose. If the patient presents with severe acidosis, he or she may need to be treated with bicarbonate replacement. This should be done carefully and slowly, preferably, by continuous infusion with a dose no greater than 1 mEq/kg/hr.

Usually, metabolic defects are not accompanied by liver failure in children, therefore if the patient is clinically stable and does not show signs of encephalopathy, the usual nonspecific treatments may be bypassed.

ADRENAL GLAND DISORDERS

Adrenal gland failure leading to adrenal insufficiency can develop primarily or from hypothalamic, pituitary failure (secondary). Adrenal insufficiency is uncommon in the general pediatric intensive care patient. Adrenal crisis (hypocortisolism) is a potentially dangerous and often unrecognized emergency requiring prompt and accurate recognition and immediate therapy. On the other hand, Cushing's syndrome (hypercortisolism) can present with hypertensive encephalopathy, leading to seizures requiring emergent treatment. Disorders of androgen production are illnesses that may be seen in the pediatric critical care setting, but are rarely acute or life-threatening. Many of the inborn errors of biosynthesis of cortisol and/or aldosterone may be grouped together under the term congenital adrenal hyperplasia (CAH). This entity may present with severe electrolyte abnormalities (low sodium, high potassium) and severe dehydration leading to shock. The initial presentation is usually in a newborn infant, but there may be similar clinical findings in an older infant or young child.

Adrenocortical insufficiency

Clinical presentation. Inadequate mineralocorticoid and glucocorticoid effects are both responsible for the clinical manifestations of a patient in acute adrenal crisis. Although these crises are uncommon in the pediatric emergency setting, the health care professional must be prepared to deal with them.

Patients commonly present with weight loss, dehydration, hypotension, or profound shock. Electrolyte abnormalities including hyponatremia, hyperkalemia, hypercalcemia, and acidosis are due to a lack of mineralocorticoid. Inspite of the loss of extracellular fluid volume, the shock or preshock state may respond poorly to volume and catecholamine infusions alone, but may require, in addition, replacement of the glucocorticoid deficit.[51,121] Patients may also present with confusion, apathy, or frank psychosis due to the lack of glucocorticoid. Abdominal pain, nausea, vomiting, and diarrhea are common complaints of patients with acute adrenal insufficiency. Sudden death has been reported in adrenal insufficiency.[75] The health care provider may be faced with a variety of clinical presentations of adrenal insufficiency. The neonate may have adrenal aplasia or perinatal adrenal hemorrhage, usually associated with a traumatic birth; both clinical situations may lead to cardiovascular collapse. A more subacute insidious onset of clinical signs is characteristic of congenital adrenal hyperplasia, a group of disorders inherited as autosomal recessive traits. These infants may present at 1 to 4 weeks of age with a salt-losing severe 21-hydroxylase deficiency producing an adrenal crisis. These patients clinically have progressive irritability or lethargy, vomiting, poor feeding, and progress to overt cardiovascular collapse. The infant who presents with severe dehydration may be suspected of having pyloric stenosis, but congenital adrenal hyperplasia must be considered in the differential diagnosis. The infant with CAH will be hyponatremic and hyperkalemic; metabolic acidosis may be present if in impending shock. In contrast, the infant with pyloric stenosis should not be hyponatremic and should present with a metabolic alkalosis due to chloride loss in the emesis. Even though sepsis, congenital heart disease, trauma and inborn errors of metabolism must be considered, CAH should not be forgotten as a possible cause of shock or neurological deterioration in an infant. These patients require urgent repletion of the intravascular volume, sodium replacement, and glucose support. As long as the sodium replacement is adequate, mineralocorticoid therapy may not be necessary. These therapies alone may correct the hyperkalemia without any further intervention.

If CAH is suspected, emergency administration of stress doses of glucocorticoids should be administered. It is unlikely to be detrimental to an infant not suffering from CAH, but it may be useful to one that does have CAH.

Acute hemorrhage into the adrenal glands as a result of a coagulopathy can appear at any age; the Waterhouse-Friderichsen syndrome is usually associated with sepsis.

It has been suggested by Knowlton[87] that the association of petechiae with meningococcemia is a sign that the adrenal glands may be at risk for developing this syndrome. Acute adrenal failure due to adrenal hemorrhage can therefore lead to cardiovascular collapse. The theory of reduced adrenal corticosteroid output due to poor adrenal perfusion during a state of shock with cardiovascular collapse[70] has been challenged by more recent data[18] demonstrating that the adrenal medulla and the adrenal cortex are protected during shock and hypoxia, respectively.

Patients with Addison's disease, a syndrome of chronic hypoadrenalism may present with a milder form of the adrenal crisis syndrome with episodes of acute life-threatening decompensation occurring occasionally.

Due to the increasing number of children with human immunodeficiency virus (HIV) infection, endocrinologic dysfunction is an ever increasing presentation with this clinical entity.[131] Histologic abnormalities and invasion of the adrenal cortex by opportunistic infections has been reported in up to 80% of HIV positive patients.[60] Currently, slightly less than 20% of Addison's disease is due to tuberculosis with the remaining 80% due to an autoimmune cause.[81,116] Some other infectious agents include: cytomegalovirus, cryptococcus, and mycobacterium avium-intracellulare.

The health care professional should also consider certain drugs that may cause inhibition of adrenal steroidogenesis including trimethoprim-sulfamethoxasole and ketoconazole. One other important case of adrenal hypofunction which should be considered is the patient who is deficient in ACTH production, secondary to either primary pituitary disease such as tumors, surgery, radiation (especially after tumor removal), infarction, or hypothalamic-pituitary-adrenal (HPA) axis suppression due to exogenous corticosteroids. Although the patient may show signs of cortisol deficiency, volume depletion may not be as much of a problem for these patients as for those with primary hypoadrenalism. These patients may develop hyponatremia secondary to ingestion of unquantified amounts of hypotonic fluids. The mineralocorticoid effect of cortisol partially controls fluid homeostasis. The health care provider must also consider the multiple hormone deficiencies which may occur in these complex patients, such as growth hormone, thyroid stimulating hormone, ACTH from the adenohypophysis, and vasopressin from the neurohypophysis.

Treatment and management. As with any patient in shock, the establishment of at least one but preferably two secure intravenous (IV) lines for fluid replacement and drug administration are necessary. Blood samples are used to determine baseline cortisol, electrolytes, BUN, glucose, and calcium (ionized calcium preferably) values. If a central line or an intraosseous (IO) line has been placed in the bone marrow, 25% dextrose may be given in a dose of 2 ml/kg, IV or IO, unless the glucose is known to be normal. If the patient only has peripheral IV access, the concentration of dextrose should be limited to 12.5%, and the dose should be doubled to 4 ml/kg IV. An infusion of 5% dextrose in normal saline at twice the maintenance rate should be started. If the patient shows signs of shock, 20 ml/kg of normal saline or lactated Ringer's solution should be infused as rapidly and as often as is necessary to reverse a state of shock. The patient should receive hydrocortisone replacement when adrenal crisis has been diagnosed at a dose equivalent to 50 to 100 mg/m^2/day IV (divided into 4 doses). This is approximately four to eight times the non-stress physiologic dose of 12 mg/m^2/day IV. If the child is stable, the dose can be tapered over several days to the physiologic dose level.

The clinician must be aware that, for the patient with known adrenal hypofunction, any stress sufficient to bring the patient to a state of severe dehydration, hypoperfusion, or frank shock will require additional emergency corticosteroid supplementation. Any patient that presents with sepsis, major trauma, or severe gastroenteritis leading to significant dehydration should be covered with a minimum of three to four times the maintenance dose of steroids. Acutely, we would rather administer an excess rather than the more dangerous inadequate dosage of corticosteroids. Physiologic stress steroid replacement doses should be considered in the patient with acute adrenal damage, such as meningococcemia.

The health care professional dealing with an acutely ill, unstable patient who had been on steroids for a chronic illness, such as asthma or collagen vascular disease, should be supplemented with stress dosage of three to four times the physiologic maintenance they have been on.

Pheochromocytoma

Pheochromocytomas are rare catecholamine secreting tumors. Children with this disorder may present with hypertension, sometimes so severe it may include hypertensive encephalopathy or cardiac failure. Unlike in adults, children will secrete primarily norepinephrine which leads to severe hypertension. These tumors are usually located within the adrenal medulla but may be found elsewhere in the body.[150]

Clinical presentation and treatment. Children usually do not present with palpitations, headache, and paroxysmal sweating as the adult patient. They usually have sustained symptoms rather than intermittent. Children usually present with sustained hypertension, headaches, sweating, nausea, vomiting, visual disturbances, and weight loss. They also present with tachycardia, polydipsia, polyuria, abdominal pain, and tremors. It is not uncommon for these patients to be volume contracted and therefore present with polycythemia and an elevated hematocrit. These patients may develop hypertensive encephalopathy and cardiac failure. The usual peak incidence occurs in children between 9 and 12 years of age, but all ages have been reported. It is more common in boys, and malignancies, although rare, are reportedly bilateral and multiple.

Patients with multiple endocrine adenomatoses, Cushing's syndrome, and neurofibromatosis should be seriously considered for pheochromocytoma if they present with hypertension. If the patient develops uncontrolled hypertension while awaiting the transport team or during transport, a sodium nitroprusside infusion may be started at a low dose (0.25-1.0 mcg/kg/min), and continuous cardiac and hemodynamic monitoring (at least by automatic inflating cuff placed at one minute intervals for recording of blood pressure) should be instituted. Should tachydysrhythmias develop, they would be best managed with lidocaine (1-2 mg/kg IV bolus and continuous infusion at 20-80 mcg/kg/minute). If control is not achieved, then the clinician should consider intravenous propranolol (0.01 to 0.1 mg/kg IV slowly; maximum of 1 mg/dose) or esmolol (0.3-0.5 mg/kg over 5 min and an infusion at 0.025-0.1 mg/kg/min titrated to effect). If hypotension should develop, this is best managed with crystalloid infusion.

Medical personnel caring for patients who have suffered chronic severe hypertension and require acute therapy must keep in mind that there has been an upward shift in the lower limit of the autoregulatory curve for cerebral blood flow.[6,56,123] Therefore, even though there is no such data on chronically hypertensive children, one should consider a fall of 20 to 40 mm Hg to be the maximum for patients receiving acute treatment for chronic hypertension and pheochromocytoma.

THYROID DISORDERS

Even though thyroid storms are rare amongst pediatric critically ill children, it represents a rare form of acute multisystem failure in children, and since this disorder is not easily recognized, it carries a high mortality rate unless it is diagnosed early and treated aggressively.

Pathophysiology

The pathogenesis of thyrotoxicosis, also known as Grave's disease is based on an autoimmune and a genetic etiologies. Thyroid function is regulated by hypothalamic-pituitary control and intrathyroidal autoregulation. Thyrotropin releasing hormone (TRH) is produced in the hypothalamus, stimulating thyrotropin [thyroid-stimulating hormone (TSH)] production once it reaches the anterior pituitary. TSH is then secreted, facilitating the secretion of thyroid hormone by direct action on thyroid follicular cells. Alterations in the supply of iodine may cause a dysfunction in the autoregulation of the thyroid. The thyroid becomes more responsive to TSH when the iodide supply is low.

The cellular effects of thyroid hormones remain unclear. There is an increase in adrenergic receptor sites in myocardial cells due to thyroid hormone and an increase in glucocorticoid lung tissue. Although oxygen consumption is not influenced, chronotropic and inotropic effects of thyroid hormones can be reversed by beta adrenergic blockade.[84] The metabolism of various hormones (insulin, cortisol, etc.) can be accelerated by thyroid hormone, bone turnover,[34,100] and hematopoiesis.[74] Maturation of many systems in the early neonatal period,[110] various endocrine functions such as normal luteinizing hormone, follicle-stimulating hormone, growth hormone,[64] and normal hypoxic and hypercapnic drives need thyroid hormone for normal function.

Clinical presentation. Since most of the signs and symptoms produced by an excess of thyroid hormone would be similar to a hypermetabolic state with a particular emphasis on the cardiovascular system, it is not a surprise that the most commonly reported symptoms in childhood thyrotoxicosis are autonomic in nature. Tachycardia,[126] nervousness,[126] increased pulse pressure, increased appetite, proptosis, tremors, weight loss, and heat intolerance[30] are the most commonly reported signs and symptoms in childhood thyrotoxicosis. Less frequently, dysrhythmias, psychosis, congestive heart failure, shock, coma, and seizures may also present.[1]

There are other disorders associated with thyrotoxicosis including diabetes mellitus,[32] Down's syndrome, juvenile rheumatoid arthritis, Addison's disease, myasthenia gravis, Hashimoto's thyroiditis, the nephrotic syndrome, chronic active hepatitis, and possibly systemic lupus erythematosus. Thyroid storms usually have an abrupt onset and almost always follow an acute stress situation. Any child known to have one or more endocrinopathies or autoimmune disease should alert the clinician that they are at higher risk for developing thyroid disease. These patients may present with confusion, lethargy, weakness, diaphoresis, cutaneous flushing, fever, and tachycardia. In extreme cases, these patients may have hepatomegaly, jaundice, nausea, and vomiting. If left untreated this illness will progress to extreme hyperpyrexia, coma, and death.[30] In addition to the usual manifestations of thyroid hormone excess, patients in thyroid storm will have an altered mental status, fever, and tachycardia out of proportion to the fever. Agitation, psychosis, stupor, or coma may present as the central nervous system manifestations.[117]

The differential diagnosis of thyrotoxic crisis includes sepsis, malignant hyperthermia, anticholinergic poisoning transfusion reactions, and adrenal crisis. The health care provider should be alerted to the possibility of thyroid storm in a patient with no known thyroid disease or familial thyroid disease or a patient known to have multiple endocrinopathies.

The medical team at the referring institution, as well as the transport team, will not have the benefits of diagnostic tests, since definitive serum concentrations of triiodothyronine (T^3) and tetraiodothyronine (T^4 or thyroxine) would take too long to establish a definitive diagnosis by laboratory values. Therefore, the diagnosis of thyroid storm is reached tentatively based on the patient history and physical examination, and treatment should not be held up awaiting the results of thyroid hormone levels.

Management. Thyrotoxic patients in crisis, with major organ system dysfunction induced by excessive thyroid hormone, need to be stabilized to achieve a euthyroid state as soon as possible to prevent worsening of an altered hemodynamic state. Secondly, effective treatment for the condition that is causing the significant morbidity should be established. The hyperdynamic cardiovascular state and the effects of the accelerated metabolic state must be addressed initially. As with all life-threatening illnesses the ABCs must be followed, and attention must be given to the airway first. Supplemental oxygen should be provided, but most children will maintain intact airway reflexes and not require airway intervention. At least one large bore IV catheter, preferably two, should be secured and hypovolemia corrected rapidly with 20 ml/kg of crystalloid solution. This should be delivered as rapidly as possible and as often as necessary. A rapid bedside glucose determination should be performed, and if the patient develops hypoglycemia, dextrose 0.5-1 gm/kg IV should be administered and a glucose/crystalloid containing solution should then be infused. External cooling and nonaspirin antipyretics (aspirin may displace thyroid hormone from binding proteins and increase free hormone levels,[153] should be administered for fever. If the patient's hyperdynamic cardiovascular state is so severe prior to transport, IV propranolol (0.01 mg/kg) should be administered by slow IV push every 10 minutes until improved or until a total of 5 mg has been given. One should be careful with patients who have a history of reactive airway disease, since this may be exacerbated by the administration of beta-blockers. In patients with Grave's disease, glucocorticoids may inhibit the release of thyroid hormone from the thyroid[4] and may inhibit the conversion of T^4 to T^3 (0.1 mg/kg dexamethasone).[30,135] The clinician should be aware that, in the event of induced bradycardia secondary to beta blockers, atropine and ultimately isoproterenol may be required to reverse this process. Thyroid stimulating immunoglobulins may have transplacental passage in mothers with Grave's disease. Some of the drugs which the mother may be required to take may cross the placenta. Even though the infant may appear euthyroid at birth, as the bloodstream levels of these antithyroid drugs fall, the infant will become progressively more hyperthyroid. Neonatal thyrotoxicosis may present at 1 to 2 weeks of age with symptoms similar to neonatal sepsis. These patients will appear febrile, irritable, and will require appropriate treatment for sepsis, including as full septic workup. They may present with failure to thrive, diarrhea, thrombocytopenia, feeding intolerance hepatosplenomegaly, and seizures in which the treating team must consider other neonatal differential diagnoses, including congenital and acquired infections, congenital heart disease, or the possibility of a drug-abusing mother.[114] These patients should be treated with the same consideration and priority and the same treatment methods as for older children with thyroid storm.

Hypothyroidism

Infants and children with hypothyroidism are usually asymptomatic or minimally symptomatic, and the diagnosis may be easily missed. The most severe clinical presentation is myxedema, and this is extremely rare in children. These patients usually present with all the symptoms of a severe hypometabolic state, including sluggishness, hypothermia, constipation, and bradycardia. Patients may present with the most severe form which is coma with congestive heart failure and tachycardia; not infrequently pericardial effusion may be present. Many factors may precipitate myxedema in an already hypothyroid patient (see Box 27-2). In adults, pulmonary infections[48] have been reported as the most common precipitating factor. This has not been the case in children.

Physical examination. Vital signs may be important diagnostic clues, including body temperature below normal in cases of myxedema.[48] These patients will generally have a regular, but bradycardic pulse, and the blood pressure will often be elevated.[48] With longstanding hypothyroidism, patients may present with characteristic skin findings including thick and doughy appearance, orange or yellow tint without scleral icterus indicating carotenemia. Dry and brittle hair and periorbital edema or other cutaneous signs. These patients may present with respiratory compromise (upper airway obstruction) secondary to macroglossia.

Cardiac examination may reveal muffled heart sounds, decreased intensity of the point of maximum impulse and cardiomegaly consistent with a pericardial effusion. These patients rarely, if ever, suffer pericardial tamponade.[147] Patients may present with abdominal findings consistent with decreased bowel sounds and distention indicative of an ileus or a pseudoobstruction.

Diagnosis and treatment. Again as in other thyroid states, it is important to recognize that immediate diagnosis will only be by clinical findings, since confirmation with serum thyroid function tests are not laboratory tests which would be readily available.

Successful treatment of infants and chil-

BOX 27-2 FACTORS THAT MAY PRECIPITATE MYXEDEMA

Surgery
Anesthesia
Myocardial insufficiency
Sedatives and narcotics
Gastrointestinal bleeding
Intracerebral bleeding
Hyponatremia
Injections
Exposure to cold

dren with myxedema includes treating the metabolic complications, infections, life-threatening emergencies, and supportive care (see Box 27-3). Emergent treatment, as in all thyroid disorders, includes establishing an adequate airway and ensuring breathing and circulation. When presenting with hypothermia, these patients are best treated with passive rewarming. Active rewarming such as warm baths has shown a lack of efficacy[141] and may in fact represent a hazard by causing peripheral vasodilation worsening preexisting shock.[12,141] Hyponatremia generally responds well to fluid restriction, since these patients may present with a syndrome of inappropriate antidiuretic hormone. Most authors recommend judicious use of hypertonic saline when the serum sodium concentration falls below 120 mEq/L, since infants and children may suffer seizures if the serum sodium is allowed to go below this level.[12,152] Treatment with IV glucose may be indicated, and seizures may be treated with standard anticonvulsants once correction of hyponatremia, hypoglycemia, and hypoxia have been instituted. These patients may not present with fever, sweating, or leukocytosis, and therefore the identification of infections may be difficult.[103]

Supportive care. Since these patients may present with hypercarbia, hypoxia, or decreased airway reflexes, intubation and assisted ventilation should be carried out immediately when indicated.[163] Hypotension should be treated aggressively with fluid and inotropic support if indicated. Dopamine may be preferable to other inotropic agents in order to maintain coronary blood flow in these patients.[152] Stress dose glucocorticoids (12 mg/m²/day in four divided doses) may be beneficial, since these patients may have multiple endocrinopathies, including adrenal disease.

Myxedema is a rare condition which, if untreated, carries a high mortality. The pathophysiology is complex and often involves profound hypothyroidism as well as an inciting event. The diagnosis should be based on the clinical presentation, and treatment should not be delayed while awaiting confirmatory laboratory data.

BOX 27-3 TREATMENT FOR MYXEDEMA

- Correction of electrolyte imbalance
- Passive rewarming
- Antibiotics for underlying infections
- Respiratory support
  - Endotracheal intubation (if indicated)
- Hemodynamic support
  - Dopamine 5-15 mcg/kg/min (better for coronary flow)
  - Crystalloid boluses 20 ml/kg (until refill <2 sec)
- Treat hypoglycemia
  - Dextrose 25%—0.5-1.0 gm/kg *bolus*
- Stress dose steroid therapy
  - Hydrocortisone

ELECTROLYTE DISORDERS

Potassium

Pathophysiology. The serum potassium concentration is regulated more tightly than any other ion, and minor changes in extracellular potassium concentration could lead to increase morbidity and potentially life-threatening consequences. Neuromuscular transmission is dependent on the ratio of intracellular to extracellular potassium.

The treating team must keep in mind that alterations in acid-base balance could cause potassium shifts into and out of cells. Some examples of various illnesses or injuries include alkalemia, which leads to hypokalemia as potassium enters cells in exchange for hydrogen ions and thereby minimizes changes in extracellular pH. It can be misleading, since the measured pH change is not predictive of the change in serum potassium concentration. Certain patients may be susceptible to unpredictable potassium shifts which may be associated with profound muscle weakness or significant periodic paralysis as hypokalemia exists. Hypothermia will induce intracellular potassium shifts, and subsequent rewarming will lead to efflux of potassium from the intracellular space into the intravascular space. Potassium supplementation in these cases must be done cautiously, since it may cause severe hyperkalemia in patients who are rewarmed too quickly.

In the adult population, hypokalemia has

been associated with an increased frequency of atrial and ventricular ectopy, including atrial tachycardia, atrial ventricular blocks, premature ventricular contractions, ventricular tachycardia, and fibrillation. This is not commonly seen in the pediatric population, unless either these patients had congenital heart disease (CHD), are experiencing presurgical or postsurgical repair for CHD, or had a history of atrial or ventricular dysrhythmias. In known cardiac patients the arrhythmias of digitalis intoxication are worsened by hypokalemia and hypercalcemia; therefore, serum potassium levels should be monitored carefully, especially if they are also receiving diuretic therapy.

One of the first manifestations of potassium depletion is muscle weakness which can lead to paralysis if treatment is delayed; in severe cases, respiratory muscle paralysis may occur. Cramping pain, swelling, and paresthesias are common complaints of patients with hypokalemia. Muscle ischemia has been reported as the cause of rhabdomyolysis leading to hypokalemia.[86] Patients may suffer a paralytic ileus due to impaired gastric motility which leads to nausea, vomiting, and constipation. Autonomic smooth muscle is usually the primary affected site.

Treatment of hypokalemic emergencies. If arrhythmias, respiratory muscle paralysis, or severe muscle weakness are believed to be secondary to hypokalemia, the IV route for rapid correction is required. Intravenous potassium chloride is the preferred medication for most emergencies except those involving concomitant phosphate depletion, such as diabetic ketoacidosis, where potassium phosphate may be indicated. Intravenous potassium should be administered through a large peripheral or central vein or via IO line to diminish the risk of causing sclerosis in smaller vessels. Intravenous potassium infusions should be mixed in solutions that do not contain dextrose, since this may stimulate endogenous insulin release with subsequent potassium shift intracellularly. The maximum recommended rate of IV potassium replacement ranges from 0.5 to 1 mEq/kg/hr. These doses must be given carefully, since they can rapidly lead to hyperkalemia, especially in the patients with concurrent acidemia, diabetes mellitus, and renal tubular acidosis. Other medications that may prevent potassium from entering the cell include: nonsteroidal antiinflammatory agents, angiotensin converting enzyme inhibitors, or beta-blockers.

Hyperkalemia

In the steady state, serum potassium levels are regulated by renal clearance which provides the ultimate defense against hyperkalemia. This state may be altered by either external or internal causes which may affect directly or indirectly the kidney. Other factors include hyperosmolarity which produces cellular contraction, increased cellular potassium levels, and potassium efflux from cells.[109] Skeletal muscle injury is a common source of elevated serum potassium following motor vehicle accidents or catabolic states such as major surgery, sepsis, or burns. Transient hyperkalemia may also occur during hemolytic states.[111] Other disorders include; various forms of urinary obstruction,[8] lupus nephritis,[35] patients with sickle cell nephropathy,[7] and patients on cyclosporine.[120] A rare cause of hyperkalemia is primary adrenal insufficiency (Addison's disease).[116] One of the most common causes of hyperkalemia is drug induced, secondary to a number of medications which may disturb the potassium balance. These include nonsteroidal antiinflammatory drugs, cyclosporine, potassium sparing diuretics, and angiotensin converting enzyme inhibitors such as captopril and enalapril.[103,143] Another cause of hyperkalemia which is often overlooked is excessive potassium intake in the form of either oral ingestion of potassium supplements or the dependent portion of unmixed parenteral fluid containers such as the potassium salts of penicillins and other IV medications.[89]

Clinical manifestations. Unless hyperkalemia is severe, it is usually asymptomatic. It is the effect on the electrical conduction of the heartbeat that forces prompt clinical attention to the imminent danger of cardiac arrest or arrhythmia. Levels of 6 mEq/L or less have insignificant effects on the heart. The appearance of tall peaked T-waves, especially in the precordial leads, is the initial change in the electrocardiogram as the levels of potassium increase. Unless treated, this finding may be the beginning of more serious electrocardiographic changes which may be manifested as merging of the normal U and T waves.[43] The Q-T interval is normal or diminished in hyperkalemia.[142] As the intraventricular conduction becomes further delayed, the PR interval becomes prolonged and then the P wave amplitude decreases; the QRS complexes widen into a sine wave pattern. This may represent a form of ventricular flutter which finally leads to the stages of cardiac standstill.[93] Other concomitant electrolyte abnormalities, such as hyponatremia, hypocalcemia, acidosis, or hypermagnesemia, may exaggerate these electrocardiographic changes.

Patients may present with pseudohyperkalemia which is a condition presenting with high serum levels invitro in normokalemic subjects who have markedly elevated platelet (greater than 10^6 platelets/mm^3) or white blood cell (greater than 50,000/mm^3) counts.[109] Obviously, hemolysis from phlebotomizing a patient may also create hyperkalemia when potassium is released from ischemic muscle distal to a tourniquet.[37]

Management. In the pretransport or transport setting, a critically ill patient may need to have treatment initiated before the cause is certain. Treatment choices include agents to antagonize the effect of potassium directly on membrane potentials, redistribute potassium internally into cells, or remove it from the body.

If electrocardiographic changes show a loss of P waves or widening of QRS complexes, this denotes cardiac toxicity and requires administration of intravenous calcium to reduce the membrane threshold potential so that normal membrane excitability is restored. Calcium will neither lower serum potassium levels nor remove it from the body. In patients with circulatory compromise, calcium chloride 25-50 mg/kg given IV over 1 hour will improve and protect cardiac conduction. It is appropriate to administer calcium if the serum level of potassium is greater than 7 mEq/L, since cardiac toxicity is imminent. The duration of action of calcium is so short that it must be combined with therapy to lower potassium levels; if the serum level is under 7 mEq/L, treatment may begin with measures to redistribute or rid the body of potassium. Regular insulin 0.1 U/kg IV will mobilize potassium into cells and should be given with glucose to avoid hypoglycemia, unless the blood sugar is substantially elevated (greater than 300 mg/dl). Repeated insulin doses may be administered combined with glucose infusion as needed.

Alkalinization therapy with sodium bicarbonate will also promote cellular uptake of potassium. This is most effective when acidosis is a contributing factor and may be used even in the absence of a low pH. It should be avoided in patients with hypernatremia, and if the serum calcium is low, as in uremic acidosis, calcium should also be given to avoid hypocalcemic tetany during alkali therapy.

While the above therapies are undertaken, measures to remove potassium from the body should also begin promptly once the patient is stabilized. Unless end-stage renal failure is present, powerful loop diuretics, such as furosemide, should be administered to promote kaliuresis. These patients should be given adequate amounts of normal saline to avoid volume depletion. Kayexalate may be administered if renal failure is severe, since potassium clearance by the colon can be augmented with this substance. This is a cation exchange resin which increases stool potassium in exchange for sodium. It can be given orally with 20% sorbitol to avoid constipation, and for a more rapid effect, or if ileus is present, a retention enema in a slurry of kayexalate and sorbitol is preferable. The clinician should be cautious of sodium overload which may occur if the patient has significantly compromised renal clearance.

Clinical disorders causing hypokalemia and hyperkalemia require a basic understanding of normal potassium homeostasis consisting of external and internal causes of potassium balance and imbalance. The renal system is primary in maintaining the external balance of potassium, likewise several factors are known to modulate the internal potassium balance, such as its distribution within the body.

Calcium homeostasis

The clinician must be aware of the important differences between calcium bound to albumin versus free, unbound ionized calcium (Ca^{2+}). Direct measurement of ionized serum calcium instead of total serum calcium is the most accurate and therefore should be employed whenever possible. The sarcoplasmic reticulum is less extensive in cardiac muscle, therefore Ca^{2+} release and reuptake are very slow. Hence, cardiac contractions are enhanced by factors which increase intracellular Ca^{2+} concentration, such as cardiac glycosides, beta-adrenergic agents, and calcium infusions. Conversely, hypocalcemia, calcium channel blocking drugs, ATP depletion by ischemia (such as in shock), or phosphate depletion can impair the influence that calcium exerts on myocardial contractility.

The clinician must not forget that calcium is also important in causing profound central nervous system derangement in abnormally high or abnormally low concentrations in the extracellular fluid. Central nervous system involvement may include a wide spectrum of clinical findings from hypercalcemic coma to hypocalcemic seizures and tetany.

Hypocalcemia. There is significant neuromuscular and cardiovascular involvement when a patient presents with hypocalcemia. Tetany is the most common symptom associated with hypocalcemia, other common physical signs include Chvostek's and Trousseau's signs (facial stimulation of neuromuscular plates causing significant spasm). Depressed calcium levels impede acetylcholine release and deplete cellular stores needed for effective muscular contraction. Clinical pathologic states caused by hypocalcemia include heart failure,[57] cardiac dysrhythmias,[76] hypotension,[24] ineffective digitalization,[28] urinary retention,[85] infantile apnea,[55] papilledema,[62] seizures,[29] and prolonged curarization.[112]

There are many causes of hypocalcemia (Table 27-1) which may be due to a number of clinical entities. Specifically, these may be hormonal, dietary, or as a result of a number of other processes. Usually the mechanisms of many of the known causes of hypocalcemia may be mixed.[3,25,27,68] Severely reduced total calcium and phosphate levels and ionized calcium can be seen in a hyperventilating patient with respiratory alkalosis.[155] It is likely that most critically ill children are at risk to develop hypocalcemia, since a great diversity of causes exist. Calcium binding to albumin changes with pH, free fatty acid concentration, and osmolarity; therefore, the clinician

TABLE 27-1 CAUSES OF HYPOCALCEMIA

Parathyroid hormone insufficiency	*Calcitriol insufficiency*	*Chelation or precipitation*
Hypoparathyroidism	Inadequate production	Hyperphosphatemia
Primary	Malabsorption of vitamin D	Citrate infusion
Acquired—Trauma	Lack of sunlight	Tumor lysis syndrome
Sepsis	Advanced hepatic disease	Toxic shock syndrome
Autoimmune	Advanced renal disease	Drug toxicity
Burns	Advanced bone disease	Ethylene glycol
Surgery	Drugs	Sodium sulfate
Tumor	Cisplatin	EDTA
	Mithramycin	Sodium fluoride
	Phenytoin	
Hypomagnesemia		Diffuse muscle necrosis
Hypermagnesemia	Nephrotic syndrome	
Advanced metabolic bone disease		
Hypothyroidism		
Drugs: Beta-adrenergic blockers		
Cimetidine		
Aminoglycosides		

must recognize the variability of calcium levels from one individual to another and between one disease entity and another. Acidosis decreases calcium binding to albumin, and alkalosis increases its binding. Rapid infusion of concentrated albumin solutions can transiently lower the ionized calcium levels.[26]

Clinical presentation. Although it is common for critically ill patients to present with mild hypocalcemia, they rarely have associated clinical manifestations.[159] Neurologic and cardiovascular functions are usually intact.[20]

When patients are symptomatic, neuromuscular and cardiovascular abnormalities are the most common presenting features of hypocalcemia (Table 27-2). Neuronal irritability including tetany, muscle spasms, hyperreflexia, seizures, and paresthesias are common.[161] Vascular manifestations of hypocalcemia include hypotension due to a decreased smooth muscle contraction in vascular tissues.[20]

Treatment. Along with serum calcium levels (preferably ionized), magnesium and phosphorus levels should be evaluated. The transport team should collect and save blood samples for plasma parathormone (PTH) and calcitriol for further specific diagnostic testing.

The patient with impending neuromuscular and/or cardiovascular collapse should have prompt restoration of serum calcium.[69,106] Caution must be taken in hyperphosphatemic patients when administering calcium, since this may result in calcium precipitation, organ injury, and possible death. These patients may be best treated by lowering the phosphorus level.[160] Hypomagnesemic and hypermagnesemic patients respond poorly to calcium therapy and therefore should have normalization of the serum magnesium level first.[162]

Severe or symptomatic hypocalcemia is a medical emergency and should be treated with intravenous calcium. Calcium chloride may have a slightly more predictable rise in calcium than the other salts. The recommended dose is 20 to 30 mg/kg/dose of a 10% calcium chloride solution infused over 1 hour. The advantage of this salt over the other salts is probably very slight.[156]

Intravenous calcium is irritating to veins, and care should be taken by securing a large vein, central venous line, or an IO line to avoid causing tissue damage with extravasation. Calcium chloride and other calcium salts should be diluted in dextrose water or normal saline prior to administration. Care should be taken that the infusion of the calcium salt is not administered too rapidly, since it can be dysrhythmogenic in which patients, digitalized or not, may suffer life-threatening arrhythmias. Bradycardia and asystole may result from an intravenous calcium infusion if given too rapidly. Patients should be on a cardiac monitor, and resuscitative drugs (atropine) should be readily available.

Hypercalcemia. Patients with mild hypercalcemia are usually asymptomatic. Hypercalcemia is an infrequently encountered problem in the pediatric population. Patients

TABLE 27-2 CLINICAL FEATURES OF HYPOCALCEMIA

Neuromuscular	*Cardiovascular*	*Respiratory*
Increased neuronal irritability	Hypotension	Laryngeal spasm
Tetany	Bradycardia	Bronchospasm
Chvostek's and Trousseau's signs	Asystole	
Hyperreflexia	Dysrhythmia	
Paresthesia	Impaired cardiac contractility	
Weakness	ECG abnormalities	
Seizures	QT and ST prolongation	
Muscle spasms	Asystole	
	Bradycardia	
	Decreased catecholamine response	
	Decreased digitalis response	

with systemic hypercalcemia may present with anorexia, nausea, polyuria, and lassitude. Lethargy and dehydration may be associated with deteriorating renal function if the hypercalcemia is severe (greater than 14 mg/dl).

Hyperthyroidism, pheochromocytoma,[139] malignancies,[2] hypervitaminosis A and D, familial hypocalciuric hypercalcemia,[91] loop diuretics, granulomatous disease (tuberculosis, sarcoidosis), Addison's disease, and William's syndrome[54] may cause hypercalcemia in children. Approximately 20% of children with hypercalcemia may present with hypertension. Therefore, the health care provider caring for a critically ill child with a possible endocrinopathy and hypertension should consider hypercalcemia as the etiology for the elevated blood pressure. Concentrations below 15 mg/dl are generally not regarded as acute or life-threatening, and therefore, any therapeutic efforts should be directed to the primary cause. Due to the severe water and sodium depletion associated with severe hypercalcemia, volume expansion with isotonic saline solution is the primary first step of any therapeutic regimen. By expanding extracellular volume and diluting extracellular fluid calcium, there is an increase in the excretion of calcium in the urine. Volume expansion should be performed using normal saline solution (10-20 ml/kg/hr) and, if followed by a loop diuretic, will produce a brisk calciuresis. Potassium and magnesium supplementation should be considered, since patients with hypercalcemia may present with hypokalemia. Hypomagnesemia may be aggravated by volume expansion.

There is no quick therapeutic modality to decrease serum calcium levels. The clinician and transport team should consider the various diagnostic possibilities, since this will impact the time and length of recuperation of a patient who presents with hypocalcemia. This should be considered a temporary measure until specific treatment directed at the primary disease takes effect. Appropriate emergent treatment would include IV fluids to correct volume depletion, dilution of extracellular fluid calcium, and promoting renal calcium excretion.

Phosphate

In the normal child, serum phosphate concentration ranges from 4.0 to 7.1 mg/dl. Various physiologic events such as carbohydrate or fat ingestion, exercise, and acid/base changes may alter the serum phosphate concentration through transcellular shifts. Since the majority of phosphate is intracellular, serum phosphate concentrations are unreliable as a guide to total body phosphate stores. The kidneys excrete approximately 90% of a daily phosphate load, while the other 10% is excreted by the gastrointestinal tract.

Phosphorus is a vital constituent of nucleic acids, nucleal proteins, and membrane phospholipids. Phosphate metabolism is of importance in critically ill children because phosphate is an essential element for the proper maintenance of many biologic functions such as normal modulation of oxygen-hemoglobin dissociation and tissue oxygenation, cell membrane integrity, neurologic function, and skeletal, diaphragmatic and cardiac muscle function.

Hypophosphatemia. Some disease states, such as diabetic ketoacidosis (DKS), may invoke all three mechanisms which constitute the causes of hypophosphatemia[90] (reduced intake, increased excretion, and shift from extracellular fluid to intracellular fluid). A child in DKA may arrive at the hospital with depleted body phosphate stores, since there is an excess, initially in hyperphosphaturia. When insulin therapy begins, this further increases the drive of serum phosphate, along with glucose and potassium, into the cells and produces a more profound hypophosphatemia. Acidosis, heavy metal poisoning, hypocalcemia, paint and glue sniffing,[140] renal tubular disorders, and Reye's syndrome[22] also reduce serum phosphate levels. The clinician must keep in mind that correcting states of low cardiac output by saline infusion or the use of inotropic agents may result in increased urinary losses of phosphate due to improvement in the glomerular filtration rate. Patients with persistent gastrointestinal dysfunction, such as emesis, diarrhea, and malabsorption, and patients with severe malnutrition must be considered as being at risk.

There may be depressed leukocyte phagocytosis, muscular weakness, respiratory failure,[148] platelet and increased red blood cell destruction[15] from rhabdomyolysis, sinus node dysfunction, depressed myocardial function,[118] and liver failure.

In spite of these significant complications, the treatment of hypophosphatemia and the phosphate repletion is not to be undertaken under a rapid infusion, although replacement should begin at the referring institution or during transport. Intravenous correction of severe hypophosphatemia (serum phosphate $\leq$ 1 mg/dl) is necessary to avoid major clinical sequelae. If the patient's phosphorus levels are between 0.5 to 1.0 mg/dl, diaphragmatic contractility may be depressed, thereby creating a state of respiratory distress or frank acute respiratory failure.[5,63]

Replacement of phosphorus at these levels is suggested in doses from 0.05 to 0.25 mmol of PO_4/kg given intravenously over a 4 to 12 hour rate.[82] If the patient presents with a serum phosphorus concentration below 0.5 mg/dl, one should be more aggressive and administer 0.09 to 0.5 mmol of PO_4/kg over a 4 to 12 hour rate.[95] When acutely treating hypophosphatemia, caution must be taken to avoid hypocalcemia, hypomagnesemia, hyperphosphatemia, hypotension, and acute renal failure. The lower end of the dosage ranges should always be administered in the presence of hypocalcemia or renal failure. If the patient has severe hypocalcemia, phosphate should not be administered until the serum calcium has been corrected.

Hyperphosphatemia. There are three causes of hyperphosphatemia: inadequate excretion, excessive intake, and intracellular fluid to extracellular fluid shifts. Usually, massive intake is due to a child receiving excessive vitamin D or oral or rectal phosphate supplementation. Inadequate excretion is usually due to any decrease in glomerular filtration rate, such as volume depletion, renal failure, and myocardial failure. Shifts of phosphate from the intracellular to the extracellular fluid are seen in a variety of clinical situations which share a common pathway, such as patients who have received cytotoxic therapy for acute lymphoblastic leukemia and Burkitt's lymphoma as part of the tumor lysis syndrome.[14,108] Also, lactic acidosis has been associated with hyperphosphatemia[16] as well as a state of hypoperfusion secondary to shock. There may be lysis of red blood cells during blood drawing which may produce a spurious hyperphosphatemia.[133]

Aggressive intravenous administration of phosphate for treatment of hypophosphatemia has been reported to cause hyperphosphatemia.[26] One must remember that hyperphosphatemia in concentrations greater than 10 mg/dl will cause concomitant serum ionized calcium concentrations below 1.5 mEq/L.[26] These patients may show clinical signs of hypocalcemia, including prolonged QT intervals, tetany, and frank seizure activity. Phosphate containing laxatives and the administration of oral or rectal containing solutions[11,154] may cause severe hyperphosphatemia and concomitant hypocalcemia.

Acutely, the clinician may treat the patient with restitution of plasma volume with saline 20 ml/kg, and if the patients show symptomatic hypocalcemia replacement, with calcium chloride (10% solution), 20-30 mg/kg/dose IV slowly. A nasogastric tube may be placed, and an antacid containing aluminum hydroxide may be administered (1 ml/kg) recognizing that this process of phosphate binding will take many hours.

Magnesium

Magnesium is a cofactor for many enzymatic processes using ATP. The kidney is the primary affector of serum magnesium. Plasma magnesium is approximately 65-85% bound to protein. In the light of the fact that most of the body's magnesium is tissue bound, (50% to bone, 25% to muscle, 1% to extracellular fluids, and 24% to body's other soft tissues) one should view serum magnesium levels with caution. Normal total plasma magnesium concentration is 1.4 to 2.0 mmol/l (1.7 to 2.4 mg/dl). All body processes which utilize ATP require magnesium. Normal renal function readily avoids hypermagnesemia, but hypomagnesemia is much more common and requires careful attention.

Hypomagnesemia. The causes of hypomagnesemia can be divided into three basic concepts: 1) increased magnesium losses, 2) decreased magnesium intake, and 3) alterations in the distribution of magnesium. Studies of critically ill patients have found that 20 to 50% of patients are hypomagnesemic, with the lowest incidence in the patients with the worst renal function.[128] There are many causes of symptomatic hypomagnesemia. Some of them are listed in Box 27-4.

Many patients will present with multiple electrolyte disturbances in association with hypomagnesemia including hypokalemia, hypocalcemia, hyponatremia, hypophosphatemia, and distal tubular acidosis.[128] Patients on diuretic agents such as furosemide, thiazides, and ethacrynic acid present with hypomagnesemia due to increasing magnesium excretion.[71]

Children with known congenital heart disease, either preoperative or postoperative and on digoxin may be at a higher risk if associated with hypomagnesemia, this has been reported in adult patients on cardiac glycosides.[101] These patients may be at a higher risk for myocardial sensitivity to digoxin induced dysrhythmias.[136] Other cardiovascular manifestations of hypomagnesemia may include increased PR and QT intervals, flat broad T-Waves, and ventricular tachydysrhythmias.[94] Neuromuscular and behavioral clinical manifestations of hypomagnesemia include muscle fasciculations, cramps, paresthesias, spasticity, convulsions, delirium, hyperirritability, and frank tetany.[41] Hypomagnesemic neonates may present with clinical symptoms of gitteriness, hyperalertness, weakness, poor feeding, and other similar adult manifestations.[115] Hypomagnesemic neonates and adults have been reported to have skeletal and respiratory smooth muscle weakness.[107]

Treatment. The primary cause of increased loss of magnesium must be identified and treated appropriately, with current renal function being assessed and included as an integral part of the management. Usually, magnesium replacement is done over a period of 3 to 5 days to achieve normomagnesemia. A transport team or an emergency medicine physician awaiting to transfer a patient to a tertiary care institution will require immediate attention to a critically low magnesium level (less than 1.8 mg/dl) which may present with the above mentioned manifestations. Treatment consists of 25-50 mg/kg/dose (0.2-0.4 mEq/kg/dose) over 1 to 2 hours. These patients should be placed on a cardiorespiratory monitor, and neurologic evaluation should be performed serially.

Magnesium is involved in a number of important physiologic functions and in all intracellular energy metabolism utilizing ATP, therefore, the clinician must keep in mind the need for supplementation of this most important intracellular cation when patients present with symptomatology consistent with magnesium deficiency.

Syndrome of inappropriate antidiuretic hormone

A decrease in effective arterial blood volume or a rise in plasma osmolarity will induce the release of antidiuretic hormone (ADH). When the serum sodium concentration becomes subnormal in a critically ill patient, we find this to be inappropriate. The initial presentation is a relative concentrated urine within a clinical setting of euvolemia, normal serum sodium, and normal urine output; this is considered the syndrome of inappropriate antidiuretic hormone (SIADH). This diagnosis cannot be made until other causes of salt wasting have been ruled out such as sweat, stool, renal dysfunction, or water intoxication.[73]

The treating team should be acutely aware of the possibility of SIADH developing in certain clinical situations, such as head injury and subarachnoid hemorrhage.[36] Other patients at risk of developing SIADH are those who have undergone neurosurgery, especially for tumors,[33] those presenting with meningitis and meningoencephalitis,[104] patients who have suffered burns,[138] and those with respiratory infections.[125] There are certain conditions which may mimic SIADH, including adrenal insufficiency, hypopituitarism, hypothyroidism, renal dysfunction, and diuretic use.

Treatment. Therapy for SIADH should begin either in the referring institution or during transport. This anticipatory action provides a head start in attempting to slow

BOX 27-4 COMMON CAUSES OF HYPOMAGNESEMIA

Decreased Intake
- Protein calorie malnutrition
- Prolonged parenteral nutrition

Alternation in Distribution
- Sepsis syndrome
- Transfusion therapy
- Alkalemia
- Thermal injury
- Catecholamine

Increased Losses
- Gastrointestinal
  - Pancreatitis
  - Malabsorption syndromes
  - Laxative abuse
- Renal
  - Glomerulonephritis
  - Renal tubular acidosis
  - SIADH
  - Acidemia
  - Diabetic ketoacidosis
- Drug induced
  - Loop diuretics
  - Mannitol
  - Digoxin
  - Aminoglycosides
  - Calcium
  - Ethanol

down, reverse, or arrest the process.

If a patient is suffering from an illness known to cause SIADH, the treatment of choice would be fluid restriction. If the patient remains hemodynamically stable, fluid restriction, anywhere from two-thirds to 25% of total maintenance, is recommended. If the patient shows asymptomatic hyponatremia, simple fluid restriction will usually correct this problem. Patients who display symptomatic hyponatremia should be treated aggressively with osmotic diuretics (mannitol .250-1.0 gm/kg/dose) and/or loop diuretics (furosemide at 0.5-1.0 mg/kg/dose). If the patient shows severe obtundation, coma, and/or seizures, 3% normal saline (0.513 mEq per ml) should be administered in an amount calculated to restore the serum sodium to a level greater than 120 to 125 mEq/L:

$$(\text{desired Na} - \text{actual Na}) \times 0.6 \times \text{Kg} = \text{mEqs of Na needed to raise plasma Na concentration}$$

Half of this amount can be infused over 5 to 10 minutes or until symptoms subside, and the remainder may be administered over 2 to 4 hours or until the plasma sodium concentration has reached the desired level. Care must be taken if this solution is administered into a peripheral vessel, since it may cause significant injury to the surrounding tissues if extravasation occurs. It is administered preferably in a large vessel, a central venous line, or an IO line.

If a child is hypovolemic as well as hyponatremic, in spite of perhaps presenting with SIADH, blood volume must be corrected.[127] The IV fluids of choice would be normal saline or blood products, if clinically indicated. The clinician should see an increase in urinary output within a relative short period of time (1 to 3 hours) after fluid restriction therapy has begun. If the transport team recognizes the patient with hyponatremia, the clinician must decide whether this finding is dilutional. This decision will then dictate the course of the treatment, and fluid restriction will improve the patient's electrolyte imbalance.

DIABETES INSIPIDUS

Patients with diabetes insipidus (DI) manifest an inability to conserve water. These patients will then be subject to polyuria and polydypsia as the primary clinical features. Critically ill children may present with a variety of illnesses which may have DI as a component. These patients will present with hypertonic serums (hypernatremia by laboratory findings). Usually there is a history of impaired thirst mechanism, impaired state of responsiveness, or a breakdown in the water delivery system.

Hypotonic polyuria is usually associated with a low urine osmolality (less than 200 mOsm/kg) with an increased urine volume. Three causes can be attributed to this: 1) inadequate secretion of ADH (central or neurogenic DI), 2) impaired renal response to ADH (nephrogenic DI), and 3) an increase in water intake (primary polydypsia). Regardless of which of these three causes exist, they will all produce a high urine volume, a low urine osmolality, and typically, a near normal or slightly elevated plasma osmolality. Injuries which cause cerebral ischemia, such as global hypoxia, infections, and severe trauma, may include injury to the anterior hypothalamus and produce DI secondary to the global insult.[80,122] Some other reported causes of DI in pediatric patients include acute tubular necrosis (ATN), obstructive uropathy, pyelonephritis, polycystic kidney disease, sickle cell anemia, protein starvation, and hypercalcemia.[122]

Physiologic diagnosis of diabetes insipidus

After documentation of hypotonic polyuria (the hallmark of the diagnosis is an excessive flow of dilute urine), the establishment of the physiologic cause becomes essential for appropriate management of this entity. The urine osmolality is generally less than 200 mOsm/L corresponding to a specific gravity less than 1.005. If a patient presents with a urine osmolality ≤200 mOsm/L and the patient has not received an osmotic diuretic (glucose, mannitol, glycerol, or x-ray contrast materials), then the patient can be safely diagnosed with DI.

Excessive fluid intake and osmotic diuresis are two of the most common causes of DI in critically ill children. The clinician must not forget that in developed countries the most common causes of diabetes insipidus are head trauma and neurosurgery.[149] In children, 10% of cases are caused by tumors prior to any surgical intervention, 37% of cases are related to postsurgical intervention for intracranial tumors, and 3% are related to nonsurgical trauma.[65]

There is a rare entity known as hereditary DI which appears to be autosomal dominant with incomplete penetration. Autopsy findings suggest a congenital defect in ADH synthesis.[113] Other rare causes of DI in children include histiocytosis X, with a higher percentage in those with multisystem involvement.[40,65] Septo-optic dysplasia and other intracranial defects and central nervous system infections are responsible for over 20% of cases of diabetes insipidus in children.[65]

Studies have shown that global brain injury associated with DI has a near 100% mortality within 1 to 5 days after the injury.[80]

Treatment

As in all cases of critically ill patients, especially severe head injury patients, the ABCs should be achieved and stabilized. Specifically, if volume losses are significant, these patients may enter a state of hemodynamic instability. For the patients who present with shock, 20 ml/kg of an isotonic solution, such as lactated Ringer's or isotonic saline, is indicated (as often and as rapidly as necessary). Once shock is treated, solutions should ideally not contain more than 37 mEq of sodium/L (relatively hypotonic solutions), so as to avoid excessive sodium loading of the patient. In other words, it is necessary to add dextrose to maintain the osmolality of the infusate of the solution. On the other hand, the transport team must be careful not to deliver large volumes of fluid containing dextrose, since this may induce hyperglycemia and thereby produce an osmotic diuresis. The transport team should have a recent set of electrolytes, paying special attention to the serum sodium concentration. If the patient is hypernatremic, care should be taken that full correction of the abnormality is done over an extended period of time (calculate IV fluids and divide over 48 hours).[132] During the initial stabilization of a patient in acute DI, fluid replacement with hypotonic solutions should be sufficient until the patient arrives at the tertiary care institution. If the transport team is aware that they will be transporting a patient with acute diabetes insipidus, they may prepare a vasopressin infusion (0.5 to 15 mU/kg/hr), thereby obviating the need for large volumes of fluid to be administered and avoiding the risk of rapid electrolyte shifts. The usual starting dose is 0.5 mU/kg/hr, and if no effect is seen within 30 minutes, the infusion is doubled every 30 minutes thereafter. It is rare that a patient will need more than 10 mU/kg/hr, with the average patient responding in the 2 to 4 mU/kg/hr range. Success is considered establishing a urine output rate less than 2 ml/kg/hr. The clinician must be careful, since vasopressin is a potent vasoconstrictor, and its most extreme effect is seen in patients with severe CNS injury. Patients may show severe systemic vasoconstriction leading to tissue ischemia, profound lactic acidosis, and may actually lead to infarction of skin over extremities. It is for these reasons that extremely high rates of vasopressin infusion should be avoided. Diabetes insipidus is effectively treated with replacement of free water deficits and exogenous vasopressin replacement.

DIABETIC KETOACIDOSIS

Diabetic ketoacidosis (DKA) is one of the most frequently encountered metabolic disorders in the intensive care unit.[42,67,83] The metabolic abnormalities which precipitate DKA are multifaceted. In spite of advances in the treatment of diabetes mellitus, DKA remains a significant source of morbidity and mortality in all age groups. Children represent approximately 1.6% of all DKA deaths,[72] and mortality is especially high in the elderly. The mortality rate for DKA ranges from 3 to 17%.[72,134]

Pathophysiology

Three major tissues in the body (liver, fat, and muscle) convert from a normal state to a catabolic state during DKA. Inadequate amounts of insulin give rise to diabetes mellitus. The byproducts of these tissues (liver, fat, muscle) are utilized by the liver to promote gluconeogenesis and ketogenesis, which essentially make up the entity called DKA.[9] Insulin is necessary to prevent ketone formation and inhibit mobilization of peripheral triglycerides and amino acids. It also inhibits glycogenolysis, gluconeogenesis, proteolysis, lipolysis, and ketogenesis.[78]

The main reasons for an increasing hyperglycemia, are not just insulin deficiency, since after the first few hours, glucose production falls significantly.[105] Impaired glucose utilization and slowed urinary excretion secondary to hypovolemia and low glomerular filtration rate then become the main factors in maintaining elevated glucose levels.

There is marked overproduction of acetoacetate, betahydroxybutyrate, and acetone. These, along with an elevated blood glucose concentration due to insulin deficiency, are responsible for the biochemical alteration of increased acid production in DKA. Very often, infectious, emotional, or traumatic causes are identified as the precipitating factors in DKA. Stress hormones such as cortisol, growth hormone, epinephrine, and norepinephrine are all present in excess quantities in patients in DKA.[88,96]

The health care provider must not forget that there are a number of other hormonal and biochemical changes occurring in patients suffering from DKA, such as changes in cortisol levels, which enhance gluconeogenesis, block glucose uptake by muscle, and support lipolysis.[88,96] Growth hormone appears to have a similar effect on these patients. Epinephrine impedes the release of insulin and blocks glucose uptake by muscle and inhibits glycolysis. Patients with DKA have also been noted to have elevated levels of vasopressin, plasma renin activity, and aldosterone.[146] It seems that these patients respond to volume depletion and a hypertonic state by elevating their vasopressin levels. It has been suggested that these elevated vasopressin levels may increase the risk of cerebral herniation in patients who have been aggressively rehydrated.[39] The transport team must also keep in mind that a newborn suffering from cyanotic congenital heart disease requiring prostaglandin E_1 infusion may present with hyperglycemia and ketosis after the infusion has been instituted.[31] Prostaglandins can stimulate glucagon release and inhibit insulin release.

Ketogenesis and acidosis

When a patient becomes hypovolemic due to osmotic diuresis, hypoperfused tissues will turn to anaerobic glycolysis which, in turn, will produce lactic acidosis in DKA.

Hyperchloremic acidosis[119] may present on admission and may be common during initial therapy. If the patient is able to maintain salt and water intake for a significant period of time, they will potentially waste bicarbonate possibly resulting in an acidosis out of proportion to the measured anion gap. The potentiation of this effect will be further seen when patients are resuscitated with solutions containing large amounts of chloride, such as normal saline. If a patient presents with DKA and a small anion gap, they may recover from acidosis more rapidly if bicarbonate is used in the resuscitating intravenous fluid in place of chloride. Patients with DKA have associated ongoing continuous fluid losses (osmotic diuresis which leads to intravascular volume depletion). This loss of volume is by far the most dangerous process brought on by DKA, since shock will invariably occur when dehydration is severe. Therefore, hyperglycemia and dehydration will contribute to the hyperosmolality. The glomerular filtration rate will be affected when the fluid loss is severe enough, and subsequently, the excretion of excess glucose will be tapered, thereby promoting further hyperglycemia. It is very helpful when body weights are known, since this can estimate the degree of dehydration. More often than not, body weights are not always known, therefore, estimations are usually made based on physical findings and clinical presentation. A safe estimation of the degree of dehydration in a child with DKA is a water deficit of 15-20% of body weight. There have been clinical reports correlating the level of obtundation and electroencephalogram changes to the degree of hyperosmolality in patients with DKA.[144]

Electrolyte imbalance

Potassium. There is a major deficit in total body potassium in DKA due to osmotic diuresis and recurrent vomiting.[9,50,151] Although total body stores are depleted, plasma values may be normal or even high at presentation.[52] This may be due to elevated extracellular hydrogen ions being exchanged for intracellular potassium. In spite of a patient presenting with hyperkalemia and DKA, or for that matter (more seriously), if the patient presents with a serum potassium concentration below the normal level in the face of severe metabolic acidosis, immediate institution of intravenous potassium is required. Potassium administration should begin immediately after the patient has received fluid resuscitation, and it should be added to the maintenance IV fluids. Hypokalemia is likely to result when insulin is administered to the patient with acute DKA, therefore, the clinician must be keenly aware and replenish potassium from the beginning. In DKA serum potassium levels do not correlate well with either lactic acidosis or ketoacidosis. It is very important to accurately monitor potassium supplementation and potassium levels, given the rapid decline in potassium concentration immediately after the institution of insulin therapy.[10] Patients who suffer from hypokalemia may have cardiac arrhythmias and respiratory failure.[129]

Phosphate. Although it is well established that total body phosphate stores may be markedly depleted in cases of DKA, phosphate therapy continues to remain an unclear and controversial issue in the treatment of acute DKA. There has been no evidence that phosphate therapy contributes significantly to the patient's clinical outcome.[47,161] In theory, profound hypophosphatemia is due to osmotic diuresis and competition with glucose for reabsorption at the renal tubules. Depressed levels of 2,3-diphosphoglycerate (2,3-DPG) has been described in DKA.[77] There has been no conclusive evidence that phosphate repletion has had a significant effect on 2,3-DPG.[79] Some authors claim there is little urgency to replace the deficits of phosphate.[47,157,161] Regardless of the controversy, serum phosphate levels should be obtained, and phosphate therapy should be replaced even though it may be of theoretical benefit. There may be an advantage to using potassium phosphate and reducing the amount of chloride delivered and perhaps avoiding hyperchloremic acidosis during therapy. A combination of 50% potassium chloride and 50% potassium phosphate administered according to weight (in the IV maintenance fluids) will achieve the goal of normalizing potassium serum levels.

Bicarbonate. Of all the electrolyte replacement therapies, bicarbonate remains the most controversial in the management of DKA. Severe acidosis is of no doubt a dangerous consequence of DKA and may result in a negative inotropic effect on the myocardium.[124,129] Patients may present with confusion, stupor, arrhythmias, and coma when severe acidosis is present. There is no question that treatment of severe acidosis (pH less than 7.1) should be undertaken. There is also no question that the treatment of DKA with fluid and insulin will improve this acidosis. The use of sodium bicarbonate in the care of a child with DKA must be done carefully and closely monitored. Acid/base status must be closely monitored, and the transport environment may not be the most suitable for this type of electrolyte monitoring. Risks of alkali therapy include tissue hypoxia due to increased hemoglobin-oxygen affinity, paradoxic CNS acidosis, and potential reduction of serum potassium and calcium levels. Rapid infusion of bicarbonate should be avoided and is preferably administered by a continuous infusion with a delivered concentration of 1 mEq/kg/hr. Arterial blood gases should be monitored as an indicator of acid/base status on an hourly basis (if possible), and when the patient has reached a pH of 7.2 to 7.25, the bicarbonate infusion should be discontinued. The replacement of fluids and insulin will continue to reverse the acidotic state. This may be a recommendation that can be given to the referring physician while the transport team is en route.

Laboratory abnormalities. Patients in DKA should have a number of laboratory examinations performed including arterial blood gas, pH, electrolytes, BUN, glucose, creatinine, osmolality, ketones, lactate, calcium, magnesium, and phosphate. The interval can be lengthened to hourly for pH, PCO_2, sodium, potassium, glucose, and ketones, and thereafter, if the patient shows stable control, the interval may be lengthened. Obviously, the transport team can not perform hourly serum chemistries, but prior to the transport, a recent set of chemistries is desirable. If the patient presents with severe potassium and calcium alterations, a lead II ECG strip should be monitored hourly. Patients who present in shock should have close monitoring of their urinary output, and a urinary bladder catheter should be placed. The patients neurologic status should be assessed at least hourly initially, and if obtunded, a Glasgow coma score should be documented.

Patients may present with extreme lipemia due to hypertriglyceridemia,[151] and it is not uncommon for hyponatremia to be reported by the laboratory due to this lipemia which can decrease the measured sodium value by decreasing the aqueous phase of blood. Also, the degree of hyperglycemia influences the measured sodium concentration by including water movement from the intracellular to the extracellular space, thereby diluting the sodium concentration. The shift in sodium concentration is approximately 1.6 mEq/dl for every elevation in glucose concentration of 100 mg/dl above a serum level of 200 mg/dl.

Treatment of complications requiring critical care transport

The successful treatment of DKA revolves around identifying the precipitating factor and reversing the metabolic and hormonal abnormalities which characterize such a clinical state. Life-threatening complications must be addressed immediately by the health care provider caring for the critically ill child in DKA. Management must be prioritized and, as in all life-threatening entities, the establishment of airway, breathing, and circulation (ABCs) must be first and foremost.

Cardiac dysrhythmias. Electrolyte abnormalities are seen in patients being treated for DKA including hyperkalemia, hypokalemia, or hypocalcemia. These patients may have a potential for life-threatening or fatal cardiac dysrhythmias. Patients in DKA should be placed on an ECG monitor throughout the transport as with all other patients. Peaked T-waves may provide an early evidence of hyperkalemia. A lead II ECG strip provides a quick and reliable source of information in patients of all ages for this specific cardiac dysrhythmia.[98]

Cerebral edema. There are two states of altered sensorium in patients with DKA.[158] Uncommonly, one may see progressive cerebral edema which begins during the treatment of DKA, and the other is the altered sensorium seen commonly in patients who present with DKA due to decreased intravascular volume and perfusion pressure. The mechanisms for altered consciousness in the diabetic hyperosmolar state is not clear.[53] Although unproven, it must be considered that there is an increased risk for cerebral edema and herniation with rapid rehydration.[39] If a patient with DKA presents with a progressively deteriorating Glasgow coma score and a state of deepening coma, it is more likely to occur in the pediatric diabetic and may be almost always fatal.[38] Animal studies have shown that cerebrospinal fluid pressure rises during the phase of isotonic saline rehydration in subjects with acute hyperglycemic hyperosmotic diuresis. There is no hard scientific data which explains the etiology of cerebral edema in DKA, however, most clinicians seem to agree that euglycemia and rehydration should be performed in a cautious and controlled manner.[42] Therefore, it is imperative that the transport team be cautious and prudent in their rehydrating efforts of the child presenting in DKA. If a child presents with fever and a clouded sensorium and the question whether this patient may have sepsis or meningoencephalitis exists, the next question the health care provider will have is whether a lumbar puncture should be performed or not. If the patient presents with shock and acidosis and the possibility of significant cerebral edema, then antibiotics should be administered during the initial resuscitation. The lumbar puncture should be waived until the patient shows signs of stability. Compromising respiration and venous return to the heart to perform the lumbar puncture may have a severe adverse effect on the patient, and if the patient has cerebrospinal fluid withdrawn in the presence of cerebral edema, there may be downward herniation of the intracranial contents. Antigenic evidence of the common bacterial infections will be able to be recovered after the patient has shown signs of stability inspite of appropriate antibiotic therapy.

If the child is comatose and has a Glasgow coma score less than 8, the patient should be intubated to prevent aspiration and also to assist in hyperventilation in the treatment of cerebral edema. These patients benefit from a pharmacologic "cocktail" as adjuncts in endotracheal intubation. Barbiturates should be avoided, since these may produce hypotension in an already hypovolemic and potentially hypotensive patient. The drugs of choice for intubating the comatose child in DKA are 1) atropine (0.02 mg/kg IV, minimum dose 0.1 mg), 2) fentanyl (5 mcg/kg IV) or lidocaine (1 to 2 mg/kg IV) 3) pancuronium bromide (0.01 mg/kg IV defasciculating dose) and succinylcholine (1 mg/kg IV).[66] This rapid sequence intubation is indicated to prevent cerebral compromise in a patient with DKA and progressive neurologic deterioration.

Pulmonary edema. Pulmonary edema, albeit an unusual finding in DKA, may present with increasing oxygen requirements and little or no radiographic changes. Some of the possible causes include low plasma oncotic pressure,[137] increased pulmonary capillary permeability,[19] myocardial failure,[9] and a neurogenic basis for the pulmonary edema.[97] If the patient presents with opacification on the chest x-ray, without overt signs of pulmonary edema, there may have been aspiration of gastric contents due to decreased level of consciousness. Adequate arterial blood oxygenation must be maintained to avoid further tissue injury and prolonged acidosis.

Insulin therapy. The next consideration in the treatment of DKA should be the administration of insulin. Because of increased counter-regulatory hormones, insulin resistance is universally present in all patients with ketoacidosis.[58] Therefore, in the first 24 hours of DKA, there may be an increase in the number of units of insulin required to control the hyperglycemia. Once the hyperglycemia and ketosis have been documented, a continuous IV infusion of regular insulin is established at a rate of 0.1 U/kg/hr. A previously established practice (and now controversial tissue) to provide the patient with an initial bolus of IV insulin has fallen out of practice.[49] The serum glucose should be checked hourly, (depending on how long the transport lasts) and when the serum glucose falls to 300 mg/dl, 5% dextrose should be added to the intravenous fluids while continuing with the insulin infusion. Ketoacidosis takes longer to correct than the elevated blood glucose, and insulin therapy is essential for this process.[151] If the patient's serum glucose falls to less than or equal to 150 mg/dl, 10% dextrose should be added to the IV fluids.

Diabetic ketoacidosis remains a significant cause of morbidity and mortality in pediatric endocrinology. The transport team and the team caring for the patient at the referring institution must have training in the management of the child with DKA so as to rapidly stabilize, begin therapy, and maintain complications to a minimum in these patients.

Hyperosmolar hyperglycemic non-ketotic coma. Patients who present with this entity usually have marked hyperglycemia, dehydration, hyperosmolality, decreased sensorium, and absence of ketosis or acidosis. Of note, is the fact that this is an extremely unusual occurrence in childhood. This entity is more common in the elderly patient rather than the pediatric patient.[21] The mortality rate in adults is very high (40 to 60%).[92] Some of the causes of hyperosmolar hyperglycemic nonketotic coma (HHNC) at any age include infection, severe trauma, exogenous steroids, exogenous catecholamines, hyperalimentation, anticonvulsants (phenytoin), and thiazide diuretics.

Treatment. These patients may present in severe shock, and fluid replacement is the herald basis of treatment with 20 ml/kg of isotonic crystalloid infused as rapidly and as frequently as needed to reverse shock. Once shock has been reversed and treated, intravenous fluids should be changed to 0.45% NaCl to continue cautious correction of the hyperosmolar state. Potassium chloride should be replaced and supplemented as needed by serum levels. Fluids should be infused as in DKA at a 24 to 48 hour rate allowing for maintenance needs and replacement of ongoing losses. Insulin therapy must be administered cautiously, since serum glucose levels can fall precipitously. As in DKA, a continuous IV infusion of regular insulin should be started at 0.05 U/kg/hr (half the dose of the DKA patient), which may be enough to decrease serum glucose levels. This infusion should be adjusted based on serum glucose levels and should be monitored closely. When blood glucose levels reach 300 mg/dl (which may have occurred prior to the transport team's arrival), 5% dextrose is added to the IV fluids. Since these patients do not have ketosis or acidemia, if the serum glucose continues to fall, the insulin drip should be reduced by half or discontinued before the patients become hypoglycemic.[13,39]

Hypoglycemia

Pathophysiology. Hypoglycemia is defined as a plasma glucose less than 45 mg/dl, even in the absence of symptoms. In critically ill children, hypoglycemia is viewed either when CNS hypoglycemia produces seizures or coma[23] or when hypoglycemia is part of an illness that is life-threatening in itself. There are many etiologies of hypoglycemia in pediatric patients. Some of them include lack of available glucose or its precursors, increased peripheral glucose utilization (such as in tumors), deficiency in gluconeogenesis, and glycogenolysis, deficiencies in hormonal regulation, inborn errors of amino acid metabolism, idiopathic hypoglycemia, and ingestion of drugs or toxins which may lead to hypoglycemia.

Signs and symptoms. During an episode of hypoglycemia, the symptoms are due to adrenergic nervous system discharge and neuroglycopenia.[45] These symptoms include sweating palpitations and anxiety and result in manifestations such as changes in pupillary size and increased oral secretions. Hypothermia or hyperthermia may occur during hypoglycemia. Neuroglycopenic symptoms occur when glucose levels are approximately 36 mg/dl and below with changes in the electroencephalogram and patient behavior. The cerebral cortex is the most susceptible to the effects of hypoglycemia followed by the cerebellum, basal ganglia, thalamus, hypothalamus, midbrain, brain stem, spinal cord, ganglia, and finally, peripheral nerves. Children commonly present with seizures associated with hypoglycemia. Various mechanisms have been proposed including insufficient glucose metabolism and increased sodium, potassium, and water content in the brain.[45,99] Other causes of hypoglycemia include hepatic disease, renal disease, sepsis, total parenteral nutrition, insulin treatment of hyperglycemia, extensive thermal burns, and starvation.[44,46]

Treatment. Regardless of the etiology, if the patient's glucose level is critically low, treatment should begin. This level of glucose should be treated with IV dextrose (0.5-1.0 gm/kg). This can be achieved with a 25% dextrose solution, if the patient has either central venous access or an IO line in place, otherwise this high concentration of dextrose may sclerose peripheral vessels. It is preferable to administer no higher than 12.5% dextrose into a peripheral IV. A dextrose containing solution will be required as maintenance fluids (5% or 10% as indicated).

DISCUSSION

Endocrine disorders can cause significant morbidity and mortality in the critically ill pediatric patient. Delayed treatment may create a potentially harmful clinical setting. This chapter is intended to provide the health care professional caring for critically ill children with an endocrine emergency with a rational, concise, and potentially aggressive approach to the management, stabilization, and transport of the child with life-threatening endocrine and electrolyte disorders.

The author wishes to thank Ms. Gerri Walsh in the preparation of this manuscript.

REFERENCES

1. Aiello D and others: Thyroid storm: presenting with coma and seizures, *Clin Pediatr* 28:571, 1989.
2. Al-Rashid R, Cress C: Hypercalcemia associated with neuroblastoma, *Am J Dis Child* 133:838, 1979.
3. Arnaud C, Kolb F: The calcitropic hormones & metabolic bone disease. In Greenspan F, editor: *Basic and clinical endocrinology,* Norwalk, CT, 1991, Appleton & Lange.
4. Arteaga E and others: Effect of the combination of dexamethasone and sodium ipodate on serum thyroid hormones in Graves's disease, *Clin Endocrinol* 19:619, 1983.
5. Aubier M and others: Effect of hypophosphatemia on diaphragmatic contractility in patients with acute respiratory failure, *N Engl J Med* 313:420-4, 1985.
6. Barry D and others: Cerebral blood flow in rats with renal and spontaneous hypertension: resetting of the lower limit of autoregulation, *J Cereb Blood Flow Metab* 2:347, 1982.
7. Batlle D and others: Hyperkalemic hyperchloremic metabolic acidosis in sickle cell hemoglobinopathies, *Am J Med* 72:188, 1982.
8. Batlle DC, Arruda JAL, Kurtzman NA: Hyperkalemic distal renal tubular acidosis associated with obstructive uropathy, *N Engl J Med* 304:373, 1981.
9. Beigelman P: Severe diabetic ketoacidosis (diabetic "coma") 482 episodes in 257 patients: experience of three years, *Diabetes* 20:490, 1971.
10. Beigelman PM: Potassium in severe diabetic ketoacidosis, *Am J Med* 54:419-20, 1973.
11. Biberstein M, Parker BA: Enema-induced hyperphosphatemia, *Am J Med* 79:645-6, 1985.
12. Blum M: Myxedema coma, *Am J Med Sci* 264:432, 1972.
13. Boehme W and others: Low-dose insulin for diabetic nonketotic hyperosmolar coma, *JAMA* 242:1260, 1979.
14. Boles J-M and others: Acute renal failure caused by extreme hyperphosphatemia after chemotherapy of an acute lymphoblastic leukemia, *Cancer* 53:2425-9, 1984.
15. Borghi L, Canali M, Sani E: Erythrocyte sodium transport in acute hypophosphatemia in man, *Miner Electrolyte Metab* 10:26, 1984.
16. Brautbar N, Kleeman CR: Hypophosphatemia and hyperphosphatemia: clinical pathophysiologic aspect. In *Clinical disorders of fluid and electrolyte metabolism,* ed 4, New York, 1987, McGraw Hill.
17. Breningstall GN: Carnitine deficiency syndromes, *Pediatr Neurol* 6(2):75-81, 1990.
18. Breslow M and others: Adrenal medullary and cortical blood flow during hemorrhage, *Am J Physiol* 250:H954, 1986.
19. Brun-Buisson C, Bonnet F, Bergeret S: Recurrent high-permeability pulmonary edema associated with diabetic ketoacidosis, *Crit Care Med* 13:55, 1985.
20. Butterworth JF, Strickland RA, Zaloga GP: Hemodynamic actions and drug interactions of calcium and magnesium. In Zaloga GP, editor: *Endocrine emergencies, problems in critical care,* Philadelphia, 1990, JB Lippincott.
21. Cahill GJ: Hyperglycemic hyperosmolar coma: a syndrome almost unique to the elderly, *J Am Geriatr Soc* 31:103, 1983.
22. Carroll J, Kanter R: Hypophosphatemia and Reye's syndrome, *Crit Care Med* 13:480, 1985.
23. Carter WJ Jr: Hypothermia—a sign of hypoglycemia, *JACEP* 5:594, 1976.
24. Chaimovitz C and others: Hypocalcemia hypotension, *JAMA* 222:86, 1972.
25. Chan J and others: Calcium and phosphate metabolism in children with idiopathic hypoparathyroidism or pseudohypoparathyroidism: effects of 1,25-dihydroxy vitamin D_3, *J Pediatr* 106:421, 1985.
26. Chernow B and others: Iatrogenic hyperphosphatemia: a metabolic consideration in critical care medicine, *Crit Care Med* 9(11):772-4, 1981.
27. Chesney R, Rosen J, DeLuca H. Disorders of calcium metabolism in children. In Collu R and others, editors, *Recent progress in pediatric endocrinology,* New York, 1983, Raven Press.
28. Chopra D, Janson P, Sawin C: Insensitivity to digoxin associated with hypocalcemia, *N Engl J Med* 296:917, 1977.
29. Clarke P, Carre I: Hypocalcemia, hypomagnesemic convulsions, *J Pediatr* 70:806, 1967.
30. Clayton G and others: Disorders of the thyroid. In Kaplan S, editors: *Clinical pediatric and adolescent endocrinology,* Philadelphia, 1982, WB Saunders.
31. Cohen M, Nihill M: Postoperative ketotic hyperglycemia during prostaglandin el infusion in infancy, *Pediatrics* 71:842, 1983.
32. Cooppan R, Kozak GP: Hyperthyroidism and diabetes mellitus, *Arch Intern Med* 140:370, 1980.
33. Cusick J, Hagen T, Findling J: Inappropriate secretion of antidiuretic hormone after trans-sphenoidal surgery for pituitary tumors, *N Engl J Med* 311:36, 1984.

34. Daly J, Greenwood R, Himsworth R: Serum calcium concentration in hyperthyroidism at diagnosis and after treatment, *Clin Endocrinol* 19:397, 1983.
35. DeFronzo RA and others: Impaired rental tubular potassium secretion in systemic lupus erythematosus, *Ann Intern Med* 86:268, 1977.
36. Doczi T and others: Syndrome of inappropriate secretion of antidiuretic hormone after subarachnoid hemorrhage, *Neurosurgery* 9:394, 1981.
37. Don BR and others: Pseudohyperkalemia caused by fist clenching during phlebotomy, *N Engl J Med* 322:1290, 1990.
38. Duck S, Kohler E: Cerebral edema in diabetic ketoacidosis, *J Pediatr* 98:674, 1981.
39. Duck SC, Wyatt DT: Factors associated with brain herniation in the treatment of diabetic ketoacidosis, *J Pediatr* 113:10, 1988.
40. Dunger DB and others: The frequency and natural history of diabetes insipidus in children with Langerhans' cell histiocytosis, *N Engl J Med* 321:1157, 1989.
41. Elin RJ: Mg metabolism in health and disease, *Dis Mon* 34:166-218, 1988.
42. Ellis EN: Concepts of fluid therapy in diabetic ketoacidosis and hyperosmolar hyperglycemic nonketotic coma, *Pediatr Clin North Am* 37(2):313-21, 1990.
43. Ettinger PO, Regan TJ, Oldewartel HA: Hyperkalemia, cardiac conduction, and the electrocardiogram: a review, *Am Heart J* 88:360, 1974
44. Felig P, Lynch V: Starvation in human pregnancy: Hypoglycemia, hypoinsulinemia, and hyperketonemia, *Science* 170:990, 1970.
45. Field JB: Hypoglycemia, definition, clinical presentations, classification, and laboratory tests, *Clin Endocrinol Metab* 18:27, 1989.
46. Fischer KF, Lees JA, Newman JH: Hypoglycemia in hospitalized patients: causes and outcomes, *N Engl J Med* 315:1245, 1986.
47. Fischer JN, Kitabchi AE: A randomized study of phosphate therapy in the treatment of diabetic ketoacidosis, *J Clin Endocrinol Metab* 57:177-80, 1983.
48. Forester CF: Coma in myxedema, *Arch Intern Med* 111:100, 1963
49. Fort P. Waters S, Lifshitz F: Low-dose insulin infusion in the treatment of diabetic ketoacidosis: bolus versus no bolus, *J Pediatr* 96:36, 1980.
50. Foster DW, McGarry JD: The metabolic derangements and treatment of diabetic ketoacidosis, *N Engl J Med* 309:159-69, 1983.
51. Fritz I, Levine R: Action of adrenal cortical steroids and norepinephrine on vascular responses of stress in adrenalectomized rats, *Am J Physiol* 165:456, 1951.
52. Fulop M: Serum potassium in lactic acidosis and ketoacidosis, *N Engl J Med* 300:1087, 1979.
53. Fulop M and others: Hyperosmolar nature of diabetic coma, *Diabetes* 24:594, 1975.
54. Garabedian M and others: Elevated plasma 1,25-dihydroxy vitamin D concentrations in infants with hypercalcemia and an elfin facies, *N Engl J Med* 312:948, 1985.
55. Gershanik J, Levkoff A, Duncan R: The association of hypocalcemia and recurrent apnea in premature infants, *Am J Obstet Gynecol* 113:646, 1978.
56. Gifford RWJ: Effect of reducing elevated blood pressure on cerebral circulation, *Hypertension* 5:17, 1983.
57. Giles T, Iteld B, Rives K: The cardiomyopathy of hypoparathyroidism, *Chest* 79:225, 1981.
58. Ginsberg HN: Investigation of insulin resistance during diabetic ketoacidosis: role of counter-regulatory substances and effect of insulin therapy, *Metabolism* 26:1135-46, 1977.
59. Glasgow A and others: Hypoglycemia, hepatic dysfunction, muscle weakness, cardiomyopathy, free carnitine deficiency and long-chain acyl-carnitine excess responsive to medium chain triglyceride diet, Pediatr Res 17:319, 1983.
60. Glasgow B and others: Adrenal pathology in the acquired immune deficiency syndrome, *Am J Clin Pathol* 84:594, 1985.
61. Goodman S: Inherited metabolic disease in the newborn: approach to diagnosis and treatment, *Adv Pediatr* 33:197, 1986.
62. Grant D: Papilloedema and fits in hypoparathyroidism with a report of three cases, *O J Med* 22:243, 1953.
63. Gravelyn TR and others: Hypophosphatemia-associated respiratory muscle weakness in a general inpatient population, *Am J Med* 84:870-6, 1988
64. Greenspan F, Rappaport B: Thyroid gland. In Greenspan F, editor, *Basic and clinical endocrinology*, Norwalk, CT, 1 1991, Appleton & Lange.
65. Greger NG and others: Central diabetes insipidus, 22 years' experience, *Am J Dis Child* 140:551, 1986.
66. Gregory G: Induction of anesthesia. In Gregory G, editor: *Pediatric anesthesia*, New York, 1989, Churchill Livingstone.
67. Hanley RM: 'Diabetic' emergencies: they happen with or without diabetes, *Posgrad Med* 88(3):90-6, 1990.
68. Harrigan C, Lucas C, Ledgerwood A: Significance of hypocalcemia following hypovolemic shock, *J Trauma* 23:488, 1983.
69. Henrich W, Hunt J, Nixon J: Increased ionized calcium and left ventricular contractility during hemodialysis, *N Engl J Med* 310:19, 1984.
70. Herman A, Mack E, Egdahl R: The relationship of adrenal perfusion to corticosteroid secretion in prolonged hemorrhagic shock, *Surg Gynecol Obstet* 132:795, 1971.
71. Hollifield JW: Potassium and Mg abnormalities: Diuretics and arrhythmias in hypertension, *Am J Med* 28-32, 1984.
72. Holman R, Herron C, Sinnock P: Epidemiologic characteristics of mortality from diabetes with acidosis or coma, United States, 1970-, *Am J Public Health* 73:1169, 1983.
73. Househam K, Vermeulen J, Klein M: Early clinical diagnosis of the syndrome of inappropriate secretions of antidiuretic hormone, *S Afr Med J* 63:498, 1983.
74. How J, Davidson R, Bewsher P: Red cell changes in hyperthyroidism, *Scand J Haematol* 23:323, 1979.

75. Jindrich E: Adrenal hypofunction and sudden death, *Forensic Sci* 29:930, 1984.
76. Johnson J, Jennings R: Hypocalcemia and cardiac arrhythmias, *Am J Dis Child* 115:373, 1968.
77. Kanter Y, Gerson A, Bessman A: 2,3-Diphosphoglycerate, nucleotide phosphate, and organic and inorganic phosphate levels during the early phases of diabetic ketoacidosis, *Diabetes* 24:429, 1977.
78. Karam J Salber P, Forsham P: Pancreatic hormones & diabetes mellitus. In Greenspan F, editor, *Basic and clinical endocrinology,* Norwalk, CT, 1991, Appleton & Lange.
79. Keller U, Berger W: Prevention of hypophosphatemia by phosphate infusion during treatment of diabetic ketoacidosis and hyperosmolar coma, *Diabetes* 29:87, 1980.
80. Keren G and others: Diabetes insipidus indicating a dying brain, *Crit Care Med* 10:798, 1982.
81. Ketchum C, William J, Maclaren N: Adrenal dysfunction in asymptomatic patients with adrenocortical autoantibodies, *J Clin Endocrinol Metab* 58:1166, 1984.
82. Kingston M, Ali-Sibai MB: Treatment of severe hypophosphatemia, *Crit Care Med* 13(1):16-8, 1985.
83. Kitabchi AE, Murphy MB: Diabetic ketoacidosis and hyperosmolar hyperglycemic nonketotic coma, *Med Clin North Am* 72(6):1545-63, 1988.
84. Klein I, Levey G: New perspectives on thyroid hormone, catecholamines, and the heart, *Am J Med* 76:167, 1984.
85. Knapp M. Gough K: An unusual neurological manifestation of hypocalcemia, *Lancet* 1:475, 1967.
86. Knochel J, Schlein E: On the mechanism of rhabdomyolysis in potassium depletion, *J Clin Invest* 51:1750, 1972.
87. Knowlton A: Adrenal insufficiency in the intensive care setting, *J Intensive Care Med* 4:35, 1989.
88. Krane EJ: Diabetic ketoacidosis: biochemistry, physiology, treatment, and prevention, *Pediatr Clin North Am* 34(4):817-34, 1987.
89. Lankton JW, Siler JN, Neigh JL: Hyperkalemia after administration of potassium from nonrigid parenteral-fluid containers, *Anesthesia* 39:660, 1973.
90. Lau K: Phosphate disorders. In Kokko J, Tannen R, editors: *Fluids and electrolytes,* Philadelphia, 1990, WB Saunders.
91. Law W, Health H: Familial benign hypercalcemia, *Ann Intern Med* 102:511, 1985.
92. Leske J: Hyperglycemic hyperosmolar nonketotic coma, *J Emerg Nurs* 10:145, 1984.
93. Levine HD: Electrolyte imbalance and the ECG, *Mod Conc Cardiovas Dis* 23:246, 1954.
94. Levine S, Crowley T, Hai H: Hypomagnesemia and ventricular tachycardia, *Chest* 81:244, 1982.
95. Lloyd CW. Johnson CE: Management of hypophosphatemia, *Clin Pharm* 7(2)123-8, 1988.
96. MacGillivray M, Bruck E, Voorhees M: Acute diabetic ketoacidosis in children: role of the stress hormones, *Pediatr Res* 15:99, 1981.
97. Malik A: Mechanisms of neurogenic pulmonary edema, *J Am Heart Assoc* 57:1, 1985.
98. Malone J, Brodsky S: The value of electrocardiogram monitoring in diabetic ketoacidosis, *Diabetes Care* 3:543-7, 1980
99. Malouf R, Brust JCM: Hypoglycemia: causes, neurological manifestations, and outcome, *Ann Neurol* 17:421, 1985.
100. Manicourt D and others: Disturbed mineral metabolism in hyperthyroidism: good correlation with triiodothyronine, *Clin Endocrinol* 10:407, 1979.
101. Martin BJ, McAlpine JK, Devine BL: Hypomagnesaemia in elderly digitalized patients, *Scott Med J* 33:273-4, 1988.
102. Maslowski AH and others: Haemodynamic, hormonal, and electrolyte responses to captopril in resistant heart failure, *Lancet* 1:71, 1981.
103. Menendez CE, Rivlin RS: Thyrotoxic crisis and myxedema coma, *Med Clin North Am* 57:1463, 1973.
104. Menon R, et al: Syndrome of inappropriate secretion of antidiuretic hormone (SIADH) in children with meningoencephalitis, *Indian J Med Res* 77:373, 1983.
105. Miles J, Gerich J: Glucose and ketone body kinetics in diabetic ketoacidosis, *Clin Endocrinol Metab* 12:303, 1983.
106. Mirro R, Brown D: Parenteral calcium treatment shortens the left ventricular systolic time intervals of hypocalcemia neonates, *Pediatr Res* 18:71, 1984.
107. Molloy DW and others: Hypomagnesemia and respiratory muscle power, *Am Rev Respir Dis* 129:497-8, 1984.
108. Monballyu J and others: Transient acute renal failure due to tumor lysis-induced severe phosphate load in a patient with Burkitt's lymphoma, *Clin Nephrol* 22(1):47-50, 1984.
109. Moreno M, Murphy C, Goldsmith C: Increase in serum potassium resulting from the administration of hypertonic mannitol and other solutions, *J Lab Clin Med* 73:291, 1968.
110. Morishige W: Thyroid hormone influences glucocorticoid receptor levels in the neonatal rat lung, *Endocrinology* 11:1017, 1982.
111. Mulligan I and others: Acute haemolysis due to concentrated dialysis fluid, *Br Med J* 284:1151, 1982.
112. McKie B: Hypocalcaemia and prolonged curarization; a case report, *Br J Anaesth* 41:1091, 1969.
113. Nagai I, and others: Two cases of heriditary diabetes insipidus, with an autopsy finding in one, *Acta Endocrinol* 105:318, 1984.
114. Neal P and others: Unusual manifestations of neonatal hyperthyroidism, *Am J Perinatol* 2:231, 1985.
115. Nelson N, Finnstrom O, Larsson L: Neonatal hyperexcitability in relation to plasma ionized calcium, Mg, phosphate and glucose, *Acta Pediatr Scand* 76:579-84, 1987.
116. Nerup J: Addison's disease: a report of 108 cases, *Acta Endocrinol* 76:127, 1974.
117. Newcomer J, Haire W, Hartman C: Coma and thyrotoxicosis, *Ann Neurol* 14:689, 1983
118. O'Connor L, Wheeler W, Buthune J: Effect of hypophosphatemia on myocardial performance in man, *N Engl J Med* 297:901, 1977.
119. Oh M and others: Hyperchloremic acidosis during the recovery phase of diabetic ketosis, *Ann Intern Med* 89:925, 1978.

120. Peterson KC, Silberman H, Berne TV: Hyperkalemia after cyclosporine therapy, *Lancet* 1:1470, 1984.
121. Ramey E, Goldstein M, Levine R: Action of norepinephrine and adrenal cortical steroids on blood pressure and work performance of adrenalectomized dogs, *Am J Physiol* 165:450, 1951.
122. Ramsay D: Posterior pituitary gland. In Greenspan F, editor: *Basic and clinical endocrinology*, Norwalk, CT, 1991, Appleton & Lange.
123. Reed G, Devous M: Cerebral blood flow autoregulation and hypertension, *Am J Med Sci* 289:37, 1985.
124. Riley LJ Jr, Cooper M, Narins RG: Alkali therapy of diabetic ketoacidosis: biochemical, physiologic, and clinical perspectives, *Diabetes Metab Rev* 5(8):627-39, 1989.
125. Rivers R, Forsling M, Olver R: Inappropriate secretion of antidiuretic hormone in infants with respiratory infections, *Arch Dis Child* 56:358, 1981.
126. Rockey P, Griep R: Behavioral dysfunction in hyperthyroidism, *Arch Intern Med* 140:1194, 1980.
127. Rose B: *Clinical physiology of acid-base and electrolyte disorders*, New York, 1984, McGraw-Hill.
128. Ryzen E and others: Magnesium deficiency in a medical ICU population, *Crit Care Med* 13:19, 1985.
129. Sanson TH, Levine SN: Management of diabetic ketoacidosis, *Drugs* 38(2):289-300, 1989.
130. Saudubray J and others: Clinical approach to inherited metabolic diseases in the neonatal period: a 10-year survey, *J Inherited Metab Dis* 12(Suppl 1):25-41, 1989.
131. Schwartz LJ and others: Endocrine Function in children with human immunodeficiency virus infection, *Am J Dis Child* 145:330, 1991.
132. Shalhoub R: Correcting disorders of serum sodium concentration, *Drug Ther* 59, 1979.
133. Slatopolsky E and others: Hyperphosphatemia, *Clin Nephrol* 7(4):138-46, 1977.
134. Snorgaard O and others: Diabetic ketoacidosis in Denmark: epidemiology, incidence rates, precipitating factors and mortality rates, *J Intern Med* 226(4)223-8, 1989.
135. Solomon, DH: Treatment of Graves' hyperthyroidism. In Ingbar SH, Braverman LE, editors: *The thyroid*, ed 5, Philadelphia, 1986, JB Lippincott.
136. Specter MJ, Schwizer E, Goldman R: Studies on Mg mechanism of action in digitalis-induced arrhythmias, *Circulation* 52:1001-5, 1975.
137. Sprung C, Rackow E, Fein I: Pulmonary edema: a complication of diabetic ketoacidosis, *Chest* 77:687, 1980.
138. Stark H, Weinberger A, Ben-Bassat M: Persistent hyponatremia and inappropriate antidiuretic hormone secretion in children with extensive burns, *J Pediatr Surg* 14:149, 1979.
139. Stewart A and others: Hypercalcemia in pheochromocytoma, *Ann Intern Med* 102:776, 1985.
140. Streicher Z and others: Syndromes of toluene sniffing in adults, *Ann Intern Med* 94:758, 1981.
141. Summers VK: Myxedema coma, *Br Med J* 2:366, 1953.
142. Surawicz B: Relationship between electrocardiogram and electrolytes, *Am Heart J* 73:814, 1967.
143. Textor SC and others: Hyperkalemia in azotemic patients during angiotensin converting enzyme inhibition and aldosterone reduction with captopril, *Am J Med* 73:719, 1982.
144. Tsalikian E, Becker D, Crumrine P: Electroencephalographic changes in diabetic ketosis in children with newly and previously diagnosed insulin-dependent diabetes mellitus, *J Pediatr* 98:355, 1988.
145. Tsau YK and others: Renal tubular acidosis in childhood. *Acta Paediatr Scand* 31(4):205-13, 1990.
146. Tulassay T and others: Atrial natriuretic peptide and other vasoactive hormones during treatment of severe diabetic ketoacidosis in children, *J Pediatr* 11(3)329-34, 1987.
147. Urbanic RC, Mazzaferri EL: Thyrotoxic crisis and myxedema coma, *Heart Lung* 7:435, 1978.
148. Varsano S and others: Hypophosphatemia as a reversible cause of refractory ventilatory failure, *Crit Care Med* 11:908, 1983.
149. Verbalis JG, K Robinson AG, Moses AM: Postoperative and post-traumatic diabetes insipidus, *Front Horm Res* 13:247, 1985.
150. Voorhees M: Disorders of the adrenal medulla; multiple endocrine adenomatosis syndromes. In Kaplan S editor: *Clinical pediatric and adolescent endocrinology*, 1982 Philadelphia, WB Saunders.
151. Walker M, Marshall SM, Alberti KGMM: Clinical aspects of diabetic ketoacidosis, *Diabetes Metab Rev* 5(8):651-63, 1989.
152. Wartofsky L: Myxedema coma. In Ingbar SH, Braverman LE, editors: Werner's *The Thyroid, a fundamental and clinical text*, ed 5, Philadelphia, 1986, JB Lippincott.
153. Wartofsky L: Thyrotoxic storm. In Ingbar SH, Braverman LE, editors: *The Thyroid*, ed 5, Philadelphia, 1986, JB Lippincott.
154. Wason S, Tiller T, Cunha C: Severe hyperphosphatemia, hypocalcemia, acidosis, and shock in a 5-month old child following the administration of an adult Fleet enema, *Ann Emerg Med* 18:696-700, 1989.
155. Watchko J, Bifano E, Bergstrom W: Effect of hyperventilation on total calcium, ionized calcium, and serum phosphorus in neonates, *Crit Care Med* 12:1055, 1984.
156. White R and others: Plasma ionic calcium levels following injection of chloride, gluconate, and gluceptate salts of calcium, *J Thorac Cardiovasc Surg* 71:609, 1978.
157. Wilson HK and others: Phosphate therapy in diabetic ketoacidosis, *Arch Intern Med* 142:517-20, 1982.
158. Winegrad A, Kern E, Simmons D: Cerebral edema in diabetic ketoacidosis, *N Engl J Med* 312:1184, 1985.
159. Zaloga GP: Calcium homeostasis in the critically ill patient, *Magnesium* 8:190, 1989.

160. Zaloga GP: Phosphate disorders. In Zaloga GP, editor: *Endocrine emergiencies, problems in critical care,* Philadelphia, 1990, JB Lippincott.
161. Zaloga GP, Chernow B: Divalent ions: calcium, magnesium and phosphorus. In Chernow B, editor: *The pharmacologic approach to the critically ill patient,* ed 2. Baltimore, 1988, Williams and Wilkins.
162. Zaloga GP, Roberts JE: Magnesium disorders. In Zaloga GP, editors: *Endocrine emergencies, problems in critical care,* Philadelphia, 1990, JB Lippincott.
163. Zwillich CW and others: Ventilatory control in myxedema and hypothyroidism, *N Engl J Med* 292:662, 1975.

28

TRANSPORT HEMATOLOGY

ANTHONY L. PEARSON-SHAVER

Because pediatric transport teams care for patients referred to pediatric tertiary care centers, it is within reason to suspect that some patients will have hematologic problems. While hematologic problems may affect morbidity and mortality, their consequences during transport are frequently limited to their affects on the team's ability to stabilize the patient. Hematologic emergencies, which require immediate evaluation and therapy, occur during pediatric transports. However, definitive evaluation of hematologic disorders can usually await arrival at the referral facility. This chapter will discuss common hematologic problems in children and, where appropriate, identify conditions that require evaluation or therapy while the transport team stabilizes the patient or during transfer to the base facility.

ANEMIA

Anemia, defined as a reduction in either red cell volume or the concentration of hemoglobin, is classified morphologically on the basis of cellular size and the estimated cellular content of hemoglobin. While anemia is frequently not a cause for concern to members of a transport team, situations may arise that favor an optimal hemoglobin concentration before transport. Severely anemic patients may present with signs of congestive heart failure and shock and may require transfusion during the initial resuscitation. Likewise, anemic patients with shock may require transfusion to maintain adequate oxygen delivery before transport.

Oxygen transport

Oxygen is carried most efficiently by hemoglobin. Each hemoglobin molecule carries two oxygen atoms ($Hgb + O_2 \rightarrow HgbO_2$). When fully saturated, 1 gram of pure hemoglobin carries 1.39 ml of oxygen. Therefore, the amount of oxygen carried by hemoglobin in the blood is dependent on hemoglobin concentration and saturation. Though transported most efficiently by hemoglobin, small amounts of oxygen are dissolved in the aqueous portion of blood as a function of the partial pressure of oxygen. Only 0.003 ml of oxygen per 100 ml per mm Hg of oxygen is transported in aqueous form. Therefore, the hemoglobin concentration and the oxygen saturation of hemoglobin are responsible for nearly all of the oxygen which is carried in the blood. While minimally important to the actual transportation of oxygen, the partial pressure of dissolved oxygen creates a pressure gradient between the blood and red blood cells. A reduction in either hemoglobin concentration, oxygen saturation, or the partial pressure of oxygen will lead to a decrease in oxygen carrying capacity.

Circumstances will dictate the patient's need to be treated and the method of treatment. With an anemic patient whose blood is fully saturated and hemodynamically stable, the risk of hypoxia is low when transported at sea level. When a patient presents with anemia, hypoxemia, acidosis, and hemodynamic instability, the transport team should consider transfusion as part of the initial stabilization. The method of transport and the topography of the land are important factors to consider as the partial pressure of oxygen decreases with altitude. Therefore, patients transported at high altitudes will have a decreased partial pressure of oxygen (PO_2) and decreased oxygen saturation of hemoglobin. Anemic patients requiring transport at high altitude should at least be given supplemental oxygen to improve oxygen delivery.

The oxygen content in the blood is a function of the patient's hemoglobin, the saturation of hemoglobin with oxygen, and the amount of oxygen dissolved in the aqueous portion of blood. Expressed as an equation:

$$\text{Oxygen content} = 1.39 \times \text{Hgb} \times \text{arterial oxygen saturation} + 0.003 \times PaO_2$$

Assuming the patient's hemoglobin is 15, arterial oxygen saturation is 100%, and PaO_2 is 100 mm Hg, the oxygen content is approximately 20. Transfusion should be considered if the oxygen content is 14 or less. Transfusion is particularly helpful in patients who are hemodynamically compromised or those who are not fully saturated.

Classification of anemia

Anemia is classified on the basis of the red blood cell morphology indices: mean corpuscular volume and mean corpuscular hemoglobin concentration (Table 28-1). When examined microscopically, the red blood cell is about the size of the nucleus of a small lymphocyte. Smaller red cells are microcytic, and larger red cells macrocytic. Red blood cell size analysis is frequently automated and performed by a cell counter which reports average values. The reports from an automated counter are most reliable when the red cells are all about the same size, this is reflected in mean corpuscular volume (MCV). The red cell distribution width is a calculated index that reflects variation in red blood cell size. A large red blood cell distribution width suggests variability in cell size and renders the automated MCV unreliable. Anemias classified by MCV are microcytic (low MCV), normocytic (normal MCV), or macrocytic (high MCV). Normal MCVs are listed in the table (Table 28-2).

TABLE 28-1 MORPHOLOGIC CLASSIFICATION OF ANEMIA

Microcytic anemias
- Iron deficiency
- Chronic disease (late)
- Thalassemia
- Lead toxicity

Normocytic anemias
- Chronic disease (early)
- Hemorrhage

Macrocytic anemias
- Folate deficiency
- B12 deficiency

TABLE 28-2 NORMAL HEMATOLOGIC VALES BY AGE

Age	*Hemoglobin (g/dL) mean (−2 SD)*	*Hematocrit (%) mean (−2 SD)*	*MCV (fl) mean (−2 SD)*
1-3 days	18.0 (14.0)	54 (42)	108 (95)
6 mo-2 yr	12.0 (10.5)	36 (32)	78 (70)
12-18			
Male	14.5 (13.0)	43 (38)	86 (77)
Female	14.0 (12.0)	41 (36)	88 (78)
Adult			
Male	15.5 (13.5)	47 (40)	88 (78)
Female	14.0 (12.0)	41 (36)	88 (78)

Brown RG: Determining the cause of anemia, *Postgraduate Medicine* 89:161, 1991.

Mean Corpuscular Hemoglobin Concentration (MCHC) is a derived red blood cell index that estimates red blood cell hemoglobin content. Normal values range from 32 to 36 gm/dl. MCHC represents a derived average and as such it may not reflect heterogeneity noted in any particular patient. Specimens which fall within the range of normal values are considered to be normochromic and those below normal values are hypochromic. Increased MCHC values have been noted only in spherocytic disorders, and automated cell counters are relatively insensitive to the increased MCHC.[17] The MCHC like the MCV should be evaluated in light of the blood smear. Upon microscopic examination the pallor noted at the center of the red cells should have a diameter approximately equal to one third of the cellular diameter. If the area of central pallor is larger, the cell is said to be hypochromic.

The Red Cell Distribution Width (RDW), as mentioned earlier, is a calculated index that reflects the variation in red cell size.[17,26] It has been suggested that RDW provides useful information when evaluating the cause of anemias because the increased heterogeneity is the result of abnormal erythropoiesis which produces a variation in the size and shape of red blood cells.[38] When considered together, RDW, MCV, and MCHC are the values which are typically used to define anemic syndromes.

Though anemia may cause significant morbidity, it does not frequently require therapy during the stabilization phase of transport. Red blood cell transfusion should be used to replace blood volume lost in patients who have sustained hemorrhage or to treat shock and maintain oxygen delivery in patients whose hemodynamic status is marginal. In patients who require volume resuscitation following blood loss, anemia is better tolerated than hypovolemia. Therefore, aggressive volume resuscitation must be the initial priority.[24]

APLASTIC ANEMIA

Aplastic anemia is a rare failure of hematopoiesis characterized by pancytopenia and bone marrow hypoplasia. In the general public, three to six cases occur per million, and two to four children per million under fifteen years of age are affected.[31,64] There is a male predominance, and the age distribution of aplastic anemia is bimodal. Peak occurrence is noted in patients under twenty years of age and over forty years of age. The failure of hematopoiesis may be constitutional or acquired. Viruses, particularly hepatitis C and Epstein-Barr viruses, cause aplastic anemia. Chloramphenicol, nonsteroidal anti-inflammatory agents, gold, and environmental toxins have been implicated as well. Over 70% of acquired cases of aplastic anemia are idiopathic.[3]

Attempts should be made to identify the cause of the condition when evaluating patients suspected of being aplastic. When taking a history, specific questions should be asked regarding drug exposure, toxins, recurring infections, and hepatitis. Blood smears reveal variable degrees of pancytopenia, and one or more hematopoietic lines of cell development may be disproportionately affected. On physical examination, pallor and bruising may be present. The presence of infection and hemorrhage indicate a poor prognosis. Children with severe aplastic anemia do not respond well to supportive therapy alone, and only 20% of these patients survive.[9]

Patients with neutropenia and fever require urgent broad spectrum antibiotic therapy that treats common pathogens. Intravenous vancomycin 10 mg/kg/dose every 6 or 8 hours will provide good gram positive therapy. An aminoglycoside (i.e., gentamicin 2.5 mg/kg/dose IV every 8 hours) or a third generation cephalosporin (ceftazidime 50 mg/kg IV every 6 hours) will provide adequate coverage for gram negative organisms. All blood products given to patients with aplastic anemia should be leukocyte depleted to reduce HLA sensitization, and CMV negative patients should receive only CMV negative blood products. The options for cure in affected children lies between bone marrow transplantation for those with an HLA full match family donor and immunosuppressive therapy for those who do not.

SICKLE CELL ANEMIA

Sickle cell anemia is a hemoglobinopathy that results from a single base substitution at the sixth position of nuclear DNA that causes valine to be substituted for glutamic acid on the beta-globin chain of the hemoglobin molecule.[35] When deoxygenated the sickle hemoglobin polymerizes and forms long rods that distort the normal biconcave shape of the RBC into a sickle. Sickling is reversed in young red cells when their hemoglobin is reoxygenated. As cells age, repeated cycles of sickling and unsickling damage the cell membrane. Spectrin and actin become permanently polymerized and return to a normal shape is hampered. Sickling results in stasis and hypoxemia which causes more sickling, tissue necrosis, pain, and tissue infarction. Pathophysiologic consequences of sickle cell disease are due to cellular hypoxia secondary to repetitive vasoocclusive episodes and chronic anemia.

In the United States sickle cell disease occurs primarily in African Americans, although it is noted in many races throughout the world. It has been suggested that the base substitution in the hemoglobin molecule protects heterozygotes from malaria, therefore sickle cell disease is prevalent in the indigenous population areas where malaria is endemic.[2]

The diagnosis of sickle cell disease is inclusive of patients with homozygous hemoglobin S (SS disease), hemoglobin S and hemoglobin C (S-C disease), and hemoglobin S and beta thalessemia (S-B thalessemia).[68] Because patients with sickle cell disease have no hemoglobin A in cord blood, an electrophoretic diagnosis can be made in newborns. Newborn patients homozygous for hemoglobin S have hemoglobin FS in cord blood. As the patient grows older, hemoglobin S predominates. The presence of hemoglobins SA, and F in cord blood is consistent with sickle cell trait and sickle cell-beta thalessemia. Solubility testing and peripheral smears for sickle cell disease may not be helpful in the newborn period. Fetal hemoglobin causes false positive solubility tests and fetal hemoglobin inhibits sickling on peripheral smears by inhibiting polymerization in sickle hemoglobin.[51]

The anemia seen in patients with sickle cell disease is due to increased red cell destruction by the reticuloendothelial system. This fact and the fact that sickle cells are more fragile and lack the deformability of normal RBCs explain the short life span (as short as 20 days) of sickle cells in the circulation.

Clinical manifestations of sickle cell disease

Patients with sickle cell disease come to medical attention for different reasons, depending on their age. Young patients commonly present with vasoocclusive and anemic crises while older patients present more frequently with the effects of chronic anemia and organ failure. Vasoocclusive crises are painful, transient, and result in ischemic damage to organs. Crises are precipitated by infection, fever, acidosis, and dehydration. As the concentration of fetal hemoglobin falls, infants as young as 3 months of age[51] begin to present with pain crises. Musculoskeletal pain is most common, and dactylitis and the hand/foot syndrome are frequent early presentations. Juvenile rheumatoid arthritis is a frequent presumptive diagnosis in infants and toddlers who present with musculoskeletal pain. Older children frequently present with extremity pain without swelling or low back pain. As one might expect the child in crisis cries due to pain and guards the affected area. If extremities are involved the differential diagnosis must include osteomyelitis. Abdominal crises are often indistinguishable from an acute abdomen and causes of an acute abdomen must be diligently sought.

Patients who present in uncomplicated sickle crises tend to have stable hemoglobins, white counts, and reticulocyte values. Anemia in sickle cell disease is a chronic condition (hemoglobin during periods of stability may range from 7 to 9 gm/dl) characterized by macrocytosis and ongoing hemolysis. Despite continual red cell destruction, hemoglobin and reticulocyte values may remain stable for significant periods of time.

Three types of life-threatening anemic crises are seen in sickle cell patients. Splenic sequestration is seen in young patients before the involution of the spleen as it attempts to eliminate the deformed cells. Sequestration crises are often preceded by a viral illness, and patients present with weakness, pallor, and abdominal enlargement due to splenomegaly. As the anemia progresses, tachycardia ensues and the patient may develop congestive heart failure. Hemoglobin may drop as much as 10 percent from the patient's normally low hemoglobin levels. Hypotension and hypovolemic shock may occur if the crisis is severe enough.

Aplastic crises are frequently seen during or following infections.[42,56] The short life span of the red cells in addition to the inhibition of erythroid production by the bone marrow during an infection are responsible for the anemia that occurs. Monitoring of the reticulocyte count in these patients may assist in the prediction of the fall in hemoglobin.

Hyperhemolytic crises are the least common type of anemic crises. The hemoglobin falls despite an increased reticulocyte count. Acute bacterial infections, exposure to oxidant drugs, and red cell glucose-6-dehydrogenase deficiency have all been implicated. Hyperhemolytic crises tend to be self-limited.[68]

The acute chest syndrome (ACS) is an acute febrile episode associated with pulmonary infiltrates, chest pain, cough, dyspnea and hypoxemia in patients with sickle cell disease.[41] As hypoxia develops, red cells sickle. Sickling causes decreased blood flow to the area resulting in localized alveolar damage and local hypoxia. Increased local hypoxia then leads to further injury. The ACS occurs commonly in sickle cell patients. One center reported that the acute chest syndrome occurred in 17% of its pediatric sickle cell patients over a two year period of time.[54] Another reported that the acute chest syndrome occurs in as many as 50% of sickle cell patients at one time or another.[11] Patients with sickle cell anemia who present with ACS are sicker than normal children with pneumonia.[11] Patients with ACS require longer hospitalizations and, following the initiation of therapy, are febrile longer than patients with pneumonia.[54]

Infection has long been thought to be an important cause of the acute chest syndrome[11,12] and *Pneumococcus, H. influenza, S. aureus* and mycoplasma have been isolated from patients with ACS. The literature suggests that infection is a less important etiologic factor in adults than in children. A recent study in adult patients with the acute chest syndrome showed infection to be a cause of ACS in only 21% of patients who were studied.[41] These results suggest that infection causes fewer cases of ACS than once thought. Poncz and others[54] found an identifiable infectious cause of ACS in only 38 of 102 patients. Bacterial infection was found in 12 patients, viral infection in 10 patients, and mycosplasma in 16 patients.

The clinical course of ACS appears to be affected by its etiology. Patients with ACS due to bacterial and mycoplasma pneumonia were sicker than those with ACS of either undetermined or viral cause.[54] When considering antibiotic therapy for ACS, mycoplasma must be covered as well as commonly occurring bacteria.

Invasive infections due to *Streptococcus pneumoniae* occur 30 to 100 times more frequently in children with sickle cell anemia than in healthy children.[76] The spleen normally acts to filter organisms and to aid in opsonization to increase bacterial killing.[51,55,72] Functional asplenia is the primary reason that patients with sickle cell disease are more susceptible to infection. Other proposed immunologic abnormalities include suspected defects in the complement alternate pathway,[37,71] defects in the synthesis of IgG and IgM, and impaired T cell and B cell interaction.[72] While infection with *Streptococcus pneumoniae* is common, infections due to *Hemophilus influenzae, Escherichia coli,* and *Staphylococcus aureus* also occur.[60]

Chronic cardiac and pulmonary changes have been noted in sickle cell disease. Cardiac enlargement and systolic ejection murmurs are common in patients with sickle cell anemia, and acute congestive heart failure develops in patients during anemic crises. Pulmonary function may be impaired in patients with sickle cell disease. Investigators have described reductions in total lung capacity, vital capacity, and forced vital capacity.[14,63] A recent report by Pianosi and others[87] stated that patients with sickle cell disease had lower static lung volumes, lower dynamic lung volumes, and lower flow rates than age, sex, and race matched subjects. None of the subjects tested had values abnormal for age, sex or race. The investigators further noted expiratory flow patterns consistent with both obstructive and restrictive pulmonary injury in sickle cell patients. Prior episodes of the acute chest syndrome were not associated with an increased frequency of abnormalities in pulmonary functions. Pianosi concluded that patients with sickle cell disease may have small lungs due to poor growth.

Neurologic complications are commonly seen in sickle cell patients. While aneurysms, subdural hematomas, and meningitis have all been described, strokes cause significant morbidity and mortality. Initial strokes in sickle cell patients occur at a mean age of 10 years. Following the initial stroke, patients tend to have a good functional recovery. Strokes recur frequently in sickle patients (the recurrence rate is as high as 50%), and recovery following recurrent strokes is not as favorable. With each successive stroke, neurologic function deteriorates.

Treatment of Sickle cell disease

The patient must be adequately evaluated and causes of pain, fever, and dehydration other than sickle cell disease eliminated (see Box 28-1). Pain should be adequately treated. Opioid analgesics are appropriate therapy for pain. Care must be taken to ensure that airway compromise does not occur. Because patients are more difficult to assess and treat in a moving environment, airway stability should be established and the patient's response to analgesia understood before leaving the referring hospital. Rehydration is an important aspect of pain crisis therapy. Vascular access should be established and adequate fluids given early in the resuscitation. One must maintain a high index of suspicion for infection in patients with sickle cell disease. When

BOX 28-1 GUIDELINES FOR TREATING PATIENTS WITH SICKLE CELL ANEMIA

Maintain airway patency
- If the patient cannot maintain the airway without assistance, intubation is in order.
- Reevaluate the patient's airway after analgesics have been given to ensure that airway patency is maintained.

During the transport, supplemental oxygen should be given. An F_iO_2 of 1.0 is recommended.
- Monitor arterial oxygen saturations.
- Maintain an arterial oxygen saturation greater than 95%.

Adequate ventilation must be ensured.
- Check breath sounds for air movement.
- Observe chest rise.
- Intubate if the patient is not ventilating.
- Evaluate ventilation after analgesics are administered.

Fluid resuscitate the patient.
- Give 20 cc/kg boluses of isotonic fluid if patients are hypovolemic. (As with shock, the patient may initially require 80-100 cc/kg fluid).
- Maintenance fluids should be ordered to meet the patient's maintenance fluid requirements plus 50%.

Antibiotics should be given to treat possible bacterial infection.
- Penicillin G (100,000 to 200,000 units/kg/day IV) will treat S. *pneumoniae.*
- Cephalosporin provides coverage for S. *pneumoniae, H. influenzae,* and E. *Coli.*
  - Cefuroxime 75-150 mg/kg/day IV
  - Ceftriaxone 50-100 mg/kg/day IV
- If E. *Coli* is strongly suspected, an aminoglycoside should be added.
  - Gentamicin 7.5 mg/kg/day IV
- If S. *aureus* is suspected.
  - Nafcillin 50-100 mg/kg/day IV

Analgesia should be offered.
- Meperidine 1 mg/kg/dose every 4 hours
- Morphine 0.1 mg/kg/dose every 4 hours
- Fentanyl 3 mcg/kg/dose every 2 hours

antibiotics are administered, care should be taken to treat for *S. pneumoniae, H. influenzae, E. coli,* and *S. aureus*. If a patient is suspected of having the acute chest syndrome, mycoplasma should be treated as well as the bacteria previously mentioned. Supplemental oxygen should be administered to prevent hypoxemia, particularly in those patients with the acute chest syndrome.

NEUTROPENIA

Neutropenia is an absolute decrease in the number of circulating polymorphonuclear leukocytes (PMNs). As children grow, neutrophils represent a smaller percentage of white cells,[69,75] and the mean neutrophil count falls with age. Neutrophils represent as much as 60% of the white blood cells in the periphery during the first few days of life, and by two weeks of age, neutrophils represent only 40% of the white blood cells seen on a peripheral smear. Lymphocytes predominate in the blood from 2 weeks to 8 years of age when PMNs again become the dominant peripheral white blood cell. Neutropenia in adults and older children is defined as a white blood cell count less than 1500 PMNs/mm^3, and in infants 1 to 2 months of age less than 2500 PMNs/mm^3.

Neutropenia results from decreased bone marrow production or increased peripheral destruction of PMNs. Decreased production occurs as a result of abnormalities in the marrow stem cell development. PMNs are derived from committed stem cells in the bone marrow. Precursors undergo four to five mitotic divisions through the myelocytic stage which requires 7 to 8 days. Functional maturation requires another 3 to 5 days. Upon completion of maturation the PMN resides in the bone marrow storage compartment for 1 to 2 days.[69] Factors which modulate PMN production and maturation are poorly understood, but humoral positive and negative feedback mechanisms and the glycoprotein colony stimulating factor appear to increase PMN proliferation.[69] Prostaglandin E, produced by monocyte-macrophages in response to increased colony stimulated factor levels, appears to inhibit PMN committed stem cell proliferation.[52] Under stressful conditions, cell divisions may be skipped, maturation may be shortened, and cells may be released into the periphery prematurely.

The half-life of circulating PMNs in the vasculature is 6 to 7 hours. Half of the available PMNs circulate, and the remainder adhere to vascular endothelium.[7] Circulating neutrophils leave the vasculature randomly and survive in tissues which are in direct contact with the outside environment (GI tract, cervical canal, and tracheobronchial tree, 1 to 4 days). Studies of the granulocytopoietic process suggest that decreased or ineffective production of neutrophils may be the principal mechanism of neutropenia in severely affected patients.[23] Increased margination is postulated as the mechanism responsible for neutropenia in less severely affected patients.[23]

Several neutropenia syndromes have been described and are listed in Table 28-3. Acquired neutropenia has been noted as a result of bone marrow infiltration by malignant cells, nutritional deficiencies (i.e., B12 and folate), toxic injury (following exposure to chemotherapy, radiation therapy, and heavy metals), infections (Table 28-4), and exposure to drugs (Table 28-5).

Patients with absolute PMN counts less than 1000/mm^3 appear to be more susceptible to infection,[69] and cutaneous infections such as stomatitis, gingivitis, and skin infections predominate. When the absolute PMN decreases to less than 500/mm^3 patients develop more severe infections. While these facts are generally accepted, neutropenic patients are often remarkably free of infection and do not require corticosteroid therapy, androgenic steroid therapy, splenectomy, or cytotoxic therapy.[23] The elevated monocyte count frequently seen in neutropenic patients would appear to explain the low rate of infection, but monocytes respond slower than PMNs to chemotactic stimuli and have a slower rate of ingestion.[69,23] Monocytes appear to offer little protection against pyogenic organisms during the early stages of exposure but are delivered to infection sites as exposure continues in adequate numbers to induce inflammatory lesions.[23]

TABLE 28-3 NEUTROPENIA SYNDROMES

Cyclic neutropenia
A disorder characterized by repetitive episodes of neutropenia occurring every 14 to 24 days. Ulceration of mucous membranes, lymphadenopathy, skin, and respiratory infections are common, but life-threatening infections are rare. Cyclic neutropenia is believed to be due to a defect in the regulation of the uncommitted stem cells.

Benign neutropenia
PMN counts vary from 200 to 1500/mm^3. Patients usually develop only mild infections of the skin and mucous membranes. Benign neutropenia occurs as the result of a defect in the regulation of mitosis in PMN precursors. Patients require only symptomatic treatment.

Severe congenital neutropenia
PMN counts frequently are less than 200/mm^3. Patients are predisposed to life-threatening infections, and episodes of pneumonitis are frequent. The bone marrow is depleted of mature PMNs and no cell lines appear to develop beyond promyelocytes and myelocytes. Bone marrow transplantation may be required in some patients.

Neutropenia associated with phenotypic abnormalities
Neutropenia has been associated with a number of phenotypic abnormalities such as Schwachman-Diamon syndrome, Fanconi's pancytopenia, and Chediak-Higashi syndrome

Bone marrow storage pool disorders
PMN counts less than 300/mm^3 have been noted in 30% of healthy black and 7% of healthy white patients. It has been suggested that neutropenia in these patients is due to an inability to mobilize PMNs into the circulation from the bone marrow storage pool.

Acquired neutropenia
Caused by bone marrow infiltration by malignant cells, nutritional deficiencies, toxic injury (chemotherapy, radiation therapy, heavy metal poisoning), infection, and drugs.

Isoimmune neonatal neutropenia
This syndrome occurs as the result of maternal sensitization of fetal neutrophil antigens. Maternal IgG crosses the placenta and destroys the infant's neutrophils. The infant's PMN count usually recovers within 7 weeks of birth as maternal IgG titers decrease. Cutaneous infections predominate, and antibiotics should be prescribed as required for specific infections.

Autoimmune neutropenia
Occurs as a result of autoantibodies directed against PMNs. Neutropenia is seen in infants with a median age of 12 months. Benign infections of the skin, upper respiratory tract, and ear predominate, though more severe infections have been noted.

Neutropenia has been demonstrated in 3% of in-patients and 7% of out-patients when CBCs were retrospectively examined.[1] Studies of otherwise healthy children with neutropenia (absolute neutrophil counts less than 500 PMNs/mm^3) have shown the incidence of infection to range from 6% to 15%.[1,19,66] In a series of 119 children followed serially for neutropenia (PMN $<$ 1500 PMNs/mm^3), 47% had neutrophil counts less than 1000 WBCs/mm^3 and only 4 patients developed infections.[1] None of those patients who developed infections had neutrophil counts less than 500 PMNs/mm^3, though all 4 patients were neutropenic for more than 30 days. The documented nadir was not associated with the onset of the infectious complication in any of the patients who developed infections. Another recent study of patients without underlying malignancy who presented with neutropenia and fever suggests that the overall rate of serious bacterial infection in neutropenic

TABLE 28-4 INFECTIONS ASSOCIATED WITH NEUTROPENIA

Bacterial	**Rickettsial**
Typhoid fever	Rocky Mountain spotted fever
Paratyphoid fever	Typhus fever
Tuberculosis (disseminated)	Rickettsial pox
Brucellosis	
Gram-negative sepsis	**Fungal**
	Histoplasmosis
Viral	
Infectious hepatitis	**Protozoal**
Infectious mononucleosis	Malaria
	Leishmaniasis (Kala-azar)
Influenza	
Measles	
Rubella	
Roseola	
Varicella	
Dengue fever	
Colorado tick fever	
Smallpox	
Poliomyelitis	
Yellow fever	
Sand-fly fever	
Psittacosis	
Mumps	
Cytomegalovirus	
Lymphocytic choriomeningitis virus	

Weetman RM, Boxer LA: Childhood neutropenia: symposium on pediatric hematology, *Pediatric Clinics of North America* 27(2):361, 1980.

patients with fever was only 8%.[19] The authors identified severe neutropenia (PMN < 500 PMNs/mm³) in several children older than two years of age who presented with fever but were ultimately culture negative. Clinical presentation was an important factor in distinguishing culture negative patients from those with systemic bacterial infections. Approximately 30% of those who were irritable or had a toxic appearance were culture positive (bacterial meningitis or sepsis). No child who was febrile with a newly discovered neutropenia and appeared well had evidence of systemic bacterial infection. Observation was recommended for neutropenic febrile patients who appear well and are older than two months of age. Sepsis should be assumed in neutropenic patients with fever who are less than 2 months of age.

Children with malignancy who present with fever and neutropenia are considered to be immunocompromised.[89] Similarly, previously well children who present with overwhelming sepsis, neutropenia and fever should be considered to be immunocompromised.[26] These children require aggressive antibiotic therapy covering for age and condition appropriate pathogens.

As part of their assessment the transport team must decide whether the neutropenic patient should receive antibiotics. As in all patients it will be necessary to consider the patient's history with special attention to previous illnesses (unusual recurrence of infections or malignancy), drugs, and exposure. A thorough physical examination will reveal the presence of toxicity, irritability, or hemodynamic compromise. The literature would suggest that previously well patients who have unremarkable physical examinations and fever can be safely observed. Neutro-

TABLE 28-5 DRUGS ASSOCIATED WITH NEUTROPENIA

Antibacterial drugs	
Carbenicillin	Sulfonamide
Cephalosporins	Vancomycin
Chloramphenicol	
Penicillins, including semi-synthetic penicillins	
Antipsychotic drugs	
Aminopyrin	Dipyone
Phenylbutazone	
Antithyroid and antirheumatic drugs	
Propylthiouracil	Gold thiomalate
Tranquilizing drugs	
Chlorpromazine	Mepazine
Meprobamate	Promazine hydrochloride
Cytotoxic agents	
Cyclophosphamide	Cytosine arabinoside
Methotrexate	6-Mercaptopurine
6-Thioguanine	Adriamycin

Weetman RM, Boxer LA: Childhood Neutropenia: symposium on pediatric hematology, *Pediatric Clinics of North America* 27(2):361, 1980.

TABLE 28-6 TREATMENT GUIDELINES FOR PATIENTS WITH NEUTROPENIA

Pathogens	*Therapy*
Gram-positive bacteria	
S. aureus	IV naficillin 50 mg/kg/dose every 6 hours
S. pneumoniae	or
	IV vancomycin 10 mg/kg/dose every 6 hours
Gram-negative bacteria	
H. influenzae	gentamicin 2.5 mg/kg/dose every 8 hours
Escherichia coli	or
	ceftazidime 50 mg/kg/dose every 8 hours
P. aeruginosa	

penic patients who are febrile and appear ill and patients with a history of malignancy who are febrile should receive aggressive antibiotic therapy. In the latter situation, antibiotics should be given early.

Until specific bacteria are identified, broad spectrum antibiotics should be given (Table 28-6). Patients should be treated for infections caused by gram-positive bacteria including *Staphylococcus aureus* and *Streptococcus pneumoniae.* Potential gram-negative bacteria that should be treated include *Hemophilus influenzae, Escherichia coli,* and *Pseudomonas aeruginosa.* Intravenous naficillin 50 mg/kg/dose every 6 hours provide coverage for gram-positive bacteria. Either gentamicin 2.5 mg/kg/dose or ceftazidime 50 mg/kg/dose given intravenously every 8 hours will treat most suspected gram-negative bacteria. In patients who have been hospitalized or those colonized with methicillin resistant *S. aureus,* vancomycin 10 mg/kg/dose every 6 hours should replace naficillin as gram positive coverage.

THROMBOCYTOPENIA

Platelets are cytoplasmic fragments of bone marrow megakaryocytes which circulate in the vascular space and assist in the maintenance of vascular integrity. When vascular interruption occurs, platelets interact with blood vessels and coagulation proteins to form a mechanical seal that prevents blood from leaving the intravascular space. Production begins in the bone where megakaryocytes, large granulate polypoid cells with increased cytoplasmic volume, and large lobulated nuclei, shed cytoplasmic fragments which circulate as platelets. Megakaryocytes normally constitute about 0.3% nucleated bone marrow cells[47] and are produced by the same stem cells that produce erythroid and myeloid lines. Smaller in size than other bone marrow products, platelets are one quarter of the diameter of the normal red blood cells. Following release from bone marrow sinusoids, platelets circulate for a mean life-span of 8 to 10 days. Aging platelets are removed by reticuloendothelial cells of the liver and spleen. Approximately two-thirds of the platelet mass circulates, and the remaining one-third resides in the spleen forming two interchangeable pools of platelets.[46] Normal children and adults have a platelet count of 150 to 400 $\times$ 10^9 platelets/liter. A decrease in the quantity of circulating platelets is termed thrombocytopenia. Disorders which cause thrombocytopenia are characterized by suboptimal production, abnormal distribution, or increased destruction.

Classic symptoms of thrombocytopenia are bleeding into skin and mucus membranes, particularly in the form of petechiae. Less commonly, thrombocytopenia presents with microcirculatory bleeding manifested as epistaxis, oozing from the gums, hematuria, melena, or menorrhea. Rare presentations of thrombocytopenia include catastrophic hemorrhages of the gastrointestinal system or the central nervous system. Usually symptomatic children have lower platelet counts than asymptomatic children, but the severity of hemorrhage in thrombocytopenia does not always correlate with the platelet count. Evaluation of children with thrombocytopenia should include a complete blood count, a platelet count, and a peripheral blood sphere. Before gamma globulin therapy is started examination of the bone marrow is indicated.

Thrombocytopenic syndromes are classified by etiology or age of occurrence, and several have been described. When thrombocytopenia is noted in well neonates, immune mechanisms are frequently responsible for reductions in the platelet count. Maternal isoimmune antibodies and maternal autoimmune antibodies have both been described as causes of neonatal thrombocytopenia. Thrombocytopenia in sick neonates is frequently secondary to sepsis or gestational infections. Several drugs that cause thrombocytopenia are listed in Table 28-7. Immune-mediated mechanisms, direct toxicity to circulating platelets, and direct injury to megakaryocytes have been offered as explanations for the occurrence of thrombocytopenia with drug therapy.

Microangiopathic disease such as hemolytic anemia, hemolytic uremic syndrome, thrombotic thrombocytopenic purpura and disseminated intravascular coagulation present with thrombocytopenia due to increased platelet destruction that occurs when platelets circulate through small blood vessels affected by vasculitis. An interesting phenomenon, the "wearing blender syndrome," occurs following repair of congenital heart lesions with prosthetic valves and patches. Microangiopathic hemolytic anemia and thrombocytopenia occur as a result of red blood cells and platelets coming in contact with these artificial surfaces.

In hypersplenism up to 90% of the total platelet mass may be sequestered in an enlarged spleen.[36,49] Though circulating platelet counts are low, patients with splenomegaly rarely have episodes of significant bleeding. Thrombocytopenia is seen in patients infected with a wide variety of microorganisms, and common viral illnesses and vaccines are frequently responsible. Disorders of the autoimmune system and malignant infiltrative processes cause thrombocytopenia as well.

Acute therapy for thrombocytopenia is not required unless patients are bleeding, the platelet count is less than 50,000, or invasive procedures are anticipated. Invasive procedures such as central venous catheter placement, nasotracheal intubation, and chest tube insertion are not uncommon during transports. Transport team members should consider platelet transfusion before performing these procedures, if the procedures are absolutely necessary and the delay is appropriate. If procedures are not required and patients are not bleeding, platelet transfusion can occur after the team arrives at the pediatric center.

TABLE 28-7 DRUGS ASSOCIATED WITH THROMBOCYTOPENIA IN CHILDREN

Anticonvulsants, sedatives	Miscellaneous
Diphenylhydantoin	Cytotoxic agents
Carbamazepine	Sulfonylureas
Clonazepam	Gold salts
Sodium valproate	Penicillamine
Primidone	Quinidine
Antibiotics	
Sulfisoxazole	
Trimethoprim-sulfamethoxazole	
Para-aminosalicylate	
Rifampin	
Pentamidine	
Chloramphenicol	

Lightsey AL: Thrombocytopenia in Children, *Pediatric Clinics of North America* 27:293, 1980.

COAGULATION DISORDERS

Disseminated Intravascular Coagulation

Disseminated Intravascular Coagulation (DIC) is a dynamic process triggered by activation of the clotting cascade that results in generation of excess thrombin, further activation of the coagulation cascade, shortened survival of hemostatic elements, deposition of fibrin in the microcirculation, and activation of the fibrinolytic system. DIC is associated with a number of illnesses and conditions (see Box 28-2). The spectrum of manifestations range from purpura and overt bleeding to mild clotting abnormalities with a minimal decrease in platelet number. As one might suspect, therapy for DIC is as variable as its presentation. Some patients require only monitoring, some require platelet transfusion and factor replacement, and yet others require heparin therapy and factor replacement.[28]

The clinical constellation that is seen when DIC develops is thrombocytopenia, prolonged clotting times (prothrombin and partial thromboplastin times), low fibrinogen levels, and elevated fibrin degradation products. DIC is noted in a number of clinical conditions, and the clinician must maintain a high

BOX 28-2 CONDITIONS ASSOCIATED WITH DISSEMINATED INTRAVASCULAR COAGULATION

Bacterial sepsis
Disseminated fungal infections
Systemic viral infections
Shock
  Hypovolemic shock
Head trauma (penetrating trauma)
Multiple trauma with shock
Burns
Septic abortions
Rhabdomyolysis
Heat stroke
Snake envenomation
Hemolytic transfusion reaction

index of suspicion. In evaluating a patient with suspected DIC, one must consider the patient's underlying condition because it may alter the classic DIC criteria. For example, fibrinogen has been shown to be an acute phase reactant in infection and as many as 57% of patients with DIC may have normal fibrinogen levels.[62]

The cornerstone of therapy for DIC is treatment of the underlying condition. Understanding the pathophysiology of the disease process in question will frequently assist the clinician by allowing the development of a rational management plan. Patients with platelet, fibrin, or clotting factor deficiency may require replacement therapy if there is evidence of bleeding or invasive procedures are required. Cryoprecipitate, fresh frozen plasma, and platelets are appropriate, and large replacement volumes must frequently be given due to bleeding or ongoing consumption. Whenever replacement therapy is initiated, fibrinogen and platelet survival should be monitored by checking levels 30 to 60 minutes after the initial transfusion and every 6 hours thereafter. The transport team will not be able to monitor replacement therapy in this fashion. If replacement therapy is provided by the transport team, levels should be checked on arrival at the base hospital. Heparin infusion may be useful in patients with signs of fibrin deposition, such as dermal necrosis in purpura fulminans, acral and dermal ischemia, or venous thromboembolism. In the treatment of DIC, heparin inhibits the activation of thrombin and fibrin deposition.

Hemophilia

Over 95% of inherited blood coagulation disorders can be collectively termed hemophilia, and are secondary to deficiencies of factor VIII (Hemophilia A) or factor IX (Hemophilia B or Christmas disease). Factors VIII and IX are plasma proteins involved in the intrinsic pathway of blood coagulation and are necessary for generation of an insoluble fibrin clot at the site of vascular injury. Therefore, when factors VIII and IX are deficient, partial thromboplastin time (PTT) will be prolonged but bleeding time and prothrombin time (PT) remain normal. Factor VIII is a complex high molecular weight protein with a half-life of approximately 12 hours and is consumed during the clotting process. Factor IX is a vitamin K dependent factor synthesized in the liver with a half-life in the circulation of 24 hours, but unlike factor VIII it is not consumed during the clotting process. If either factor VIII or IX is present in a concentration less than 20 to 30 percent of normal, generation of thrombin and subsequent fibrin formation will be impaired.

Hemophilia occurs in one in ten thousand male births, and there are approximately twenty-five thousand severely affected hemophiliacs in the United States.[32] Clinical manifestations depend upon patient age and the severity of the factor deficiency. Factor VIII and IX levels are less than one percent of normal in patients who are severely affected, and recurrent hemorrhages occur spontaneously or follow extremely minor injury in severely affected patients. Prolonged bleeding occurs following circumcision, subcutaneous ecchymoses are noted over bony provinces by three to four months of age, and large hematomas following intramuscular injection are noted in infants with severe hemophilia. Hemarthroses and intramuscular bleeds are noted in toddlers and preschool children who present with limping and pseudoparalysis. Patients with moderate factor deficiency present only after identifiable injury and do not have episodes of spontaneous bleeding. Mild hemophilia can be clinically silent presenting only with significant trauma later in life.

In making the diagnosis of hemophilia, history provides more valuable information than laboratory tests. The location and type of bleeding often identify the disorder and can differentiate between problems with platelet function and coagulation protein deficiency.[13] For instance, patients with hemophilia never have petechiae, and spontaneous bleeding from the mucosal membranes is rare because platelet number and function are normal.

Family history reveals the x-linked pattern of inheritance. Mothers are usually asymptomatic carriers, and male members of a mother's family will manifest a similar pattern of hemorrhage as the severity of hemophilia is constant within one family. In approximately one-third of cases the family history of hemophilia is negative, suggesting spontaneous mutations.[49] As expected, hemophilia occurs rarely in females.[45]

When evaluating a patient with hemophilia, platelet count, prothrombin time (PT), partial thromboplastin time (PTT), and bleeding time are all important. The prothrombin and bleeding times are normal, while the partial thromboplastin time is prolonged. Bleeding time can be affected by the ingestion of aspirin. Partial thromboplastin time is usually two to three times the normal values. In some laboratories, factor VIII and IX levels 5% to 10% of normal, will yield only slightly prolonged partial thromboplastin times and normal partial thromboplastin times at levels 20 to 25% of normal. Factor levels less than 25% are insufficient to prevent hemorrhage following surgery. Factor assays are important as they allow one to determine the amount of factor replacement required.

Patients with von Willebrand's disease will present with symptoms that suggest hemophilia, but the pattern of bleeding and the family history will be different. Von Willebrand's disease follows a pattern of autosomal inheritance, and the pattern of bleeding suggests platelet dysfunction with mucosal bleeding and petechiae. In addition to prolonged partial thromboplastin times, patients with von Willebrand's disease present with a prolonged bleeding time.

Hemorrhage in patients with hemophilia may occur anywhere in the body, but commonly within joint cavities[6,13,25] and muscles. Vigorous therapy is required as permanent joint damage and nerve compression secondary to intramuscular bleeding may occur. Although it only occurs in three percent of patients with hemophilia, central nervous system bleeding is a significant cause of morbidity and the leading cause of death in patients with hemophilia.

Hemorrhage within a muscle or joint presents with pain followed by swelling and warmth. The decreased morbidity noted in some patients is due to muscle spasms.[6] Immediate factor replacement is the most important therapeutic intervention to stop bleeding, pain, and swelling (see Box 28-3). Fresh-frozen plasma, cryoprecipitate, and Factor VIII and IX concentrates are available for replacement. The use of fresh-frozen plasma to replace factors is currently limited in children. Though it contains all coagulation factors, large volumes are required for adequate replacement. Cryoprecipitate can be used to treat von Willebrand's disease and for Factor VIII replacement but contains no Factor IX. Though expensive, Factor VIII and IX concentrates give reliable amounts of factor per vial and are the preferred sources of replacement factors.

Pain can be controlled with either acetaminophen (15 mg/kg) or narcotic analgesics (Fentanyl 3-5 mcg/kg, Morphine 0.1 mg/kg or Demerol 1 mg/kg), but aspirin and aspirin containing products should never be used in hemophiliacs because the inhibition of platelet function will prolong the bleeding time. Aminocaproic acid (Amicar), an inhibitor of fibrinolysis, is extremely useful for treating bleeding in the oral cavity following tooth extraction or after local trauma.[22,50] When Amicar is used, large doses (100 mg/kg) must be administered every 6 hours for 7 to 10 days.

When treating patients with hemophilia, two basic assumptions must always be made:

1. The patient and his parents know when bleeding occurs. Believe the patient and/

BOX 28-3 FACTOR REPLACEMENT THERAPY FOR HEMOPHILIA:[18]

One unit of factor equals the amount of Factor VIII or IX in 1 ml of normal pooled anticoagulated plasma.
Infusion of 1 unit/kg raises the Factor VIII level by two percent with a subsequent half-life of 12 hours.
Infusion of 1 unit/kg raises the Factor IX level by 1 percent with a subsequent half-life of 24 hours.
Desired factor levels (Factor VIII and Factor IX deficiency):
- In soft tissue and joint bleeds, an activity level of 50% should be achieved through factor transfusion.
- When life threatening bleeds (surgery, CNS) occur, an activity level of 100% should be achieved through transfusion.

Treatment of soft tissue and joint bleeds:
- Factor VIII deficiency:
  - Transfuse 25 units/kg factor VIII concentrate
  - Factor VIII concentrate contains 250-400 units/vial
  - Cryoprecipitate contains 100 units/bag
- Factor IX deficiency:
  - Transfuse 50 units/kg of factor IX concentrate
  - Factor IX concentrate contains 500 units/vial

Treatment of life threatening bleeds:
- Factor VIII deficiency
  - Transfuse 50 units/kg factor VIII
- Factor IX deficiency
  - Transfuse 100 units/kg factor IX

or his parent(s) if he thinks he's bleeding, though physical signs are not evident.

2. If uncertain about the occurrence of a bleed, assume it has happened. When in doubt, infuse.

TRANSFUSION OF BLOOD PRODUCTS

Red blood cell transfusion

One unit of whole blood contains approximately 450 ml of blood collected from a healthy adult donor. Packed red blood cells are the cellular sediment that remains after whole blood is centrifuged. The resultant unit of packed red blood cells has a hematocrit of 70% to 80% and a volume of 250 ml. Though most of the plasma is removed, 70 to 100 ml of plasma remains in each unit of packed red blood cells. Packed red blood cells are usually anticoagulated with citrate phosphate dextrose adenine solution and stored at 1 to 6°C for up to 35 days. When indicated, red blood cell transfusion increases hemoglobin, hematocrit, and the oxygen carrying capacity of blood (see Box 28-4 and Table 28-8).

The storage of blood causes several metabolic derangements that impact either the recipient or the function of the transfused red cells. The potassium concentration of stored blood increases with prolonged storage due to decreased activity of the red cell ionic pumps.[65] Following transfusion the activity of the ionic pumps is reestablished. Both hyperkalemia and hypokalemia have been noted following transfusion. Hypokalemia is noted most commonly following transfusion,[70] but hyperkalemia can occur as a result of rapid

BOX 28-4 RED CELL TRANSFUSION FORMULAS

When transfusion is indicated, several formulas can be used to determine the amount of whole blood or red blood cells to be given.
- 10 ml/kg of packed red blood cells increase the hemoglobin by 2.5 to 3 gm/dl and the hemoglobin concentration by 10% (31)
- 6 ml/kg of whole blood increases the hemoglobin by 1 gm/dl (30)
- 3 ml/kg of packed red cells increases the hemoglobin by 1 gm/dl (30)

TABLE 28-8 VOLUME, WBC CONTENT, AND EXPIRATION OF DIFFERENT BLOOD COMPONENTS

	Storage (°C)	*Volume in ml*	*Average total WBC content*	*Expiration*
Whole blood	−1-−6	45	1-2 × 10⁹	Variable*
Red blood cells	−1-−6	250	2-2 × 10⁹	Variable*
Washed red blood cells	−1-−6	Variable	<5 × 10⁸†	24 hr
Deglycerolized red	Frozen < −65, or < −120	250		Frozen up to 10 cerolized 24 hr
Platelet concentrate	−20-−24 with agitation	50-75	4 × 10⁷	24 hr or 5 days‡ 4 hr after pooling
Plateletpheresis unit	−20-−24 with agitation	200-500	3 × 10⁸	24 hr or 5 days§
Cryoprecipitate	Frozen < −18 Thawed −1-−6	25	0	12 mo frozen 6 hr after defrost or 4 hr after pooling
Fresh-frozen plasma	Frozen < −18 Thawed −1-−6	125	0	12 mo frozen 24 hr after defrosting
Pediatric-frozen plasma	Frozen < −18 Thawed −1-−6	Variable	0	12 mo frozen 24 hr after defrosting
Liquid plasma	As liquid −1-−6	125	1.5 × 10⁵	5 days after whole blood expiration
Single-donor plasma	Frozen < −18 As liquid −1-−6	125	0	5 yr frozen 24 hr after defrosting
Granulocyte concentrate	−20-−40, no agitation	200-500	1 × 10¹⁰	24 hr

All products should be transfused within 4 hours of spiking of bag.
* Variable depletion; depends on methods and starting volume.
† See text for anticoagulants.
‡ Depends on method of collection.
§ May also be contained 20 to 100 × 10¹⁰ platelets.
Luban NL: Basic transfusion medicine. In Fuhrman B, Zimmerman J, editors, *Pediatric Critical Care*, St Louis, 1992, Mosby-Year Book.

red cell infusion.[43] Blood stored 3 weeks may contain an acid load as high as 30 to 40 mmol/liter due to citric acid from the anticoagulant and lactic acid produced by the red cells themselves. Citrate is metabolized by the liver to bicarbonate and may cause a profound alkalosis, but the impact of red cells transfusion on a patient's acid-base status depends on the rate of administration, the rate of citrate metabolism by the liver, and the patient's hemodynamic status.

Red cell function following transfusion requires time to recover. Cellular ionic pumps require time to reestablish their normal intracellular potassium concentration. Hypothermia causes abnormalities in red cell citrate and lactate metabolism, red cell deformability, platelet function, and hemoglobin oxygen affinity. The affinity of hemoglobin for oxygen is also affected by the concentration of 2,3-diphosphoglycerate (2,3 DPG) in the red cell. Following transfusion the oxygen dissociation curve is shifted to the left due to low concentrations of 2,3 DPG.[67] Recovery may take several hours, and as one might suspect, during that time oxygen availability to the tissues is decreased. If citrate glucose is used as the anticoagulant, 2,3 DPG concentrations may be low enough to cause a shift in the oxygen dissociation curve after 1 week, however newer anticoagulant preservatives containing citrate, glucose, adenine, and phosphorus can preserve red cell 2,3 DPG up to 14 days.

Massive transfusion is defined as transfusion of 1.5 times the patient's estimated blood volume or replacement of the patient's blood volume in less than 24 hours.[24] Blood losses requiring massive transfusion can occur as a result of traumatic injury or surgery and will acutely cause hypovolemia. Hemorrhage that leads to acute hypovolemia is a medical emergency requiring an aggressive resuscitation to replace the patient's circulating volume. Because anemia is better tolerated than hypovolemia, volume resuscitation is the first priority. Dilutional coagulation defects have been described when volume losses were replaced with red cell concentrates or cells suspended in additive solutions.[24] Transfusion with massive amounts of whole blood does not result in a reduction in coagulation factors because Factors I, II, VII, IX, X, XI, and XII are available in adequate concentrations. If red cell concentrates are used to replace massive blood losses, one unit of whole blood is recommended after the first four units of red cells are transfused.[24]

Complications of red blood cell transfusion include: ABO incompatibility hemolytic transfusion reactions, hepatitis, transmission of CMV and HIV viruses, hypocalcemia, potassium disturbances, and alkalosis.[24,29] ABO incompatibility hemolytic transfusion reactions are the most common cause of acute mortality due to transfusion and occur most frequently in the emergency setting due to clerical errors.[24,34] Cytomegalovirus is the most commonly transmitted viral agent and in the United States. Blood is not routinely tested for CMV as cytomegalovirus is endemic only causing significant pathology in immunocompromised transfusion recipients. The prevalence of CMV is age-dependent, and 20% of the blood donating population is infected by 20 years of age. The most frequent infectious complication of blood transfusion continues to be transmission of hepatitis C, though hepatitis B, and the Human Immunodeficiency Virus have been transmitted by transfusion as well. With massive transfusion, large quantities of the anticoagulant sodium citrate can be infused, causing metabolic alkalosis and ionized hypocalcemia.

Platelet transfusion

Random donor platelet concentrates are prepared by centrifugation of whole blood units. The platelet rich plasma which results is spun again to produce the cell-free plasma used to provide the component. The yield of platelets in a platelet concentrate should equal at least 5.5×10^{10} and more commonly yields are as high as 7.0×10^{10} platelets per concentrate.[58] The yield of platelets is affected by the time and force of centrifugation used to separate platelet rich plasma from whole blood,[59] the number of white cells contaminating the platelet concentrate[46,79] and storage conditions. Platelets are sensitive to pH changes which occur in the storage package, the type of container used to store the platelets, the storage temperature, and the method of agitation used during storage.[58] Viability is best preserved when platelets are stored at room temperature (22 degrees Centigrade)[73,98] using a mechanical rotator.[33]

Apheresis platelets are harvested from a single donor using an in-line centrifuge. The yield of apheresis is directly related to the donor's platelet count, and the final product usually contains the equivalent of at least 6 units of platelet concentrates. Although there is less information available concerning viability in function of apheresis platelets, it appears that apheresis platelets are viable and functional immediately after collection.[19,39,57] Apheresis donors are often specially selected HLA compatible donors who support patients refractory to pooled random donor concentrates.

Patients who are thrombocytopenic due to problems with platelet production may benefit from prophylactic platelet transfusions to maintain platelet counts greater than 50,000. If platelet counts are greater than 50,000, clinical judgment should be used taking into consideration the severity of bleeding and the risk of further bleeding. When significant bleeding is noted in a patient with a platelet count higher than 100,000, platelet dysfunction must be entertained when the patient has longer than expected bleeding times for the platelet count. Indeed, it may be impossible to precisely define solely on the basis of platelet count the indications for platelet transfusions to prevent bleeding because platelet dysfunction is so frequent. Platelet dysfunction in thrombocytopenic patients is most commonly related to drugs [anti-inflammatory drugs including aspirin and semisynthetic penicillins[15,16,61]] and the patient's primary disorder.

In monitoring the response to platelet transfusion, one must examine the incremental increase in platelet count, platelet survival, platelet function, and the degree of improvement in hemostasis. The incremental increase in platelet number can be calculated by comparing the pretransfusion platelet count to the platelet count 1 hour after transfusion. One unit of platelets per 10 kg body weight should raise the platelet count by 10,000 platelets/microliter, or 1 unit of platelets/m^2 should raise the platelet count 12,000. Platelet survival will be indicated by serial platelet counts and will determine the transfusion frequency required. Survival of transfused platelets appears to be dependent on the patients initial platelet count. The lower the platelet count, the shorter the survival time due to platelet participation in the maintenance of vascular integrity.[58] At lower levels a larger percentage of platelets line the vascular epithelium. Platelet function is inferred by the resolution of bleeding, which suggests a shorter bleeding time and the development of hemostasis.

Refractoriness to platelet transfusion is signified by a lack of increase in platelet number 1 hour after transfusion. Patients can become refractory to platelet transfusion in several clinical scenarios including DIC, hemorrhage, drug administration (amphotericin and amrinone), splenic hyperfunction, and the presence of HLA and platelet specific antibodies. When patients are refractory to platelet transfusion, ABO-matching of platelets, single donor platelets, and ultraviolet irradiation of platelets are options to reduce the antigenicity of the platelet concentrate.[40]

Though the prophylactic platelet transfusion for low platelet counts is a common practice, there is little evidence to support its use in a patient who is not bleeding. Before administering a platelet transfusion the clinician must evaluate the patient's diagnosis, condition, and the suspected cause of thrombocytopenia.[40] One should consider whether the moving environment common to transport will justify platelet transfusion in patients who are to be transported. See Box 28-5 for guidelines for platelet transfusion.

BOX 28-5 GUIDELINES FOR PLATELET TRANSFUSION

Indications for platelet transfusion:
- Prophylactic platelet transfusion of platelets may be useful if platelet count is less than 50,000.
- If the platelet count is 50,000 to 100,000, use clinical judgment as to the need for transfusion.
- If the platelet count is greater than 100,000, platelets should be transfused only if active bleeding is noted.

Transfusion formulas:
- One unit of platelets per 10 kg body weight should raise the platelet count by 10,000 platelets/microliter.
- One unit of platelets/m^2 should raise the platelet count by 12,000 platelets/microliter.

Fresh frozen plasma

Fresh-frozen plasma is the liquid portion of a unit of human blood that has been centrifuged, separated, and frozen solid at −18°C within 6 hours of collection.[21] Fresh-frozen plasma is a single donor plasma donor unit product and contains labile and stable components of the coagulation, fibrinolytic, and complement systems. A number of proteins are found in FFP which have diverse activities, including maintenance of oncotic pressure and modulation of immunity. Due to its potential risks, the use of FFP as a volume expander is discouraged. While rich in protein content, FFP is not the ideal colloid volume expander and its use should be confined to the treatment of specific coagulation disorders (see Box 28-6).

Patients with diagnosed factor deficiencies should not be treated with FFP because low factor concentrations require large volume transfusions.[18] If specific factors are available, their use is preferred. Cryoprecipitate contains fibrinogen and factor VIII and can be used to treat patients with Hemophilia A and von Willebrand's disease. Concentrates of Factors VIII and IX are available for treatment of patients with Hemophilia A and Christmas disease.

Infections (hepatitis) and allergic reactions

BOX 28-6 INDICATIONS FOR THE USE OF FRESH-FROZEN PLASMA

Replacement of Factors II, V, VII, IX, XI

Emergent (active bleeding or required surgery) or urgent reversal of warfarin effect. Patients treated with warfarin are deficient in Factors II, V, VII, IX, XI. If routine reversal is required, vitamin K can be used.

Correction of documented coagulation defects associated with massive transfusion.

Treatment of thrombotic thrombocytopenic purpura.

Because FFP is a source of antithrombin III, it can be used to treat patients deficient in antithrombin III who require surgery or heparin therapy for treatment of thrombosis.

Before the availability of intravenous gamma globulin, FFP was used as a source of immunoglobulins in patients who required immunoglobulins to treat humoral immunodeficiencies.

complicate therapy with FFP. The incidence nonicteric or icteric hepatitis is 3% to 10% following multiple transfusions FFP. As in red cell transfusion, non-A, non-B hepatitis is the most common infection transmitted, but CMV and hepatitis B are transmitted as well. The HIV virus may be transmitted in FFP as well. Allergic and anaphylactic reactions also occur following FFP transfusion, and presentation varies from hives to pulmonary edema. Alloimmunization has been noted and is manifested by the development of Rh antibodies in some patients following FFP infusion.[21]

REFERENCES

1. Alario AJ, O'Shea JS: Risk of infectious complications in well-appearing children with transient neutropenia, *AJDC* 143:973, 1989.
2. Allison AC: The distribution of the sickle cell trait in East Africa and elsewhere, and its apparent relationship to the incidence of subterian malaria, *Trans Voy Soc Trop Med Hyg* 48:312, 1954.
3. Alter BP, Potter NU, Li FP: Classification of the aplastic anemias, *Clin Haematol* 7:431-65, 1978.
4. Altman PL, Dittmer DS: *Blood and other body fluids*, Washington, DC, 1961, Federation of American Societies for Experimental Biology.
5. Ariyan S, Shessel FS, Picket LK: Cholecystitis and cholelithiasis masking as abdominal crises in sickle cell disease, *Pediatrics* 58:252, 1976.
6. Arnold WD, Hilgartner MW: Hemophiliac arthropathy: Current concepts of pathogenesis and management, *J Bone Joint Drug* 59A:287-305, 1977.
7. Athens JW and others: Leukokinetic studies: III. the distribution of granulocytes in the blood of normal subjects, *J Clin Invest* 40:159-64, 1961.
8. Austen DEG: The structure and function of factors VIII and IX, *Clin Haematol* 8:31-52, 1979.
9. Bacigalupo A and others: Treatment of SAA in Europe 1970-1985: a report of the SAA Working Party, *Bone Marrow Transplantation* 1(suppl 1):19-21, 1986.
10. Baehner RL, Strauss HS: Hemophilia in the first year of life, *N Engl J Med* 275:524-8, 1966.
11. Barrett-Connor E: Acute pulmonary disease and sickle cell anemia, *Am Rev Resp. Dis* 104:159, 1971.
12. Barrett-Connor E: Pneumonia and pulmonary infarction in sickle cell anemia, *JAMA* 224:997-1000, 1973.
13. Biggs R, editor: *Human blood coagulation: haemostasis and thrombosis*, ed 2, Oxford, Blackwell Scientific Publications, 1976.
14. Bromberg PA: Pulmonary aspects of sickle cell disease, *Arch Intern Med* 133:652, 1974.
15. Brown CH and others: Effect on platelet function following the administration of penicillin compounds, *Blood* 47:949, 1976.
16. Brown CH and others: The hemostatic defect produced by carbenicillin, *N Engl J Med* 291:265, 1974.
17. Brown RG: Determining the cause of anemia: general approach, with emphasis on microcytic hypochromic anemia, *Post Graduate Medicine* 89:161, 1991.
18. Buchanan GR: Hemophilia, *Ped Clin N Am* 27:309, 1980.
19. Buchholz DH and others: Description and use of the CS-3000 blood cell separator for single-donor platelet collection, *Transfusion* 23:190, 1983.
20. Bussel JB: Thrombocytopenia in newborns, infants, and children: *Pediatr Ann* 19:181, 1990.
21. Consensus Conference: Fresh-frozen plasma: indications and risk, *JAMA* 253:551, 1985.
22. Corrigan JJ Jr: Oral bleeding in hemophilia: treatment with epsilon aminocaproic acid and replacement therapy, *J Pediatr* 80:124-8, 1972.
23. Dale DC and others: Chronic neutropenia, *Medicine* 58:128-44, 1979.
24. Donaldson MDJ, Seaman MJ, Park GR: Massive blood transfusion, *Br J Anaest* 69:621-30, 1992.
25. Duthie RB and others: *The management of musculoskeletal problems in the haemophilias*, Oxford, Blackwell Scientific Publications, 1972.
26. Evans TC, Jehle D: The red blood cell distribution width, 9:71-4, 1991.
27. Fagiolo E, D'Addosis AM: Post-transfusion graft-vs-host disease (GVHD): immunopathology and prevention, *Haematologica* 70:62-74, 1985.
28. Feinstein DI: Treatment of disseminated intravascular coagulation: seminars in thrombosis and hemostasis, 14:351, 1988.

29. Goodnough LT, Shuck JM: Risks, options, and informed consent for blood transfusion in elective surgery, *Am J of Surg* 159:602, 1990.
30. Gottschall TL and others: Importance of white blood cells in platelet storage, *Vox Sang* 47:101, 1984.
31. Halperin DS and others: Severe acquired aplastic anemia in children: 11 years experience with bone marrow transplantation and immunosuppressive therapy, *Am J Pediatr Hematol Oncol* 11:304-9, 1989.
32. Hilgartner MW, editor: Hemophilia in children, Littleton, Massachusetts, 1976, Publishing Sciences Group, Inc.
33. Holme S, Vaidja K, Murphy S: Platelet storage at 22°C: effect of type of agitation on platelet morphology, viability and function in vivo, *Blood* 52:425, 1979.
34. Honig CL, Bove JR: Transfusion-associated fatalities: review of Bureau of Biologics reports 1976-1978, *Transfusion* 20:653-61, 1980.
35. Hunt JA, Ingram VM: a terminal peptide sequence of human hemoglobin, *Nature* 194:640, 1959.
36. Jandl JH, Aster RH: Increased splenic pooling and the pathogenesis of hypersplenism, *Am J Med Sci* 253:383, 1967.
37. Johnson CS, Tegos C, Butler E: Thalassemia minor: routine erythrocyte measurements and differentiation from iron deficiency, *Am J Clin Pathol* 80:31-86, 1983.
38. Johnston RB Jr, Newman SL, Struth AG: An abnormality of the alternate pathway of complement activation of sickle cell diseases, *N Engl J Med* 288:803, 1973.
39. Katz AJ and others: Platelet collection and transfusion using the Fenwal CS-3000 cell separator, *Transfusion* 21:560, 1981.
40. King DJ: Transfusion and the use of blood products, *Bailliere's Clinical Hematology* 4:545, 1991.
41. Kirkpatrick MB, Haynes J Jr, Basso JB Jr: Results of bronchoscopically obtained lower airway cultures from adult sickle cell disease patients with the acute chest syndrome, *Am J Med* 90:206, 1991.
42. Leikin SL: The aplastic crisis of sickle cell disease occurrence in several members of families within a short period of time, *Am J Dis Child* 93:128, 1957.
43. Linko K, Tigerstedt I: Hyperpotassaemia during massive blood transfusions, *Acta anaesthesiologica Scandinavia* 28:220-1, 1984.
44. Luban NLC: Basics of transfusion medicine. In Fuhrman BP, Zimmerman JJ, editors, *Pediatric critical care*, 1992, St. Louis, Mosby-Year Book.
45. Lusher J, McMillian CW, The Hemophilia Study Group: Severe Factor VIII and Factor IX deficiency in females, *Am J Med* 65:637-48, 1978.
46. McClure PD: Idiopathic thrombocytopenic purpura in children: should steroids be given, *Pediatrics* 55:68-74, 1975.
47. McMillan CW: Platelet and vascular disorder. In Mill DR and others, editors: Blood disease in infancy and childhood, 1978, St. Louis, CV Mosby Co.
48. Moroff G, Friedman A, Robkin-Kline L: Factors influencing changes in pH during storage of platelet concentrates at 20-24°C, *Vox Sang* 42:33, 1982.
49. Naiman JL, Bergman GE: Hematologic clues to systemic disease in children, *Sem Hematol* 12:287, 1975.
50. Needleman HL, Kaban LB, Kevy SV: The use of epsilon-aminocaproic acid for the management of hemophilia in dental and oral surgery patients, *J Am Dent Assoc* 93:586-90, 1976.
51. O'Brien RT and others: Prospective study of sickle cell anemia in infancy, *J Pediatr* 89:205, 1976.
52. Pelus LM and others: Regulation of macrophage and granulocyte proliferation, *J Exp Med* 150:277-92, 1979.
53. Pianosi P and others: Pulmonary function abnormalities in childhood sickle cell disease, *J Pediatr* 122:366, 1993
54. Pizzo PA and others: Fever in the pediatric and young adult patient with cancer; a prospective study of 1001 episodes, *Medicine* 61:153-6, 1983.
55. Powars DR, Pegelow CH: The spleen in sickle cell disease and thalassemia, *Am J Pediatr Hematol Oncol* 1:343-53, 1979.
56. Singer K, Motulsky AG, Wile SA: Aplastic crisis in sickle cell anemia, *J Lab Clin Med* 33:721, 1950.
57. Slichter SJ: Efficacy of platelets collected by semi-continuous flow centrifugation (Haemonetics Model 30), *Br J Haematol* 38:131, 1978.
58. Slichter SJ: Platelet transfusion therapy, *Hem/Onc Clin N Am* 4:291, 1990.
59. Slichter SJ, Harker LA: Preparation and storage of platelet concentrates: I. factors influencing the harvest of viable platelets from whole blood, *Br J Haematol* 34:393, 1976.
60. Smith JA: The natural history of sickle cell disease, Ann NY Acad Sci, 565:104-8, 1989.
61. Snyder EL and others: Extended storage of platelets in a new plastic container: II. in vivo response to infusion of platelets stored for 5 days, *Transfusion* 25:209, 1985.
62. Spero JA, Lewis U, Hasiba: Disseminated intravascular coagulation, *Thromb Haemost* 38:33, 1980.
63. Sproule BJ, Halden ER, Miller WF: A study of cardiopulmonary alterations in patients with sickle cell disease and it variants, *J Clin Invest* 37:486, 1958.
64. Szklo M and others: Incidence of aplastic anemia in metropolitan Baltimore: a population based study, *Blood* 66:116-9, 1985.
65. Valeri CR: Viability and function of preserved red cells, *N Engl J Med* 284:81-8, 1971.
66. Valiaveeden R and others: Transient neutropenia in childhood, *Clin Pediatr* 12:639-42, 1987.
67. Valtis DJ, Kennedy AC: Defective gas transport function of stored red blood cells, *Lancet* 1:119-24, 1954.
68. Vichinsky EP, Lubin BH: Sickle cell anemia and related hemoglobinopathies, *Pediatr Clin of North Am* 27:429, 1980.
69. Weetman RM, Laurence AB: Childhood Neutropenia, *Ped Clin N Am* 27:261, 1980.

70. Wilson R, Mammen R, Walt AJ: Eight years experience with massive blood transfusions, *J of Trauma* 11:275-85, 1971.
71. Winkelstein JA, Drachman RH: Deficiency of pneumococcal serum opsonizing activity of sickle cell disease, *N Engl J Med* 279:459, 1968.
72. Wong W, Overturf GD, Powars DR: Infection caused by *Streptococcus pneumoniae* in children with sickle cell disease: epidemiology, immunologic mechanisms, prophylaxis, and vaccination, *Clin Infect Dis* 14:1124-36, 1992.
73. Xanthou M: Leukocyte blood picture in healthy full-term and premature babies during the neonatal period, *Arch Dis Child* 45:242, 1970.
74. Young NS and others: Aplastic anemia in the Orient, *Br J Haematol* 62:1-6, 1986.
75. Zacharsk LKR, Elveback LR, Linman JW: Leukocyte counts in healthy adults, *Am J Clin Pathol* 56:148, 1971.
76. Zarkowsky HS and others: Bacteremia in sickle hemoglobinopathies, *J Pediatr* 109:579-85, 1985.

29

TRANSPORT OF A PATIENT WITH GASTROINTESTINAL BLEEDING

WILLIAM E. HARDWICK, JR.

The diagnosis and the management of gastrointestinal (GI) tract hemorrhage in infants and children has advanced dramatically in recent years. Reports from the 1960s and 1970s demonstrate a failure to diagnose the site of bleeding in 30 to 50% of GI patients.[2,20] At present, however, a bleeding source can be established in more than 95% of pediatric GI hemorrhage patients.[14] This improvement is due largely to technical advances in fiberoptic endoscopy and imaging techniques (arteriography, red blood cell labeling), usually only available in tertiary centers. Therefore, the need for transportation of GI hemorrhage patients to these institutions with definitive diagnostic and therapeutic capabilities has increased. The ability to diagnose and treat GI bleeding is an essential skill for all transport physicians.

The causes of GI hemorrhage are extensive and vary greatly with patient age. It is necessary to have a systematic approach for organizing information from the history/physical examination into a plan of action. Particular emphasis should be placed on 1) the initial assessment of the severity of bleeding and appropriate resuscitation, and 2) minor treatment differences based on general classification of bleeding source.

DIAGNOSIS/RECOGNITION

The first question the transport physician must ask in the diagnosis and management of a patient with a suspected GI tract hemorrhage is whether the patient has indeed bled. It is essential to verify that the material in the vomitus, aspirate, or stool is blood. Certain fruits and fruit juices such as beets, tomatoes, and cranberry juices, as well as red food coloring (Koolaid®, Hawaiian Punch®, Jello®) and antibiotic syrups may resemble blood when vomited or expelled in a stool. The ingestion of spinach, blueberries, grapes, licorice, charcoal as well as bismuth (Pepto-Bismo®) and iron preparations can result in dark stools which resemble melena.[21] The presence of blood in stool can be verified by the Hemoccult (guaiac) or Hematest (toluidine blue O) assay, although iron supplements, red meats, and iodide may cause false positive results.[7,12] False negative results may be seen with dehydrated stool specimens or with the ingestion of ascorbic acid (Vitamin C).[10,23] Gastric fluid is particularly difficult to test for occult blood because of the acidic pH; therefore, gastroccult (test cards specifically for gastric aspirates) should be used.[17] The transport physician must also entertain the possibility that blood which is vomited or passed in stool may have its origins outside of the GI tract (i.e., epistaxis, hematuria, menses). For example, a newborn may swallow maternal blood during delivery which is then vomited or passed in the stool simulating hemorrhage. The Kleihauer or Apt Test can distinguish between maternal and fetal red blood cells and help exclude true GI hemorrhage.[9]

If a gastrointestinal (GI) tract hemorrhage is diagnosed, the next logical question (although not the most important in determining initial therapy), is "where is the source of the bleeding." Evaluation and treatment of GI bleeding during transport usually does not require that an exact source be diagnosed, but some distinctions may be helpful in determining ongoing therapy after initial resuscitation or in determining the need for surgical consult at the receiving hospital. Pediatric GI hemorrhage has historically been classified by the site of bleeding: upper GI tract (UGI) versus lower GI tract (LGI). With UGI hemorrhage the bleeding site is proximal to the ligament of Treitz (esophagus, stomach, or proximal duodenum), and with LGI hemorrhage, bleeding is distal to the ligament of Treitz.

Most episodes of GI hemorrhage are due to UGI bleeding, and almost all cases of UGI bleeding can be further grouped into two meaningful categories: mucosal lesions or esophageal varices.[1] Most pediatric UGI hemorrhages occur secondary to damaged GI tract mucosa or erosion extending to the mucosal vasculature. Mucosal lesions (esophagitis, Mallory-Weiss tear, gastritis, duodenitis, gastric ulcer, or duodenal ulcer) may be caused by varied insults including chemical irritants, drugs, and stress-related processes.[1] Although bleeding from both mucosal lesions and esophageal varices usually ceases spontaneously, varices carry a worse prognosis and require more invasive treatment.

LGI mucosal lesions may be caused by infection (bacterial colitis), structural abnormalities (Meckel's diverticulum), allergic disorders (protein sensitive allergy), and ischemic injuries (intussusception, necrotizing enterocolitis). Lesions causing significant LGI hemorrhage require surgical intervention more often than UGI lesions.

Characteristics of the bleeding episode will often help determine the site of the bleeding lesion. Hematemesis, or vomited blood, is the hallmark of UGI hemorrhage. Melena or black, tarry stool (denatured blood) also suggests a lesion high in the gastrointestinal tract. Hematochezia or bright red/maroon blood mixed with the stool indicates a lower bleeding source in the distal half of the colon. The presence of mucus or pus points to an inflammatory etiology, either infectious or nonspecific, as in inflammatory bowel disease. Currant jelly stools are ominous signs of vascular compromise, as is seen in intussusception. Loose stool or blood without stool is suggestive of diffuse disease.[5] Bright red blood only on the outside of a formed stool or on the toilet paper following a formed stool suggests an anorectal lesion.

Other clues from the history and physical examination may help direct the physician to the source of bleeding. Pain with an episode of GI bleeding suggests a peptic lesion (gastritis or ulcer) or ischemic bowel. When the pain is accompanied by the signs and symptoms of intestinal obstruction, the need for surgical consult and definitive diagnosis is urgent.[14] Preceding vomiting suggests a Mallory-Weiss tear. Concurrent CNS disorders, recent surgery, or burns may indicate a stress ulcer. Fever, tenesmus, and diarrhea suggest colitis. Alcohol and medications such as aspirin, nonsteroidal anti-inflammatory agents, anti-coagulants, and steroids may be contributing factors.[6] If physical examination of the skin reveals petechiae, unexplained bruising, hemarthroses, gum bleeding, or oozing at a venipuncture site consider a systemic bleeding disorder. Examination of the oropharynx and nasopharynx may reveal an extra-gastrointestinal source of bleeding (i.e., epistaxis). Signs of liver disease or portal hypertension such as hepatosplenomegaly, jaundice, ascites, and spider nevi are seen with esophageal varices. Since fresh blood in the GI tract acts as an irritant/cathartic, the presence of hyperactive bowel sounds in a hemodynamically unstable patient suggests GI bleeding despite absence of outward signs. With decreased or absent bowel sounds in a patient with significant GI hemorrhage, consider a surgical etiology.[13]

The last and most important question the transport physician must ask on initial evaluation is, if bleeding has been confirmed, "how much blood has been lost." The magnitude of blood loss is crucial in determining initial therapy and predicting needs on transport. Fortunately, in the pediatric population exsanguinating GI hemorrhage from any source is uncommon.[14] Unfortunately, because of the resiliency of the pediatric cardiovascular system, it may take as much as 20% of acute blood loss in children before they start to show clinical signs.[11] Clinical signs include postural hypotension, age-matched tachycardia, tachypnea (secondary to tissue acidosis), narrowed pulse pressure, poor capillary refill, mental confusion, and pallor (Table 29-1).

Indications for transfer

If the history and physical examination reveal hemodynamic stability and a relatively minor bleeding site (anorectal lesion or minor bleeding due to infection), the pediatric patient usually can be safely treated outside of a tertiary center. Any infant or child with hemodynamic instability, an ongoing major GI bleed, history or physical examination suggestive of a significant GI bleed (≥85 ml/kg blood loss; low initial hematocrit level < 25%), coexisting medical disorder, or coagulopathy should be transferred to a tertiary pediatric center for intensive care monitoring, further therapy, and diagnostic evaluation.[19] A clear nasogastric aspirate should never be used as an indicator to discharge or not transfer a patient if the history is suggestive of significant GI bleed. In a hemodynamically unstable patient, transfer should not take precedence over the initial volume resuscitation and ABCs.

Emergency treatment

Since most episodes of pediatric GI bleeding will stop spontaneously, regardless of source, the major immediate concern is cardiovascular restoration and airway protection. Investigation for source of bleeding should not preclude resuscitation. Aspiration, one of the complications of major upper GI hemorrhage, is associated with great morbidity and mortality. Consider intubation (cuffed endotracheal tube) to protect the airway under these circumstances.[14]

Intravenous access should be obtained early in all but the most minor episodes of GI hemorrhage. Circulatory collapse with vasoconstriction may make future attempts at peripheral IV access more difficult. Resuscitation in the pediatric population can usually be conducted admirably with peripheral IV access alone. With major bleeding, two large bore IV lines (14 to 18 gauge in a child; 22 gauge in an infant) are essential, and in children under six years of age, intraosseous infusions may be used if venous access is difficult.[1,13] The goals of intravenous therapy are two-fold: replenishing intravascular volume and restoring oxygen-carrying capacity (reflected in hemoglobin and hematocrit values). The transport physician can accomplish this first goal with crystalloid solution, colloid solution, or blood products; the second goal can be achieved only with blood. If there is evidence of hypovolemia (tachycardia, diminished pulses, delayed capillary re-

TABLE 29-1 CLINICAL PARAMETERS FOR ESTIMATING BLOOD LOSS IN CHILDREN*

	% Blood loss		
	15-25%	*25-40%*	*>40%*
Sensorium	Irritable poor feeding	Lethargic	Unresponsive or responsive to pain only
Skin	Capillary refill delayed	Pale, capillary refill delayed	Pale, capillary refill delay
Heart rate	Increased	Increased	±
Systolic blood pressure	NL	NL/Decreased	Decreased
Urine output	±	Decreased	Decreased

* Adapted from Advanced Pediatric Life Support (APLS): The pediatric emergency medicine course handbook, ed 2, 1993.

fill or hypotension), immediate intervention is necessary.

On the basis of existing evidence, one cannot be dogmatic about which resuscitation fluid to choose. Replacement of blood with blood is the ideal therapy, but delays associated with cross-matching, as well as risk of transfusion reactions, limit its usefulness in early resuscitation. With massive blood loss, O-negative or Rh type-specific blood can be given with less delay to maintain intravascular volume and to replace red blood cells, accepting the accompanying risk of a transfusion reaction.

The same hemodynamic end-points can be achieved during resuscitation with both crystalloid and colloid solutions; crystalloid will require more volume and will result in greater interstitial compartment expansion.[16,18,22] Since there is interstitial depletion as well as intravascular depletion in hemorrhagic shock, crystalloids can be used logically in the initial resuscitation. A bolus of 20 ml/kg of normal saline or lactated Ringer's solution should be infused rapidly. Additional fluid boluses should be given as indicated by frequent reevaluations. Reevaluation after each intervention is crucial, since overexpansion of the intravascular volume may be detrimental and too rapid expansion may aggravate bleeding from esophageal varices. After bleeding has stabilized, packed red blood cells can be used for replacement. For underlying coagulation disorders, vitamin K (1 mg/yr of age — maximum 10 mg given IM), platelets, or fresh-frozen plasma can be given as needed.[9]

Initial laboratory studies in any patient with a severe GI bleed should include 1) type and crossmatch, 2) complete blood count (CBC), 3) platelet count, 4) prothrombin time (PT), and 5) a partial thromboplastin time (PTT). An isolated hematocrit value is an unreliable indicator of acute blood loss, but serial measurements may be useful in following ongoing bleeding. Arterial blood gases and pH may also be important parameters to follow in severe blood loss associated with shock. The patient should also receive supplemental oxygen (because of decreased oxygen carrying capacity) and have a urinary catheter inserted to accurately measure urine output.

UPPER GASTROINTESTINAL (GI) TRACT BLEED

If significant upper GI bleeding is suspected, aspiration of the stomach through an oral or nasogastric (NG) tube should be performed. Although the therapeutic effectiveness of gastric lavage is still unknown, this procedure does aid in the diagnosis, evacuates clots from the stomach (allowing endoscopic exam), relieves distention, and lessens the risk of aspiration. A 12F NG tube is usually appropriate in small children, while a 14F to 16F tube is used in older children. Volume of single infusion is also age-dependent: 50 ml in infants, 100-200 ml in older children.[1] Esophageal varices are not a contraindication for the placement of a NG tube. The NG tube can be left in place and used to monitor subsequent bleeding.

Mucosal lesions in an upper GI hemorrhage are chronically treated with antacids and H_2 receptor antagonists, with the aim of therapy being to neutralize gastric acid or suppress production. However, there is no evidence that either are beneficial with active bleeding. Antacids are used to maintain the gastric pH at 5 or higher. In acute mucosal hemorrhage, the recommended dose of antacids is 0.5 ml/kg up to a maximum of 30 ml/dose given every 1-2 hrs. to maintain gastric pH $\geq$ 5.[9,15] The H_2 antagonist, cimetidine, has been used in children. The suggested dosage is 7.5 mg/kg/dose Q6°, orally or IV.[8] Whether combined therapy is better than antacids alone is not known.

With variceal bleeding, vasopressin may prevent the need for more invasive measures. Vasopressin is a nonselective, short-acting vasoconstrictor which decreases blood flow and pressure through the portal circulation. Its major complications include arrhythmias, hypertension, myocardial ischemia, peripheral ischemia, and hyponatremia. An initial intravenous bolus of 0.3 U/kg (up to a maximum of 20 U) is given over 20 minutes followed by a continuous drip at 0.2-0.4 U/1.73m^2/min.[9] Peripheral infusion is as effective as selective infusion into the superior mesenteric artery.[3] Other therapeutic options include balloon tamponade. The use of a Sengstaken-Blakemore tube is a high-risk procedure with serious complications, including esophageal rupture, airway occlusion and pulmonary aspiration.[4] Its use should be limited to endoscopically proven varices after pharmacological measures have failed.

LOWER GASTROINTESTINAL (GI) TRACT BLEEDING

The initial treatment of LGI bleeding uses the same stabilization, monitoring and volume replacement techniques seen in UGI hemorrhage. Management of LGI hemorrhage differs in that it requires more rapid surgical consultation as the necessity for surgical intervention is a greater possibility. A major priority for transport is to identify the cases of lower tract hemorrhage associated with intestinal obstruction or vascular compromise and arrange for expedient surgical evaluation on arrival to the receiving hospital. Urgent laparotomy is indicated in intussusception (after failed air or barium enema reduction), midgut volvulus, intestinal obstruction, perforation or vascular compromise.[6]

Potential complications, adverse effects to anticipate

The primary adverse events to prevent/anticipate while transporting a GI hemorrhage patient are the complications of hypovolemic shock (decreased volume, decreased oxygen carrying capacity). With volume loss expect a metabolic acidosis secondary to lactic acid production. Heat loss with hypothermia can occur rapidly in exposed children, worsening perfusion and acidosis. With severe volume loss expect profound multisystem organ failure. As mentioned previously, significant upper GI bleeding carries the potential for aspiration. Intubation to protect the airway is justifiable. Also, as stated previously, the use of blood products carries the inherent risk of transfusion reaction. These risks can be decreased by using packed red blood cells instead of whole blood (when possible), fresh-frozen plasma, filters, and blood warmers. Complications of massive blood replacement include hypercitraemia, hyperlactacidemia, hypocalcemia, diminished clotting factors, and decreased platelets. Intravenous calcium and fresh-frozen plasma (10 ml/kg) should be given after every 40-50 ml/kg of packed cells or whole blood. Platelets should be checked after every 40 ml/kg of blood and transfused as needed.[1]

REFERENCES

1. Boyle JT: Gastrointestinal bleeding. In Fleisher G, Ludwig S, editors: *Textbook of pediatric emergency medicine*, ed 2, Baltimore, 1988, Williams & Wilkins.
2. Brayton D: Gastrointestinal bleeding of "unknown origin," *Surgery* 107:288, 1964
3. Chojkier M, Conn HO: Esophageal tamponade in the treatment of bleeding varices: a decadal progress report, *Dig Dis Sci* 25:267, 1980.
4. Chojkier M and others: A controlled comparison of continuous intra-arterial and intravenous infusions of vasopressin in hemorrhage from esophageal varices, *Gastroenterology* 77:540, 1979.
5. Fitzgerald JF: Gastrointestinal bleeding in infants and children. In Sugawa C, Schuman BM, Lucas CE, editors: *Gastrointestinal bleeding*, New York, 1992, Igaku-Shoin.
6. Fontanarosa PB: Gastrointestinal hemorrhage. In Reisdorff EJ, Roberts MR, Wiegenstein JG, editors: *Pediatric emergency medicine*, Philadelphia, 1993, W. B. Saunders.
7. Gogel HK, Tandberg D, Strickland RG: Substances that interfere with guiac card tests, *Am J Emerg Med* 7:474, 1989.
8. Goudsouzian N and others: The dose-response effects of oral cimetidine on gastric pH and volume in children, *Anesthesiology* 55:533, 1981.
9. Hyams JS, Leichtner AM, Schwartz AN: Recent advances in diagnosis and treatment of gastrointestinal hemorrhage in infants and children, *J Pediatr* 106:1:1, 1985.
10. Jaffe RM and others: False-negative stool occult blood test caused by ingestion of ascorbic acid (vitamin C), *Ann Intern Med* 83:824, 1975.
11. Jorden RC, Barkin RM: Multiple trauma. In Rosen P and others, editors: *Emergency medicine—concepts and clinical practice*, ed 2, St. Louis, 1988, CV Mosby.
12. Lifton LJ, Kreiser J: False positive stool occult blood tests caused by iron preparations: a controlled study and review of the literature, *Gastroenterology* 83:860, 1982.
13. Ochsenschlager DW: Gastrointestinal bleeding. In Barkin RM, editor: *Pediatric emergency medicine—concepts and clinical practice*, St. Louis, 1992, Mosby-Year Book, Inc.
14. Oldham KT, Lobe TE: Gastrointestinal hemorrhage in children: a pragmatic update, *Pediatr Clin North Am* 32:5:1247, 1985.
15. Peterson WL and others: Healing of duodenal ulcer with an antacid regimen, *N Engl J Med* 297:341, 1977.
16. Rackow EC and others: Fluid resuscitation in circulatory shock: A comparison of the cardiorespiratory effects of albumin, hetastarch and saline solutions in patients with hypovolemic and septic shock, *Crit Care Med* 11:839-850, 1983.

17. Rosenthal P, Thompson J, Singh M: Detection of occult blood in gastric juice, *J Clin Gastro Enterol* 6:119, 1984.
18. Scheinkestel CD and others: Fluid management of shock in critically-ill patients, *Med J Australia* 150:508-17, 1989.
19. Shandling B: The gastrointestinal tract. In Nelson WE, Behrman RE, Vaughan VC, editors: *Nelson textbook of pediatrics*, ed 13, Philadelphia, 1987, W. B. Saunders.
20. Spencer R: Gastrointestinal hemorrhage in infancy and childhood: 476 cases, *Surgery* 55:718, 1964.
21. Stillman AE: Black heme-positive stools without gastrointestinal hemorrhage, *J Pediatr* 100:414, 1982.
22. Virgilio RW, Smith DE, Zarins CK: Balanced electrolyte solutions: experimental and clinical studies, *Crit Care Med* 7:98-106, 1979.
23. Wells HJ, Pagno JF: "Hemoccult" test: reversal of false-negative results due to storage, *Gastroenterology* 72:1148, 1977.

30

ENVIRONMENTAL EMERGENCIES

CARDEN JOHNSTON
LAURA PHILLIPS
MADELINE JOSEPH

CARBON MONOXIDE/SMOKE INHALATION

Carbon monoxide (CO) is a tasteless, colorless, odorless, and nonirritating gas produced by the incomplete combustion of carbonaceous material.[25] An estimated 5,000 deaths from carbon monoxide occur annually in the United States.[14] As fire-related exposure accounts for two-thirds of carbon monoxide deaths, CO poisoning and smoke inhalation are often concurrent problems. Additional sources of carbon monoxide inhalation include automobile exhaust and defective ventilation systems on kerosene and gasoline stoves.

Carbon monoxide includes tissue hypoxia by reversibly binding to hemoglobin, producing carboxyhemoglobin and a leftward shift of the oxyhemoglobin curve. The affinity of carbon monoxide to hemoglobin is 250 times that of oxygen to hemoglobin. In addition, carbon monoxide inhibits cellular metabolism by binding to cytochrome oxidase and complexing with myglobin in muscle cells. Smoke is a combination of fine particles, toxic gases, and irritant chemicals which may include nitrogen oxides, aldehydes, phosgene, sulphur dioxide, hydrogen chloride, hydrogen cyanide, and carbon dioxide.[12] Smoke inhalation injury results either from inhalation of these substances, or from direct thermal injury to the upper airway.[27] The lower airway is usually spared from thermal injury by the efficient heat exchanging tissues of the upper airway, but bronchospasm, mucosal injury, and pulmonary edema may occur from inhalation of pulmonary irritants and carbonaceous particulate matter.[12]

Diagnosis

The classical presentation of mild carbon monoxide exposure is an afebrile patient with influenza-like symptoms that rapidly improve when the patient is removed from the source of CO exposure. In cases of severe exposure, confusion, syncope, seizures, arrhythmias, hypotension, and death may occur. Red discoloration of the skin and retinal hemorrhages have been described, but are not common findings and are often associated only with very high carboxyhemoglobin levels.[36] Patients more commonly have a cyanotic or pale appearance (See Table 30-1). In addition to the above signs, the patient who is also suffering from smoke inhalation may show signs of direct thermal injury to the upper airway such as stridor, hoarseness, and mucosal edema. Laryngeal edema peaks at 2 to 8 hours after injury.[27] Signs of pulmonary injury include tachypnea, wheezing, rales, rhonchi, and severe respiratory distress.

Emergency treatment

The approach to the patient with carbon monoxide and/or smoke exposure begins with removing the patient from the exposure source and limiting his or her activity to decrease metabolic demand.[25] The airway,

TABLE 30-1[4,6,8,12] SIGNS AND SYMPTOMS OF SMOKE INHALATION

% HbCO	Signs and symptoms
0-10	None, slight headache or angina in patients with coronary artery disease
10-20	Headache, dyspnea or exertion, exercise-induced angina, nausea, vomiting, mildly impaired judgement
20-30	Worsening headache and dyspnea, gastrointestinal signs and symptoms, altered mental status
30-40	Severe headache and gastrointestinal complaints, visual changes
40-50	Syncope, tachypnea, tachycardia
50-60	Seizures, coma, Cheyne-Stokes respirations
60-70	Hypotension, respiratory failure
70-80	Weak pulse, death

breathing, and circulation should be quickly assessed. Any child with signs of significant airway obstruction will require immediate intubation. Indications of potential airway compromise that should prompt early intubation include stridor, hoarseness, respiratory depression, apnea, coma, oropharyngeal edema, full thickness nasolabial burns, and circumferential neck or chest burns. Any patient with suspected carbon monoxide exposure should immediately receive 100% oxygen with high flows via a tight-fitting face mask, a mask with a reservoir (nonrebreather), or an endotracheal tube. Treatment with 100% oxygen reduces the half-life of carbon monoxide from six hours to 60 to 90 minutes.[25] A carboxyhemoglobin level should be drawn upon arrival at a medical facility. Carboxyhemoglobin levels, which are expressed as the percent of hemoglobin saturated by CO (% HbCO), may not always correlate with clinical symptoms.[34,35,49] Decisions about therapy should be based upon the clinical appearance of the patient as well as the carboxyhemoglobin level. Patients who have been treated with 100% oxygen prior to obtaining a carboxyhemoglobin level may have normal to low levels with symptoms consistent with significant carbon monoxide exposure. Patients should receive 100% oxygen until all acute symptoms have resolved, and the carboxyhemoglobin level is well below usual symptomatic levels.

Pulse oximetry may be falsely normal in the patient with carbon monoxide poisoning because the oximeter does not detect the presence of HbCO or other abnormal hemoglobins.[27] The normal hemoglobin may be 100% saturated with oxygen, but a high percentage of abnormal hemoglobin means inadequate oxygen available for delivery to tissues. The arterial blood gas PO_2 may also be normal, as it is a measure of dissolved oxygen and is not affected by hemoglobin saturation.[36]

Other labwork that may be helpful includes a complete blood count, urine for myoglobin and hemoglobin, electrolytes, blood urea nitrogen, and a serum creatinine. A baseline electrocardiogram and chest x-ray should be obtained. Intravenous fluids should be started and delivered at maintenance rates. A urethral catheter should be placed to measure urine output and the adequacy of volume replacement.[47]

Indications for transport

Patients with any degree of neurologic or cardiac dysfunction and patients with carbon monoxide levels greater than 25% are potential candidates for hyperbaric oxygen therapy (HBO), and consultation should be obtained with centers able to provide such therapy.[25,27,69] HBO provides efficient oxygen delivery at pressures of 2 to 3 atmospheres and reduces the half-life of carbon monoxide to 23 minutes.[4] Uncontrolled studies suggest that early treatment with HBO decreases mortality and decreases neurologic morbidity.[18,35,59] Pregnant females with carbon monoxide exposure should also be considered candidates for hyperbaric oxygen treatment as fetal levels may be 10 to 15% greater than maternal levels.[49] The fetus is especially at risk because carbon monoxide exacerbates the innate leftward shift of the fetal oxygen hemoglobin dissociation curve. Smoke inhalation victims with any signs of airway obstruction should also be transported, after intubation, to a tertiary care center for bronchoscopy and management of potential upper and lower airway disease.

Stabilization for transport

Patients with smoke inhalation should be assessed for impending airway obstruction. Any sign of clinical deterioration necessitates intubation, as loss of the airway in transport could be disastrous. Patients with carbon monoxide exposure should remain on 100% oxygen until all acute symptoms have resolved and a HbCO level of less than 5% has been obtained.[27] An arterial blood gas measurement prior to transport will help to direct adequate ventilation. Patients with bronchospasm should be treated with bronchodilator aerosols. The patency of intravenous lines should be ensured. Other fire or trauma related injuries should be investigated and appropriate treatment initiated. The cervical spine should be immobilized in any patient with a history of falling, jumping from a height or other trauma.

Potential problems in transport

Patients with inhalation injury may have reduced pulmonary compliance early after lung injury because of parenchymal injury, pulmonary edema, pleural effusions, or constricting eschars from chest wall burns. High peak inspiratory pressures and the addition of positive end-expiratory pressure may be required to maintain oxygenation and ventilation and to treat adult respiratory syndrome (ARDS).[47] These patients are also at risk of pneumothorax as a complication of pulmonary edema and high airway pressures. Fluid management should be balanced between maintaining adequate cardiac output and preventing exacerbation of pulmonary edema. Potential immediate complications of carbon monoxide exposure should be anticipated and include seizures, coma, cerebral edema, pulmonary edema, myoglobinuria, and arrhythmias. Patients should have continuous cardiac monitoring and a patent intravenous line to deliver anticonvulsants and antiarrhythmics as needed. Immediate suction availability is imperative as the unconscious patient with a suppressed gag reflex may vomit and aspirate.

HYPERTHERMIA

Heat illness is a spectrum of disease processes ranging from the minor heat syndromes of heat edema, heat cramps, and heat syncope to the major syndromes of heat exhaustion and heat stroke. Heat-related syndromes are more common in the humid, summer months and are responsible for thousands of deaths in the United States annually.[8,55] Patients with minor heat illnesses usually respond to cooler environments and oral rehydration and are unlikely to need transport. Heat exhaustion and heat stroke, however, due to their potential for death or serious morbidity, must be promptly recognized and treated. These patients may require transport to a tertiary care center.

Risk factors for heat illness include age (infants and the elderly), obesity, dehydration, heart disease, skin disorders, medication or drug use, lack of acclimatization, fatigue, excessive or restrictive clothing, infection, and a previous episode of heat stroke.[4,26,55] Infants and small children are predisposed to serious heat illness because of less effective thermoregulatory mechanisms. Children with cystic fibrosis are another at-risk population. Adolescents, with their interest in outdoor sports, their response to peer pressure and their possible experimentation with judgement impairing drugs, are also at risk for thermal illnesses.[31]

In response to increased heat exposure, the thermoregulatory center in the hypothalamus triggers heat-losing mechanisms, resulting in an increased cardiac output, increased sweating, and vasodilation.[26] With vasodilation, large volumes of blood are shunted peripherally in an effort to dissipate heat. When these heat-losing mechanisms cannot match the rate of heat production, the core body temperature rises and heat illness occurs. Relative to an adult, a child's slower rate of acclimatization and larger surface area per unit of body weight increase the risk of heat illness.[26] In addition, children produce more heat for a given exercise and sweat at higher temperatures than do adults.[26]

Diagnosis

A thermometer which measures extremes of temperature is essential for making the diagnosis of heat exhaustion and heat stroke. *Heat exhaustion* is a vague syndrome which may be a precursor to heat stroke. Patients have a temperature up to 39°C (102.2°F) with a variety of signs and symptoms including malaise, headache, nausea, vomiting, irritability, tachycardia, and dehydration. Mental status changes are mild, and the liver is not affected. In heat exhaustion, the peripheral circulation vasodilates in response to temperature elevation, shunting large blood volumes peripherally and causing sodium and water losses. With the decrease in central circulating blood volume, a compensatory increase in heart rate and stroke volume occur. Temperature regulatory mechanisms remain intact. If these patients are left unattended, they can develop heat stroke.

Heat stroke is a life-threatening emergency recognized by hyperpyrexia (>41°C or >106°F) and altered mental status. Thermoregulatory mechanisms are no longer functioning, and the patient is at risk for multiorgan tissue destruction. Myocardial infarction, hepatocellular necrosis, disseminated intravascular coagulation, pulmonary edema, rhabdomyolysis, renal failure, seizures, and coma have all been described with heat stroke.[55]

There are two types of heat stroke: exertional and nonexertional (or classic).[16] Exertional heat stroke typically occurs in the unacclimatized adolescent athlete. Dehydration, heavy clothing, extreme exertion, peer pressure and extreme temperatures are predisposing factors. These patients have an acute onset of neurologic symptoms including headache, ataxia, syncope, confusion, seizures, delirium, and coma. Tachycardia, hyperventilation, and hypotension are present. The sweating mechanism is usually intact.

Nonexertional or classic heat stroke is defined by hyperpyrexia, hot dry skin, and altered mental status. However, strict adherence to these three criteria may lead to under-diagnosis and delays in treatment. The aged and infants are more at risk for this form of heatstroke. Other signs and symptoms include marked dehydration, anorexia, vomiting, malaise, dizziness, tachycardia, tachypnea, and hypotension. Mental status alterations may range from confusion to seizures or coma.

Indications for transport

Any patient with a history of heat stress and alteration in mental status should be evaluated as a heat stroke patient. Because of the risk of mortality and neurologic morbidity, these patients should be transported to a pediatric tertiary care facility.

Emergency treatment

Patients with heat exhaustion should initially be placed in a cool environment. Mild cases can be treated with oral rehydration with salty drinks such as tomato juice or Gatorade.® More severe cases require intravenous fluids with an initial 20 cc/kg bolus of normal saline followed by replacement of estimated losses. Helpful laboratory studies include a complete blood count, electrolytes, blood urea nitrogen, creatinine, and a urinalysis. Vital signs should be closely monitored. If there is any doubt of the diagnosis, the patient should be treated for heat stroke.

Emergency management of the patient with heat stroke begins with assessment of airway, breathing, and circulation. Patients in the field should have their clothing removed and be removed from bright sunlight. Alert patients can be orally hydrated. Cooling should begin with the application of cool or ice water to the trunk and extremities. Upon arrival to a medical facility, a rectal temperature should be continuously monitored, and cooling should be performed as fast as 0.1°C/min. Labwork and procedures should never delay cooling efforts. Consideration of the mechanisms for heat loss (i.e. radiation, evaporation, conduction, and convection) leads to successful methods of lowering body temperature. One of the most effective and practical ways to cool a patient is to continuously spray water over the body surface (aids evaporation and conduction) and create air movement with fans (improves convective heat loss) while maintaining a cool environment (radiation).[50,53] Cold intravenous fluids add little to the cooling process and can cause arrhythmias. Pertioneal lavage, iced water enemas, and iced gastric lavage have not been well studied in humans, and the latter therapy also carries a potential risk for cardiac arrhythmias.[9,58] Submersion in cold water has been used by the military with excellent success but is not recommended in an unstable patient.[16] Constriction of small peripheral blood vessels may actually lead to reduction of heat dissipating capabilities. Antipyretics are ineffective in the treatment of heat stroke. Ice packs applied to major arterial flow points (carotids, femoral arteries, and axillae) can accelerate the cooling process.[8] Severe shivering should be avoided as it may actually raise body temperature. Chlorpromazine (.05 mg/kg IV) can be used to abate the shivering response.[50]

Along with cooling, intravenous fluid replacement should begin with a bolus of 20 cc/kg of normal saline or Ringer's lactate which may be repeated as needed to restore perfusion and urine output. A central venous line should be placed in hypotensive patients. Due to the potential for renal failure, a urethral catheter can be placed to monitor urine output. Hypoglycemia should be considered and, if present, treated with a 1-2 cc/kg of D_{25}.

Laboratory evaluation of the hyperthermic patient includes a complete blood count, urinalysis, urine for myoglobin and protein, electrolytes, blood urea nitrogen, creatinine, lactate, glucose, calcium, liver function tests, coagulation studies, CPK, arterial blood gas, and a blood culture (if sepsis is suspected).

Stabilization for transport

Many of the above methods may be impractical in the transport environment. At a minimum, the patient's skin should be kept wet and exposed. Dynamic air circulation in a swift open vehicle has a favorable effect on cooling. Bedside fans accomplish the same purpose. In addition, ice packs can be applied to the groin and axillae.[8] Patients should not be placed in unairconditioned vehicles where the cooling process cannot be continued. Air transport in a cool environment will also help facilitate the cooling process.

Benzodiazepines have been advocated by some for the anxious, uncomfortable patient during the cooling process. Chlorpromazine has also been used to depress the shivering response and to prevent an increase in heat production. Its use should be reserved for the patient in whom shivering interferes with cooling, as its anticholinergic effects may inhibit sweating.

Dantrolene, a muscle relaxant which slows the release of calcium from the sarcoplasmic reticulum, should be considered in the hyperthermic patient who is not responsive to conventional cooling measures. Although one study showed a faster rate of cooling in dantrolene-treated patients (2.45 mg/kg) as compared to controls, the occurrence of neurologic sequelae was the same in the two groups. The starting dose for dantrolene is 1 mg/kg. Side effects (muscle weakness, nausea) usually manifest at 2.5 mg/kg.[55]

Potential complications during transport

Complications from heat stroke are numerous and may include hypoglycemia (especially in infants and children), electrolyte disturbances, acidosis, alkalosis, myocardial ischemia, cerebral edema, disseminated intravascular coagulation, thrombocytopenia, hepatocellular degeneration, cholestasis, acute tubular necrosis, interstitial nephritis, and myoglobinuria.[55]

Seizures are common in heat stroke patients and may be treated with benzodiazepines or phenobarbital.[26] Because seizures can exacerbate hyperthermia, patients with status epilepticus should be intubated and paralyzed with muscle relaxants. Hypotension that is unresponsive to adequate fluids and cooling should be treated with dobutamine because of its beneficial effect on myocardial contractility and peripheral vasodilation.[60] Epinephrine and norepinephrine should be avoided because of their peripheral vasoconstrictor effects.[60]

Once treatment of the hyperthermic patient has been initiated, a differential diagnosis can be considered. Head trauma, cerebral vascular accident, thyrotoxicosis, malignant hyperthermia, neuroleptic malignant syndrome, drug ingestion, and heat exhaustion with syncope must all be considered. Drugs associated with hyperthermia include anticholinergics, cocaine, amphetamines, and salicylates. Infections such as meningitis, encephalitis, malaria, and Rocky Mountain Spotted Fever all may present with fever and mental status changes.[55]

Prognosis of the patient with heat stroke is dependent upon duration of coma and hyperpyrexia, the severity of coagulopathy, liver function abnormalities and renal failure, and the presence of preexisting or concurrent illness.[11,50,51]

HYPOTHERMIA

Hypothermia, defined as a core body temperature of less than 35°C (95°F), is a common entity that is easily unrecognized. Infants are particularly at risk for hypothermia because of a large surface area to weight ratio, a lack of subcutaneous fat, and a failure to produce heat by shivering.[46,54] Children may rapidly become hypothermic during near-drowning events even in water of 70°F.[22,32] Other predisposing conditions for hypothermia include advanced age, environmental extremes, alcohol and drug consumption, endocrinopathies, head and spine trauma, and infection.[46,54] While hypothermia is associated with exposure to cold ambient temperatures, other factors such as wind velocity, exposure to moisture, lack of protective clothing, and duration of exposure influence extent of decreased body temperature.

In response to cold stress the hypothalamus stimulates the sympathetic nervous system, initiating catecholamine release, peripheral vasoconstriction, and shunting of blood centrally.[26,44] Increases in both metabolic rate and muscle tone (shivering) also occur to prevent further heat loss.[26,54,67] As temperatures drop, the body's metabolic rate slows, reflected by a reduction in cardiac output, respiratory effort, and central nervous system function.

Diagnosis

Classically, hypothermia is defined by temperature as mild (32-35°C or 89.6-95°F), moderate (28-32°C or 82-89.6°F), and severe (<28°C or <82°F). Core body temperature is best measured with a low reading rectal thermometer. However, in the severely hypothermic patient in extreme conditions, measurement of a rectal temperature may be difficult.[64] For this reason, hypothermia can be classified on the basis of the neurologic exam, with all comatose patients viewed as severely hypothermic, and patients with confusion, combativeness, or ataxia as moderately hypothermic.[64]

The mildly hypothermic patient will have an intact shivering mechanism and few alterations in sensorium. Mild bradycardia and respiratory depression may also exist. In more severely hypothermic patients, shivering is replaced by muscle rigidity. Faint or absent heart sounds, hypotension, and a variety of ECG changes may exist, including a low voltage QRS, prolongation of PR, QRS, and QT intervals, and ST-T wave changes. The classic "J" or "Osborn" wave (a positive deflection of the RT segment) is pathognomonic for hypothermia and may signal ventricular fibrillation.[28,38,67] While ventricular fibrillation is more common in the older patient, cardiac standstill is seen more frequently in children. Respiratory depression to the point of apnea and central nervous system depression resembling brain death may occur.

Indications for transport

Any patient with severe hypothermia and the moderately hypothermic patient who is unresponsive to passive rewarming will require transport to a tertiary care center for continuation of core rewarming.

Emergency management

In the process of rewarming a patient with hypothermia, consideration should be given to avoiding the four mechanisms of heat loss: radiation (maintain a warm environment), evaporation (keep the patient dry), conduction (remove obvious sources of circulating air), and convection (do not place cool objects on or near the patient).

Patients with hypothermia should be handled gently and removed from any source of cold exposure as quickly as possible. In the mildly or moderately hypothermic patient, any cold, wet clothing should be removed and passive rewarming should be initiated with warm blankets, a warm environment, and warmed, humidified oxygen. A cardiac monitor should be placed. Intravenous fluids, warmed to 40-42°C, do not significantly warm the patient at pediatric maintenance rates but are better than cold intravenous fluids.[20] The cervical spine should be immobilized in the patient with a history of falling, diving or other potentially traumatic events.

Patients with severe hypothermia will require more aggressive intervention. Shallow respirations may provide adequate ventilation in patients with temperatures less than 28°C. Apneic patients will require tracheal intubation and mechanical ventilation. Patients with severe hypothermia may be bradycardic and hypotensive but have adequate circulation to meet their physiologic needs, the so-called "metabolic icebox."[28] Pulses may be difficult to assess and should be palpated for a full minute. CPR should be avoided in patients with temperatures below 28°C if any pulse is present or if narrow QRS complexes are present by cardiac monitoring. Standard CPR should be initiated for the usual indications in patients in which the core temperature is unknown, the temperature is greater than 28°C or with asystole or ventricular fibrillation.[26,68] Cardioversion and antiarrythmics should be withheld until a body temperature of 30°C is obtained, at which point standard resuscitation protocols should be followed.[26,68]

Severely hypothermic patients may be volume depleted secondary to fluid sequestration, and fluid resuscitation should begin with a 20 cc/kg bolus of warmed normal saline.[26] Warmed $D_5\frac{1}{2}$ NS should be used for maintenance intravenous fluids. Lactated Ringer's solution should be withheld as the hypothermic liver cannot metabolize lactate.[68]

Stabilization for transport

Numerous techniques of active external rewarming have been used with hypothermic patients. Their use should be tailored to the individual patient, the risk of adverse effects, and the practicality and availability of these techniques in individual emergency departments and during transport. External warming techniques include warm baths, thermal blankets and pads, heat lamps, hot packs, radiant heat warmers, and maintenance of a high ambient air temperature. These techniques are not appropriate for the severely hypothermic patient but may be helpful in preschool-aged patients with acute hypothermia and in mildly to moderately hypothermic patients.[29,52] Concerns over the use of these techniques include the risk of afterdrop[17] (the admixture of cold, acidotic blood from the vasodilated peripheral circulation into the central circulation), increasing oxygen consumption before cardiac output is restored, and skin burns which may occur when topical devices are hotter than 45°C.[21] Active external rewarming, if used, should be restricted to the thorax and abdomen. Vasodilation of small peripheral vessels can contribute to loss of body heat.

The most severely hypothermic patient, especially one who has suffered a cardiopulmonary arrest, will require one or more core rewarming techniques. These include peritoneal dialysis, hemodialysis, mediastinal irrigation, and gastric or rectal lavage with warmed fluids. Extracorporeal blood rewarming is considered the ultimate therapy for arrested hypothermic patients experiencing cardiopulmonary arrest.[1,68]

Delivery of humidified warmed oxygen is practical in the transport setting. In intubated, ventilated patients, the humidifier temperature of the ventilator should be maintained at 44°C.[32] Simple measures such as removal of wet, cold clothing, the use of warm blankets, and maximizing temperature in the transport vehicle should be followed. A rectal temperature should be frequently monitored, and body temperature should be raised by 1°C per hour.

Frozen extremities should not be thawed until core temperatures reach 32-34°C.[28] Because refreezing causes increased tissue damage, thawing should not be attempted in the transport environment. Intravenous catheters should never be placed in frozen extremities.

In addition to a serum glucose to screen for hypoglycemia (common in infants and young children), labwork should include serum electrolytes, complete blood count, amylase, arterial blood gas, serum creatinine, urinalysis, and liver function tests. Additional labwork may be indicated to delineate the etiology if endocrine disturbances, drug exposure, alcohol use, or infection are suspected. Due to the risk of sepsis, blood and urine cultures should be obtained in hypothermic patients without a history of environmental exposure. Patients with a history of trauma should undergo cervical spine immobilization and should have appropriate radiographic studies performed. Blood and urine samples for toxicologic screening should be obtained if an ingestion is suspected.

A urethral catheter should be placed because hypothermic patients may have polyuria or oliguria. Continuous monitoring of heart rate, blood pressure, respiratory rate, temperature, and arterial blood gases should be performed. Corrections of arterial pH should not be made for temperature. Pharmacologic agents should be used cautiously as drug metabolism is unpredictable in hypothermic states. Exceptions to this include glucose, lidocaine, and bretylium.[54] Insulin should be avoided as endogenous stores will become effective with rewarming.[44] Steroids have not been shown to be useful. Antibiotics should be administered to all hypothermic newborn infants and should be strongly considered in all other children with nonexposure hypothermia.

Potential complications

A potential complication of hypothermia to anticipate during transport is arrhythmias, particularly ventricular fibrillation, as the cold myocardium is sensitive. While many antiarrhythmics have been used, bretylium appears to be the drug of choice. Although the optimal dose and rate of infusion are unresearched, the drug should be withheld until a temperature of 28-30°C has been obtained. Another worrisome complication is "afterdrop," defined as the maximum drop in temperature that occurs with rewarming, particularly with external rewarming techniques. With afterdrop, peripheral potassium-laden blood moves into the central circulation. Patients should be closely monitored for electrocardiographic signs of hyperkalemia, and the transport team should anticipate the most practical methods of lowering serum potassium levels (see Chapter 27).

At present, no clear criteria exist for withdrawing support from the hypothermic patient exist. Successful resuscitations have occurred in patients with severe hypothermia and prolonged periods of cardiopulmonary arrest, especially small children cooled rapidly in near-freezing water. Absence of cardiac function after resuscitation and warming to 32°C remains the only valid criteria for withdrawing support in the severely hypothermic patient.[28]

SNAKE BITES

Pathophysiology

Although about 8,000 venomous snake bites are reported in the United States each year, there are fewer than 12 fatalities.[23] There are two families of poisonous snakes: crotalidae, or pit vipers, and elapidae. Rattlesnakes, a member of the crotalidae or pit viper family, account for about 65% percent of venomous snake bites and for almost all deaths. Other pit vipers include the copperhead and the cottonmouth. Pit vipers have anterior fangs, a triangular shaped head, and a thermoreceptor pit on each side of the face. The coral snake belongs to the elapidae family and is the only other native poisonous snake, inflicting less than 1% of all bites. Up to 50% of all snakebites are actually nonvenomous. Although current antivenins are fairly effective in preventing morbidity and mortality, their side effects combined with the possible low dose and potency of snake venom allow most patients to be treated only with observation.

Crotalidae venoms are complex mixtures, chiefly proteins, having enzymatic activity, including proteases, phospholipase and hyaluronidases. The proteases primarily cause tissue necrosis at the site of injection of venom. The hyaluronidases break down cell junctions, thereby spreading the venom. The phospholipase destroy cell wall and capillary membranes allowing serum protein and plasma to leak into the interstitial tissues causing local edema. Venoms include polypeptides which appear to have specific chemical and physiologic receptor sites. Elapidae venom is neurotoxic causing paresthesia and eventually respiratory paralysis.[56]

Recognition

Although some pit viper bites may not be recognized immediately, those serious enough to require transport will have rapid swelling, ecchymosis, pain, and at least one puncture wound. Most of these serious snake bites will be from eastern or western dia-

TABLE 30-2 CATEGORIES OF ENVENOMATION

Degree	*Pit viper bites* *Signs and symptoms*
No envenomation	No fang marks, or fang marks are present with less than 1 inch of edema. No local or systemic signs or sytmptoms. Laboratory data are essentially normal.
Minimal	Fang marks, pain, edema and erythema confined to the surrounding area (to 5 inches). No systemic or laboratory abnormalities.
Moderate	Edema, erythema, bullae, or ecchymoses progress beyond the area of the bite (6 to 12 inches). Tender adenopathy, systemic reactions and laboratory abnormalities may be present.
Severe	Rapid extension of edema, pain, bullae or ecchymoses to involve entire extremity. Serious systemic reactions such as shock are present. Laboratory abnormalities reflect coagulation defect or elevation in serum creatinine occur. Bites on thorax, head, and neck should be considered to be severe envenomation.

mondback rattlesnakes, as they are capable of delivering a large dose of potent venom.[48]

Coral snake bites cause more of a diagnostic problem. The bite marks, resembling small horseshoe shapes with minimal swelling, are difficult to see, and the paresthesia that develops requires a high index of suspicion especially in children too young to describe the symptoms.

Indications for transfer

A child with a moderate or severe (see Table 30-2) pit viper or coral snake bite will need antivenin. If enough antivenin is not available or if the primary hospital is not equipped with staff and equipment to manage a child with anaphylaxis, the child should be transferred as soon as possible. Also, the child with a bite on the trunk, neck, or face or having a serious envenomation will need treatment in a pediatric intensive care environment.

Emergency treatment

As in all emergencies, the first priority is to ensure adequacy of the respiratory and circulatory systems. In the absence of immediate life-threatening symptoms, information regarding the size and species of the snake, circumstances related to the bite, number of bites inflicted, and type of field therapy (e.g., tourniquet, incision, and suction) administered should be obtained.

Pit viper

A preliminary physical examination should include recording vital signs, evaluation of neurologic status, and classification of severity of envenomation (see Table 30-2). A circumferential measurement of the bitten extremity(ies) should be recorded and repeated periodically as described below. Baseline laboratory data should include a complete blood count, platelet count, electrolytes, blood urea nitrogen, serum creatinine, and urinalysis. Due to high frequency of coagulopathies associated with snake bite, it is appropriate to evaluate prothrombin time and to quantify fibrinogen degradation products. Blood for typing and cross-matching should be obtained, as the hemolysin in the venom can make the process impossible later.

Offer comfort to the child in order to lessen venom dissemination resulting from excitement and movement. Rings, watches, and all other potentially restrictive items should be removed. The area of the bite should be immobilized at heart level in a functional position. The use of arterial tourniquets, incisions, suction, and local ice application are not recommended.[30] Lymphatic constriction bands (wide piece of rubber tubing) that lightly compress the skin enough to occlude lymph flow but not tight enough to impede venous or arterial flow may be beneficial, especially with viper bites. Most authorities agree that antibiotics which offer coverage for both aerobic and anaerobic organisms are indicated.[24,39]

Measure the extremity circumference at a marked location and recheck every 15 to 30 minutes for six hours, then at least every four hours. In moderate to severe envenomation, polyvalent (crotalidae) antivenin should be given. While copperhead bites are often treated without antivenin,[62] diamondback rattlesnake envenomations are very dangerous and may require extra antivenin. A 50% increase in the adult dose is given in children because of the relatively larger amount of venom delivered in relation to weight. If there are multiple bites, antivenin should be increased by another 50%.

After the decision has been made to initiate antivenin therapy, the patient should be skin tested using the provided material intradermally. The intradermal skin test should be administered by giving 0.02 cc of a 1 : 10 dilution of antivenin. Always have resuscitation equipment close at hand. In the event of a positive skin test, treatment with antivenin should be initiated in an environment fully prepared to treat anaphylaxis. Whether or not the skin test is positive, corticosteroids or diphenhydramine may be given before the administration of antivenin to attempt to diminish any adverse reactions. Two IV sites are recommended in case one is needed to administer epinephrine and corticosteroids. The initial dose of antivenin is based on the envenomation ranking (see Table 30-2).[65]

No envenomation	No antivenin
Mild envenomation	0 to 5 vials
Moderate envenomation	10 vials
Severe envenomation	15 or more vials

For rattlesnake bites, each vial of antivenin is initially mixed with 10 ml of saline. In an adolescent or adult the antivenin may be further diluted 1 : 4 with saline or Lactated Ringer's solution. For the child, this volume may be excessive, so antivenin may be administered without further dilution. Begin to administer the antivenin at rates of 1 to 2 ml/hr and observe reactions. If no adverse reactions occur, increase the rate over a 30 minute period. Antivenin produces its greatest effects when given within the first 4 hours of a bite, but in severe envenomation it may be effective even after 24 hours. Antivenin should be administered until the pain, edema, and other systemic reactions have ceased. The clinician titrates the antivenin to the venom's clinical effects. The diminution of pain while using antivenin is an endpoint some clinicians use, and therefore opioids and other pain relievers are not commonly used.[65]

Coral snake

Supportive care is of the utmost importance. Neither constriction bands nor suction will slow the absorption of venom. If a documented or highly probable coral snake bite has occurred, the patient should be treated prophylactically before more symptoms develop. The antivenin will prevent but not reverse paralysis. The recommended dose is 3-5 vials of coral antivenin. An additional 3-5 vials may be given if further signs of toxicity develop. Antivenin should ideally be given in the first 4 to 6 hours.[57]

Preparation for transport

Secure the two IV lines. Prepare a flow sheet including amount of antivenin administered, amount of fluids given, vital signs, circumferential measurements of extremities, and amount of pain the child is experiencing. Label and sign tubes of blood drawn early for possible cross-matching. Copy all medical records. A urethral catheter should be seriously considered as urine output is an important monitor of the patient's volume status and renal function.

Complications en route

Transport itself should not add to complications of snakes or spider bites. Complications of the bite itself should be anticipated and appropriate preparations made. The venom can have toxic effects on the heart. Tissue necrosis can lead to acute tubular necrosis, so urine output must be maintained. Vital signs must be monitored frequently. Fluid loss may be significant enough in the area of the bite to lead to signs of shock. The antivenin can cause allergic reactions, including anaphylaxis. An appropriate dose of epinephrine should be immediately available to be given intravenously. Dosages of diphenhydramine, steroids, and fluids for volume resuscitation should be calculated in advance. Potentially needed medications and equipment should be prepared for easy access during transport.

SPIDER BITES

Among 20,000 species of spiders in the United States, the most dangerous venomous spiders are Latrodectus species (the black widow) and Loxosceles species (the brown recluse).

Black widow spider

The mature female black widow is glossy black, gray, or brown with a red, orange, or yellow hourglass-shaped marking on the ventral abdomen. Its venom contains a powerful neurotoxin which acts at the neuromuscular junction by binding to glycoproteins or gangliosides on the presynaptic membrane and opening cation channels, resulting in release of acetylcholine and norepinephrine, causing muscular cramps, hypertension and cholinergic effects.[3]

Clinical presentation. Pain may begin immediately at the site of the bite, followed by erythema, itching, and swelling. Two red puncture marks are often present surrounded by an area of blanching and an outer bluish erythematous border called a "target" or "halo" lesion.[61] Spasm of large muscle groups and severe pain usually begin within 30-60 minutes after the bite, peak in 1 to 6 hours, and may persist for several days.

Consider a child with a sudden onset of irritability, hypertension, and muscle rigidity, particularly of the abdominal musculature, as possibly having black widow spider envenomation. Diagnostic procedures such as complete blood count, abdominal radiographs, and lumbar puncture may be required to exclude the possibility of central nervous system infection or an acute intra-abdominal process unless a history of contact with black widow spider is obtained. Nausea, vomiting, headache, weakness, increased salivation, and anxiety are common. Severe envenomation may produce shock, coma, or respiratory failure. These severe cases may also have ECG changes that are similar to those of digitalis overdose. Deaths are usually due to respiratory or cardiac failure or to a hypertensive crisis. Deaths are infrequent, particularly now that antivenin is available.

Management. Benzodiazepines or calcium gluconate have been used to ease muscle rigidity and pain. Hypertension usually resolves with pain control, but a hypertensive crisis may require anti-hypertensive drugs. The use of latrodectus-specific antivenin is recommended for severe envenomation in children who have no allergic contraindication and in whom analgesics were unsuccessful for pain relief.[13]

Patients requiring advanced life support or the administration on antivenin should be admitted to a tertiary care facility. Most patients have a relatively benign course and can be managed with in-patient observation in a monitored setting.

Brown recluse spider

The brown recluse spider is characterized by a violin-like marking on the cephalothorax. Brown recluse bites usually occur indoors. The venom is a complex mixture of at least nine proteins among which hyaluronidase, protease, hemolysins, and sphingomyelinase have been identified. The venom attaches to red blood cells, setting off a cascade of events leading to local and systemic hemolysis, complement activation, and intravascular coagulation.[42]

Clinical presentation. Local effect: Initially the bite site is painless. Within a few hours the area becomes indurated, erythematous, and painful. A bleb may develop over the bite site. The central portion is surrounded by halos of blanching and rings of erythema resembling a bull's eye target. A necrotic black center is highly characteristic of a brown recluse bite. Systemic reactions usually occur within 24-48 hours and range from fever, chills, nausea, vomiting, and arthralgia to symptoms of hemolysis, disseminated intravascular coagulopathies (DIC), renal failure, and rarely, death.

Management. Severe systemic effects such as hemolysis, DIC, and renal failure should be assessed both clinically and by obtaining appropriate laboratory tests such as complete blood count, reticulocyte count, serum haptoglobin, bilirubin, urine analysis, and tests for myoglobinums, renal profile, platelet count, PT, PTT, fibrin split products, and electrolytes. Children should be in a center able to treat renal failure and/or DIC.

Transport considerations. During transport, management includes immobilization of the bite site. Diphenhydramine may be used for pruritus. For severe pain, narcotic analgesics are indicated. With severe hemolysis, platelets and packed red blood cells may be required. If hemoglobinuria is present, fluids and alkalinization of urine are required to prevent acute tubular necrosis. Dapsone has been used in the treatment of brown recluse spider bites after evaluating the child for glucose 6-phosphate dehydrogenase deficiency.

Disposition. Consider transfer to an ICU or tertiary facility in the following cases of spider bites:

1. Requirement for advanced life support in patients with black widow and brown recluse spider bites.
2. Requirement for antivenin administration when the primary facility is not staffed or equipped to manage a child with anaphylaxis.
3. The presence of severe hemolysis or renal failure in patients with brown recluse spider bites.

Regional poison control centers have current information on snake and spider bites.

SUBMERSION INJURIES

Drowning, the third leading cause of death in the United States for children ages 1 to 14 claims more than eight thousand lives per year overall, with the worldwide fatality rate at approximately 3.5 per 100,000 population.[37] The incidence of drowning by year of age follows a bimodal distribution with one peak in the toddler age group and another in adolescence. Male children drown in higher proportion to female children in all age groups.[5,66] Up to 80% of childhood drowning occurs in swimming pools, which are described in the legal literature as "attractive nuisances."[19] Bathtub, mop bucket, and more recently, the 5-gallon plastic industrial buckets have been documented as locations for drowning, especially for toddlers.[7,63] Children with a seizure disorder have a four-fold increased risk of drowning.[40,66] Abuse or neglect should be considered in all drowning related incidents in young children.

Near drowning is an incident of being submerged in a liquid leading to asphyxia with at least a temporary loss of consciousness and with subsequent survival for at least 24 to 48 hours. The chance of the submerged child surviving is most dependent on the immediate recognition and appropriate airway management. Outcome correlates more with the care given at the scene of the injury than with the care given in the pediatric intensive care unit. Appropriate levels of care during community hospital stabilization and interhospital transport could reasonably be considered to have a positive impact on outcome.

Pathophysiology

Following an initial struggle to reach the surface, during which the victim consciously controls the urge to breathe, a submerged person will be forced to inspire. When liquid enters the larynx, spasm occurs, preventing liquid from entering the lungs. The swallowing mechanism tries to clear the oral cavity, as the mouth is full of water. As asphyxia worsens and the laryngospasm relaxes, the diaphragm contracts, pulling water into the lungs in about 85% of cases ("wet" drowning). Although the amount of aspirated fluid is often emphasized, the amount of water swallowed is usually both greater and more potentially dangerous. Gastric distension, resulting in respiratory mechanical obstruction, and vomiting with aspiration can be chemically disastrous. The patient becomes more hypoxic as the duration of submersion continues, initially affecting the brain and heart. The primary insult demanding treatment by emergency medicine personnel is hypoxia. The most important factor in neurologic outcome is the extent of anoxic and ischemic central nervous system injury.[15] Other systems injured include: 1) pulmonary: adult respiratory distress syndrome (ARDS), 2) cardiac: myocardial ischemia, arrhythmias, cardiovascular collapse, 3) renal: acute tubular and/or cortical necrosis, 4) gastrointestinal: mucosal sloughing with profuse bloody diarrhea, 5) hematologic: disseminated intravascular coagulation.

Emergency scene treatment

Stabilize the cervical spine if there is a chance of diving injury, but the treatment for near drowning is securing an airway and delivering oxygen, often beginning while the patient is still in the water. Clean debris from the mouth and begin breathing with supplemental oxygen. The child will vomit often before the first breath. Clear the airway and continue treatment with ventilation and oxygen. Unless the hospital is just across the street, ensure airway management before transport.

If cardiac function does not return within 25 minutes of advanced life support and if the child was submerged over 25 minutes in water over 5°C, the outcome can be predicted to be death or severe neurologic sequelae.[45]

Emergency department management

A. Patient with spontaneous respirations. This child requires assessment of vital signs, a complete physical exam, and possibly a check of the metabolic status, including glucose. Observation for 12 to 24 hours is needed because of the potential for the development of adult respiratory distress syndrome or other organ failure.

B. Patient with no spontaneous respirations. Ensure airway patency and oxygenation, and hyperoxygenate the patient, obtain vital signs, monitor the cardiac rate and rhythm, and oxygen saturation. Regularly recheck the endotracheal tube placement and auscultate for pneumothoraces. The use of positive-end respiratory pressure may be required to decrease the amount of pulmonary edema and to maintain alveolar patency. Check metabolic status, especially glucose. In experimental animal models, elevated blood and brain glucose levels increased neurologic damage during hypoxic-ischemic injury.[43] Ashwal and others reported that an elevated initial blood glucose was highly predictive of death or vegetative survival.[2] Glucose should be kept within the physiologic range, so do not use intravenous fluids with (hyperosmolar) glucose unless hypoglycemia occurs. Placement of a nasogastric tube should be done early, as the stomach is usually full of swallowed liquid.

The most likely reason for the patient's unconsciousness is hypoxic injury, but other possibilities should be considered. Toxic ingestion (legal or illegal drugs, alcohol), head and spinal cord trauma, hypovolemic shock, and hypothermia may cause altered mental status, and any possibility should be appropriately investigated.

Indications and considerations for transfer to tertiary care

A. Patient with spontaneous respirations. The majority of near drowning patients will, despite great parental and patient anxiety, have maintained spontaneous respirations and normal mental status throughout. They will be able to be discharged from the emergency department after a thorough exam. Children with a history of asphyxia should be observed for 12 to 24 hours for organ failure, especially of the lungs.[41] The observation should be done in a setting with personnel who can recognize deteriorating pulmonary function and provide a continuum of appropriate intensive care including transport. If the child had a momentary period of asphyxia and is ambulatory in the emergency department, admission to the local hospital may be appropriate. If the child was submerged longer than five minutes or did not respond with consciousness immediately at the scene, observation close to a pediatric intensive care unit is suggested. Consult with your PICU about optimal care for the individual child, and consult with your transport team to ensure availability, if needed. Initial chest radiography does not correlate with outcome, as hypoxia can be severe without significant fluid aspiration and pulmonary edema may be present in a child who has had relatively little anoxic damage.

B. Patient without spontaneous respirations. The decision to transfer a patient who has been treated aggressively in an emergency department setting and does not have spontaneous respirations is problematic. The child who only has a heartbeat return and/or has no apparent neurologic function has a very high chance of death or severe neurological impairment. The prognosis should be communicated to the family prior to transport. Too often the family feels that if the child has a heartbeat at the time of arrival to the pediatric intensive care unit, the child's prognosis will markedly improve. The few children with a positive outcome, despite poor prognostic indicators, have been those submerged in water temperatures less than 5°C and those with a large surface area and small body mass.[6]

Children who do not have spontaneous respirations, but have other causes of altered mental status, such as a drug overdose, may have a better outcome and should be transferred to the PICU. Another reason to transfer the child is if the parents are willing for their child to be considered for organ donation. The organ bank would most likely want the child in the PICU to coordinate all of the complex technical and emotional challenges. If the child does not yet have serious pulmonary complications, he or she may soon require fine tuning of ventilator and respiratory management.

Stabilization

Maintain PaO_2 at normal levels or above by increasing PEEP, FiO_2, and inspiratory time and pressure as needed. Warm the patient as necessary, and provide maximal cerebral perfusion pressure. Maintain glucose at physiologic levels. Although aspiration and absorption of salt and fresh water can transiently alter serum electrolytes, this is rarely of any long-term clinical significance. Correct abnormalities only if clinically symptomatic. The end tidal CO_2 monitor on the endotracheal tube may not be accurate if it was a "wet" drowning and there was pulmonary damage. Be sure to calibrate the end tidal CO_2 monitor.

If the patient is in shock and not responding to oxygen therapy, fluid boluses should be minimized unless ongoing losses are occurring. Early use of ionotopic agents such as dopamine or dobutamine to maintain adequate cardiac output may prevent excessive fluid administration leading to worsened cerebral edema. Monitor the liver size clinically, cardiac size via x-ray, and observe urine output until a central line can be placed to judge volume.

When at least 20 ml of fluid per pound is aspirated, fibrillation occurs in 80 percent of animals. But because approximately 85 percent of human immersion victims aspire less than 10 ml per pound, fibrillation is rare.[33] However, myocardial failure secondary to asphyxia is seen and should be investigated with an ECG.

Transportation: anticipation and complications

Transport with an endotracheal tube securely in place if the Glasgow Coma Scale is less than 8, there is an absent or weak gag reflex, the child is hemodynamically unstable, or the child is inadequately oxygenated. Transport with oxygen saturations as close to 100% as possible. Mark the position of the point of maximum impulse of the heart, so if the patient suddenly deteriorates, a shift may be detected. If a shift occurs, check for a pneumothorax on the opposite side.

Although cuffed endotracheal tubes are seldom used in children, the child developing ARDS or pulmonary edema may require enough pressure that the cuff should be inflated. Consider intubating with a cuffed tube and even leaving it deflated until needed. This is important if there is a long transport during which the lung compliance is anticipated to increase. The cuff will expand if it is filled with air when the airplane or helicopter flies at high altitudes. The pilot should be asked to keep cabin pressure high (at a low altitude) or the cuff should be adjusted during ascent and descent. Simply deflate the cuff and reinflate with the same number of cc used originally. Check for leaks frequently if the transport vehicle is quiet enough for auscultation. Normally, there should be just a small leakage of air at maximal inspiration.

If the patient is cold, the transport team should provide humidified oxygen warmed to 98°F-105°F for the duration of the transport. Sedation and neuromuscular blockade in the agitated, intubated, ventilated patient may help prevent increased intracranial pressure.

Prevention

Transport team members should join groups such as the American Red Cross, American Heart Association, American Academy of Pediatrics, or Safe Kids to educate lay people, legislators, and professionals about water safety and should also set an example by practicing safety. Prevention of a submersion injury is much easier than treatment.

REFERENCES

1. Althaus U, Aeberhard P, Schüpbach P: Management of profound accidental hypothermia with cardiorespiratory arrest, *Ann Surg* 195:492-5, 1982.
2. Ashwal S and others: Prognostic indications of hyperglycemia and reduced cerebral blood flow in childhood near-drowning, *Neurology* 40:820-3, 1990.
3. Baba A, Cooper JR: The action of black widow spider venom on cholinergic mechanisms in synaptosomes, *J Neurochem* 34:1369-79, 1980.
4. Bacon C, Scott D, Jones P: Heatstroke in well-wrapped infants, *Lancet* 2:422-5, 1979.
5. Baker SP: *Drowning: injury fact book,* 1984, Lexington Books.
6. Bolte RG, Black PG, Bowers RS: The use of extracorporeal rewarming in a child submerged for 66 minutes, *JAMA* 260:377-9, 1988.
7. Bundick LD, Ross DA: Bathtub-related drownings in the United States, 1979-1981, *Am J Public Health* 75:630-3, 1985.
8. Buss DD and others: Heat illness, *Minnesota Medicine* 73:33-5, 1990.
9. Bynum G, Patton J, Bowers W: Performed lavage cooling in an anesthetized dog heatstroke model, *Aviat Space Environ Med* 49:779-84, 1978.
10. Channa AB and others: Is dantrolene effective in heat stroke patients?, *Crit Care Med* 18(30):290-2, 1990.
11. Choo MH: Clinical presentation of heat disorders, In Yeo PPB and Lin MK, editors: *Heat disorders,* Singapore, 1968, Headquarters Medical Services.
12. Clark R, Beeley JM: Smoke inhalation, *British J Hosp Med* 41:252-9, 1989.
13. Clark FR and others: Clinical presentation and treatment of black widow spider envenomation: a review of 163 cases, *Ann Emerg Med* 21(7):782-7, 1992.
14. Cobb N, Etzel RA: Unintentional carbon monoxide-related deaths in the United States: 1979 through 1988, *JAMA* 266(5):659-63, 1991.
15. Conn AW, Edmonds JF, Barker GA: Cerebral resuscitation in near-drowning, *Pediatr Clinics of North America* 26:691-701, 1979.
16. Costrini A: Emergency treatment of heatstroke and comparison of whole body cooling techniques, *Medicine and Science in Sports and Exercise* 22(1):15-8, 1990.
17. Davies DM, Millar EJ, Miller IA: Accidental hypothermia treated by extracorporeal blood warming, *Lancet* 1:1036-7, 1967.
18. Dean BS, Verdile VP, Krenzelok EP: Coma reversal with cerebral dysfunction recovery after repetitive hyperbaric oxygen therapy for severe carbon monoxide poisoning, *Am J Emerg Med* 11(6):616-8, 1993.
19. Dean J, Setzer NA: Near drowning. In Rogers MC, editor: *Textbook of Pediatric Intensive Care,* ed 1, Baltimore, 1987, Williams & Wilkins.
20. Faries G and others: Temperature relationship to distance and flow rate on warmed iv fluids, *Ann Emerg Med* 20:1198-1200, 1991.
21. Feldman KW, Morray JP, Schaller RT: Thermal injury caused by hot pack application in hypothermic children, *Amer J Emerg Med* 3(1):38-41, 1985.
22. Fitzgerald FJ, Jessup C: Accidental hypothermia: a report of 22 cases and reviews of the literature, *Yearbook Medical Publishers* 27:127-150, 1982.
23. Gold BS, Barish RA: Venomous snakebites, *Emerg Med Clin North Am* 10(2):249-67, 1992.
24. Gold BS, Barish RA: Venomous snakebites, *Maryland Med J* 9:833-42, 1990.
25. Goldfrank LR and others: Carbon monoxide. In Goldfrank LR, editor: *Goldfrank's toxicologic emergencies,* Norwalk, CT, 1990, Appleton and Lange.
26. Haller A and others: Body temperature disturbances. In Silverman BK, editor: *APLS: The pediatric emergency medicine course,* Elk Grove Village, IL, 1993, American Academy of Pediatrics.
27. Haller A and others: Toxic injuries. In Silverman BK, editor: *APLS: the pediatric emergency medicine course,* Elk Grove Village, IL, 1993, American Academy of Pediatrics.
28. Hotstrand HT: Accidental hypothermia and frostbite. In Barkin RM, editor: *Pediatric emergency medicine: concepts and clinical practice,* St. Louis, 1982, Mosby-Yearbook.
29. Kaplan M, Eidelman AI: Improved prognosis in severely hypothermic newborn infants treated by rapid rewarming, *J Ped* 105(3):470-4, 1984.
30. Kunkel DB: Bites of venomous reptiles, *Emerg Med Clin North Am* 2:563-77, 1984.
31. Lee RP, Bishop GF, Ashton CM: Severe heat stroke in an experienced athlete, *Med J Aust,* 153:100-3, 1990.
32. Medical News: Boy drowns in cold water for 38 minutes and lives, *JAMA* 238:302, 1987.
33. Modell JH, Davis JH: Electrolyte changes in human drowning victims, *Anesthesiology,* April, 414-20, 1969.
34. Mofenson HC, Caraccio TR, Brody GM: Carbon monoxide poisoning, *Am J Emerg Med* 2(3):254-61, 1984.
35. Norkool DM, Kirkpatrick JN: Treatment of acute carbon monoxide poisoning with hyperbaric oxygen: a review of 115 cases, *Ann Emerg Med* 14(12): 1168-71, 1985.
36. Olson KR: Carbon monoxide poisoning: mechanisms, presentation, and controversies in management, *J Emerg Med* 1:233-47, 1983.
37. Orlowski JP: Drowning, near drowning, and ice-water submersions, *Pediatric Clinic of North America* 34:75-91, 1987.
38. Osborne JJ: Experimental hypothermia: respiratory and blood pH changes in relationship to cardiac function, *Am J Physiol* 175:389-98, 1953.
39. Parrish HM: Letter to editor, *Missouri Med* 60:240, 1963.

40. Pearn JH: Epilepsy and drowning in childhood, *Br Med J* 1:1510, 1977.
41. Pearn JH: Secondary drowning in children, *Br Med J* 281:1103-5, 1980.
42. Pitts RM and others: Tough spiders: identifying and treating their bites, *Emerg Ped* 5:72-5, 1992.
43. Pulsinelli WA and others: Moderate hyperglycemia augments ischemic brain damage: a neuropathic study in the rat, *Neurology* 32:1239-46, 1982.
44. Purdue GF, Hunt JL: Cold injury: a collective review, *JBCR* 7(4):331-42, 1986.
45. Quan L, Kinder D: Pediatric submersions: prehospital predictors of outcome, *Pediatrics* 90:909-13, 1992.
46. Reuler JB: Hypothermia: pathophysiology, clinical settings, and management, *Ann Int Med* 89:519-27, 1978.
47. Reynolds EM, Ryan DP, Doody DP: Mortality and respiratory failure in a pediatric burn population, *J Ped Surg* 28(10):1326-31, 1993.
48. Russell FE: *Snake venom poisoning,* Great Neck, NY, 1983, Scholicum International.
49. Sanchez R and others: Carbon monoxide poisoning due to automobile exposure: disparity between carboxyhemoglobin levels and symptoms of victims, *Pediatrics* 82(4):663-5, 1988.
50. Shapiro Y, Seidman DS: Field and clinical observations of exertional heat stroke patients, *Medicine and Science in Sports and Exercise* 22(1):6-14, 1990.
51. Shapiro Y, Rosenthal T, Sohar E: Experimental heatstroke: a model in dogs, *Arch Intern Med* 131:688-92, 1973.
52. Sheilds CP, Sixsmith DM: Treatment of moderate to severe hypothermia in an urban setting, *Ann Emerg Med* 19(10):1093-7, 1990.
53. Simon HB: Hyperthermia, *New Eng J Med* 329(7):483-7, 1993.
54. Stewart C: Generalized hypothermia. In Stewart C, editor: *Environmental emergencies,* Baltimore, 1990, Williams and Wilkins.
55. Stewart C: The spectrum of heat illness. In Stewart C, editor: *Environmental emergencies,* Baltimore, 1990, Williams and Wilkins.
56. Stewart CE: *Environmental emergencies, bites and stings,* Baltimore, MD, 1990, Williams & Wilkins.
57. Sullivan JB, Wingert WA: *Reptile bites.* In Auerbach PS, Geehr EC, editors: *Management of wilderness and environmental emergencies,* St. Louis, 1989, Mosby Company.
58. Syverud SA, Barber WJ, Amsterdam JT: Iced gastric lavage for treatment of heatstroke efficacy in a canine model, *Ann Emerg Med* 14:424-32, 1985.
59. Thom SR, Kein LW: Carbon monoxide poisoning: a review, epidemiology, pathophysiology, clinical findings, and treatment options including hyperbaric oxygen therapy, *Clin Tox J* 27(3):141-156, 1989.
60. Thompson AE: Environmental emergencies. In Fleisher D, Ludwig S, editors: *Textbook of pediatric emergency medicine,* Baltimore, 1993, Williams & Wilkins.
61. Vance M and others: The target lesion: a pathognomonic sign of black widow spider envenomation, *Vet Hum toxicol* 28:485, 1986.
62. Wagner CW, Golladay ES. Crotalid envenomation in children: selective conservative management, *J Ped Surg* 24:128-31, 1989.
63. Walker S, Middelkamp JN: Pail immersion accidents, *Clin Pediatr* 20:341-3, 1981.
64. Wilkerson J: Hypothermia update: 1992 Mt. Hood Conference Proceedings, *Wilderness Medicine Letter* 10(3):1-10, 1993.
65. Wingert WA, Chan L: Rattlesnake bites in Southern California and rationale for recommended treatment, *West J Med* 148:37-44, 1988.
66. Wintemute GJ: Childhood drowning and near drowning in the United States, *AJDC* 144:663-9, 1990.
67. Wong KC: Physiology and pharmacology of hypothermia, *West J Med* 138(2):227-32, 1983.
68. Zell SC, Kurtz KJ: Severe exposure hypothermia: a resuscitation protocol, *Ann Emerg Med* 14(4):339-45, 1985.
69. Zimmerman SS, Truxal B: Carbon monoxide poisoning, *Pediatrics* 68(2):215-24, 1981.

31

TRANSPORT OF THE POISONED CHILD

DONALD D. VERNON
MITCHELL P. ROSS

Poisoning remains a common problem, with 1.8 million exposures reported to U.S. poison control centers during 1991, and estimates of total poisonings ranging as high as 4.4 million.[69] As many as 60% of poisoning victims (more than one million per year) are children under 6 years of age.[69] In young children (<6 years) poisoning is accidental, often not serious, and usually does not present diagnostic difficulties, since the young child does not attempt to disguise his or her actions.[56,69] The older child or teenager is more likely to poison himself in an attempt at suicide or while using recreational drugs such as cocaine or alcohol.[69] Although many teenage suicide attempts are not serious attempts to terminate existence, they may nonetheless present a threat to life if a potentially lethal substance is ingested (such as acetaminophen or tricyclic antidepressants).[58]

At least two-thirds of all reported poison exposures are asymptomatic, and accidental poisonings, the most common sort in young children, are often trivial.[69] Patients with significant signs and symptoms of poisoning still number in the many thousands yearly in the United States, however, and surveys suggest that 3-4.5% of all admissions to a pediatric intensive care unit are due to intoxication.[32,33,63,69,108] Indications for transport of the poisoned child include severity of illness beyond the scope of the referring hospital or a requirement for specialized services (e.g. dialysis, hyperbaric chamber, specific antidotal therapies) which are unavailable at the referring hospital.

INITIAL APPROACH TO POISONED PATIENT

Although specific antidotes and treatments exist for a number of substances causing poisoning, basic supportive measures including airway management, evaluation and support of breathing, and assessment and maintenance of adequate circulation are of primary importance in initial management. A careful history, directed physical examination, and laboratory evaluation should be used to identify the reason for the patient's illness. Upon making a diagnosis of intoxication, measures aimed at decreasing drug absorption and hastening drug elimination are initiated. Finally, one may undertake specific or antidotal treatment. Transport of the poisoned patient will often take place in the initial hours after the poisoning event when medical effects of intoxication may still be evolving, meaning that patient status may deteriorate during transport; thus, one is required to anticipate developments for the transport period.

Respiratory abnormalities are the most common life-threatening manifestations of severe poisoning, and therefore, airway management and maintenance of oxygenation and ventilation are of primary importance in the transportation of poisoned patients. Impairment of respiratory drive may occur associated with central nervous system depression or seizures, both common in intoxication.[122] Airway obstruction may occur from loss of muscular tone due to central nervous system depression or seizures, from mucosal edema from ingestion of caustic or corrosive substances, or from thermal injury. Pulmonary aspiration is a risk in many poisonings for several reasons. There may be a combination of emesis and depressed level of consciousness and associated depression of airway protective reflexes. Aspiration is also a risk during gastric evacuation, either by induced emesis or by gastric tube. Endotracheal intubation is the most practical and reliable way of ventilatory assistance for transport and should be performed prior to transport, both for airway protection during gastric decontamination and because symptoms may progress rapidly in the hours immediately following a poisoning event.

Close attention to hemodynamic status is integral to the care of the severely poisoned patient during transport. Causes of poisoning-related shock include hypovolemia, such as is seen in patients following iron ingestions with fluid loss into the bowel, vasodilatation with distributive shock following ingestions of phenothiazines, and in cardiogenic shock, as is seen following tricyclic antidepressant overdoses. Shock due to poisoning, as for other causes, is usually best treated by intravenous fluid administration, and isotonic fluids such as Ringer's lactate should be given liberally. Inotropic drugs are not commonly needed but can be life-saving in intoxications which depress myocardial performance (i.e., tricyclic antidepressants).

Alteration in mental status may not be a direct result of the toxic exposure, and metabolic considerations such as hypoglycemia and hypoxia must be addressed. All obtunded patients should receive glucose (0.5-1.0 g/kg) and naloxone (0.1 mg/kg) empirically. In evaluation of the unconscious patient, one must consider head trauma, central nervous system infection, or seizures as possible causes of central nervous system depression.

Following the initial resuscitation of the intoxicated patient, decontamination must be initiated. In addition to gastrointestinal decontamination, respiratory and surface decontamination may be required. In cutaneous exposures it is necessary to remove all contaminated clothing and wash or rinse the patient with copious amounts of clear water or saline, followed by thorough cleansing with a nongermicidal soap. All cutaneous decontamination should be completed prior to transport because accumulation of volatile fumes in the closed cabin of an airplane or helicopter are a risk to the health and safety of the transport team and pilot.

Decontamination of the gastrointestinal tract usually involves the use of forced emesis or gastric lavage to empty the stomach, followed by instillation of activated charcoal (usually mixed with a cathartic agent such as sorbitol) into the gastrointestinal tract to prevent absorption of any remaining toxin. The utility of gastric emptying versus activated charcoal administration is currently undergoing reevaluation, and in some experimental ingestions, activated charcoal was deemed superior in preventing absorption.[33] Clearly, such decisions must be made for each clinical situation; for instance, gastric emptying seems reasonable when one is faced with a massive ingestion of a highly toxic substance.

Induction of emesis is contraindicated in patients with depressed mentation, who may rapidly develop depressed mentation or seizures (as in tricyclic antidepressant ingestions), or who have ingested caustic agents or hydrocarbons, and in children under 6 months of age in whom safety of emetic agents has not been demonstrated. Induction of emesis may be relatively contraindicated for transport; protection of the airway for an actively vomiting child may be difficult to ensure in a cramped transport vehicle or aircraft. A dose of 5-10 ml of syrup of ipecac for children ages 6-12 months, 15-30 ml in children 1-12 years, and 30 ml in older children and adults, accompanied by up to 8 ounces of clear fluids will induce vomiting within 15-30 minutes for up to 60 minutes.

Gastric lavage can be managed more easily in the transport situation and is preferable in any event for patients with depressed mental status. In obtunded patients, endotracheal intubation must be performed before gastric lavage to protect the airway. A large bore (30-34 French) orogastric tube is recommended to provide a sufficient diameter for return of tablet fragments. Several liters of warmed saline lavage fluid are often required to return a clear effluent. Lavage should be used with caution in patients having ingested hydrocarbons, as passage of the orogastric or nasogastric tube may induce emesis. Lavage is also contraindicated in patients with significant caustic injury due to concerns about possible emesis or perforation of the esophagus or stomach.

An alternative mode of gastric emptying is whole bowel irrigation using an osmotically stable fluid such as polyethylene glycol-electrolyte solution (GoLytely, Braintree, MA), administered orally or via nasogastric tube. Large volumes of the fluid are administered (up to 25-35 ml/kg/hour),[31] and the fluid lavages the entire gastrointestinal tract to flush out ingested poisons.[111] Use on transport might be impractical, however, and efficacy is unproved.

Activated charcoal effectively binds many ingested toxins, preventing absorption and facilitating passage from the body. Some toxins are not bound, however, including alcohols, ethylene glycol, certain organophosphate and carbamate pesticides, and acids and alkali.[41] Activated charcoal is at worst benign, and is probably worth giving in most poisonings. Charcoal is usually administered with a cathartic, most commonly sorbitol.

Poisoning-induced agitation or psychosis may present serious dangers on transport, particularly air transport, if a wild, uncontrolled patient should interfere with the pilot. Substances which may result in such behavior are largely drugs of abuse, such as cocaine, amphetamines, and phencyclidine.[51] Patients must be made sufficiently calm to ensure safe transport; inability to do so is a legitimate ground on which to cancel or postpone the trip. Judicious use of sedative drugs, such as benzodiazepines, may be necessary, and in extreme cases, neuromuscular blockade and endotracheal intubation may be justifiable for transport purposes alone.

DIAGNOSIS OF UNKNOWN INTOXICATION

Poisoning is often considered in diagnosing coma of unknown cause but might also be considered when there are prominent gastrointestinal signs such as vomiting, metabolic signs such as metabolic acidosis, or rapid onset of multisystems dysfunction. The neurological examination which suggests poisoning has depression of consciousness as the major feature, while cranial nerve reflexes are preserved. Signs such as asymmetry, abnormal motor posturing, or marked pupillary dilatation suggest structural brain lesions and virtually exclude intoxication.

The laboratory toxicology screen is frequently ordered to evaluate such patients. This seems like the ideal tool, but its diagnostic power is disappointingly feeble. Such screens influence medical management in as few as 4.4% of cases.[59,83,119] Test results may be slow in coming, and many substances are not detected by currently used screening methods. Therefore, identification of an unknown poisoning is based on the history of illness and on clinical manifestations of poisoning, with specific tests for poisons as confirmation.

Many substances responsible for poisoning produce characteristic groups of clinical signs, sometimes termed "toxidromes." These toxidromes can suggest specific agents or classes of agents.[33,83] A list of some of these toxidromes is provided in Table 31-1. For instance, anticholinergic signs (mydriasis, tachycardia, dry mouth and eyes, etc.) combined with coma, seizures, and cardiac rhythm disturbances, suggest intoxication with tricyclic antidepressants. Hyperventilation and metabolic acidosis without gross changes in sensorium are consistent with salicylate poisoning. However, with the addition of depressed level of consciousness, intoxication with methanol or ethylene glycol is possible. The former can be detected with the ferric chloride test performed on urine, while presence of an osmolal gap suggests the latter two. In this fashion, one can attempt to identify the offending poison or at least guide subsequent specific (rather than screening) laboratory testing.[83] Unfortunately, many intoxications do not produce typical toxidromes. Additionally, in the transport setting, the specific toxin is often unknown. Therefore, general supportive care must then suffice.

TABLE 31-1 DIAGNOSIS OF UNKNOWN INTOXICATION

Symptoms/signs	*Possible toxins*
Altered consciousness, delirium, coma	Benzodiazepines, other sedatives, opiates, alcohols, neuroleptics, tricyclic antidepressants; almost any poison in large overdosage
Respiratory depression	Any substance which alters sensorium (benzodiazepines, other sedatives, opiates, alcohols, neuroleptics, tricyclic antidepressants); almost any drug in large overdosage
Hypotension	Most substances which depress sensorium (see above); also β-blockers, theophylline, iron
Opiate Depression of consciousness, miosis, hypotension, hypoventilation	Codeine, meperidine, etc.
Anticholinergic Dry skin, decreased secretions, tachycardia, mydriasis	Tricyclic antidepressants (with EKG abnormalities), neuroleptics, antihistamines
Sympathetic overactivity Agitation, hypertension, seizures	Sympathomimetics, cocaine, theophylline, amphetamines, phenylpropanolamine
Metabolic acidosis	Methanol, ethylene glycol, salicylates (with hyperventilation)
Gastrointestinal Nausea, vomiting, diarrhea	Most substances in overdose; especially salicylates, theophylline, iron
No signs or symptoms	Any substance—many purported accidental ingestions are trivial or nonexistent

SPECIFIC AGENTS

Clonidine

Clonidine is a widely prescribed imidazoline derivative used for chronic control of hypertension and treatment of narcotic and tobacco withdrawal.[82] It is available in oral form and a transdermal delivery system which contain as much as 7.5 mg of clonidine and maybe potentially lethal to a small child.[6,16,19,45,46]

At therapeutic doses, clonidine is an alpha-2 adrenergic agonist at presynaptic receptors in the central nervous system where it inhibits sympathetic outflow, thus decreasing systemic vascular resistance, heart rate, and cardiac output.[15,74] In overdose, clonidine may stimulate peripheral alpha-1 adrenergic receptors with a resulting increase in peripheral vascular resistance and blood pressure.[25]

The cardiovascular effects of clonidine in overdose are dose-dependent, with centrally mediated cardiovascular effects including hypotension and bradycardia in modest ingestions.[18,25] In massive overdose, peripheral alpha adrenergic effects may predominate, resulting in severe hypertension with reflex bradycardia.[25] Central nervous system effects include miosis, lethargy, hypotonia, hyporeflexia, and drowsiness which may progress to coma. Seizures have also been reported, often occurring without warning in the first few hours after ingestion.[50] Waxing and waning depression of consciousness, with unpredictable respiratory depression and resulting apnea, are typical[4] and may be primary reasons for admission in a patient with clonidine poisoning.

Treatment of clonidine is mostly supportive. Decontamination must be done early on because absorption is rapid, and gastric lavage is preferred as unconsciousness may develop. Activated charcoal appears useful. Endotracheal intubation should be strongly considered for transport if mental status depression is present. Hypertension early in the course of large ingestions may be substantial; systolic blood pressures in excess of 200 mmHg have been reported.[25] The hypertensive phase is usually relatively short-lived and is best managed by short-acting antihypertensive agents such as sublingual nifedipine or intravenous nitroprusside.[24] Following the hypertensive phase, hypotension and bradycardia commonly occur, often requiring treatment with intravenous fluid administration and sometimes vasopressor agents such as dopamine.

Seizures associated with clonidine poisoning should be manageable with benzodiazepines. Initial enthusiasm for narcotic antagonists such as naloxone, based on clinical similarity between clonidine and narcotic overdoses, has not been supported by clinical experience.[8,42,62,120]

Digoxin

Digoxin, the digitalis preparation primarily used in the United States, remains one of the most frequently prescribed medications. Digoxin is an inhibitor of the Na+/K+ exchange pump in cell membranes throughout the body. Its therapeutic effect is mediated through an increase in sodium and calcium concentration in myocardial cells, resulting in an increase in the force of myocardial contraction. Digoxin increases vagal tone, decreases heart rate, and decreases cardiac impulse conduction. A decrease in refractory period coupled with an increase in automaticity result in an increased risk of dysrhythmia. In evaluation of digoxin intoxication, digoxin serum concentrations (therapeutic range 0.5 to 2.0 ng/mL) may be misleading because during distribution (within 6 hours of ingestion) digoxin concentrations may be substantially elevated.[107] Children, in general, are more resistant to the effects of digoxin and tolerate much higher serum digoxin concentrations than adults.

The toxic effects of digoxin can be divided into cardiac and extracardiac effects. Extracardiac effects include fatigue, changes in color vision, weakness, anorexia, nausea, and abdominal pain.[104] Electrolyte abnormalities are common. Hyperkalemia is a result of inhibition of the Na+/K+ pump at the cell membrane, resulting in accumulation of potassium in the extracellular fluid space, and may worsen arrhythmias. Hypokalemia (seen in chronic intoxication associated with diuretic use) increases myocardial sensitivity to the cardiac effects of high digoxin concentrations and should be carefully corrected.[106] Hypercalcemia and hypomagnesemia may also cause an increased sensitivity to digoxin effect.[91,106] Cardiac effects of digoxin toxicity include heart block, severe sinus bradycardia, and premature atrial and ventricular contractions, which may progress to atrial or ventricular fibrillation. Ventricular tachyarrhythmias are grave prognostic signs which are associated with a 50% risk of mortality.

Conventional treatment of digoxin intoxication is supportive. Digoxin is slowly absorbed from the gastrointestinal tract, and gastric emptying should be useful. Activated charcoal given immediately following ingestion binds up to 98% of an administered dose of digoxin.[77] Intravenous lidocaine or use of a transvenous or transthoracic pacemaker may be necessary to control ectopy. Bradyarrhythmias may respond to treatment with atropine. Hypokalemia and hypomagnesemia should be judiciously corrected.

Recently, sheep-derived, digoxin-specific antibody fragments (Fab) have become available for treatment of digoxin poisoning. Digoxin Fab avidly binds digoxin with subsequent complete inactivation of both cardiac and extracardiac digoxin effects and resolution of dysrhythmias and hyperkalemia within minutes.[105] The digoxin-Fab complex is eliminated in the urine. Indications for the use of digoxin Fab include the presence of life-threatening arrhythmias, serum potassium greater than 5.5 mEq/L, or history of large ingestion.[30] Thus, most patients ill enough to be transported probably should receive digoxin Fab.

Digoxin Fab binds an equivalent molar amount of digoxin. Dosing can be based upon estimation of the amount of digoxin ingested with administration of 40 mg (one vial) of Fab for each 0.6 mg digoxin. Alternatively, the serum digoxin concentration (SDC) may be used to calculate the body burden of digoxin with subsequent dosing of Fab in the same fashion.

$$\text{Digoxin body burden (mg)} = \text{SDC} \times 5.6 \times \text{Wt (kg)}/1000$$

Iron

A recent survey of childhood poisoning hazards suggested that iron intoxication presents the single greatest risk of death in the pediatric patient, as it is both toxic and readily available.[68] Many formulations of therapeutic iron and iron-containing multivitamins exist, with widely varying contents of elemental iron. Ingestions of less than 20 mg elemental iron/kg body weight are nontoxic, ingestions of 30-60 mg/kg are possibly toxic, while ingestions in excess of 150-200 mg/kg are potentially fatal. Iron sulfate or iron fumarate tablets (rather than multivitamins) present in the gut are sufficiently dense to be seen on abdominal radiographs.

The historical description of iron intoxication as four distinct stages has no physiological basis and is not very useful clinically. Immediately after iron ingestion there are prominent gastrointestinal symptoms including nausea, vomiting, and diarrhea which is often bloody, due to the corrosive effect of iron on the gastrointestinal mucosa. There is loss of intravascular fluid into the lumen of the bowel, due to the loss of mucosal and vascular integrity and weeping of fluid from submucosal capillaries. In severe intoxication, there is progressive hemodynamic compromise (largely from intravascular fluid depletion but also due to vasodilatation from ferritin and histamine release) and occasionally myocardial dysfunction, frank shock may occur.[94,115] Late sequelae include gastrointestinal stricture formation and hepatic injury.

Peak serum iron concentration measured 3-5 hours after ingestion is useful in evaluation of iron poisoning. Concentrations less than 300 μg/dL are normal, while concentrations greater than 500 μg/dL indicate intoxication. Laboratory correlates of serious iron intoxication include leukocytosis (white blood cell count in excess of 15,000 cells/μL) and serum glucose greater than 150 mg/dL.

Treatment of iron poisoning is largely supportive. Gastric emptying may be followed in severe cases by whole bowel irrigation, or rarely, gastrotomy.[64,112] Activated charcoal binds insignificant amounts of iron. Aggressive treatment of shock is critical and may require massive fluid resuscitation, often in excess of 100 mL/kg.[115] In massive overdose, direct cardiotoxic effects of iron may necessitate inotropic drugs such as dopamine.

The specific iron chelating agent deferoxamine binds free iron in the blood. The resulting ferrioxamine complex is eliminated in the urine, but the amount of iron removed is a small fraction of the ingested dose, suggesting that any protective effect is independent iron elimination. Deferoxamine is given by continuous infusion at 15 mg/kg/hour; hypotension may occur at higher doses. Indications for deferoxamine include 1) serum iron concentration greater than 500 μg/dL; 2) symptomatic ingestion with severe vomiting or bloody diarrhea and serum iron concentration greater than 300 μg/dL; 3) evidence of cardiovascular compromise, and 4) white blood cell count in excess of 15,000 cells/μL or serum glucose greater than 150 mg/dL. Ferrioxamine colors the urine a characteristic red-orange, and chelation should be continued until the color has disappeared. Although the use of deferoxamine has an intuitive appeal, a beneficial effect on outcome has not been proven.

Narcotics

Pure opiate receptor agonists (heroin, morphine, methadone, and codeine) have predictable effects in overdose, including miosis, sedation, cardiovascular depression (primarily orthostatic hypotension and syncope), and respiratory depression. The single most serious effect of narcotics is respiratory depression, resulting in hypoxia and hypercapnia. In addition, in overdose the development of noncardiogenic pulmonary edema (via an unknown mechanism) may compound the hypoxic effects of respiratory depression.[10,73,109] Less commonly considered drugs, such as diphenoxylate (Lomotil), propoxyphene (Darvon), pentazocine (Talwin), and meperidine (Demerol), may have somewhat different effects, including seizures (propoxyphene and meperidine), hallucinations, and dysphoria (partial narcotic agonists such as pentazocine).[28,48] Diphenoxylate, used in combination with atropine as Lomotil for control of diarrhea, is not very toxic in adults, but small doses may be fatal for young children.[21]

Most effects of narcotic overdose are effectively treated with maintenance of ventilation and general supportive care. Specific treatment of narcotic overdose involves reversal of the respiratory depressant effects of the narcotic with either a pure opiate antagonist such as naloxone, or partial agonist-antagonist such as nalbuphine. Dosing of naloxone or nalbuphine is empirical. A starting dose of 0.1 mg/kg of either drug is a reasonable starting point, followed by titration to effect. Both naloxone and nalbuphine have relatively short half-lives, significantly shorter than most narcotics. Both require either repeated dose or continuous infusion to maintain reversal of effect.

Tricyclic antidepressants

Ingestion of tricyclic antidepressants is a significant toxicological problem both because it is common (18,000 ingestions in 1991)[69] and because these compounds possess severe neurological and cardiovascular toxicity.[20,63] Toxicity is encountered at 10-30 mg/kg, and fatality is possible at 50 mg/kg. Toxicity has, however, been reported at smaller doses. Tricyclic antidepressants are rapidly and completely absorbed from the gut, metabolized slowly ($T_{1/2}$ 16-80 hours), and are extensively protein-bound (volumes of distribution 10-50 L/kg).[7]

Overdose with tricyclic antidepressants is characterized by rapid progression of signs and symptoms of intoxication. Central nervous signs include depression of consciousness (the sole sign of intoxication in as many as 50% of patients) and seizures, which are common.[20] Anticholinergic effects may produce mydriasis, dry mouth and eyes, and tachycardia. Tricyclic antidepressants in overdose possess severe cardiac toxicity, probably due to a quinidine-like effect on sodium transport in the myocardium, with resultant rhythm disturbances, including both atrial and ventricular dysrhythmias, and a depression of myocardial function,[88,116] the most life-threatening aspect of tricyclic antidepressant poisoning.

Gastric decontamination seems warranted, given the considerable toxicity of these drugs. This should not be delayed for transport unless it is impossible at the referring site or unless the trip is very brief. Activated charcoal is useful[78] and should be administered only after protecting the airway. Serious consideration should be given to intubation prior to transport for any tricyclic poisoning case which shows significant signs of intoxication, in case there is rapid progression of intoxication en route. Plasma concentrations of tricyclic antidepressants ≥1000 ng/mL are roughly associated with severe poisoning, although the electrocardiogram may be a more useful assessment. QRS duration ≥0.1 seconds is associated with signs of severe intoxication, including seizures and myocardial compromise.[12]

Anticholinergic signs of tricyclic antidepressant poisoning may be prominent but rarely or never require treatment. Respiratory depression occurs about as often with tricyclic antidepressants as with any other CNS depressant.[20] Seizures may be resistant to treatment; benzodiazepines have been used, although some have argued for phenytoin.[44] When seizures are resistant to treatment it may be reasonable to induce neuromuscular blockade prior to transport, to stop the adverse metabolic effects of excessive muscle activity and because it is difficult and unsafe to transport a vigorously convulsing child.

The cardiovascular alterations seen in tricyclic antidepressant poisoning include rhythm disturbances and circulatory shock. Sodium bicarbonate is the most effective treatment, particularly for the rhythm disturbance, and should be given as a bolus of 2-4 mEq/kg and then supplied as a constant infusion. The goal of administering sodium bicarbonate being to increase the blood pH to 7.5-7.55.[13,20] Proposed mechanisms of action for sodium bicarbonate include the pH-dependent increase in the degree of protein binding of the tricyclic antidepressants and antagonism of the effects on the inward sodium current in the cardiac myocytes.[20,98] Alkalinization via hyperventilation is also effective, although probably to a lesser extent.[88] Antidysrhythmic drugs have been used with varying degrees of success, and lidocaine and particularly phenytoin have been suggested.[44] Type Ia antidysrhythmic agents, such as quinidine and procainamide, have effects on the myocardium basically identical to those of the tricyclic antidepressants and are absolutely contraindicated.

Shock in tricyclic antidepressant poisoning is due largely to a decrement in myocardial performance, and administration of inotropic drugs may be life-saving.[13,57,116] Effects of tricyclic antidepressants on cellular transport of neurotransmitters (dopamine, norepinephrine) have suggested that direct-acting inotropes such as norepinephrine would be most effective,[53] but a recent study of experimental amitriptyline poisoning demonstrated that dopamine was also effective in reversing the shock of tricyclic antidepressant poisoning.[88,92,116]

The anticholinesterase drug physostigmine has been suggested as a specific antidote for tricyclic poisoning, but its use must be condemned.[79,87] Despite the presence of anticholinergic signs, the major toxic effects of tricyclic antidepressants are not related to the atropine-like effects, and it is illogical to presume that physostigmine would reverse them.[20,79] Reported adverse effects of physostigmine in tricyclic poisoning include sudden death from cardiac asystole.[87]

Theophylline

Despite current controversy about the role of theophylline in the management of asthma it remains widely prescribed, particularly in sustained-release forms. Theophylline, a methylxanthine closely related to caffeine, possesses a narrow margin of safety and is capable of severe toxicity in overdose (39 fatalities reported in 1991).[36,69,100] Its half-life varies from 3.5 hrs in young children to 8 hours in adults, with first-order kinetics at therapeutic doses approaching zero-order kinetics in severe intoxication.[22,36,47,89] Actions include inhibition of phosphodiesterase, inhibition of calcium uptake, blockade of adenosine receptors, and increase in blood catecholamine concentrations by inducing release of endogenous stores, but the relationship between these properties and the pharmacological and toxicological effects of theophylline is unclear.[22,30,36,89]

In overdose, theophylline exerts toxic effects on several organ systems. Nausea and vomiting occur both from gastric irritation (in an oral overdose) and from stimulation of the central nervous system.[22,36] Cardiovascular effects include tachycardia and a variety of supraventricular and ventricular dysrhythmias; these tend to be worse in older adults than in children.[22,36] In severe intoxication, there may be hypotension from vasodilatation despite an increase in cardiac output.[22] Central nervous system signs are prominent, including tremors and agitation. Seizures are common and indicate severe intoxication.[22,36] There may be a variety of electrolyte and acid-base disturbances, including hypokalemia (most commonly), hypercalcemia, hypophosphatemia, hyperglycemia, and metabolic acidosis.[22,36,47,100]

Theophylline plasma concentrations above 20 μg/mL are considered toxic; coincidentally, this is also the top of the usual therapeutic range.[100] Significant toxicity becomes likely at plasma concentrations greater than 35 μg/mL in older adults and greater than 50 μg/mL in children. Toxic doses may be a small as 10-20 mg/kg, but the acute toxicity of a dose may be difficult to predict because sustained-release preparations may result in somewhat delayed toxicity.[22,30] Plasma theophylline concentrations provide only a rough indication of toxicity because some patients (especially children) being only mildly affected at blood concentrations of 100 μg/mL, while others are severely intoxicated with blood concentrations as low as 40 μg/mL.[100]

Given the considerable toxicity of theophylline, gastric evacuation is of obvious value.[36,47] Theophylline is avidly bound by activated charcoal, and volunteer studies have shown a significant reduction in theophylline half-life with multiple-dose activated charcoal.[36,47] Since theophylline intoxication tends to induce vomiting, however, there may be practical difficulties in activated charcoal administration and gastric lavage, especially during transport.

Consideration should be given to endotracheal intubation prior to transport, because theophylline-poisoned patients are prone to both seizures and vomiting, presenting obvious risks for pulmonary aspiration. Rhythm disturbances and the hypotension occasionally seen in severe intoxication are believed to be due to beta-2 adrenoreceptor stimulation, and successful use of propranolol has been reported.[22,36,85,86] The ultra short acting cardioselective beta-blocker esmolol has been used to good effect in an animal model of theophylline poisoning.[35] Inotropic/pressor agents may be useful for treating severe hypotension, and drugs such as norepinephrine with prominent alpha-agonist activity would seem better choices.

Seizures due to theophylline intoxication can reasonably be treated with benzodiazepines or barbiturates, while phenytoin appears to be less effective.[36,37,86] However, seizures may be resistant to drug therapy and serve as a marker of clinically severe poisoning and increased risk of mortality.[36,37,85,100] For transport purposes, they should be considered an indication for intubation and control of the airway. It may be necessary to induce neuromuscular blockade for safe transport and to ablate the adverse metabolic effects of excess seizure activity until definitive therapy can be provided at the receiving institution.[37]

Theophylline is efficiently removed via extracorporeal blood-cleansing techniques, and charcoal hemoperfusion yields a 4- to 6-fold increase in theophylline clearance.[36,47] Standard hemodialysis is roughly half as effective.[85,86] Decisions and preparations for these procedures should be made while the patient is en route, since they may dictate the destination of the transport. Suggested indications vary but include plasma theophylline concentration ≥100 μg/mL in an acute overdose, ≥60 μg/mL in chronic intoxication, or levels ≥20 μg/mL in patients with signs of severe toxicity (intractable seizures, cardiac rhythm disturbances).[37,47,86,100]

Cocaine

Cocaine abuse has increased greatly following the introduction of the cheap, smokable, highly addictive "crack" form of the drug about 10 years ago, although intravenous injection and "snorting" of cocaine are still practiced.[71,76] The recent much-publicized deaths of prominent sports figures following cocaine abuse serves to illustrate the dangers of this drug.[23,70]

The pediatric transport team might encounter cocaine intoxication in several guises. Adolescents may intentionally abuse cocaine.[71,121] Presence of cocaine in the home is an obvious risk factor for accidental poisoning, and passive inhalation of crack smoke has apparently caused seizures and sudden death in infants and young children who appear to be highly susceptible to this form of cocaine.[71,121] Finally, cocaine passes readily into breast milk, and intoxication of an infant in this fashion has been reported.[71,121]

Cocaine has three pharmacological effects. It is a local anesthetic, a potent central nervous system stimulant, and inhibits reuptake of neurotransmitters including norepinephrine and dopamine, leading to catecholamine excess.[11,39,76] The neurological and cardiovascular toxicity of cocaine is thought to be related to the latter two effects. An excessive dose of cocaine induces marked neural stimulation manifested by agitation, restlessness, tremors, anxiety, and occasional paranoid ideation.[11,39] Seizures are the most common serious effect.[70,76] Cardiovascular effects are presumably due to adrenergic overdrive and include hypertension, rhythm disturbances, and intense vasoconstriction.[11,39,70,76] Chest pain is common, and myocardial infarction has been reported in individuals without underlying coronary artery disease.[11,39,70]

The most common manifestation of severe acute cocaine toxicity is sudden death, presumably due to cardiac rhythm disturbances or convulsions with resultant respiratory arrest; some acutely intoxicated patients do arrive at medical facilities alive.[11,70,76] Treatment of cocaine intoxication is symptomatic and reactive in nature, and there is no specific antidote. Gastric decontamination is rarely indicated because ingestion is not a common mode of abuse. The patient with depressed consciousness may reasonably be given naloxone, since coadministration of cocaine with opiates ("speedball") is occasionally practiced.[76] Signs of intoxication abate rapidly, owing to the rapid metabolism of cocaine. Even severely affected individuals may recover quickly enough so that hospital admission is unnecessary.[23] Sedation may be necessary prior to initiating transport, since cocaine-intoxicated individuals will not likely be calmed by the noisy, stimulus-rich transport environment.[39] Seizures can be treated with benzodiazepines, but sustained seizures may require endotracheal intubation and controlled ventilation, which as always should be considered before transport proper begins.[39,76]

Hypertension can often be managed expectantly with sedation only because the time course of intoxication is only a few hours.[11] Should drug therapy of blood pressure be necessary, propranolol has been used successfully,[23] although others state that this may be harmful and may actually worsen hypertension.[70,76,90] Vasodilators, such as nitroprusside, or an alpha-adrenergic blocking agent, such as phentolamine, might also be rational choices.[70,76] Case reports exist of the successful use of labetolol,[70] but the relatively weak alpha-adrenergic blocking effect of this agent would argue against its use.[23,39]

Ethanol

Ethanol, present in alcoholic beverages and in products such as mouthwash, cologne, and medications, possesses considerable toxicity at excessive doses.[49] It is rapidly absorbed from the stomach and small intestine,[3,30] has a modest volume of distribution of 0.7 L/kg for children, and is eliminated according to zero-order kinetics.[3,30] Ethanol is primarily a CNS depressant, although at large doses there may be vasodilatation, myocardial depression, and occasionally cardiac rhythm disturbances.[30] Hypoglycemia is common in children and was seen in 24% of a series of pediatric patients; it is probably the cause of enthanol-related seizures.[49,65] For children, ingestion of roughly 0.4 mL/kg of absolute ethanol will yield a plasma concentration of 50 mg/dL (0.05%).[30] Plasma concentrations of 50 mg/dL or less are typically asymptomatic, with euphoria and excitement occuring at 100-250 mg/dL.[3] At higher concentrations there is progressive interference with mentation. Coma occurs at concentrations greater than roughly 400 mg/dL, and death from respiratory depression is possible beyond about 500 mg/dL.[3,30] In adults, blood ethanol concentrations fall at roughly 15 mg/dL/hr, however, in children blood ethanol levels fall much more rapidly, 28 mg/dL/hr.[65] The relationship between blood concentrations and clinical toxicity is inconstant, however, and children may have exaggerated signs and symptoms of intoxication, as they are usually ethanol-naive.[3]

Even severely intoxicated patients should improve with basic cardiopulmonary supportive care. Naloxone is useful only if opiates are also present.[3] Gastric decontamination is not usually of value because ethanol is so rapidly absorbed. Activated charcoal appears to be ineffective.[30] Close attention should be paid to fluid and electrolyte status and particularly to blood glucose; 50% dextrose should be given to patients with altered mental status.[65] For comatose patients, respiratory depression is possible and protection of the airway is paramount, since vomiting is common in acute ethanol ingestion. Chronic alcoholics may manifest a number of life-threatening problems, including abstinence syndromes, hepatic cirrhosis, and delirium tremens, but these are of no concern in acute intoxication in a child.[3]

Methanol

Methanol may be found in most households, usually in windshield washing and deicing solutions for automotive use. Childhood ingestions are usually accidental, but mass poisonings have occurred in adults, when methanol has contaminated or been substituted for ethanol-containing beverages.

Methanol is rapidly absorbed from the gastrointestinal tract, with peak plasma concentrations occurring within 30 minutes to several hours; vapor inhalation and dermal absorption occasionally cause intoxication.[1,14,30,67] Methanol is slowly cleared from the circulation with a half-life of 14-20 hours, increasing to perhaps 24-30 hours in severe intoxication and 30-35 hours with ethanol therapy.[30] It is oxidized by the enzyme alcohol dehydrogenase to formaldehyde with rapid subsequent conversion to formic acid,[1,67] which is primarily responsible for methanol toxicity.[1,110] There is severe metabolic acidosis with formate as the principal abnormal anion. Lactic acidosis may occur late in severe methanol poisoning, possibly due to interference with oxidative metabolism.[54,67]

Methanol is extremely toxic, and there does not appear to be any safe dose. Death in an adult has resulted from ingestion of 15 ml of a 40% solution, although even a 500 ml ingestion may be survivable with prompt, aggressive care.[30] Significant toxicity is said to correlate with a blood concentration ≥50 mg/dL, but patients who present to medical care late may have severe acidosis and toxicity despite lower levels, as the methanol may have been largely converted to its toxic metabolites. On ingestion methanol is said to have central nervous system depressant effects somewhat similar to those of ethanol with clouding of the sensorium.[1,110] There is then characteristically a variable latent period of perhaps 12-24 hours before symptoms of methanol toxicity manifest which is believed to correspond to the slow metabolic conversion of methanol to formic acid.[110] Initial symptoms include headache, nausea, epigastric pain, and a feeling of general unwellness.[14,110] The patient may become agitated and combative. Vital signs are frequently normal, and there are no severe cardiopulmonary effects, although pulmonary edema has been reported as an autopsy finding.[1] Ocular damage is a prominent and serious effect. Visual symptoms are prominent and include blurred vision, double vision, and occasionally total loss of vision. Fundoscopic findings are frequently abnormal,[14,110] and ocular toxicity is apparently mediated by formate.[54,67,110] In severe cases, there may be permanent visual changes even with proper treatment.[30,110] Metabolic acidosis is prominent and severe.[110] In fatal cases there is progressive onset of coma with death resulting from respiratory arrest. There may be permanent neurological impairment in survivors. Necrosis of the putamen and cerebral edema may be found on autopsy.[110]

Treatment of methanol poisoning is aimed at preventing the formation of toxic metabolic products. Gastric decontamination via lavage may be useful if it can be performed within 2 hours of ingestion, while charcoal appears ineffective.[30] Central nervous system depression and respiratory compromise are possible, and airway protection and ventilation must be ensured. Ethanol is an effective antidote because its affinity for alcohol dehydrogenase is as much as 9-fold greater than that of methanol,[1] so that the oxidation of methanol to toxic metabolites can be effectively blocked.[84,110] Indications for ethanol therapy include significant methanol ingestion (≥0.4 mL/kg) pending measurement of blood methanol concentration, metabolic acidosis, methanol blood concentration ≥50 mg/dL, and any symptoms referable to methanol toxicity.[54,110] Adequate protection is provided by plasma ethanol concentration of 100 mg/dL, and this can be achieved by giving 0.6 g/kg ethanol loading dose followed by 66-154 mg/kg/hr maintenance.[54] Oral administration of ethanol is effective, but in children intravenous administration will likely be easier; a 10% solution can be prepared by addition of 60 ml absolute ethanol to 500 ml 5% dextrose.[54] Ethanol should be continued until the blood methanol concentration is below 20-30 mg/dL.[30,54] Since ethanol is also a central nervous system depressant, close attention must be paid to respiratory status during ethanol therapy. At the time they undergo interhospital transport, many children who have ingested methanol may be asymptomatic; however, a lack of symptoms should not dissuade one from beginning ethanol therapy in this setting.[1] Formic acid is metabolized to carbon dioxide and water via a folate-dependent mechanism. As a result some have suggested high-dose folate administration to encourage this process.[1,67] Patients with severe acidosis should undergo alkali therapy for correction, since correction of pH to values ≥7.35 often results in marked improvement in visual symptoms.[54,110]

Hemodialysis is accepted therapy for methanol poisoning, since methanol has a long half-life which is further prolonged by ethanol therapy and formate is also removed.[110] Hemodialysis is indicated for patients with methanol blood concentrations ≥50 mg/dL or other signs of significant toxicity, including visual disturbances and acidosis. Hemodialysis should be initiated as soon as possible, so it may be wise to begin arrangements for this as the transport is in progress.

Ethylene glycol

Ethylene glycol is a sweet-tasting substance that is most commonly found as the major component of antifreeze for the cooling systems of motor vehicles. From the toxicological standpoint, it is similar to methanol, being a central nervous system depressant that is metabolized by alcohol dehydrogenase to toxic products, and can be treated by ethanol administration and hemodialysis.[117]

Ethylene glycol is rapidly absorbed from the gastrointestinal tract with peak levels occurring in 1-4 hours. The minimal lethal dose is said to be 1-1.5 mL/kg.[30,117] The half-life of ethylene glycol in blood is approximate 3-5 hours, but is greatly prolonged during ethanol therapy.[30] Ethylene glycol is initially oxidized via alcohol dehydrogenase to glycoaldehyde, but its further metabolism is not well characterized; glycolate and oxalate are formed, however.[54] Metabolic acidosis occurs largely due to glycolate, although there is some contribution of lactic acidosis due to interference in cellular metabolism.[54] The role of oxalate in ethylene glycol intoxication is less clear. Calcium oxalate is insoluble, and calcium oxalate crystals can be found in many tissues at autopsy. The contribution of calcium oxalate to overall toxicity is uncertain, although deposition in the kidneys may be the cause of renal failure observed in this condition.[54]

The initial signs of ethylene glycol ingestion are disturbances in central nervous system function similar to those of ethanol intoxication, followed in 4-12 hours by signs and symptoms related to toxic metabolic products.[117] Metabolic acidosis results in hyperventilation.[14,117] Chelation of calcium by oxalate may lead to signs of hypocalcemia, including neuromuscular irritability and cardiac rhythm disturbances.[54] Myocardial failure and pulmonary involvement have been reported in severe cases, although the mechanisms of these effects is unknown.[14,54,117] Twenty-four to 72 hours after ingestion, signs of renal involvement appear, including oliguria, acute tubular necrosis, and frank renal failure, which may be permanent.[30,54,117]

As ethylene glycol poisoning may result in central nervous system depression and respiratory compromise, management of the airway must be ensured. Gastric decontamination should be assayed, given the considerable toxicity of ethylene glycol.[117] Activated charcoal administration also seems reasonable, although there is no general agreement on its usefulness.[14,30,117] As noted above for methanol, ethanol treatment (plasma concentration of 100 mg/dL) is effective in preventing the formation of the toxic metabolic products of ethylene glycol, again based on the greater affinity of ethanol for alcohol dehydrogenase (100-fold vs. ethylene glycol). Good urine output must be ensured by adequate fluid administration. Acidosis is thought to worsen the effects of ethylene glycol poisoning, and some recommend aggressive alkali treatment to correct pH, although massive doses may be required.[54] Calcium can be given to correct symptomatic hypocalcemia but should be used cautiously to avoid excessive calcium oxalate deposition in the kidney and other tissues.[54]

Hemodialysis effectively removes ethylene glycol and its metabolites, as well as effectively correcting many of the metabolic abnormalities such as acidosis and hypocalcemia; it should be combined with ethanol treatment. Hemodialysis has been recommended for every patient with confirmed ethylene glycol poisoning. If such patients initially present to an institution which does not offer this service for children, transfer to a hospital where hemodialysis is performed with ongoing ethanol treatment, is an appropriate use of transport services.[54]

Salicylates

Salicylates, principally aspirin, are cheap and useful analgesic, antipyretic, and antiinflammatory drugs, and as such are found in most homes. The use of aspirin for children and the number of childhood aspirin poisonings have decreased in recent years, as acetaminophen has become more popular. However, salicylate poisoning remains a relatively common event, and fatalities continue to occur.[17,75] Although aspirin is the most obvious source of salicylates, other forms may contain dangerous concentrations; as little as 4 ml of methyl salicylate (oil of wintergreen) may be fatal to a child.[30]

Salicylates are readily absorbed from the gastrointestinal tract, although absorption may be slowed in overdose.[81] The volume of distribution is small at 0.1-0.2 L/kg, but may be increased in overdose.[30,81] Metabolism is first-order at therapeutic doses with a plasma half-life of 2-4.5 hours, but half-life can be greatly prolonged in overdose due to saturation of major metabolic pathways.[30,81]

Salicylates in overdose have prominent toxic metabolic effects, and may result in severe electrolyte and acid-base disturbances, as well as effects on central nervous system function. Early in an acute overdose there is nausea and vomiting from gastrointestinal irritation. There is direct stimulation of the respiratory centers, and hyperventilation with respiratory alkalosis is the first sign of mild salicylate poisoning. Hyperthermia is common in children and, in combination with hyperventilation, results in dehydration.[17,81] Tinnitus is common. Coma and convulsions are seen in severe intoxication and are grave prognostic indicators.[30,81] Noncardiogenic pulmonary edema may be seen in severe cases and may be more common in children than adults; the mechanism is unknown.[30,81] There is uncoupling of oxidative phosphorylation with resultant derangements of substrate metabolism and defective cellular energy production.[17] Metabolic acidosis is prominent in severe cases and is presumably related to excessive production of organic acids from interference in cellular metabolism.[17,30,81]

Chronic intoxication may result from salicylate doses only modestly greater than proper therapeutic doses, given over several days. Such patients may have clinically severe toxicity at rather modest plasma salicylate concentrations. Assessment of toxicity is based on the history, clinical signs, and plasma salicylate intoxication. Acute ingestion of 150 mg/kg is generally nontoxic, with mild toxicity expected in the range 150-300 mg/kg. Three hundred to 500 mg/kg of salicylate will result in serious toxicity, and fatality is possible at doses in excess of 500 mg/kg.[81] Children are more susceptible than adults to salicylate intoxication, with greater likelihood of severe metabolic acidosis and pulmonary edema. Plasma concentrations are routinely measured and are of assistance in management.[17] Mild intoxication, characterized by hyperventilation and respiratory alkalosis, is seen at plasma concentrations of up to 25 mg/dL.[81] The appearance of metabolic acidosis indicates a moderately severe intoxication, commonly with plasma concentrations in excess of 35 mg/dL.[81] Severe central nervous systems signs, including coma and seizures, are correlated with plasma concentrations ≥60-75 mg/dL and signal a worrisome prognosis.[81] The Done nomogram relates severity to plasma salicylate concentration and time after ingestion,[26] but unfortunately tends to overestimate toxicity, is not useful until 6 hours after ingestion, and cannot be used for a chronic or sustained-release ingestion.[29] (Figure 31-1)

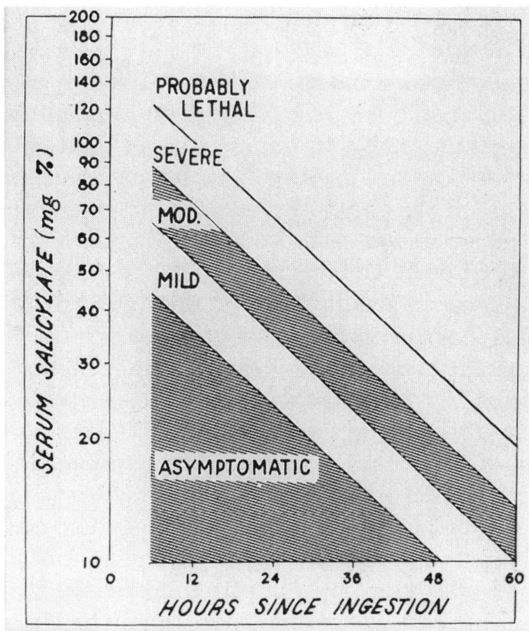

Fig. 31-1. Nomogram relating serum salicylate level to severity of intoxication at varying intervals after acute ingestion of single doses of aspirin. Nomogram starts at six hours to ensure that levels will not be interpreted before they have reached their peak; it can be used earlier if more than one level is obtained to establish that level is on decline. From: Done AK: Aspirin overdosage: incidence, diagnosis, and management, *Pediatrics* 62:890-7, 1978.

Because salicylate absorption may be prolonged in overdose, patients will frequently arrive with unabsorbed drug in the gastrointestinal tract. Gastric decontamination via lavage or induced emesis is thus useful, although many patients will already be vomiting. Salicylates are moderately bound by activated charcoal, and multiple-dose charcoal is reportedly beneficial, since there may be ongoing absorption for some time after ingestion.[61,78,81] Airway protection for transport is important because vomiting may occur along with seizures and coma.

Management of fluid and electrolyte balance is of primary importance in salicylate intoxication. The various metabolic effects frequently combine to cause dehydration, and fluid should be generously given to result in good urine flow for elimination of the toxin (2 mL/kg/hr, or 50 mL/hr for an adult).[81] Forced diuresis, however, does not appear to appreciably enhance salicylate elimination.[81] Bicarbonate administration is the mainstay of treatment; alkalinization of the urine (pH ≥ 7.4) greatly enhances the elimination of salicylate owing to an ion-trapping mechanism.[30,81] Also, uncorrected acidosis leads to increased penetration of salicylate into tissues, particularly the brain, with resultant accentuation of the central nervous system and metabolic abnormalities. Alkalinization can be accomplished by rapid administration of 1-2 mEq/kg of bicarbonate followed by 0.5 mEq/kg/hr. Bicarbonate dose should be initiated prior to transport and ongoing during the transport proper.

Hemodialysis is effective in removing salicylate, although the majority of patients respond to more conservative methods. Suggested indications include plasma concentration ≥ 100mg/dL or clinically severe intoxication,[55] although some have suggested that it be used more liberally.[17]

Carbon monoxide

Carbon monoxide, an odorless, colorless gas which is a product of incomplete combustion, is the leading cause of poisoning fatality in the U.S., with some estimating up to 4,000 deaths yearly.[30,97,114] Daily low-level exposure is largely from cigarette smoke and automobile exhaust, but poisoning results mostly from dwelling fires and defective home heating devices. Methylene chloride, a common component of paint removal compounds, is metabolized to carbon monoxide and is an occasional cause of intoxication.[93]

Carbon monoxide binds to hemoglobin with an avidity 200-240 times that of oxygen, so that breathing air with a even small proportion of carbon monoxide may rapidly result in a large proportion of carboxyhemoglobin, which is then unavailable for oxygen transport.[30,52,114] Ambient carbon monoxide levels as low as 100 parts per million can result in detectable symptoms and significant carboxyhemoglobin levels within 2 hours.[30]

It has become clear that the toxicity of carbon monoxide is not adequately explained by its binding to hemoglobin and interference with oxygen transport.[2,40,114] Carboxyhemoglobin levels are useful in confirming the diagnosis of carbon monoxide poisoning and correlate to some extent with minor symptoms such as headache and nausea, but are not useful in predicting severe toxicity.[40] Carbon monoxide does bind to proteins other than hemoglobin, including myoglobin and cytochrome oxidase, and there is speculation that it may thus interfere with cellular metabolism.[40,97,114] Also, there is some evidence that the neurological toxicity of carbon monoxide is mediated by lipid peroxidation of cell membranes in the brain.[40,114] However, the contributions of these putative mechanisms of carbon monoxide toxicity are not currently known.

The organs most affected by carbon monoxide poisoning are the central nervous system and the heart, the latter less so in children because they lack preexisting coronary artery disease. The signs and symptoms of mild poisoning are not specific and suggest vague unwellness, including headache, nausea, and malaise. Carboxyhemoglobin levels of 20% are typical.[52,97] Poisoning of moderate severity, characterized by visual changes and altered mentation, is associated with carboxyhemoglobin levels of 30-40%.[52,97] Higher carboxyhemoglobin levels are associated with seizures and frank coma, with lethality associated with levels in excess of 50-70%.[52,97] As noted above there is only a loose relationship between carboxyhemoglobin levels and clinical status. Because the clinical signs of carbon monoxide poisoning are nonspecific, diagnosis may require some index of suspicion.

Oxygen administration is the traditional mainstay of therapy for carbon monoxide poisoning. The half-life of carboxyhemoglobin, 4-5 hours in air, is markedly reduced in 100% oxygen for 50-90 minutes.[52,97] All patients with confirmed or possible carbon monoxide exposure should have 100% oxygen applied by face mask immediately and during transport until proper evaluation can be completed. Patients who have altered sensorium should be electively intubated for this purpose as soon as possible. The elimination of carboxyhemoglobin can be further speeded by hyperbaric oxygen therapy; the half-life is 23 minutes at 3 atmospheres pure oxygen. The efficacy and mechanism of action of hyperbaric oxygen for carbon monoxide poisoning has not been proven, although there are numerous anecdotal reports of its benefit,[114] and it has become an accepted treatment for this condition.[2,40,60,118] Since hyperbaric oxygen therapy is not widely available, a decision on its use must be made as arrangements for transport are underway, since this will often determine the destination of the transport. Hyperbaric oxygen treatment is advised for any patient who has significant central nervous system toxicity, such as altered mentation or coma, as well as cardiovascular signs, although these would likely be less common in children.[97] Although it would seem to be most useful in the first hours after intoxication, some have claimed it may still be beneficial as many as 20 hours later.[52]

Carbon monoxide poisoning often does not occur in isolation. Many patients who are in house fires will have burns and severe pulmonary injury from inhalation of other toxic gases including hydrogen cyanide, and hypoxemic respiratory failure and the adult respiratory distress syndrome may be seen.[40,113]

Carbon monoxide poisoning may have a grave prognosis. Most fatalities occur at the scene, but there is significant mortality and morbidity even in patients who reach the hospital alive. As many as 11-40% may have permanent neurological sequelae, particularly neuropsychiatric abnormalities.[30,97,118] Reports of patients who seemingly recover fully, only to have late neurological deterioration several days or even weeks later, are puzzling and worrisome.

Acetaminophen

Acetaminophen has become the most widely analgesic/antipyretic for children. Along with this widespread use has come increased incidence of overdosage, with over 100,000 exposures in 1991.[30,58,69] The major toxicity of acetaminophen is hepatic necrosis. Acetaminophen is readily absorbed from the stomach, with peak levels at 1 hour at therapeutic doses. Overdose may prolong absorption so that peak levels may not occur for as long as 4 hours.[30] The volume of distribution is roughly 0.75-1.0 L/kg, and elimination half-life at therapeutic doses is approximately 2-3 hours. At therapeutic doses, acetaminophen is primarily metabolized by sulfation and glucuronide formation (the former predominates in children, while the latter pathway predominates in adults). Perhaps 5% is oxidized by P450 mixed-function oxidases to a reactive metabolite which is rapidly detoxified by conjugation with glutathione.[30,58,96] In overdose, relatively larger amounts are thought to be shunted through the P450 pathway, with resultant depletion of glutathione stores and subsequent accumulation of the reactive intermediate which then damages hepatocytes via covalent bonding with cell components.[34,58,66,96,103]

Liver toxicity may be expected with acute ingestions of more than 150 mg/kg; children appear to be less susceptible than adults.[34,66] Initial clinical symptoms of acetaminophen overdose may be relatively mild, including mild gastric upset, nausea, and malaise. Usually there is no cardiopulmonary compromise, although central nervous system depression, frank coma, and circulatory shock have been reported in massive overdoses.[66] Following this, there is generally a period of 1-2 days without symptoms, even in cases in which severe liver toxicity will subsequently develop, although there may be elevation in transaminase values. Beginning about 3-4 days post-ingestion there may be signs of progressive liver involvement, including jaundice and coagulopathy and signs of hepatic encephalopathy such as confusion, lethargy, and coma. Patients who recover after hepatic toxicity generally do so completely, and signs of chronic liver dysfunction are unusual.

Several antidotes have been studied, including methionine, cysteamine, and N-acetylcystine, which is the only antidote approved for use in the U.S.[58,96] (Table 31-2). It evidently serves as a sulfur donor to replenish glutathione and thus prevent formation of the toxic metabolite.[34,58,96,103] The prescribed dosage regimen is a loading dose of 140 mg/kg, followed by 17 doses of 70 mg/kg, given every 4 hours so that the treatment requires 72 hours.[96] A number of studies have demon-

TABLE 31-2 ANTIDOTES

Agent	Antidote	Other specific treatment
Tricyclic antidepressants	Fab antibody fragments (investigational) (physostigmine is *not* antidotal)	Alkalinization
Organophosphate insecticides	Atropine, pralidoxime	
Methanol	Ethanol	Hemodialysis
Ethylene glycol	Ethanol	Hemodialysis
Digoxin	Digibind® Fab fragments	
Acetaminophen	N-acetyl cysteine	
Iron	Deferoxamine (efficacy not clear)	
Lead (acute)	2,3-dimercaptosuccinic acid (DMSA, succimer)	
	EDTA (Ethylenediamine-tetraacetate)	
Cyanide	cyanide antidote kit (sodium nitrite/sodium thiosulfate)	
Opiates	Naloxone	
Benzodiazepines	Flumazenil	

strated virtually total protection against hepatotoxicity if N-acetyl cysteine is given within 8-10 hours of acetaminophen ingestion, with some benefit at 16 hours and possibly as far as 24 hours from ingestion.[58,95,96,103] Although N-acetyl cysteine is quite nontoxic, its tendency to cause nausea and vomiting is a significant practical problem in oral administration. Intravenous N-acetyl cysteine is used in Europe and Canada and appears to be effective but is not currently approved in the U.S.[58,102] There may be some benefit from N-acetyl cysteine up to 36 hours after ingestion. Given its minimal toxicity and the grim prospect of hepatic necrosis, one can easily justify its administration even late in the course of acute poisoning.[34]

Treatment of acetaminophen poisoning involves the usual decontamination measures, but with an eye toward the administration of the specific antidote N-N-acetyl cysteine. Gastric lavage should be attempted if the patient presents within 4 hours or so. Induced emesis probably should not be done, since nausea is already a problem with N-acetyl cysteine administration. Administration of charcoal is a bit controversial. Activated charcoal does effectively bind acetaminophen, but there has been concern that it might also bind N-acetyl cysteine, thus rendering the antidote ineffective. Recent data suggests that the effectiveness of N-acetyl cysteine is only somewhat reduced in the presence of activate charcoal, so that some references do recommend concurrent activated charcoal administration.[78] Given the excellent effectiveness of N-acetyl cysteine in preventing hepatotoxicity, its administration should assume top priority (compared with gastric emptying and charcoal administration) in early management of acetaminophen poisoning.

A nomogram has been constructed by Rumack and others to aid in assessing acetaminophen toxicity which predicts hepatotoxicity based on the plasma acetaminophen concentration and the time elapsed since ingestion.[96] The nomogram begins at 4 hours postingestion and is not useful before that time. A fair number of patients, particularly young children, manifest no hepatotoxicity despite plasma concentrations in the toxic range.[34,95]

Many, perhaps most, patients will undergo transport before acetaminophen plasma concentration is known (Figure 31-2). N-acetyl cysteine administration should begin while awaiting this initial value in most cases because of the effect of time on the efficacy of this treatment, unless one is sure that the result can be reported well before 8 hours have elapsed since ingestion.

Phenothiazines and other neuroleptics

The term neuroleptics is used to denote several classes of drugs useful in the treatment of psychoses; they are also known as major tran-

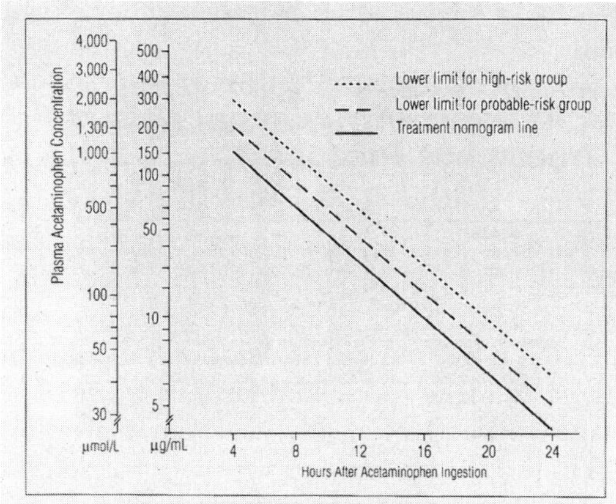

Fig. 31-2. Nomogram lines used to define risk groups, according to initial plasma concentrations. From: Smilkstein MJ and others: Acetaminophen overdose: a 48-hour intravenous N-acetylcysteine treatment protocol, *Ann Emerg Med* 20:1058–63, 1991.

quilizers and antipsychotic drugs. Based on their chemical structure, these agents are divided into several classes, including the prototypic phenothiazines (chlorpromazine, thioridazine), the structurally similar thioxanthines (thiothixene), and the structurally dissimilar butryophenones (haloperidol), as well as others. Despite structural variations, these agents have common effects both therapeutically and in overdose. As these drugs are widely used, poisoning exposures are fairly common (11,000 in 1991), however 80% of reported ingestions occur outside the pediatric age group and are commonly suicidal gestures or attempts.[9,69] When they are taken in isolation, lethality of neuroleptic overdosage is fairly low.[9] Most reported deaths (21 in 1991)[69] have resulted when other substances were taken in combination with the neuroleptic agent.

Pharmacokinetics of these agents is complex, but there is similarity amongst the group. Oral absorption is incomplete (32% for chlorpromazine), with large volumes of distribution (20 L/kg) and extensive protein binding.[43] Elimination half-lives are long (18 hours for chlorpromazine), and there are many active metabolites.[30]

The neuroleptics have a variety of pharmacological activities important in overdose. They are known to be dopaminergic receptor blockers in the central nervous system, although the importance of this action in overdose is unclear. They resemble the tricyclic antidepressants in that they exert both anticholinergic effects and a quinidine-like membrane depressant effect;[72] however, the severity of these effects seems much less than with the tricyclic antidepressants. There is also peripheral blockade of the α-adrenoreceptor, resulting in vasodilatation. In the central nervous system, the neuroleptics depress the reticular activating system and cause sedation.

As noted above, pure neuroleptic overdose is rarely fatal, especially in children.[5,72] In the clinical presentation of neuroleptic overdose, central nervous system depression is prominent. However, respiratory depression sufficient to require assisted ventilation is unusual unless there is coingestion of another central nervous system depressant. Children may be more likely to manifest this. Seizures may occur but are most common in patients with a preexisting seizure disorder. Anticholinergic effects may result in pupillary dilatation and sinus tachycardia, and these are a clue to the diagnosis in an unknown but suspected neuroleptic overdose. However, in many cases of severe phenothiazine intoxication the pupils are actually small, possible related to α-blockade.[9,72] The most frequent cardiovascular sign is hypotension, especially with the phenothiazines, and is largely due to vasodilatation related to α-adrenergic blockade. Changes in the ECG are related to conduction delays and include QRS and QT prolongation. These are most common with thioridazine, less so with chlorpromazine, and rare with haloperidol.[9,30,72,80] Ventricular dysrhythmias have been reported, most commonly with thioridazine.[27,30,80] However, cardiac rhythm disturbances are neither as predictable nor as severe as those seen with the tricyclic antidepressants, despite the pharmacological similarities notes above. Most cases in the literature are anecdotal case reports. Although fatalities have been reported,[27] serious cardiotoxicity is actually infrequent even in massive neuroleptic overdose and is difficult to predict.[9,43]

In addition to the above noted effects of

overdose, neuroleptics cause a variety of other adverse effects which may occur with either therapeutic or excessive doses, but which nonetheless are important events requiring therapy. Most important among these are acute dystonic reactions which children are particularly susceptible to, including torticollis, upward gaze (oculogyric crisis), grimacing, or opisthotonus.[30] Acute dystonic reactions may occur with all classes of neuroleptics but are most common with agents having the least anticholinergic effects (such as haloperidol).[99] Acute dystonia as a presenting sign in a child should strongly suggest neuroleptic exposure.[38,101] Other motor manifestations such as hyperkinesia may be seen but would not likely be a reason for patient transport. Similarly, adverse effects such as neuroleptic-induced Parkinson's-like syndrome or extrapyramidal reactions (tardive dyskinesia) may be most troublesome in patients receiving neuroleptics therapeutically, but are not immediately life-threatening and thus probably will not motivate transport of the patient. The neuroleptic malignant syndrome is an unusual but potentially fatal complication of neuroleptic agents characterized by increased muscle tone, altered consciousness, hyperthermia, and autonomic abnormalities (labile blood pressure, flushing, incontinence). It is an idiosyncratic reaction rather than one related to overdose.[30,43]

As the potency of the various drugs varies (haloperidol is roughly 20 times as potent on a milligram basis as is chlorpromazine), so do toxic doses. Toxicity is difficult to predict in any event from a given exposure, but may result from ingestions of 3-5 times the usual daily dose. For instance, 200-1000 mg of chlorpromazine or 50-150 mg of haloperidol may be toxic for a small child. Plasma concentration correlate poorly with clinical effects and are not routinely available in any case. Therefore, treatment is based primarily on clinical manifestations.

Treatment of neuroleptic overdosage in the main consists of basic supportive care. There is no specific antidote. Physostigmine has been used to counteract the anticholinergic effects but probably does not treat the most severe manifestations of neuroleptic overdose. Extracorporeal drug removal techniques, such as hemodialysis or hemoperfusion, will be ineffective owing to the large volumes of distribution characteristic of these agents. Gastric decontamination may be especially important in neuroleptic intoxication because the anticholinergic effects may slow gut motility, and gastric emptying may thus be effective up to 4-6 hours postingestion.[9] Since seizures and unconsciousness may occur, however, consideration should be given to forgo induced emesis in favor of lavage and activated charcoal administration. As noted above, assisted ventilation is seldom required in pure neuroleptic ingestion but may be necessary when there is coingestion of other substances or for control and protection of the airway. Seizures may be treated with standard anticonvulsants. Hypotension usually improves with fluid administration. If inotropic/vasopressor agents become necessary, drugs with pure alpha-adrenoreceptor agonist activity are usually recommended (norepinephrine).[9] Agents such as dopamine and epinephrine, which possess both α- and β-adrenoreceptor agonist activity, could possibly worsen hypotension, since in the presence of neuroleptic-induced α-blockade, unopposed β-adrenoreceptor activation might increase vasodilatation. Lidocaine and phenytoin are first-line treatments for ventricular dysrhythmias; sodium bicarbonate has been suggested (analogous to its use in tricyclic antidepressant cardiotoxicity), but its effectiveness is unproved. Ventricular pacing has been used with success.[72]

Acute dystonic reactions in children usually improve with intravenous diphenhydramine administration (2 mg/kg) within 5-10 minutes.[99] Oral diphenhydramine should then be used to prevent their recurrence.

REFERENCES

1. Adinoff B, Bone GH, Linnoila M: Acute ethanol poisoning and the ethanol withdrawal syndrome, *Medical Toxicology* 3:172-96, 1988.
2. Agency for Toxic Substances and Disease Registry: Methanol toxicity, *Am Fam Physician* 47:163-71, 1993.
3. Algren JT, Rodgers GC: Hypertension associated with clonidine ingestion, *Vet Hum Toxicol* 2:32-5, 1984.
4. Allen MD, Greenblatt DJ, Noel BJ: Overdosage with antipsychotic agents, *Am J Psychiatry* 137: 234-5, 1980.

5. Artman M, Boerth RC: Clonidine poisoning: a complex problem, *Am J Dis Child* 137:171-4, 1983.
6. Baldessarini RJ: Drugs and the treatment of psychiatric disorders. In Gilman AG and others, editors, *Goodman & Gilman's the pharmacological basis of therapeutics,* ed 8, New York, 1990, Pergamon Press.
7. Banner WJ, Lund ME, Clawson L: Failure of naloxone to reverse clonidine toxic effect, *Am J Dis Child* 137:1170-1, 1983.
8. Barry D, Meyskens FL, Becker CE: Phenothiazine poisoning: a review of 48 cases, *California Medicine* 118:1-5, 1973.
9. Benowitz NK, Rosenberg J, Becker CE: Cardiopulmonary catastrophes in drug-overdosed patients, *Med Clin North Am* 63:278, 1979.
10. Benowitz NL: Clinical pharmacology and toxicology of cocaine, *Pharmacol Toxicol* 72:3-12, 1993.
11. Boehnert MT, Lovejoy FH: Value of the QRS duration versus the serum drug level in predicting seizures and ventricular arrythmias after an acute overdose of tricyclic antidepressants, *N Engl J Med* 313:474-9, 1985.
12. Brown TCK: Tricyclic antidepresant overdosage: experimental studies on the management of circulatory complications, *Clin Toxicol* 9:255-72, 1976.
13. Burkhart KK, Kulig KW: The other alcohols: methanol, ethylene glycol, and isopropanol, *Emerg Med Clin North Am* 8:913-28, 1990.
14. Campese VM and others: Role of sympathetic nerve inhibition and body sodium-volume state in the antihypertensive action of clonidine in essential hypertension, *Kidney Int* 18:351-7, 1980.
15. Caravati EM, Bennett DL: Clonidine transdermal patch poisoning, *Ann Emerg Med* 17:175-6, 1988.
16. Chapman BJ, Proudfoot AT: Adult salicylate poisoning: deaths and outcome in patients with high plasma salicylate concentrations, *Q J Med* 72: 699-707, 1989.
17. Conner CS, Watanabe AS: Clonidine overdose: a review, *Am J Hosp Pharm* 36:906-11, 1979.
18. Corneli HM and others: Toddler eats clonidine patch and nearly quits smoking for life [letter], *JAMA* 261:42, 1989.
19. Crome P: Poisoning due to tricyclic antidepressant overdosage, clinical presentation and treatment, *Med Toxicol* 1:261-85, 1986.
20. Curtis JA, Goel KM: Lomotil poisoning in children, *Arch Dis Child* 54:222-5, 1979.
21. Dawson AH, Whyte IM: The assessment and treatment of theophylline poisoning, *Med J Aust* 151: 689-93, 1989.
22. Derlet RW: Cocaine intoxication, *Postgrad Med* 86:245-8, 1989.
23. Dire DJ, Kuhns DW: The use of sublingual nifedipine in a patient with a clonidine overdose, *J Emerg Med* 6:125-8, 1988.
24. Domino LE, Domino SE, Stockstill MS: Relationship between plasma concentrations of clonidine and mean arterial pressure during an accidental clonidine overdose, *Br J Clin Pharmacol* 21:71-4, 1986.
25. Done AK: Aspirin overdosage: incidence, diagnosis, and management, *Pediatrics* 62:890-7, 1978.
26. Donlon PT, Tupin JP: Successful suicides with thioridazine and mesoridazine, *Arch Gen Psychiatry* 34:955-7, 1977.
27. Dougherty RJ: Propoxyphene-overdose deaths, *JAMA* 235:2716, 1976.
28. Dugandzic RM and others: Evaluation of the validity of the Done nomogram in the management of acute salicylate intoxication, *Ann Emerg Med* 18:1186-90, 1989.
29. Ellenhorn MJ, Barceloux DG: *Medical Toxicology,* New York, 1988, Elsevier Science Publishing Company, Inc.
30. Everson GW, Bertaccini EJ, OLeary J: Use of whole bowel irrigation in an infant following iron overdose, *Am J Emerg Med* 9:366-9, 1991.
31. Fazen LE, Lovejoy FH: Acute poisoning in a children's hospital: a 2-year experience, *Pediatrics* 77:144-51, 1986.
32. Fine JS, Goldfrank LR: Update in medical toxicology, *Pediatr Clin N Am* 39:1031-51, 1992.
33. Flanagan RJ, Meredith TJ: Use of N-acetylcysteine in clinical toxicology, *Am J Med* 91(3C):131S-39S, 1991.
34. Garr GG, Banner W, Laddu AR: The effects of esmolol on the hemodynamics of acute theophylline toxicity, *Ann Emerg Med* 16:1334-9, 1987.
35. Gaudreault P, Guay J: Theophylline poisoning: pharmacological considerations and clinical management, *Med Toxicol* 1:169-91, 1986.
36. Goldberg MJ, Park GD, Berlinger WG: Treatment of theophylline intoxication, *J Allergy Clin Immunol* 78(4Pt2):811-17, 1986.
37. Goldfrank LR and others, editors: *Goldfrank's Toxicologic Emergencies,* ed 4, Norwalk, CT, 1990, Appleton & Lange.
38. Goldfrank LR, Hoffman RS: The cardiovascular effects of cocaine, *Ann Emerg Med* 20:165-75, 1991.
39. Gorman DF, Runciman WB: Carbon monoxide poisoning [see comments], *Anaesth Intensive Care* 19:506-11, 1991.
40. Greensher J, Mofenson HC, Caraccio TR: Ascendency of the black bottle (activated charcoal), *Pediatrics* 80:949-51, 1987.
41. Gremse DA, Artman M, Boerth RC: Hypertension associated with naloxone treatment for clonidine poisoning, *J Pediatr* 108(5Pt1):776-78, 1986.
42. Haddad LM, Winchester JF, editors: Clinical management of poisoning and drug overdose, ed 2, Philadelphia, 1990, W.B. Saunders Company.
43. Hagerman GA: PKH reversal of tricyclic-antidepressant-induced cardiac conduction abnormalities by phenytoin, *Ann Emerg Med* 10:82-6, 1981.
44. Hamblin JE, Martin CA: Transdermal patch poisoning [letter], *Pediatrics* 79:161, 1987.
45. Harris JM: Clonidine patch toxicity [published erratum appears in DICP 1991 Jun;25(6):682] [see comments], *DICP* 24:1191-4, 1990.
46. Heath A, Knudsen K: Role of extracorporeal drug removal in acute theophylline poisoning: a review, *Med Toxicol Adverse Drug Exp* 2:294-308, 1987.

47. Hershey LA: Meperidine and central neurotoxicity, *Ann Intern Med* 98:548-9, 1983.
48. Hornfeldt CS: A report of acute ethanol poisoning in a child: mouthwash versus cologne, perfume and after-shave, *J Toxicol Clin Toxicol* 30:115-21, 1992.
49. Hunyor SN and others: Clonidine overdose, *Br Med J* 4:23, 1975.
50. Hurlbut KM: Drug-induced psychoses, *Emerg Med Clin North Am* 9:31-52, 1991.
51. Ilano AL, Raffin TA: Management of carbon monoxide poisoning, *Chest* 97:165-9, 1990.
52. Jackson JE, Banner W: Tricyclic antidepressant overdose: cardiovascular responses to catecholamines, *Vet Hum Toxicol* 23:361, 1981.
53. Jacobsen D, McMartin KE: Methanol and ethylene glycol poisonings: mechanism of toxicity, clinical course, diagnosis and treatment, *Med Toxicol* 1:309-34, 1986.
54. Jacobsen D, Wiik LE, Bredesen JE: Haemodialysis or haemoperfusion in severe salicylate poisoning, *Hum Toxicol* 7:161-3, 1988.
55. Jaimovich DG: Transport management of the patient with acute poisoning, *Pediatr Clin N Am* 40:407-30, 1993.
56. Jandhyala BS and others: Effects of several tricyclic antidepressants on the hemodynamics and myocardial contractility of the dog, *Eur J Pharmacol* 12:403-10, 1977.
57. Janes J, Routledge PA: Recent developments in the management of paracetamol (acetaminophen) poisoning, *Drug Saf* 7:170-7, 1992.
58. Kellerman AL and others: Impact of drug screening in suspected overdose, *Ann Emerg Med* 16:1206-16, 1987.
59. Kindwall EP: Uses of hyperbaric oxygen therapy in the 1990s, *Cleve Clin J Med* 59:517-28, 1992.
60. Kirshenbaum LA and others: Does multiple-dose charcoal therapy enhance salicylate excretion, *Arch Intern Med* 150:1281-3, 1990.
61. Kulig K, Rumack BH: Efficacy of naloxone in clonidine poisoning [letter], *Am J Dis Child* 137:807-8, 1983.
62. Lacroix J, Gaudreault P, Gauthier M: Admission to a pediatric intensive care unit for poisoning: a review of 105 cases [see comments], *Crit Care Med* 17:748-50, 1989.
63. Landsman I and others: Emergency gastrotomy: treatment of choice for iron bezoar, *J Pediatr Surg* 22:184-5, 1987.
64. Leung AK: Ethyl alcohol ingestion in children: a 15-year review, *Clin Pediatr (Phila)* 25:617-9, 1986.
65. Lieh-Lai MW and others: Metabolism and pharmacokinetics of acetaminophen in a severely poisoned young child, *J Pediatr* 105:125-8, 1984.
66. Leisivuori J, Savolainen H: Methanol and formic acid toxicity: biochemical mechanisms, *Pharmacol Toxicol* 69:157-63, 1991.
67. Litovitz T, Manoguerra A: Comparison of pediatric poisoning hazards: an analysis of 3.8 million exposure incidents: a report from the American Association of Poison Control Centers, *Pediatrics* 89(6Pt1):999-1006, 1992.
68. Litovitz TL and others: 1991 annual report of the American Association of Poison Control Centers National Data Collection System, *Am J Emerg Med* 10:452-509, 1992.
69. Lobl JK, Carbone LD: Emergency management of cocaine intoxication: counteracting the effects of today's 'favorite drug,' *Postgrad Med* 91:161-2, 1992.
70. Lovejoy FHJ, Shannon M, Woolf AD: Recent advances in clinical toxicology, *Curr Probl Pediatr* 22:119-29, 1992.
71. Lumpkin J and others: Phenothiazine-induced ventricular tachycardia following acute overdose, *JACEP* 8:476-8, 1979.
72. Master K: Narcotics and pulmonary edema, *Ann Intern Med* 77:817, 1972.
73. Mathias CJ: Role of sympathetic efferent nerves in blood pressure regulation and in hypertension, *Hypertension* 18(5Suppl)III22-30, 1991.
74. McGuigan MA: A two-year review of salicylate deaths in Ontario, *Arch Intern Med* 147:510-2, 1987.
75. Mofenson HC, Caraccio TR: Cocaine, *Pediatr Ann* 16:864-74, 1987.
76. National Heart, Lung and Blood Institute workshop: Hyperbaric oxygenation therapy, *Am Rev Respir Dis* 144:1414-21, 1991.
77. Neuvonen PJ, Elfving SM, Elonen E: Reduction of absorption of digoxin, phenytoin, and aspirin by activated charcoal in man, *Europ J Clin Pharmacol* 13:213-8, 1978.
78. Neuvonen PJ, Olkkola KT: Oral activated charcoal in the treatment of intoxications: role of single and repeated doses, *Med Toxicol Adverse Drug Exp* 3:33-58, 1988.
79. Newton RW: Physostigmine salicylate in the treatment of tricyclic antidepressant overdosage, *JAMA* 231:941-3, 1975.
80. Niemann JT and others: Cardiac conduction and rhythm disturbances following suicidal ingestion of mesoridazine, *Ann Emerg Med* 10:585-8, 1981.
81. Notarianni L: A reassessment of the treatment of salicylate poisoning, *Drug Saf* 7:292-303, 1992.
82. Nunn TCL, Simon PA: Pharmacotherapy for smoking cessation, *Clin Pharm* 8:710-20, 1989.
83. Osterloh JD: Utility and reliability of emergency toxicologic testing, *Emerg Med Clin North Am* 8:693-723, 1990.
84. Palmisano J, Gruver C, Adams ND: Absence of anion gap metabolic acidosis in severe methanol poisoning: a case report and review of the literature, *Am J Kidney Dis* 9:441-4, 1987.
85. Paloucek FP, Rodvold KA: Evaluation of theophylline overdoses and toxicities [see comments], *Ann Emerg Med* 17:135-44, 1988.
86. Parr MJ and others: Theophylline poisoning—a review of 64 cases, *Intensive Care Med* 16:394-8, 1990.
87. Pentel P, Peterson CD: asystole complicating physostigmine treatment of tricyclic antidepressant overdose, *Ann Emerg Med* 9:588-90, 1980.
88. Pentel P, Peterson CD: Tricyclic antidepressant overdosage: management of arrythmias, *Med Toxicol* 1:101-21, 1986.

89. Rall TW: Drugs used in the treatment of asthma. In Gilman AG and others, editors, *Goodman and Gilman's the pharmacological basis of therapeutics*, ed 8, New York, 1990, Pergamon Press, Inc.
90. Ramoska E, Sacchetti AD: Propranolol-induced hypertension in treatment of cocaine intoxication, *Ann Emerg Med* 14:1112-13, 1985.
91. Reisdorff EJ, Clark MR, Walters BL: Acute digitalis poisoning: the role of intravenous magnesium sulfate, *J Emerg Med* 4:463, 1986.
92. Richelson E, Pfenning M: Blockade by antidepressants and related compounds of biogenic amine uptake into rat brain synaptosomes: most antidepressants selectively block norepinephrine uptake, *Eur J Pharmacol* 104:277-86, 1984.
93. Rioux JP, Myers RA: Methylene chloride poisoning: a paradigmatic review, *J Emerg Med* 6: 227-38, 1988.
94. Robotham JL, Lietman PS: Acute iron poisoning: a review, *Am J Dis Child* 134:875-9, 1980.
95. Rumack BH and others: Acetaminophen overdose 662 cases with evaluation of oral acetylcysteine treatment, *Arch Intern Med* 141:380-5, 1981.
96. Rumack BH, Peterson RG: Acetaminophen overdose: incidence, diagnosis, and management in 416 patients, *Pediatrics* 62(suppl):898-903, 1978.
97. Sadovnikoff N, Varon J, Sternbach GL: Carbon monoxide poisoning: an occult epidemic, *Postgrad Med* 92:86-8, 1992.
98. Sasyniuk BI, Jhamandas V: Mechanism of reversal of toxic effects of amitriptyline on cardiac purkinje fibers by sodium bicarbonate, *J Pharmacol Exp Ther* 231:387-94, 1984.
99. Scialli JVK, Thornton WE: Toxic reactions from a haloperidol overdose in two children, *JAMA* 239:48-50, 1978.
100. Sessler CN: Theophylline toxicity: clinical features of 116 consecutive cases, *Am J Med* 88:567-76, 1990.
101. Sinaniotis CA and others: Acute haloperidol poisoning in children, *J Pediatr* 92:1038-39, 1978.
102. Smilkstein MJ and others: Acetaminophen overdose: a 48-hour intravenous N-acetylcysteine treatment protocol, *Ann Emerg Med* 20:1058-63, 1991.
103. Smilkstein MJ and others: Efficacy of oral N-acetylcysteine in the treatment of acetaminophen overdose, *N Engl J Med* 319:1557-62, 1988.
104. Smith TW and others: Digitalis glycosides: mechanisms and manifestations of toxicity, Part III, *Prog Cardiovasc Dis* 27:26, 1984.
105. Smith TW and others: Treatment of life-threatening digitalis intoxication with digoxin-specific Fab antibody fragments: experience in 26 cases, *N Engl J Med* 307:1357-62, 1982.
106. Sonnenblick M and others: Correlation between manifestations of digoxin toxicity and serum digoxin, calcium, potassium, and magnesium concentrations and arterial pH, *Br Med J (Clin Res Ed)* 286:1089-91, 1983.
107. Springer M, Olson KR, Feaster W: Acute massive digoxin overdose: survival without use of digitalis-specific antibodies, *Am J Emerg Med* 4:364-8, 1986.
108. Steinhart CM, Pearson SAL: Poisoning, *Crit Care Clin* 4:845-72, 1988.
109. Sternbach G, William Osler: Narcotic-induced pulmonary edema, *J Emerg Med* 1:165-7, 1983.
110. Suit PF, Estes ML: Methanol intoxication: clinical features and differential diagnosis, *Cleve Clin J Med* 57:464-71, 1990.
111. Tenenbein M: Whole bowel irrigation for toxic ingestions, *J Toxicol Clin Toxicol* 23:177-84, 1985.
112. Tennebein M, Wiseman N, Yatscoff RW: Gastrotomy and whole bowel irrigation in iron poisoning, *Pediatr Emerg Care* 7:286-8, 1991.
113. Thom SR: Smoke inhalation, *Emerg Med Clin North Am* 7:371-87, 1989.
114. Thom SR, Keim LW: Carbon monoxide poisoning: a review epidemiology, pathophysiology, clinical findings, and treatment options including hyperbaric oxygen therapy, *J Toxicol Clin Toxicol* 27:141-56, 1989.
115. Vernon DD, Banner W, Dean JM: Hemodynamic effects of experimental iron poisoning, *Ann Emerg Med* 18:863-6, 1989.
116. Vernon DD and others: Efficacy of dopamine and norepinephrine for treatment of hemodynamic compromise in amitriptyline intoxication, *Crit Care Med* 19:544-9, 1991.
117. Verrilli MR and others: Fatal ethylene glycol intoxication, report of a case and review of the literature, *Cleve Clin J Med* 54:289-95, 1987.
118. Weiss LD, Van MKW: The applications of hyperbaric oxygen therapy in emergency medicine, *Am J Emerg Med* 10:558-68, 1992.
119. Wiley J, 2d F: Difficult diagnoses in toxicology: poisons not detected by the comprehensive drug screen, *Pediatr Clin North Am* 38:725-37, 1991.
120. Wiley JF2 and others: Clonidine poisoning in young children, *J Pediatr* 116:654-8, 1990.
121. Young SL, Vosper HJ, Phillips SA: Cocaine: its effects on maternal and child health, *Pharmacotherapy* 12:2-17, 1992.
122. Zaccara G, Muscas GC, Messori A: Clinical features, pathogenesis and management of drug-induced seizures, *Drug Saf* 5:109-51, 1990.

32

NEONATAL TRANSPORT

Resuscitation and Documentation
MARY BUSER-GILLS
JONATHAN M. WHITFIELD

Special Considerations in the Transport of the Extremely Low Birth Weight Infant (The Infant Less Than 1000 g)
DEBORA TRALMER
JONATHAN M. WHITFIELD

Sepsis
JONATHAN M. WHITFIELD

Respiratory Problems of the Neonate
DANIEL M. HALL

Congenital Heart Disease
MARY BUSER-GILLS

Perinatal Asphyxia and Seizures
JOHN P. KINSELLA

Transport of the Dysmorphic Infant
ELIZABETH KIRBY

Perinatal Substance Abuse—Transport of the Drug-Addicted Infant
BARBARA GOLZ

Surgical Conditions of the Neonate
JAY S. RODEN

Resuscitation and Documentation

While neonatal transports may take place in the Emergency Medical Services (EMS) setting, the majority of neonatal transports are interfacility. The EMS focus is on immediate stabilization in order to transfer the infant as quickly as possible to the nearest medical facility. During interfacility transport, the neonate should receive care at the level available at the receiving institution. Stabilization of the neonate in preparation for transport begins with the initial resuscitation and patient management at the referring institution and continues with the care provided by the transport team before departure. Because the presence of hypothermia, hypotension, and acidosis before transport has a significant negative impact on patient outcomes, the initial resuscitation and stabilization are critical to successful transport.[8]

HISTORY OF NEONATAL TRANSPORT

The modern era of neonatal transport began in North America with the publication of a paper titled "Transfer of a Premature or Other High-Risk Newborn Infant to a Referral Hospital" by Sydney Segal in 1966.[9] In this paper the essential elements of a system of neonatal transfer were articulated, including organization, communications, personnel, equipment, and ground and air ambulances. Sporadic but nonsystem transfer of neonates occurred before publication of this paper.[3] The organization of a system dedicated to the safe transfer of the neonate was articulated by Segal in a later Canadian Pediatric Society publication titled "Manual for the Transport of High Risk Newborn Infants" in 1972.[3] The essential elements of a neonatal transport system have not changed since that time.

The dangers of a nonsystem approach to transfer of the neonate were documented by Chance and others.[5] The importance of skilled care by individuals trained specifically in newborn care during transfer of the premature neonate was shown in a controlled study.[6] Mortality and length of subsequent hospital stay were improved in the infants who had skilled transport. Wide acceptance of the concept of regionalization of perinatal care led to the development of many transport systems throughout the United States in the 1970s. Neonatal transport must have a continuum of intensive care from the moment of recognition of illness in a newborn to the request for transport from the referring hospital to the stabilization process, transport, and final arrival at the receiving hospital.

INITIAL RESUSCITATION

The American Heart Association and American Academy of Pediatrics have developed the Neonatal Resuscitation Program (NRP), a standardized program for delivery room resuscitation of the neonate.[2] An abbreviated approach follows below. An equipment list is shown in Appendix 1.

Clear the airway

The first goal must be to establish a clear airway. Personnel present at the delivery must evaluate the need for suctioning, oxygen delivery, and artificial airways. The neonate should have the nose, mouth, and oropharynx cleared of fluid and secretions by bulb, DeLee® or mechanical suction as soon as the head is delivered, particularly if meconium-stained amniotic fluid is present. The aspiration of meconium-stained fluid contributes to significant morbidity and mortality in the neonate. Adequate suctioning at this time will reduce the chances of aspiration occurring with the delivery of the thorax and the infant's first breaths.[4] After delivery, if the infant has respiratory depression or distress, the oropharynx and trachea should be suctioned under direct visualization before the use of positive-pressure ventilation is used.

Dry the infant

As soon as possible after delivery, the infant should be dried and placed near a heat source. An open-bed radiant warmer provides an appropriate heat source and easy access to the infant for further care. The use of a stocking cap can significantly decrease heat loss. Only a few seconds are needed to dry the infant; drying should be delayed only in the infant born through meconium-stained amniotic fluid. In this instance, drying the infant may stimulate respiratory effort and should be postponed until the airway has been cleared.

Initiate breathing

Once the airway is clear, the infant's airway should be optimized by maintaining the head in the sniffing position. Blow-by oxygen may be administered until the infant is pink. During the initial stabilization, 100% oxygen should be used and then weaned as indicated by physical examination and monitoring of oxygenation. If the heart rate remains below 100 or respirations are inadequate after clearing the airway and providing stimulation, positive-pressure ventilation should be initiated. Face-mask ventilation should be attempted initially. Adequate ventilation should be evaluated by assessing chest excursion and breath sounds. Ventilating pressures should always be monitored with a manome-

TABLE 32-1 ENDOTRACHEAL TUBE SIZE SELECTION

Weight (kg)	*ET tube (size)*	*Depth of insertion (cm from upper lip)*	*Suction catheter size (F)*
<1	2.5	7	5
1-2	3.0	8	6
3-4	3.5	9	8
>4	4.0	10	8-10

ter. Pressures up to 30 to 40 centimeters of water may be required for the initial opening breaths. Pressures should then be reduced to the minimum required to maintain adequate ventilation. The infant will respond to adequate ventilation with rising heart rate, improved color, and improved tone. The level of respiratory support may be decreased to continuous positive airway pressure or blow-by oxygen.

If the infant does not respond with improved heart rate and color after 30 seconds to 1 minute of bag and mask ventilation, an endotracheal tube should be placed (Table 32-1). Evaluation for right main stem intubation, esophageal placement, and adequate ventilation should be completed immediately following intubation. Ventilation must be continued until spontaneous respirations are established.

Circulation

If the heart rate remains below 60 beats per minute or between 60 and 80 beats per minute without rising despite adequate ventilation, cardiac massage should be instituted. The lower third of the sternum should be depressed 1.5 to 2.0 centimeters ($\frac{1}{2}$-1 inch) at a rate of 120 times per minute. Effectiveness should be evaluated, including heart rate, systolic pressure, ECG, and pupil size. Cardiac massage should be continued until the heart rate is over 80 beats per minute.

Drug support

Drugs rarely are needed in the delivery room once adequate ventilation has been established. However, if the heart rate remains below 80 despite adequate ventilation and cardiac massage for 30 seconds, or if there is no heart rate, epinephrine should be instilled down the endotracheal tube (Table 32-2). To ensure that the epinephrine reaches the lungs, it may be diluted in or flushed with 1 to 2 ml of normal saline. The most immediate vascular access in the delivery room is the umbilical vein; the needle should be inserted just far enough to obtain blood return. If fur-

TABLE 32-2 NEONATAL EMERGENCY DRUG DOSAGES

Drug	*Indication*	*Dose*	*Route**
Naloxone (Hydrochloride)	Narcotic depression	0.1/mg/kg	IV/ETT preferred, IM/SC acceptable
Epinephrine (1:10,000)	Bradycardia, cardiac arrest	0.1-0.3 ml/kg	ETT/IV
Sodium bicarbonate 4.2% (0.5 mEq/ml)	Metabolic acidosis	2 mEq/kg slowly over at least 2 to 3 minutes	IV (always clear line before and after administration)
5% Albumin Normal saline Whole blood Lactated Ringer's Solution	Hypotension, volume restoration	10 ml/kg over 5 to 10 minutes	IV
Dextrose 10%	Hypoglycemia	2 to 4 ml/kg	IV

* IV = intravenous; IM = intramuscular; ETT = endotracheal tube; SC = subcutaneous

ther pharmaceutical resuscitation is required, recommended drugs, dosages, routes, and indications are outlined in Table 32-2.

PRETRANSPORT STABILIZATION

Once the initial resuscitation has been completed, the infant must be stabilized for transport. Unless the transport team attends, the delivery management of the high-risk neonate begins *before* the arrival of the transport team. The transport team must balance anticipated clinical complications, the time and distance of the transport, the need for reaching definitive care, and the benefits of further stabilization in each case. These factors will determine the extent of pretransport stabilization. While not always attainable, the goal of stabilization is an infant with normal vital signs, normal blood pressure and perfusion, normal blood gases, and normal glucose and electrolytes.

THERMOREGULATION

The goal of thermoregulation is to maintain the infant in a neutral thermal environment. The neutral thermal environment is that range of ambient temperature within which the baby can maintain normal body temperature with a minimum metabolic rate and oxygen consumption.[1,9] The infant is at high-risk for hypothermia due to a large surface area-to-body mass ratio. In addition, the low birth weight baby has decreased subcutaneous fat. Hypothermia and hyperthermia usually are iatrogenic and increase the metabolic demands on an already stressed infant. Management of the infant's environment must include both ambient temperature control and reduction of heat loss. Heat losses occur through convection, conduction, evaporation, and radiation (see Special Considerations in the Transport of the Extremely Low Birth Weight Infant, discussed later in this chapter).

The infant is at increased risk of poor temperature regulation in the transport environment. The wide range of weather conditions and outside temperatures impacts control of incubator temperature. The use of double walled incubators, heat shields, insulating incubator covers, and heating mattresses can improve thermal stability. Other interventions that may decrease heat loss include the placing of stocking caps; swaddling in blankets, foil, or plastic; keeping the infant dry; and preventing drafts.

The optimal temperature ranges for the newborn are skin temperature of 36.0° to 36.5°C (96.8°-97.7°F), axillary temperature of 36.5° to 37.0°C (97.7°-98.6°F), and rectal temperature of 36.5° to 37.0°C (97.7°-98.6°F). Both the skin and axillary temperatures should be monitored. An infant can have a normal core temperature as measured by axillary or rectal temperature and still be cold-stressed, as indicated by a low skin temperature. Skin temperature should be monitored continuously throughout transport by a skin-temperature probe attached to the infant's abdomen.

FLUID AND ELECTROLYTES

The goal of fluid management is to maintain normal hydration while avoiding fluid overload. Primary fluid losses in the neonate occur through urine output and insensible water losses (IWL) of the skin and respiratory tract. Other mechanisms of loss include stool, gastric drainage, ostomies, and surgical wounds. The premature infant has increased fluid requirements to compensate for high transepidermal water loss. Because the epidermal barrier of the preterm infant's skin is poor, insensible water losses (IWL) can be as low as 40 to over 150 ml/kg/day. A number of conditions can increase insensible water losses, while specific interventions can decrease the losses (Box 32-1).

Fluids for the first day of life are normally 60 to 100 ml/kg/day, based on the evaluation of the infant's anticipated maintenance needs and fluid losses. Fluid requirements normally increase by 10 to 30 ml/kg/day on subsequent days during the first week, based on careful monitoring of the infant's hydration status. Monitoring includes measuring weight, urine output, specific gravities, and serum electrolyte levels.

Addition of electrolytes to intravenous fluids usually is not necessary in the first day. Serum electrolytes and urine output should be evaluated before initiating IV additives. Potassium should not be added until the infant is voiding. Normal electrolyte supple-

BOX 32-1 FACTORS IMPACTING INSENSIBLE WATER LOSS (IWL)

Factors increasing IWL
- Prematurity
- Radiant warmers
- Elevated environmental temperatures
- Respiratory distress
- Hyperthermia
- Phototherapy
- Ventilation with dry gases

Factors decreasing IWL
- Heat shields or plastic film blanket
- Ventilation with warm, humidified gases
- Warm humidified environment
- Neutral thermal environment
- Preventing drafts

mentation is 3 to 4 mEq/kg/day of sodium and 2 to 3 mEq/kg/day of potassium.

Certain infants may have special requirements for either increased or restricted fluid therapy. Infants with the following complications must be evaluated carefully for fluid balance: preterm infants <1500 grams; infants with birth asphyxia and potential renal injury, cerebral edema, or cardiac dysfunction; surgical patients with exposed bowel, third spacing, and nasogastric losses; infants with congestive heart failure; or infants with electrolyte imbalance.

GLUCOSE MANAGEMENT

The neonate is susceptible to hypoglycemia caused by immature glucose control mechanisms or decreased glucose stores, or both. At birth, the infant's glucose level is 70% to 80% of the mother's serum glucose. During the next 1 to 3 hours, the neonate's glucose level will fall to its nadir. In the absence of factors interfering with normal glucose metabolism, the baby's glucose level will rise progressively during the first days of life. The definition of hypoglycemia based on normative data has been described as being less than 25 mg/dl in the preterm infant, less than 35 mg/dl in the term infant less than 72 hours of age, and less than 45 mg/dl in the term infant greater than 72 hours of age.[7] Many clinicians define hypoglycemia as less than 40 mg/dl for all infants, thus providing a safe margin for error. Infants with inadequate intake, inadequate glucose stores, or increased glucose utilization should be considered at risk for hypoglycemia. Glucose screening should begin in the first $\frac{1}{2}$ to 1 hour and continue at least hourly until stable, maintaining levels between 40 and 130 mg/dl. Bedside testing with enzymatic reagent strips is convenient to use during transport. One should confirm abnormal values with a laboratory sample when possible.

Infants weighing more than 1000 grams usually can be maintained on 10% dextrose in water (D/W) at 4 to 6 mg/kg/minute. Infants weighing less than 1000 grams may become hyperglycemic on glucose administered at these rates and are therefore frequently started on 5 to 7.5% D/W (D_5-$D_{7.5}W$). Careful screening of blood glucose must be continued until stable levels are achieved.

Infants with mild hypoglycemia may respond to increasing the glucose infusion to a rate of 8 to 10 mg/kg/minute. If the hypoglycemia is profound or not responding to the increased infusion rate, or if the infant is symptomatic, a 2 ml/kg bolus of 10% D/W (200 mg/kg) may be given, followed by the higher glucose infusion rate (6 to 8 mg/kg/minute). Infants with refractory hypoglycemia may require higher concentrations of IV glucose. A central line should be used to administer concentrations greater than 12.5% dextrose/water.

RESPIRATORY MANAGEMENT

Once the airway has been established during initial resuscitation, the transport team must assess the need for ongoing respiratory support. Oxygen can be delivered by a number of methods. Blow-by or free-flow oxygen can be used on a short-term basis but is subject to wide swings in oxygen concentration when the incubator is accessed. The use of an oxygen headbox will allow the delivery of measurable, stable concentrations of oxygen. Oxygen flow rates of 5 to 10 liters/minute will ensure adequate flow and prevent the accumulation of CO_2. Continuous positive airway pressure can be delivered by various methods, including nasal prongs, nasopharyngeal tube, or endotracheal tube. A differential diagnosis should be developed, and risks should be determined for the anticipated duration of the transport. Because of the uncontrolled transport environment, the endotracheal tube should be placed electively at the referring facility, if the team anticipates the need for endotracheal intubation before arrival at the receiving institution (see Table 32-1).

Monitoring of the infant's respiratory status continues throughout transport, allowing adjustments in treatment en route. The development of portable monitors has made possible the monitoring of oxygen concentration, transcutaneous PO_2, PCO_2, and oxygen saturation. Use of these monitors decreases the need for multiple blood gases in the referring facility and increases the number of neonates admitted to the receiving center with PO_2 levels within the normal range.[10]

BLOOD PRESSURE/PERFUSION

Assessment of the infant for hypovolemia and decreased tissue perfusion begins with the perinatal history. A history of placenta previa, abruptio placentae, third trimester bleeding, or blood loss during delivery places the infant at risk for hypovolemia and anemia. A history of perinatal asphyxia increases the risk of myocardial dysfunction. Assessment of the infant who has hypovolemia may reveal tachycardia, color which is pale or gray, prolonged capillary refill time, and decreased pulse volume and urinary output. The infant's extremities may be cool when compared with the central temperature. The blood pressure may be misleading, because infants frequently are able to maintain a normal pressure initially. Similarly, the hematocrit may not reflect the amount of blood loss until the volume loss has been partially replaced by internal fluid shifts.

Treatment is aimed at restoring normal intravascular volume and perfusion. If hypovolemia is suspected, volume may be increased with whole blood, fresh-frozen plasma, 5% albumin, lactated Ringer's solution or normal saline. Further treatment with packed cells may be necessary to relieve anemia. Vasoactive drugs may be indicated if myocardial dysfunction is suspected. Careful monitoring must be maintained throughout transport to evaluate the infant's response to therapy and titrate further volume or vasoactive support. A pretransport checklist is shown in Table 32-3.

DOCUMENTATION

To achieve continuity of care for the transported infant the receiving staff must be given copies of the perinatal history, the mother's labor and delivery record, and the infant's medical chart. The care provided during transport also must be documented carefully, and a copy of the transport record must be given to the receiving staff. Important documentation points for the transport team include the following:

Logistical documentation

1. Name of referring physician.
2. Name and location of referral facility.
3. Time of referral call.
4. Time transport team notified.
5. Time of departure en route to referral facility.
6. Time of arrival at referral facility.
7. Time of departure from referral facility.
8. Time of arrival at receiving facility.
9. Transport delays.
10. Mode of transport.

Patient care documentation (see Appendix 2)

1. Significant previous medical history; history of prenatal care, labor and delivery.
2. Date and time of birth.
3. Delivery room resuscitation, including interventions and Apgar scores.
4. Care provided before arrival of the transport team, including significant laboratory data and radiographic studies.
5. Patient condition on arrival of the transport team, assessment, plan of care, interventions, patient response, and consultations with referring physicians and medical control physician.
6. Ongoing assessments, management, and patient responses throughout transport.
7. Patient assessment and current treatment at time of transfer of care to receiving staff.

TABLE 32-3 PRETRANSPORT STABILIZATION CHECKLIST

A irway	• Patent? Place endotracheal tube if needed.
B reathing	• Record respiratory rate. • Provide oxygen to keep pink (pulse oximeter 86% to 95% saturated). Mechanical ventilation as needed. • ABG. • Chest radiograph. Endotracheal tube position above carina?
C ardiovascular	• Record heart rate/blood pressure. • Obtain IV access (5% or 10% dextrose solution at 60 to 80 cc/kg/day). • *Careful* volume expansion to support blood volume. Consider inotropes if no response, e.g., dopamine.†
D rugs	• Antibiotics. After CBC and blood culture, other drugs as needed (all drug dosages calculated on per kg basis). Glucose if hypoglycemia is present.
D ocumentation	• Record full history, examination, and laboratory results.†† Memorandum of transfer. Copy of infant and mother's chart.
E nvironment	• Ensure thermoneutrality and safety.
E vacuation	• Continuously monitor heart rate, blood pressure, respiration and oxygen saturation. • OG for gastric decompression.

ABG = arterial blood gas
CBC = complete blood count
OG = Orogastric tube
† Weight in Kg × 60 = milligrams of drug mixed in 100 cc of IV solution. 1 cc per hour infusion rate delivers 10 micrograms per kg per minute.
†† Example of transport documentation form shown in Appendix 32-2.

REFERENCES

1. Buetow KC, Klein SW: Effect of maintenance of normal skin temperature on survival of infants of low birthweight, *Pediatrics* 34:163-70, 1964.
2. Bloom RS, Cropley C: *Textbook of neonatal resuscitation,* Elk Grove Village, Illinois, 1990, American Heart Association and American Academy of Pediatrics.
3. Butterfield LJ: Intensive care for newborns, *Rocky Mtn Med Journal* 65:85-90, 1968.
4. Carson BS and others: Combined obstetric and pediatric approach to prevent meconium aspiration syndrome, *Am J Obstet Gynecol* 126:712-5, 1976.
5. Chance GW, O'Brien MJ, Swyer PR: Transportation of sick neonates 1972: an unsatisfactory aspect of neonatal care, *Can Med Assoc J* 109:847, 1973.
6. Chance GW and others: Neonatal transport: a controlled study of skilled assistance, *J Pediatr* 93:662-6, 1978.
7. Cornblath M and others: Hypoglycemia in infancy: the need for a rational definition, *Pediatrics* 85:834-7, 1990.
8. Ferrara A: Evaluation of efficacy of regional perinatal programs. *Semin Perinatol* 1:303-8, 1977.
9. Hey EN: The relationship between environmental temperature and oxygen consumption in the newborn baby, *J Physiol* 200:589-95, 1969.
10. Miller C and others: Control of oxygenation during the transport of sick neonates, *Pediatrics* 66:117-9, 1980.

Special Considerations in the Transport of the Extremely Low Birth Weight Infant (The Infant Less Than 1000 g)

Transporting the extremely low birth weight (ELBW) infant can be challenging, even to the most experienced transport team. Overall mortality for infants weighing less than 1,000 grams is greatest during the first 72 hours. The outcome of the ELBW infant born outside a perinatal facility is critically dependent on the resuscitation, stabilization, and overall quality of care performed by the transport team.

To successfully transport the ELBW infant, transport team members must be knowledgeable of both physiologic and clinical characteristics specific to these vulnerable infants. Of particular importance are the risks for 1) hypotension, 2) hypothermia, 3) hypoglycemia, and 4) respiratory distress with associated hypoxia. The goal of the transport team must be prevention of these complications.[1,5,6,7]

HYPOTENSION

An infant with a mean blood pressure less than the gestational age in weeks expressed in mm Hg is hypotensive.[2,8] If an ELBW infant is hypotensive, volume expansion with colloid (5% albumin or plasmanate) or crystalloid (if colloid is not available) is recommended (5 to 10 cc/kg colloid or 10 to 20 cc/kg crystalloid). Initiation of inotropes should be considered (e.g., dopamine at 5 mcg/kg per minute) if myocardial dysfunction is suspected.[4] Caretakers must understand the extreme vulnerability of the vascular supply to the subependymal matrix of the immature brain. Cerebral blood flow can be blood pressure passive (absence of autoregulation).[13] Episodes of low blood pressure will result in ischemia, and episodes of elevated blood pressure will result in excessive blood flow. These mechanisms are believed to increase risk of hemorrhage. Intraventricular hemorrhage is associated with high mortality and morbidity in these infants.[10] For these reasons, hypotension as well as sudden changes in blood pressure must be avoided. In the ELBW infant, volume replacement must always be done slowly (e.g., a maximum infusion of a 10 ml/kg bolus of colloid should be given over 5 to 10 minutes and preferably over 10 to 20 minutes if the clinical situation permits). (See discussion of Blood Pressure and Perfusion earlier in this chapter.)

HYPOTHERMIA

A neutral thermal environment is defined as an environmental temperature at which an infant can sustain a normal body temperature with minimal metabolic activity and oxygen consumption.[12]

The ELBW infant, as compared with the full-term infant or older child, has certain characteristics that contribute to thermal instability:

1. Relatively large body surface as compared with weight.
2. Decreased subcutaneous stores of fat.
3. Greater body water content and very immature skin, increase evaporative water losses.
4. Ineffective positioning ability (related to poorly developed flexor tone) prevents the infant from reducing body surface area in response to cold stress.
5. Poorly developed metabolic mechanisms for responding to thermal stress, such as mobilization of brown fat (nonshivering thermogenesis).

To provide a thermally neutral environment and prevent hypothermia, the transport team must be aware of these characteristics and understand the potential mechanisms of heat loss, for example, evaporation, convection, conduction, and radiation (Table 32-4). Minimizing heat loss during transport is essential. Appropriate interventions to accomplish this are illustrated in Fig. 32-1.

The ELBW infant must be dried immediately after birth (reduces evaporative losses) and placed in a preheated radiant warmer or

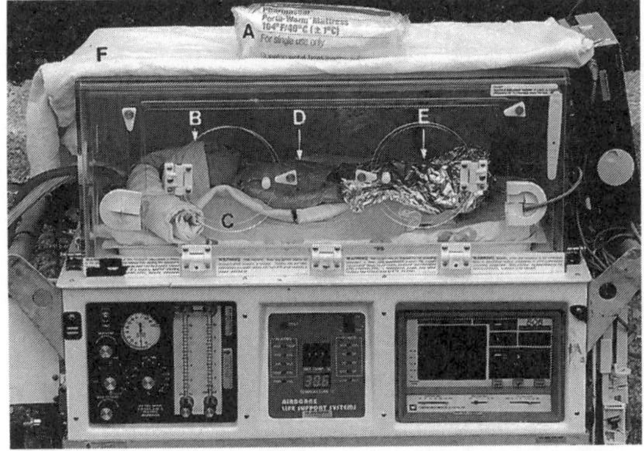

Fig. 32-1. *Interventions to maintain a neutral thermal environment during transport* (A. Portawarm® mattress (Baxter). This can be placed under the infant in the incubator as a supplemental heat source. B. Hat. C. Water-filled gloves. D. Plastic wrap. E. Aluminum foil [silver swaddler]. F. Blanket over isolette. Courtesy of Marcia Schrader, NNP, Baylor University Medical Center, Dallas, Texas.

TABLE 32-4 MECHANISMS OF HEAT LOSS AND RECOMMENDED INTERVENTIONS TO PREVENT OR MINIMIZE THEIR EFFECT

Heat loss mechanism	*Intervention*
Evaporation H_2O evaporates from the skin and respiratory tract.	• Immediately dry infant. • Place in prewarmed environment. • Wrap in warm, dry blankets. • Plastic heat shield • Cotton-lined cap
Convection Heat is lost to moving air or fluid around the baby.	• Prewarm environment (i.e., transport incubator and vehicle). • Avoid opening door or portholes on incubator. • Drape blanket over incubator.
Radiation Infant radiates heat to surrounding colder solid objects.	• Use plastic heat shield or plastic wrap. • Warm water-filled gloves, chemical heat packs. • Aluminum foil
Conduction Heat is conducted to cold objects in direct contact with infant.	• Portable warming mattress • Preheat all surfaces and objects in direct contact with infant.

incubator (reduces radiant and conductive heat loss). Additional warming devices may be necessary, including chemical heat packs (decreases conduction loss), plastic wrap, plastic heat shields, warmed blankets, silver swaddlers, hats, and even water-filled gloves. Transport incubator doors and portholes must be kept closed as much as possible (reduces convective losses). Covering the outside of the incubator and preheating the transport vehicle are additional means of preventing hypothermia during transport (reduces radiant losses). Transport team members should note that the difficulty in maintaining thermoneutrality is exacerbated during air transport because of marked reduction in ambient temperature with increasing altitudes (4°F drop in temperature per 1,000 feet) with resultant cooling of the fuselage (increased radiant losses).[10]

HYPOGLYCEMIA

ELBW infants experience significant perinatal stress resulting in increases in metabolic rate, oxygen consumption, and glucose consumption. A functionally immature gluconeogenic and glycogenolytic enzyme system and minimal glycogen stores make the ELBW infant reliant upon exogenous sources of glucose. Hypoglycemia is common in the first 24 to 72 hours of life, thereby warranting early glucose screening (see glucose management above). Hypoglycemia in the ELBW infant should be defined as a blood glucose value less than 40 mg/dl. Prevention of hypoglycemia may be accomplished by starting a glucose infusion with 5% dextrose at a rate of 80 to 100 cc/kg/day. Treatment of hypoglycemia requires an immediate bolus of 10% dextrose at 1 to 2 cc/kg (100 to 200 mg/kg) followed by a continuous IV infusion of glucose (5 cc per kg per hour or 8 mg/kg per minute). Rescreening should be done 30 minutes after initiating this therapy, and another bolus of 10% dextrose should be administered, if warranted. Because of the difficulty of starting and maintaining intravenous access, especially in the transport environment, the ELBW infant may benefit from having an umbilical arterial or centrally placed umbilical venous catheter placed for administration of fluids before transport.

RESPIRATORY DISTRESS AND HYPOXIA

The respiratory care needs of the ELBW infant are complex and require thorough and constant assessment during transport. Respiratory distress in these infants commonly is caused by surfactant deficiency but also may be caused by respiratory insufficiency secondary to anatomical immaturity of the lung (canalicular stage of lung development).[3] ELBW infants have weak and fatiguable respiratory muscles and a very compliant chest wall. Both factors cause additional difficulty in the ELBW infant and adversely affect the ability to generate the necessary lung opening pressures to recruit and then maintain adequate lung volumes.[11] Mechanical ventilatory assistance is often required as a routine part of resuscitation. Thus, if the ELBW infant shows signs of respiratory distress, supplemental oxygen should be administered and, if necessary, the infant should be intubated. The decision to intubate in the transport setting is based upon both clinical assessment ("work of breathing") and arterial blood gas assessment. After intubation, excessive pressures and overventilation must be avoided because of the associated risks of barotrauma and hyperoxia.[9]

Recently, the wide availability of surfactant preparations for clinical use has changed the approach used to manage the ELBW infant during transport. In the transport setting, early intubation is recommended prior to transport, before the infant deteriorates. Many centers now advocate the use of surfactant before transport. In any event, stabilization of the airway by elective intubation and provision of continuous positive airway pressure will establish lung volume more effectively and should be considered in all ELBW infants.

REFERENCES

1. Buser MK: Care and transport of the neonate. In Lee G, editor: *Flight nursing: principles and practice,* St. Louis, 1991, Mosby-Year Book.
2. Cabel LA, Larrazabal C, Siassi B: Hemodynamic variables in infants weighing less than 1000 grams, *Clin Perinatol* 6:327-38, 1986.
3. Chernick V, Kendig EL, editors: *Disorders of the respiratory tract in children,* Philadelphia, 1990, WB Saunders.
4. Gill AB, Weindling AM: Randomized controlled trial of plasma protein fraction versus dopamine in hypotensive very low birthweight infants, *Arch Dis Child* 69:284-7, 1993.
5. Gunderson LP, Kenner C, editors: *Care of the 24-25 week gestational age infant (small baby protocol),* Petaluma, CA, 1990, Neonatal Network.
6. Horgan M and others: Morbidity and mortality in infants with birth weights between 501 and 1000 grams, *Perinatol* 6:243-50, 1986.
7. Jain L, Vidyasagar D: Cardiopulmonary resuscitation of newborns: its application to transport medicine, *Pediatr Clin North Am* 40:287-302, 1993.
8. Joint working party of the British Association of Perinatal Medicine and Research Unit of the Royal College of Physicians: development of audit measures and guidelines for good practice in the management of neonatal respiratory distress syndrome, *Arch Dis Child* 67:1221-7, 1992.
9. Klaus MH, Fanaroff AA: *Care of the high-risk neonate,* Philadelphia, 1993, WB Saunders.
10. LeBlanc MH: Evaluation of two devices for improving thermal control of premature infants in transport, *Crit Care Med* 12:593, 1984.
11. Polin RA, Fox WW: *Fetal and neonatal physiology,* Vol 1, Philadelphia, 1992, WB Saunders.
12. Sauer PJ, Visser HK: The neutral temperature of very low birth weight infants, *Pediatrics* 78:288, 1984.
13. Volpe JJ: *Neurology of the newborn,* Philadelphia, 1987, WB Saunders.

Sepsis

The newborn infant has a limited repertoire of responses to a variety of illnesses and conditions; thus, the presenting signs in many disease states, including sepsis, may be very similar (Table 32-5). The newborn (especially the preterm infant) generally has limited physiologic reserve, and it is therefore essential that the caretaker perform a rapid but thoughtful examination to determine the cause of abnormal signs and begin treatment expeditiously. In the transport setting, initiation of this process must *not* await arrival of a tertiary care transport service. If assistance is needed, the tertiary care center should be contacted by phone, and treatment should begin after phone consultation so that valuable time is not lost.

Any full-term or preterm neonatal patient who appears ill, should be assumed to have an infection as causing the symptoms until proved otherwise. Sepsis can be caused by bacteria, viruses, or fungi (Table 32-6). Onset of sepsis may be classified as early (<4 days) or late (4 days) (Table 32-7). Although the laboratory studies used to evaluate a potentially septic infant are sensitive, few have

TABLE 32-5 CLINICAL SIGNS OF NEONATAL SEPSIS

General:
a) Lethargy/irritability
b) Hypothermia (<36.0°C)
c) Hyperthermia (>37.8°C)
d) Petechiae/purpura
e) Jaundice

Respiratory:
f) Respiratory distress
g) Apnea

Cardiovascular:
h) Tachycardia (>160 beats per minute)
i) Hypotension (mean BP < GA* in weeks expressed as mm Hg)
j) Pale and/or mottled appearance
k) Poor capillary refill > 3 seconds

Gastrointestinal:
l) Emesis
m) Feeding difficulties
n) Abdominal distention
o) Diarrhea
p) Hepatosplenomegaly

Other:
q) Hypoglycemia (<40 mg/dl)

* GA = Gestational age expressed in weeks, i.e., at 28 weeks' gestation the infant should have a mean BP ≥ 28 mm Hg.

good positive or negative predictive value (Table 32-8).

In evaluating the infant, a history that identifies risk factors for sepsis is helpful (Box 32-2). The most useful application of laboratory studies evaluating the potentially septic infant is a study repeated during a period of 6 to 12 hours, such as a complete blood count with demonstration of persistent normal values. For example, a normal white blood cell count on two occasions 6 to 24 hours apart in a patient whose signs of illness are improving has excellent negative predictive power for the *absence* of infection.

Broad-spectrum antibiotics should be administered to any neonate who appears ill, only *after* appropriate specimens (including blood, spinal fluid, and urine) are obtained. This approach may be a counsel of perfection in the transport setting. In the first four days of life with early-onset disease, a blood culture followed by initiation of antibiotics takes priority over obtaining spinal fluid in the transport setting. Urine is never a primary source of infection with early-onset disease

TABLE 32-6 MICROBIOLOGY OF NEONATAL SEPSIS AT YALE-NEW HAVEN HOSPITAL (1979 TO 1988)*

Organism (%)	*No. of isolates*
1. Gram-positive aerobic bacteria (41%)	
β-Hemolytic streptococci group B	64
Coagulase-negative staphylococci	36
β-Hemolytic streptococci group D	
Enterococcus sp.	18
Staphylococcus aureus	14
Viriidans streptococci	11
Streptococcus pneumoniae	2
Listeria monocytogenes	2
Bacillus aereus	1
2. Gram-negative aerobic bacteria (54%)	
Escherichia coli	46
Klebsiella pneumoniae	18
Haemophilus influenzae	8
Enterobacter cloacae	7
Pseudomonas aeruginosa	6
Klebsiella oxytoca	5
Serratia marcescens	3
Enterobacter agglomerans	2
Acinetobacter anitratums	2
Pseudomonas cepacia	2
Pseudomonas fluorescens	1
Arizona hinshawii	1
Morganella morganii	1
Salmonella C-2	1
Haemophilus parainfluenzae	1
3. Gram-negative anaerobic bacteria (2%)	
Bacteroides fragilis	4
Bacteroides thetaiotaomicron	1
Fusobacterium necrophorum	1
4. Fungi (3%)	
Candida albicans	10
Candida lusitaniae	1

* Modified from Gladstone IM and others: A ten year review of neonatal sepsis and comparison with fifty year experience, *Pediatr Infect Dis J* 9(11):821, 1990. © by Williams & Wilkins, 1990.[1]

TABLE 32-7 DISTRIBUTION BY AGE OF 270 POSITIVE CULTURES AT YALE-NEW HAVEN HOSPITAL (1979 TO 1988)*

Birth location	*No. of positive cultures (% of total)*
Inborn (age when cultured, days)	
Early (0-4)	93 (35)
Late (5-30)	54 (20)
Postneonatal (>30)	56 (21)
Outborn	67 (25)
Total	270 (100)

* Modified from Gladstone IM and others: A ten year review of neonatal sepsis and comparison with fifty year experience, *Pediatr Infect Dis J* 9(11):821, 1990. © by Williams & Wilkins, 1990.[1]

BOX 32-2 MATERNAL RISK FACTORS FOR NEONATAL SEPSIS

Premature labor (before 37 weeks' gestation)
Prolonged rupture of membranes (>12-24 hr)
Maternal fever
Chorioamnionitis
Maternal group B streptococcus carriage (as many as 30% of pregnant mothers)

but can be obtained in this setting and sent for latex agglutination for group B streptococcus.

Several important conditions can masquerade as infection in the newborn.[2] Some of these disorders require specific and life-saving treatment, for example, coarctation of the aorta requires administration of PGE_1. Other masqueraders of neonatal sepsis are shown in Table 32-9. Table 32-10 shows the appropriate antibiotic drug dosages.

TABLE 32-8 INTERPRETATION OF LABORATORY TESTS IN THE SEPTIC-APPEARING NEONATE

Laboratory test	*Positive predictive value**	*Negative predictive value†*
I/T ratio > 0.2‡	++	++
WBC < 5,000/mm³§	++	++++
CRP + ‖	+	++++
ESR > 15 mm/hr¶	++	++++
Neutrophil morphology**	++	+
Platelets < 150,000/mm³	+	+
Fibronectin	++	++++
Any 2 tests or more	++	++++
(gastric aspirate/external ear aspirate)	+	+
Clinical impression	++++	++++
Fever > 100°F	+++	++++
CIE (or latex agglutination)	++++	++++
Blood culture	++++	++++

* Test is positive *only* when infection is present.
† Test is negative *only* when infection is absent.
‡ Immature neutrophils ÷ total neutrophil count.
§ White blood cells.
‖ C-reactive protein, qualitative or quantitative.
¶ Micro Erythrocyte Sedimentation Rate (ESR) (age in days + 2 to 3 mm/hr; maximum of 20 mm/hr is normal).
** Toxic granulations, Dohle bodies, vacuolization.
CIE = Counterimmune Electrophoresis

+ = 0% to 25%;
++ = 25% to 50%;
+++ = 50% to 75%;
++++ = 75% to 100%.

TABLE 32-9 MASQUERADERS OF NEONATAL SEPSIS AND EMERGENCY TREATMENT

Diagnosis	Treatment
1. Cardiac disease:	
a. Ductal-dependent structural heart disease (e.g., coarctation, interruption of aorta, hypoplastic left heart)	PGE, 0.05 to 0.1 μg/kg/min
b. Paroxysmal atrial tachycardia	Synchronized DC (0.5 to 1 joules/kg) cardioversion IV adenosine (50 to 100 μg/kg)
c. Myocarditis	Supportive
d. Myocardial infarction	Supportive
2. Nonbacterial infections:	
Viral (e.g., HSV/varicella/RSV)	Acyclovir 10 mg/kg q 8 h VZIG 125 units IM RSVIG* 10 ml/kg IV
3. Respiratory distress (e.g., HMD, TTN)	Supportive
4. Endocrine/metabolic	
a. Hypoglycemia	10% glucose IV 2 ml/kg as a bolus, then 5 ml/kg/hr
b. Lactic acidosis Organic acidosis Urea cycle defects Congenital adrenal hyperplasia	See ref. 5
5. Other:	
a. Gastrointestinal (e.g., NEC, volvulus, appendicitis, toxic megacolon, gastroenteritis with dehydration)	May require urgent laparotomy.
b. Methemoglobinemia	IV methylene blue 1-2 ml/kg

NEC = necrotizing enterocolitis
PGEI = prostaglandin E (Prostin, Upjohn Co.)
RSVIG = respiratory syncytial virus immunoglobulin
VZIG = varicella zoster immune globulin
HSV = herpes simplex virus
HMD = hyaline membrane disease
TTN = transient tachypnea of newborn

TABLE 32-10 INITIAL ANTIBIOTIC DOSAGES FOR TERM NEONATES

		Dosages (mg/kg/day) and intervals of administration	
Antibiotics	*Routes of administration*	*Age 0 to 7 days*	*Age >7 days*
Amikacin	IM, IV	20 div q 12 hr	30 div q 8 hr
Ampicillin	IV, IM		
Meningitis		150 div q 8 hr	200 div q 6 hr
Other diseases		75 div q 8 hr	100 div q 6 hr
Aztreonam	IV, IM	90 div q 8 hr	120 div q 6 hr
Cefazolin	IV, IM	40 div q 12 hr	60 div q 8 hr
Cefotaxime	IV, IM	100 div q 12 hr	150 div q 8 hr
Ceftazidime	IV, IM	90 div q 8 hr	150 div q 8 hr
Ceftriaxone	IV, IM	50 once daily	75 once daily
Cephalothin	IV	60 div q 8 hr	80 div q 6 hr
Chloramphenicol	IV, PO	25 once daily	50 div q 12 hr
Clindamycin	IV, IM, PO	15 div q 8 hr	20 div q 6 hr
Erythromycin estolate	PO	20 div q 12 hr	30 div q 8 hr
Gentamicin	IM, IV		7.5 div q 8 hr
Kanamycin	IM, IV	150 div q 8 hr	30 div q 8 hr
Methicillin	IV, IM	75 div q 8 hr	
Meningitis		15 div q 12 hr	200 div q 6 hr
Other diseases		150 div q 12 hr	100 div q 6 hr
Metronidazole	IV, PO	75 div q 8 hr	30 div q 12 hr
Mezlocillin	IV, IM	60 div q 8 hr	225 div q 8 hr
Oxacillin	IV, IM	5 div q 12 hr	150 div q 6 hr
Nafcillin	IV		75 div q 6 hr
Netilmicin	IM, IV	150,000 units div q 8 hr	7.5 div q 8 hr
Penicillin G	IV (units/kg/day)	60,000 units div q 8 hr	
Meningitis			200,000 U div q 6 hr
Other diseases		50,000 units (one dose)	100,000 U div q 6 hr
Penicillin G	IM (units/kg/day)	50,000 units once daily	
Benzathine		225 div q 8 hr	50,000 U (one dose)
Procaine		5 div q 12 hr	50,000 U once daily
Ticarcillin	IV, IM	30 div q 12 hr	300 div q 6 hr
Tobramycin	IM, IV		7.5 div q 8 hr
Vancomycin	IV		45 div q 8 hr
Antiviral:			
Acyclovir	IV	30 div q 8 hr	30 div q 8 hr
Antifungal:			
Amphotericin	IV	0.5 q day	0.5 q day (test dose required)

* Adapted from Nelson JD: *1993-1994 Pocketbook of pediatric antimicrobial therapy,* ed 10, Baltimore, 1993, Williams & Wilkins.
Note: Four infants <2,000 g. See reference pages 16, 17.[3]

REFERENCES

1. Gladstone IM and others: A ten year review of neonatal sepsis and comparison with fifty year experience, *Pediatr Infect Dis J* 9(11):821, 1990.
2. Holbrook PR: *Textbook of pediatric critical care,* Philadelphia, 1993, WB Saunders.
3. Nelson JD: *1993-1994 Pocketbook of pediatric antimicrobial therapy,* ed 10, Baltimore, 1993, Williams & Wilkins.

Respiratory Problems of the Neonate

BACKGROUND

Even though guidelines for perinatal care increasingly call for maternal-fetal referral when a high-risk delivery is anticipated,[4] large numbers of newborn infants still require interhospital transport to access a higher level of care. The majority of these transfers involve some form of respiratory distress. In fact, 56% of neonatal transports to The Children's Hospital in Denver require assisted ventilation.

GENERAL PRINCIPLES

The safe and effective transport of neonates with respiratory distress requires accurate diagnosis and an understanding of pulmonary pathophysiology, physical principles of oxygen tension, and gas expansion, as well as the appropriate monitoring of oxygenation, ventilation, and circulatory status. Important aspects of interhospital care include assessment, diagnosis, anticipation, and stabilization. The clinical condition of the infant will continue to evolve during and after transport; consequently, excessive time should not be wasted attempting to "cure" the patient. Only enough time should be spent to ensure a safe move.

A critical decision to be made before transport is whether to initiate distending airway pressure by CPAP or IPPV. While benefiting many, others may worsen because of complications of overinflation. Important factors in this decision process are the gestational age, postnatal age, diagnosis, progression of the disease, and anticipated duration of transport. Near-term infants with good lung compliance and normal inflation who are well oxygenated with supplemental oxygen of less than 0.60 FiO_2 often may be moved over short distances in warmed, humidified oxygen. It is important to remember that during air transport, alveolar partial pressure of oxygen may fall by as much as 150 mm Hg depending on altitude, aircraft pressurization, and elevation gained (Fig. 32-2).

Very low birth weight infants and those with rapidly progressing or advanced disease characterized by apnea and diminished lung compliance and volume will require stabilization and transport on distending pressure.

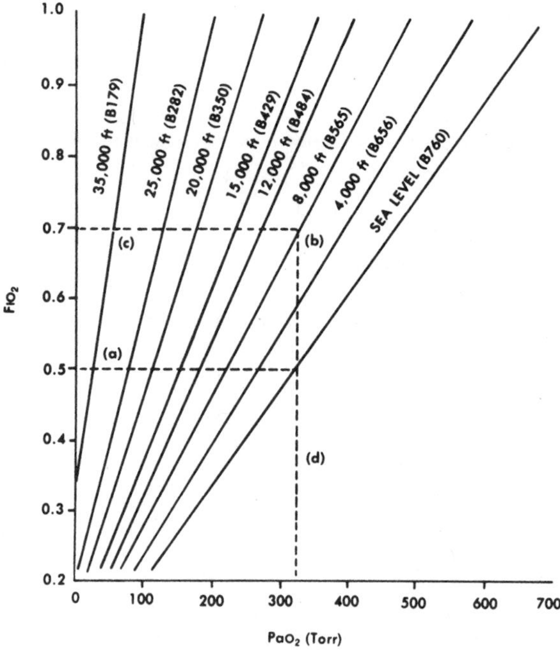

Fig. 32-2. From Merenstein GB, Pettett G: Transport of ventilated infants. In Goldsmith P, Karotkin EH, editors: Assisted ventilation of the neonate, Philadelphia, 1988, WB Saunders Company.

TABLE 32-11 RESPIRATORY CARE DURING TRANSPORT

	Hood oxygen	*Distending airway pressure*
Gestational age		
<34 weeks		x
>34 weeks	x	
Examination		
Tachypnea	x	
Retractions		x
Diminished air entry		x
Apnea		x
Chest x-ray		
Clear	x	
Streaky, normal inflation	x	
Granular, reduced inflation		x
Dense infiltrates		x
Air trapping, extrapulmonary air	x	
Disease course		
Stable	x	
Rapidly progressive		x
Advanced		x
FiO_2		
<0.60	x	
>0.60		x

TABLE 32-12 CHARACTERISTICS OF PORTABLE GAS CYLINDERS

	Volume and flow duration of oxygen in three cylinder sizes											
	Full			¾			½			¼		
Cylinder type	*E*	*M*	*H*	*E*	*M*	*H*	*E*	*M*	*H*	*E*	*M*	*H*
Contents (cu. ft.)	22	107	244	16.5	80.2	193	11	53.5	122	5.5	26.8	61
Liters	622	3028	6900	466.5	2271	5175	311	1514	3450	155.5	757	1724
Pressure (psi)		2000			1500			1000			500	

	Approximate number of hours of flow in three cylinder sizes											
	Full			¾			½			¼		
Cylinder type	*E*	*M*	*H*	*E*	*M*	*H*	*E*	*M*	*H*	*E*	*M*	*H*
Flow rate (liters/min)												
2	5.1	25	56	3.8	18.5	42	2.5	12.5	28	1.3	6	14
4	2.5	12.6	28	1.8	10.4	21	1.2	6.3	14	0.6	3.1	7
6	1.7	8.4	18.5	1.3	6.3	13.7	0.9	4.2	9.2	0.4	2.1	4.5
8	1.2	6.3	14	0.9	4.6	10.5	0.6	3.1	7	0.3	1.5	3.5
10	1	5	11	0.7	3.7	8.2	0.5	2.5	5.5	0.2	1.2	2.7
12	0.8	4.2	9.2	0.6	3	6.7	0.4	2.1	4.5	0.2	1	2.2
15	0.6	3.4	7.2	0.4	2.5	5.5	0.3	1.7	3.5	0.1	0.8	1.7

From Merenstein GB, Pettett G: Transport of ventilated infants. In Goldsmith JP, Karotkin EH, editors: Assisted ventilation of the neonate, Philadelphia, 1988, WB Saunders Company.

While the decision must be individualized for each transport, Table 32-11 lists some generalizations that may be useful. A bedside trial of distending airway pressure can be attempted with tight fitting, hand-held mask CPAP. If air entry and oxygenation (PO_2, $TcSaO_2$) improve while retractions lessen, pressure may be beneficial during transport.

Before transporting a patient on distending airway pressure, complete stabilization must be undertaken. Because nonintubated CPAP can be unstable, a securely taped endotracheal tube is preferred. If it is anticipated that intubation and ventilation might be necessary during transport, these steps should be performed during stabilization in the referring hospital. Turbulence, small space, and poor lighting can make these procedures difficult in transit.

EQUIPMENT

Proper equipment is essential for transport of the neonate with respiratory disease. Equipment should include the following:

1. Oxygen hood
2. Oxygen analyzer
3. Self-inflating or anesthesia bag
4. Ventilator
    - Compact, light-weight
    - Gas driven
    - Pressure-limited, time-cycled
5. Portable air and oxygen cylinders (Table 32-12)
6. Battery-powered monitoring equipment
7. Suction

VENTILATOR STABILIZATION

Because transport ventilators will generate wave forms and pressures that are different from NICU devices, the patient must be stabilized on the transport ventilator before departure. This stabilization will include many or all of the following:

- Examination of chest wall movement
- Auscultation of air entry
- Chest x-ray measure of inflation
- Arterial blood gases
- Transcutaneous PO_2, PCO_2, SaO_2

Ventilator settings should be chosen to optimize oxygenation and ventilation, minimize gas consumption, and reduce risks of complications.

High flow, rapid rates, and high pressures generally increase gas consumption and dictate the cylinder sizes required in transport.

Battery powered monitoring is essential to assess the patient adequately in a transport setting. Monitoring should include heart rate, rhythm, respiratory rate, blood pressure, and noninvasive PO_2, PCO_2, SaO_2 measurements.

Ease of application and reliable correlation favor pulse oximetry over transcutaneous PO_2 monitoring. Given the oxygen affinity of fetal hemoglobin, saturations of approximately 94%[6] should be targeted to encourage pulmonary vascular dilation and ductal closure while minimizing toxicity.

Because acute lung disease in the newborn often is characterized by an intrapulmonary shunt, normal oxygenation usually is associated with adequate ventilation. As such, PCO_2 monitoring is less critical. While end-tidal CO_2 monitoring has been used in infants during transport to assess endotracheal tube placement and ventilation, it requires intubation, and the correlation with PCO_2 is variable, particularly in the presence of respiratory acidosis.[1,5]

RESPIRATORY CONDITIONS REQUIRING TRANSPORT

While the above general principles apply to most newborns with respiratory distress in transport, the many pulmonary conditions can be grouped into the following disease categories.

Homogeneous, granular, low-volume lungs
Normal-volume lungs
Space-occupying mass effects
Patchy or dense infiltrates
Clear, underperfused lungs

HOMOGENEOUS, GRANULAR, LOW-VOLUME LUNGS

This group consists mostly of patients with hyaline membrane disease. These patients usually are premature (<34 weeks) and demonstrate grunting, flaring, retracting, and diminished air entry on examination. The x-ray shows a diffusely granular appearance with decreased lung volumes (Fig. 32-3). Arterial blood gases usually will show comparable deterioration in oxygenation and ventilation.

If transported early in the course when oxygen requirement is modest (FiO_2 0.40-0.50), distending airway pressure may not be necessary or beneficial. On the other hand, progressive disease characterized by increasing FiO_2, work of breathing and loss of volume will require intubation and ventilation. In general, higher mean airway pressures (↑PIP, ↑PEEP, ↑Inspiratory Time) should improve oxygenation. The administration of exogenous surfactant may be beneficial, but also can result in rapidly changing functional re-

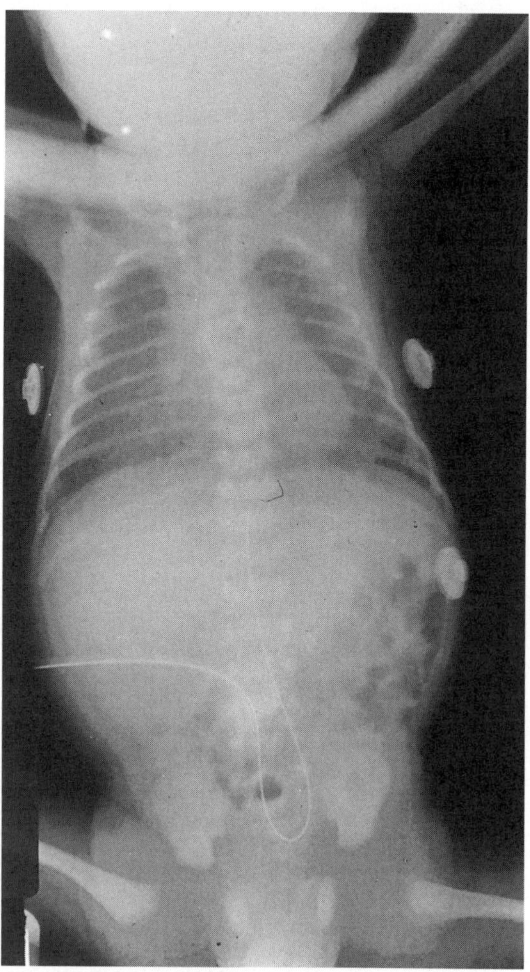

Fig. 32-3. Respiratory distress syndrome.

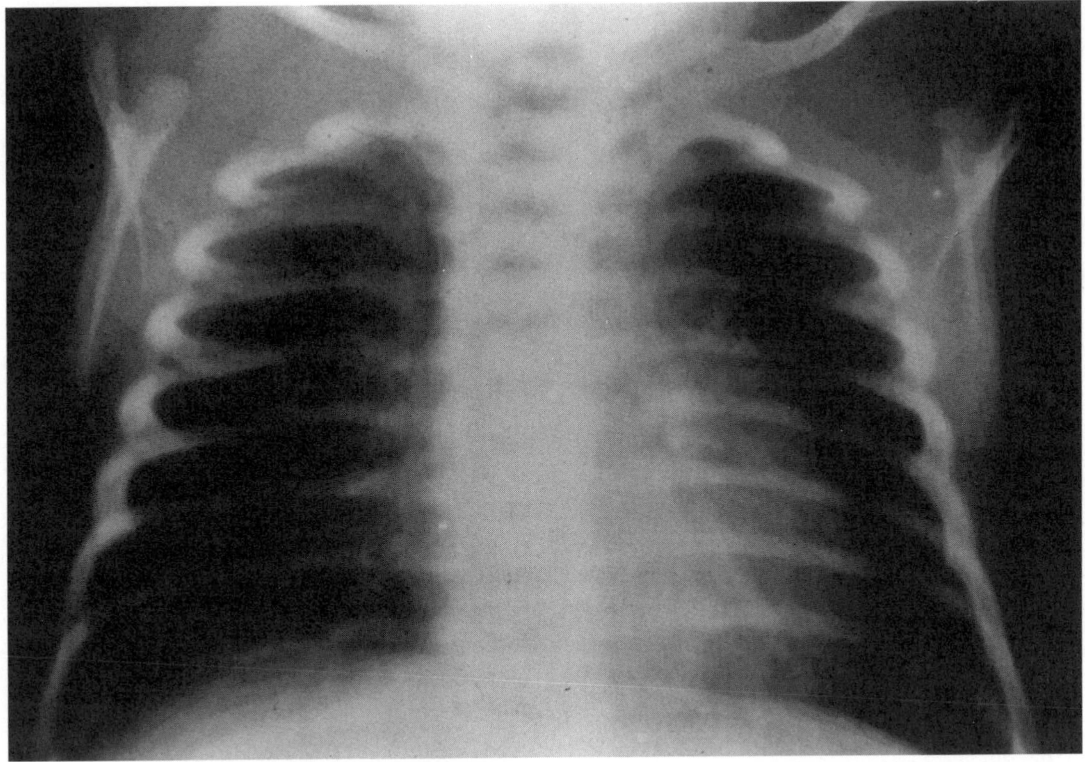

Fig. 32-4. Retained lung fluid.

sidual capacity and compliance,[3,8] thus increasing the risk of lung overdistention and air leak. Consequently, the clinician should choose accordingly and allow stabilization time between surfactant administration and transport departure.

NORMAL-VOLUME LUNGS

This group of patients is typified by retained lung fluid, wet lung, and transient tachypnea of the newborn (Fig. 32-4). These are usually near-term or term infants born following rapid labor and delivery or Cesarean section. These infants present with rapid breathing, good air exchange, and streaky, well-inflated chest x-rays. Ventilation usually is normal or increased, but oxygenation is moderately impaired. Transport usually can be accomplished with warmed, humidified hood oxygen and peripheral intravenous access.

SPACE-OCCUPYING MASS EFFECTS

Space-occupying mass effects are uncommon entities but present special challenges in recognition, stabilization, and transport.[1] Included are diaphragmatic hernias (Fig. 32-5), lobar emphysema, cystic adenomatoid malformations, pneumothorax (Fig. 32-6), and restrictive abdominal distention (Fig. 32-7). Diagnosis is best made by x-ray.

These mass effects can profoundly affect oxygenation, ventilation, venous return, and cardiac output. Physical examination often will show asymmetric breath sounds, shifted heart tones, and poor skin perfusion. Arterial blood gases will show significant elevation of PCO_2 and depression of PO_2. Stabilization should include efforts to reduce the mass effect through thoracentesis, thoracostomy, paracentesis, and gastric decompression. Positioning the patient with the less-affected side upward may be helpful. Intubation and controlled ventilation with heavy sedation or neuromuscular blockade is required in many cases.

PATCHY OR DENSE INFILTRATES

These patients usually are born near-term and have pneumonia or aspiration (see Fig.

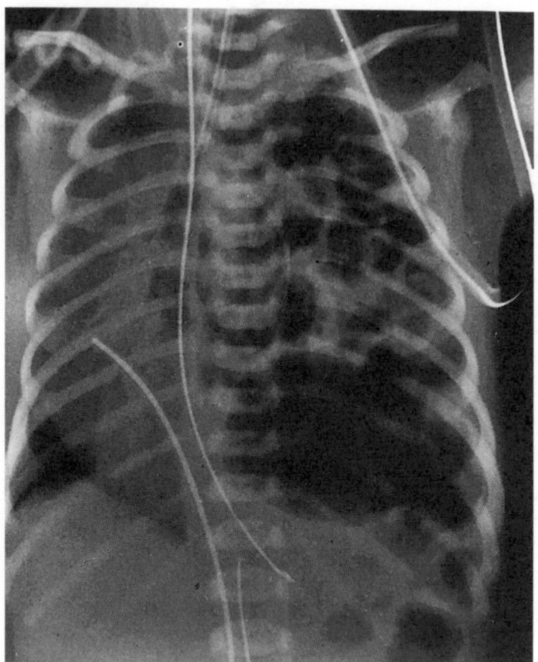

Fig. 32-5. Diaphragmatic hernia.

32-8). Physical examination will reveal tachypnea, increased work of breathing, retractions, unequal air entry, and rales. Arterial blood gases demonstrate comparable disturbances in PO_2 and PCO_2. The chest x-ray shows patchy infiltrates, often with unequal inflation and air trapping.

The risk of air leak is increased because of unequal inflation, and distending airway pressure should be used cautiously in transport. Hood oxygen is safest if the oxygenation and ventilation deficits are modest. During assisted ventilation, it is essential to avoid the air trapping sometimes seen with long inspiratory times, high end pressures, and inadvertent PEEP generated by very-high-rate conventional ventilation.

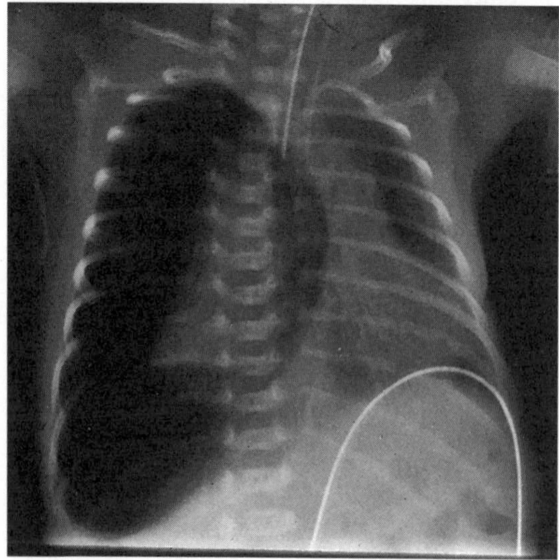

Fig. 32-6. Pneumothorax.

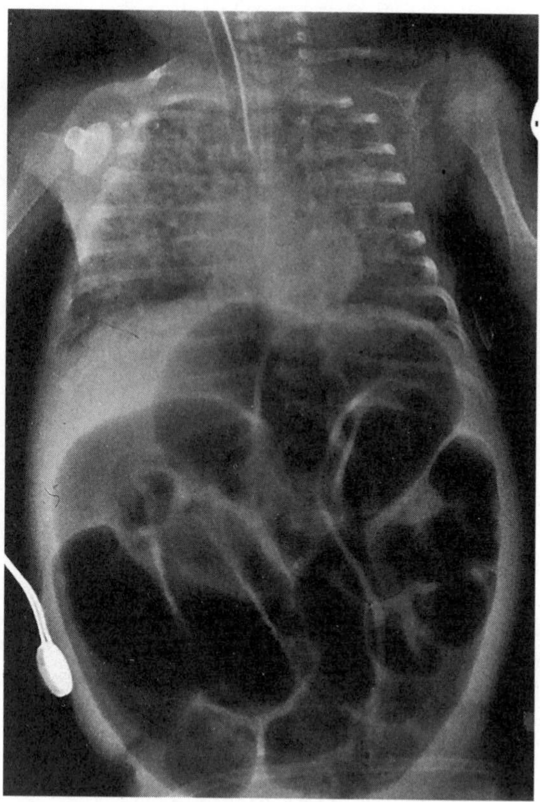

Fig. 32-7. Abdominal distention.

CLEAR, UNDERPERFUSED LUNGS

Persistent pulmonary hypertension of the newborn (PPHN) usually occurs at term and can be seen with minimal or extensive lung disease (Fig. 32-9). It is characterized by oxygenation being worse than ventilation as a result of diminished pulmonary perfusion. While the findings are determined largely by the underlying disease, these infants are often cyanotic and tachypneic but have good air entry. Cardiac auscultation may reveal findings of pulmonary hypertension, such as a lower sternal border tricuspid insufficiency murmur and accentuated second heart sound. The chest x-ray is often nearly clear or may be characteristic of the primary process.

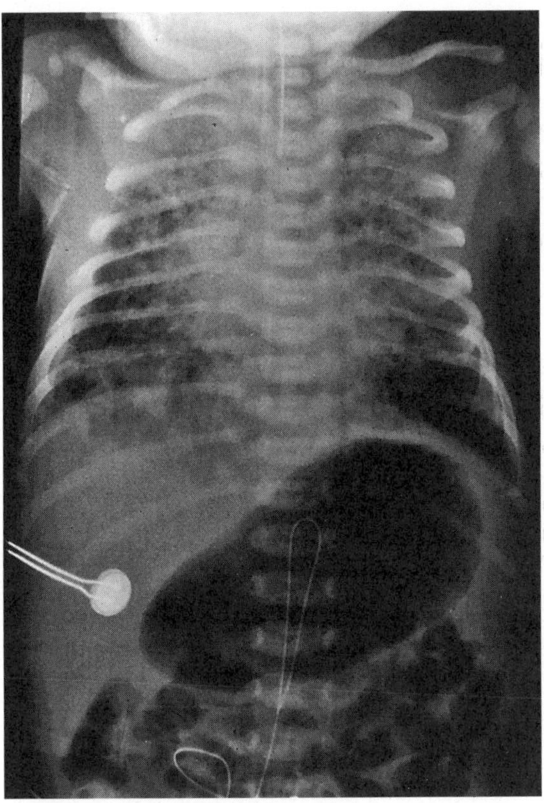

Fig. 32-8. Meconium aspiration.

Therapy should be aimed at maintaining high alveolar and arterial oxygen levels to promote pulmonary vasodilatation. High-inspired hood oxygen may be adequate. If not, rapid rate hyperventilation to achieve respiratory alkalosis is often effective. To achieve this synchronously, heavy sedation or paralysis often is needed.

COMPLICATIONS

Complications can arise during transport; these complications must be prevented where possible and rapidly corrected when present. Mechanical problems such as endotracheal tube plugging or dislodging can be prevented by using warm (35-37° C), humidified (70% saturation) gases, proper tube affixing, and suctioning.

Perhaps the most life-threatening complication that can develop is extrapulmonary air. The use of time-cycled, pressure-limited ventilators with changing lung compliance in an asynchronously breathing patient can result in overdistention and air leak. This extrapulmonary air compromises oxygenation, ventilation, systemic venous return, and cardiac output. Its volume can expand with increases in altitude and should be evacuated before transport when possible (Table 32-13) (Fig. 32-10).

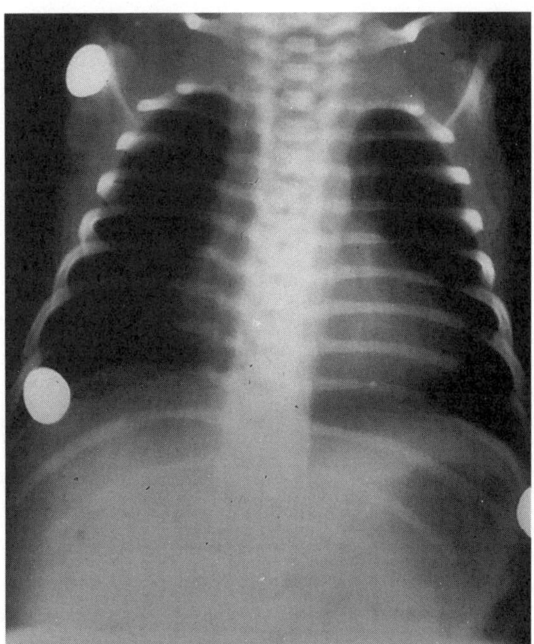

Fig. 32-9. Pulmonary hypertension.

Air leak may be prevented by close monitoring, careful choice of ventilator settings, and patient sedation or paralysis. Chest wall excursion and breath sounds should be assessed as frequently as possible throughout transport. In general, lower flow rates, shorter inspiratory times, and lower pressures may reduce the risk of lung injury from assisted ventilation. More synchronous venti-

TABLE 32-13 EFFECTS OF ALTITUDE ON EXPANSION OF ENCLOSED GAS

Altitude (feet)	*Expansion factor of trapped gas*
Sea level	×1
10,000	×1.5
18,000	×2
27,000	×3
33,400	×4
38,500	×5

From Merenstein BG, Pettett G: Transport of ventilated infants. In Goldsmith JP, Karotkin EH, editors: Assisted ventilation of the neonate, Philadelphia, 1988, WB Saunders Company.

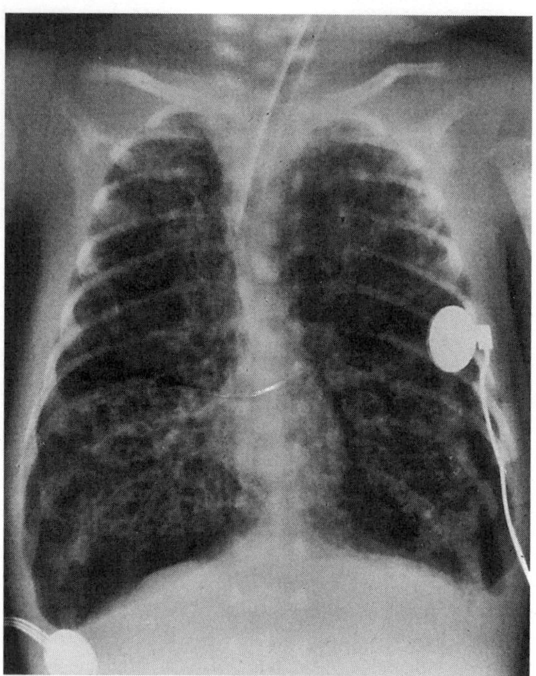

Fig. 32-10. Pulmonary interstitial emphysema with pneumothorax.

lation may be achieved with drug therapy which may include the following: anxiolytics (diazepam, lorazepam, midazolam), narcotics (morphine, fentanyl), or neuromuscular blockers (pancuronium, vecuronium).

Clinical signs of air leak include worsening oxygenation, bradycardia, hypotension, diminished breath sounds, muffled or shifted heart tones, and positive transillumination. Such free air should be evacuated with needle thoracentesis through the third intercostal space in the midclavicular line.

FUTURE CONSIDERATIONS

While the vast majority of newborns with pulmonary disease can be effectively transported with hood oxygen, intubated CPAP, or pressure-limited, assisted ventilation, complex therapies for severe pulmonary hypertension are being applied with the limited use of extracorporeal membrane oxygenation (ECMO)[2] and inhaled nitric oxide (NO)[7] as part of interhospital care.

REFERENCES

1. Bhende MS, Thompson AE, Orr RA: Utility of an end-tidal carbon dioxide detector during stabilization and transport of critically ill children, *Pediatrics* 89:1042, 1992.
2. Cornish ID: Extracorporeal membrane oxygenation as a means of stabilizing and transporting high risk neonates, *ASAIO Trans:* 37:564, 1991.
3. Cotton and others: Differential effects of synthetic and bovine surfactants on lung volume and oxygenation in premature infants with RDS, *Pediatric Res* 31:304A, 1992.
4. Freeman RK, Poland RL: *Guidelines for perinatal care,* ed 3, Elk Grove Village, IL, 1992, American Academy of Pediatrics, The American College of Obstetricians and Gynecologists.
5. Hand and others: Discrepancies between transcutaneous and end-tidal carbon dioxide monitoring in the critically ill neonate with respiratory distress syndrome, *Crit Care Med* 17:556, 1989.
6. Hay WW, Thilo E, Curlander JB: Pulse oximetry in neonatal medicine. In Brans YW, editor: *Clinics in perinatology,* Philadelphia, 1991, WB Saunders Company.
7. Kinsella JP: Inhaled nitric oxide in transport of neonates with pulmonary hypertension, unpublished experience, 1993.
8. Milner AD: How does exogenous surfactant work, *Arch Dis Child* 68:253, 1993.

Congenital Heart Disease

RECOGNITION

Congenital heart disease of the newborn generally presents with cyanosis, congestive heart failure, arrhythmias, or cardiogenic shock, with cyanosis and congestive failure being the most common presentations. The approach to the infant with congenital heart disease may be divided into those with cyanotic or acyanotic lesions. These two groups frequently present with different constellations of signs.

CYANOTIC LESIONS

The primary physical manifestation is central cyanosis. These infants may have no respiratory distress or may be tachypneic without dyspnea. The precordium is normally quiet, and a murmur may or may not be present. Arterial blood gases document hypoxemia despite an oxygen-enriched environment. In addition, the infant may respond to the hypoxemia with hyperpnea resulting in a respiratory alkalosis. Severe hypoxemia may force the infant to convert to anaerobic metabolism, thus developing a metabolic acidosis. While sometimes difficult to interpret, chest radiographs may reveal dark lung fields because of decreased pulmonary blood flow.

ACYANOTIC LESIONS

Infants with acyanotic lesions who present in the nursery usually manifest signs of congestive heart failure. The earliest sign may be tachypnea that progresses to significant respiratory distress with retractions and grunting. The infant's color may range from pallor to ashen or grey. The extremities are frequently cool to the touch. The precordial activity is usually increased, while the pulses are diminished and/or unequal. Murmurs and hepatomegaly are common. Arterial blood gases frequently reveal metabolic acidosis because of poor systemic perfusion. In the presence of pulmonary edema, this may be compounded by a respiratory acidosis. Hypoxemia, if present, usually will respond to increased provision of inspired oxygen. Chest radiographs may reveal increased vascularity and cardiomegaly.

EVALUATION

The infant with early signs of congestive heart failure, tachypnea, and tachycardia in combination with cyanosis presents the clinician with the difficulty of differentiating pulmonary, pulmonary vascular, and cardiac etiologies. The approach to this clinical dilemma includes careful consideration of the clinical history and evaluation of physical findings.

CLINICAL HISTORY

A clinical history may reveal risk factors for pulmonary or pulmonary vascular etiologies. Risk factors would include prematurity, postmaturity, meconium-stained fluid, prolonged rupture of membranes, neonatal asphyxia, or Cesarean delivery. In the presence of severe respiratory distress or intense cyanosis, the chest radiograph could be expected to reveal corresponding abnormalities in the case of pulmonary etiologies. Persistent pulmonary hypertension of the newborn (PPHN) frequently occurs in association with underlying respiratory disease but may present with a deceptively unremarkable chest film. A history of normal oxygenation levels is also helpful in decreasing the likelihood of a diagnosis of cyanotic heart disease.

PHYSICAL EVALUATION

Infants with cyanosis on the basis of pulmonary disease will normally improve oxygenation in an oxygen-enriched environment. A hyperoxia test may be useful in demonstrating the infant's ability to significantly improve oxygenation in the presence of high levels of inspired oxygen. This can be accomplished by monitoring the infant's arterial oxygen saturation using pulse oximetry. Simultaneous monitoring of preductal (right arm) and postductal (lower extremity sites will allow the evaluation of oxygenation response to changes in inspired oxygen as well as information about right-to-left shunting of blood across the ductus arteriosus. Preductal and postductal blood gases also may be measured. A difference of 3% to 4% in oxygen saturation or 15 to 20 torr in PaO_2 is significant. Infants with severe respiratory compromise may require positive end expiratory pressure to produce a measurable increase in oxygenation. Lack of response to the hyperoxia test does not eliminate PPHN as the etiology of central cyanosis. For severe distress, further steps may be taken to induce pulmonary vasodilatation. These might include the development of a respiratory alkalosis through hyperventilation, a metabolic alkalosis through administration of sodium bicarbonate or THAM, or the use of vasodilator drug therapy. Although usually unavailable at the referring institution, echocardiography can be performed to determine the presence of congenital heart disease and evaluate the contribution of pulmonary hypertension to systemic hypertension.

In addition to a complete physical examination of the cardiovascular system, a full set of vital signs and blood pressures should be obtained. Blood pressures should be obtained in at least the right arm and a lower extremity. A leg pressure 15 to 20 torr lower than the right arm pressure may indicate the presence of coarctation of the aorta.

Immediate onset of respiratory distress at

delivery is most consistent with a pulmonary etiology. However, the presence of clear signs of congestive heart failure at birth may indicate severe in utero anemia, critical aortic stenosis, critical coarctation of the aorta, interrupted aortic arch, Ebstein's malformation, or severe fetal bradycardia or tachyarrhythmia.

Complete evaluation of the infant would include laboratory studies for hypoglycemia, hypocalcemia, and sepsis.

PRETRANSPORT STABILIZATION

Supportive care

Oxygen should be administered to produce an FiO_2 of approximately 0.40. In addition to congenital heart disease, infants may have respiratory compromise secondary to pulmonary disease or congestive heart failure and may benefit from the administration of low concentrations of oxygen.

Ventilatory support may be required for the infant with severe respiratory distress or shock. The use of positive end-expiratory pressure may be beneficial in the management of the infant with pulmonary edema. Elective intubation should be completed before transport, if the need for airway intervention is anticipated before arrival at the receiving center.

During acute management, fluids should be administered with caution. In severe congestive heart failure, the use of diuretics may be considered.

Pharmaceutical support

Ductal-dependent lesions, including cyanotic defects with restricted pulmonary flow, acyanotic defects with left heart obstruction, and defects dependent on blood mixing across the ductus, benefit from the intravenous administration of prostaglandin E_1 (PGE_1).[1] PGE_1 will open a closed ductus arteriosus or maintain the patency of the ductus. Side effects of PGE_1 use include apnea, vasodilation with flushing, fever and local erythema. Because apnea may develop during transport, elective intubation before departure from the referring institution should be considered.

Infants with congestive heart failure and shock may require the use of inotropic agents to improve cardiac output and improve circulation. Metabolic acidosis may be buffered with sodium bicarbonate or THAM.

TRANSPORT MANAGEMENT

Management of the infant with congenital heart disease during transport requires vigilance in monitoring for changes in cardiac output, oxygenation and respiratory status. The use of pulse oximetry, transcutaneous oxygen and carbon dioxide monitors, and invasive aortic pressure monitoring are helpful in evaluating the effectiveness of PGE_1 therapy and respiratory management. The infant receiving PGE_1 must also be carefully monitored for apnea or hypoventilation.

REFERENCES

1. Freed MD and others: Prostaglandin E_1 in infants with ductus arteriosus-dependent congenital heart disease, *Circulation* 64:899-905, 1981.

Perinatal Asphyxia and Seizures

Perinatal asphyxia is a condition marked by severe fetal or neonatal hypoxic-ischemic injury leading to decreased tissue substrate delivery and metabolic acidosis. Perinatal asphyxia frequently affects multiple organ systems, resulting in hypoxic-ischemic encephalopathy with seizures, myocardial dysfunction, systemic hypotension, meconium aspiration, hepatic dysfunction, disseminated intravascular coagulation, and acute renal failure. The term "birth depression" is often more appropriate when initially describing the newborn with low Apgar scores who requires resuscitation in the delivery room.

This section will focus on the neurologic sequelae of hypoxic-ischemic encephalopathy (HIE) and the relevant clinical issues relating to transport of the asphyxiated newborn.

INITIAL EVALUATION

Most perinatal hypoxic-ischemic cerebral insults occur before (antepartum) or during (intrapartum) birth.[5] Antepartum asphyxia may be caused by altered placental gas exchange and acute or chronic uteroplacental insufficiency. Antepartum asphyxia is more likely to occur in pregnancies complicated by maternal diabetes, preeclampsia, or intrauterine growth retardation. Severe asphyxia may result from interruption of the umbilical circulation caused by placental and umbilical cord accidents (e.g., abruption, placenta previa, prolapsed cord, or nuchal cord). Other factors that may place the newborn at risk for asphyxia include maternal hypotension, maternal cardiopulmonary disease or severe anemia, and transitional neonatal pulmonary hypertension causing critical hypoxemia. Signs of intrapartum fetal distress include fetal heart rate alterations (particularly late decelerations and decreased variability), acid-base disturbances on umbilical cord blood gas analysis, and meconium staining of the amniotic fluid.

The Apgar score is a useful indicator of the response to resuscitation in the delivery room; however, the predictive value of this score at 1 and 5 minutes is limited. For example, in full-term neonates with an Apgar score of 0-3 at 5 minutes, the incidence of cerebral palsy (CP) is approximately 1%. The longer the score is low, the greater is its significance in predicting an adverse neurologic outcome. Nine percent of survivors with an Apgar score of 0-3 at 15 minutes will have CP, and 57% of infants with this score at 20 minutes will demonstrate CP (Table 32-14).[1,3] A low umbilical cord pH (<7.00) is also suggestive of severe fetal compromise but is less predictive of ultimate outcome.[2]

The initial evaluation of the neonate with suspected HIE can yield useful clues to the severity of the insult and may correlate well with outcome.[4] As outlined in Table 32-15, HIE may be divided into mild, moderate, and severe categories. Mild HIE is not associated with long-term sequelae. However, 20% to 40% of all infants with moderate HIE will suffer neurologic sequelae, and major sequelae likely will affect all infants with severe HIE.

TABLE 32-14 INCIDENCE OF DEATH AND CEREBRAL PALSY BASED ON APGAR SCORE

APGAR score 0 to 3	*% Death in 1st year*	*% Cerebral palsy in survivors*
1 minute	3	1
5 minutes	8	1
10 minutes	18	5
15 minutes	48	9
20 minutes	59	57

TABLE 32-15 CATEGORIES OF HYPOXIC-ISCHEMI ENCEPHALOPATHY

Mild	Hyperalertness, uninhibited reflexes, sympathetic overactivity, duration <24 hours
Moderate	Lethargy, hypotonia, seizures
Severe	Coma, flaccid tone, suppressed brain-stem function, seizures

PRINCIPLES OF MANAGEMENT

Although the insult causing HIE may have occurred in utero, the ultimate severity of the neurologic sequelae also will be affected by early neonatal management. The basic components of the management of HIE are outlined in Table 32-16.

Maintenance of adequate ventilation is essential following an asphyxial insult, with emphasis on avoiding hypercarbia (cerebral acidosis) and severe hypocarbia, which can decrease cerebral blood flow. A reasonable range for $PaCO_2$ is 20 to 35 torr. Adequate oxygenation should be maintained ($PaO_2 >$ 50 torr), but marked hyperoxia should be avoided to minimize additional neuronal injury.

TABLE 32-16 ESSENTIAL COMPONENTS IN THE MANAGEMENT OF HYPOXIC-ISCHEMIC ENCEPHALOPATHY

Maintenance of adequate ventilation (avoid hypercarbia, hypocarbia).
Maintenance of adequate blood pressure and perfusion.
Maintenance of adequate blood glucose levels.
Prevention of fluid overload-recognize SIADH.
Control of seizures.

Modified from Volpe JJ, Neurology of the Newborn, WB Saunders, Philadelphia, 1987.
SIADH = Syndrome of Inappropriate AntiDiuretic Hormone

Maintaining adequate blood pressure is critically important in the immediate neonatal period after asphyxial insult. Autoregulation of the cerebral circulation frequently is compromised, and cerebral blood flow tends to be "pressure-passive." Systemic hypotension may lead to further ischemic injury, while systemic hypertension may cause intracranial hemorrhage. Therefore, after adequate volume resuscitation and cardiotonic support to establish normal systemic blood pressure and tissue perfusion, particular attention should be given to minimizing interventions which can cause abrupt increases in blood pressure. Volume resuscitation also-should be guided by the recognition that cerebral edema frequently complicates HIE, and fluid overload may exacerbate the brain injury (particularly in the presence of SIADH).

Adequate supplies of glucose are essential to meet cerebral energy demands. Glucose levels should be carefully monitored to avoid hypo- and hyperglycemia. Intravenous glucose supplementation should be adjusted to maintain blood glucose in the 75 to 100 mg/dl range[5]. Calcium levels should be monitored, and hypocalcemia should be treated promptly.

IDENTIFICATION AND MANAGEMENT OF SEIZURES

Seizures occur in the majority of cases of severe HIE and may contribute to additional central nervous system injury. Seizures are associated with hypoventilation, leading to hypoxemia and hypercarbia. Moreover, marked increases in cerebral metabolism and systemic arterial pressure can have adverse CNS effects, as noted above.

Seizure activity in the newborn may not be readily apparent. The most common types of seizure are subtle and involve paroxysms such as repetitive blinking, sucking, or "rowing" movements of the upper extremities. The five major varieties of neonatal seizures are listed in Table 32-17. Jitteriness must be distinguished from seizure activity (Table 32-18).

Initial management of seizures should focus on maintaining adequate oxygenation and ventilation. Blood should be drawn for determination of glucose, calcium, magnesium, electrolytes, and blood gases. If the seizure activity is sustained or recurrent, and if no-correctable metabolic cause is identified (e.g., hypoglycemia, hypocalcemia, or hypomagnesemia), phenobarbital should be administered in a dose of 20 to 30 mg/kg. Seizures refractory to treatment with phenobarbital may require additional anticonvulsants as outlined in Table 32-19.

TABLE 32-17 CATEGORIES OF NEONATAL SEIZURES

Subtle	Tonic deviation of eyes, sustained eye opening, eyelid blinking, sucking, "swimming rowing pedaling" movements, apneic spells.
Generalized tonic	Tonic extension or flexion of upper limbs, tonic extension of lower limbs.
Multifocal clonic	Migratory clonic limb movements.
Focal clonic	Well-localized clonic jerking movements.
Myoclonic	Synchronous jerks of flexion of upper limbs.

TABLE 32-18 JITTERINESS VERSUS SEIZURES

Clinical features	*Jitteriness*	*Seizures*
Eye deviation, abnormal gaze	–	+
Stimulus sensitive	+	–
Predominant movement	Tremor	Clonic, jerking
Movements cease with passive flexion	+	–

TABLE 32-19 TREATMENT OF SEIZURES

Glucose	10% solution (D10), 2ml/kg IV
Phenobarbital	20-30 mg/kg IV
Phenytoin	20 mg/kg IV (0.5-1.5 mg/kg/minute)
Diazepam	0.3 mg/kg IV
Calcium gluconate	100-200 mg/kg/dose IV, over 5-10 minutes
Magnesium sulfate	20-40 mg/kg IM

SUMMARY

Perinatal asphyxia is characterized by multisystem hypoxic-ischemic injury and seizures. Acute management during transport must focus on cardiopulmonary stabilization and minimizing additional central nervous system injury. Careful management of hemodynamic and pulmonary variables, rapid correction of metabolic derangements, and appropriate treatment of seizures will reduce the likelihood of additional injury during neonatal transport.

REFERENCES

1. Brann AW: Hypoxic ischemic encephalopathy (asphyxia), *Pediatric Clinics of North America,* 33:451-64, 1986.
2. Carter BS, Haverkamp AD, Merenstein GB: The definition of acute perinatal asphyxia, *Clin Perinatol* 20:287-304, 1993.
3. Nelson KB, Ellenberg JH: Apgar scores as predictors of chronic neurologic disability, *Pediatrics,* 68:36-44, 1981.
4. Robertson C, Finer N: Term infants with hypoxic-ischemic encephalopathy: outcome at 3.5 years, *Dev Child Neurol* 27:473, 1985.
5. Volpe JJ: *Neurology of the newborn,* Philadelphia, 1987, WB Saunders.

Transport of the Dysmorphic Infant

Transport of the dysmorphic infant requires that the clinician pay special attention to data collection and physical examination.[7,8,12] Information gained at the time of transfer may be of significance to consultants at the receiving institution.[1]

When an infant has an anatomic anomaly the family and parental medical history, along with past and current obstetric history, acquire additional importance.[2-6,10,11] It may be impractical at the time of transport to gather a complete family pedigree, but information regarding other family members with malformations may provide clues to a pattern of inheritance. Past obstetric history, especially early fetal losses, are suggestive of genetic errors. Some recurrent anomalies, such as polydactyly, may be autosomal dominant.[1]

All unusual features should be noted when a dysmorphic infant is assessed.[6] Minor anomalies (those of little cosmetic or functional consequence) noted on physical examination are of special significance because there is a relationship between their occurrence and the possibility of a major anomaly. A major anomaly is a defect that causes significant cosmetic or functional deficit and requires medical or surgical intervention. A study by Marden in 1964 revealed this association.[9] An infant with no visible minor anomaly has a 1.4% risk of having a major anomaly, and an infant with one minor anomaly has a 3% risk of having a major anomaly. When two minor anomalies are noted on examination, the risk of a major anomaly increases to 11%. Infants whose physical examinations reveal three or more minor anomalies have a 90% probability of also having a major anomaly.

The transport of an infant who has an anomaly often requires special attention to avoid further morbidity. An anomaly can complicate management of the airway, thermoregulation, and positioning of the infant. There also may be an increased risk of infection and the possibility of compounding the insult to the newborn, for example, recurrent aspiration with a tracheoesophageal fistula (Table 32-20).

Airway management in the dysmorphic infant may be complicated by upper airway obstruction, as in choanal atresia.[7] Newborns are obligate nose breathers, and an oral airway may be all that is needed. If the tongue is the cause of the obstruction (as in macroglossia or micrognathia), an oral airway may not be sufficient. If the infant is placed in a prone position, the tongue can fall forward, away from the oropharynx, and allow air passage. Occasionally, the disparity of the relative size of the tongue and the mandible is so great that intubation is required.

Esophageal atresia with or without tracheoesophageal fistula increases the risk of aspiration. Isolated esophageal atresia increases the possibility of aspiration of oral secretions. Before transport, a large-bore suction catheter should be placed in the pouch and intermittent suctioning used to help control the accumulation of secretions. Also, the infant should be placed in a prone position with the head of the bed down to allow excess saliva to fall out of the mouth. If esophageal atresia is

TABLE 32-20 TRANSPORT OF INFANTS WITH ANOMALIES: COMPLICATIONS AND INTERVENTIONS

Anomaly	*Transport complication*	*Intervention*
Encephalocele	Increased heat loss due to increased surface area.	• Neutral thermal environment. • Cover/drape head with hat, blanket, or towel. • Use of a chemical heat source. • Continuous monitoring of skin temperature. • Monitor axillary temperature frequently.
	Increased risk of morbidity.	• Care in handling and positioning. • Provide appropriate support for the defect.
Macrocephaly	Increased heat loss due to increased surface area.	• Neutral thermal environment. • Cover/drape head with hat, blanket, or towel. • Use of a chemical heat source. • Continuous monitoring of skin temperature. • Monitor axillary temperature frequently.
Choanal atresia	Upper airway obstruction.	• Use oral airway.
Cleft palate	Occlusion of airway with tongue.	• Position prone. • Intubation, if needed.
Macroglossia	Occlusion of airway with tongue.	• Position prone. • Use of an oral airway. • Intubation, if needed.
Micrognathia	Occlusion of airway with tongue.	• Position prone. • Use of an oral airway. • Intubation, if needed.
Esophageal atresia	Aspiration of oral secretions.	• Position prone. • Head of bed down. • Large-bore suction catheter in pouch with intermittent suction.
Esophageal atresia with tracheo-esophageal fistula	Aspiration of gastric contents.	• Position prone. • Head of bed up. • Large-bore suction catheter in pouch with intermittent suction.
Neck mass	External compression of the trachea.	• Intubation as needed.
Externalized viscera	Increased heat loss due to increased surface area and evaporative losses.	• Neutral thermal environment. • Use of a chemical heat source. • Continuous monitoring of skin temperature. • Monitor axillary temperature frequently. • Use of a "bowel bag." • Wet-to-dry dressing with normal saline covered with plastic wrap. • Place an Orogastric tube in the dressing for irrigation during transport.
	Increased risk of infection.	• Use sterile technique to examine and wrap the defect. • Broad-spectrum antibiotic coverage.
Prune-belly syndrome	Increased risk of injury to abdominal organs.	• Large rolls at the flanks to allow belt to be placed above abdomen.

complicated by tracheoesophageal fistula, the gastric contents may be aspirated through the fistula. The morbidity associated with aspiration of gastric contents exceeds that of aspiration of saliva. Stabilization still includes a large-bore catheter placed in the esophageal pouch for suctioning as well as prone positioning, but the head of the bed should be *elevated* to avoid gastric content aspiration.

Some anomalies may exert external pressure on the trachea. Large masses such as giant hemangiomas may require intubation to ensure patency of the airway.

Thermoregulation also may be more difficult when a child has an anomaly. Provision of a neutral thermal environment is important but may not be adequate when an anomaly increases heat loss. Infants lose much of their body heat from their scalps; thus, infants with macrocephaly from malformations such as hydrocephaly and hydranencephaly will have increased heat loss because of the increased surface area of the cranium. Some of these babies have such large heads that stockinette caps will not fit. In these instances, a blanket or towel may be draped around the baby's head to provide a barrier to heat loss. Use of a chemical heat source, such as a Portawarm®, may also be necessary. Evaporative heat losses are associated with exposure of highly perfused organs that are externalized and do not have the normal insulation of the integument. Cordis ectopia, omphalocele, gastroschisis, exstrophy of the bladder, and meningoceles all cause difficulty in management of heat loss. Thermoregulation requires a moisture barrier such as a "bowel bag" or wet-to-dry dressings covered by plastic wrap. If using a wet-to-dry dressing, a gavage tube may be curled in the dressing to irrigate the dressing as needed during the transport. Additional heat sources (such as a Portawarm) also may be needed.

Positioning of the dysmorphic infant may become very complex, as demonstrated by the head up head down recommendations for the infant who has esophageal atresia with or without tracheoesophageal fistula. Many anomalies create complications because the normal protective/supportive mechanisms of the body do not exist. Malformations such as meningoceles require prone positioning with the head slightly down to reduce the pressure of cerebrospinal fluid at the site of the defect. Contractures of the hips in these infants may require an additional roll at the hip to support the pelvis and hips. Infants with gastroschisis should be positioned with their right side down to minimize ischemic effects to the bowel.

Infants with prune-belly syndrome are difficult to secure in the isolette without strapping across their unsupported abdominal organs. Placing two large rolls along each flank allows the safety belt to be secured above the abdomen.

Externalized visceral and other breaks in the integument increase the risk of infection. Inspection of these types of defects should be done with sterile technique, and any dressing or equipment that comes into contact with the defect should be sterile. Appropriate antibiotic therapy with broad-spectrum coverage should be initiated before transport (see the Section on Sepsis).

REFERENCES

1. Aase JM: *Diagnostic dysmorphology,* New York, 1992, Plenum Medical Book.
2. Avery G: *Neonatology, pathophysiology and management of the newborn,* ed 3, Philadelphia, 1987, JB Lippincott.
3. Avery M: *Schaffer's diseases of the newborn,* ed 6, Philadelphia, 1988, WB Saunders.
4. Bankier A: Annotation: approach to the dysmorphic child, *Journal of Pediatric Child Health* 26:69-70, 1990.
5. Benson RC: *Handbook of obstetrics and gynecology,* ed 8, Los Altos, California, 1983, Lange Medical Publications.
6. Cohen MM: Syndromology: an updated conceptual overview, *Int J Oral Maxillofac Surg* 19:81-8, 1990.
7. Graham JM: *Smith's recognizable patterns of human deformation,* ed 2, Philadelphia, 1988, WB Saunders.
8. Jones K: *Smith's recognizable patterns of human malformation,* ed 4, Philadelphia, 1988, WB Saunders.
9. Marden PM, Smith DW, MacDonald MJ: Congenital anomalies in the newborn infant, including minor variations, *J Pediat* 64:357, 1964.
10. Miller ME: Approach to the dysmorphic newborn. In Ziai M, Clarke TA, Merritt TA, editors: *Assessment of the newborn,* Boston, 1984, Little, Brown and Company.
11. Moore KL: *The developing human,* ed 4, Philadelphia, 1992, WB Saunders.
12. Scanlon JW and others: *A system of newborn physical examination,* Baltimore, 1979, University Park Press.

Perinatal Substance Abuse — Transport of the Drug-Addicted Infant

Rapid recognition, complete assessment, and appropriate pharmacological treatment of the drug-addicted infant must begin at transport.

Perinatal addiction is a major concern for clinicians in the fields of maternal-fetal and neonatal medicine. Studies have noted that as many as 15% of newborns in large urban centers are affected by drug abuse, with minorities disproportionately affected.[3] A multidisciplinary approach, beginning at delivery, will facilitate the best intervention and development for the newborn.

Recognition of the drug-addicted newborn is based on maternal history or recognition of adverse obstetrical or neonatal consequences, or both (Table 32-21). Suspected substance abuse generally is confirmed by urine or meconium toxicology screens.

Symptoms and effects may be associated with specific substances of abuse. Some of the more common symptoms and effects to be noted on transport are:

A. Alcohol[4,10]
   1. Growth retardation
   2. Characteristic facial dysmorphology, including flattening of facial features, short palpebral fissures, and smooth philtrum with thin, smooth upper lip.
   3. Heart defects, especially septal defects
   4. Mild/moderate microcephaly
   5. Neural tube defects
   6. Breech presentation

B. Tobacco[8,16,17]
   1. Growth retardation
   2. Hypoglycemia
   3. Hypothermia
   4. Polycythemia

C. Cocaine[1,5,9,13-15]
   1. Apnea
   2. Irritability, jitteriness, and inconsolability
   3. Intolerance to stimuli or change
   4. Seizures/intracranial hemorrhages
   5. Hypertension/stroke
   6. Possible birth defects
   7. Necrotizing enterocolitis or other infections
   8. Meconium-stained amniotic fluid
   9. Abruption
   10. Premature labor or delivery, or both

D. Heroin/Methadone[7]
   1. Respiratory distress, especially tachypnea
   2. Growth retardation
   3. Seizures
   4. Anemia
   5. Meconium staining
   6. Spontaneous abortions
   7. Increase in infection risk, especially sexually transmitted diseases.

In infants whose mothers are receiving methadone treatment, 60% require pharmacologic treatment for drug withdrawal.[7]

After drug addiction is identified in the infants, the degree of neonatal abstinence syndrome (NAS) must be evaluated.[2] This evaluation will determine the need for pharmacologic intervention. Any seizure activity should be noted. The neonatal abstinence scoring system[6] assists in the detection of addiction and pharmacologic response to NAS[6] (Table 32-22).

Infants with NAS exhibit respiratory symptoms as well as metabolic and central nervous system symptoms. Analysis should include serum glucose, calcium, magnesium, electrolytes, complete blood count with differential, blood culture, arterial blood gases, urine for group B streptococcus antigen, and a chest x-ray. A cranial ultrasound also may be helpful (if available), and a urine or meconium toxicology screen may be useful when the infant urinates or defecates.

Assessment and pretransport management of the drug addicted newborn must consist of:

A. Obtaining a complete family, maternal, and perinatal history, especially as it relates to substance abuse and drugs in-labor. Maternal drug use patterns should be documented (remember that drugs given during labor can cause a positive drug screen).

B. Performing a complete physical and neurologic examination. Any seizure activity or malformations should be described. Be aware that many addicts are polysubstance abusers.[11,12]

TABLE 32-21 EFFECTS OF PRENATAL DRUG EXPOSURE

	CNS depressants						*CNS stimulants*	
	Alcohol	*Narcotics*	*Barbiturates*	*Tranquilizers*	*Marijuana*	*Toluene (glue, paint)*	*Cocaine (crack) or amphetamines*	*Cigarette smoking*
Miscarriage	+	+					++	++
Premature labor & delivery		+					++	++
Placental abruption							++	+
Fetal distress in labor		+			+		++	+
Asphyxia/strokes							++	
IUGR	+	+			+	+	++	+
Poor brain growth	++	+				+	+	
Dysmorphic facial features	+				°	+		
Increased birth defects	+	+				+	+	
NAS	+	++	+	+	+	+	+	
Abnormal parent-infant interaction	+	+	+	+	+	+	+	
Chronic feeding problems	+	+	+	+	+	+	+	
Developmental delays	+	+	+			+	+	
Cerebral palsy							+	
Lower I.Q.	+	+	+			+	+	
Behavior problems/attention deficit	+	+	+			+	+	
Increased SIDS risk		+					+	°
Drug exposure after birth					+	+	+	+
Abuse/neglect	+	+	+	+		+	+	

° Possible association
\+ Associated
++ Strongly associated
NAS Neonatal Abstinence Syndrome
Courtesy of S Langendoerfer, MD, Denver, CO.

TABLE 32-22 NEONATAL ABSTINENCE SCORING SYSTEM

Signs and symptoms	*Score*
Excessive high-pitched cry	2
Continuous high-pitched cry	3
Sleeps < 1 hour after feeding	3
Sleeps < 2 hours after feeding	2
Sleeps < 3 hours after feeding	1
Hyperactive moro reflex	2
Markedly hyperactive moro reflex	3
Mild tremors disturbed	1
Moderate-severe tremors disturbed	4
Increased muscle tone	2
Excoriation (specify area)	1
Myoclonic jerks	3
Generalized convulsions	5
Sweating	1
Fever < 38.2°C (37.2 to 38.2°C)	1
Fever > 38.2°C	2
Frequent yawning > 3-4 times/interval	1
Mottling	1
Nasal stuffiness	2
Sneezing (>3-4 times/interval)	1
Nasal flaring	2
Respiratory rate > 60/minute	1
Respiratory rate > 60/minute with GFR	2
Excessive sucking	1
Poor feeding	2
Regurgitation	2
Projectile vomiting	3
Loose stools	2
Watery stools	3

From Finnegan LP: Neonatal abstinence syndrome. In Nelson N, editor: *Current therapy in neonatal perinatal medicine,* ed 2, Toronto, 1990, D.C. Decker. Reprinted by permission.

Score can be totaled and followed over time to evaluate response to treatment.

C. Assessing all current laboratory results and obtaining any further laboratory work as early as possible, before pharmacologic intervention.
D. Establishing IV access as needed. Assess perfusion and capillary refill time.
E. Ensuring adequate airway for transport, especially when the infant has a history of seizures. (Be aware that Narcan can cause possible acute drug withdrawal if given to addicted infants.)
F. Monitoring the infant with a cardiorespiratory monitor, pulse oximeter, and skin probe (for temperature control).
G. Speaking with the parents—be clear, honest and nonjudgmental. Inform the mother that breastfeeding is harmful to infants when illicit drugs are used.

After this initial evaluation and assessment, the transport team and attending physician should discuss the need for immediate treatment. Phenobarbital is the drug of choice when the infant has been exposed to multiple drugs. A loading dose of 20 mg/kg should be given before transport, with subsequent doses dependent on the abstinence score and clinical condition 12 hours later.[6]

Care in transport will consist of careful observation for phenobarbital toxicity:

A. CNS depression and absent reflexes
B. Respiratory depression/apnea
C. Pupillary constriction/dilation
D. Temperature instability
E. Perfusion/capillary refill changes or other cardiac alterations
F. Acute neurogenic bladder with urinary retention

Supportive care in these infants also is essential. Stimulation of any kind can result in physiologic instability:

A. Place the infant in the darkest, quietest environment the clinical status will allow. (Even the motor from the isolette can be very disturbing.)
B. Swaddle the infant in a flexed position and monitor temperature. Increased movement and irritability can increase temperature.
C. Attempt to calm the infant with a pacifier.
D. Monitor vital signs closely, using monitors (decrease stimulation).
E. If feeding on transport is possible and considered safe, these infants often do best with small, frequent feedings.

REFERENCES

1. Bandstra ES, Burkett G: Maternal-fetal and neonatal effects of in utero cocaine exposure, *Semin Perinatol* 15(4):288-301, 1991.
2. Chasnoff IJ: Newborn infants with drug withdrawal symptoms, *Pediatr Rev* 9(9):273-7, 1988.
3. Chasnoff IJ, Landress H, Barrett M: The prevalence of illicit drug or alcohol use during pregnancy and discrepancies in mandatory reporting in Pinellas county, Florida, *N Engl J Med* 322:1202-6, 1990.
4. Coles CD: Impact of prenatal alcohol exposure of the newborn and the child, *Clin Obstet Gynecol* 36(2):255-6, 1993.

5. Dusick AM and others: Risk of intracranial hemorrhage and other adverse outcomes after cocaine exposure in a cohort of 323 very low birth weight infants, *J Pediatr* 122(3):438-45, 1993.
6. Finnegan LP: Neonatal abstinence syndrome. In Nelson N, editor: *Current therapy in neonatal perinatal medicine,* ed 2, Toronto, 1990, DC Decker.
7. Finnegan LP: Perinatal substance abuse: comments and perspectives, *Semin Perinatol* 15(4):331-9, 1991.
8. Gorrella TL, editor: *Neonatology basic management, on-call problems, diseases, drugs,* 1988, Appleton & Lange.
9. Horn PT: Persistent hypertension after prenatal cocaine exposure, *J Pediatr* 121(2):288-91, 1992.
10. Jones KL and others: Pattern of malformation in offspring of chronic alcoholic mothers, *Lancet* 1:1267, 1973.
11. Jorgensen KM: The drug-exposed infant, *Critical care nursing clinics of North America* 4(3):481-5, 1992.
12. Khalsa JH, Gfroerer J: Epidemiology and health consequences of drug abuse among pregnant women, *Semin Perinatol* 15(4):265-70, 1992.
13. Little BB and others: Cocaine abuse during pregnancy: maternal and fetal implications, *Obstet Gynecol* 73:157-60, 1989.
14. McClenny R: Cocaine: a brief history, *Neonatal Network* 10(4):53-7, 1991.
15. Mehata SK and others: Transport myocardial ischemia in infants prenatally exposed to cocaine, *J Pediatr* 122(6):945-9, 1993.
16. Schonberg SK and others, editors: *Substance abuse: a guide for health professionals,* Elk Grove Village, IL, 1988, American Academy of Pediatrics.
17. Sham B: Perinatal substance abuse. In Beachy P, Deacon J, editors: *Care curriculum for neonatal intensive care nursing,* 1993, NAACOG, WB Saunders.

Surgical Conditions of the Neonate

CHEST CONDITIONS

Congenital Diaphragmatic Hernia (CDH)[10,12]

CDH presenting in the newborn period is of several types, but the posterolateral defect described by Bochdalek is most common and requires urgent intervention. The defect may be a small slit or a virtual absence of the diaphragmatic substance. CDH occurs on the left side in 85% of cases, and approximately 1% of cases are bilateral. CDH causes pulmonary hypoplasia and underdevelopment of the small pulmonary arteries, especially if the herniation occurs early in gestation.

Recognition. CDH frequently is diagnosed prenatally with ultrasound. Polyhydramnios is found in 75% of CDH cases and has been associated with an increased mortality rate. Physical examination of the newborn having CDH typically reveals a scaphoid abdomen, decreased breath sounds on the side of the hernia, and a shift of the heart sounds from the normal position. The infant may exhibit severe respiratory distress and cyanosis. A chest x-ray usually confirms the diagnosis, and the nasogastric tube may be seen to enter the stomach in its herniated location (Fig. 32-11).

Evaluation. The infant should be checked for other organ system abnormalities. Nervous system abnormalities (including anencephaly, myelomeningocele, hydrocephalus, and encephalocele) may be apparent. Cardiac abnormalities as well as trisomy 13 and 18 are reported with CDH.[2]

Stabilization. Stabilization of an infant with CDH requires 1) a focus on the mechanical forces that allow ventilation and decrease distention of the herniated abdominal viscera

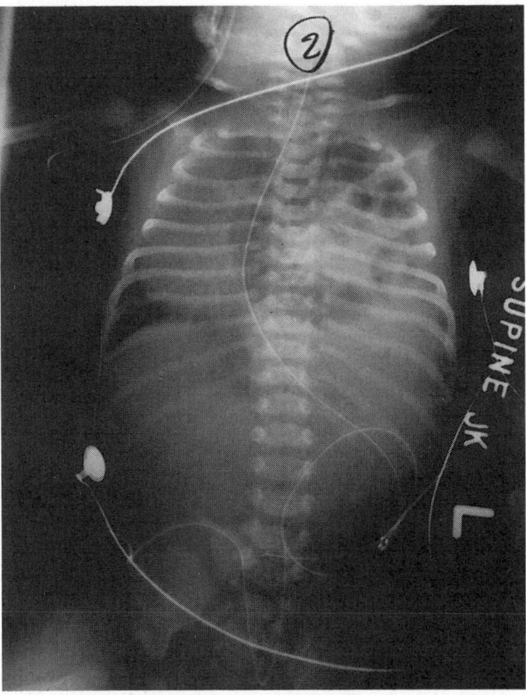

Fig. 32-11. Left congenital diaphragmatic hernia with shift of the heart and mediastinum into the right chest.

with gas, and 2) medical management to lower pulmonary vascular resistance, thus decreasing right-to-left shunting at the foramen ovale and the ductus arteriosus. Infants with respiratory distress require prompt endotracheal intubation and ventilation. Muscle paralysis facilitates hyperventilation and decreases the amount of swallowed gas. Ventilation with a mask should be avoided, as this insufflates the intestine. The PaO_2 should be maintained above 100 if possible, and the $PaCO_2$ between 30 and 35. The pH should be maintained at 7.45 to 7.50. The use of tolazoline is advocated by some to reduce pulmonary hypertension, though its effect is not selective for the pulmonary vasculature and may cause hypotension. The systolic pressure should be maintained, if possible, above pulmonary artery pressures, and this may require volume infusion, the administration of dobutamine/dopamine, or both.

Transport. Transport should be performed in an environment that allows optimal monitoring. Pulse oximetry in the right upper extremity allows preductal monitoring, and pulse oximetry in the lower extremity allows postductal monitoring. Typically, arterial catheters are placed in the umbilical artery either before or after transport, and a right radial arterial line allows preductal monitoring as well. These infants should be transported to a center prepared for advanced forms of support before or after the repair. Forms of support considered to be beneficial include extracorporeal membrane oxygenation (ECMO),[7] high-frequency ventilation,[2] and administration of nitric oxide.[3] Of all infants with CDH, 36% die before reaching a neonatal treatment center.

Congenital lobar emphysema[5]

Congenital lobar emphysema results from the trapping of air, usually in an upper lobe. This trapping of air may lead to significant overdistention of the lobe, causing a shift away from the mediastinum towards the contralateral lung.

Recognition and evaluation. Congenital lobar emphysema usually is diagnosed with a chest x-ray. Because of hyperlucency this condition may be confused with a pneumothorax (Fig. 32-12). Congenital heart disease may be associated.

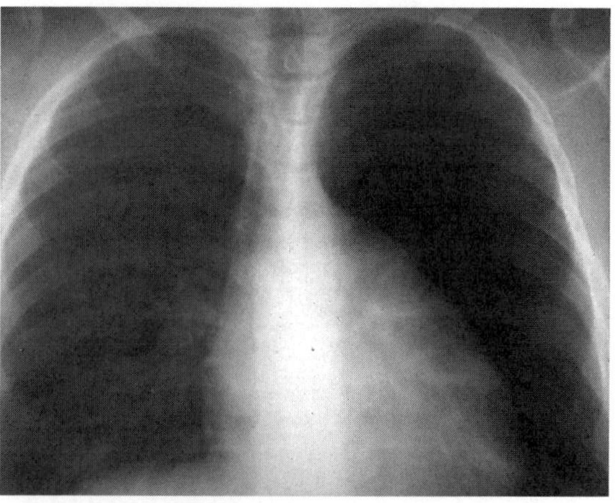

Fig. 32-12. *Congenital lobar emphysema.* Note hyperlucency in left upper lobe.

Stabilization. If possible, patients with congenital lobar emphysema should not be treated with endotracheal intubation, as this may lead to further overdistention of the emphysematous lobe. Selective intubation of the uninvolved lung may allow improved ventilation.

Transport. Transport should be accomplished with the usual hemodynamic and pulmonary neonatal monitoring. In the rare event of sudden unmanageable collapse of the patient, emergency thoracotomy will allow the lung to herniate from the chest cavity and improve ventilation and hemodynamics (Fig. 32-13).

Cystic adenomatoid malformation[4]

Cystic adenomatoid malformation is a multicystic mass of pulmonary tissue that is a proliferation of bronchial structures. Three types exist: Type 1 with multiple cysts greater than 2 cm in diameter, Type 2 with smaller cysts less than 1 cm in diameter, and Type 3, which is noncystic and frequently produces mediastinal shift.

Recognition. Cystic adenomatoid malformation usually is apparent on chest x-ray, but it may be confused with congenital diaphragmatic hernia. The bowel gas pattern is usually normal, and the stomach and nasogastric tube appear below the diaphragm. Contrast studies of the gastrointestinal tract or ultrasound examinations help to differentiate these conditions as well.

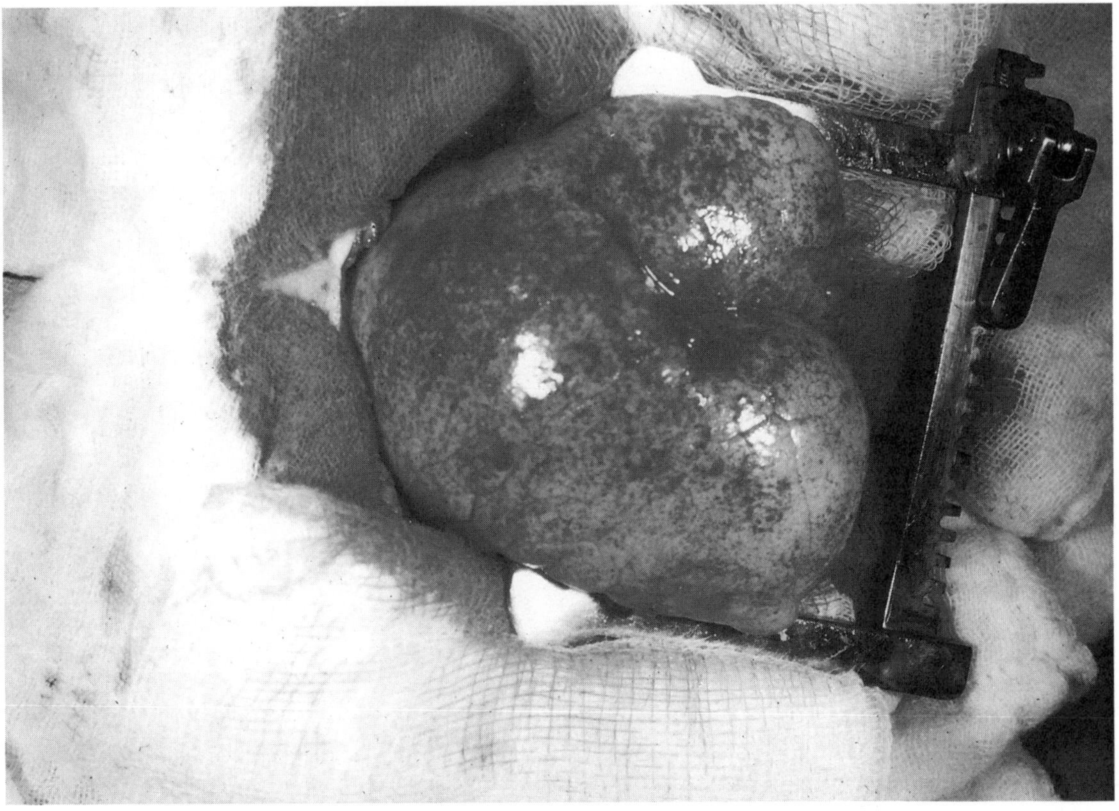

Fig. 32-13. *Congenital lobar emphysema.* Note emphysematous lobe protruding from chest wound.

Evaluation. Types 2 and 3 are associated most frequently with respiratory distress in the newborn.

Stabilization. The patient should be ventilated and managed as a patient with a congenital diaphragmatic hernia.

Transport. The patient should be transported to a center which has surgeons capable of resecting the malformation. These patients also may benefit from support techniques described in the section of congenital diaphragmatic hernia.

Esophageal Atresia (EA) and Tracheoesophageal Fistula (TEF)

These abnormalities develop in the first month of gestation when the foregut separates into esophageal and respiratory structures. The etiology is unknown. The incidence of this anomaly is 1 in 3,000 live births.

Recognition. The most common form encountered is that of a blind-ending proximal esophageal atresia with a distal tracheoesophageal fistula (Fig. 32-14). EA is diagnosed when the infant is unable to eat and produces excessive saliva. On x-ray the nasogastric tube does not pass below the upper chest. Gas present in the GI tract implies that there is a TEF. An isolated TEF is diagnosed after repeated bouts of aspiration by using contrast esophagram.

Evaluation. Evaluation should include a search for any associated anomalies of the vertebrae, anus, heart, kidney, or limbs. Particular care should be taken to evaluate for imperforate anus (Fig. 32-15).

Stabilization. A soft suction tube should be maintained in the proximal esophageal pouch to help prevent aspiration of saliva. A slightly head-up position is recommended to avoid aspiration of gastric contents into the trachea via the fistula. Added oxygen or mechanical ventilation may be required but may lead to insufflation of the gastrointestinal tract via the fistula. A gastrostomy tube may decompress the stomach when this occurs but

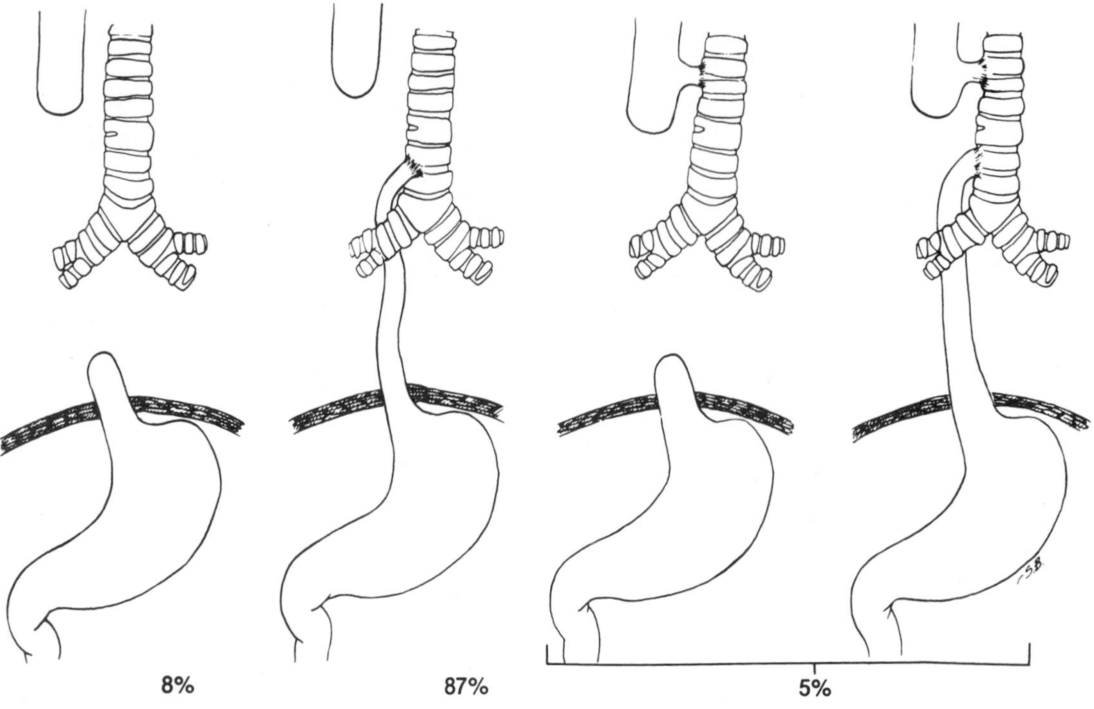

Fig. 32-14. Patterns of esophageal atresia and tracheoesophageal fistula.

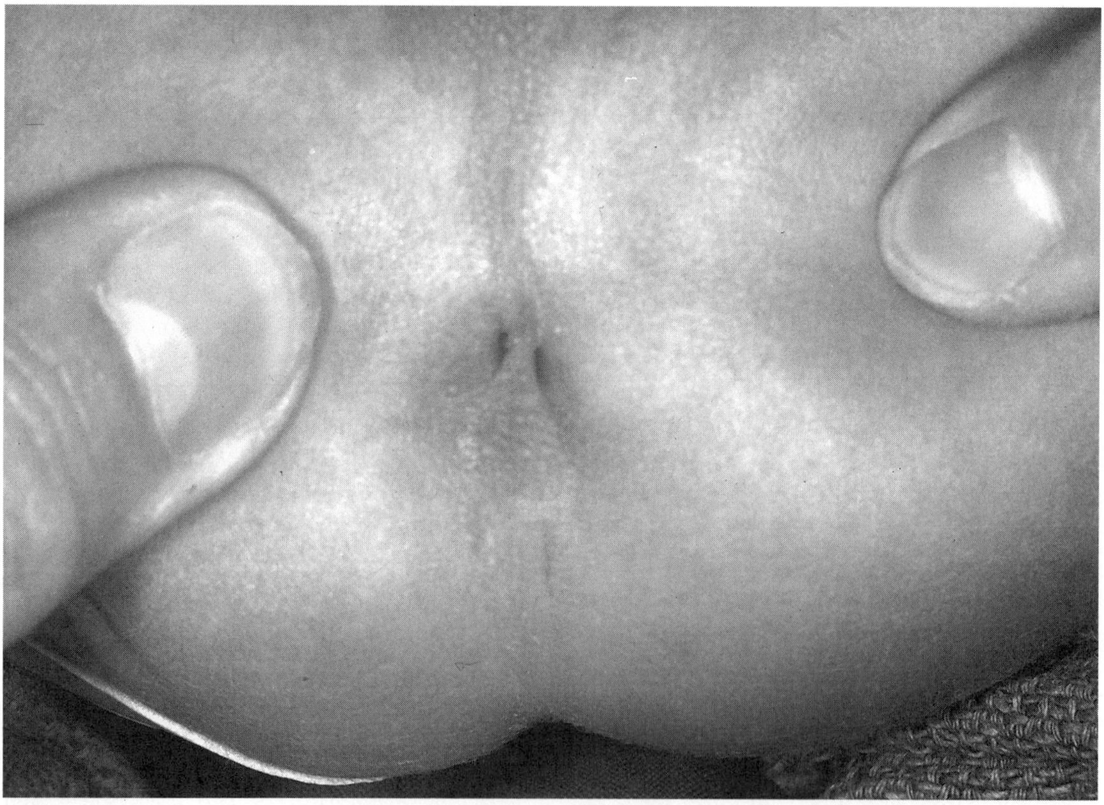

Fig. 32-15. Imperforate anus.

also may be a source of air leak. This air leak may be managed by placing the gastrostomy tube to water seal with a chest tube-type setup, or the fistula may be temporarily occluded with a Fogarty balloon catheter via the gastrostomy tube or may be placed with a bronchoscope.

Transport. The patient should be managed with ventilatory support, and the considerations described above should be noted. The most common cause of death in these patients relates to significant cardiac disease; pharmacologic management of these problems should be provided.

ABDOMINAL CONDITIONS

Abdominal wall defects[9]

Omphalocele.

Recognition. An omphalocele is an abdominal wall defect in which the abdominal structures are covered by a membrane or sac from which the umbilical cord arises (Fig. 32-16). The sac may vary greatly in size and contain any abdominal structure. Upper abdominal omphaloceles may even contain the heart. Lower abdominal omphaloceles may be associated with exstrophy of the bladder.

Evaluation. One third of patients with omphaloceles have associated chromosomal abnormalities, including trisomy 13, 18, and 21.[8] Omphalocele may be associated with Beckwith-Wiedemann syndrome (exophthalmos-macroglossia-gigantism), which may be recognized by the presence of a large tongue (Fig. 32-17). Significant hypoglycemia occurs in as many as 50% of these patients. The coexistence of severe cardiac disease contributes to mortality in these patients.[6]

Stabilization. Acute management of these patients primarily focuses on associated cardiac anomalies and hypoglycemia. Fluid loss from the exposed sac is not a significant problem.

Transport. The exposed sac usually is covered with a sterile dressing. Transport should be to a center equipped to deal not only with

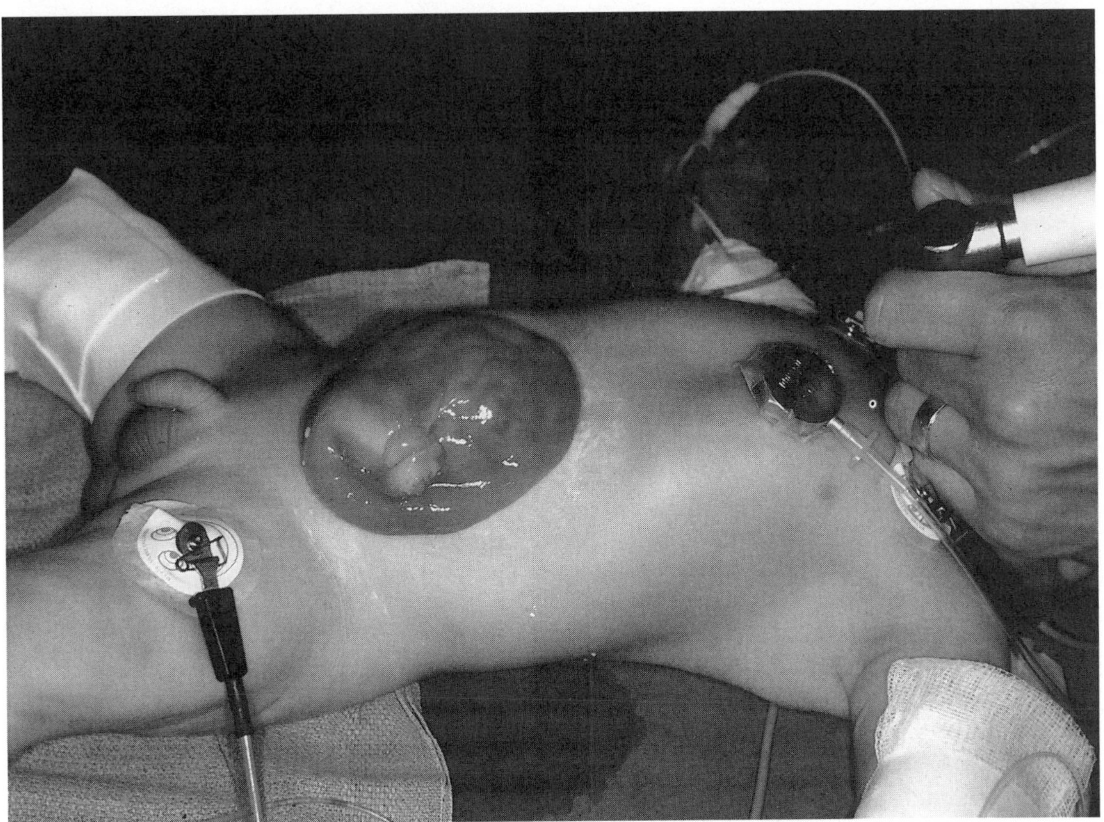

Fig. 32-16. Typical moderate-sized omphalocele.

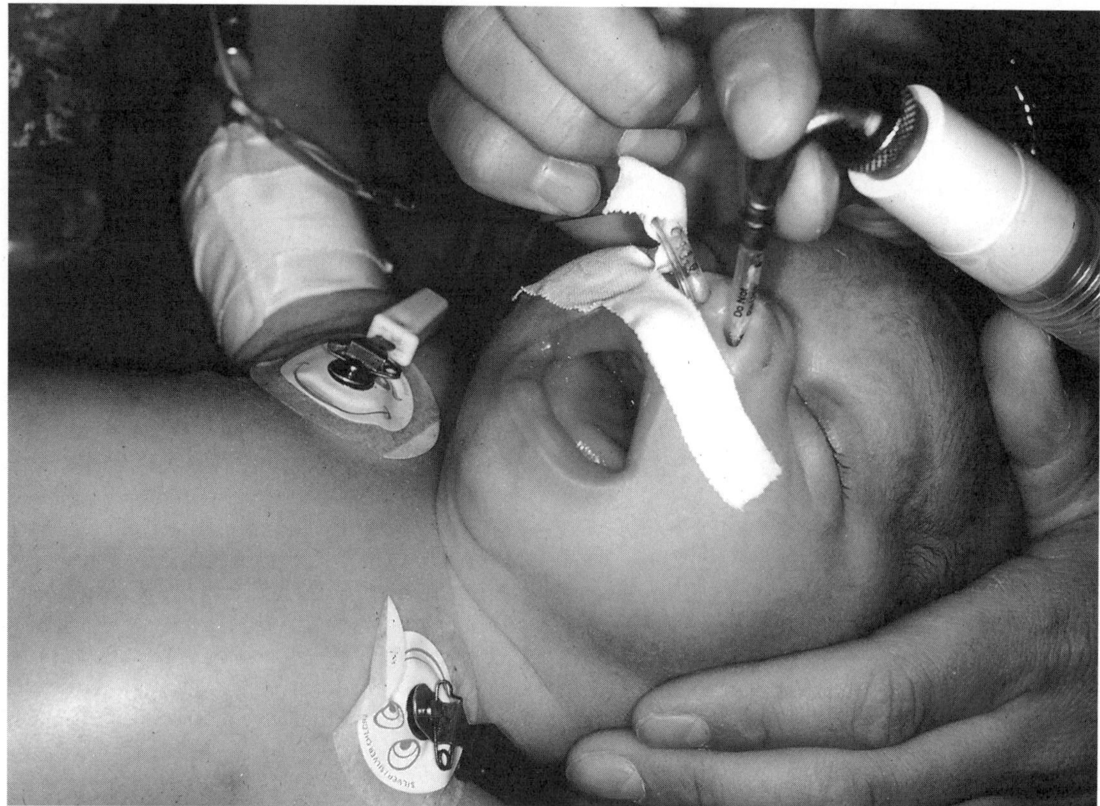

Fig. 32-17. Large tongue associated with Beckwith-Wiedemann syndrome.

the omphalocele but also with the frequently associated cardiac anomalies.

Gastroschisis.[9]

Recognition. The abdominal wall defect of gastroschisis is usually 2 to 4 cm in diameter and located to the right of the umbilical cord (Fig. 32-18). No sac is present, and the exposed viscera are most commonly those located in the gastrointestinal tract. The serosal surface typically is thickened and may be stained with meconium. The diagnosis of gastroschisis, as with omphalocele, is frequently made by using ultrasound during pregnancy.

Evaluation. Few life-threatening anomalies are associated with gastroschisis. The majority of associated anomalies are of gastrointestinal origin and may be recognized by inspection of the herniated viscera.

Stabilization. Fluid loss from the exposed viscera requires increased fluid and electrolyte replacement. Broad-spectrum antibiotic coverage should be initiated after delivery.[9]

Transport. The exposed viscera should be dressed in a manner that minimizes fluid and heat loss. This may be accomplished using moist, saline-soaked dressings next to the viscera covered by dry gauze and a water-impervious material such as cellophane. An important consideration is to dress and position the viscera so that the vascular supply is not compromised through the small abdominal wall defect (Fig. 32-19).

Intestinal atresia.[14] Intestinal atresia is the most common cause of intestinal obstruction in the newborn. The incidence of intestinal atresia is estimated at 1 per 2,500 live births. The most common site of obstruction is the duodenum, followed by the jejunum, ileum, and colon. The obstruction may be caused by a blind-ending atretic segment (Fig. 32-20) or an intrinsic web-type blockage.

Recognition. The diagnosis usually is suggested by poor feeding, bilious vomiting, and abdominal distention, particularly with more distal obstruction. Plain x-ray of the abdomen reveals markedly dilated loops of intestine with a paucity of gas distally. A contrast enema may help rule out other forms of ob-

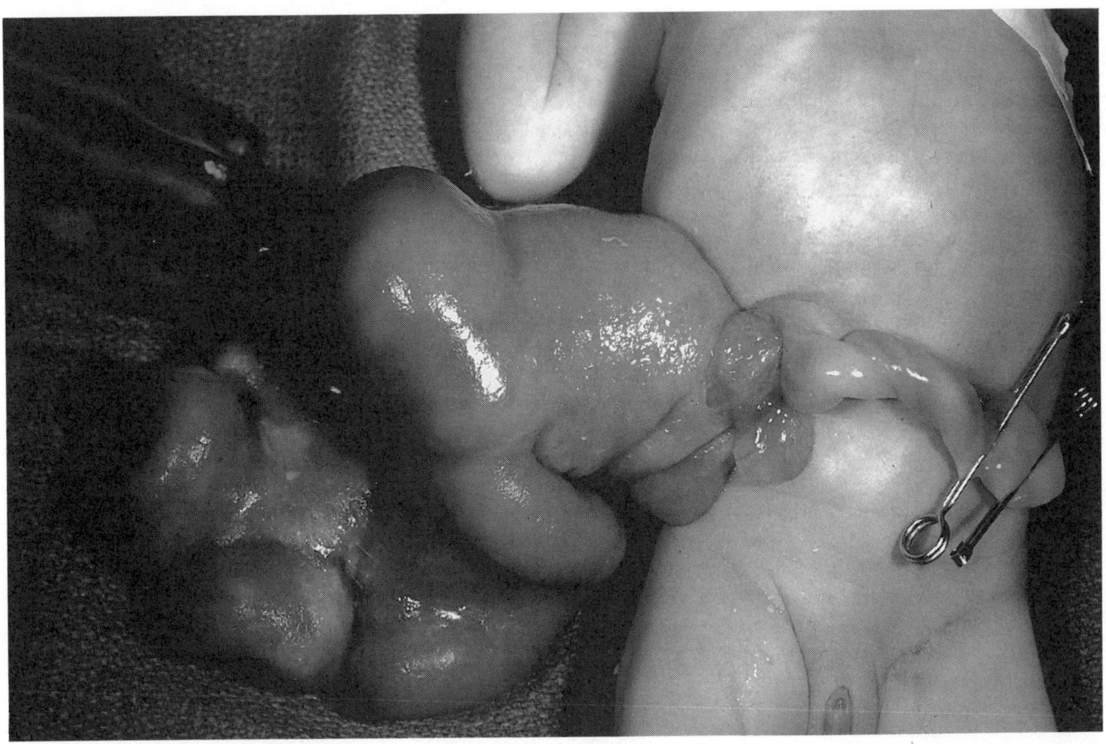

Fig. 32-18. Typical gastroschisis.

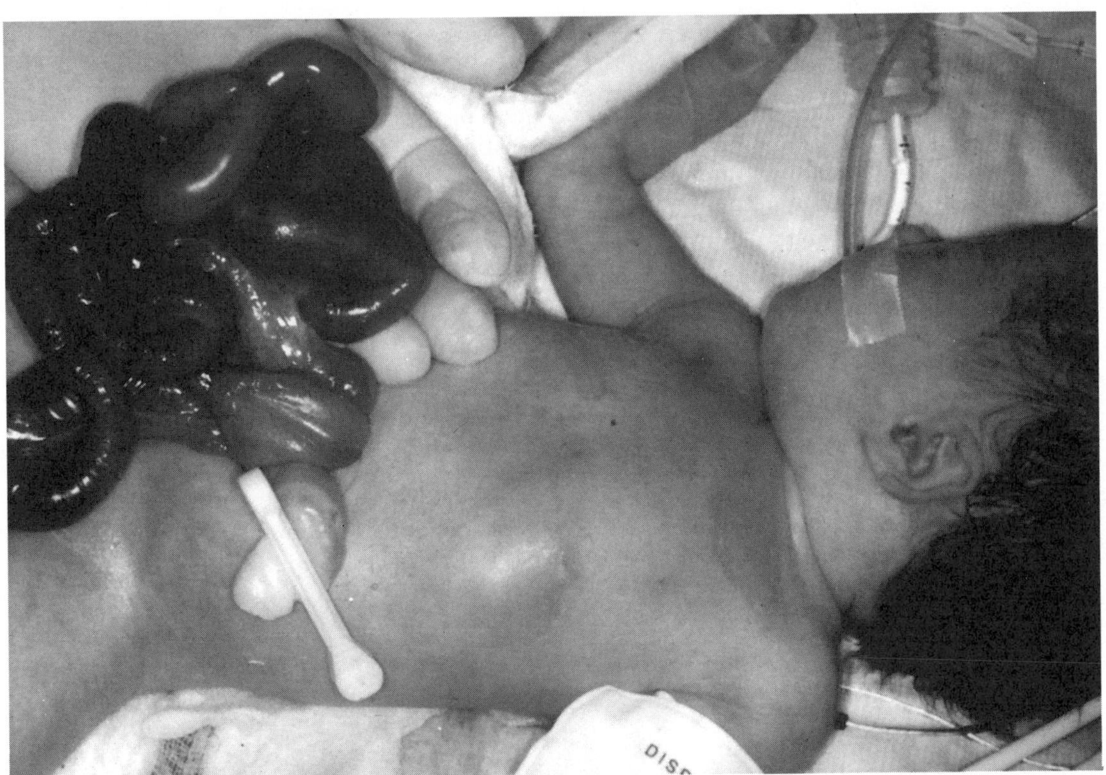

Fig. 32-19. Gastroschisis with intestinal infarction due to kinking of mesenteric blood supply.

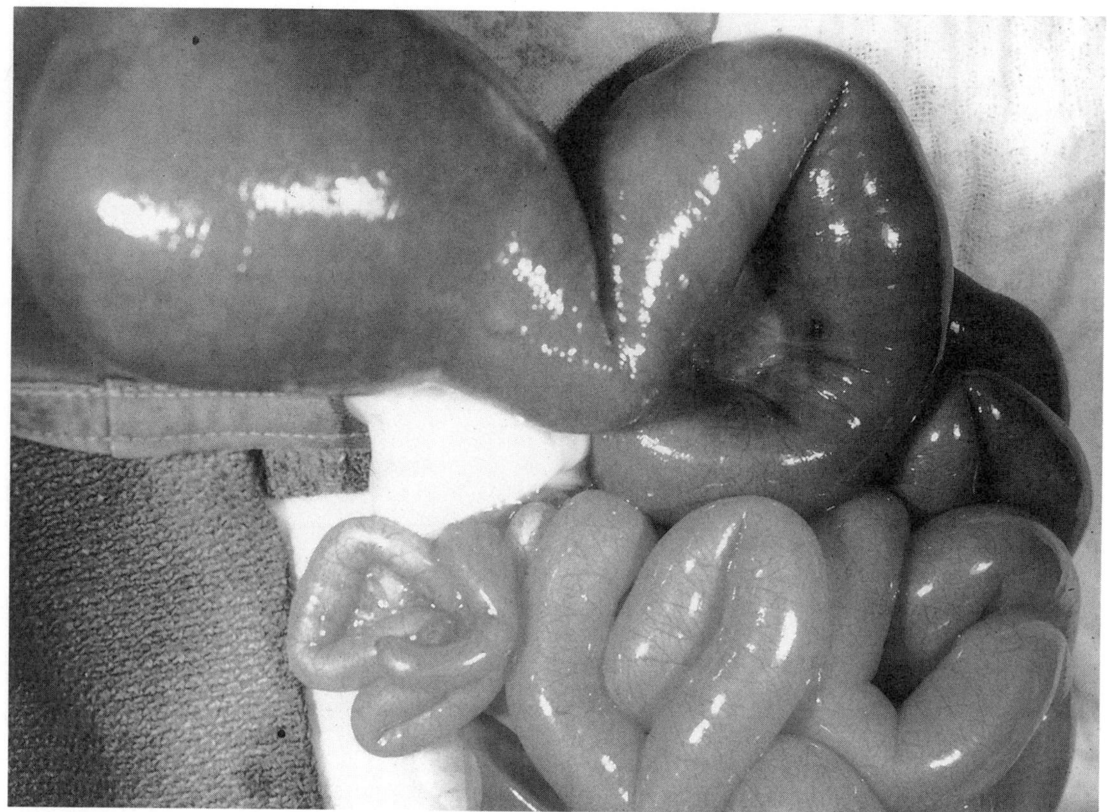

Fig. 32-20. Typical appearance of jejunal atresia.

struction. The diagnosis is frequently established by ultrasound before delivery.

Evaluation. Duodenal obstruction may be associated with trisomy 21 and other anomalies, most notably of the heart. More distal obstructions rarely are associated with major anomalies. Jejunal and ileal atresia occasionally are associated with cystic fibrosis.

Stabilization and transport. The gastrointestinal tract should be decompressed using nasogastric suction, with care taken to replace GI fluid loss. Transport may proceed in a nonemergent fashion.

Malrotation.[1] Malrotation results from improper return of the developing intestine to the abdominal cavity during the late first trimester. This may result in upper intestinal obstruction caused by abnormal bands or volvulus, which also may compromise the intestinal blood supply.

Recognition. Malrotation with or without volvulus should be suspected with the sudden onset of bilious vomiting. Abdominal distention or abdominal mass may be present. If intestinal compromise has occurred, the stools may be grossly bloody. In the presence of midgut volvulus, the patient may deteriorate rapidly with onset of shock and respiratory distress. The condition should be suspected clinically by the mode of presentation and is best confirmed with a limited upper GI x-ray showing the abnormal rotation pattern (Fig. 32-21).

Evaluation. Once the diagnosis of malrotation is established, little evaluation of the patient is needed. During the diagnostic workup, patients should be examined for the presence of necrotizing enterocolitis or a source of sepsis that could lead to a similar deterioration.

Stabilization. Rapid volume resuscitation and attempts to correct acid-base abnormalities are important. Blood should be made available and antibiotics started. Preparation should be made for prompt surgical exploration.

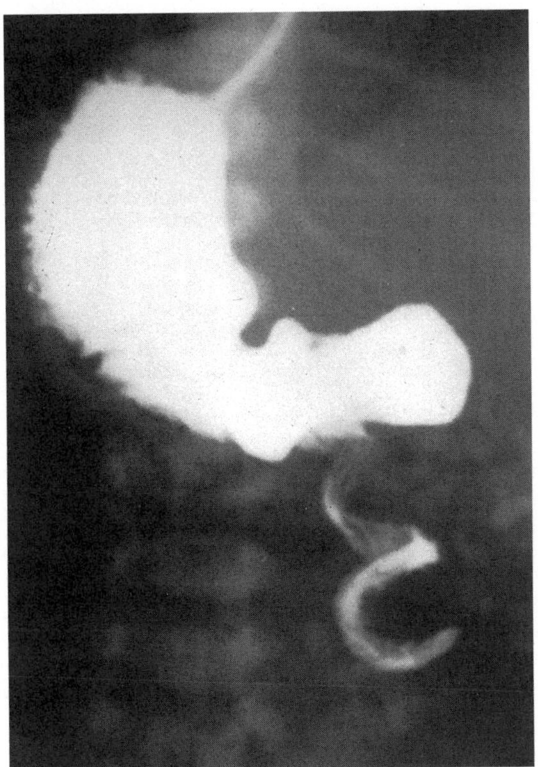

Fig. 32-21. Upper GI series with malrotation and volvulus.

Transport. A suspicion of midgut volvulus should prompt emergent transport. Volume resuscitation can be accomplished en route. The accepting institution should be advised of this suspicion so that arrangements for an operating room can be made in advance of arrival.

Meconium ileus/peritonitis.[8] Cystic fibrosis is a disease of the exocrine glands. Fifteen percent of infants with cystic fibrosis are born with an intrauterine intestinal obstruction caused by thickened meconium plugging the intestine. In some cases, the large inspissated meconium mass may have provoked a volvulus and may occasionally be associated with perforation. Meconium ileus accounts for approximately 15% of neonatal intestinal obstructions.

Recognition. The condition presents with intestinal obstruction during the first few days of life and initially may be indistinguishable from intestinal atresia. In the presence of a family history of cystic fibrosis, meconium ileus should be suspected. When an intrauterine perforation has occurred, abdominal calcification may be seen on an abdominal radiograph. A contrast enema may demonstrate a microcolon and distal small intestine with plugs of meconium present (Fig. 32-22).

Evaluation. Meconium ileus may be confused with meconium plug syndrome, which is differentiated by contrast enema and usually resolves with nonoperative management. When intestinal perforation is associated with meconium ileus, a large, fluid-filled pseudocyst may be present.

Stabilization. Patients with meconium ileus typically are stable and require only nasogastric decompression and fluid replacement. Enemas of 5% Mucomyst or normal saline may help relieve some of the obstruction. Large meconium pseudocysts may cause enough abdominal distention to compromise ventilation, thus requiring emergent aspiration of some of the fluid.

Transport. Lung problems directly related to cystic fibrosis are not common in the newborn. These infants can be transported with standard neonatal techniques.

Hirschsprung's disease.[11] Hirschsprung's disease is a functional obstruction of the intestine, most commonly in the sigmoid colon (Fig. 32-23), that results from improper mi-

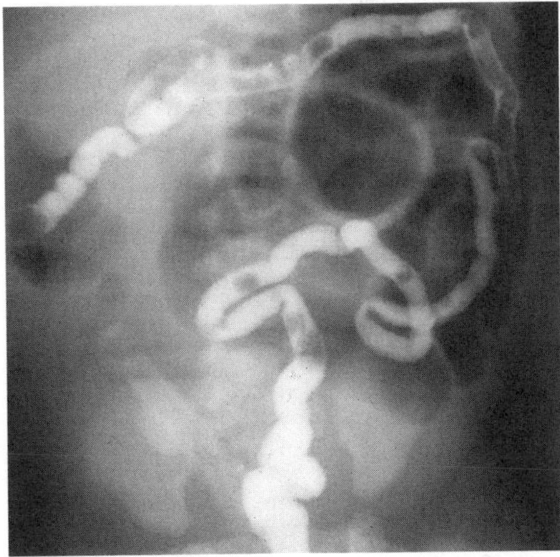

Fig. 32-22. Contrast enema showing small colon and plugs of meconium.

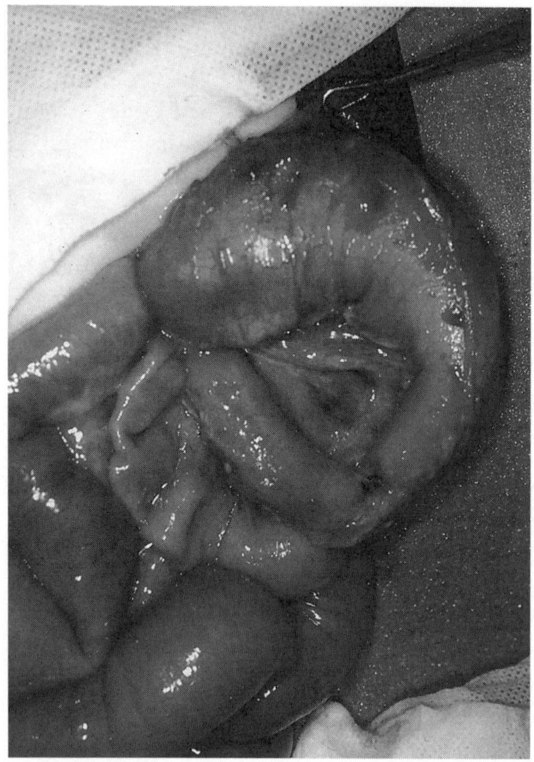

Fig. 32-23. Hirschsprung's disease with level of involvement at sigmoid colon.

gration of intramural ganglion cells.

Recognition. The condition usually presents during the first few days of life with abdominal distention and failure to spontaneously pass meconium during the first 48 hours. A barium enema usually is suggestive and may help define the level of disease involvement in the intestine. The definitive diagnosis is made by suction rectal biopsy to search for ganglion cells in the rectum.[13]

Evaluation. Trisomy 21 is seen frequently with this disease, and features of this anomaly should be sought.

Stabilization. Most patients diagnosed as having Hirschsprung's disease are in no acute distress, however, a septic state associated with toxic megacolon may be seen. In these patients, IV antibiotics and attempted decompression of the colon with a soft rubber catheter and saline irrigations may be helpful. Aggressive IV fluid resuscitation is warranted.

Transport. The majority of patients with Hirschsprung's disease are in no distress and may be transported electively. The receiving institution must have pathologists who are experienced in interpreting intraoperative frozen section biopsies for correct placement of the site of colostomy.

Necrotizing enterocolitis (NEC).[13] NEC is most frequently seen in preterm, stressed infants and may occur in the first days of life or may be delayed by several weeks. The cause appears to be a microvascular ischemic event that occurs in part or all of the intestines.

Recognition. NEC typically presents with abdominal distention, gastric residuals, vomiting, bloody diarrhea, increasing ventilatory requirements, and abdominal tenderness and discoloration (Fig. 32-24). Radiographic findings include pneumatosis intestinalis or free intraperitoneal air (if perforation has occurred).

Evaluation. Infants with NEC may become ill very rapidly with thrombocytopenia, neutropenia, and cardiovascular collapse or may

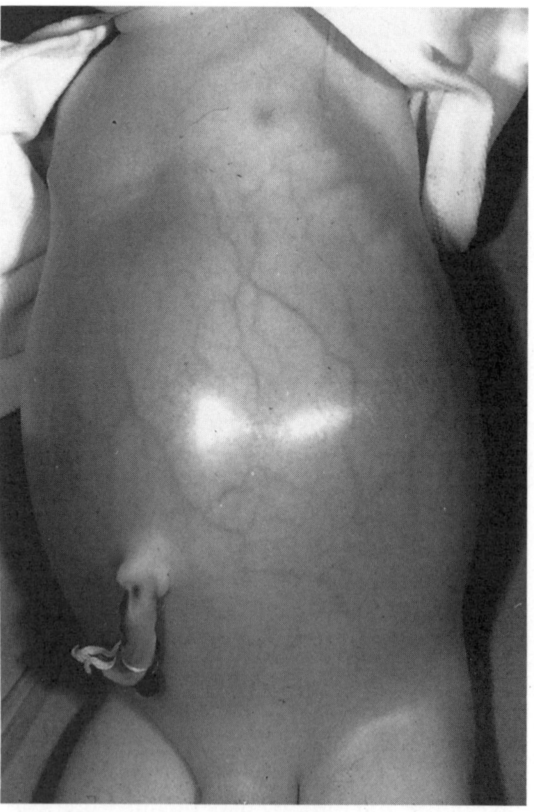

Fig. 32-24. Necrotizing enterocolitis with distended, discolored abdomen.

have a milder course of disease with less pronounced findings.

Stabilization. Initiation of antibiotic therapy, cessation of enteral feedings, gastric suction, and fluid and acid-base correction are important measures.

Transport. Infants with NEC require prompt but careful transport with an effort to minimize stress. Packed red blood cells, platelets, and colloid infusions may be required en route to a center with pediatric surgical capabilities.

REFERENCES

1. Andrassy RJ, Mahour GH: Malrotation of the midgut in infants and children, *Arch Surg* 116:158-60, 1981.
2. Boros SJ, Mammel MC: A practical guide to HFV, *Ann Pediatr* 17:508-16, 1988.
3. Frostell C and others: Inhaled nitric oxide: a selective pulmonary vasodilator reversing hypoxic pulmonary vasoconstriction, *Circulation* 83:2038, 1991.
4. Gwinn JL, Barnes GR, Kaufman HJ: Radiological case of the month: cystic adenomatoid malformation, *Am J Dis Child* 112:61-2, 1966.
5. Jones HC and others: Lobar emphysema and congenital heart disease in infancy, *J Thorac Cardiovasc Surg* 49:1, 1965.
6. Knight PJ, Sommer A, Clatworthy HW: Omphalocele: a prognostic classification, *J Pediatr Surg* 16:599-604, 1981.
7. Langham M and others: Mortality with ECMO and congenital diaphragmatic hernia in 93 infants, *J Pediatr Surg* 22:1150-4, 1987.
8. Mobogunje OA, Mang CI, Mahor GH: Improved survival of neonates with meconium ileus, *Arch Surg* 117:37-40, 1982.
9. Nakayama DK and others: Management of the fetus with an abdominal wall defect, *J Pediatr Surg* 19:408-13, 1984.
10. Nakayama DK and others: Prenatal diagnosis and management of the fetus with congenital diaphragmatic hernia: initial clinical experience, *J Pediatr Surg* 20:118-24, 1985.
11. Nixon HH: Hirschsprung's disease: progress in management and diagnostics, *World J Surg* 9:189, 1985.
12. Puri P: Epidemiology of congenital diaphragmatic hernia. In Puri P, editor: *Congenital diaphragmatic hernia*, vol 24, Basel, Germany 1989, Karger.
13. Stoll BJ and others: Epidemiology of necrotizing enterocolitis: a case control study, *J Pediatr* 96:447-51, 1980.
14. Touloukian RJ: Intestinal atresia, *Clin Perinatol* 5:3, 1978.

APPENDIX 32-1

NEONATAL EQUIPMENT INVENTORY

This equipment is designed for critical-care, interfacility, neonatal transport.

Respiratory equipment

Laryngoscope handle with blades size Miller 0 and Miller 1
Spare laryngoscope bulbs and batteries
ET tube stylette
Anesthesia bag (500 ml) with manometer/self-inflating bag with manometer
Face mask sizes 0 and 1
ET tube sizes 2.5, 3.0, and 3.5
Suction catheter and glove sets, sized 5/6F, 8F, and 10F
Thoracentesis setups:
- 60cc syringe
- 3-way stopcock
- 23 gauge butterfly
- Alcohol and povidone-iodine (Betadine)
- Heimlich valve setups
- Argyle trocar cannula, 10F and 12F

Intravenous therapy equipment

250-cc bags of D_5W and $D_{10}W$
IV pump tubing
IV filters
Platelet and blood infusion sets
UAC catheters sized 3.5F and 5F
IV extension tubing
T-connectors, multiport connectors
Steri drape
Syringes, sizes from 1 cc through 60 cc
Needles, assorted sizes 18 gauge through 25 gauge
3-way stopcock and stopcock plugs
Betadine and alcohol wipes
Scalp vein needles, sizes 23 and 25 gauge
Quick catheters, sizes 22, 24, and 26 gauge
Medication additive labels
Disposable razors
Paper tape measure
Tongue blades
Armboards, sizes premature and infant
Assorted tape
Umbilical tape
Betadine and alcohol, one bottle each
4.0 silk suture with curved needle
Assorted tape
Umbilical tape
Betadine and alcohol, one bottle each
4.0 silk suture with curved needle
Umbilical artery catheterization/thoracotomy set, including:
- 2 sterile drapes, iris forceps, needle holders, scissors, curved forceps, tongue tissue forceps, sterile 2 × 2s, umbilical tape, scalpel, and blade

Blunt end adapters, sizes 17, 18, and 20 gauge

Thermoregulation and monitoring equipment

Stocking cap
Plastic wrap/bubble wrap
Portawarm
Silver swaddler
Thermometers
Limb leads
Chest electrodes
Heart monitor lead wires
Capillary tubes

Glucose screening strips
Lancets
Arterial transducer tubing

Miscellaneous

Blood culture bottles
Scissors and hemostat
Flashlight
2 × 2 gauze pads
Limb restraints
Safety pins
Rubber bands
Pacifier
Cotton balls
Benzoin/liquid adhesive tape
"Christmas tree" adapters
5F and 8F feeding tubes
Germicidal cleaning cloth
Salem sump tubes, 10F, and 12F
Repogle tube, 10F
Sterile glove packs
Sphygmomanometer with cuffs sizes premature, newborn, and infant
Neonatal stethoscope
Trash bag/needle disposal system

Medications

Epinephrine 1:10,000
$NaHCO_3$, 4.2%
$NaHCO_3$, 8.4%
Naloxone hydrochloride (Narcan)
Atropine
Calcium gluconate 10%
Glass filter needles
Dopamine
Dobutamine
Isoproterenol (Isuprel)
Tolazoline (Priscoline)
Prostaglandins E_1
Phenobarbital
Phenytoin (Dilantin)
Diazepam (Valium)
Fentanyl
Pancuronium bromide (Pavulon)
Chloral hydrate
Morphine sulfate
Concentrated sodium chloride and potassium acetate
Lidocaine (Xylocaine) 1%
Heparin, 1000 U/ml
0.9% normal saline diluent
Sterile water diluent
Flush solution
Antibiotics
5% albumin
$D_{50}W$
Hyaluronidase (Wyadase)

APPENDIX 32-2

An example of transport documentation is shown on the following three pages. (Adapted from the transport form used by Utah Valley Medical Center, Provo, Utah. Courtesy, Steve Minton, MD.)

NEONATAL TRANSPORT/ADMISSION HISTORY

DATE ____________

MOTHER'S LAST NAME	FIRST	AGE	FATHER'S LAST NAME	FIRST	MARITAL STATUS ☐ M ☐ S ☐ D ☐ Sep ☐ Wid
MOTHER'S SS#			MOTHER'S MR#		RACE ☐ Hispanic Origin ☐ Mexican ☐ Puerto Rican ☐ American Indian ☐ White ☐ Black ☐ Asian ☐ Samoa ☐ ______
STREET ADDRESS	STATE	ZIP	PHONE #		
PRENATAL CARE WK INITIATED ____	PRENATAL MD	GRAVIDA ____ PARITY ____ F P A L Including this Pregnancy / / / AB SPON ____ AB THER ____	LMP	EDC/LMP	EDC/US

FAMILIAL CONDITIONS

Mother ....

Father ....

Sibling ....

PREVIOUS PREGNANCIES

☐ No Problems
☐ Premature Delivery
☐ Hx Infertility
☐ Pre-eclampsia
☐ Eclampsia
☐ Gestational Diabetes
☐ Diabetes
☐ Neural Tube Defects
☐ Hx Infant Congenital Anomalies
☐ Term Infants <5 lbs
☐ Infants >9 lbs
☐ >42 Weeks
☐ Neonatal Deaths Before Age 1 mo.
☐ ....

CURRENT PREGNANCY

☐ No Problems
☐ Premature Labor
☐ prom
☐ Oligohdramnios
☐ Polyhydramnios
☐ Vaginal Bleeding
☐ 1st ☐ 2nd ☐ 3rd Trimester
☐ Diabetes Class A B C D R
☐ Placenta Previa
☐ Placenta Abruptio
☐ Essential Hypertension
☐ Pre-Eclampsia ☐ Eclampsia
☐ HELLP
☐ Incompetent Cervix ☐ Cerclage
☐ Rh Incompatibility
☐ Infection
....
☐ Chromosomal-Fetal Anomalies:
....
☐ Height ...... ft ...... in
☐ Weight Gain During Preg .... lbs
☐ ....

SIGNATURE

PRENATAL LABS

Blood Type and Rh ....
Rubella Imm ☐ Non ☐
RPR Reac ☐ Non ☐ Unk ☐
Hepatitis B Pos ☐ Neg ☐ Unk ☐
MSAFP ☐ Normal ☐ Abn Unk ☐
Maternal/Fetal Ultrasound
☐ Date ....
Results ....
☐ Date ....
Results ....
☐ Not Done ☐ Unk
Amniocentesis
☐ Date ....
Results ....
☐ Not Done ☐ Unk

MEDICATIONS DURING PRENANCY

☐ Vitamins ☐ Iron
☐ Cigarettes ppd ....
☐ Alcohol ....
☐ Social Drugs ....
☐ RhoGam ....
☐ Antibiotics ....

ADMISSION CRITERIA

Date .... Time ....
☐ Laboring ☐ rom
☐ Bleeding ☐ Planned C-Section
☐ Elective Induction
☐ Indicated Induction ....

ONSET OF LABOR

Date .... Time ....
☐ Prior to rom, Not Augmented
☐ Prior to rom, Augmented
☐ After rom, Not Augmented
☐ After rom, Augmented Successfully
☐ After rom, Unsuccessful Augmen.
☐ No labor
☐ Unknown
☐ ....

RUPTURE OF MEMBRANES

Date .... Time ....
Duration ....
☐ Spontaneous ☐ Artificial
☐ Meconium Stained
☐ ....

SIGNATURE

FETAL MONITORING

☐ Internal ☐ External
☐ Auscultation
☐ None ☐ Unk

INTRAPARTUM INFECTION

☐ Chorioamnionitis
☐ Active Genital Herpes
Cultures:
☐ GBS ☐ P ☐ N ☐ Pend
☐ Herpes ☐ P ☐ N ☐ Pend
☐ Chlamydia ☐ P ☐ N ☐ Pend

LABOR & DELIVERY DRUGS

☐ Epidural Block
☐ General Anesthesia
☐ Sedative/Analgesic
☐ Betamimetics
☐ Steroids
☐ Mag Sulfate
☐ ....
☐ None ☐ Unknown

TYPE OF DELIVERY

☐ Vaginal
☐ Vertex ☐ Breech
☐ Assistance
☐ Forceps ☐ Low ☐ Mid
☐ Vacuum
☐ Other
☐ C Section
☐ Elective
☐ Emergency
☐ Indication

INFANT

Name .... ☐ M ☐ F ☐ Unk
Birthdate .... Time ....
Birthwt. .... ☐ AGA ☐ SGA ☐ LGA
Cord Gas PH / PCO_2 / PO_2 / BXS
Source ☐ Art ☐ Ven ☐ Unk
Delivering MD ....
Delivering hospital ....
City & State ....
Transfer Hospital ....

SIGNATURE

APGARS

	1	5	10	15
Heart Rate				
Respiratory Effort				
Muscle Tone				
Reflex Irritability				
Color				
Total	__	__	__	__

RESUSCITATION

☐ Suction ☐ Bulb ☐ Cath ☐ ETT
☐ O_2
☐ Bag & Mask
☐ intubation
☐ Chest Compressions
☐ PIV ☐ UAC ☐ UVC
☐ Volume Expander
☐ Narcan ☐ Epi ☐ $NaHCO_3$
☐ Exosurf ☐ Survanta ☐ Other Surf
☐ ....

FEEDINGS

☐ Breast ☐ Formula ☐ Unknown
☐ Formula Intolerance in Siblings

PSYCHOSOCIAL

☐ No Problems Identified
☐ Language Barrier
☐ Relinquishing Baby
☐ Hx Family Alcohol and/or Drug Abuse
☐ Support Person ....
☐ Other ....

RELIGIOUS

Religious Preference ....
Religious Requests ....

REFERRING PHYSICIAN

....

FOLLOW-UP PHYSICIAN

....

ADDITIONAL COMMENTS

....

SIGNATURE MD

MED REC NO. ....
PATIENT ....
PHYSICIAN ....
BILLING NO. ....

BAYLOR UNIVERSITY MEDICAL CENTER
DALLAS, TEXAS

NEONATAL TRANSPORT/ADMISSION HISTORY
PAGE 1 OF 3

H-360

NEONATAL TRANSPORT RECORD

DATE ______________________

ETT # _____ , _____ CM

UAC ________ FR ________ CM

UVC ________ FR ________ CM

PATIENT IDENTIFICATION

Name: ______________________

Hospital Transported

From: ______________________

To: ______________________

ID Verified ______________________

VENTILATION / BLOOD GASES

TIME	FiO_2	Mode / IMV	PIP / PEEP	I-time / MAP		O_2 Sat / Color	TC PO_2 / TC CO_2	Source	pO_2	pCO_2	pH	HCO_3 / BE	Hct / Hgb	Glucose / Dextrose

VITAL SIGNS / IN / OUT

STATUS (KEY BELOW)	TIME	TEMP (C°) R/A/S	ISOLETTE TEMP (C°)	HEART RATE	RESP RATE	PERIPHERAL BP	ARTERIAL BP	CAP REFILL		IN: IV 1 INT / CUM	IN: IV 2 INT / CUM	IN: IV 3 INT / CUM		OUT: URINE / STOOL	OUT: BLOOD OUT

STATUS(ES):
1=Arrive Hospital
2=Depart Hospital
3=Arrive Destination

COLOR
1. Deeply Cyanotic, Dark or Dusky
2. Mildly Cyanotic
3. Pink
4. Red or Plethoric
5. Pale/Mottled

VENT MODE
1. Bagging
2. Ventilator
3. Headbox
4. Isolette
5. Face Mask
6. Nasal Cannula
7. Nasal CPAP

SOURCE
A = Arterial
V = Venous
C = Capillary

TIME

SKIN
- ☐ Unremarkable
- ☐ Peeling
- ☐ Pale
- ☐ Plethoric
- ☐ Meconium stained
- ☐ Central Cyanosis
- ☐ Acrocyanosis
- ☐ Jaundice
- ☐ Forceps marks
- ☐ Vacuum marks
- ☐ Bruising
- ☐ Laceration/Abrasion
- ☐ Scalp lead lesion

HEENT
- ☐ Unremarkable
- ☐ Molding
- ☐ Caput
- ☐ Cephalohematoma

HEENT (cont.)
- ☐ Sutures separated
- ☐ Sutures overriding
- ☐ Fontanelles-large
- ☐ Fontenelles-bulging
- ☐ Eye discharge
- ☐ Eyes fused
- ☐ Ears abnormal shape/position
- ☐ Nares not patent
- ☐ Cleft lip/palate
- ☐ Neck masses
- ☐ ____________
- ☐ ____________
- ☐ ____________
- ☐ ____________

CARDIOVASCULAR
- ☐ Unremarkable
- ☐ Tones diminished
- ☐ Rhythm irregular
- ☐ Murmur

CARDIOVASCULAR (cont.)
- ☐ Pulses decreased
- ☐ Pulses increased
- ☐ PMI shift
- ☐ ____________
- ☐ ____________

RESPIRATORY
- ☐ Unremarkable
- ☐ Grunting
- ☐ Flaring
- ☐ Retracting
- ☐ Rales
- ☐ Rhonchi
- ☐ Barrel Chest
- ☐ Breath sounds R>L
- ☐ Breath sounds L>R
- ☐ Breath sounds decreased
- ☐ ____________
- ☐ ____________

ABDOMEN/GU
- ☐ Unremarkable
- ☐ Distended
- ☐ Scaphoid
- ☐ Discolored
- ☐ Hepatomegaly
- ☐ Abdominal wall defect
- ☐ Imperforate anus
- ☐ Hypospadias
- ☐ ____________

EXTREMITIES
- ☐ Unremarkable
- ☐ Fractures
- ☐ Extra digits
- ☐ Deformity
- ☐ Edema
- ☐ ____________
- ☐ ____________
- ☐ ____________
- ☐ ____________

SPINE
- ☐ Unremarkable
- ☐ Neural tube defect
- ☐ ____________
- ☐ ____________
- ☐ ____________

CARDIOVASCULAR
- ☐ Unremarkable
- ☐ Hypertonia
- ☐ Hypotonia
- ☐ Lethargic/unresponsive
- ☐ Irritable
- ☐ High pitched cry
- ☐ Clonus sustained
- ☐ Facial weakness
- ☐ Arm weakness ☐ R ☐ L
- ☐ ____________
- ☐ ____________
- ☐ ____________
- ☐ ____________
- ☐ ____________

Date		
Time		
Source		
Na		
K		
Cl		
Ca		
WBC		
PMNs		
Bands		
META / MYELO		
I/T		
ANC		
Plts		
Hct		

URINE CX ☐ ● Rd ☐ ● Rec
TRACH ASP CX ☐ ● Rd ☐ ● Rec
BLOOD CX ☐ ● Rd ☐ ● Rec
GASTRIC CX ☐ ● Rd ☐ ● Rec

SIGNATURE ____________ SIGNATURE ____________ SIGNATURE ____________ SIGNATURE ____________ MD

MED REC NO. ______________________

PATIENT ______________________

PHYSICIAN ______________________

BILLING NO. ______________________

BAYLOR UNIVERSITY MEDICAL CENTER
DALLAS, TEXAS

NEONATAL TRANSPORT RECORD
PAGE 2 OF 3

H-360

NEONATAL TRANSPORT RECORD

DATE ____________________

INFANT HISTORY

Date of Birth __________ Time __________

EGA: __________ (dates) __________ (exam)

Weight: BW __________ Cur __________

PROBLEM LIST

MAJOR CARRIER TYPE

☐ 1. Helicopter
☐ 2. Fixed Wing
☐ 3. Ambulance
☐ 4. Other __________

TYPE OF TRANSPORT

☐ 1. Forward
☐ 2. Back Transport
☐ 3. Procedure __________

CARRIER: __________

Call Received		Arrive Referral
Dispatch Notified		Depart Referral
Time Out		Time Out
Lift Off		Land
Land		Time In
Comments:		Complete Restock

NURSING PROCEDURES

MEDICATIONS (drug, dose, route, time) — GIVEN BY R/TT

☐ Eye Prophylaxis ☐ Aquamephyton

FLUIDS (total Fluids __________ cc/kg/24°)

IV Site	Solution	Rate

X-RAYS:

☐ Parent Teaching ☐ Consents Signed ☐ Parent Visit
☐ Maternal Blood

Comments: __________

PROCEDURES: ☐ Intubation ☐ Reintubation ☐ UAC ☐ UAC Replaced ☐ UVC ☐ PIV ☐ IO
☐ Needle Asp. ☐ Chest Tube ☐ Chest Compression ☐ Attended Delivery ☐ __________

SIGNATURE	SIGNATURE	SIGNATURE	SIGNATURE MD

MED REC NO. __________

PATIENT __________

PHYSICIAN __________

BILLING NO. __________

BAYLOR UNIVERSITY MEDICAL CENTER
DALLAS, TEXAS

NEONATAL TRANSPORT RECORD
PAGE 3 OF 3

H-360

33

THE ECMO CANDIDATE

SUSAN E. DAY

Extracorporeal membrane oxygenation (ECMO) is a therapy which combines extracorporeal circulation and gas exchange through an artificial lung to support patients with reversible cardiorespiratory failure. The procedure is accomplished by draining central venous blood from the right atrium, usually through a cannula placed in the right internal jugular vein, and circulating the blood through the extracorporeal circuit using a servocontrolled roller pump or centrifugal pump. The blood passes through a silicon membrane oxygenator, where carbon dioxide is removed and oxygen is added, and then through a heat exchanger, where the blood is warmed to room temperature before being returned to the body. The arterial cannula is usually passed via the right common carotid artery. The neck vessels are usually ligated permanently. During the ECMO procedure the patient's blood is anticoagulated with heparin.

The extracorporeal circulation supplements the cardiac output of the ailing heart and enables inotropic support to be decreased or discontinued. The artificial lung can provide total gas exchange, allowing mechanical ventilator settings to be reduced to minimal support and allow parenchymal lung disease to heal without added barotrauma. In patients who have reversible pulmonary hypertension, the pulmonary vascular resistance can fall during several days of ECMO therapy.

PATIENTS WHO ARE REFERRED FOR ECMO

The patients who are most often referred to medical centers that offer ECMO are newborns with severe respiratory failure who have failed to respond or who no longer respond to conventional mechanical ventilation. Many of them will have some element of either primary or secondary persistent pulmonary hypertension of the newborn (PPHN). In this condition the pulmonary vascular resistance remains high, preventing normal transition to adult circulation pathways. Transient pulmonary hypertension is associated with polycythemia, hypoglycemia, hypothermia, and hypoxia. Persistent pulmonary hypertension is associated with syndromes of active vasoconstriction, such as bacterial sepsis and pneumonia. It also is associated with underdevelopment of the lung, as in congenital diaphragmatic hernia, and maldevelopment of pulmonary vessels, such as with chronic intrauterine asphyxia or meconium aspiration pneumonitis.[27]

Among older children and adults, some causes of respiratory failure which have been successfully treated with ECMO include bacterial and viral pneumonia, intrapulmonary hemorrhage, aspiration, infection with Pneumocystis carinii, and adult respiratory distress syndrome.[2,4,23,49,54] ECMO has also been used successfully to support the failing heart following repair of congenital heart lesions, in patients with myocarditis or cardiomyopathy, and as a bridge to cardiac transplantation.[33,37,49,50,57,60]

OVERVIEW OF THE HISTORY OF EXTRACORPOREAL LIFE SUPPORT

In the early and mid 1970s there were several case reports of patients who were successfully treated with ECMO for severe respiratory failure.[15,28,32] In 1979, Zapol and others reported the results of an NIH-sponsored randomized study on the use of ECMO in adults.[62] For a variety of reasons related to study design and patient selection, the trial failed to show improved survival in adults with severe respiratory failure using ECMO plus mechanical ventilation over ventilation alone. After this study, clinical use of prolonged extracorporeal support for adults decreased in the United States.

In the 1980s Gattinoni and others in Europe revived extracorporeal life support (ECLS) for adults.[21,25] A variation of ECMO, extracorporeal CO_2 removal ($ECCO_2R$) provided partial bypass using venovenous rather than venoarterial access. Pulmonary blood flow was preserved, and low rate, low pressure ventilation decreased ventilator-induced lung injury. Since reports of success using ECLS appeared, the use of variations of ECMO and $ECCO_2R$ has resumed in North America.[1,5,24,34,48,53]

To date, the most successful application of ECMO continues to be in newborns with severe respiratory or cardiac failure. In 1976 the first successful use of ECMO in a newborn was reported by Bartlett and others.[8] Multiple clinical series followed, showing survival rates of 54 to 90% among patients who had a predicted mortality of 80 to 100%.[9,11,29,38,41,44,56,59] Two controversial randomized controlled studies demonstrated improved survival with ECMO and lung rest over conventional ventilatory and pharmacologic management in patients with predicted 80 to 85% mortality.[10,46] The most commonly utilized technique in newborns, as described before, is venoarterial access using the right carotid and internal jugular vessels. Venovenous ECMO was described in early series[6,36] and originally involved cannulation of the right internal jugular vein for blood drainage and a femoral vein for return of oxygenated blood. Venovenous ECMO has been used more in recent years for patients who do not require as much hemodynamic support from the extracorporeal circulation. A double lumen cannula is now available for venovenous access in neonates, requiring only the right internal jugular vein, thereby sparing the carotid artery.[3]

In 1989 the Extracorporeal Life Support Organization (ELSO), an international consortion of health care professionals and scientists, was formed. Based at the University of Michigan, its goals include education and multicenter research in ECLS and maintaining a registry of patients who have been treated with ECMO and other forms of ECLS. As of July 1994 there were 88 active ECLS centers in North America and 21 centers in Europe, Australia, and Japan (see Box 33-1). Also as of July 1994, 11364 patients had undergone ECLS. Overall survival was as follows: 81% survival among 9258 neonates, 49% survival for 754 pediatric patients with respiratory failure, 44% survival for 1222 pediatric patients with cardiac failure, and 38% survival among 130 adults with cardiac or respiratory failure.[23]

GENERAL PRINCIPLES FOR TRANSPORTING PATIENTS FOR ECLS

Communication

Critical care providers who wish to offer extracorporeal life support to their patients should contact the staff of ECLS centers in their region and familiarize themselves with referral procedures and transport resources. The ECLS center's indications for transfer should be discussed.

When a particular patient is identified who may require extracorporeal support, early contact with the ECLS physician is recommended. The receiving physician will require complete and accurate information on the patient's medical history and hospital course. Further stabilization measures and diagnostic procedures to rule out any contraindications may be recommended at the time of initial contact.

Patient preparation

The referring physician should discuss all therapeutic options and risks, including the

BOX 33-1 ACTIVE EXTRACORPOREAL LIFE SUPPORT CENTERS

Alabama
- Children's Hospital of Alabama, Birmingham

Arizona
- Phoenix Children's Hospital, Phoenix
- St. Joseph's Hospital and Medical Center, Phoenix

Arkansas
- Arkansas Children's Hospital, Little Rock

California
- Children's Hospital of Los Angeles, Los Angeles
- Children's Hospital of Oakland, Oakland
- Children's Hospital of Orange County, Orange
- Lucille Salter Packard Children's Hospital, Palo Alto
- Huntington Memorial Hospital, Pasadena
- Sutter Center for Women's Health, Sacramento
- San Diego Regional ECMO Program, San Diego
- Sharp Memorial Hospital, San Diego
- University of California, San Francisco

Colorado
- Children's Hospital, Denver

Connecticut
- Yale University School of Medicine

District of Columbia
- Children's National Medical Center
- Georgetown University Hospital

Florida
- Shands Hospital, University of Florida, Gainesville
- Joe DiMaggio Children's Hospital at Memorial, Hollywood
- Miami Children's Hospital, Miami
- Arnold Palmer Hospital for Children and Women, Orlando
- Tampa General Hospital, Tampa

Georgia
- Egleston Children's Hospital, Atlanta
- Medical College of Georgia, Augusta

Idaho
- St. Luke's Hospital, Boise

Illinois
- Children's Memorial Hospital, Chicago
- University of Chicago Hospitals, Chicago
- Christ Hospital and Medical Center, Oak Lawn
- Lutheran General Hospital, Park Ridge
- St. Francis Medical Center, Peoria
- Rockford Memorial Children's Hospital, Rockford

Indiana
- James Whitcomb Riley Hospital, Indianapolis

Kentucky
- University of Kentucky Medical Center, Lexington
- Kosair Children's Hospital, Louisville

Louisiana
- Ochsner Foundation Hospital, New Orleans
- Tulane University Medical Center, New Orleans

Maryland
- Johns Hopkins Hospital, Baltimore
- Shock Trauma Center, Baltimore

Massachusetts
- Children's Hospital, Boston
- Massachusetts General Hospital, Boston

Michigan
- University of Michigan Medical Center, Ann Arbor
- Children's Hospital of Michigan, Detroit
- Butterworth Hospital, Grand Rapids

Minnesota
- Minnesota Regional ECMO Program, Minneapolis

Missouri
- Children's Mercy Hospital, Kansas City
- Cardinal Glennon Children's Hospital, St. Louis
- St. Louis Children's Hospital, St. Louis

Nebraska
- University of Nebraska Medical Center, Omaha

New Jersey
- Cooper Hospital University and Medical Center, Camden
- Newark Beth Israel Medical Center, Newark
- United Hospitals Medical Center, Newark

New Mexico
- University of New Mexico, Albuquerque

New York
- Children's Hospital, Buffalo
- Columbia Presbyterian Medical Center, New York

North Carolina
- Carolinas Medical Center, Charlotte
- Duke University Medical Center, Durham

Ohio
- Children's Hospital Medical Center, Akron
- Children's Hospital Medical Center, Cincinnati

BOX 33-1 ACTIVE EXTRACORPOREAL LIFE SUPPORT CENTERS—cont'd

Ohio (cont'd)
- Rainbow Babies and Children's Hospital, Cleveland
- Children's Hospital, Columbus
- Miami Valley Hospital, Dayton

Oklahoma
- Children's Hospital of Oklahoma, Oklahoma City
- Saint Francis Hospital, Tulsa

Oregon
- Emanuel Hospital and Health Center, Portland

Pennsylvania
- Hershey Medical Center, Hershey
- Children's Hospital of Philadelphia, Philadelphia
- St. Christopher's Hospital, Philadelphia
- Thomas Jefferson University Hospital, Philadelphia
- Children's Hospital of Pittsburgh, Pittsburgh
- Guthrie Clinic, Sayre

South Carolina
- Medical University of South Carolina, Charleston
- University of South Carolina, Columbia

Tennessee
- LeBonheur Children's Medical Center, Memphis
- Vanderbilt University Medical Center, Nashville

Texas
- Driscoll Children's Hospital, Corpus Christi
- Children's Medical Center, Dallas
- Presbyterian Hospital, Dallas
- Cook-Fort Worth Children's Medical Center, Fort Worth
- University of Texas—Medical Branch, Galveston
- Hermann Children's Hospital, Houston
- Texas Children's Hospital, Houston
- Wilford Hall Medical Center, Lackland Air Force Base
- University Medical Center, Lubbock
- Santa Rosa Children's Hospital, San Antonio

Virginia
- University of Virginia Medical Center, Charlottesville
- Medical College of Virginia, Richmond

Washington
- Children's Hospital Medical Center, Seattle

Wisconsin
- Children's Hospital of Wisconsin, Milwaukee

Australia
- Royal Children's Hospital, Melbourne
- Prince of Wales Children's Hospital, New South Wales

Austria
- Universitat Kinderklinik, Graz

Canada
- Royal Alexandra Hospital, Edmonton, Alberta
- Hospital for Sick Children, Toronto, Ontario
- Montreal Children's Hospital, Quebec

England
- Groby Road Hospital, Leicester
- Hospital for Sick Children, London
- Freeman Hospital, Newcastle upon Tyne

France
- Hospital Robert-Debre, Paris

Germany
- Free University of Berlin
- Universitats-Kinderklinik, Mannheim

Italy
- Salesi Children's Hospital, Ancona
- Ospedali Riuniti Di Bergamo, Bergamo

Japan
- Central Hospital, Aichi
- National Children's Hospital, Tokyo

The Netherlands
- Academisch Hospital, Maastricht
- St. Radoud Hospital, Nijmegen
- Sophia's Children's Hospital, Rotterdam

Scotland
- Yorkhill ECMO Center, Glasgow

Sweden
- St. Goran's Children's Hospital, Stockholm

From the Extracorporeal Life Support Organization, Ann Arbor, Michigan, April, 1993.

risks of transfer, with the patient's family and, if possible, with the patient. A copy of the medical record including radiographs and other imaging should be prepared. Any other necessary diagnostic procedures should be performed. The receiving center may request that additional monitoring catheters be placed or changed to alternate sites because of the vascular access requirements for bypass.

The meticulous planning and attention to detail required to successfully transfer a candidate for ECLS cannot be emphasized too strongly. A patient who has suffered a severe hypoxic or ischemic insult before or during transfer may no longer be a candidate for ECLS after arrival at the receiving hospital.

TRANSPORT OF NEONATES FOR ECMO

Newborn infants who are referred for ECMO will probably have received intensive therapy to reverse the hypoxemia associated with persistent pulmonary hypertension, which causes right-to-left shunting at the level of the ductus arteriosus or foramen ovale or both. Therapy is complicated by the decreased lung compliance from pulmonary parenchymal disease or pulmonary hypoplasia. Conventional management often includes mechanical hyperventilation, alkalosis, sedation, neuromuscular blockade, volume boluses, inotropic medications, and antibiotics.[19,20,26] Optimal ventilatory management is controversial, with some reports of success allowing $PaCO_2$ levels as high as 60 mm Hg and PaO_2 levels between 50 and 70 mm Hg, without the use of hyperventilation or neuromuscular blockade.[22,61] Some patients may receive exogenous surfactant or high frequency oscillatory ventilation.[17] Selective pulmonary vasodilatation using medications such as tolazoline may be tried with variable success.[39] These medications can also cause systemic hypotension. By the time of request for transfer to an ECMO center, these modalities will probably have failed to maintain adequate gas exchange or hemodynamic stability.

Criteria for initiation of ECMO therapy vary among ECMO centers based on each center's estimated mortality of 80% or greater without ECMO therapy. Frequently used criteria include alveolar-arterial oxygen difference (A-aDO_2), oxygenation index (OI = [mean airway pressure $\times$ FiO_2 $\times$ 100/ postductal PaO_2]), acute deterioration, or barotrauma. Exclusion criteria often include birth weight less than 2,000 grams, gestational age less than 35 weeks, intracranial hemorrhage, uncorrectable coagulopathy, or presence of other fatal anomalies. The etiology of the respiratory failure is expected to be reversible within a finite period of time, approximately 10 days. Prolonged mechanical ventilation at high pressures and FiO_2 for more than 7 to 10 days or the presence of a severe congenital heart lesion are relative contraindications.

Infants who are ill enough to require ECMO therapy are also most likely to tolerate transfer poorly. The optimal time to refer to an ECMO center is before the patient has actually met criteria for the procedure. Boedy and others have noted that of all accepted referrals for ECMO to their center, 11% of the patients died before, during, or as a consequence of transport.[12] These transport-related deaths comprised 39% of all deaths in their ECMO program. The Extracorporeal Life Support Organization developed Guidelines for Neonatal ECMO Consultation, which recommended that "the referring physician should begin to consider the need for ECMO when a patient who has received appropriate medical management has a PaO_2 of 50 to 60 mm Hg, when the PIP is greater than 35 cm H_2O, and FiO_2 is 1.00. After consultation with an ECMO physician the time of transfer can be determined through a team approach taking into account such items as transport time, type of transport needed, and regional availability of 'ECMO beds.' "*

Critical care transport teams who will transport ECMO patients should receive education in the diseases and the pathophysiology involved. Protocols should be developed with regard to equipment, personnel, and procedures. At the time of the initial referral contact, the referring and receiving physicians discuss the patient's course, recommended stabilization, and any tests that may be done at the referring hospital to rule out any contraindications to transfer or ECMO therapy. The transport team should ask the referring nursing staff which medications and intravenous solutions the patient is receiving and how many intravascular catheters are in place.

The equipment necessary for transfer includes an ample number of battery-powered syringe pumps that can operate at rates as low as 0.1 ml per hour. Medication-containing solutions for inotropes, neuromuscular blocker, sedation, buffer, vasodilators, and mainte-

* From Extracorporeal Life Support Organization: ELSO guidelines for neonatal consultation, Ann Arbor, Mich., 1992.

nance fluid can be mixed in advance. Several doses of resuscitation drugs and fluid for volume expansion can be prepared.

Other essential equipment includes an isolette for maintaining a neutral thermal environment and an ECG monitor with capability to monitor temperature and at least one intravascular pressure. Two pulse oximeters are used to measure both preductal and postductal oxygen saturations to detect right-to-left shunting at the ductus arteriosus. Transcutaneous PO_2 and PCO_2 monitors are helpful. A portable end-tidal CO_2 monitor can assess adequacy of ventilation and detect a displaced or obstructed endotracheal tube.

The transport ventilator should have the capability to ventilate a 2 to 5 kg infant with rates as high as 100 breaths per minute. It may be necessary for the transport personnel to hand ventilate the patient. A controlled rebreathing circuit of the Mapleson type with adjustable pressure-limiting valve and airway pressure manometer is recommended. Because the patient's lungs are often poorly compliant, a spare bag for the circuit should be taken because of the possibility of rupture. A self-inflating ventilating bag should also be immediately available in case of loss of gas flow. Since most of these patients will be transported with an FiO_2 of 1.0, a supply of oxygen sufficient to provide fresh gas flow at 2 to 3 times the patient's minute ventilation is necessary. Other equipment which should be at hand include suction, portable illuminator, and instruments for needle thoracentesis, chest tube placement, and umbilical vessel catheterization. All electrical equipment should have a battery life of several hours and be fully charged. The function of all equipment should have been tested previously in the vibrating environments of air and ground vehicles.[52]

The transport vehicle should have an inverter for electrical power while in transit. All fixed wing aircraft should be pressurized. Since the ability to assess and treat patients for deterioration is severely limited by noise and vibration, the selection of helicopters to transport infants for ECMO should be done very carefully. The transport team should be aware of the effects of altitude on oxygenation and gas field spaces, including pneumothoraces.[42] Optimally, ground transport is preferred when time, distance, and the patient's condition permit.

The optimal team composition for transporting patients for ECMO includes a physician, nurse, and respiratory therapist, if possible. The combined skills of the team members should include neonatal resuscitation, endotracheal intubation, venous and arterial excess, treatment of pneumothoraces, radiograph interpretation, and operation and maintenance of all monitoring equipment, pumps, and ventilators. It may be advisable for the transport team to take with them consent forms for ECMO and the cannulation procedure, depending on the distance of family from the ECMO center and the mother's postpartum condition.

When the transport team arrives at the referral center, they should receive updated information on the patient's condition from the patient's caretakers and confirm the medications, fluids, and ventilator settings in use. The most recent chest radiographs, blood gases, and other lab work should be reviewed. The positions of all catheters should be confirmed and secured. Infants with persistent pulmonary hypertension respond adversely to touch, noise, change in temperature, hypoxia, acidosis, hypercapnia, and hypotension. The IV fluids and continuous infusions are transferred to the transport syringe pumps one at a time, allowing for the patient to be stabilized in between for any changes in blood pressure. Before the patient is moved, ventilation should be transferred to the transport ventilator to allow time for stabilization. If the patient requires manual ventilation, the transport personnel take over ventilation as the last step. Before transferring the patient to the transport incubator, the transport team personnel should discuss with the patient's parents the plans for transport and therapy at the receiving center, and, if necessary, obtain consent for ECMO. The transport team should confirm that all of the patient's medical records and imaging studies are copied and available. The team should call the receiving staff and update them on the patient's status, needs for equipment on arrival, and estimated time of return.

Patients with congenital diaphragmatic hernia

The use of ECMO therapy has had a variable effect on the mortality from congenital diaphragmatic hernia (CDH).[7,31,40,47] Some centers have demonstrated improved survival in patients formerly considered in the highest risk category.[58] Overall, patients with congenital diaphragmatic hernia continue to have the lowest survival rate (58%) among neonatal ECMO patients, however, due to the irreversibility of hypoplasia in the most severely effected infants.[23]

Patients with congenital diaphragmatic hernia may be referred for ECMO therapy before or after surgical repair. There have been some indications that patients may be better candidates for surgical repair after a period of stabilization using either conventional mechanical ventilation or ECMO.[13,30,45,61] Each center performing ECMO for neonates may have its own criteria for timing of referral of patients with congenital diaphragmatic hernia and recommendations for resuscitation and stabilization once a CDH has been recognized. In severely affected infants, those who present within the first 24 hours of life, stabilization will usually include endotracheal intubation, mechanical ventilation, and hemodynamic stabilization with special attention to acid-base status. A large nasogastric or orogastric tube should be placed with intermittent suction to prevent inflation of the gastrointestinal tract and further compression of the lung and shift of the mediastinum.

The management of the CDH patient during transport includes the same interventions as those for other ECMO patients, with attention to GI decompression and positioning the patient with the head elevated and the affected hemithorax down. Patients who are referred for ECMO after surgical repair of CDH are among the most unstable patients. Their gas exchange and hemodynamic status may be extremely labile. They are at very high risk for development of pneumothoraces. Broedy and others found that postoperative CDH patients represented 28% of transport-related deaths and recommended that they be transported in utero or in the early postoperative period.[12] A regional ECMO center may recommend that infants undergo the surgical repair at an institution where ECMO is available.

TRANSPORT OF OLDER CHILDREN AND ADULTS FOR ECLS

As compared with neonates with severe respiratory insufficiency, adults, children and older infants with acute respiratory failure are a very heterogeneous group. Multiple organ system failure is common, and risk of mortality increases with each additional system failure. Before referral for ECMO or other rescue therapy, such as high frequency ventilation, many intensive therapies will have been initiated to maximize O_2 delivery and metabolic CO_2 removal and minimize interstitial edema. These include endotracheal intubation and mechanical ventilation with increasing levels of positive end expiratory pressure (PEEP), pulmonary artery catheterization and use of fluids and inotropes to optimize cardiac output, diuresis or hemofiltration, transfusion, antibiotics, and nutrition. Sedation and neuromuscular blockade are added for worsening pulmonary compliance. The patient's risk for air leaks is very high, and many patients will have already undergone tube thoracostomies. Bronchoscopy or open lung biopsy may have been performed for diagnostic purposes.[14]

Criteria for initiating ECMO or $ECCO_2R$ therapy for pediatric and adult patients are not uniform, and again, it is best for referring and receiving staff to discuss criteria for potential ECLS patients before the need arises. The goal of criteria is to select patients with acute, severe, potentially fatal respiratory failure at a point where the disease is still reversible. Some centers use variations of the criteria used in the NIH adult ECMO study[62] (transpulmonary shunt greater than 30% after a period of maximal medical therapy) with an additional criterion for static compliance or PAO_2. For children, some centers use variations of neonatal entry criteria.[2] Not uncommonly some patients are selected for ECLS, primarily because death is considered imminent.

Reversibility of the primary process is more difficult to determine than mortality risk. The extent of pulmonary fibrosis may be determined by an open lung biopsy. The best candidates for ECLS are those who are still on the acute phase of disease, having undergone mechanical ventilation for fewer than 6 days.

Criteria for exclusion from ECLS are often easier to identify than those for inclusion. Exclusion criteria may include ventilator therapy longer than 10 days, cardiac arrest, major brain injury, active bleeding, or underlying terminal disease.

When critically ill adults and children are referred for transport to an ECLS center, the same principles for communication and preparation of the patient apply as for neonatal transports. Transfer of complete and accurate information is essential. Equipment, fluids, and medications are prepared to maintain the current level of support and treat potential complications. Because of extremely poor lung compliance, the greatest challenge is maintaining adequate gas exchange. Continuous monitoring with end-tidal CO_2 and pulse oximetry should be done. Both mechanical and manual ventilation with airway pressure monitoring should be available with back-up resuscitation bags in case of rupture. McQuillan and others described a modification of a transport ventilator which provides continuous O_2 flow during transport for patients who require high levels of PEEP or have air leaks.[43] For management of pneumothoraces, Heimlich valves may be attached to the end of thoracostomy tubes. If a repeat chest radiograph demonstrates reaccumulation of pleural air, the distal end of the Heimlich valve can be attached to a portal suction machine.

TRANSPORT OF PATIENTS DURING EXTRACORPOREAL SUPPORT

More than 1,000 infants per year now undergo ECMO therapy. As of 1989, 97% of neonates undergoing ECMO were born outside of ECMO centers.[55] Although the numbers of ECMO centers is increasing, there will continue to be a large number of infants who must be transported to a regional ECMO center, sometimes over a distance of several hundred miles. Because of the high risk of mortality from respiratory failure, in addition to the risk of transport over the time and distances involved, some ECLS centers have developed the capability to initiate ECMO for selected patients at the referring hospital and transport the patient to the ECMO center on bypass.[36]

The decision to develop an ECMO transport team should not be made lightly. Months of planning are required. Team members should be thoroughly familiar with the pathophysiology and management of respiratory and cardiac failure in all age groups of the patients to be transported. The transport team will need to include members who are proficient in the management of the patient on bypass and the ECMO equipment itself. The team also will need to include surgeons who can perform cannulation at the referring hospital.

The team needs to be entirely self-sufficient with regard to durable and disposable equipment, monitors, and medications. The referring center cannot be expected to provide any back-up supplies. There should be enough equipment and spare components to maintain bypass for 24 hours, should weather interfere with the return to the ECMO center. All transport vehicles must have inverters for electrical power, and all battery-powered equipment should be fully charged. Checklists and protocols should be developed to ensure correct placement of all equipment in transport vehicles and assignments of roles to team members.

Cornish and others from Wilford Hall U.S. Air Force Medical Center described a modified ECMO circuit with a cart developed to transport equipment and an isolette.[16,18] This system was designed to be conveyed on a United States Air Force C-9 aircraft. Every detail of this system was tested by medical, nursing, and engineering personnel. Each component had to withstand the stresses of flight, including acceleration-deceleration forces, vibration, turbulence, temperature, altitude, and barometric pressure. A mobile ECMO transport team has also been developed at Arkansas Children's Hospital using a Sikorsky S-76 helicopter as the preferred vehicle (Mark Heulitt, M.D., personal communication).

A program for transporting adult patients during ECMO was developed at the University of Michigan after some patients who had been referred for ECLS died before bypass could be initiated. A sturdy, easily maneuverable transport cart was designed with a locking mechanism, handles for lifting, an extension cord, and straps for securing equipment. Other equipment prepared for transport included tools, priming supplies, backup circuit components, cannulation equipment, and 18 different types of catheters. The estimated combined cost to duplicate this system from new equipment with the additional supplies is over $26,000. The personnel of the Michigan ECLS Transport Team includes two ECMO specialists, two surgeons, one or two ambulance drivers, and a transport nurse. Protocols are written for each member of the team in each stage of the process, including pretransport telephone arrangements, assembly of equipment, loading and unloading of the patient and equipment, and assignment of responsibilities during cannulation and travel and upon return to the receiving unit. Separate additional protocols were prepared for ground vehicles, helicopter and fixed wing aircraft.

Among the important details to be considered when planning to perform ECMO during transport include selection of vehicles for both transporting the team and equipment to the referring hospital and for return of the patient with the team and supplies. The communication with the referring hospital needs to convey the transport team's requirements for blood products, space, operating room personnel, oxygen, medical records, radiographs, and availability of the patient's family for consent. Arrangements need to be made to obtain emergency privileges at the referring hospital for ECLS surgeons. Pretransport communication also includes instructions for changing the sites of invasive monitoring catheters to allow for placement of the ECMO cannulae.

Staff at a regional ECMO center who are considering developing a program for ECLS during transport must weigh the potential benefit against tremendous risks and costs. An ECLS transport service may deprive the ECLS center of critical staff for many hours at a time. The dedicated equipment and vehicles needed are very expensive. The process is physically and emotionally taxing for team members. If the regional need merits the costs, then the importance of extensive preparation, rehearsal, and compliance with protocols can not be exaggerated. Ongoing review of all ECLS transports should be done so that all incidents and complications can result in revision of protocols. In most cases the need for ECLS transport can be obviated by education and communication with potential referring staff, resulting in timely referral before a patient is too unstable to transport.

REFERENCES

1. Abrams JH and others: Low-frequency positive-pressure ventilation with extracorporeal carbon dioxide removal, *Crit Care Med* 18:218, 1990.
2. Adolph V and others: Extracorporeal membrane oxygenation for nonneonatal respiratory failure, *J Pediatr Surg* 26:326, 1991.
3. Anderson HL and others: Venovenous extracorporeal life support in neonates using a double lumen catheter, *Trans Am Soc Artif Intern Organs* 35:650, 1989.
4. Anderson HL and others: Extracorporeal membrane oxygenation for pediatric cardiopulmonary failure, *J Thorac Cardiovasc Surg* 99:1011, 1990.
5. Anderson HL and others: Early experience with adult extracorporeal membrane oxygenation in the modern era, *Ann Thorac Surg* 53:553, 1992.
6. Andrews AF and others: Venovenous extracorporeal membrane oxygenation in neonates with respiratory failure, *J Pediatr Surg* 18:339, 1983.
7. Atkinson JB and others: The impact of extracorporeal membrane support in the treatment of congenital diaphragmatic hernia, *J Pediatr Surg* 26:791, 1991.
8. Bartlett RH and others: Extracorporeal membrane oxygenation (ECMO) cardiopulmonary support in infancy, *Trans Am Soc Artif Intern Organs* 22:80, 1976.
9. Bartlett RH and others: Extracorporeal membrane oxygenation for newborn respiratory failure: forty-five cases, *Surgery* 92:425, 1982.
10. Bartlett RH and others: Extracorporeal circulation in neonatal respiratory failure: prospective randomized study, *Pediatrics* 76:479, 1985.
11. Bartlett RH and others; Extracorporeal membrane oxygenation (ECMO) in neonatal respiratory failure: 100 cases, *Ann Surg* 204:236, 1986.
12. Boedy RF, Howell CG, Kanto WP: Hidden mortality rate associated with extracorporeal membrane oxygenation, *J Pediatr* 117:462, 1990.
13. Breaux CW and others: Improvement in survival of patients with congenital diaphragmatic hernia utilizing a strategy of delayed repair after medical and/or extracorporeal membrane oxygenation stabilization, *J Pediatr Surg* 26:333, 1991.

14. Chapman RA, Bartlett RH: *Extracorporeal life support manual for adult and pediatric patients*, ed 1, Ann Arbor, MI, 1991, University of Michigan Medical Center.
15. Cooper JD and others: Cardiorespiratory failure secondary to peripheral pulmonary emboli survival following a combination of prolonged extracorporeal membrane oxygenator support and pulmonary embolectomy, *J Thorac Cardiovasc Surg* 71:872, 1976.
16. Cornish JD and others: Inflight use of extracorporeal membrane oxygenation for severe neonatal respiratory failure, *Perfusion* 1:281, 1986.
17. Cornish JD and others: Extracorporeal membrane oxygenation and high-frequency oscillatory ventilation: potential therapeutic relationships, *Crit Care Med* 15:831, 1987.
18. Cornish JD and others: Extracorporeal membrane oxygenation as a means of stabilizing and transporting high risk neonates, *Trans Am Soc Artif Intern Organs* 37:564, 1991.
19. Drummond WH and others: The independent effects of hyperventilation, tolazoline, and dopamine on infants with persistent pulmonary hypertension, *J Pediatr* 98:603, 1981.
20. Duara S, Gewitz MH, Fox WW: Use of mechanical ventilation for clinical management of persistent pulmonary hypertension of the newborn, *Clin Perinatol* 11:641, 1984.
21. Durandy Y, Chevalier JY, Lecompte Y: Single-cannula venovenous bypass for respiratory membrane lung support, *J Thorac Cardiovasc Surg* 99:404, 1990.
22. Dworetz AR, et al: Survival of infants with persistent pulmonary hypertension without extracorporeal membrane oxygenation, *Pediatrics* 84:1, 1989.
23. ECMO Registry of the Extracorporeal Life Support Organization (ELSO), Ann Arbor, Michigan, July 1994.
24. Egan TM and others: Ten-year experience with extracorporeal membrane oxygenation for severe respiratory failure, *Chest* 94:681, 1988.
25. Gattinoni L and others: Low-frequency positive-pressure ventilation with extracorporeal CO_2 removal in severe acute respiratory failure, *JAMA* 256:881, 1986.
26. Hageman JR, Adams MA, Gardner TH: Persistent pulmonary hypertension of the newborn: trends in incidence, diagnosis, and management, *Am J Dis Child* 138:592, 1984.
27. Hansen T, Corbet A: Disorders of the transition. In Taeusch HW, Ballard RA, Avery ME, editors: *Diseases of the newborn,* Philadelphia, 1991, W.B. Saunders Co.
28. Hanson EL and others: Venoarterial bypass with a membrane oxygenator: successful respiratory support in a woman following pulmonary hemorrhage secondary to renal failure, *Surgery* 75:557, 1974.
29. Hardesty RL and others: Extracorporeal membrane oxygenation: successful treatment of persistent fetal circulation following repair of congenital diaphragmatic hernia, *J Thorac Cardiovasc Surg* 81:556, 1981.
30. Hazebroek FWJ and others: Congenital diaphragmatic hernia: Impact of preoperative stabilization: a prospective pilot study in 13 patients, *J Pediatr Surg* 23:1139, 1988.
31. Heiss K and others: Reversal of mortality for congenital diaphragmatic hernia with ECMO, *Ann Surg* 209:225, 1989.
32. Hill JD and others: Prolonged extracorporeal oxygenation for acute post-traumatic respiratory failure (shock-lung syndrome), *N Engl J Med* 286:629, 1972.
33. Kanter KR and others: Extracorporeal membrane oxygenation for postoperative cardiac support in children, *J Thorac Cardiovasc Surg* 93:27, 1987.
34. Katz NM and others: Venovenous extracorporeal membrane oxygenation for noncardiogenic pulmonary edema after coronary bypass surgery, *Ann Thorac Surg* 46:462, 1988.
35. Kee SS, Sedgwick J, Bristow A: Interhospital transfer of a patient undergoing extracorporeal carbon dioxide removal, *Br J Anaesth* 66:141, 1991.
36. Klein MD and others: Venovenous perfusion in ECMO for newborn respiratory insufficiency: a clinical comparison with venoarterial perfusion, *Ann Surg* 201:520, 1985.
37. Klein MD and others: Extracorporeal membrane oxygenation for the circulatory support of children after repair of congenital heart disease, *J Thorac Cardiovasc Surg* 100:498, 1990.
38. Krummel TM and others: Clinical use of an extracorporeal membrane oxygenator in neonatal pulmonary failure, *J Pediatr Surg* 17:525, 1982.
39. Kulik TJ, Lock JE: Pulmonary vasodilator therapy in persistent pulmonary hypertension of the newborn, *Clin Perinatol* 11:693, 1984.
40. Langham MR and others: Mortality with extracorporeal membrane oxygenation following repair of congenital diaphragmatic hernia in 93 infants, *J Pediatr Surg* 22:1150, 1987.
41. Loe WA and others: Extracorporeal membrane oxygenation for newborn respiratory failure, *J Pediatr Surg* 20:684, 1985.
42. Macnab AJ and others: In-flight stabilization of oxygen saturation by control of altitude for severe respiratory insufficiency, *Aviat Space Environ Med* 61:829, 1990.
43. McQuillan PJ, Hillman DR, Woods WPD: Positive end expiratory pressure and critical oxygenation during transport in ventilated patients, *Intensive Care Med* 16:513, 1990.
44. Moront MG and others: Extracorporeal membrane oxygenation for neonatal respiratory failure: a report of 50 cases, *J Thorac Cardiovasc Surg* 97:706, 1989.
45. Nakayama DK, Motoyama EK, Tagge EM: Effect of preoperative stabilization on respiratory system compliance and outcome in newborn infants with congenital diaphragmatic hernia, *J Pediatr* 118:793, 1991.
46. O'Rourke PP and others: Extracorporeal membrane oxygenation and conventional medical therapy in neonates with persistent pulmonary hypertension of the newborn: a prospective randomized study, *Pediatrics* 84:957, 1989.

47. O'Rourke PP and others: The effect of extracorporeal membrane oxygenation on the survival of neonates with high-risk congenital diaphragmatic hernia: 45 cases from a single institution, *J. Pediatr Surg* 26:147, 1991.
48. Pilato MA and others: Treatment of non-cardiogenic pulmonary edema following cardiopulmonary bypass with veno-venous extracorporeal membrane oxygenation, *Anesthesiology* 69:609, 1988.
49. Redmond CR and others: Extracorporeal membrane oxygenation for respiratory and cardiac failure in infants and children, *J Thorac Cardiovasc Surg* 93:199, 1987.
50. Rogers AJ and others: Extracorporeal membrane oxygenation for postcardiotomy cardiogenic shock in children, *Ann Thorac Surg* 47:903, 1989.
51. Sakai H and others: Effect of surgical repair on respiratory mechanics in congenital diaphragmatic hernia, *J Pediatr* 111:432, 1987.
52. Short L and others: A comparison of pulse oximeters during helicopter flight, *J Emerg Med* 7:639, 1989.
53. Snider MT and others: Venovenous perfusion of adults and children with severe acute respiratory distress syndrome: the Pennsylvania State University experience from 1982-1987, *Trans Am Soc Artif Intern Organs* 34:1014, 1988.
54. Steinhorn RH, Green TP: Use of extracorporeal membrane oxyygenation in the treatment of respiratory syncytial virus bronchiolitis: the national experience, 1983 to 1988, *J Pediatr* 116:338, 1990.
55. Stolar CJH, Snedecor SM, Bartlett RH: Extracorporeal membrane oxygenation and neonatal respiratory failure: experience from the Extracorporeal Life Support Organization, *J Pediatr Surg* 26:563, 1991.
56. Trento A, Griffith B, Hardesty RL: Extracorporeal membrane oxygenation experience at the University of Pittsburgh, *Ann Thorac Surg* 42:56, 1986.
57. Trento A and others: Extracorporeal membrane oxygenation in children: new trends, *J Thorac Cardiovasc Surg* 96:542, 1988.
58. Van Meurs KP and others: Effect of extracorporeal membrane oxygenation on survival of infants with congenital diaphragmatic hernia, *J Pediatr* 117:954, 1990.
59. Weber TR and others: Extracorporeal membrane oxygenation for newborn respiratory failure, *Ann Thorac Surg* 42:529, 1986.
60. Weinhaus L and others: Extracorporeal membrane oxygenation for circulatory support after repair of congenital heart defects, *Ann Thorac Surg* 48:206, 1989.
61. Wung JT and others: Management of infants with severe respiratory failure and persistence of the fetal circulation, without hyperventilation, *Pediatrics* 76:488, 1985.
62. Zapol WM and others: Extracorporeal membrane oxygenation in severe acute respiratory failure: a randomized prospective study, *JAMA* 242:2193, 1979.

34

TRANSPORT PROTOCOLS

ARTHUR COOPER
GEORGE L. FOLTIN

Whether engaged in pediatric prehospital transport or assisting with pediatric interhospital transport, the protocols under which emergency medical technicians and paramedics are permitted to function provide written guidelines to be followed in the event of identifiable pediatric emergencies. In essence, their protocols define these providers' scope of practice with respect to infants and young children. In reality, they are a set of "doctor's orders" to emergency medical technicians and paramedics functioning as physician extenders, but are developed by a consensus panel of regional experts in pediatric emergency and critical care medicine and approved by the regional medical control authority. As such, they carry the same weight as direct physician orders to other types of health professionals, such as nurses and respiratory therapists.

At the basic life support (BLS) level, these protocols should stress rapid pediatric assessment, oxygen administration, expeditious transport, keeping the child warm, and other components of BLS (foreign-body-in-airway clearing maneuvers, use of airway adjuncts and ventilation devices, cardiopulmonary resuscitation, and extrication, immobilization, and splinting), as necessary. At the advanced life support (ALS) level, these protocols should additionally permit definitive management of airway and breathing (including endotracheal intubation, nasogastric decompression, laryngoscopic foreign-body-in-airway retrieval, and in some systems, needle decompression of tension pneumothorax), reserving the use of drugs (inhaled β-agonists and injected sympathomimetics, anticonvulsants, and blood-glucose-elevating agents), fluids (dextrose in water and balanced salt solution), and cardioversion and defibrillation as specifically indicated, usually upon the direct order of an on-line medical control physician. Yet, such protocols must reflect sound operational policy as well as current medical therapy with respect both to treatment and to triage, and must be continuously revised to prescribe optimal patient management. To realize these goals, they must artfully blend the realities of pediatric practice with the capabilities of the regional emergency medical system and the peculiarities of its geography to ensure swift, safe transport to definitive care.[2,3,8]

Modifications in this general approach may be required in rural areas where lengthy transport times are anticipated. For example, investing time in optimally stabilizing the patient before transport is more likely to be beneficial in areas where long ambulance trips are the norm than in areas where running times are typically short. Yet, the vast majority of prehospital providers in rural and frontier areas are BLS providers, with ALS providers being concentrated in urban and suburban communities. Protocols designed for use in remote areas may therefore require 1) interface with ALS providers dispatched by helicopter, or 2) specialized training in intermediate levels of ALS care which permit providers with limited education in pediatrics to obtain definitive airway control and establish venous access prior to transport.

To the extent possible, resuscitation and stabilization at the scene or in transport should reflect actual clinical practice in the emergency department or critical care unit. However, it is unwise, in the opinion of the authors, for protocols under which emergency medical technicians and paramedics will provide or support patient care to emphasize life support modalities which do not directly affect maintenance of ventilation, oxygenation, and perfusion. This is not to suggest that other modalities are not important or do not impact upon the provider's ability to maintain airway, breathing, and circulation. Yet, the provider's time is usually better spent in direct visual monitoring of the child and in technical support of airway and breathing, given the limited space and personnel that are generally available to attend to the patient in the back of a moving ambulance.

The protocols that follow represent the New York City Regional Emergency Medical Advisory Committee's[5,6,7] attempt to guide the prehospital emergency care and critical interhospital management received by pediatric patients transported under the aegis of the New York City Emergency Medical Service 911 System. Initially developed and periodically updated by the American Academy of Pediatrics District II Committee on Emergency Medical Services for Children, they were recently merged with protocols developed by the New York City Emergency Medical Service Medical Advisory Committee, predecessor of the newly established New York City Regional Emergency Medical Advisory Committee. The protocols then underwent extensive editorial revision to ensure consistency between adult and pediatric protocols to the extent feasible without substantively compromising optimal patient care, prior to their formal adoption by the Regional Emergency Medical Advisory Committee, the legally constituted medical control authority for New York City. As such, they represent a true regional consensus of physician experts in pediatric and adult prehospital emergency medicine and critical interhospital transport and are utilized by all ambulances that are dispatched through the New York City Emergency Medical Service 911 System.

PEDIATRIC PREHOSPITAL PROTOCOLS

Unlike adults, children do not normally sustain cardiorespiratory arrest as the result of a sudden cardiac event, but rather as the result of progressive respiratory deterioration. Nor is the effect of trauma in the child chiefly hemodynamic, but rather neuroventilatory: only 10% of children with significant mortality risk are hypotensive at the time of admission to the trauma center, although some 50% present with an altered level of consciousness due to head trauma, with concomitant derangements in airway and breathing. Thus, pediatric prehospital emergencies more frequently involve respiratory insufficiency than circulatory failure, regardless of underlying cause. Hence, the benchmark of pediatric prehospital care is neither rapid defibrillation and cardiopulmonary resuscitation (as it is for the adult cardiac patient) nor is it rapid transport and treatment of shock (as it is for the adult trauma patient). Ideally, effective management of airway and breathing followed by rapid transport (keeping the child warm) to an emergency department that is specifically equipped and staffed for pediatric resuscitation (an "emergency department approved for pediatrics" or "EDAP") is best.

Yet, few prehospital pediatric emergencies are critical emergencies requiring advanced life support, and most therefore require either basic life support (chiefly supplemental oxygen), or a less acute mode of care. For this reason, and because the unique presentations of most serious pediatric illnesses relate chiefly to complications that result in respiratory failure and shock, separate pediatric BLS protocols are needed only for a core group of critical pediatric conditions. Ideally, such protocols should stress directed assessments as the means to facilitate timely interventions. Moreover, they are designed not so much to provide definitive treatment as prevent further deterioration en route to the primary receiving hospital.

Regardless, a child should be not denied advanced life support if it is within the capabilities of the regional emergency medical services (EMS) system to provide this level of care. However, although more numerous because of the greater scope of paramedic practice, ALS protocols should ideally reflect an approach to pediatric prehospital emergency medicine that is conservative yet permissive. The ALS protocols should be conservative in that, as with BLS protocols, maintenance of airway, breathing, and circulation and rapid transport to an appropriate facility, keeping the child warm, are stressed as the primary priorities, particularly in short-transport (less than 20 minutes) urban EMS systems. These protocols should also be permissive, however, in that intubation is allowed in the field based on paramedic judgment. In the absence of data to support prolonged on-scene time for other ALS interventions, such treatments are administered either en route or in situations of unavoidable transport delay, except in long-transport (greater than 20 minutes) suburban and rural EMS systems where pretransport stabilization may be desirable. Yet, however the regional EMS system is configured, steps must be taken to ensure that online medical control is provided by bona fide experts in pediatric emergency medicine, trauma surgery, and critical care, and that it is readily available to BLS and ALS personnel alike.

Responsibilities of prehospital professionals

The first responsibility of prehospital professionals is to evaluate the scene with respect to safety. Such evaluation should include environmental conditions, the emotional state of involved patient(s) or family members, contact with hazardous materials, and exposure to infectious pathogens. Conditions that may pose a direct threat to health or safety of providers, patients, and other persons at the scene require the immediate involvement of appropriate public health or safety officers. Prehospital professionals should use caution in circumstances for which they have not been specifically trained.

Once the scene has been judged to be safe, attention is directed immediately to the expanded primary survey. Medical care is then immediately provided as indicated by the patient's condition or complaint, in accordance with the appropriate prehospital care protocol(s) and the provider's capabilities and certification. Emergency medical technicians should request paramedic assistance as soon as possible after it is determined that circumstances require advanced life support decisions or interventions. However, neither treatment nor transport should be delayed pending arrival of advanced life support personnel or equipment, particularly when the estimated travel time of paramedics to the scene exceeds the estimated transport time to the hospital.

Medical authority at the scene

Medical control at the scene should be the responsibility of the highest qualified medical authority on site. The designated medical control physician will be in charge whenever physically present. Paramedics will be in charge whenever both ALS and BLS personnel are present, while emergency medical technicians will be responsible for patient care at the scene of an emergency if paramedics are not present. However, no on-scene provider may be considered relieved of direct patient care responsibilities unless these are expressly assumed by a provider of equal or higher level of training—although paramedics may release patients not requiring ALS care to BLS personnel for transport to the nearest appropriate receiving facility.

If a physician with appropriate qualifications is present at the scene and attempts to direct or assist with patient care, the designated medical control physician should be contacted for approval. If granted, the physician's requests concerning emergency medical care and the movement of the patient should be honored, provided they do not conflict with standard operating procedures. If the designated medical control physician cannot be contacted, field personnel may accept direction from the on-scene physician within the context of their protocols. However, under no circumstances should emergency medical technicians or paramedics exceed the scope of practice defined by their protocols, even upon the direct order of a physician.

Communications with medical control facilities

Protocols are guidelines that itemize and prioritize the steps which should be followed to treat a typical patient under normal circumstances. However, situations may arise which do not fit neatly into the usual pattern. The designated medical control physician should be contacted whenever the emergency medical technician or paramedic is in doubt about how to proceed. The on-line medical control physician will then order the most appropriate treatment for that patient, consistent with the protocols and the on-scene provider's scope of practice.

Because few emergency medical technicians will have ready access to an on-line medical control physician, BLS protocols are usually designed to be used in the absence of physician input and consist solely of standing orders. By their very nature, the decisions made and interventions performed by paramedics are far more complex and frequently require the input of an on-line medical control physician. For this reason, ALS protocols typically begin with standing orders but conclude with one or more medical control options that cannot be implemented without first contacting medical control. However, medical control may be used as resource at any time prior to the implementation or completion of standing orders.

If there is no applicable ALS protocol in spite of a clear need for advanced life support exists, operating procedures should allow the paramedic to initiate airway control (including endotracheal intubation), oxygen administration, cardiac monitoring, and intravenous infusion (to keep the vein open), as necessary and pending contact with medical control. The on-line medical control physician will then define the emergent clinical problem and determine the most suitable therapy. Contact with an on-line medical control physician should ordinarily be made within 20 minutes of the time the paramedic arrives upon the scene. In the event contact with an on-line medical control physician cannot be established, paramedics cannot be authorized to administer optional treatment and should perform only those procedures which fall under standing orders, either before or during transport.

Transportation decisions made by prehospital professionals in consultation with the designated on-line medical control physician may encompass the following areas: manner of extrication, when required, and preparation of the patient for transport; safe conveyence of the patient from the scene to the ambulance on appropriate equipment in an appropriate position; designation of a different provider level to transport the patient; and transportation of the patient to the nearest appropriate hospital in accordance with regional guidelines. Of these, the most important is the last, as hospitals may vary in their capabilities with respect to the care of pediatric patients. Ideally, regional medical control authorities will have decided in advance which hospitals may be designated to receive pediatric patients via ambulance by virtue of having emergency departments approved for pediatrics, known as EDAPs, and will have incorporated ambulance destination within their pediatric protocols. At a minimum, such hospitals should be fully equipped for the simultaneous emergency resuscitation of two pediatric patients, be staffed by physicians and nurses who have successfully completed appropriate training in pediatric advanced life support and the early care of the injured child, and have made prior arrangements with the regional pediatric critical care center (PCCC) for transfer of children whose illnesses and injuries may require this level of care.

Legal issues affecting pediatric prehospital transport (see Chapter 36 on Legal Issues)

The doctrine of implied consent is the basis for medical intervention in situations which pose an immediate threat to life, and this doctrine supersedes other concerns.[4] In situations which do not pose an immediate threat to life, consent for routine treatment is presumed to exist whenever a direct request for medical assistance is made by a responsible caretaker. Only those caretakers with full parental rights may refuse medical assistance for a child once it has been requested. However, in most jurisdictions, the law protects prehospital providers who proceed in good faith to render medical assistance to a child if they perceive a potential threat to life or limb, even when permission is denied by the child's legal guardian.

Prehospital providers are clearly obligated to treat and transport any child whose life or limb(s) may be in jeopardy as a result of suspected child abuse, including physical neglect. If abuse is judged likely, but no life-threatening emergency appears to exist, prehospital providers should request police assistance in consultation with a medical control physician, if available, as in most jurisdictions, police officers are vested with the final decision-making responsibility with respect to public intervention in private matters. In such circumstances, the prehospital provider should also perform a brief visual survey of the immediate surroundings for evidence of abuse in addition to the usual patient assessment. All pertinent findings should be recorded on the prehospital care report. This information should also be verbally transmitted to the physician or nurse on duty at the receiving hospital.

Cardiopulmonary resuscitation is indicated whenever prehospital providers encounter an unresponsive, pulseless, apneic patient, whether child or adult. However, prehospital providers usually are permitted by protocol not to institute resuscitative measures in cases where there is rigor mortis, extreme dependent lividity, tissue decomposition, obvious mortal injury, or a properly executed "do not resuscitate" order that conforms to the laws of the jurisdiction within which death occurs. None of these is typically present in circumstances surrounding the death of a child. By contrast, the most common fatal illnesses encountered by prehospital providers in the field are sudden infant death syndrome (SIDS) and traumatic cardiac arrest following blunt injury.

The outcome associated with these conditions is so dismal that some authorities believe neither time nor effort should be expended in attempting to resuscitate such children. Yet, in the authors' view, attempts at resuscitation of such children are justified despite the near-certainty of failure. Distraught parents will know, at the very least, that everything possible was done to revive their previously healthy child. Similarly, distressed prehospital providers will be reassured that their failure to intervene did not contribute to the child's ultimate demise, thereby minimizing the psychic impact of the critical incident and the subsequent development of posttraumatic stress disorder.

Principles of pediatric prehospital care

Patients under 16 years of age should be treated as pediatric patients, and the appropriate protocols should be used. It is best to avoid agitating pediatric patients, as an assessment or treatment which is not tolerated by the patient may provoke or increase respiratory distress. Obtaining a blood pressure reading, for example, may be counterproductive if it agitates the patient or delays transport. Every attempt should also be made to keep pediatric patients warm during transport.

All children require continuous monitoring of their airways to ensure airway patency. Such monitoring should include the position of the patient's head as well as determination of the need for oropharyngeal suctioning, airway adjuncts, and advanced life support airway management techniques. The correct position for airway maintenance is age-dependent. In pediatric patients with suspected trauma, the airway maneuver of choice is the modified jaw thrust with in-line cervical stabilization.

There are no contraindications to high concentration oxygen in the prehospital environment in any pediatric patients. Pediatric patients who require supplemental oxygen should receive high concentration oxygen via the mask that best fits around the mouth and nose without pressing on the eyes, preferably a partial nonrebreathing mask. Humidified oxygen is preferred, but dry oxygen is better than no oxygen. If a partial nonrebreathing mask is not well tolerated, blow-by oxygen is acceptable.

Pediatric patients exhibiting signs of respiratory failure require assisted ventilation via a mask which completely covers the mouth and nose but not the eyes. This should be done using a pocket mask and supplemental oxygen or pediatric or adult bag-valve-mask and reservoir with flow set at 10-15 lpm. Mouth-to-mouth or mouth-to-mouth and nose ventilation should be used only when airway adjuncts are not available. Use of either the esophageal gastric tube airway or the oxygen powered breathing device is contraindicated in pediatric patients.

Control of the airway and rapid transport are the underlying principles of pediatric prehospital protocols and best serve the needs of the pediatric patient. Intubation should be attempted when other maneuvers used to ventilate the pediatric patient are inadequate, unless croup or epiglottitis is suspected. However, since intravenous or intraosseous access are more difficult in small children, these and other advanced life support interventions are carried out en route or during a transport delay. Intravenous access should precede intraosseous access, and each should be limited to a single attempt, although intraosseous access should not be used in patients over 6 years of age.

The need for definitive treatment in the field or in transport, other than invasive airway management techniques, is infrequent. Length-based resuscitation tapes should be used for calculation of all fluid, drug, and defibrillation doses in pediatric patients. The initial rate of fluid administration should not exceed 20 ml/kg. Currently available length-based resuscitation tapes also provide average weight, heart rate, respiratory rate, and blood pressure for age, as well as proper equipment sizes and fluid, drug, and defibrillation dosages.

The protocols developed for use by emergency medical technicians and paramedics in the New York City region who perform pediatric prehospital transport may be found in Appendix 34-1.

PEDIATRIC INTERHOSPITAL PROTOCOLS

The needs of patients requiring interhospital transport typically are quite different from the needs of those requiring prehospital care. In the latter case the call is initiated in the field by a person requesting emergency medical treatment from an ambulance service or emergency medical service agency, usually on an emergent basis (primary transport). The patient in this instance has not been assessed by a licensed health professional, and the patient's condition may be less stable than suspected on the basis of presenting symptoms. In the former case the call is initiated by a licensed health professional requesting transport to or from a medical care facility, often on a nonemergent basis (secondary transport). The patient in this instance has been assessed by a licensed health professional, and the patient's condition can be more accurately determined on the basis of professional judgment. Thus, it usually is possible to predict the physiologic status of the patient during transport with some certainty and to provide the level of care that most closely matches the perceived need.

Interhospital transports comprise the largest number of secondary transports. Certain types of interhospital transports (such as those involving high-risk neonates, unstable infants with congenital heart disease, or critically ill or injured children), typically demand a far higher level of care than others (such as those involving back transfers of stable patients to their hospitals of origin). For the former, highly sophisticated referral, hospital-based transport teams may be needed. For the latter, ambulance service-based transport crews may be sufficient to meet the needs of patient transfer. It is therefore encumbent upon the emergency medical services system to allocate its scarce resources as efficiently as possible without placing the patient at undue risk during the course of transport.

In most parts of the country, policies, protocols, and procedures for pediatric interhospital transport are based upon informal agreements between physicians in the sending and receiving hospitals and local ambulance services. Ideally, regional medical control authorities will establish formal rules, roles, and responsibilities for health care providers participating in pediatric interhospital transport, in collaboration with regional experts in pediatric emergency medicine, pediatric surgery, pediatric anesthesiology, and pediatric critical care medicine. Yet, the majority of pediatric interhospital transports nationwide are high-risk transports of critically ill or injured children, conducted by physicians and nurses for whom specific patient care protocols may be unnecessary, as treatments normally required by pediatric patients during such transports are within their established scope of practice. This is not so for emergency medical technicians and paramedics called upon to participate in pediatric interhospital transports, for whom it is necessary not only to develop specific patient care protocols that define the expanded scope of practice demanded by such transports, but also to provide the additional training that will allow these transports to be conducted smoothly and safely.

While emergency medical technicians and paramedics are frequently involved in patient care during secondary transport, they do not play the leading role required of them during primary transport. Instead, the patient remains the ultimate medical responsibility of the sending physician and facility, until such time as ultimate medical responsibility is passed to a receiving physician and facility. The transport vehicle should be viewed as a movable platform upon which appropriate functions of the sending or receiving facility may be carried out. Thus, the role of emergency medical technicians and paramedics is to assist with, rather than perform, patient care upon the request of properly credentialed physicians or physician surrogates based in the sending or receiving facility, according to advance directive of the medical control physician to whom they are responsible.

Responsibilities of sending and receiving physicians

It is the responsibility of the sending physician, in consultation with the receiving physician, to determine the level of care required for each interhospital transport. This decision is based upon perceived need, and when appropriate and available, the advice of the medical directors of the referral hospital transport service or the medical director of the ambulance service providing the transport vehicle. In cases of high-risk transports involving the use of a referral hospital-based, physician or nurse-led transport team, the receiving physician will usually assume responsibility for arranging for transport. In cases of medium- and low-risk transports not involving the use of a referral hospital-based, physician or nurse-led transport team, the sending physician will usually assume responsibility for arranging for transport by a paramedic or emergency medical technician-staffed transport crew, but may in certain cases personally accompany the patient during transport. In neither case, however, will the receiving physician have had the personal opportunity to examine the patient prior to dispatch of the transport team or crew. Thus, while the sending physician and receiving physician share responsibility for determining the level of care that may be required during transport, the receiving physician's ability to share in the responsibility for this decision can extend only so far as the sending physician's description of the patient's condition is accurate.

In cases of critical or acute transports where a patient requires transfer from a facility unable to provide definitive care for an (emergency) condition, the receiving physician should also advise the sending physician regarding any critical medical interventions that may be necessary to support the patient prior to the arrival of the transport team or crew, within the limits of good medical judgment. The sending physician should ensure that these recommendations are followed, within the limits of good medical judgment and professional and institutional capability. Again, however, the receiving physician will not have had the opportunity to personally examine the patient to determine if the recommended interventions in fact are warranted. Thus, direct responsibility for the emergency management of the patient cannot be accepted by the receiving physician until personally examined by that physician or a physician surrogate directly responsible to that physician.

Medical authority during transport

Good medical practice dictates that every patient receive the level of care most appropriate to the condition(s) for which that patient is being treated. This requires at any given moment that the immediate treatment of any patient be supervised by a licensed physician who is both knowledgeable about that phase of treatment and immediately available in person, by telephone, or through properly trained and credentialed physician surrogates. Medical authority for the care of an individual patient during transport must therefore rest with the attending physician(s) in the sending or receiving facility who are most knowledgeable about and familiar with the care that a patient has received prior to and during transport. Ultimate responsibility can be shared with other attending physicians who are more knowledgeable about specific treatments a patient may require during transport but cannot be delegated to physicians who possess inadequate knowledge of the definitive care a patient may require during transport or physician surrogates (including physicians-in-training), regardless of their level of expertise.

Emergency medical technicians assisting with the care of patients during transport must therefore be informed not only of the exact nature of the transport and the level of care that will be required, but also should be in possession of an order from the responsible sending physician or properly credentialed designee which authorizes transport. This order should state which physician or physician surrogate will be responsible for each element of the care the patient may require while en route. This order should also indicate what procedures emergency medical technicians assisting with the care of patients during transport will be allowed to perform or assist with en route, under what circumstances, and at whose specific request. Emergency medical technicians will be allowed only to assist in performing procedures that are either within their defined scope of practice or in which they have received special additional training and are specifically permitted by advance direction of their medical control physician or properly credentialed designee.

Note that emergency medical technicians must at all times remain under the direct and indirect medical control of their medical control physician or properly credentialed designee, even when requested by physician(s) attending the transport to perform or assist with procedures during the course of a secondary transport. The patient, however, will at all times remain under the medical authority of the sending or receiving physician.

Transfer of medical authority

It is the responsibility of health care professionals in the sending facility to assist transport providers in initiating transport and assuming medical responsibility for the safe, smooth, and expeditious patient transport. This should include assistance in stabilizing and securing the airway for transport, assistance in determining mechanical ventilator settings and vasoactive infusion rates that will be required during transport, assistance in preparing for continuation of whatever other pharmacologic agents or therapeutic interventions that may be required en route, assistance in providing and preparing medications that may be required en route, assembling copies of all necessary patient records (including a copy of the hospital chart and copies of all pertinent x-ray films), preparing a written transfer note, arranging for informed consent for transport, and meeting other reasonable requests of the transport team or crew. In addition, the sending physician should sign an order authorizing transfer from the sending facility to the receiving facility. The sending physician should also sign an order authorizing transport of the patient by the transport team or crew which describes the nature of the transport, the level of care required, and the responsibilities of nonphysician transport providers.

In cases of high-risk transports, the very act of requesting transport constitutes a declaration by the sending facility that the patient requires a higher level of care than it is capable of providing. In such circumstances, there exists a duty on the part of the receiving facility to assume responsibility for the patient as soon after the arrival of its transport team as is feasible, within the limits of the capabilities of the transport team. Upon the request of the physician leader of the transport team, providers responsible to the sending physician should also assist the transport team in preparing for transport in ways described in the preceding paragraph. However, the patient must be considered to be under the medical authority of the receiving facility once primary responsibility for management of the airway is assumed by its agents.

In cases of medium-risk and low-risk transports that are accompanied by the attending or other credentialed physician from the referring hospital, ongoing medical treatment should be the immediate responsibility of the attending physician(s) or properly trained, credentialed, and supervised physician surrogate(s) from the sending facility, assisted by the transport crew (within the limits of their scope of practice and special additional training). In cases of medium-risk and low-risk transports not accompanied by the attending or other properly credentialed physician(s), the sending physician should also sign an order authorizing ongoing medical treatment by the transport crew (within the limits of their scope of practice and special additional training), including ongoing administration of whatever medications and treatments begun in the sending facility that are expected to be continued en route. Transfer of medical authority for conduct of the transport itself, from the sending physician to the physician responsible for supervising the providers caring for the patient during transport, formally occurs once all parties agree that the patient is ready for transport. Primary responsibility for management of the airway is then passed from providers responsible to the sending physician to providers responsible to the physician who is supervising transport personnel. However, transfer of medical authority for the overall care of the patient from the sending physician to the receiving physician does not formally occur until the patient arrives at the receiving facility and is accepted by the receiving physician.

Transport begins the moment transfer of primary responsibility for management of the airway is actually effected. This does not ordinarily take place until the patient has been optimally prepared for transport, within the limits of the sending facility's ability to assist the transport team or crew in doing so. Transport ends the moment primary responsibility for management of the airway is accepted by health professionals assigned to the patient care unit within the receiving facility that has accepted the transfer. This should be accomplished as soon after the arrival of the patient at the designated patient care unit as is feasible, within the limits of the receiving facility's ability to relieve the transport team or crew of immediate responsibility for management of vital life support(s).

Legal issues affecting pediatric interhospital transport

Section 9121(b) of the Consolidated Omnibus Budget Reconciliation Act (COBRA) of 1985, otherwise known as the Emergency Medical Treatment and Active Labor Act (PL 99-272), and all subsequent amendments,[1] have the strongest impact on medical providers when it comes to interhospital transfer. They mandate that all institutional participants in the Medicare program rendering treatment to any patient in an emergency room for any emergency medical condition or to a woman in active labor, first stabilize the patient prior to transfer. Exceptions are only permitted by written certification of the treating physician, or a "medical person" acting as the agent for that physician, that the medical benefits of immediate transfer reasonably outweigh the risks of ongoing medical treatment in the sending facility. The provisions of the law pertain specifically only to patients in the categories stated above and apply irrespective of those patients' ability to pay. However, these provisions should be applied to all patients in designated, licensed, health care facilities who may require interfacility transfer. Further, such transfer is allowed only if:

- the transferring hospital provides the medical treatment within its capacity that minimizes the risks to the individual's health, and, in the case of a woman in labor, the unborn child;
- the receiving facility has available space and qualified personnel for the treatment of the patient;
- the receiving facility has agreed to accept the patient and provide appropriate treatment;
- the transferring hospital sends to the receiving facility all medical records (or copies thereof), related to the individual's emergency condition, available at the time of transfer, . . . ;
- the transfer is effected through qualified personnel and transportation equipment, including the use of necessary and medically appropriate life-support measures during the transfer; and
- the transfer meets other requirements that the Secretary of Health and Human Services may find necessary.

Sections 1866 and 1867 of the Social Security Act, enacted in 1986, extend the transfer requirements initially mandated under the "anti-dumping" provisions of COBRA. They mandate that both informed consent for transfer by the patient or health care proxy and a written order for transfer by the treating physician (or a "medical person" acting as the agent of that physician) be obtained prior to transfer. They further mandate immediate transfer to a facility "appropriate" for the patient's needs if the patient has not been stabilized, either because the patient requests it or the patient cannot be medically stabilized, provided the sending facility has first done all within its capacity to minimize the risk to the patient during transfer, and the sending physician makes written documentation of the above. Hospitals that have specialized capabilities or facilities (such as trauma centers, burn centers, neonatal intensive care units) may not refuse to accept appropriate transfer if they have the capacity to treat the individual(s) requiring transfer.

Principles of pediatric interhospital transport

Most children needing interhospital transport are critically ill or injured children requiring specialized treatment in a pediatric intensive care unit, trauma center, or burn center located in a tertiary referral hospital some miles distant from the primary receiving hospital. In an ideal world the majority of such patients would undergo primary transport to the tertiary referral hospital, based upon pediatric field triage criteria established by the regional medical control authority, obviating the need for secondary transport whenever logistically possible. However, few emergency medical services (EMS) systems nationwide possess this level of organization, except in metropolitan areas served by children's hospitals that are universally recognized as the pediatric referral centers for the regions in which they are located. Secondary transport, therefore, should be viewed as a necessary component of any regionalized system of pediatric care, and formal agreements structured to ensure its proper execution.

The key issue in pediatric interhospital transport is avoidance of physiologic deterioration through maintenance of the critical environment. To achieve this goal, the patient must be optimally stabilized by physicians and nurses in the transferring hospital prior to transport, and the ambulance must be equipped and staffed to perform whatever life-sustaining interventions may be required en route. The vehicle must therefore be outfitted as if it were a fully monitored patient bed in a pediatric intensive care unit, and the patient attended during transport by providers capable of supporting the patient's airway, breathing, and circulation in an optimal manner, within the limits imposed by the available space. Whenever possible therefore physicians and nurses familiar with the critical care of the pediatric patient should conduct these transports in accordance with accepted standards of critical medical and nursing practice, assisted as necessary by providers such as emergency medical technicians or paramedics who have received additional training in the principles and practices of pediatric interhospital transport which are within their scope of practice.

Transporting emergency medical technicians and paramedics should render patient care, or assist physician and nurse members of pediatric interhospital transport teams in rendering patient care only upon request, only by advance directive of their medical control physician, and only if they have been trained and credentialed to perform all required task(s) in accordance with standards established by the medical director of the ambulance service providing the transport vehicle and the medical director of the pediatric interhospital transport service. The medical director of the ambulance service providing the transport vehicle should be maintaining records documenting compliance with the above, and should furnish medical directors of pediatric interhospital transport services they assist with evidence of the above.

Transporting emergency medical technicians and paramedics should render care involving the use of specialized equipment only if they have been specifically trained in the use of the make and model of specialized equipment to be utilized during transport. Such training should be conducted only by individuals authorized to operate such equipment, such as critical care physicians, critical care nurses, or life support technologists (respiratory therapists or cardiopulmonary perfusionists). Following initial didactic and laboratory training, clinical training of sufficient length to assure clinical competency must be provided by an appropriate preceptor. Continuing education in the operation of all such equipment must also be provided to assure clinical competency is fully maintained.

The protocols developed for use by emergency medical technicians and paramedics in the New York City region who assist with pediatric interhospital transport are shown in Appendix 34-2.

REFERENCES

1. Consolidated Omnibus Budget Reconciliation Act of 1985, S.9121(b) (Emergency Medical Treatment and Active Labor Act), P.L. 99-272, 100 Stat. 165, 42 U.S.C. 1395dd(c) (2), as amended by the Omnibus Budget Reconciliation Act of 1989, S.6211(c) (5) and (d), P.L. 101-239, 103 Stat. 2246 and 2247.
2. Dieckmann RA: Prehospital policies and procedures. In Dieckmann RA: *Pediatric emergency care systems: planning and management,* Baltimore, 1992, Williams and Wilkins.
3. Hoffman SH, Dieckmann RA: Prehospital illness treatment. In Dieckmann RA: *Pediatric emergency care systems: planning and management,* Baltimore, 1992, Williams and Wilkins.
4. Lazar RA: *EMS law: a guide for EMS professionals,* Rockville, 1989, Aspen Publications.
5. New York City Regional Emergency Medical Advisory Committee: *New York City Regional Emergency Medical Advisory Committee pre-hospital basic life support treatment protocols,* New York, 1995, Regional E.M.S. Council of New York City, Inc.
6. New York City Regional Emergency Medical Advisory Committee: *New York City Regional Emergency Medical Advisory Committee pre-hospital advanced life support treatment protocols,* New York, 1995, Regional E.M.S. Council of New York City, Inc.
7. New York City Regional Emergency Medical Advisory Committee: *New York City Regional Emergency Medical Advisory Committee combined basic and advanced life support interfacility treatment protocols,* New York, 1994, Regional E.M.S. Council of New York City, Inc.
8. Tunik M, Foltin G: Prehospital protocols. In Luten R, Foltin G: *Pediatric resources for prehospital care,* ed 3, Arlington, National Center for Education in Maternal and Child Health, 1993.

APPENDIX 34-1

TABLE 34-A1 NYC REMAC GENERAL PREHOSPITAL TREATMENT PROTOCOL 400 (©Copyright Regional E.M.S. Council of N.Y.C., Inc., 1995)

Standard approach to the patient

Perform Initial Scene Survey.
Note: Refrain from making direct contact with patients exposed to hazardous materials until they have been decontaminated.

Initiate Basic Cardiac Life Support if indicated.

Perform Expanded Primary Survey.

Administer oxygen if indicated.

Determine if Advanced Life Support is required.

Obtain at least two sets of vital signs and monitor as necessary.
Note: Obtaining vital signs should *not* interfere with treatment or delay transport of the critically ill or injured patient.

Obtain a complete medical history.

Complete the physical examination as the patient's condition dictates.

Treat the patient according to the appropriate protocol(s).

Provide continuous psychological first aid.

Maintain body temperature.

Transport the patient as soon as possible to the nearest appropriate hospital. Patients may be removed to the ambulance by stair chair, scoop stretcher, long board, ambulance cot, or other appropriate means.
Note: The method of transportation should *not* aggravate the patient's condition or injuries.
Note: For trauma patients, transport is a priority!

Monitor and continue patient care en route to the hospital.

Document all findings and information, as they pertain to patient condition or care, on the Prehospital Care Report.

TABLE 34-A2 NYC REMAC PEDIATRIC PREHOSPITAL BLS PROTOCOL 442 (©Copyright Regional E.M.S. Council of N.Y.C., Inc., 1995)

Care of the newborn

Monitor the newborn's airway.

Administer oxygen if the newborn is cyanotic.
Note: If the newborn has persistent central cyanosis (longer than 15 to 30 seconds); hypoventilation (respiratory rate less than 30 breaths per minute); or bradycardia (heart rate less than 100 beats per minute), see newborn resuscitation protocol.

Assess for shock and treat if indicated. (See pediatric shock protocol.)

Monitor the umbilical cord for bleeding.

Dry and wrap the newborn in a silver swaddler, clean sheet, and/or a blanket.

Keep the head covered, with only the face exposed.

Provide a warm, draft-free environment.
Note: Newborns are susceptible to hypothermia. Maintain body temperature at all times.

Determine the Apgar Score at 1 and 5 minutes.
Note: Do *not* delay transport or the immediate care of respiratory or cardiovascular distress in order to obtain an Apgar Score.

Transport, keeping the newborn warm.

TABLE 34-A3 NYC REMAC PEDIATRIC PREHOSPITAL BLS PROTOCOL 443

(©Copyright Regional E.M.S. Council of N.Y.C., Inc., 1995)

Newborn resuscitation

A newborn requires resuscitation if there is:
- Persistent central cyanosis (longer than 15 to 30 seconds);
- Hypoventilation (respiratory rate less than 30 breaths per minute);
- Bradycardia (heart rate less than 100 beats per minuts), or
- Breathlessness and pulselessness.

Initiate Neonatal Resuscitation procedures (See guidelines below.)

Request Advanced Life Support Assistance.

Transport, keeping the newborn warm.

Guidelines for Newborn Resuscitation

Note: Newborns are characterized as under thirty (30) days of age. For infants thirty (30) days to one (1) year of age, see pediatric nontraumatic cardiac arrest protocol.

If the newborn has persistent central cyanosis *and/or* hypoventilation:
- Assist ventilations at a rate of 40 to 60 breaths per minute.
- Switch to high concentration mask or "blow by" oxygen once the respiratory rate is greater than 30 breaths per minute and central cyanosis disappears.

If the newborn has bradycardia:

Heart Rate Greater than 80 but Less than 100
- Assist ventilations at a rate of 40 to 60 breaths per minute.
- Switch to high concentration mask or "blow by" oxygen once the heart rate is greater than 120 beats per minute, the respiratory rate is greater than 30 breaths per minute, and central cyanosis disappears.

Heart Rate Greater than 60 but Less than 80
- Assist ventilations at a rate of 40 to 60 breaths per minute.
- Begin chest compressions with interposed breaths in a ratio of 3 : 1 at a combined rate of 120 per minute if the heart rate does not increase to 80 beats per minute after one minute.
- Stop chest compressions once the heart rate increases to 100 beats per minute, and assist ventilations at a rate of 40 to 60 breaths per minute.
- Switch to high concentration mask or "blow by" oxygen once the heart rate is greater than 120 beats per minute, the respiratory rate is greater than 30 breaths per minute, and central cyanosis disappears.

Heart Rate 60 or Less
- Assist ventilations at a rate of 40 to 60 breaths per minute.
- Begin chest compressions with interposed breaths in a ratio of 3 : 1 at a combined rate of 120 per minute if the heart rate does not increase to 80 beats per minute after one minute.
- Stop chest compressions once the heart rate increases to 100 beats per minute, and assist ventilations at a rate of 40 to 60 breaths per minute.
- Switch to high concentration mask or "blow by" oxygen once the heart rate is greater than 120 beats per minute, the respiratory rate is greater than 30 breaths per minute, and central cyanosis disappears.

Heart Rate 60 or Less
- Assist ventilations at a rate of 40 to 60 breaths per minute.
- Begin chest compressions with interposed breaths in a ratio of 3 : 1 at a combined rate of 120 per minute if the heart rate does not increase to 80 beats per minute after 15 seconds.
- Stop chest compressions once the heart rate increases to 100 beats per minute, and assist ventilations at a rate of 40 to 60 breaths per minute.
- Switch to high concentration mask or "blow by" oxygen once the heart rate is greater than 120 beats per minute, the respiratory rate is greater than 30 breaths per minute, and central cyanosis disappears.

If the newborn is breathless and pulseless:
- Initiate CPR with chest compressions and interposed breaths in a ratio of 3 : 1 at a combined rate of 120 per minute.
- Continue CPR until spontaneous circulation has been restored or resuscitative efforts have been transferred to persons of equal or higher level of training.

TABLE 34-A4 NYC REMAC PEDIATRIC PREHOSPITAL BLS PROTOCOL 450

(©Copyright Regional E.M.S. Council of N.Y.C., Inc., 1995)

Pediatric respiratory distress/failure

Note: Respiratory *distress* in a child is characterized by *increased* respiratory effort, i.e., anxiety, tachypnea, nasal flaring, and intercostal retractions, *without* central cyanosis.

Note: Respiratory *failure* in a child is characterized by *ineffective* respiratory effort, i.e., agitation or lethargy, severe dyspnea or labored breathing, bobbing or grunting, and marked intercostal and parasternal retractions, *with* central cyanosis.

Continued.

TABLE 34-A4 NYC REMAC PEDIATRIC PREHOSPITAL BLS PROTOCOL 450—cont'd

Pediatric respiratory distress/failure
Note: Bradycardia is an ominous sign that indicates hypoxic cardiac arrest is imminent.
Monitor the airway.
If an obstructed airway is suspected, see Pediatric Obstructed Airway Protocol.
If croup or epiglottitis is suspected, see Pediatric Croup/Epiglottitis Protocol.
If respiratory distress is present: Administer oxygen and allow patient to maintain a comfortable, upright position. **Note:** There are *no contraindications* to high concentration oxygen in the prehospital setting, even in pediatric patients. Do *not* allow the mask to press against the eyes.
If respiratory failure is present: *Age Less than 2 Years* Assist ventilations at a rate of 20 to 30 breaths per minute. *Age 2 Years or Greater* Assist ventilations at a rate of 15 to 20 breaths per minute. **Note:** Do *not* use a demand valve resuscitator. **Note:** Chest rise is the best indication of adequate ventilation in the prehospital setting.
Request Advanced Life Support assistance.
Transport, keeping the child warm.

TABLE 34-A5 NYC REMAC PEDIATRIC PREHOSPITAL BLS PROTOCOL 451

Pediatric obstructed airway
If the patient is conscious and *can* breathe, cough, speak, or cry: Administer oxygen. **Note:** Avoid agitating the patient.
If the patient is unconscious or *cannot* breathe, cough, speak, or cry: Perform obstructed airway clearing maneuvers appropriate for age. **Note:** If an enlarged epiglottis is seen when attempting to clear the airway, see Pediatric Croup/Epiglottitis Protocol.
Request Advanced Life Support assistance.
Transport, keeping the child warm.
Continue obstructed airway clearing maneuvers en route to the hospital until the foreign body is dislodged. **Note:** The patient must be taken to the hospital for evaluation even if the airway obstruction is cleared.
If the airway obstruction is cleared: Monitor the airway. Initiate CPR if indicated. (See Pediatric Nontraumatic Cardiac Arrest Protocol.) Administer oxygen. Continue transport, keeping the child warm.

TABLE 34-A6 NYC REMAC PEDIATRIC PREHOSPITAL BLS PROTOCOL 452

Pediatric croup/epiglottitis

Note: *Croup* should be suspected in a child with stridor, retractions, barking cough, normal or slightly elevated temperature, and a history of upper airway infection.

Note: *Epiglottitis* should be suspected in a child with stridor, retractions, muffled voice, high fever, and drooling.

If the child is conscious:
Administer oxygen.
Request Advanced Life Support assistance.
Transport in a sitting position, keeping the child warm. When feasible, allow a parent to accompany the child in the patient compartment.
Note: Avoid agitating the patient. Do *not* examine oropharynx. Allow saliva to drain from the mouth. Do *not* place patient in a supine position.

If the child is unconscious:
Assist ventilations.
Note: High pressure bag-valve-mask, mouth-to-mask, or mouth-to-mouth ventilation may be required.
Request Advanced Life Support assistance.
Transport, keeping the child warm.

TABLE 34-A7 NYC REMAC PEDIATRIC PREHOSPITAL BLS PROTOCOL 453

Pediatric nontraumatic cardiac arrest

Initiate Basic Cardiac Life Support procedures. (For infants, see guidelines below.)

Request Advanced Life Support Assistance.

Transport, keeping the child warm.
Note: Use of the semi-automatic defibrillator is *not* indicated for patients less than ten (10) years of age.

Guidelines for Infant Cardiopulmonary Resuscitation
Note: Infants are categorized as thirty (30) days to one (1) year of age. For newborns less than thirty (30) days of age, see newborn resuscitation protocol.

If the infant has severe bradycardia:
Assist ventilations at a rate of 20 to 30 breaths per minute.
Begin chest compressions with interposed breaths in a ratio of 5 : 1 at a combined rate of 120 per minute if the heart rate does not increase to 80 beats per minute after 15 seconds.
Stop chest compressions once the heart rate increases to 100 beats per minute, and assist ventilations at a rate of 20 to 30 breaths per minute.
Switch to high concentration mask or "blow by" oxygen once the heart rate is greater than 120 beats per minute, the respiratory rate is greater than 30 breaths per minute, and central cyanosis disappears.

If the infant is breathless and pulseless:
Initiate CPR with chest compressions and interposed breaths in a ratio of 5 : 1 at a combined rate of 120 per minute.
Continue CPR until spontaneous circulation has been restored or resuscitative efforts have been transferred to persons of equal or higher level of training.

TABLE 34-A8 NYC REMAC PEDIATRIC PREHOSPITAL BLS PROTOCOL 458

Pediatric shock

Note: Shock in the child is characterized by signs of inadequate peripheral perfusion, which may include altered mental status; tachycardia; pallor; cool, cyanotic lower extremities; delayed capillary refill; weak or absent peripheral pulses.

Note: The definition of shock in the child does *not* depend upon blood pressure.

Monitor the airway.

Assess the need for spinal immobilization.

Administer oxygen.
Note: There are *no contraindications* to high concentration oxygen in the prehospital setting, even in pediatric patients.

If the patient has an altered mental status, ventilate at a rate of 25 breaths per minute by a Bag-Valve-Mask, if tolerated.

Control external bleeding.

Request Advanced Life Support assistance.

Transport, keeping the child warm.

Apply MAST and inflate if appropriate.
Do *not* delay transport.
Note: Inflation of the abdominal compartment is contraindicated in patients less than ten (10) years of age.

Elevate the legs.

Treat all injuries as appropriate.

TABLE 34-A9 NYC REMAC PEDIATRIC PREHOSPITAL ALS PROTOCOL 550

Pediatric respiratory arrest

For pediatric patients in actual or impending respiratory arrest or who are unconscious and cannot be ventilated:
1. Begin Basic Life Support Pediatric Respiratory Distress/Failure procedures.
   Note: Do *not* overextend neck. If an obstructed airway is suspected, see Pediatric Obstructed Airway Protocol.
2. Begin assisted ventilation.
3. Perform endotracheal intubation.

During transport, or if transport is delayed:
4. Administer Naloxone 2.0 mg, IM, or via the endotracheal tube, in patients two (2) years of age or older. Use half the amount (1.0 mg) of this drug in patients less than two (2) years of age.
5. If abdominal distension occurs, pass a Nasogastric Tube. Pass an orogastric tube in patients less than two (2) years of age.
6. Contact Medical Control for implementation of one or more of the following options:

Medical control options:
Option A: Begin an IV (IO) infusion of Ringer's Lactate (RL), to keep vein open. Attempt IV or IO only once each.
Option B: Administer Naloxone 2.0 mg, IV (IO) bolus, or via the Endotracheal Tube, in patients two (2) years of age or older. Use half the amount (1.0 mg) of this drug in patients less than two (2) years of age.
Option C: Transportation decision.

TABLE 34-A10 NYC REMAC PEDIATRIC PREHOSPITAL ALS PROTOCOL 551

Pediatric obstructed airway

For pediatric patients who are unconscious or *cannot* breathe, cough, speak, or cry:
1. Begin Basic Life Support Pediatric Obstructed Airway procedures.
2. Perform Direct Larygoscopy. Attempt to remove the foreign body with appropriate sized Magill Forceps.
   Note: If an enlarged epiglottis is visualized, see Pediatric Croup/Epiglottitis Protocol.
3. Perform Endotracheal Intubation.
4. Transportation decision.

TABLE 34-A11 NYC REMAC PEDIATRIC PREHOSPITAL ALS PROTOCOL 552

Pediatric croup/epiglottitis

1. Begin Basic Life Support Pediatric Croup/Epiglottitis procedures.
   Note: Do *not* attempt endotracheal intubation. Use high pressure bag-valve-mask, mouth-to-mask, or mouth-to-mouth ventilation.

During transport, or if transport is delayed:

2. If abdominal distension occurs, pass a Nasogastric Tube. Pass an orogastric tube in patients less than two (2) years of age.
   Note: Do *not* attempt to pass a nasogastric or orogastric tube in a conscious patient.
3. Transportation decision.

TABLE 34-A12 NYC REMAC PEDIATRIC PREHOSPITAL ALS PROTOCOL 553

Pediatric nontraumatic cardiac arrest

1. Begin Basic Life Support Pediatric Non-traumatic Cardiac Arrest procedures.
2. Perform Endotracheal Intubation.

During transport, or if transport is delayed:

3. Administer Epinephrine 0.1 mg/kg (0.1 ml/kg of a 1 : 1,000 solution), via the Endotracheal Tube. (See Broselow Tape.)
4. If abdominal distension occurs, pass a Nasogastric Tube. Pass an orogastric tube in patients less than two (2) years of age.
5. Begin Cardiac Monitoring, record and evaluate ECG strip.
   a. If in ventricular fibrillation, immediately defibrillate at 2 joules/kg, using paddles of appropriate size. (See Broselow Tape.) If the defibrillator is unable to deliver calculated dose, use the table below:

Age	*Energy*
0-3 years	20 joules
4-9 years	50 joules

   b. If still in ventricular fibrillation, immediately repeat defibrillation at 2 joules/kg, using paddles of appropriate size. (See Broselow Tape.) If the defibrillator is unable to deliver calculated dose, use the table below:

Age	*Energy*
0-3 years	20 joules
4-7 years	50 joules
8-9 years	100 joules

   Note: If the defibrillator is unable to deliver as low a dose as recommended, use the lowest available setting.

6. Begin an IV (IO) infusion of Ringer's Lactate (RL), to keep vein open. Attempt IV or IO only once each.

Continued.

TABLE 34-A12 NYC REMAC PEDIATRIC PREHOSPITAL ALS PROTOCOL 553—cont'd

Pediatric nontraumatic cardiac arrest

7. Administer Epinephrine 0.01 mg/kg (0.1 ml/kg of a 1 : 10,000 solution), IV (IO). Repeat as necessary, increasing the dose to 0.1 mg/kg (0.1 ml/kg of a 1 : 1,000 solution. (See Broselow Tape.)
8. Contact Medical Control for implementation of one or more of the following options:

Medical control options:

Option A:	Repeat any of the above standing orders.
Option B:	Administer Lidocaine 0.1 mg/kg, IV(10) bolus, or via the Endotracheal Tube. (See Broselow Tape.)
Option C:	Administer Atropine Sulfate 0.02 mg/kg, IV (IO) bolus, or via the Endotracheal Tube. Minimum dose is 0.10 mg, maximum dose is 1.0 mg. (See Broselow Tape.)
Option D:	Administer Naloxone 2.0 mg IV (IO) bolus, via the Endotracheal Tube, or IM in patients two (2) years of age or older. Use half the amount (1.0 mg) of this drug in patients less than two (2) years of age.
Option E:	Administer 50% Dextrose 0.5 gm/kg, IV (IO) bolus, in patients two (2) years of age or older. Use 25% Dextrose in patients less than two (2) years of age. Maximum dose is 25 gm. (See Broselow Tape.)
Option F:	Administer Sodium Bicarbonate 1.0 mEg/kg, IV (IO) bolus. (See Broselow Tape.)
Option G:	Begin rapid IV (IO) infusion of Ringer's Lactate (RL), 20 ml/kg. (See Broselow Tape.)
Option H:	Transportation decision.

TABLE 34-A13 NYC REMAC PEDIATRIC PREHOSPITAL ALS PROTOCOL 554

Pediatric asthma

For pediatric patients with acute asthma and/or active wheezing:

1. Begin Basic Life Support Pediatric Respiratory Distress/Failure procedures.
2. Administer Metaproteronol 5% (0.3 ml in 2.5-5.0 ml of 0.9% Saline Solution) OR Albuterol Sulfate (one unit dose bottle of 3.0 ml), by nebulizer, at a flow rate that will deliver the solution over 5 to 15 minutes, in patients six (6) years of age or older. Use half the amount of either drug in patients less than six (6) years of age.
3. In patients one (1) year of age or older with severe respiratory distress, respiratory failure, and/or decreased breath sounds, administer Epinephrine 0.01 ml/kg (0.01 ml/kg of a 1 : 1,000 solution), subcutaneously. Maximum dose is 0.3 mg (0.3 ml of a 1 : 1,000 solution).

   Note: Severe respiratory distress in a child is characterized by markedly increased respiratory effort, i.e., severe agitation, dyspnea, tripod position, and intercostal and parasternal retractions.

   A silent chest is an ominous sign that indicates respiratory failure is advanced and respiratory arrest is imminent.

During transport, or if transport is delayed:

4. If the patient develops or remains in severe respiratory distress or respiratory failure, contact Medical Control for implementation of one or more of the following options:

Medical control options:

Option A:	Repeat Epinephrine 0.01 ml/kg (0.01 ml/kg of a 1 : 1,000 solution), subcutaneously, 20 minutes after the first dose. Maximum dose is 0.3 mg (0.3 ml of a 1 : 1,000 solution).
Option B:	Repeat Metaproteronol 5% (0.3 ml in 2.5-5.0 ml of 0.9% Saline Solution) OR Albuterol Sulfate (one unit dose bottle of 3.0 ml), by nebulizer, at a flow rate that will deliver the solution over 5 to 15 minutes, in patients six (6) years of age or older. Use half the amount of either drug in patients less than six (6) years of age.
Option C:	Begin an IV infusion of Ringer's Lactate (RL), to keep vein open. Attempt IV only once.
Option D:	Transportation decision.

TABLE 34-A14 NYC REMAC PEDIATRIC PREHOSPITAL ALS PROTOCOL 555

Pediatric anaphylactic reaction

1. Begin Basic Life Support Anaphylactic Reaction procedures.
2. If the patient develops signs of respiratory failure, airway obstruction, or decompensated shock, perform Endotracheal Intubation, and administer Epinephrine 0.1 mg/kg (0.1 ml/kg of a 1 : 1,000 solution), via the Endotracheal Tube. (See Broselow Tape.)
3. If Endotracheal Intubation cannot be accomplished, administer Epinephrine 0.01 mg/kg (0.01 ml/kg of a 1 : 1,000 solution), subcutaneously. Maximum dose is 0.3 mg (0.3 ml of a 1 : 1,000 solution).

During transport, or if transport is delayed:

4. If abdominal distension occurs, pass a Nasogastric Tube. Pass an orogastric tube in patients less than two (2) years of age.
5. Contact Medical Control for implementation of one or more of the following options:

Medical control options:

Option A: Repeat any of the above Standing Orders.

Option B: Begin an IV (IO) infusion of Ringer's Lactate (RL) via a large bore IV (18-22 gauge) or IO catheter to keep vein open. Attempt IV or IO only once each.

Option C: If the patient has signs of shock, begin rapid IV (IO) infusion of Ringer's Lactate 20 ml/kg. Repeat as necessary. (See Broselow Tape.)

Option D: Administer Epinephrine 0.5 mcg/kg (0.1 ml/kg of a 1 : 100,000 solution), IV (IO) bolus, cautiously. Repeat as necessary, using the same dose.

Option E: Transportation decision.

TABLE 34-A15 NYC REMAC PEDIATRIC PREHOSPITAL ALS PROTOCOL 556

Pediatric altered mental status

Note: Maintenance of normal respiratory and circulatory function is always the first priority. Patients with altered mental status due to respiratory failure or arrest, shock, trauma, near drowning or other anoxic injury should be treated under other protocols.

For pediatric patients in coma, with evolving neurological deficit, or with altered mental status of unknown etiology:

1. Begin Basic Life Support Altered Mental Status procedures.

During transport, or if transport is delayed:

2. Administer Glucagon 1.0 mg, IM.
3. Begin an IV (IO) infusion of Ringer's Lactate (RL), to keep vein open. Attempt IV or IO only once each.
4. Administer 50% Dextrose 0.5 gm/kg IV (IO) bolus, in patients two (2) years of age or older. Use 25% Dextrose in patients less than two (2) years of age. Maximum dose is 25 gm. (See Broselow Tape.)
5. If there is no change in mental status, administer Naloxone 2.0 mg, IV (IO) bolus, in patients two (2) years of age or older. Use half the amount (1.0 mg) of this drug in patients less than two (2) years of age.
6. If there is still no change in mental status, repeat Naloxone 2.0 mg, IV (IO) bolus, in patients two (2) years of age or older. Use half the amount (1.0 mg) of this drug in patients less than two (2) years of age.
7. If IV (IO) access has not been established, administer Naloxone 2.0 mg, IM, in patients two (2) years of age or older. Use half the amount (1.0 mg) of this drug in patients less than two (2) years of age.
8. If the patient continues to have an altered mental status, contact Medical Control for implementation of one or more of the following options:

Medical control options:

Option A: Repeat any of the above standing orders.

Option B: Transportation decision.

TABLE 34-A16 NYC REMAC PEDIATRIC PREHOSPITAL ALS PROTOCOL 557

Pediatric status epilepticus

For pediatric patients in Status Epilepticus (seizure remains ongoing at the time of arrival of EMS):

1. Begin Basic Life Support Seizures procedures.

During transport, or if transport is delayed:

2. Administer Diazepam 0.5 mg/kg, via rectum. (See Broselow Tape.)

Continued.

TABLE 34-A16 NYC REMAC PEDIATRIC PREHOSPITAL ALS PROTOCOL 557—cont'd

Pediatric status epilepticus

3. Administer Glucagon 1.0 mg, IM.
4. Begin an IV (IO) infusion of Ringer's Lactate (RL), to keep vein open. Attempt IV or IO only once each.
5. Administer 25% Dextrose 0.5 gm/kg, IV (IO) bolus. (See Broselow Tape.)
6. If seizure persists, contact Medical Control for implementation of one or more of the following options:

Medical control options:

Option A: Repeat 25% Dextrose 0.5 gm/kg, IV (IO) bolus. (See Broselow Tape.)

Option B: Administer Diazepam 0.2 mg/kg, IV (IO) bolus. Rate of administration may not exceed 1.0 mg/min.
Note: Do *not* attempt to start IV (IO) administration of diazepam if the seizures have stopped.

Option C: Transportation decision.

TABLE 34-A17 NYC REMAC PEDIATRIC PREHOSPITAL ALS PROTOCOL 558

Pediatric/hypovolemic shock

For pediatric patients in decompensated/hypovolemic shock:
Note: Patients in compensated hypovolemic shock should *not* be treated under this protocol.

1. Begin Basic Life Support Pediatric Shock procedures.

During transport, or if transport is delayed:

2. Begin rapid IV (IO) infusion of Ringer's Lactate (RL) 20 ml/kg via a large bore IV (18-22 gauge) or IO catheter. Attempt IV or IO only once each. (See Broselow Tape.)
3. Repeat Ringer's Lactate (RL) 20 ml/kg rapid IV (IO) infusion if the patient remains in decompensated hypovolemic shock. (See Broselow Tape.)
4. Contact Medical Control for implementation of one or more of the following options:

Medical control options:

Option A: Begin rapid IV (IO) infusion of Ringer's Lactate (RL), via a second large bore IV (18-22 gauge) or IO catheter. Attempt second IV or IO only once each. (See Broselow Tape.)

Option B: Transportation decision.

TABLE 34-A18 NYC REMAC PEDIATRIC PREHOSPITAL ALS PROTOCOL 559

Pediatric traumatic/hypovolemic cardiac arrest

1. Begin transportation of the patient and other Basic Life Support Traumatic Cardiac Arrest procedures.

During transport, or if transport is delayed:

2. Perform Endotracheal Intubation.
3. Begin rapid IV (IO) infusion of Ringer's Lactate (RL) 20 ml/kg, via a large bore IV (18-22 gauge) or IO catheter. Attempt IV or IO only once each. (See Broselow Tape.)
4. If abdominal distension occurs, pass a nasogastric tube. Pass an orogastric tube in patients less than two (2) years of age.
Note: Do *not* pass a nasogastric tube in patients with craniofacial trauma.
5. Repeat Ringer's Lactate (RL) 20 ml/kg rapid IV (IO) infusion if the patient remains in traumatic cardiac arrest.
6. Contact Medical Control for implementation of one or more of the following options:

Option A: Begin rapid IV (IO) infusion of Ringer's Lactate (RL), via a second large bore IV (18-22 gauge) or IO catheter. Attempt second IV or IO only once each. (See Broselow Tape.)

Option B: Transportation decision.

APPENDIX 34-2

TABLE 34-A19 NYC REMAC GENERAL INTERHOSPITAL TRANSFER PROTOCOL 600 (©Copyright Regional E.M.S. Council of N.Y.C., Inc., 1994)

Standard approach to the patient

For special conditions, see additional protocols below.

Prior to transport:
- Review written orders to transport.
- Confirm destination accommodations.
- Perform extended primary assessment.
- **Note:** If the patient is found to be unstable or unsuitable for interfacility transport, or appears to require a higher level of care than was anticipated at the time transport was arranged, do *not* attempt transport. Contact medical control (or duly authorized agent) for further instructions.
- Measure and record vital signs.
- Initiate EKG monitoring as necessary.
- Obtain signature of accompanying physician or nurse for all medications to be carried en route on the Interfacility Transfer Report, noting routes of administration. Where possible, medications being infused by electrical pump should be converted to alternate administration systems.
- Notify medical control that transport is underway.
- Initiate and record appropriate oxygen therapy.

During transport:
- Monitor the airway.
- Continue appropriate oxygen therapy.
- Monitor and record vital signs as necessary.
- Perform or assist in performing those procedures allowed by specific advance direction of medical control, as necessary.
- In the event of a clinical emergency, and a physician, nurse practitioner, or physician surrogate is present, assist with allowed procedures on request and contact medical control.
- In the event of a clinical emergency, and a physician, nurse practitioner, or physician surrogate is *not* present, revert to pre-hospital standing orders and contact medical control.

After transport:
- Notify medical control that transport has been accomplished. Complete and sign the Interfacility Transfer Report, recording all measurements of vital signs made during transport, and describing in detail any changes in patient condition or unusual incidents occurring en route.

TABLE 34-A20 NYC REMAC GENERAL INTERFACILITY TREATMENT PROTOCOL 601 (©Copyright Regional E.M.S. Council of N.Y.C., Inc., 1994)

Ventilator management

Note: Paramedics may provide, or assist in providing, mechanical ventilatory support during interfacility transport only if they have completed special additional training in the use of transport ventilators, including appropriate continuing education, and are properly credentialed by the ambulance service medical director to operate such equipment.

Before transport:

Together with physician, nursing, and respiratory therapy staff (as appropriate), ensure that the endotracheal tube is patent, intact, properly positioned, and securely taped.

If the transport is not accompanied by a physician or nurse, obtain written order for ventilator settings to be used en route.

Note: If you are not familiar with the type of transport ventilator being used, or do not feel comfortable with the ventilator settings prescribed by the sending physician, do *not* attempt transport. Contact medical control (or duly authorized agent) for further instructions.

For Special Considerations, see below.

Place patient on pulse oximeter if not already done.

Ensure that the transport ventilator is properly functioning, that its settings are correct, and that it is ready to be attached to the endotracheal tube.

Assist physician, nursing, or respiratory therapy staff (as appropriate) detach endotracheal tube from hospital ventilator and hyperventilate patient with 100% oxygen via bag-valve device in preparation for transport, then attach endotracheal tube to transport ventilator.

Verify that breath sounds and chest rise remain present bilaterally and that vital signs remain unchanged.

During transport:

Continuously monitor airway, breath sounds, chest rise, vital signs, oxygen saturation, and ventilator function.

In the event of mechanical failure which cannot readily be corrected, detach endotracheal tube from ventilator, and perform manual ventilation with bag-valve device.

In the event of a clinical emergency, and a physician, nurse practitioner, or physician surrogate IS present, assist with ventilator management on request, and contact medical control (or duly authorized agent) as soon as possible (without compromising patient safety).

In the event of a clinical emergency, and a physician, nurse practitioner, or physician surrogate is NOT present, detach endotracheal tube from ventilator, perform manual ventilation with bag-valve device, and contact medical control (or duly authorized agent) as soon as possible (without compromising patient safety).

Note: Do *not* adjust prescribed ventilator settings. If the patient becomes unstable or needs resuscitation, detach endotracheal tube from ventilator, perform manual ventilation with bag-value device, and contact medical control (or duly authorized agent) as soon as possible (without compromising patient safety).

After transport:

Together with physician, nurse, or respiratory therapy staff (as appropriate), ensure that hospital ventilator is properly functioning, that its settings are correct, and that it is ready to be attached to the endotracheal tube.

Detach endotracheal tube from transport ventilator and hyperventilate patient with 100% oxygen via bag-value device, then assist physician, nursing, or respiratory therapy staff (as appropriate) attach endotracheal tube to hospital ventilator.

Record type and model of transport ventilator used, ventilator settings employed, and the oxygen saturation measurements obtained during transport, as well as any changes in patient condition, modifications in ventilator settings, and unusual incidents occurring en route, on Interfacility Transfer Report.

Special Considerations

Pediatric Patients

Do NOT use a volume-cycled transport ventilator for an infant or small child who requires a pressure-cycled ventilator. If a pressure-cycled transport ventilator is indicated but unavailable, perform manual ventilation via a bag-valve device during transport.

Note: Uncuffed endotracheal tubes are used in ventilating infants and small children, increasing the risk of dislodgement during transport.

Tracheostomy Tubes

In patients being ventilated via tracheostomy tubes rather than endotracheal tubes, exercise special care in detachment and attachment of ventilator circuits to avoid dislodgement of cannulas.

Note: Thick secretions are typically present in patients being ventilated via tracheostomy tubes, which may require that saline solution be used when suctioning.

Home Ventilators

If the patient is stable, without evidence of respiratory distress or respiratory failure, review written home ventilator orders (if available) and duplicate indicated home ventilator settings (as appropriate), with assistance of family member who is responsible for ventilator.

Note: If you are in doubt about the ventilator settings being used, perform manual ventilation with bag-valve device, or contact medical control (or duly authorized agent).

TABLE 34-A21 NYC REMAC GENERAL INTERFACILITY TREATMENT PROTOCOL 615 (©Copyright Regional E.M.S. Council of N.Y.C., Inc., 1994)

Continuous medication/fluid administration

Note: Paramedics may provide, or assist in providing, continuous medication or fluid administration during interfacility transport only if they have completed special additional training in the use of infusion devices, including appropriate continuing education, and are properly credentialed by the ambulance service medical director to operate such equipment.

Before transport:

Together with nursing staff, ensure that all IV/IO device(s) are patent and securely taped, that all connections are secure and watertight, that all tubing is compatible with the type(s) of medication(s) or fluid(s) being administered, and that all infusion device(s) are properly functioning.

If the transport is not accompanied by a physician or nurse, obtain written order(s) for the dosage(s), volume(s), and concentration(s) of medication(s) and fluid(s), as well as infusion rate(s), to be used en route.

Note: If you are not familiar with the type of infusion device(s) being used, or do not feel comfortable with the dosage(s), volume(s), or concentrations(s) of medication(s) or fluid(s), or infusion rate(s), prescribed by the sending physician, do *not* attempt transport. Contact medical control (or duly authorized agent) for further instructions.

Set each transport infusion device to be used at the prescribed volume and rate of infusion.

Clear each line of air pockets prior to infusion.

Switch each infusion from hospital infusion device to transport infusion device.

Note: Do *not* open stopcocks when switching between infusion devices.

Continue each infusion with transport infusion device.

Note: Protect each line from sunlight as appropriate.

During Transport:

Continuously monitor vital signs, tissue perfusion, IV/IO access site, and infusion device function.

In the event of mechanical failure which cannot readily be corrected, detach tubing from infusion device, and continue infusion by gravity drip, carefully monitoring the infusion rate by direct observation.

In the event of a clinical emergency, and a physician, nurse practitioner, or physician surrogate IS present, assist with infusion management on request, and contact medical control (or duly authorized agent) as soon as possible (without compromising patient safety).

In the event of a clinical emergency, and a physician, nurse practitioner, or physician surrogate is NOT present, adjust rate(s) of infusion as appropriate within prescribed dose range(s), and contact medical control (or duly authorized agent) as soon as possible (without compromising patient safety).

Note: If it becomes necessary to stop an infusion entirely, begin an infusion or dextrose 5% in water (D5W) to keep vein open.

After Transport:

Record type and model of infusion device(s) used, and the dosage(s), volume(s), and concentration(s) of medication(s) and fluid(s) administered, as well as any changes in patient condition, modifications in infusion device settings, and unusual incidents occurring en route, on Interfacility Transfer Report.

TABLE 34-A22 NYC REMAC GENERAL INTERFACILITY TREATMENT PROTOCOL 620 (©Copyright Regional E.M.S. Council of N.Y.C., Inc., 1994)

Major trauma transport

Major trauma patients include patients with life-threatening traumatic injuries requiring onward transport from a 911 receiving hospital emergency department to a 911 receiving hospital trauma center.

Major trauma transports shall be classified as critical transports (Segment 1 or Segment 2) when accompanied by a physician or nurse or acute transports (Segment 3 or Segment 4) when not accompanied by a physician or nurse. By definition, major trauma transports are onward transports, therefore cannot be classified as routine transports (Segment 5 or Segment 6) requiring only basic life support care. Major trauma transports shall be conducted in accordance with all applicable policies and procedures of the EMS 911 System Trauma Center Advisory Committee. Major trauma transports in patients less than fourteen (14) years of age shall also be considered high-risk pediatric transports. (See Protocol #650.)

Transporting paramedics may, if properly trained and credentialed to do so, operate under all applicable prehospital and interfacility protocols, or upon request of the designated direct medical control physician, may assist physician and nurse members of a high-risk transport team with the following tasks:

Note: Those marked with an asterisk(*) require special training.

1. Airway maintenance/suctioning.
2. Oxygen administration.
3. Airway/breathing adjuncts (OPA/NPA).
4. Assisted ventilation (BVM).
5. Endotracheal intubation (OT/NT).
6. Gastric intubation (NG/OG).
7. Vascular access (IV/IO).
8. Fluid medication/administration (IV/IO/ET/infusion device*).
9. Ventilator management.*
10. Chest tube management.*
11. Vital monitoring (EKG, S_aO_2,* $ETCO_2$*).
12. Fracture/wound management.*
13. Needle decompression of tension pneumothorax.
14. Needle cricothryotomy.

TABLE 34-A23 NYC REMAC GENERAL INTERFACILITY TREATMENT PROTOCOL 623 (©Copyright Regional E.M.S. Council of N.Y.C., Inc., 1994)

Chest tube management

Note: Parametics may provide, or assist in providing, thoracic drainage and suction during interfacility transport only if they have completed special additional training in the use of chest tubes and collection devices, including appropriate continuing education, and are properly credentialed by the ambulance service medical director to operate such equipment.

Prior to transport:

Together with nursing staff, ensure that the chest tube is patent and securely taped, and that all connections are secure and airtight, and that the collection device is properly functioning.

If the transport is not accompanied by a physician or nurse, obtain written order to clamp chest tube, or for the amount of negative pressure to be applied to thoracic cavity while en route.

During transport:

Ensure that collection device remains upright.

If chest tube remains unclamped, provide sufficient suction to collection device to maintain prescribed amount of negative pressure to thoracic cavity. If collection device falls on its side and water seal is lost, clamp chest tube.

If chest tube becomes dislodged while en route, seal wound with an occlusive dressing and tape on all four sides. If a tension pneumothorax subsequently develops, unseal one side of the occlusive dressing to vent the pressure as the patient exhales, and reseal after exhalation.

Monitor continuously for signs of tension pneumothorax.

After transport:

Record volume and character of drainage on Interfacility Transfer Report.

TABLE 34-A24 NYC REMAC GENERAL INTERFACILITY TREATMENT PROTOCOL 628 (©Copyright Regional E.M.S. Council of N.Y.C., Inc., 1994)

Major burn transport

Major burn patients include patients with life-threatening thermal, chemical, or electrical injuries requiring onward transport from a 911 receiving hospital emergency department to a 911 receiving hospital burn center.

Major burn transports shall be classified as critical transports (Segment 1 or Segment 2) when accompanied by a physician or nurse or acute transports (Segment 3 or Segment 4) when not accompanied by a physician or nurse. By definition, major burn transports are onward transports, therefore cannot be classified as routine transports (Segment 5 or Segment 6) requiring only basic life support care. Major burn transports shall be conducted in accordance with all applicable policies and procedures of the EMS 911 System Burn Center Advisory Committee. Major burn transports in patients less than fourteen (14) years of age shall also be considered high-risk pediatric transports. (See Protocol #650.)

Transporting paramedics may, if properly trained and credentialed to do so, operate under all applicable prehospital and interfacility protocols, or upon request of the designated direct medical control physician, may assist physician and nurse members of a high-risk transport team with the following tasks:

Note: Those marked with an asterisk(*) require special training.

1. Airway maintenance/suctioning.
2. Oxygen administration.
3. Airway/breathing adjuncts (OPA/NPA).
4. Assisted ventilation (BVM).
5. Endotracheal intubation (OT/NT).
6. Gastric intubation (NG/OG).
7. Vascular access (IV/IO).
8. Fluid medication/administration (IV/IO/ET/infusion device*).
9. Ventilator management.*
10. Chest tube management.*
11. Vital monitoring (EKG, S_aO_2,* $ETCO_2$*).
12. Burn wound management.*
13. Needle decompression of tension pneumothorax.
14. Needle cricothryotomy.

TABLE 34-A25 NYC REMAC PEDIATRIC INTERFACILITY TREATMENT PROTOCOL 642 (©Copyright Regional E.M.S. Council of N.Y.C., Inc., 1994)

High-risk neonatal transport

High-risk neonates include, but are not limited to, infants less than one month old born with prematurity, low birth weight, or life-threatening respiratory/circulatory illnesses, infections, congenital anomalies, or metabolic disorders.

High-risk neonatal transports shall be classified as critical transports (Segment 1 or Segment 2), and should be conducted in accordance with all applicable policies and procedures of the New York City Department of Health Perinatal Advisory Committee.

Physicians and nurses rendering interfacility treatment shall do so in accordance with accepted standards of medical and nursing practice to the extent permitted by their professional licenses, shall be trained and credentialed in high-risk neonatal transport by their base hospitals for this purpose, and shall be chiefly responsible for patient care, by written agreement of the medical directors of the high-risk neonatal transport service and the ambulance service providing the transport vehicle.

Transporting paramedics may assist physician and nurse members of the transport team in rendering patient care upon request, provided they have been trained and credentialed to perform all extraordinary task(s) in accordance with standards established jointly by the medical director of the high-risk neonatal transport service and the medical director of the ambulance service providing the transport vehicle. The medical director of the ambulance service providing the transport vehicle shall be responsible for maintaining records documenting compliance with the above, and shall furnish the medical director of the high-risk neonatal transport service with a document attesting to the above. Direct medical control during transport shall be provided by the medical director of the high-risk neonatal transport service or properly credentialed designee. Indirect medical control shall be provided jointly by the medical directors of the high-risk neonatal transport service and the ambulance service providing the transport vehicle.

Continued.

TABLE 34-A25 NYC REMAC PEDIATRIC INTERFACILITY TREATMENT 642—cont'd

High-risk neonatal transport

Transporting paramedics may assist with the following tasks:

Note: Those marked with an asterisk(*) require special training.

1. Airway maintenance/suctioning.
2. Oxygen/compressed air* administration.
3. Airway/breathing adjuncts (OPA/CPAP*).
4. Assisted ventilation (BVM).
5. Endotracheal intubation (OT/NT).
6. Gastric intubation (NG/OG).
7. Vascular access (IV/IO).
8. Fluid/medication administration (IV/IO/ET/infusion devise*).
9. Ventilator management.*
10. Chest tube management.*
11. Vital monitoring (EKG, S_aO_2,* $ETCO_2$*).
12. Transport environment (ambulance, isolette,* warming devices*).

TABLE 34-A26 NYC REMAC PEDIATRIC INTERFACILITY TREATMENT PROTOCOL 650 (©Copyright Regional E.M.S. Council of N.Y.C., Inc., 1994)

High-risk pediatric transport

High-risk pediatric patients include, but are not limited to, infants and children, newborn to 18 years of age, with life-threatening respiratory, circulatory, neurologic, metabolic, infectious, or traumatic illnesses.

High-risk pediatric transports shall be classified as critical transports (Segment 1 or Segment 2), and should be conducted in accordance with the American Academy of Pediatrics' "Guidelines for Air and Ground Transport of Pediatric Patients."

Physicians and nurses rendering interfacility treatment shall do so in accordance with accepted standards of medical and nursing practice to the extent permitted by their professional licenses, shall be trained and credentialed in high-risk pediatric transport by their base hospitals for this purpose, and shall be chiefly responsible for patient care, by written agreement of the medical directors of the high-risk pediatric transport service and the ambulance service providing the transport vehicle.

Transporting paramedics may assist physician and nurse members of the transport team in rendering patient care upon request, provided they have been trained and credentialed to perform all extraordinary task(s) in accordance with standards established jointly by the medical director of the high-risk pediatric transport service and the medical director of the ambulance service providing the transport vehicle. The medical director of the ambulance service providing the transport vehicle shall be responsible for maintaining records documenting compliance with the above, and shall furnish the medical director of the high-risk pediatric transport service with a document attesting to the above. Direct medical control during transport shall be provided by the medical director of the high-risk pediatric transport service or properly credentialed designee. Indirect medical control shall be provided jointly by the medical directors of the high-risk pediatric transport service and the ambulance service providing the transport vehicle.

Transporting paramedics may assist with the following tasks:

Note: Those marked with an asterisk(*) require special training.

1. Airway maintenance/suctioning.
2. Oxygen/compressed air* administration.
3. Airway/breathing adjuncts (OPA/NPA).
4. Assisted ventilation (BVM).
5. Endotracheal intubation (OT/NT).
6. Gastric intubation (NG/OG).
7. Vascular access (IV/IO).
8. Fluid/medication administration (IV/IO/ET/infusion device*).
9. Ventilator management.*
10. Chest tube management.*
11. Vital monitoring (EKG, S_aO_2,* $ETCO_2$*).
12. Transport environment (ambulance, isolette,* warming devices*).

Part III

MISCELLANEOUS ISSUES

35

HOUSESTAFF EDUCATION

DENNIS R. DURBIN
ANGELO P. GIARDINO

Time spent on a pediatric emergency transport team offers pediatric residents and fellows a unique opportunity to develop skills and abilities that are valuable in a wide variety of clinical practices. Residency and fellowship training comprise phases in a physician's education where skills and knowledge are both learned and applied to patient care and management. The hallmark of the residency, and to a greater degree of the fellowship, is a staged, ever-increasing level of independence while still receiving guidance and supervision from more senior physicians. This chapter explores how serving on a transport team can offer educational benefit to both the resident and fellow. Specifically, it addresses how the experience should be structured and planned in order to reach its full educational potential.

Pediatric residents and fellows have participated on transport teams for many years.[15,27,28,29,32,34] Recently, there has been increasing controversy about the role of pediatric housestaff on transport. In 1986 the American Academy of Pediatrics first published guidelines for the Ground and Air Transportation of Children which recommended that pediatric housestaff of at least the PL-3 level be used as transport physicians.[1] Despite this, results of a 1988 survey of critical care transport teams indicated that two-thirds of teams routinely used second year residents as the transport physician.[28] In 1990 a National Pediatric Transport Leadership Conference began to shift the focus of appropriate team composition away from published recommendations to the requirements of an individual team's "patient population, availability of personnel, and local expectations."[14] In its 1993 revised Guidelines for Air and Ground Transport of Neonatal and Pediatric Patients, the American Academy of Pediatrics focused training recommendations for team members on "skill levels needed to successfully transport pediatric patients rather than on specific educational degrees obtained."[3] Historically, the goal of transport training has been to produce team members (physicians, nurses, paramedics) who are fully trained and qualified to provide a high level of care to critically ill patients.[3,13,16] In many programs this goal may conflict with the reality of using junior or senior pediatric housestaff who have not had the necessary scope of clinical experience or transport-specific education to be fully trained team members. This has resulted in a questioning of the need for physicians to be present on transport. A number of studies have evaluated the need for a physician on transport.[11,12,21,27,29,32,34] These studies suggest that a physician may be required only for transports in which there is a high probability of either patient deterioration or need for a major intervention. However, these studies did not evaluate the potential educational benefit of transport service to the resident physicians. Reliance on physicians-in-training to staff transport teams mandates that residency programs and transport teams provide a planned, structured, educational program for the housestaff. A comprehensive educational program can both improve the preparation of housestaff for transport service and provide an environment in which housestaff can attain specific educational goals.

What role should the transport experience play in pediatric training at both the resident and fellow level? The American Medical Association has developed a policy statement regarding the role of housestaff in transport activities.[7] The AMA urges training programs in which housestaff participate on either ground or air transport "to notify applicants of that policy prior to and during the interview process," and "to include accident, disability, and life insurance as part of an available package for participating resident physicians." In addition, the AMA "encourages all teaching institutions where medical students or resident physicians participate (either compulsorily or voluntarily) in the air or ground transport of patients . . . to include in the educational curriculum formal training on general and safety issues pertaining to emergency transport before students or residents participate in such activity." The appropriateness of using residents and fellows on transport teams can be assessed by examining how the transport experience may address some of the guidelines established by the Accreditation Council on Graduate Medical Education (ACGME) for pediatric residency training[10] as well as the guidelines for pediatric fellowships in critical care,[9] emergency medicine,[2] and neonatology.[8] In defining the scope of pediatric residency training, the Accreditation Council on Graduate Medical Education guidelines state that the training program must "prepare the resident to function as a primary care specialist capable of providing comprehensive patient care," and be able to distinguish and manage "conditions ranging from minor illness to life-threatening conditions requiring intensive care."

In the context of training for comprehensive pediatric care, the transport experience provides housestaff the opportunity to participate in the entire continuum of care for acutely ill children, from initial resuscitation, reassessment and stabilization to definitive care. The guidelines for fellowship training in pediatric critical care, pediatric emergency medicine, and neonatology each explicitly refer to participation in transport medicine,[2,8,9] offering recommendations for training and experience in the unique transport environment. Additionally, the pediatric emergency medicine curriculum addresses the need to develop interpersonal leadership and prioritization skills in managing patients in emergency settings of which transport could be an example.

While the majority of this chapter pertains to the educational benefit of an interhospital transport experience, prehospital transport also provides an environment that may fulfill educational requirements of residency or fellowship training. A number of Emergency Medical Services (EMS) curricula for emergency medicine residents have been described.[23,31,35] Initial evaluations of the educational merit of EMS (in-field) rotations for emergency medicine residents have demonstrated that the field experience provides an opportunity to improve skills in a number of technical procedures, particularly endotracheal intubation and central venous line placement. Additionally, these rotations provide the residents with a more in-depth understanding of prehospital decision-making and prioritization. Faculty members feel that this is a desired educational goal of their training programs.

Embedded in the above standards for residency and fellowship training is the notion that planned, structured experiences containing a sufficient amount of clinical exposure lead to the attainment of life-long skills. These skills will equip the proficient pediatrician in their general or subspecialty practice. The residency guidelines state: "Each component of the curriculum must be a structured educational experience that reflects an appropriate balance between clinical and didactic activities."[10] This chapter outlines the steps required to develop, implement, and assess an educational program in transport medicine for pediatric residents and fellows.

DEVELOPING AN EDUCATIONAL PROGRAM FOR HOUSESTAFF

In a 1990 survey of large (greater than 35 residents) pediatric residency programs, Giardino and others found that 69% of the chief residents in programs which utilize pediatric residents on transports view the transport service as a learning experience.[20] Despite this, only 39% of residency programs provided a specific training process for the residents. An educational program can be developed to meet both educational goals and training requirements of physician team members with individual modifications to fit local needs. Important steps in the development of the program include: conducting a needs assessment, 2) identifying specific educational goals, 3) developing individual curricular components, 4) implementing the curriculum, and 5) creating a process of both program evaluation and an assessment of the participant's performance (Box 35–1).

Step 1: the needs assessment

Attaining the full educational potential of transport activities requires the input and support of a dedicated faculty member, typically the Medical Director of the program. The director should begin the development of an educational program with a needs assessment. This is a mechanism to determine targeted areas of educational intervention, outcomes to be assessed, and what resources are available or needed. The needs assessment may begin with an evaluation of the epidemiology of the patient population served by an individual program. Information about the age range of the patients, their spectrum of clinical conditions, the number and type of interventions performed by the team, and the prior training and expectations of the housestaff who will participate on the team should be determined. This information can be obtained from review of local transport data bases, surveys and interviews of the referral base and team members, or specific observation of transports. It is also necessary to assess existing resources that can support a specific educational program. Such resources as a free-standing dedicated nursing staff, a specific transport rotation for residents, interested faculty members, and access to a number of teaching aids will influence the type of program that can be developed at a given institution. The purpose of the needs assessment is to identify specific educational goals to be obtained by housestaff and practical mechanisms by which to implement the program.

BOX 35-1 STEPS INVOLVED IN PLANNING A COMPREHENSIVE EDUCATIONAL PROGRAM IN TRANSPORT

The needs assessment
Identification of specific educational goals
Development of curricular components
Implementation of program
Evaluation and outcomes assessment

Step 2: identification of specific educational goals

The educational goals of a given transport program will vary depending on the patient population served, the previous knowledge of the housestaff involved, the role of the transport team in the institution, the educational resources available, and the strengths and interests of the faculty members involved. For pediatric residents, transport offers a clinical experience and educational opportunity unlike any other in their residency program. The practice of transport medicine may provide junior and senior residents opportunity for greater independence in their patient assessment and management, as well as a unique environment in which to apply skills acquired primarily in other rotations. Transport service provides fellows, particularly in the fields of neonatology, critical care, and emergency medicine, an opportunity to further develop and refine expertise in the management of critically ill children. Transport medicine is a bridge linking the initial resuscitation and stabilization of a patient with his/her definitive diagnosis and care. Fellows with patient care experience in the transport setting will better understand all facets of care for critically ill children. Some fellows with a particular interest in transport may also develop academic skills in transport medicine related to teaching, research, and administration. Since there is considerable variety in the experiences of housestaff among residency and fellowship programs, each transport program must determine the specific educational goals that are relevant to its training program. The educational goals of a transport experience for housestaff are primarily related to the acquisition of a number of cognitive, procedural, and communications skills needed to provide patient care in the transport environment.

Cognitive skills. The transport literature has focused on training team members (including pediatric housestaff) prior to transport service.[15,28] An academic transport experience must identify the cognitive skills that housestaff should develop during the rotation. Transport service provides residents with an opportunity for greater independence in patient management. It may be the only part of their training conducted outside of a tertiary care center where 24 hour access to more experienced senior physicians and sophisticated technology is taken for granted. The transport setting can lead to more realistic expectations about the limitations of the information received during a transport call as well as the ability of referring physicians to carry out recommendations by the transport team. Residents planning careers in private practice can experience emergency medicine in more realistic settings than the tertiary care center emergency department. Because transport medicine is practiced in unfamiliar surroundings, residents are forced to rely more on their own clinical judgment while managing acutely ill patients. Therefore, a well-planned educational program should include adequate preparation and appropriate supervision to develop cognitive skills that promote confidence in independent practice. A recent assessment of the educational value of transport service at the Children's Hospital of Philadelphia revealed that the primary educational benefits of a transport rotation pertain to improving cognitive skills such as clinical judgment, ability to prioritize, and independent decision-making.[17] Additional cognitive skills as knowledge of common pediatric life-threatening illnesses or injuries, recognition of deterioration in a patient's condition, factoring time into decision-making, and appropriate use and interpretation of laboratory and radiographic data, can also be developed during a transport experience. Proficiency in these skills is generally obtained through significant experience in caring for patients on transport. It is not likely that residents with limited transport participation will fully develop all desired cognitive skills during their rotations. A transport curriculum must provide methods (outlined below in the section on curricular development) to enhance the "hands-on" clinical experience of the housestaff. In addition, intensive care unit and emergency medicine rotations may both complement the benefits of the transport rotation and better prepare the resident for their role on the transport team.

Procedural skills. Since the goal of specialized pediatric transport teams is to deliver a level of care as close as possible to that of the receiving hospital, team members should be capable of performing all procedures necessary for the stabilization and care of critically ill children.[3] The most common major procedure performed by a transport team is endotracheal intubation.[12,29,32] Other procedural skills necessary on transport include obtaining peripheral and central venous access, arterial access, intraosseous line placement, chest tube placement, defibrillation or cardioversion, and cardiopulmonary resuscitation.[29] Most orientation programs for both physicians and nurses focus on development of procedural skills to determine readiness for transport.[3,20] However, the frequency with which transport team members perform a major procedure is relatively low. Recent reviews demonstrate that only 5 to 15% of patients require a major procedure by a member of the transport team.[26,29,32] This is because referring hospital personnel frequently have performed necessary procedures prior to the arrival of the transport team. If a transport program utilizes a small number of personnel to perform necessary procedures, then those personnel must maintain proficiency in their technical skill. If, however, a large group of residents divide transport coverage throughout the year, then it cannot be expected that an individual resident will perform transport procedures with the regularity required to develop true proficiency in these skills.

Because of the relative infrequency of residents performing major procedures on transport, they are not likely to view the experience as an opportunity to enhance their technical skills.[17] Therefore, emphasizing proficiency in technical skills may not be a valuable educational goal for many transport programs that utilize a large group of residents. On the contrary, fellows with significant prior experience in these skills may find that participation on transport enhances proficiency by providing an opportunity to perform a variety of procedures under a wide range of conditions. Housestaff without a sufficient level of expertise in the necessary procedures should have access to more senior physicians who can provide on-site supervision when needed. In addition, the transport curriculum should provide opportunity for supervised practice of these procedures and a mechanism to monitor the number and success rates of procedures performed by housestaff.

Communications skills. Transport service may help residents develop communication skills that will be useful, regardless of their ultimate career path. Both primary care pediatricians and subspecialists will likely utilize transport systems in the course of their practice. Experience during residency and fellowship training with the communications involved in interhospital transport will better prepare housestaff for roles as either referring or receiving physicians. Transport situations will introduce housestaff to pediatricians, emergency medicine physicians, and family practitioners on the "front lines" which can improve communications during future phone calls and transports. In addition, the practice of interhospital transport provides pediatric housestaff with opportunities to develop skills used to communicate with other members of the transport team and members of the patient's family.

As representatives of the tertiary care center, residents are often placed in the unfamiliar role of consultant to more experienced referring hospital staff. This situation creates the potential for misunderstandings which can lead to disagreement about patient management. Resolution of differences in a manner that does not jeopardize patient care or future interactions between the referring physician and the transport team frequently challenges the diplomatic skills of housestaff on transport. Specific education and experience addressing the skills required for effective communication with other physicians can be an important benefit of the transport experience for residents.

Interactions with transport nurses are unique among those interactions which housestaff have with other nurses in the course of their training. Residents with limited transport experience typically work with nurses whose training and expertise allow a great degree of independence in their role. While a majority of transport programs view the resident, if present, as the team leader,[20] housestaff may more frequently perceive the transport nurse as a coequal partner on the team, rather than as an assistant to the resident.[17] Residents should learn to incorporate the suggestions of experienced nurses in their decision-making on transports. In addition, they should be able to communicate orders clearly, since many of them are carried out prior to being written. Curricular components which value the participation of nursing staff help develop communication skills that foster a spirit of collaboration and cooperation between team members.

Finally, housestaff are frequently challenged to communicate effectively with patients and their families during transport. The transport setting typically finds parents in the midst of an unexpected and very stressful event. Parents may have either an incomplete understanding of the need for transport or inflated expectations of the capabilities of the transport team. This may create misunderstandings between members of the team and the patient's family. Recognition of different coping mechanisms, expectations, and level of comprehension that families have about transport is the first step toward communicating effectively with families. Specific communication skills desired on transport include the ability to speak clearly and succinctly, demonstrate empathy and concern while instilling confidence, and respond to questions directly and honestly. Residents should be provided educational opportunities which allow them to practice communication methods through role-playing and to observe more experienced nurses and physicians on transport.

The transport environment enables pediatric residents to acquire and develop a number of cognitive, technical, and communications skills. Expectations about the pace and level of skills development on transport should be consistent with those of other rotations in the residency program. Placing residents in situations which require proficiency in skills they have not yet developed places patients at risk and undermines the educational potential of the experience. A curriculum which addresses the desired outcomes of the experience will educate pediatric residents and fellows while maintaining a high quality of patient care.

Step 3: development of individual curricular components

Because the spectrum of clinical experience and anticipated educational goals may vary significantly among transport programs, it is not likely that a single transport curriculum with universal application can be designed. Many different methods exist to teach transport-specific skills to residents and other personnel involved in transport. Certain educational modalities, with appropriate modifications to fit local needs, are considered central to the design of an effective transport curriculum for pediatric residents and fellows.

Specific curricular components in a comprehensive transport educational program can be implemented in three distinct phases[20] (Box 35-2). Phase I involves those curricular components utilized prior to the transport experience. These provide proper training and preparation of the physician for transport service. Phase II includes modalities employed during a transport. These provide an appropriate level of supervision and support to the team while on the transport. Phase III involves activities occurring after a transport-which provide team members with performance feedback and evaluation. Individual curricular components which may be implemented in each phase are described below, including the specific educational objectives to be accomplished by each.

BOX 35-2 SUMMARY OF INDIVIDUAL CURRICULAR COMPONENTS BY PHASE OF IMPLEMENTATION

- Phase I—Prior to Transport
  - Pretransport training and qualifications
  - Orientation course
  - Procedural skills training
  - Didactic conferences
  - Case simulations
  - Written materials
- Phase II—During the Transport
  - Supervised transports
  - On-line medical command
- Phase III—Following the Transport
  - Case review and feedback
  - Stress management seminars

Phase I: the pretransport curriculum

Pretransport training and qualifications. The minimum qualifications necessary for residents to participate on transports vary widely across programs.[15,28,31] Of those programs utilizing residents on transport, about half require neonatal intensive care unit (NICU) experience, and half require pediatric intensive care unit (PICU) experience.[15] The median amount of previous PICU time is 1 month (range 0 to 6 months), while the median amount of prior NICU and emergency department time is 2 months (range 1 to 6 months and 0 to 8 months, respectively). In addition, a number of residency programs provide and require Pediatric Advance Life Support (PALS)[6] certification or other "packaged" critical care courses for their housestaff.[15] The objective of requiring a minimum level of experience prior to transport is to provide residents with a basic introduction to the patient population, techniques involved in resuscitation, and stabilization, and priorities in the management of critically ill children.

Orientation course. Residents and fellows should have a formal orientation to their particular transport program prior to participating on the team. A comprehensive orientation should include the following features:

1. An introduction to the patient population. Residents should know the demographics of the patient population they will serve, including the age distribution and the spectrum of diagnoses and severity of illness. They should also know the types of procedures, medications, and other interventions that can be anticipated by their population.
2. An overview of the communications system. Housestaff should have a working knowledge of the communications systems utilized by their program, including how referring physicians access the system, how the team is contacted for mobilization, means of remaining in contact with both the referring and receiving hospital while enroute, and identification of the medical command physician for each transport.
3. A discussion about medical-legal responsibilities on transports, including required written records, obtaining consent, and transfer of responsibility from the referring hospital to the transport team.
4. Knowledge of the equipment commonly used on transport. Physicians should be able to recognize equipment malfunctions and trouble-shoot equipment failures.
5. Knowledge of safety on transport includes basic epidemiology of vehicular accidents, safety features of the ambulance or aircraft, and the appropriate use of lights and sirens during ground transport.

The objectives of the orientation are to introduce the resident or fellow to their role on the team, the logistics of arranging a transport, and the safe management of patients in a mobile environment.

Procedural skills training. Despite the fact that residents participating on transport may not be required to regularly perform technical procedures, every transport program should have a system to ensure that housestaff have acquired and maintained necessary procedural skills. In some systems, previous or concurrent rotations in intensive care units, the operating room, or the emergency department will provide sufficient experience to obtain required proficiency in these skills. A mechanism should exist to monitor the number and type of procedures performed during all rotations. If housestaff do not regularly perform procedures during transport or other rotations, other methods exist to provide opportunity for practice. Use of animal labs and mannequins or participation in a number of critical care courses such as Pediatric Advanced Life Support (PALS),[6] Neonatal Resuscitation Program (NRP),[5] or Advanced Trauma Life Support (ATLS)[4] can enhance a resident's procedural experience. These modalities must be used in conjunction with field experience, since they are not sufficient to guarantee an adequate level of expertise. On-site supervision of procedures performed by junior housestaff is ideal both as a quality assurance mechanism and to optimize the educational value of the experience for the resident. The overall objective of the various strategies utilized in technical skills training is to provide a structured environment with an appropriate amount of supervised practice for housestaff to develop proficiency in the skills necessary for transport.

Didactic conferences. Lecture series can provide a basic fund of knowledge about the etiology, pathogenesis, and management of a variety of conditions requiring transport. A program can highlight those conditions commonly transported by their team such as trauma, seizures, congenital heart disease, sepsis, or the problems of premature infants. For pediatric housestaff who may participate in similar lectures outside their transport experience, didactic sessions can focus more on transport-specific issues as the limitations of monitoring, immobilization of a trauma patient on transport, aviation physiology, management of infants on prostaglandin infusions, and proper stabilization prior to transport. Didactic conferences may also provide an opportunity for nursing members of the team to participate in the curriculum and provide a means of documenting to residency program directors the scope of clinical exposure provided to housestaff during a transport rotation.

Case simulations. Mock transport scenarios may be developed either as a regular (weekly or monthly) component of the transport curriculum or as part of an expanded orientation program. Cases can be designed to be comprehensive in their review of activities on transport or can emphasize specific problematic areas such as communication with referring physicians or transport nurses, technical skills, or decision-making on transport.

Computer-based simulations have been developed as an alternative means of supplementing housestaff education in a number of clinical areas.[30,33] Initial evaluations of computer-based education have demonstrated it to be an effective means of improving fund of knowledge and patient management for medical students and housestaff.[24] Transport-specific computer simulated cases have not as yet been developed. The development and use of educational software will provide an additional way of increasing a resident's exposure to patient management on transport during a limited transport rotation. The educational objectives of mock case scenarios are to enhance the exposure which residents have to transport management and to identify potential deficiencies in judgment or performance in need of further intervention.

Written materials. Generally considered central to any curriculum, written materials such as a course syllabus have been underutilized in transport medicine to date. In 1990 only 22% of transport programs which utilized pediatric housestaff provided a written transport manual or course syllabus.[20]

A comprehensive syllabus should contain clearly stated and specific educational goals and objectives. It should outline expectations of the housestaff and identify all educational materials available during their transport experience. In addition, a series of directed readings in the form of textbook chapters, review articles, and recent investigations should be provided. Those topics felt to be essential for the patient population served by the individual program should be covered. The goal of a transport syllabus is to supplement the other curricular materials which are available to the housestaff for those clinical conditions frequently encountered on transport.

Phase II: the intratransport curriculum

Supervised transports. The Phase I curricular components described above are designed to be used by the resident prior to or between actual transports. As beneficial as they are, the bulk of educational value is likely derived from the resident's participation on real transports. As with many other areas of residency and fellowship training, "on-the-job-experience" with proper supervision is an invaluable way to obtain a comprehensive education in transport medicine. Like many of the educational strategies described previously, supervised transports are currently underutilized by residency programs and transport teams. Only 50% of institutions utilizing pediatric residents on transport teams reported providing supervised initial transports.[15] Senior physicians (either attendings, fellows, or senior residents with an acceptable degree of transport experience) should directly supervise the first transports of housestaff new to the team. This provides an opportunity to reinforce desired behaviors and skills while identifying areas in need of further educational intervention. The competence of individual residents prior to and during their initial transports should be used to determine when a resident no longer requires direct supervision during routine transports. Of course, any time a transport is anticipated to require skills beyond that generally expected of the transport resident, direct supervision by a more senior and qualified physician should be available. There is little educational benefit and potential patient morbidity can be expected when an unprepared resident is placed in a situation where "trial-and-error" management is performed.

On-line medical command. Related to, but distinct from, direct supervision of transports is the availability of on-line supervision or medical command by phone during a transport. Prior to any transport, the medical command physician who is responsible for the actions of the team during the transport must be identified. On-line medical supervision is utilized by most transport programs. In 1990 over 80% of programs that utilized pediatric housestaff always identified a senior physician at the receiving hospital to field questions by phone for the transport team.[20] Availability does not always dictate utilization, however. One transport program, comparing the performance of second and third year pediatric residents on transport, found that only 26% of housestaff called a more senior physician for advice during transport.[22] Since every transport offers a unique set of circumstances in which a patient is managed, even routine clinical problems can contribute to a resident's transport education when discussed with a senior physician. In addition, medical-legal and quality assurance pressures mandate discussion of all patients with the physician of record at some time during the transport.

Phase III: following the transport

Case review and feedback. In a recent assessment of the transport curriculum at The Children's Hospital of Philadelphia, feedback and review of individual cases were judged by pediatric housestaff to be among the most valuable components of the curriculum.[17] In this system a review of transports performed by the junior residents on the transport service is conducted on a weekly basis. Less formal review on an "interesting case" basis can also be effective in programs without sufficient volume or without the resources required to support a regular formal review. Despite the effectiveness of case review, only 30% of transport programs utilizing pediatric housestaff regularly provided timely review and feedback to residents as noted in the 1990 survey by Giardino and others.[20] Case conferences provide housestaff with valuable feedback concerning alternative patient management strategies, deficits in judgement, and follow-up information concerning patient outcome. In programs which utilize a large number of residents to provide transport coverage, individual residents may not have sufficient opportunity to obtain a "critical mass" of transport experience. Including as many of these residents as possible in case review conferences broadens the exposure of an individual resident to transport-specific patient management. Because most medical directors and medical command physicians infrequently accompany the team on transports, case review conferences provide valuable insight into the performance of a resident. The information provided in these sessions can be used to improve his/her evaluation at the completion of the transport rotation.

Cases should be chosen for review that both highlight common management or communications pitfalls, as well as uncommon or complicated scenarios that present unique challenges to team members. As with many of the other curricular components described, transport nurses should be encouraged to participate in case review conferences to provide the residents with a variety of experienced opinions.

Stress management seminars. Several stresses unique to the practice of transport medicine have been recently described.[3,19,25] These include the potential for vehicular accidents, practicing medicine in an unfamiliar environment, limited access to tertiary care resources, the sense of being isolated with the responsibility for critically ill children, erratic work schedules, and the physical stress of working in a moving, vibrating, noisy environment. Even with proper preparation prior to the transport experience, these and other stresses are frequently experienced by pediatric housestaff. An assessment of second year pediatric residents at The Children's Hospital of Philadelphia found that concerns about performing technical procedures correctly, managing an acute emergency alone, and practicing medicine in a mobile environment were the most frequent anxieties expressed by residents following their transport rotation.[17]

Regular or informal opportunity to recognize and express these concerns can be beneficial to all team members. Critical Incident Stress Debriefing (CISD) is a technique that has been used effectively by prehospital emergency personnel and others involved in critical care and emergency medicine.[18] It provides an opportunity for persons involved in particularly stressful events to better understand and more effectively deal with their own response to the event. If available, this technique might prove valuable to members of a transport team following particularly stressful transports. In addition, stress reduction techniques such as relaxation training, regular physical exercise, and proper diet and sleep habits should be practiced by those members of the team who perform transports most often.

Step 4: implementation

Given unlimited resources in terms of time and personnel, any program could launch and maintain the ideal curriculum outlined above. The reality of completing education and service requirements, in addition to limited resources, time, and personnel make this ideal difficult to achieve. Issues that must be considered in implementing an individual curriculum include 1) time and availability of interested faculty, 2) scheduling priorities in the residency or fellowship program, 3) resources necessary for various curricular components, and 4) interest in and support for a nursing role in the educational program. Implementation strategies often require creativity and innovation. For example, at The Children's Hospital of Philadelphia, a didactic transport lecture series has been incorporated into the core lectures given to the entire housestaff. These presentations are given by the senior residents who under the guidance of faculty members assume responsibility for developing the lecture and an accompanying handout and for collecting representative cases to aid in the discussion.

Step 5: evaluation and outcomes assessment

No discussion of educational programming would be complete without addressing outcomes that should be monitored and assessed to determine if the program is having its desired effects. Ideally, the evaluation should provide information that can be used to modify the educational goals or to develop new curricular components based on the strengths and deficiencies of the program (See Table 35-1). As with other rotations in residency or fellowship training, a faculty member, likely the Medical Director of the transport program, should provide a timely performance evaluation to the housestaff who participate on transport. Approaching the evaluation in terms of the three general skills areas that are targeted for development seems most appropriate. Thus, cognitive, technical, and communication skills each will require their own means of assessment. Cognitive skills can be monitored using the case review conferences, mock case scenarios, or supervised transports. Cognitive outcomes to be assessed may include fund of knowledge, ability to prioritize, independence, and decision-making skills. Technical skills can be monitored by tracking total number and success rates for individual procedures. Finally, communication skills can be assessed using nursing evaluation, performance in role-playing scenarios, or through sampling the opinions of referring hospital personnel.

Evaluation of the overall educational program can be accomplished using faculty impressions, housestaff self-assessment and impressions, or characterization of the patient mix to illustrate the scope of clinical exposure for housestaff on transport. This evaluation should attempt to identify those aspects of the educational program that are unique to transport as well as those that complement other clinical rotations in the training program.

DEVELOPING A MORE ACADEMIC ENVIRONMENT

Participation in outreach education, attendance at national educational and scientific meetings in the field of pediatric transport, and participation in transport research are all activities designated by the American Academy of Pediatrics as helpful training strategies.[3] These educational activities are best used by programs which have the training of future local or national leaders in transport medicine as one of their educational goals.

Outreach educational programs can better prepare referring hospital personnel to perform the initial stabilization and resuscitation of transported patients. These activities can also improve communication between the referring hospitals and the tertiary care center. The participation of transport personnel in these activities can improve the public relations of the team in the community.

Because of its relative infancy, virtually every aspect of the practice of transport medicine requires rigorous, objective evaluation. In 1990 a National Pediatric Transport Leadership conference established priorities for future transport research.[14] Areas in need of evaluation include development of a triage tool to determine need for a physician on the transport team, examination of current practice standards, establishment of guidelines for

TABLE 35-1 DIDACTIC CONFERENCES WITH LEARNING OBJECTIVES AND SAMPLE CASES

Conference	*Objectives*	*Sample cases*
The Pediatric Airway	Knowledge of the anatomical features unique to the pediatric airway. Assessment of airway obstruction. Indications for tracheal intubation.	4 year old with epiglottitis.
Shock/Sepsis	Recognition of signs/symptoms of shock. Priorities in management. Monitoring and reassessment.	6 month old with severe diarrhea. 2 year old with meningococcemia.
Congenital Heart Disease	Evaluation of suspected congenital heart disease. Knowledge of the common physiologies. Indications for and complications of prostaglandin infusions.	Newborn with cyanosis. Newborn with a murmur.
Trauma	Proper evaluation of the trauma patient. C-spine stabilization for transport. Management of intracranial hypertension.	5 year old struck by a car.
Coma	Interpretation of the physical exam. Constructing a differential diagnosis. Priorities in management.	3 year old with fever and altered mental status (meningoencephalitis).
Seizures	Proper use of medications. Assessment of need for tracheal intubation. Diagnostic evaluation prior to transport.	3 year old in status epilepticus.
Toxicology	Knowledge of common presenting signs and symptoms of serious poisonings. Decontamination strategies. Priorities in management.	15 year old with a TCA overdose.
Common Surgical Problems	Knowledge of surgical conditions requiring emergent transport.	Newborn with an abdominal wall defect.
Multiple Congenital Anomalies	Recognition of major syndromes. Assessment of priorities in management.	Newborn with Trisomy 13
Premature Infants	Knowledge of the conditions commonly seen in premature infants. Management of Respiratory Distress Syndrome. Presentation, evaluation and management of a pneumothorax.	Newborn 28 week infant with RDS.
Near Drowning	Knowledge of the pathophysiology of drowning. Priorities in management.	7 year old submerged for 5 minutes.
Smoke Inhalation	Assessment of physical findings. Indications for tracheal intubation. Interpretation of lab values (COHb).	4 year old unconscious from a house fire.

Continued

TABLE 35-1 DIDACTIC CONFERENCES WITH LEARNING OBJECTIVES AND SAMPLE CASES—cont'd

Conference	*Objectives*	*Sample cases*
Diabetic Ketoacidosis	Knowledge of the pathophysiology of DKA. Assessment of hydration. Priorities in management.	12 year old 20% dehydrated from DKA.
Monitoring on Transport	Knowledge of the limitations of monitoring on transport. Familiarity with new technologies available for portable monitoring.	Assessment of endotracheal tube position in the ambulance.
Grief and Bereavement	Knowledge and recognition of coping mechanisms used by families and medical staff. How to give bad news to parents.	Child requiring CPR prior to transport.
In programs which utilize aeromedical transport regularly:		
Aviation Physiology	Knowledge of the effects of altitude on oxygenation. Knowledge of other physiologic effects of flight.	Newborn on mechanical ventilation with chest tubes requiring high altitude helicopter transport.

nonpediatric transport systems, and determination of a variety of factors to measure the impact of transport on patient outcome. Further development of transport medicine as an academic subspecialty will rely on the interest and commitment of future physician directors of individual programs. One strategy to identify these persons as early as possible in their training is to encourage residents and fellows, whenever possible, to participate in transport research and outreach education. Results of properly conducted research should be presented at national meetings to disseminate new information as it becomes available. Attendance at national meetings also encourages the sharing of a variety of experiences related to transport. Through participation in these activities, interested housestaff or faculty can further develop the skills required both to successfully direct local transport programs and to guide the future direction of transport medicine on a national level.

SUMMARY

Participation in transport activities can be an important part of the education of residents and fellows. Transport medicine addresses a number of the educational objectives outlined in the guidelines for pediatric residency training, as well as those for critical care medicine, emergency medicine, and neonatology fellowship programs. The first step in making a transport experience educational for housestaff is to recognize this is an important goal of the transport program in an individual institution. Suggestions for how to plan and implement a comprehensive educational program in transport medicine have been presented. The success of the program depends to a great extent upon the interest and commitment of the Medical Director of the transport team. This person is responsible for creating an academic atmosphere where residents and fellows can develop a number of cognitive, procedural, and communications skills while delivering the highest quality patient care. Educating residents and fellows in transport may stimulate some to pursue transport medicine as a subspecialty interest of either critical care, emergency medicine, or neonatology. The development of transport medicine as an academic field depends upon maintaining quality patient care in an environment of planned education and investigation.

REFERENCES

1. American Academy of Pediatrics, Committee on Hospital Care: Guidelines for air and ground transportation of pediatric patients, *Pediatrics* 78:943, 1986.
2. American Academy of Pediatrics, Section of Emergency Medicine: Pediatric emergency medicine (PEM) fellowship curriculum statement, *Ped Emerg Care* 9:60, 1993.
3. American Academy of Pediatrics, Task Force on Interhospital Transport: *Guidelines for air and ground transport of neonatal and pediatric patients,* Chicago, 1993, The Association.
4. American College of Surgeons: *Advanced trauma life support course,* Chicago, 1989, The Association.
5. American Heart Association and the American Academy of Pediatrics: *Textbook of neonatal resuscitation,* Dallas, 1987, The Association.
6. American Heart Association and the American Academy of Pediatrics: *Textbook of pediatric advanced life support,* Dallas, 1988, The Association.
7. American Medical Association: *Policy Compendium 1992,* Policy #295.943, Chicago, 1992, The Association.
8. American Medical Association: Special requirements for residency training in neonatal-perinatal medicine. In *Graduate medical education directory,* Chicago, 1993, The Association.
9. American Medical Association: Special requirements for residency training in pediatric critical care medicine. In *Graduate medical education directory,* Chicago, 1993, The Association.
10. American Medical Association: Special requirements for residency training in pediatrics. In *Graduate medical education directory,* Chicago, 1993, The Association.
11. Baxt WG, Moody P: The impact of a physician as part of the aeromedical prehospital team in patients with blunt trauma, *JAMA* 257:3246, 1987.
12. Beyer AJ, Land G, Zaritsky A: Nonphysician transport of intubated pediatric patients: a system evaluation, *Crit Care Med* 20:961, 1992.
13. Connolly HV, Fetcho S, Hageman JR: Education of personnel involved in the transport program, *Crit Care Clin* 8:481, 1992.
14. Day S and others: Pediatric interhospital critical care transport: consensus of a national leadership conference, *Pediatrics* 88:696, 1991.
15. Day S, McCloskey K, King W: Survey of pediatric critical care transport (PCCT) programs: team member training, (abstract) *Ped Emerg Care* 8:373, 1992.
16. Dobrin RS and others: The development of a pediatric emergency transport system, *Ped Clin N Amer* 27:633, 1980.
17. Durbin DR, Giardino AP, Costarino AT: The evaluation of an educational program for housestaff on transport (abstract), *Ped Emerg Care* (in press), 1993.
18. Frehill K: Critical incident stress debriefing in health care, *Crit Care Clin* 8:491, 1992.
19. Frischer L, Gutterman DL: Emotional impact on parents of transported babies, *Crit Care Clin* 8:649, 1992.
20. Giardino AP, Burns KM, Giardino, ER: The educational value of pediatric emergency transport: by design or by default? *Ped Emerg Care* (in press), 1993.
21. Hamman BC and others: Helicopter transport of trauma victims: Does a physician make a difference? *J Trauma* 31:490, 1991.
22. Hardwick W, King W, McCloskey K: Comparison of second and third year pediatric residents on critical care transports (abstract), *Ped Emerg Care* 8:372, 1992.
23. Kallsen G, Merritt-Lindgren M: An emergency medical services curriculum for emergency medicine residencies, *Ann Emerg Med* 13:912, 1984.
24. Kim SC and others: Efficacy of a computer-based tutorial for teaching students about sickle cell disease (abstract), *AJDC* 147:454, 1993.
25. Laufer MD: One resident's opinion: problems with emergency medicine transports (letter), *JAMA* 262: 1954, 1989.
26. McCloskey KA and others: Variables predicting the need for a pediatric critical care transport team, *Ped Emerg Care* 8:1, 1992.
27. McCloskey KA, Johnston C: Critical care interhospital transports: predictability of the need for a pediatrician, *Ped Emerg Care* 6:89, 1990.
28. McCloskey KA, Johnston C: Pediatric critical care transport survey: Team composition and training, mobilization time, and mode of transportation, *Ped Emerg Care* 6:1, 1990.
29. McCloskey KA, King WD, Byron C: Pediatric critical care transport: is a physician always needed on the team? *Ann Emerg Med* 18:247, 1989.
30. Piemme T: Computer-assisted learning and evaluation in medicine, *JAMA* 260:367, 1988.
31. Rose WD and others: Field experience in aeromedical transport for an emergency medicine residency (letter), *Am J Emerg Med* 6:82, 1988.
32. Rubenstein JS and others: Can the need for a physician as part of the pediatric transport team be predicted? A prospective study, *Crit Care Med* 20:1657, 1992.
33. Schwartz W: Using the computer-assisted medical problem-solving (CAMPS) system to identify students' problem-solving difficulties, *Academic Med* 67:568, 1992.
34. Smith DF, Hackel A: Selection criteria for pediatric critical care transport teams, *Crit Care Clin* 11:10, 1983.
35. Stewart RD, Paris PM, Heller MB: Design of a resident in-field experience for an emergency medicine residency curriculum, *Ann Emerg Med* 16:175, 1987.

36

LEGAL ISSUES RELATED TO TRANSPORT

BARBARA J. YOUNGBERG

(Portions of this chapter were adapted from a previous work by the author, Medical-Legal Consideration's Involved in the Transport of Critically Ill Patients. Printed in *Critical Care Clinics*, 8:501-511, 1992)

The transportation of critically ill children and neonates can give rise to a number of legal issues which may not initially seem obvious to the providers involved in planning a transport program. The purpose of this chapter is to discuss the legal theories which are often associated with medical negligence and to explain how those theories can become complicated by the very nature of the transport process. In addition, regulations which impact patient transport (such as COBRA) will be discussed with the current interpretation of the law explained. Proactive strategies will be suggested which incorporate legislative mandates, case law, and good program management into policies and procedures which define the scope of service and the method for providing and evaluating care.

The underlying premise in developing a strong transport program is that a variety of operational factors must be evaluated as potential areas of exposure for both individual providers and the facility sponsoring the transport program. Such elements might include the population to be served, who will provide the majority of care (physicians versus nurses), to whom the service will be offered, and the primary purpose of the transport program (e.g., to make available tertiary care services to patients who are located in rural areas or other locations where specialty services are not readily available, to enhance referrals, or to participate in a trauma network program). Once these elements are identified, providers must then evaluate the legislative, regulatory, and environmental factors which help to shape the provision of that care.

The liability issues generated by the transfer/transport process can be categorized into exposures faced by the referring institution, those confronted by the transporting entity, and/or receiving institution, and those issues which may arise specific to the professionals involved in the transport process. In some cases liability may extend or overlap to all areas. In addition, it is important to understand how the elements of negligence, which give rise to malpractice claims, are blurred because of the very nature of the transport process and can cause additional overlap of liability. This knowledge will guide the practitioner seeking to establish a proactive transport program which will anticipate potential problems and develop policies and other protocol which will help to ensure that legal issues do not arise.

LEGISLATIVE, REGULATORY & INSURANCE ISSUES

Understanding the law of malpractice

Medical malpractice has become an area of significant concern for health care facilities and providers. The rise of claims against both the hospital and its physicians and nurses has been the source of much controversy and is now the subject of legislative debate and tort reform. Health care attorneys and risk managers have continually worked within the health care setting to educate staff on the elements of negligence and ways to minimize the likelihood of being named in a lawsuit. Understanding the legal theories upon which liability can be based is an important first step in the tailoring of a transport program which will protect the hospital and transport staff from risk and which will allow for the provision of the highest possible care to all pediatric patients.[9]

Understanding negligence in the context of patient transport

The four elements of negligence which must be established prior to a plaintiff prevailing in a malpractice action are as follows:

- Establishing a duty to provide care.
- Determining that a provider breached that duty by providing care which was less than an agreed upon standard of care.
- Proving that the patient was injured and that the injury was proximately caused by the breach.
- Proving that measurable damages were sustained by the plaintiff/patient.

The duty to provide care

The first element of duty is always the easiest element in the hospital malpractice case. Courts agree that a duty is established as soon as the hospital agrees to treat the patient. In a transport situation this element is often considerably more difficult to prove. When a transport team arrives at the referring hospital they often find the transferring physician continuing to provide care. They may also find that orders which they gave at the time of the initial call either were not carried out, were carried out improperly, were given based on an improper assessment. Questions often arise which relate to the point at which care, responsibility, and accountability are transferred from the referring hospital to members of the transport team and/or the receiving hospital. Clarifying this issue prior to the team's arrival at the hospital is essential and should always be addressed in written agreements acknowledged by all current and future participants in the transport program. Even if formal legal contracts are not signed by the transport program and its sponsoring hospital and referral hospital, statements of policy/procedure/protocol can be developed which specifically address these issues.

Determining breach of duty

The question of breach of duty is by far the most difficult one to answer in any malpractice case. In general, a breach of duty occurs when a professional provides care which is inconsistent with the type of care which would have been provided by any reasonable practitioner with the same level of skill practicing in the same type of setting. If a professional's behavior is found to have fallen below the standard, the next question will be whether or not that breach caused the patient's injury. Questions related to the appropriate standard of care to be used often are further confused if the standards of the referring hospital are different than the standards of the receiving hospital. An example is the situation where the referring hospital is a small rural hospital with little experience in the multiple trauma patient and the receiving hospital is a major urban trauma center. In some cases the plaintiff's counsel may attempt to focus blame, or at least responsibility, on the transport team members (even if the injury occurred while the patient was being treated by the referring hospital) in order to be able to use the higher standard of care and thereby more easily establish a breach of duty.

Careful and precise documentation of all treatments rendered and names of persons performing emergent and invasive procedures should always be clearly documented in the patient's medical record. Many hospitals have agreed to document all pretransport care on their hospital's record (evidencing their full responsibility for their actions) and begin documenting on the transport team record once the duty and responsibility shifts to the transport team. This procedure can be instrumental in identifying at what point the breach of duty actually occurred.

Although this solution sounds like a simple one, in transport situations the issue may be further complicated when the plan of care and type of intervention necessary can not be agreed upon by the referring hospital and members of the transport team. In those situations transport professionals should document that their plan of care cannot be implemented due to nonconcurrence of the referring hospital, which still has physical control of the patient. They should also document instances in which the patient's condition does not warrant transport and is so determined after the team arrives on the scene. Obviously, the wishes of the patient and/or the patient's family must be considered prior to refusing transport. In another situation the establishment of a duty to treat may become an issue if the referring hospital misrepresents to the receiving hospital the condition or needs of the patient and the receiving hospital accepts transfer under a set of circumstances which change or are more clearly understood once the team arrives on the scene. In some cases the transport team may recognize that the patient's problem could be best handled in a facility other than the designated receiving hospital. Ideally, transport teams should maintain agreements with regional hospitals which provide highly specialized services (for example hyperbaric chambers) and can then make arrangements to transport the patient to the most appropriate facility. Allowing for a court determination regarding when the transport team has accepted a patient and has a duty to provide reasonable care is critical in many cases where patient transport is involved.

Establishing proximate cause

Establishment of proximate cause can be very difficult in a transport situation where a number of caregivers are involved, many providing significant intervention. Many transport cases must analyze injury in light of the continuum of care received by the patient, including care rendered by first respondents, the referring hospital upon order by their attending physician, the referring hospital at the order of the transport team, or during the period of time when the team has assumed control and responsibility for the patient.

The issue of proximate cause is also often a difficult one to establish due to the fact that the patient in need of emergent treatment is critically ill and the severity of their condition can minimize the likelihood of recovery. Delay in the performance of life-saving measures can cause irreparable harm but, given the nature of the patient's condition and the many significant problems which necessitated intervention, it may be difficult to ascertain if the injury was a result of the presenting problem or a result of a particular intervention or lack of intervention. In many medical negligence cases which deal with critically ill patients, whose condition may change rapidly, it is often difficult, if not impossible, to determine which particular activity or intervention actually caused a deterioration or worsening of the patient's condition or the time at which the patient suffers a new injury or insult due to the interventions of the health care worker which have little or no relationship to the patient's presenting condition or pre-existing problems.

Generally, in transport situations the patient's condition is at the most critical stage, and their condition is most vulnerable to error. Timely and appropriate intervention, continuous and accurate assessment, and immediate modification of the treatment plan are necessary to ensure that the patient will have the greatest opportunity for recovery. Proper documentation during initial stabilization and transport, which includes a patient's response to all treatments rendered, will assist hospital and transport staff in overcoming allegations which link the provider's actions to patient injury or exacerbation of their illness. The development of comprehensive flow records which allow for the simple recording of assessments and interventions are critical to defend the care of providers in such situations.

Calculating damages

The final element of damages is a fairly simple legal concept. When lawsuits are filed, the issues generally are related to the amount of damages and how those damages are calculated, as opposed to the fact that the payment of some damages is appropriate. Damages are usually broken down into three areas. Actual damages, the easiest to calculate, seek to compensate the injured party for those experiences which are a direct result of the injury caused by the defendant. An example of this type of damage calculation might include a request to recover the costs associated with a surgical procedure to graft skin onto a tissue injury caused by an IV infiltration. Costs of the hospitalization as well as time lost from work would represent actual damages for such an injury. In general, the amount of money which would be needed to bring the patient back to preinjury status could all be included in the actual damage category. Special damages are the second type which can be assessed against a defendant, if liability is established. Special damages include those which are the natural but not a necessary result of the injury sustained. Special damages in a medical negligence case might include the wages lost by a family member who must take time off from work to visit the patient while in the hospital or to attend to them following discharge. Punitive damages are also at times assessed against an individual or against a hospital for particularly egregious acts or omissions. Punitive damages have little relationship to the actual injury but rather are imposed upon a defendant as a form of punishment. In a recent malpractice case,[6] a jury assessed $124 million in punitive damages (the largest in history) against a pharmaceutical company for callous behavior and reckless disregard for the safety of patients taking a particular medication and failure to warn physicians of the risks of using the prescribed medication. Although this amount was later reduced by the court, punitive damages remained part of the award. In other medical negligence cases, punitive awards are often assessed against hospitals who have knowledge of dangerous situations or conditions that could lead to patient injuries, and yet the hospital fails to correct them. Punitive awards could also be awarded in cases which involve hospitals which have knowledge of negligent or impaired caregivers yet continue to allow them to practice. In addition, many states still allow for the recovery of damages for pain and suffering and emotional distress, though in most states, caps are in place to limit the amount of damages recoverable. Pain and suffering of the patient or even that of the patient's family, who may have witnessed the incident surrounding the injury, may be assessed. Obviously, these last two types of damages are extremely difficult to accurately measure and are often left to the discretion of the jury. In many cases they can add millions of dollars to a final verdict.

In many cases where multiple defendants are named, the plaintiff's counsel may attempt to apportion damages, thereby, at least in theory, allowing each named defendant to pay for only that portion of the damage associated with the injury caused by their own negligence. State legislation addresses how apportionment works and also addresses issues associated with the concept of joint and several liability which may allow for a minimally negligent caregiver to pay a disproportionate share of the damages if codefendants are uninsured or have limits on their coverage.

When planning a transport program, one should consider judicial trends relative to damages. This would obviously include the evaluation of damage caps, verdict ranges for specific types of claims, and the economic realities of the community (which might include the standard of living, the rate of unemployment, and any other factors which could inflate or deflate the value of an injury). These factors could greatly influence the limits of insurance purchased, the cost of that insurance, and/or the amount of self-insurance funded.

Tort reform and its effect of medical negligence

Tort reform has been identified as a significant method for achieving control of both the economic and psychological costs of malpractice. In actuality, tort reform has done very little to date to significantly alter the number of malpractice claims or to reduce the awards. Recently, there has been considerable discussion about state-directed tort reform with the possible linkage of such reform to reimbursement and health care appropriation.

The most successful tort reform initiatives to date include the following items.

Penalties for frivolous suits. Thirty-two states have enacted legislation which provides for penalties for any party which files a frivolous suit. Some penalties are imposed only in cases where the cases are litigated to verdict, while others apply to cases dismissed prior to trial. The penalty usually takes the form of a fine and may also require the offending party to pay the other party's attorney fees and court costs.

Immunity protection. The doctrine of charitable immunity once insulated health care providers from civil liability if care was provided free of charge. Most states have abolished charitable immunity, as health care providers now, in most instances, are compensated for the care which they provide. Although Good Samaritan statutes still exist in most jurisdictions, they generally provide immunity only in emergency situations. Many states have moved to address the access to care problems created by malpractice by developing new immunity statutes. Seventeen states and the District of Columbia have passed statutes which provide some type of immunity to health care providers, often targeting those who provide free care or care to underserved populations. One example of this is a 1991 District of Columbia statute which provides limited immunity for obstetricians providing free care at neighborhood clinics.

Pretrial screening panels. Originally recommended by the Department of Health, Education, and Welfare's Commission on Medical Malpractice in 1973, pretrial screening panels were intended to expedite the resolution of medical malpractice claims and eliminate those without merit. Thirty-five states have now enacted some type of screening panel which is typically composed of a combination of physicians, lawyers, and consumers. Panel proceedings are generally informal, in that evidentiary rules are not followed nor are the panel deliberations recorded. The panel reviews the medical evidence presented by each party to the suit and renders a decision about the merits of the case. The panel's finding is then to be taken into consideration by the parties determining the resolution of the case. In some states, those findings can also be introduced into evidence by either party at trial.

Statutes of limitations. Statutes of limitations specify the time within which a plaintiff may file a lawsuit. Typically, the statute of limitations allows adult plaintiffs between two and four years to file suit after the date of malpractice, the date the malpractice is discovered, or some combination of the two. Minors usually have a much longer time period within which to file a claim, sometimes as long as 20 years.

Standard of care. The standard of care is the criteria against which a defendant's actions are judged. Traditionally, it has been defined as the care provided by the reasonable practitioner in similar circumstances. If the defendant fails to meet the standard of care and injures the patient, malpractice has occurred. Some tort reform advocates have argued that the standard of care has become too rigorous. Defendant health care providers are required to meet national standards available only in sophisticated medical settings rather than the local standard available in the communities in which they practice. They have also argued that standards of care which are too rigorous have led to the practice of defensive medicine rather than reasonable care, thereby contributing to the escalation of health care costs. Fourteen states have addressed this problem by enacting legislation to modify the standard of care. Some states have reestablished the locality rule, which imposes a local rather than a national standard of care. Another trend is the use of practice parameters or guidelines to establish the standard of care. The most recent example is a 1992 Maine statute which provides physicians with an absolute defense to a claim of medical malpractice when they adhere to predetermined practice parameters.

Joint and several liability. This rule permits a plaintiff to collect the full amount awarded, regardless of the financial viability of the defendants, by making defendants liable for more than their share of liability. Thus, if a defendant is uninsured or underinsured, the plaintiff is assured of receiving the full amount of the verdict because the remaining defendants will contribute more than their allocated share of the award. Even defendants who have a very low percentage of liability may be forced to contribute the majority of the settlement. This doctrine promotes the practice of suing persons who purchase insurance and may have limits greater than those of other caregivers. Thirty-three states have enacted changes in the rule of joint and several liability. Some have eliminated it only for noneconomic damages, others have eliminated it for low-fault defendants, and still others have eliminated it entirely.

Periodic payments. States mandating periodic payments seek to ensure that, if a patient is injured and that injury will require long-term therapy or care, the money will be available. Generally, if a verdict is entered in an amount indicating the consideration of prolonged costs of care, the defendant will be able to purchase an annuity or other investment plan which will enable a hospital to spend less money up-front for the settlement in guarantee for a long-term stream of benefits or payments.

Arbitration. Fifteen states have statutes specifically covering voluntary arbitration of medical malpractice claims. Some of the states include a general framework for arbitration; others are more specific in their requirements.[2] Arbitration (especially non-binding arbitration) has had little impact on medical malpractice. If effective, this approach could not only limit the costs of claims and their defense but also ensure more equitable and predictable results.

A unique approach to limiting liability

A unique approach is being tested in the state of Maine which allows for the elimination of the need to establish a standard of care if a physician adheres to predetermined practice parameters and risk management protocols. The specialty of emergency medicine is one of four represented in this project. In this project physicians develop standards of care to be adhered to while treating certain types of patient. If the standards are adhered to and the patient still suffers an injury or suboptimal outcome patients will be barred from claiming negligence. Physicians should follow this project as it potentially allows for a unique way to limit liability.

How tort reform could benefit/harm transport programs

A number of the measures described above could have a beneficial impact on the professionals involved in a transport program. Obviously, a hospital considering becoming involved in a transport contract should evaluate the status of beneficial tort reform in the jurisdictions where the program will be providing care. In instances where there are discrepancies between various state laws, provisions can be added to the contract to designate the forum and law which will control.

Understanding COBRA issues associated with transport

In 1986 the Emergency Medical Treatment and Active Labor Act of 1986 (EMTALA)[1] was added to the Social Security Act as section 1867. This act was actually section 9121 of the Consolidated Omnibus Budget Reconciliation Act of 1986, commonly referred to as COBRA. COBRA was drafted to prevent hospitals from refusing, limiting, or terminating patient care for financial reasons. Although enacted in August of 1986, COBRA underwent some important revisions which became effective in 1990. The requirements of the COBRA amendments broaden who is subject to the law and now includes all participating physicians and any other physician responsible for examination, treatment, or transfer of an individual in a participating hospital. This could include a physician who is "on call" for the care of an individual. Many recent court decisions have attempted to interpret this law for health care providers, but those opinions are ambiguous and at times even contradictory. Pronouncements from the Health Care Financing Administration (HCFA) and even directives from the Internal Revenue Service (IRS) have further added to the confusion. To complicate matters even further, some of the most recent court cases have been short-lived with one court decision being withdrawn following the receipt of a flurry of Amicus briefs (briefs filed by parties with an interest in the ultimate outcome) requesting reconsideration on the opinion.[4]

For the past 6 years health care providers have been attempting to gain a clear understanding of COBRA. The Health Care Financing Administration (HCFA) has taken the position that COBRA does not apply during prehospital ambulance runs and does not affect a hospital's ability to divert prehospital emergency patients due to the lack of bed capacity.[8] In late 1991 the IRS made clear its intention to cooperate with the Department of Health and Human Services (HHS) in determining whether a hospital's violation of the anti-kickback law is grounds for the hospital's tax exempt status.[3] The IRS has taken the position that COBRA violations are a basis for revocation. The IRS, however, in its most recent field auditor training manual, instructs its auditors to interview ambulance drivers and social workers (among other methods) in order to determine whether a hospital practices "radio triage" or if emergency medical personnel are asked to radio patients' insurance information in order to reroute uninsured patients to other facilities before they reach the emergency department.[5]

This new IRS interest and increased scrutiny only serves to increase the importance of hospital's compliance with COBRA. If fines and possible exclusion from Medicare are not serious enough, now nonprofit hospitals face the possible loss of tax exempt status as an additional consequence of a violation.

The act requires that the hospital evaluate all patients arriving at the hospital with emergency conditions and determine (and document) the appropriateness of treating the patient until stabilized before transferring the patient elsewhere. The patient (or responsible person if the patient is a minor or incompetent) always maintains the right to refuse to consent to the proposed transfer or treatment. In accordance with these provisions, the act requires the hospital to obtain the patient's written informed consent to refuse the offered treatment or transfer.

Although legal problems associated with COBRA are generally experienced by referring hospitals, transport teams should familiarize themselves with the law and recognize the fact that they can receive legal protection for "whistle blowing." This occurs when a physician or facility arranges for transport and that transport is later determined to be for financial reasons only.

Penalties for hospitals which violate COBRA provisions can be as high as $50,000 if it negligently violates the law; this amount decreases to $25,000 if hospitals have less than 100 beds. Because the interpretation of the law seems unclear, transport teams and hospital administration should carefully follow COBRA-related decisions in their jurisdiction and provide education to staff regarding the best method to ensure compliance.

Transport teams might also find it helpful to draft specific consent to transfer forms which contain specific language evidencing compliance with the mandates of COBRA. Language in the form should describe the medical screening exam which was performed, the reason for the transfer, the fact that the patient's condition will safely allow for transfer, and evidence that the patient or their guardian understands the reasons for consent and agrees to them. A thorough transfer documentation form can help to alleviate any potential allegations related to violation of COBRA.

Purchasing professional liability insurance

Determining the type of insurance policy necessary to protect staff members is also critical prior to the onset of the program. Although many malpractice policies contain standard "boilerplate language," additional endorsements can be added to cover some of the unique risks which may be associated with a transport program. You should always consult your hospital counsel, risk manager, or local broker for assistance in drafting these additional endorsements. Once purchased, copies of the policies should be reviewed by all members of the transport team so that they are certain of the conditions of coverage.

Prior to purchasing coverage, you should also determine the possibility of the presence of immunity for professionals who may be employees of state institutions or agencies receiving such protection. In some instances professionals who are protected by immunity actually heighten the likelihood of being sued if they independently purchase liability insurance.

You may also wish to check the insurance policies of the referring institutions which will be participating in the program. It will be important to ensure that coverage provided to referring hospitals and their practitioners dovetails with the coverage which the receiving hospital will purchase. Many hospitals also stipulate that they will only provide transport services to those hospitals which have a mandatory one million dollar minimum insurance requirement.

CLINICAL AND OPERATIONAL ISSUES

Training of the transport team

A well-trained transport team is essential for providing high quality care and the most advanced intervention with a minimum of risk. Initially, those persons responsible for setting up a transport program will need to identify the types of professionals which they will hire to support the program. As for any other aspect of the program development, one must consider state statutes and advanced practice acts in the states to be served by the team, which might specify restrictions or enhancements to various professionals level of practice. Obviously, prior to hiring staff you would also want to identify the type of patient whom you believe will most often avail themselves to the transport program (e.g., will the program focus on neonatal transfers to the NICU, pediatric trauma, or voluntary transfers to hospitals preferred by the parents).

If a specific patient population (for example high-risk neonates) are to be the focus of the program, obviously you would wish to recruit professionals with special expertise in the care of the neonate. If the team plans to treat a variety of patients, the team could decide to hire a variety of specially trained professionals or hire staff with strong critical care skills and offer them training in relation to the specific patient populations. The use of respiratory therapists, emergency medical technicians, or paramedics should also be discussed, and if such professionals are to be a part of the team, their roles must be clearly defined.

The use of the physician is essential in the development of standing orders and in the continual assessment of the patient and initiation of the plan of care. Specific patients may be identified in advance which will always require the attendance of a physician during transport. Even if physicians are not routinely members of the transport team, they should always be available by telephone or radio communication. A system should be developed which allows for the professional delegation of responsibility. Only if the various professionals work together as a team will the quality of care provided be maximized.

Although hiring experienced and professional staff is essential to a high quality program, on-going continued education and frequent technical skills training must be part of every transport program's method for ensuring competent and capable staff. Documentation of initial verification of skills and periodic reappraisal is essential in making an argument supporting the continued competence of staff. Besides the technical knowledge which is essential for the provision of quality of care, staff should also receive information on informed consent, documentation, and new regulations and legislation which may have an impact on their practice.

Clinical indicators as a method for review

Prerequisite to establishing a proactive monitoring and evaluation program is the identification of the aspects of care to be evaluated. These aspects of care should be selected on the basis of the scope of the care which is being provided. After defining the full scope of care, it will be evident that it is impractical to monitor all services provided. To focus monitoring efforts, members of the transport team should identify those aspects which have the most significant impact on patient care. Aspects of care may be important because they involve large numbers of patients (high-volume), have significant potential for patient harm if inappropriately managed (high-risk) or have been an area of difficulty in the past for patient or transport staff (see Table 36-1).

Many transport programs have modeled their internal quality review processes to the organization wide quality improvement initiatives as prescribed by the Joint Commission on the Accreditation of Healthcare Organizations (JCAHO) and other regulatory agencies. In addition, many payors and business coalitions are now also requesting that services for which they contract provide evidence of high quality and evidence of a process which stresses systematic and continuous review of the care and service provided. Results of the analysis should be utilized by members of the transport team to refine and improve upon the transport process. Consistently favorable trends can also be very helpful in gaining a marketing advantage when competing with other transport programs for business. Prior to implementation, indicators

TABLE 36-1 EXAMPLES OF INDICATORS FOR SELECTED ASPECTS OF CARE

Indicator to be measured	*What is measured*	*Why measured*
Appropriateness of transport	Necessity	HR,HV
Patient deterioration during transport	Process & outcome	HR,PP
Initiation of invasive procedures	Process & outcome	HR,PP
Maintenance of technical skills	Process	HR
Availability of appropriate equipment and supplies	Structure	PP
Death/discharge within 48 hours	Process, outcome & necessity	HR
Team management of the neonate	Process & outcome	HR
Medication initiation	Process	HV

HR = High-risk service, HV = High-volume service, PP = Problem-prone service

should be evaluated and tested for the availability of data, practical measurability, and content validity. Thought should be given to the delegation of data collection to those who are best positioned to gather that data in a timely and accurate manner. Multidisciplinary review of the analysis of the data will help to enhance individual accountability for patient care and to maximize continuous staff education and program improvement.

Informed consent issues

A number of issues can arise related to the informed consent process in a transport situation. In general, consent provided by a competent patient or their guardian is a prerequisite to any type of medical treatment or intervention. Medical treatment without such consent constitutes battery. There are two types of consent which have been identified: express consent and implied consent. Express consent occurs when a patient or their guardian gives a health care provider explicit permission to provide care or to transfer the patient to a facility where appropriate care is available. Implied consent, on the other hand, occurs when the actions of a patient (or the guardian of the patient) are deemed to be sufficient to imply to the reasonable person that consent is not being withheld. In many emergency situations public policy and state law generally support the assumption of implied consent for medical care when the patient is unable to provide explicit consent and when there are no other persons available to speak on behalf of the patient. Individual state laws should be consulted when drafting policies related to consent and transport teams should be aware of the need to check state laws in all states wherein they may be providing care rather than only the state where the transport program is located. As a general rule, most states define emergency treatment as treatment which is necessary to prevent an immediate threat to life, limb, or health of a patient. If the condition of the patient is likely to rapidly deteriorate without treatment, such treatment can in most cases also be justified.

Transport team members should be aware that, in issues related to consent, it is the process that is important, not merely the signing of the form. Although excellent forms can be developed which provide the patient with information which is necessary to assist them in their decision-making as it relates to health care, they should not be the sole representation of the informed consent process. Interactive dialogue should also take place which will allow the patient and/or the patient's family to receive clarification about aspects of their care or transport which may not be easily understood or explained by a form.

Legal terminology defines the age of majority and the special conditions which might allow for a minor to consent for emergency treatment. Many states also define how standard consent procedures can be modified in the event of an emergency. Familiarizing transport staff with ways to handle unique situations before they become a matter of life and death will greatly reduce confusion and apprehension related to consent at the time of transport.

It is uncontroverted that each patient care situation presents the providers with unique circumstances and challenges. Tailoring the consent process to be one which takes into consideration these unique characteristics will ensure that legal issues do not arise related to the issue of consent. In general, the best rule to follow is that the safety of the patient should always be uppermost in the decision-making process, and health care professionals who remember to always put the patient's need first will be less likely to incur liability. This issue may be further clouded if the patient or the patients family refuses transfer despite the fact that transport would clearly provide the patient with the greatest chance for survival. When issues related to informed consent arise, patients or their families should be given an accurate assessment of the patient's condition and what may occur if immediate transfer is not accomplished. Once this information is provided, the team will have to abide by the patient's decision and document carefully and completely the discussions which occurred between the patient and the provider and the patient's reluctance or refusal to accept the recommended treatment.

The importance of documentation

Errors in documentation or documentation which is incomplete or poorly written can greatly hinder the ability of defense counsel to defend the care which is provided by the transport team and physicians responsible for the care of transported patients. Because cases of medical negligence often take years to reach the trial phase, providers should be advised that very often the records which reflect the care rendered to patients will be the only way to review and corroborate the testimony related to the care which you provided to a patient and could well be the sole factor which establishes or disproves your negligence.

Important case law should also be reviewed which relates to the preservation of evidence associated with the documentation of patient care and other interventions and which can now result in significant damage awards when such evidence is lost, misplaced, or destroyed. Allegations related to the spoliation of medical evidence have in recent cases[7] resulted in a punitive damage award and the presumption that such material was "lost for a reason"—that reason being the attempt to hide information which could allow the patient to establish a claim of fault against the health care provider. In those cases where spoliation of evidence is alleged, a change in trial procedure also occurs which places the burden of proving that the information was inadvertently lost and was not lost as a means of "covering up" negligence on the hospital. In cases where spoliation is not alleged, the burden of establishing a case of negligence rests with the plaintiff.

Preserving the integrity of the medical record

Hospitals setting up transport programs should recognize that simple measures can be taken by transport personnel which can be instituted to help guarantee that vital information collected at the time of transport will be retained and become a permanent part of the patient's medical record. Developing initial assessment and flow sheets which allow for the placement of check marks to evidence critical areas of assessment or changes in the patient's condition, and having a receptacle where all rhythm strips, monitoring strips, etc. can be placed will help to ensure the completeness and accuracy of the transport medical record. Transport teams should always allow themselves adequate time immediately following a transport to complete all documentation and to carefully review it to verify that all of the information is accurate and represents what occurred from the first encounter with the referring hospital to the acceptance into the unit by the receiving hospital. A health care professional who documents with the assumption that their care will be scrutinized by a third party (or a jury) will consistently write more complete and accurate notes.

Incorporating risk management strategies into a proactive quality program

Traditional systems of risk management have been based on the premise that hospitals and health care providers would respond to patient injuries after they occurred and retroactively develop systems to correct existing systems which contributed to the patient's injury. Traditional risk management programs focused more on the purchase of insurance

BOX 36-1 TIPS ON AVOIDING LIABILITY ASSOCIATED WITH TRANSPORT PROGRAMS

- Transport situations can be very tense, and rescue/stabilization can often occur in the presence of family members. Train all staff to respond professionally and avoid the use of terms and jargon which can give the family a negative impression of the transport team.
- The legal system is often very subjective (reflecting the view of the layperson who has minimal knowledge) and may include knowledge which is incorrectly fueled by sensational media or television portrayals. If transport personnel are ever involved in litigation, they should keep this in mind and present themselves in a sympathetic, professional manner. A callous or arrogant attitude during any part of the litigation process can result in a verdict for the plaintiff, even if clear liability is not established.
- Train all personnel to be very careful regarding what is said over radio/telemetry communication. These tapes may be admitted into evidence and can be very damaging.
- If you are in the business of transporting adults, children, and neonates, you should have a system which ensures that unidose drugs and equipment are always available to respond to all emergencies. Developing charts or posters which provide appropriate dose ranges and or equipment sizes can avoid liability associated with the use of improper equipment.
- If you market yourself to customers and referral physicians and hospitals based on representations about your skills and abilities you may be at fault if you do not live up to these representations. Training of the transport team should always be consistent with how the program is marketed.
- Develop and support a proactive evaluation program for all transports which allows for multidisciplinary review of high-risk or problem prone care. This will allow for the identification and resolution of potential problems before they become patient injuries.
- Proper training of the professional transport staff is essential. Many hospitals believe that hiring qualified staff assures them of high quality care. They should be advised that skills training is essential as an on-going activity and that procedures which are not used often in the field should be maintained in the lab or in the hospital setting. Including professionals (physicians and nurses) who work in the referring hospitals and who have the responsibility for initial stabilization of patients prior to transfer can also result in an improvement of patient care.
- Care should be taken, when purchasing liability insurance for the team, that all aspects of their responsibilities are covered. It may at times be necessary to work with the carrier providing coverage to negotiate for additional endorsements to the standard policy which protect all of the team members from the high-risk activities which they may be called upon to perform.
- Keep apprised of all laws which could impact the operation of the transport program. Obtain advice from in-house counsel about the impact of new laws or regulations which could impact upon the success of the program.

and the defense of the professional providing the care than on the inherent system problems which caused the patient injury to occur. Proactive risk management programs seek to identify areas of potential problems and develop system solutions to address those problems prior to the injury of a patient and dovetail quite appropriately with the type of proactive monitoring and evaluation program already described. A great part of a proactive risk management program also revolves around education and preparation of staff so that they become familiar with both the legal process and with the reasons why liability typically occurs in transport situations. Regular reviews of care which result in litigation should become part of each transport programs quality review process and should allow for and promote a multidisciplinary review of the care provided. The focus of these reviews should always be on identifying the problems within the system which prevented optimal care from being provided. Focusing fault on an individual care giver generally will do little to enhance quality and will make members of the transport team uncomfortable about the quality review/risk management process. Health care attorneys and hospital administrators should be requested to attend so that they can assist in the development of a defense strategy and so that they can be made aware of system problems which require correction to prevent additional patient or staff injuries.

It is equally important to include in the education process those professionals from the hospitals who will be referring patients to the transport program. Such outreach programs have dual benefit. First they assist in making referring hospital staff and physicians feel a part of the team which provides quality care to the critically ill or injured patient. By doing this, the stature of the staff at the referring hospital is elevated. Second, it provides the referring hospital with essential information about pretransfer stabilization and the importance of early intervention and treatment as related to successful patient outcomes. This high quality interactive type of learning activity can be one rarely offered in the small rural or community hospital setting and can greatly enhance the level of care provided upon admission and the overall quality of care which the patient receives.

In addition, a systematic review process should be developed which enables the transport staff to review the care rendered to an identified group of patients (with similar presenting problems whose outcomes often give rise to litigation in transport settings. Clinical care should be evaluated in all of the following patients because of the frequency in which these patients become the plaintiffs in malpractice litigation or the damage award which accompanies a finding of negligence:

- All patients who die during transport.
- All patients who suffer neurologic damage prior to, during, or immediately following transport.
- All patients transferred out of receiving hospital within 24 hours following transport.
- Any patient who is transferred without consent (either direct consent or consent from family member or significant other).
- Any patient who develops a significant hematoma or extravasation injury resulting from the infusion into tissue of medication.
- Injuries to patients resulting from difficult intubation.
- Pneumothoraces which develop during transport or which are undetected prior to leaving the referring hospital or scene.

In addition, review of the process of care should also be undertaken when any of the following occur (these could help prevent situations where patients are injured):

- Occurrence of lack of appropriate supplies or medications during transport (with or without patient injury).
- Equipment malfunction (with or without patient injury).
- Loss of parts of the medical record, such as ECG or fetal monitoring strips, especially if these records substantiate a change in the patients condition which is documented in the record.
- Administrative problems which arise between referring and receiving hospital which delay the appropriate intervention or the transport.
- Issues related to improper communication between members of the transport team where orders are questioned or are not carried out.
- Deviations from agreed upon policies/procedures or protocols or breaches in conditions or signed contracts between referring and receiving hospitals.

Conclusion

The successful operation of a pediatric transport program requires careful planning, meticulous attention to changes in the legislative and regulatory environment, and a proactive approach to continuously improving the structure, process, and outcomes of care. Communicating these goals to all persons who are part of the transport network will further help to ensure that all patients will receive optimum care.

REFERENCES

1. EMTALA: Consolidated Omnibus Budget Reconciliation Act of 1986, §9121, 42 U.S.C.§1395dd.
2. GAO Report: Medical malpractice; alternative to litigation, 1992, GAO/HRD.
3. IRS: General Counsel Memorandum 39862, 1991.
4. *Johnson v University of Chicago Hospitals,* WL 259404 (Ill. Cir. 7), 1992.
5. Medicare Compliance Alert, vol 4, no 21, 1992.

6. *Proctor v Upjohn Company, 284 A 578 WL (Ill. Dist. 1) 1994.*
7. *Rodger's v St. Mary's Hospital of Decatur,* 198 Ill. 3d 871, 556 NE 2d 913 (190) and *Public Health Trust of Dade County v Valcin,* 507 So 2d 596 (Fla. Sup) 1987.
8. Tirone AJ: Personal communication. August 27, 1992, January 6, 1992.
9. Youngberg BJ: Medical-legal considerations involved in the transport of critically ill patients, *Critical Care Clinics,* 8:501-511, 1992.

37

COMMUNITY OUTREACH

KARIN A. McCLOSKEY
ROBERT B. LEMBERSKY

IMPORTANCE

A community outreach program is one of the most important elements of a critical care transport program. The goal of outreach is to provide education to staff members of emergency departments which rarely treat children. The goals of the education include 1) improvement in pediatric stabilization, 2) increased comfort and confidence in managing childhood illnesses and injuries, 3) the ability to make appropriate choices for mode of transport, and hopefully, 4) improvement in long-term outcome of the patient's illness or injury. The referring hospital can also learn techniques to prepare for pediatric transport teams, thus improving efficiency. The referring hospital medical team and the transport team can get to know each other and learn each other's capabilities. A well-developed community outreach education program can create or enhance respect for a tertiary care center. If multiple competing tertiary pediatric or neonatal centers serve the same geographical area, outreach can result in increased referrals to a particular center.

One of the most important reasons for a good outreach program involves the concept of the critical care continuum. Often both the lay public and medical care professionals upon hearing the words "critical care" envision an intensive care unit. The ICU is in fact only the final step in a long series of elements of the critical care continuum. This continuum reaches from lay response to the illness or injury to prehospital care to community hospital stabilization to interhospital transport to tertiary center emergency department stabilization and then to the ICU. Optimal outcome for the critically ill or injured patient depends on appropriate care at each step of the continuum. Some steps in the process may be unnecessary (for example when prehospital systems bring a patient directly to a tertiary center emergency department), but *no* patient ever reaches the ICU without some prior medical contact. Failure of appropriate care at any step may result in an inability of the ICU to affect an optimal outcome. The critical care transport team is in the unique position of enhancing care at multiple levels of this continuum because of its direct contact with both the community hospital and the tertiary center.

The success of a critical care transport team is also affected by its relationship with the community it serves.[16] Community relations should be seen as planned, active, continuing participation with a community in order to maintain and enhance its environment to the benefit of both parties.[15] Analysis of the hospitals that a transport team serves, with an understanding of special requirements and capabilities of the facilities and staff, should be conducted periodically. Input from the hospitals should be encouraged and communication access maintained. The director of the transport team should be easily identified and should maintain an open door policy for both questions and complaints.[7]

OUTREACH EDUCATORS

Personnel who are regularly part of the transport team itself are the optimal outreach educators. These individuals are the experts on how the system actually works.[17] Outreach education should specifically not be done by administrative personnel who have never been transport team members and who cannot provide the insight that the hands-on crew has. Since, practically speaking, most outreach programs will be presented primarily to nurses, transport nurses should participate in the process. If paramedics, respiratory therapists, or physicians are routinely part of the team, they too should be represented. It is very useful for the team's medical director to participate in the program. He or she can associate a face with a name on the letterhead and can personally demonstrate (partially by virtue of presence at the program) an availability to respond to any problems encountered with the team. Too often, concerns are not forwarded to the transport leadership, preventing improvements in the system or clarification of misunderstandings.

COSTS AND BENEFITS

The costs of a community outreach program include salary for personnel as well as travel time to the referral hospital, possible overnight stays if that hospital is several hours away or is receiving multiple or prolonged programs (see below), and the cost of any printed materials or promotional items distributed (key rings, penlights, pens, etc. with the team's name and number). Relative to the cost of other hospital programs or of the transport system itself, community outreach is a bargain. The benefits of a properly developed program should far outweigh the costs.

If the team has full-time, dedicated transport personnel, they can develop the program during their downtime and can provide presentations at an hourly rate on off-time. Alternatively, outreach can be built in as a part of the job description and planned as a certain number of a team member's work hours. In addition, team members who temporarily cannot transport due to illness precluding flight, injury precluding the physical demands of transport, or the late stages of (or complications of) pregnancy can continue to perform as useful members of the system through outreach duties.

THE CUSTOMIZED PROGRAM

An outreach program will be most successful if it meets the specific needs of the referring hospital. These needs can be determined by the transport team's past experience with the hospital and/or by requests by the hospital from a menu of choices. A reasonable length of time for the program should be determined in consideration of individual work schedules. For example, personnel working an 8 hour shift will probably tolerate a longer program than those working twelve hour shifts.

An example of a customized program for a hospital with three, 8 hour daily shifts is described. A three hour program can be used which includes a standardized hour on details of accessing the transport system, choosing which patients need it, capabilities of the system, and preparing for arrival of the team. The next two hours can be, for example, four 30 minute modules on topics which the hospital has chosen from a list developed by the educators. The modules can be developed using medical management information presented in chapters of this text, in conjunction with other printed resources and in consideration of topics most relevant to the geographical region covered (i.e., heatstroke or near drowning in southern climates, hypothermia in frigid areas). The choice of modules could include such topics as cardiopulmonary resuscitation, airway management, intraosseous infusion, respiratory distress, management of the seizing child, common serious toxic ingestions, and management of the pediatric victim of multiple trauma. In contrast to a community hospital's usual predominance of adult cardiac resuscitations, most pediatric resuscitations will have an underlying respiratory cause. Reemphasis of the role of airway and ventilatory management will serve as a starting point for medical management discussion. The similarities and differences in management of pediatric (vs adult) trauma are so important that most community outreach programs should include a module on trauma.

For community hospitals which have previously referred patients, the most common local conditions requiring transport should be presented. For example, emergency department staff may be comfortable and experienced enough with pediatric seizures that they rarely need to refer patients for seizure control or for ventilatory support related to iatrogenic respiratory depression. They may, however, have to refer all patients with significant traumatic or surgical conditions because of lack of surgical facilities for children. An "adult" intensive care unit may be able to manage some children with certain conditions. A Level II nursery may manage premature infants but refer all patients with possible congenital heart disease.

The program would be offered during the three hours prior to or following the scheduled working shift of the participants (repeated for staff members on each shift). The referring hospital may request presentation of additional modules. This can be accomplished through longer programs, a second day of the program, or a return visit by the transport team.

Past experience with a hospital or specific advance questions will demonstrate that certain hospitals need very basic information on pediatric stabilization, while others will be offended or feel patronized unless the presentation goes well beyond basics already mastered. Obviously, the latter situation can have a negative impact on community relations.

PROGRAM DESIGN

In general, the program should be presented in a relaxed, informal setting to a small group. In addition to specific interactive situations, questions should be encouraged throughout the program. The group is most likely to be positive about the experience if they are treated as professional equals and feel more like a part of a discussion than the audience of a lecture. During any breaks the transport team should remain available for individual discussions. If slides are used in the presentation, they should be interspersed with frequent lights-on discussions. Any humor in the program should take into consideration the sensibilities of an audience with varied cultural experiences and should not be at the expense of any particular gender, race, religion, etc. The program duration should be tailored to a reasonable audience attention span. If the participants are entering the program just before or after a work shift, they cannot be expected to concentrate beyond 2 to 4 hours. If, however the audience is free for the day, the presentation can be considerably longer.

During the introductory portion of the program, the concept of the critical care continuum and the community hospital's role in it should be described and emphasized. This engenders in the audience a sense of participation, responsibility, and recognition of their own importance in the ultimate prognosis of the patient. They may have previously thought of their emergency department as a place for a critically ill child to be "pushed on from" as quickly as possible to definitive care, as opposed to recognizing their vital role in the overall care of the patient. In addition, the explanation of a community hospital's role in reaching out to EMS personnel and the lay public may inspire the development of new programs which benefit the educators and the students, as well as the patients. Bringing the hospital staff onto the child's team can result in substantial improvements in pediatric care at all levels of the continuum.

If the audience is available, community outreach can include such courses as Pediatric Advanced Life Support (PALS), Advanced Pediatric Life Support (APLS), or the Neonatal Resuscitation Program (NRP). However, the program should not lose track of its mission, which is to educate hospital staff about the pediatric critical care transport process. Addition of these highly structured courses will increase the length of the program considerably and may limit the number of courses and audience members because of time and funding restraints. The courses should not be used as the sole community outreach program because they have minimal emphasis on transport issues and no information on details of the individual transport program.

Provision of useful written materials concerning common pediatric emergencies is another method of preparing the hospital for a critically ill or injured child. If information presented verbally is not called into use for several months, it is unlikely that all important details will be recalled. Giving the participants cards or posters with resuscitation information and a phone number to call for help will be a powerful tool in improving future resuscitations. Confidence will also be instilled in the members of the referring hospital staff. The transport team can give out copies of pediatric resuscitation manuals and can suggest books and manuals which would be the most useful for the hospital to purchase. As descriptive and interactive computer software is developed for emergency pediatric care, those materials can also be provided or recommended.

As part of the community relations venture the tertiary hospital's name, logo, and phone number is printed on resuscitation cards, as well as on promotional materials such as lapel pins, pens, key rings, and penlights.

TRANSPORT TRIAGE: KEY POINTS

Two questions to address early in the discussion are "how do we know who to transport" and "how do we figure out the best way to transport an individual patient." The first question is the most easily answered. A child who requires or may potentially require urgent subspecialty consultation which is not available locally is a transfer candidate. A patient requiring inpatient care, either in or out of an intensive care setting, should be transferred if the hospital lacks the staff or facilities to manage the patient's condition *and* any likely clinical deterioration. This occurs, for example, when nursing staff members on all shifts are not trained or experienced in pediatric care or when the child may need skilled airway management, but personnel with that expertise are not in-house 24 hours a day. The need for transfer does not imply that the pediatrician or emergency department personnel are not competent in the patient's management; it simply means that the hospital does not have all of the complex resources necessary to manage the rare seriously ill or injured child over a long time period.

Method of transport is more difficult to determine. Until formal transport triage scores are developed and validated, each system should teach their own method of deciding when to activate the transport team.[2,3,10,11,13,14,18] Some systems, especially those devoted to neonatal transport, prefer to send a transport team for any patient being transferred. Others, especially helicopter programs, have fairly strict criteria for severity of illness in order to use the team. Future changes in health care financing are likely to significantly restrict the use of expensive critical care transport teams. If a system has an objective triage system, such as a patient status classification system,[4] it can be explained in advance during the community outreach program. In lieu of a formal scoring system, a "common sense" approach can be presented. This approach recommends a pediatric critical care transport team for 1) patients accepted to an intensive care unit (on the principle that if that level of care is anticipated at the tertiary care center, it will be needed during transport), 2) any patient with reasonable potential for pulmonary or neurologic deterioration during the anticipated time of transport (i.e., status asthmaticus, recurrent seizures, etc.), and 3) any child with a recent life-threatening event (apnea, respiratory arrest, cardiac arrest, prolonged seizures with respiratory compromise, etc.), on the principle that what happened before could happen again. If it is not clear whether the patient meets any of these criteria, the best judgement of the referring and receiving physicians should be employed. The overall priority of maintaining the best interests of the child should be noted, along with the preference for error on the side of providing a higher level of care than is actually needed.[12]

For systems which use more than one type of vehicle, the process of choosing a vehicle for an individual transport should be discussed during the outreach program. It should be emphasized that faster (i.e., helicopter) is not always better. The negative aspects of helicopters versus ground vehicles should be mentioned (i.e., smaller space, difficulty in performing procedures, weather concerns, noise/vibration, etc.) in order to alleviate the perception that the child's illness is being taken less seriously if the team travels by ground.

PREPARATION AND COMMUNICATION

Advance and immediate preparation for transport

Transport efficiency is greatly improved when the referring hospital prepares in advance for all of the issues involved in the complex process.[1] A checklist of usual advance preparations should be presented, including but not limited to the following:

1. A list of pediatric tertiary care facilities with phone numbers. If one center is used for most referrals, alternate locations, even if out of state, should be included because of the increasing frequency of overextended (i.e., "full") pediatric and neonatal intensive care units. In addition, availability of any highly specialized services such as extra corporeal membrane oxygenation (ECMO), a burn unit, or hyperbaric oxygen therapy should be noted.
2. A list of transport systems with phone numbers serving the region. Pediatric capabilities, available vehicles, and team composition for each system should be noted.
3. A list (or pack) of pediatric equipment and supplies to supplement the usual emergency department resources.
4. A list (or pack) of pediatric equipment and supplies to supplement the usual local EMS resources.
5. Suggestions for developing administrative protocols to facilitate the transport process if local, state, or hospital policies present time-consuming obstacles. Examples of these situations include the following:
    a. Determination of exactly when and how patient responsibility is assumed by the tertiary care center (especially if a team from a third hospital is performing the transport);
    b. Negotiation of responsibility for payment for transport, especially of uninsured or underinsured patients; and
    c. Resolution of issues which may arise if the patient has to cross a state line. For example, is additional licensing or certification required for transport personnel to practice medicine in a transport vehicle which is physically in a different state from the one in which a team member usually works?

Immediate preparation

A separate checklist should be presented for "immediate preparations," for example, those improving efficiency when a critically ill or injured child is being prepared for transport from the community hospital:

1. Copies of all hospital/emergency department records and radiographs. A final page of nursing notes or other last minute information can be copied just before departure of the team.
2. Consent for transport, specifying transport team and receiving hospital should be signed by the patient's guardian. Many pediatric teams request that the parents remain at the referring hospital in order to provide consent directly to the team. An explanation of the reasons for this policy is helpful, as the referring hospital may be used for transporting adult patients with different legal consent requirements. Reasons presented include the opportunity to obtain a medical history, details of the acute event, and surgical consent, and to provide maps and an explanation of ICU policies to parents who may not arrive at the receiving hospital for hours. In addition, if the transport team is from the receiving hospital, preliminary bonding can occur between the patient's parents and personnel who may be involved in patient care after the transport.
3. Securing of all lines and tubes in preparation for a mobile environment.
4. Splinting and stabilization of cervical spine and any known or suspected fractures.
5. Preparation of blood products which may be needed during transport.
6. Provision of a phone number to call for any laboratory results which may be pending at the time of transfer.

Communication

The communication network for the transport system is of paramount importance, and an explanation of its use must be included in the outreach program.[5,6] The referring hospital should be given a hotline number or instructions on how to reach the appropriate individual for accepting a patient in transfer and dispatching the transport team. Various systems are in use, and this information must be conveyed to the referring hospitals. Important details include the background of the individual who is the initial point of contact. Is it a transport dispatcher or nurse who can activate the transport team, provide an estimated time of arrival, document needed information, and direct the call to the appropriate physician for patient acceptance and treatment recommendations? Or is the initial contact with a physician, and if so, what is the nature of that physician's subspecialty and his/her responsibility in the transport process? Another important aspect of understanding the communication system is knowing how to immediately contact the receiving physician in the event of a patient emergency during the time between patient acceptance and the time the transport team leaves the referring hospital.

The outreach program should include a discussion of the patient information needed by the receiving hospital. The best way to accomplish this is to provide copies of the data form completed when the patient is initially accepted in transfer. If the referring hospital prepares the form as the patient is assessed, important details will be available, necessary information will be obtained without the need for multiple phone calls, and efficiency of the transfer will be improved. The form can even be sent via FAX to decrease telephone time. A community outreach program is an excellent forum in which to discuss the reasons why so much information is requested in order to determine optimal mode of transport, predeparture preparations by the team, and any treatment recommendations to be offered.

LIMITATIONS OF THE TRANSPORT SYSTEM AND TRANSPORT TEAM

The goal of a pediatric critical care transport system is to safely transfer a patient to a tertiary care center in an environment as close as possible to that of a pediatric intensive care unit. Obviously, the entire unit and staff cannot be duplicated, but teams with blood gas machines, FAX machines, cellular phones, and state of the art mechanical equipment are coming increasingly close.

During the outreach program, limitations of transport systems in general and the individual system in particular should be explained. One universal limitation is that no team can arrive to assume patient care in the 5-10 minute time period that may be life-saving in a critical situation. Each hospital accepting pediatric emergency patients *must* be able to provide appropriate initial stabilization.[9]

The expansion of helicopter services has led to such rapid transports that in some cases the referring hospital may come to rely excessively on receiving physical help in a short time period. Rather than pressing the team to arrive faster, hospitals need to maintain a basic level of stabilization capability. For any given transport the helicopter may be unavailable or delayed because of weather, maintenance or prior transport requests.

Limitations to helicopter management include the inability to hear breath sounds,[8] a cramped work space, and significant difficulty in performing pediatric procedures (even by a skilled pediatric team). These concerns may add to delays in departure from the referring hospital, the team may elect to further secure an airway which may be patent but could deteriorate.

Most teams do not travel with an anesthesiologist able to take a child to the referring hospital's operating room for intubation. For that reason and also because of cases in which treatment should not be delayed awaiting a team, the referring hospital may be asked to have their anesthesiologist, ENT specialist, or surgeon secure an airway prior to arrival of the team. Frequently encountered cases in which this issue arises include children with epiglottitis or severe croup. Lack of space in transport packs may cause a team to try to use referring hospital supplies (intravenous catheters, endotracheal tubes, etc.), thus saving the team's supplies for potential use during transport.

Very team-specific considerations include the ability or inability to add a physician to the crew of a nurse-led team and the ability or inability to transport multiple patients simultaneously. Discussing all of these issues during the outreach program can assist the referring hospital in making a decision about which team to use for a given patient and can alleviate, in advance, several of the areas in which misunderstandings commonly occur.

OTHER ISSUES AND CONSIDERATIONS

The major part of a community outreach program involves transport team members going to potential referring hospitals to provide education and information. An often overlooked additional option is to invite members of the referring hospital staff to the tertiary care center for tours, Continuing Medical Education programs, and even "mini-fellowships" involving, for example, a week working or observing in the emergency department or pediatric/neonatal intensive care unit. For physicians several years out of training and practicing in relatively isolated areas, the exposure to current critical care practice can be invaluable.

In many community hospitals it is the emergency department nursing staff who may know the most about the different regional transport systems and who may even make the decision about exactly which team to call. The nurses may also be helpful in encouraging early contact with the transport system. Too often the physician staff is relatively transient, for example, rotating emergency medicine physicians doing shifts, "moonlighters" from other areas and from multiple subspecialties, and pediatricians, family practitioners, and surgeons with local practices and infrequent true emergencies requiring transport. Focusing outreach education on the nursing staff gets the message to the most consistent emergency department staff members. ED nurses can have a significant impact on many areas of the transport process, and this position should be openly respected during the outreach program. Provision of Continuing Education Unit (CEU) credits for the outreach program is also a substantial incentive to participation.

As during an actual transport, the attitude of the team members must be one of respect for the referring hospital and its role in the critical care continuum and in the patient's ultimate outcome. Criticism of past situations at that hospital or any other hospital must be carefully avoided. The outreach program is also a useful opportunity to note that there is often more than one right way to treat a medical condition. Emphasis should be placed on the fact that a change in the patient's medical management upon arrival of the team is usually *not* a criticism of prior care but more likely a conformance to the team's management protocols and to the team's specific equipment.

Finally, the transport team's follow-up process should be explained, including a contact source for information (usually the Transport Coordinator or the nurse from the transport) and an explanation of any patient confidentiality issues which may prevent a detailed report on the patient's progress. The referring hospital should be strongly encouraged to contact the Transport Coordinator or the team's Medical Director (contact phone numbers should be provided) if there are concerns about any part of the transport process because problems cannot be addressed or corrected if they are not reported.

REFERENCES

1. American Academy of Pediatrics, Committee on Pediatric Emergency Medicine: *Emergency medical services for children: the role of the primary care provider*, Elk Grove Village, IL, 1992.
2. Bion JF, Edlin SA, Ramsay G: Validation of a prognostic score in critically ill patients undergoing transport, *Br Med J* 291:432-4, 1985.
3. Cullen DJ and others: Therapeutic intervention scoring system: a method for quantitative comparison of patient care, *Crit Care Med* 2:2:57-60, 1974.
4. Dorbrin RS and others: The development of a pediatric emergency transport system, *Pediatr Clin North Am* 27:633-46, 1980.
5. Forstner G, Bales J: Building dialogue into the public consultation process: part one, *Public Relations Quarterly*, 31-5, Fall 1992.
6. Forstner G, Bales J: Building dialogue into the public consultation process: part two, *Public Relations Quarterly*, 33-7, Winter 1992-1993.
7. Hoffman P and others: Six basic steps to community relations: Openness is the key, *PR Reporter* 28(12) Sept 24, 1990.
8. Hunt RC and others: Inability to assess breath sounds during air medical transport by helicopter, *JAMA* 265:1982, 1991.
9. Joint Commission for the Accreditation of Healthcare Organization, *Accreditation manual for hospitals*, Chicago: 33, 1991.
10. Mayer TA, Walker ML: Severity of illness and injury in pediatric air transport, *Ann Emerg Med* 13:108-11, 1984.
11. McCloskey K and others: Variables predicting the need for major interventions during pediatric critical care transport, *Pediatr Emerg Med* 8:1:1-3, 1992.

12. McCloskey KA, Johnston C: Critical care interhospital transports: predictability of the need for a pediatrician, *Pediatr Emerg Care* 6:89, 1990.
13. Orr and others: Predicting the need for major interventions during pediatric interhospital transport using pretransport variable, *Pediatr Emerg Care* 8:6:371, Dec 1992.
14. Orr R and others: Pretransport pediatric risk of mortality score (PRISM) underestimates the requirement care or major interventions during interhospital transport, *Crit Care Med* 22:101-7, 1994.
15. Peak WJ: Community relations. In Lesly P, editor: *Lesly's handbook of public relations and communications*, ed 4, Chicago, IL, 1991, Probus Publishing Company.
16. Seitel FP, editor: Community relations objectives. *The practice of public relations*, ed 5, New York, 1992, MacMillan Publishing Company.
17. Spragins EE: Making good. *INC*, 114-9, May 1993.
18. Walker ML, Storrs BB, Mayer T: Factors affecting outcome in the pediatric patient with multiple trauma, *Child's Brain* 11:387-97, 1984.

38

INFECTION CONTROL

FERNANDO STEIN

A nosocomial infection is defined as a localized or systemic condition resulting from the adverse reaction to the presence of an infectious agent or its toxin, with no evidence that the infection was present or incubating at the time of hospital admission. The problem of infection during transport includes considerations related to the following:

1. Prevention of nosocomial infection.
2. Prevention of transmission of infection to members of the transport team.
3. Prevention of infection to the patient from members of the transport team.
4. Anticipation of isolation for the transported patient.

Infections affect at least 6% of patients admitted to hospitals and represent one of the leading ten causes of hospital deaths.[22] The expense of hospital associated nosocomial infections in this country is 4 billion annually.[32] For hospitals in particular, the burden of this cost is becoming increasingly significant. A recent survey showed that 82 to 95% of hospital patients whose admission was complicated by nosocomial infection did not receive additional reimbursement from their perspective payment systems for the cost of their infectious complications.[23]

During transport a number of procedures need to be performed usually under the most urgent circumstances. Break down of sterile technique is common, and it is reasonable to speculate that the origin of a significant number of nosocomial infections is traceable to the urgent procedures of stabilization and transport. Bacterial infections account for the majority of nosocomial infections. Viral infections occur at a far lower rate.[19] Gram positive organisms are more common than gram negative ones (42% and 35%, respectively).[34] Of the patients that acquire nosocomial infections, 8 to 26% will have more than one infection.[33]

This chapter analyzes the site-specific morbidity and mortality of nosocomial infections as well as the risk factors and equipment related issues in the prevention of infection during transport.

MORBIDITY AND MORTALITY

A prospective analysis of nosocomial infection over a thirty month period showed that, of approximately 14,000 patients who remained in intensive care for at least 72 hours, 6% developed nosocomial infections.[34] It is difficult to extrapolate the origin of this infection to transport related issues. However, the majority of primary bacteremias have a blood born origin. The risk of nosocomial infection increased with arterial and central venous line use. These two modalities are frequently applied during stabilization and transport. The use of invasive therapies, such as intubation and mechanical ventilation, is also associated with an increase in nosocomial infection.[18,34] According to data from the National Nosocomial Infections Surveillance (NNIS), of 79 hospitals from October of 1986 to December of 1990, nosocomial infection was acquired by an average of 9.2% of admitted patients.[28]

The most reliable predictor of death related to nosocomial infection is the child's underlying disease. Overall, the mortality attributable to nosocomial infections is about 11% for both pediatric and neonatal nosocomial infections. The mortality associated with nosocomial infection is clearly multifactorial. The type of patient, the number of affected organ systems, and the microorganisms responsible are some of these factors. For example, patients with fungal bloodstream infections have a mortality of 18%, while those with bacterial infections have a lower mortality.[41] Patients with multiple bloodstream nosocomial infections have a mortality of approximately 40%.[33]

RISK FACTORS

Children under the age of two have the highest infection rates, with up to 25% of this age group affected.[34] The severity of illness and the exposure to life-saving invasive procedures are closely associated with the development of nosocomial infections.[28] Another important factor is the use of antibiotic therapy that grossly alters the patients flora. This fosters colonization and invasion of otherwise saprophytic or symbiotic organisms. In a study characterizing patients according to their pediatric-risk-of-mortality (PRISM) score and comparing patients among different institutions over time, the patients with pediatric-risk-of-mortality (PRISM) scores over 10 on admission were more likely to develop nosocomial infections than were those with PRISM scores under 10 (10.8% versus 3.4%: $P < .001$). This type of association held true for age, service, and length of stay. The sensitivity, specificity, and positive and negative predictive values of a PRISM score greater than 10 were 75%, 53%, 11%, and 97% respectively.[38] In this study, as in other studies, bacteremia accounts for the largest percentage of infections. From the available information it is difficult to determine the exact moment where a nosocomial infection was introduced to the patient. The presence of infection in other parts of the body or the presence of wounds in other parts of the body increase the risk of catheter related infections. A multiple trauma victim who has open wounds which are contaminated with soil or body fluids may receive an in-dwelling catheter at the time of injury and is therefore more likely to contract a nosocomial infection related to that catheter than is a patient without such wounds. There are predisposing factors inherent to the patient that deserve mention, as they are associated with a higher incidence of nosocomial infection.

Predisposing factors of nosocomial infection in transport

Trauma. Patients who survive the initial insult of multiple trauma have a 20 to 60% risk of developing nosocomial infection.[40] In pediatric trauma the main cause of immediate mortality is neurosurgical death. However, infection is the leading cause of death after neurosurgical trauma.[20] All aspects of the immune system are altered following severe trauma and burns. The release of kallikreins, lymphocyte levels, and lymphocyte activity is affected by multiple trauma and burns. Macrophage and lymphocyte function become abnormal.[20,35,40]

Acute viral infection. The effect of viruses on the immune system is well recognized as one that can affect the humoral and cellular component of immune function. Viruses may cause immunosuppression by a variety of mechanisms. These include immunosuppression as a result of viral replication or the activity of soluble factors of viral and host origin released from infected cells. Viral infection of macrophages affects the function of these cells in natural and acquired immunity, and immunosuppression may result from the viral triggering of an imbalance and immune regulation culminating in the over activity of suppressor cells.[39]

Malnutrition. Children in a catabolic state, as well as in a state of chronic malnutrition, have a higher incidence of infection than do children who are well nourished. Malnutrition affects all aspects of the immune system.[4,5]

Malignancy. Patients who are immunocompromised because of malignancy or treatment for malignancy are frequently neutropenic or have severely depressed bone marrows and are obviously at risk for nosocomial infection.[31,37]

EQUIPMENT RELATED ISSUES

In general, the cleaning and maintenance of equipment should be conducted according to the Joint Commission of Hospital Accreditation Standards and the standards of the Occupational Safety Health Administration. Issues related to personnel protection are discussed later in this chapter.

The equipment used for the stabilization and transport of patients can become contaminated through exposure to infected organisms from a previous patient or personnel or from the growth and colonization of organisms due to poor maintenance. Respiratory equipment used for mechanical ventilation and respiratory support, such as the face mask, Bi-Level Positive Airway Pressure (BI-PAP), or Continuous Positive Airway Pressure (CPAP), is an important source of colonization and infection in patients who require the use of such equipment. The relatively humid medium that is created by the humidification of gases used for ventilatory support facilitates the colonization and growth of potentially pathogenic bacteria.

The risk of pneumonia associated with contaminated respiratory equipment is significant and is related to the size and number of aerosolized particles that contain bacteria, the concentration of bacteria, and whether the bacteria are delivered directly into the endotracheal tube or only to the nasopharynx and oropharynx.[15] Tube colonization and condensate are often overlooked risk factors for pneumonia. The condensate formation in the ventilator is related to differences in the temperature between inspiratory phase gas and the ambient temperature. In 1984 Kraven reported a condensate formation of 30.2 ± 11.9 ml/hr in 30 different ventilator circuits.[13] Inline medication nebulizers inserted into the respiratory face of the tube may produce bacterial aerosols. In a study where 19 inline nebulizers were sampled from seven patients during the first 24 hours after ventilator tubing was changed, 15 (79%) of the nebulizers were contaminated with more than 1,000 bacteria per ml of reservoir fluid.[14] Because nebulizers with this level of contamination can produce heavy bacterial aerosols, the nebulizers may be hazardous to patients who require such therapies. This is an important issue in the transport of patients with reactive airway disease. It is crucial that respiratory equipment used for stabilization and transport of patients both interhospital and intrahospital be maintained in the most sterile of conditions. Equipment that may become contaminated with blood or other potentially infectious materials must be checked and decontaminated as necessary before servicing or shipment. When decontamination cannot be performed the equipment should be discarded.

Water bottles which are used to humidify oxygen in ambulances are notorious for facilitating the growth of potentially infectious organisms. Stagnant water can grow all kinds of organisms, preferentially gram negative rods (*Pseudomonas sp, Acinetobacter sp, Klebsiella sp, and Serratia sp*). The air conditioning system of the transport vehicle can all be potentially hazardous to patients. Health hazards are usually related to the methods of humidification used and the types of maintenance of the filter systems. For example, the spread of legionellosis by contaminated ventilation systems is well recognized. In this case the pathogens colonize the humidification unit of the system and are distributed to the whole unit.

PERSONNEL ISSUES

A number of health care delivery personnel suffer communicable diseases. Nurses, doctors, and ambulance attendants may be suffering from a common respiratory infection or one or more chronic conditions such as tuberculosis, hepatitis, or AIDS. Today, the principle of universal precautions is particularly relevant to the protection of both the personnel and the patient during stabilization and transport.

Each year the number of new infections of Hepatitis B among health care workers ranges from 6,000 to 12,000.[36] Infection occurs primarily in young adults, of whom 6 to 10% become chronic carriers. About 250 health care workers die each year from the effects of Hepatitis B virus. As a known human carcinogen, Hepatitis B virus ranks second only to tobacco smoke. The best protection against Hepatitis B virus is immunization. The decline of clinical Hepatitis B in workers has been well documented.[29] Since up to 60% of people who are Hepatitis B surface antigen positive are not known to be positive at the time, the importance of health care workers receiving Hepatitis B vaccinations cannot be overemphasized.

Acquired Immune Deficiency Syndrome (AIDS) in health care workers from exposure to patients has been documented. Health care workers in the United States incur approximately 800,000 accidental needle sticks and sharp injuries each year. Of these, 2% (16,000) are likely to be contaminated with HIV. The chances of infection with seroconversion to HIV are about 3 to 4 per thousand needle sticks. However, the risk for Hepatitis is 60 to 300 per 1,000 needle sticks.[1]

In general, the highest risk of infection to health care personnel can be traced to break downs in the appropriate technique of universal precautions and appropriate use of modern available devices to prevent injury with needle and sharp instruments.

The major health hazard from health care personnel to children who are being stabilized and/or transported is that of viral associated diseases such as upper respiratory infections.

BACTEREMIA AND FUNGEMIA

Primary bacteremia is defined as a bloodstream infection occurring in a patient with no evidence of localized infection. However, bacteremia in the presence of a peripheral intravenous line, central venous catheter, or other form of invasive monitoring is regarded as a primary event if there is evidence of local site infection. Secondary bacteremia is defined as a bloodstream infection with microbiological or clinical evidence of infection at another sight which is the source of the bloodstream infection. Fungemia refers to the presence of fungi in the bloodstream and generally does not distinguish between primary and secondary infection. About 8% of all nosocomial infections in the United States are primary bloodstream infections. In 1989 the incidence of bloodstream infections in non-teaching hospitals was less than in teaching hospitals. This data includes adults and children.[2] The most common positive organisms of bloodstream infections is coagulase negative staphylococci, followed closely by *Staphylococcus aureus*, and enterococci.[17] It is conceivable that these bacteremias occur as a result of introduction of otherwise colonizing staphylococcus into the patient's bloodstream. While attempting to save a patient's life, time to set up appropriate sterile technique cannot be spared, and some of these infections are unavoidable. Of particular concern is the issue of meningococcemia. This disease entity is discussed elsewhere in this book, but the transport and stabilization of the patient of meningococcemia needs to proceed with the due diligence necessary to prevent infection of health care personnel. The highest rates of meningococcal disease occur in infants less than 1 year of age, with a peak incidence of 26.4/100,000 population in infants less than 4 months of age. Twenty-nine percent of cases were infants less than 1 year of age, 46% of children less than 2 years of age, and 25% persons greater than 30 years of age.[25] Although, medical personnel are not frequently infected by contact with a person with meningococcal infection, careful observation of exposed individuals and chemoprophylaxis for those who develop a febrile illness is recommended by the Red Book of the American Academy of Pediatrics. Respiratory isolation is indicated in a patient suspected of meningococcal disease while the organism is identified or until 24 hours of antibiotic therapy has been administered.

UPPER RESPIRATORY INFECTIONS

The most commonly transmitted pathogens in the viral category include:

1. Respiratory Syncytial virus
2. Rhinoviruses
3. Influenza viruses
4. Parainfluenza viruses
5. Coxsackieviruses
6. Varicella-zoster virus
7. Adenoviruses

Respiratory syncytial virus infection

It is important to emphasize that humans are the only source of transmission in the case of the respiratory syncytial virus. Transmission is usually by direct or close contact, which may involve droplets. Virus can persist on environmental surfaces for many hours, thus this is an important consideration for transport. A patient who comes into contact with secretions present on the surface of a rubber mattress or a mask or contaminated equipment is likely to become infected. Virus can be identified on one half or more of the hands of medical personnel. Infection amongst hospital personnel can occur by self inoculation with contaminated infant secretions. Nosocomial infections are frequent amongst both personnel and infants. Contact isolation is recommended for young children and infants. Strict adherence to infection control procedures, such as prevention of contamination by respiratory secretion and careful hand washing or the use of gloves, will help nosocomial spread. In several studies, use of eye-nose goggles by staff has been shown to further decrease nosocomial transmission of RSV.[10]

Rhinovirus infection

Like RSV, humans are the only known host. Transmission occurs by close person-to-person contact, aerosol fomites, and self inoculation. The source of contamination through skin contact is most relevant for this condition.[11]

Influenza virus infection

Influenza is spread from person-to-person by direct contact, droplets, or by contact with articles contaminated by nasopharyngeal secretions. This highly contagious disease needs to be considered for both exposure of medical personnel and exposure of the patient. During outbreaks of influenza the highest attack rates occur amongst school-age children. Influenza is an important source of lost working days for medical personnel. Therefore, receiving a flu shot is recommended.

Parainfluenza virus infection

Parainfluenza virus infections are transmitted from person-to-person by direct contact and by spread of contaminated nasopharyngeal secretions. As for the previous diseases, infection control measures include respiratory isolation and strict hand washing.[8]

Coxsackieviruses infection

The usual spread involves secretions and blood. Parvoviruses are the most common cause of erythema infectiosum. Outbreaks frequently occur in elementary or junior high schools during the spring months. Contact isolation, including the use of gowns and gloves, is indicated for hospitalized children with immunocompromised situations. However, women who are exposed to children either at home or at work are at an increased risk of infection with parvovirus. Pregnant women members of the health care team who find that they have been in contact with children who are in the incubation period of erythema infectiosum or who are in aplastic crisis should have the relatively low potential risk explained to them. Fetal ultrasound and alpha-fetoprotein determinations are useful when assessing damage to the fetus. Transmission of infection can be lessened by routine hygenic practices for control of respiratory infections. These include hand washing and disposal of facial tissues containing respiratory secretions. The preventive effect of immunoglobulin in an exposed person is unknown.[9]

Varicella-zoster virus infection

Humans are the only source of infection for this highly contagious virus. Person-to-person spread occurs by direct contact with varicella or zoster lesions or by airborne droplet infection. This particular infection is a major concern in the admission policies and transport of patients because of its potentially long incubation period (14 days). Children in the incubation period of varicella who are admitted to units without isolation expose health care workers and other patients to the virus. Such an outbreak causes the closure of entire health care units around hospitals in the United States.

Patients are contagious for 1 to 2 days before and shortly after the onset of the rash. Contagiousness may be for as long as 5 days after the onset of lesions. Immunocompromised patients with progressive varicella are probably contagious during the entire period of eruption of new lesions.

Strict isolation is indicated for patients with varicella for at least 5 days after the onset of the rash and for the duration of the vesicular eruption. During transport, if a patient is identified as suffering from varicella, the utmost care must be exercised to decontaminate the equipment used in the transport of the patient including stretcher, vehicle, handles, etc.[12]

Adenovirus infection

Strains of adenovirus can be transmitted by the fecal-oral route. Other routes have not been clearly defined and may vary with age. Type of infection and environmental factors may also vary. Children with respiratory adenoviral infection should be isolated with respiratory and enteric precautions.[6]

PNEUMONIA

Nosocomial pneumonia is the second most common hospital acquired infection in the United States.[24] The incidence of respiratory nosocomial infection among pediatric hospital patients ranges from 16 to 29%.[19,34] Intubated patients have a 21 times higher incidence of infection than do patients without a respiratory device.[3,16] Pneumonia is the most common fatal nosocomial infection, with mortalities ranging from 20 to 70%, depending on the causative organisms.[21,26] In adult populations, nosocomial pneumonia accounted for 60% of the fatal nosocomial infections.[21] Nosocomial pneumonia in children accounts for 10 to 15% of all hospital acquired infections.[21] The prognosis for patients with gram negative bacillary pneumonia, especially those with pseudomonas infections, is worse than for those with gram positive or viral agents.[21] However, viral agents increase the mortality in a specific subset of patients. Specifically, respiratory syncytial virus has been associated with increased mortality in premature children and in children who have bronchopulmonary dysplasia or congenital heart disease.[30] Viruses are the most common cause of pediatric nosocomial respiratory tract infections. Respiratory syncytial virus, the predominant pathogen, is implicated in numerous hospital outbreaks of respiratory infections. Up to 20% of all nosocomial lower respiratory infections are of viral etiology.[27] The colonization of medical personnel, particularly of those who perform endotracheal suction, is also a potential source of respiratory tract infection in ICU patients.[21]

REFERENCES

1. APIC Governmental Affairs Committee, APIC position paper: Prevention of device medicated bloodborne infections to health care workers, *Am J Infect Control* 21:76-8, 1993.
2. Banerjee SN and others: Secular trends in nosocomial primary bloodstream infections in the United States 1980-1989, *Am J Med* 91:586-9, 1991 (Suppl 3B).
3. Celis R and others: Nosocomial pneumonia: a multivariate analysis of risk and prognosis, *Chest* 93:318-24, 1988.
4. Chandra RK: Nutritional regulation of immunity and infection in the gastrointestinal tract, *J Pediatr Gastroenterol Nutr* 2:S181-S187, 1983 (suppl I).
5. Christou NV, McLean AP, Meakins JL: Host defense in blunt trauma: interrelationships of kinetics of energy and depressed neutrophil function, nutritional status, and sepsis, *J Traum* 20:833-9, 1980.
6. Committee on Infectious Diseases, American Academy of Pediatrics, *Adenovirus red book,* Elk Grove, IL, 1991, The Association.
7. Committee on Infectious Diseases, American Academy of Pediatrics, *Influenza virus red book,* Elk Grove, IL, 1991, The Association.
8. Committee on Infectious Diseases, American Academy of Pediatrics, *Parainfluenza virus red book,* Elk Grove, IL, 1991, The Association.
9. Committee on Infectious Diseases, American Academy of Pediatrics, *Parvovirus red book,* Elk Grove, IL, 1991, The Association.
10. Committee on Infectious Diseases, American Academy of Pediatrics, *Respiratory syncytial virus red book,* Elk Grove, IL, 1991, The Association.
11. Committee on Infectious Diseases, American Academy of Pediatrics, *Rhinovirus red book,* Elk Grove, IL, 1991, The Association.
12. Committee on Infectious Diseases, American Academy of Pediatrics, *Varicella-Zoster virus red book,* Elk Grove, IL, 1991, The Association.
13. Craven DE, Goularte TA, Make BJ: Contaminated condensate in mechanical ventilator circuits: a risk factor for nosocomial pneumonia, *Am Rev Respir Dis* 129:625-8, 1984.
14. Craven DE and others: Contaminated medications nebulizers in mechanical ventilator circuits: a source of bacterial aerosol, *Am J Med* 77:834-8, 1984.
15. Craven DE, Steger KA: Nosocomial pneumonia in the intubated patient, *Infect Dis Clin North Am* 3:843-66, 1989.
16. Craven DE, Steger KA, Barber TW: Preventing nosocomial pneumonia: state of the art and perspectives for the 1990s, *Am J Med* 91:572-5, 1991 (Suppl 3B).
17. Dickson GM, Bisno AC: Infection associate with indwelling devices: concepts of pathogenesis; infections associated with intravascular devices, *Antimicrob Agents Chemother* 33:597-601, 1989.

18. Donowitz, LG: High risk of nosocomial infection in the pediatric critical care, *Crit Care Med* 14:26-8, 1986.
19. Ford-Jones EL and others: Epidemiologic study of 4,684 hospital-acquired infections in pediatric patients, *Pediatr Infec Dis J* 8:668-75, 1989.
20. Goris RJ and others: Improved survival of multiple injured patients by early internal fixation and prophylactic mechanical ventilation, *Injury* 14:39, 1982.
21. Gross PA and others: Deaths from nosocomial infections: experience in a university hospital and a community hospital, *Am J Med* 68:219-23, 1980.
22. Haley RW: *Managing hospital infection control for cost effectiveness: a strategy for reducing infectious complications,* Chicago, 1986, American Hospital Association.
23. Haley RW and others: The financial incentive for hospitals to prevent nosocomial infections under the prospective payment system, *JAMA* 257:1611-4, 1987.
24. Horan TC and others: Nosocomial infection surveillance, *MMWR (CDC Surveill Summ)* 35:SS17-SS29, 1986.
25. Jackson LA, Wenger JD: *Laboratory-based surveillance for meningococcal disease in selected areas, United States, 1989-1991, MMWR (CDC Surveill Summ),* Vol 42, No SS-2, 1993.
26. Jacobs RF: Nosocomial pneumonia in children. *Infection* 19:64-72, 1991.
27. Jarvis WR: Epidemiology of nosocomial infection in pediatric patients, *Pediatr Infect Dis Child* 6:344-51, 1987.
28. Jarvis WR and others: Nosocomial infection rates in adult and pediatric intensive care units in the United States, *Am J Med* 91:S185-S191, 1991 (Suppl 3B).
29. Lanphear BP and others: Decline of clinical Hepatitis B in workers at a general hospital: relation to increasing vaccine–induced immunity, *CID* 16:10-14, 1993.
30. MacDonald NE and others: Respiratory syncytial viral infection in infants with congenital heart disease, *N Engl J Med* 307:397-400, 1982.
31. Marina NM and others: Fungemia in children with leukemia, *Cancer* 68:594-9, 1991.
32. Miller JP, Farr BM, Gwaltney JM Jr: Economic benefits of an effective infection control program: case study and proposal, *Rev Infect Dis* 11:284-8, 1989.
33. Miller JP, Farr BM: Morbidity and mortality associated with multiple episodes of nosocomial bloodstream infection: a cohort study, *Infect Control Hosp Epidemiol* 10:216-9, 1989.
34. Milliken J and others: Nosocomial infections in a pediatric intensive care unit, *Crit Care Med* 16:233-7, 1988.
35. O'Mahony JB and others: Depression of cellular immunity after multiple injury in the abscence of sepsis, *J Trauma* 24:869-75, 1984.
36. OSHAs bloodborne pathogens standard: analysis and recommendations, *Health Devices* 22(2):35-40, 1993.
37. Pickering LK and others: Leukocyte function in children with malignancies, *Cancer* 35:1365-71, 1975.
38. Pollack E and others: Use of the pediatric risk of mortality score to predict nosocomial infection in a pediatric intensive care unit, *Crit Care Med* 19:160-5, 1991.
39. Rouse BT, Horohov DW: Immunosuppression in viral infections, *Rev Infect Dis* 8:850-73, 1986.
40. Stillwell M, Caplan ES: The septic multiple trauma patient, *Infect Dis Clin North Am* 3:155-83, 1989.
41. Turner RB, Donowitz LG, Hendley JO: Consequences of candidemia for pediatric patients, *Am J Dis Child* 139:178-80, 1985.

39

STRESS AND THE TRANSPORT TEAM

DAVID V. MYERS

Psychological, social, and physical symptoms of stress are frequent companions of workers in health-related fields.[4,22] Those who monitor the quality of life of these workers report higher than expected rates of stress-related disease (coronary heart disease, essential hypertension, peptic ulcers irritable bowel syndrome, vasospastic phenomena, etc.), suicide, drug abuse, psychiatric disorders, and marital disharmony.[6,17]

High on the lists of stressful jobs are those of the nursing staffs in intensive care units, medical personnel in emergency departments, and emergency transport workers.[3,6] Dealing repeatedly with the delicate balance of life and death with its concomitant exposure to the intense emotional upset of family members, and the striving to maintain a competent, "calm and cool" professional demeanor, are frequently listed as major sources of staff burnout, disability, excessive absenteeism, and premature retirement.

Recently, the effects of stress on emergency services providers, including medical transport teams, have been targeted for intervention.[19-21,23] With the past two decades of rapid expansion in specialized trauma and treatment centers, telemetric monitoring devices, and rapid-response ground and air transport capability, many sources of stress found in emergency departments and ICUs have been taken out of the hospital and put on the road (or in the air).

Recognition of transport situations as stressful by both administrators and transport team members is a crucial first step in appropriate and successful stress reduction. Transport related stresses include, but are not limited to the following:

1. The potential for vehicular accidents and concerns for personal safety.
2. Having to practice medicine in an unfamiliar environment, often without access to many resources available in the usual hospital setting.
3. The sense of being isolated as possibly the only one who can make certain decisions or perform life-saving procedures.
4. Erratic work schedules (e.g., when on-call one must be prepared to leave rapidly to care for a patient with numerous possible problems, or the team member may stay on alert for the entire shift without going anywhere, or may end up on a long transport that goes well beyond the scheduled end of a shift).
5. Pressure to work when off duty because of personnel shortages during periods of increased activity.
6. Equipment management.
7. Lack of understanding by nontransport colleagues of "downtime" responsibilities.
8. The need for diplomatic, calm, effective communication with colleagues, referring and receiving hospital personnel, the patient, and the patient's parents.

9. Limited resources requiring clinical skills and judgements unnecessary in a hospital setting.
10. The potential for having to work "alone out there" with other team members in whom one may not have total confidence.
11. Feelings of lack of control over many situations (vehicle or equipment breakdowns, physician noninvolvement or over involvement at the referring hospital, etc.) for the not primarily-pediatric team members.
12. The physical stress of working in a moving, vibrating, noisy environment (including motion sickness, sleep and food deprivation, etc.).
13. The additional emotions and fears involved in being responsible for a very sick child.

Two major types of stress are salient for members of the transport team: very severe, usually acute stress (which we will call autonomous stress) and milder stress, usually chronic, which is mediated by certain characteristics of the individual experiencing it (which we will call dependent stress). This chapter will explore both. Much has been written about autonomous stress, its sources, and a few remedies. Very little material, however, has focused specifically on the sources, effects, and relief from the dependent stress of team members. To investigate these issues, stress as a general concept will first be discussed. Later we will discuss research from allied fields to examine the issues related to dependent, chronic stress. Finally we will look at the acute, autonomous stress issues and intervention strategies known as "critical incident stress debriefing," a procedure that has been specifically developed to address those problems in emergency rescue and transport personnel.

CONCEPTS OF STRESS

The notion of stress as a response to threat has been around a long time. Most health-related professionals are well aware of the autonomic arousal theory of "fight or flight" first proposed by Cannon[2] and later modified and elaborated by Selye.[24] Certain theoretical and practical problems have been identified with these early formulations, however. The most important of those problems is that stress frequently is specific to the individual experiencing it. That is, people often respond differently to particular external events. This finding has lead modern researchers and clinicians[25] to view stress as a dynamic process which includes the original notion of autonomic nervous system arousal plus the processes of identification of the external stimuli and the cognitive appraisal(s) and coping resources of the individual.

Earlier notions of stress adequately explained autonomous stress: acute, very intense events affect those who are exposed to them similarly. This more modern notion of dependent stress, the stress that is less intense, and often chronic, is that such stress is a function of the unique, dynamic interplay of the external world and the individual's interpretation and response to that world. Thus "stressors" (Selye's word originally intended to identify those external things that cause stress) can be identified not only in the external world (e.g., the work setting) but also in the abiding beliefs, values, and attitudes held by people in those work settings.

Stress is also considered to be dynamic. A well-rested, healthy person may cope with a certain set of stressors very effectively. That same person in a sleep-deprived and hungry state may respond to those stressors very differently. Finally, stress is considered to be a function of the individual's response repertoire. That is, how an individual behaves when confronted with external stimuli that are perceived as threatening can reduce or magnify the impact of the external stimuli. For example, when stressed, one individual chooses to discuss the experience with a colleague, while another tries to put it out of mind. A third individual goes on a two mile jog, while a fourth person heads for the bar. The effect of the external stimulus is modified by the person's response to it.

The cause of stress can run a full range from completely autonomous to those that are almost exclusively mediated by the attitudes and behaviors of the individual (i.e., dependent stress). First, there are external stressors of extreme magnitude, such as rape and kidnapping. Such stressors are more or less universally autonomically arousing and cause predictable untoward responses. Similarly, widespread catastrophes often affect the victims and rescuers alike, such as the often-referenced and well-documented study of the Buffalo Creek Disaster.[26] In this disaster, a slag dam broke above Buffalo Creek in West Virginia, killing many residents and sending millions of tons of water and mud cascading down the creek valley. In those circumstances, where there was widespread damage, high loss of life, and human carnage was highly visible, a majority of those present suffered clear signs of stress-related disorders. Survivors and, to a lesser degree, rescuers were so traumatized that premorbid personality characteristics and coping responses were not factors in predicting who became symptomatic.

While few empirical studies of rescuer trauma exist, one researcher quantified the percentage of nurses developing stress symptoms in response to relief efforts in a hurricane disaster at approximately 40%.[13] More recently, studies estimate that acute stress reactions occur in up to 85% of emergency personnel when they are confronted with autonomous stress.[9]

Extreme situations, however, are only a part of the overall stress picture for emergency personnel. What about situations where a minority of the emergency team members have problems? What about the cumulative effects of low grade stressors on personnel? To examine these issues, the interactive concepts of dependent stress must be considered.

It is here that the ideas, beliefs, and attitudes of the individual, as well as his or her repertoire of coping skills for stressors, come into play in both identifying and assisting in stress relief. Obviously, team members are at risk if they are experiencing stress from sources outside the job such as family conflict, financial problems, or health-related concerns. But what about predisposing personality characteristics? Do certain "personality types" predispose people to respond negatively to stressors? Several theorists and researchers have attempted to address this question by studying those individuals who seem to cope with stress better than most. The most frequently noted research includes the notions of "psychological resilience"[7] and "personality hardiness."[12]

Personality and stress resistance

The concepts of hardiness and resilience with respect to stress resistance have a common source and theme. Researchers have long recognized that some individuals seem to survive stressful circumstances better than others. Various attempts have been made to quantify traits, characteristics, or personality attributes of these stress-resisting individuals so that they may be effectively applied in selecting staff for high-stress jobs.

The research of Flach[7] generated a list of attributes that is long and interesting. His list includes 13 characteristics of "resilient" individuals. The ability to learn and change from experience, insight into self and others, a "supple" sense of self-esteem, open-mindedness, self-discipline, creativity, and a keen sense of humor are some of the most important attributes listed. Other traits cited include having a personally meaningful philosophy of life, a high tolerance for uncertainty, courage, and personal integrity. Individuals possessing these traits are believed to be disturbed by stressors, but to reach a state of recovery spontaneously and quickly.

Despite the intuitive appeal of these character traits, they present certain problems when they are applied to common staff selection issues. First, they are poorly defined and lack empirical bases. Without any established methods to identify and quantify these traits, practical application is, as yet, impossible. Second, even if these traits were well-defined and quantifiable, they are, at least in combination, presumably rare in occurrence. To find a group of physicians, nurses, and emergency transport technicians possessing all of these traits would make it difficult to fill the necessary positions.

The more empirically derived concept of "personality hardiness" of Kobasa[12] is more promising. She lists only three variables associated with resistance to stress: a high level of commitment or involvement in major personal activities; a high but not absolute sense of personal control over life events; and the belief that change is normal and represents a challenge. Research among individuals possessing these traits has shown that even when living in high-stress environments, those possessing "hardiness" have significantly fewer stress-related symptoms.

This research is not, however, without criticism. Lazarus and Folkman,[15] for example, argue that prospective studies and more precise measurements are needed before this research concept can be utilized effectively. To date, this has not been done using these three variables in combination.

Much compelling research has been conducted to assess the positive impact of one of Kobasa's variables, a personal sense of control, on mediating stress and stress-related illness. Studies from the disciples of neuroendocrinology, immunology, and cognitive-behavioral psychology have independently supported this variable as a significant mediator of stress responsiveness. Thus, it is likely that despite the criticisms leveled at Kobasa, her research findings will be further substantiated by additional investigations. The reader interested in a detailed description of the neuroendocrinological, immunological, and behavioral research on control issues should read the thorough review by Everly.[5]

Cognitive and affective variables

Research aimed at understanding why some people react to stressors with physical symptoms (e.g., migraine headaches), psychological symptoms (e.g., anxiety attacks), or behavioral symptoms (e.g., marital conflict) while others develop no symptoms at all, is both complex and incomplete. At this point in the research process, complicated personality variables are clearly at play. The well-known research on the coronary disease-prone "Type-A" personality, for example, has lead to remarkable predictions of disease-proneness in both cancer and coronary heart disease from personality factors alone.[10] For our purposes there are several interesting findings from this research. First, the personality variables associated with disease-proneness themselves produced stress. These variables were related to interpersonal style, which in turn, resulted in less than satisfying relationships. This dissatisfaction lead to increased stress. Additionally, the type of stress produced determined the type of disease manifested. For instance, cancer patients consistently sought relationships that were clearly unobtainable and in the process idealized others and diminished themselves. Intervention aimed at changing the attitudes and behaviors of these disease-prone groups reduced the mortality rates among these groups.

From this research, we can learn several important generalizations about stress:

1. Enduring, powerful emotions associated with unmet and unattainable needs for emotional closeness or other goal attainment are precursors of helplessness, hopelessness, and depression.
2. Powerful feelings associated with an unrealizable need to distance from disturbing persons or objects leads to ongoing experience of irritation, anger, and agitated helplessness.

This research, in addition to highlighting the importance of a personal sense of control, strongly suggests that perceptions and attitudes giving rise to chronic feelings of anger and hopelessness are associated with interpersonal dysfunction, stress and, ultimately, with debilitating disease and premature death. Additionally, specific attempts to alter such perceptions and their subsequent feelings, along with attempts to increase a realistic sense of personal control over life events, reduce stress and act prophylactically against enervating disease processes.

STRESS PREVENTION

What do we know from the experimental and clinical research on stress that translates into useful tools for prevention of as well as intervention into both autonomous and dependent stress? From the previous research, it is apparent that developing and maintaining healthy attitudes are essential to stress prevention. Of primary importance is the notion of personal control. An old but succinct synopsis of a healthy sense of personal control is contained in the "serenity prayer" of Alcoholics Anonymous:

> . . . God grant me the strength to change the things I can, the courage to bear the things I cannot

change, and the wisdom to know the difference. . . .

All of the critical elements for a realistic sense of personal control are contained in this short prayer. When people strive to identify elements in their lives over which they have control and effectively engage these elements, they see themselves as effective and powerful. When these same people differentiate for themselves those elements over which they have little or no control, and disengage from these elements, they reduce or eliminate feelings of frustration, irritability, and helplessness.

Certainly, were it so simple, we would all make these discriminations and never experience the negative effects of stress. Establishing and maintaining realistic perceptions of personal control is a difficult and constantly changing proposition. It is, however, the one personality variable that stands out above all in predicting the effects of stress. Individuals with a high sense of personal control typically, albeit often automatically, invoke a strategy such as follows:

1. "Can I personally be effective in this particular circumstance?"
2. "Do I care to be effective in this circumstance?"
3. If the answer to both of the above is "yes," a plan will follow fairly easily. If no plan is forthcoming, the answer to one or both of the first two questions was probably not a "yes"; further investigation, skill-building, consultation and education will provide clarification.
4. If the answer is "yes" to the first question, but "no" to the second, I am choosing where not to put my energies.
5. If the answer is "no" to the first question, but "yes" to the second, I may choose to join forces with others to form a more powerful group.
6. If the answer to the first and second questions is "no," obviously, no further effort is required.

Persons without similar strategies are plagued with doubt, guilt, frustration, and other untoward emotions. Certainly, personal emphasis on making effective discriminations regarding personal control should be a top and continuing priority.

Although we can concentrate on increasing our sense of personal control, we will never be totally effective in preventing the subjective experience of stress and its' concomitant nervous system arousal. Dealing with arousal, then, while not primary prevention, must be looked at as prevention of the long-term effects of stress. Two avenues of arousal reduction have been heavily researched and clinically applied: physical exercise and relaxation training.

STRESS INTERVENTION

Experimental and clinical research have well established that stimulation of various sites in the central nervous system (e.g., the limbic system) and that of the autonomic nervous system are central to the development of stress-related diseases. In our sedentary life styles, the effects of this arousal build up over time, without dissipation. In antiquity, such build up in preparation for action (i.e., "the old fight or flight"), was necessary for survival. Presumably, when this aggression or egression occurred, dissipation of the untoward effects of arousal also occurred. Modern civilization has removed many of these options, requiring less naturally occurring modes of dissipation.

Relaxation training

The opposite of sympathetic excitement is parasympathetic dominance. In this physiological state we find a lowering of pulse and blood pressure, decreased muscle tone, slower and deeper respirations, and other events associated with a state of quiescence. When this physiological state can be reliably and frequently induced, researchers have documented that many untoward effects of stress can be reduced or eliminated. Procedures to effect the parasympathetic dominance have been developed from many perspectives. The "reductionists" on one end of the treatment continuum have focused on the pharmacological effects of the benzodiazepines and similar anxiolytic drugs. The "holistic" therapists at the other extreme of the continuum have explored the benefits of "transcendental meditation" and self-hypnosis. Despite there being such different avenues to achieve similar results, outcome research strongly suggests that regardless of the route, the systematic application of anti-arousal procedures, from drugs to self-hypnosis and the many other middle of the road variants such as biofeedback and cognitive-behavioral relaxation, are similar and effective. Since the psychological routes have many fewer side effects and are more frequently the focus of rigorous outcome research, we will present a brief description of a generic relaxation program.

First, it is important to remember that relaxation training and its attendant benefits must be learned and deepened through practice. Most experts recommend practicing the procedures twice daily for 20-30 minutes each. In 7 to 10 days, most individuals can achieve a state of quiescence sufficient to be therapeutic.

Most relaxation programs have three areas of focus: striated muscle tone reduction, deepening and slowing of respirations, and positive mental imagery, each receiving approximately 10 minutes of focus each.

1. Skeletal muscle relaxation is usually achieved through alternately tensing and relaxing large muscle groups while seated or reclining. Hands, arms, thighs, shoulders, and facial muscles are usually the primary muscles of focus.
2. Interspersed with or following the tensing and relaxing of the large muscle groups is the training to breathe diaphragmatically and slowly. Concentration on the rhythmic and slow movement of the naval while the upper chest is motionless is usually emphasized. Most people find that it is almost impossible to focus on "deep breathing" and maintain a high state of arousal.
3. After physically relaxing and breathing "like a person who is asleep," the emphasis moves to constructing a positive, peaceful mental image while maintaining the previously attained level of relaxation. The mental image is multimodal, including visual, auditory, kinesthetic, and proprioceptive elements. During this phase, the individuals focus on experiencing fully this mental image. If or when distractions occur, trainees are taught to refocus on breathing and tensed muscle groups after which they return to their positive image.

Although this brief description sounds simplistic, it is quite powerful in application. Many clinicians who are unfamiliar with the impressive research on relaxation-type therapies overlook these procedures or fail to generalize their use. For example, after many repetitions, the positive mental imagery acquires relaxing properties of its own through classical conditioning. The image can then be employed in fairly public places for tension, anger, or anxiety control. Trained deep breathing is an excellent intervention for sleep onset difficulties. Relaxation, in conjunction with certain behavioral skills, such as assertiveness training and "stress inoculation" procedures,[18] has proven to be highly effective in combating the effects of dependent stress. For those interested in a thorough description of the relaxation response and its underlying neurophysiological substrata, see both Smith[25] and Everly.[5]

Physical exercise

Starting in the early 1960s, jogging and other forms of aerobic exercise began receiving recognition for their ability to counteract fatigue, increase mental alertness, and positively affect mood. Interestingly, research on moderate physical exercise began to find many of the stress reduction effects associated with meditation, relaxation training, and self-hypnosis. Such research on the effectiveness of even moderate exercise in reducing susceptibility to stress has led several theorists to conclude that stress itself should not be the focus, but rather the active release of that stress. For exercise to be effective as a stress reliever and preventer, it should be aerobic, noncompetitive, and regular. In general, the guidelines associated with exercise aimed at increasing cardiovascular efficiency also appear to work well for those individuals with a personal preference for active tension reduction. Walking at a brisk pace or jogging for 20 to 45 minutes 3 to 5 times per week is normally sufficient to achieve positive results. Swimming and cycling, if they are noncompetitive, are also useful. It should, of course, also be well within the physical capability of the individual as determined by an appropriate health professional. Several other physical variables warrant mentioning, especially diet and sleep.

Diet and sleep

It stands to reason that foods and chemicals that activate or further stimulate those centers of arousal associated with stress responses should be avoided by individuals seeking to reduce their overall stress levels and improve their stress tolerances. Caffeine, found not only in coffee and soft drinks but also in cocoa, chocolate, and various headache preparations, is well documented as a sympathetic stimulant. Refined sugars are less well known for their sympathetic stimulation, but some researchers and clinicians implicate large quantities of sucrose through the mechanism of "insulin overshoot" in which overproduction of insulin lowers glucose levels. This reactive hypoglycemia, especially in certain individuals, generates alarm/arousal responses.[8] Likewise, alcohol, often consumed to combat tension, has the opposite effect. Following moderate to large amounts of alcohol, there is a significant interference with restorative sleep. "Morning after" levels of tension and anxiety are much higher than prior to consumption.

Adequate sleep is often overlooked when enumerating stress-resistant variables. Although sleep deprivation is not itself directly related to tension, the effects of deprivation clearly are related. For example, we know that poor or restricted sleep depletes energy levels and increases irritability. Motivation is reduced and concentration and memory function are negatively affected.[14] Under these circumstances, and when faced with a challenge, our personal sense of competency (i.e., personal control) will be at risk. The probability of experiencing stress is clearly increased when individuals are thus deprived.

Clearly, many options exist to improve one's ability to handle stress of the dependent variety. Examining and reevaluating one's sense of personal control should be a priority, along with choosing and working in a field in which one is invested and competent. Developing effective stress interventions, whether active, as in physical exercise, or more passive, as in relaxation training, is also a must. And, of course, these intervention strategies must be in place and well-established before they can be effective. Finally, diet, alcohol use, and sleep should be reassessed and altered as necessary. If in spite of this work, an individual continues to feel anger and/or helplessness much of the time, professional consultation and/or a change of career responsibilities should be strongly considered.

CRITICAL INCIDENT STRESS

Regardless of all efforts at controlling dependent stress, emergency medical service workers, by the very nature of their jobs, maintain a high state of physiological arousal when on duty awaiting a call or during an actual emergency.[16] Added to this elevated base rate of stress, emergency transport personnel and other emergency workers will occasionally be exposed to events that will generate concentrated increases in stress, owing solely to the intensity or magnitude of the emergency. This autonomous stress will affect most all emergency workers involved and will reduce their effectiveness on the job and in other areas of their lives.[11] Examples of this type of emergency range from those of great magnitude, like an earthquake, to small but intensely negative events such as brutal abuse or murders of children. Additionally, the loss of or serious injury to an emergency team member is always traumatizing to the team. Likewise, emergencies that resonate deeply with a team member's present life circumstance, such as a pregnant physician or nurse dealing with a sudden infant death, may be particularly difficult to handle. Transport and emergency department personnel are also occasionally threatened or physically assaulted by victims and relatives of victims. Many emergency service experts consider the effects of such exposure to be cumulative when not dissipated, and it is not uncommon for emergency workers to leave this type of work after experiencing one or more occurrences of autonomous stress. Fortunately, a process known as Critical Incident Stress Debriefing (CISD) has been developed and implemented for such circumstances.

CISD was originally developed by Mitchell[19,21] to reduce the number of psychological insults to emergency service workers. CISD spread quickly and widely and is regularly utilized in many urban and suburban areas of the United States and elsewhere.

Mitchell's approach is based on psychological crisis intervention theory that holds that when individuals or groups suffer psychological trauma, and are disorganized by that trauma, there exists a window of opportunity for positive reorganization. If that window is missed, reorganization of some kind, perhaps less positive than prior to the trauma, will occur. The key, then, to effective crisis intervention, and effective CISD, is timely availability of the CISD team.

CISD is set up to respond quickly, usually within 72 hours of a critical incident, to help alleviate or reduce the psychological impact of the emergency on the service workers. Common signs and symptoms among workers exposed to intense trauma include denial and psychological numbing, guilt and shame, grief and loss, irritability, and outright displays of anger. Other symptoms include anxiety, a pervasive sense of helplessness, depression, sleep and diet disruption, and flashbacks. The discerning reader will recognize the symptoms listed here as similar to the psychiatric diagnosis of "Post-Traumatic Stress Disorder" and indeed these are very similar if not identical notions. Physiological manifestations, such as extreme fatigue, nausea, tremors, and diarrhea also may be present.

The debriefing process itself is a seven step group format that allows those present at the incident to experience the support of others who understand "what it was like" to have been there, as well as to express thoughts, emotions, and conflicts associated with the crisis. The goals of the debriefing are not only to return the team members to as high or higher level of functioning as before the incident, but also to educate and insulate them from additional stress.

The leaders for these debriefings usually come from two groups: local mental health professionals and specially trained peers from the emergency service community, all of whom are trained according to the procedures outlined by Mitchell and others.[9,16] The most effective CISD teams have drawn peer leaders from the widest array of service agencies available in the community, and include not only surface and air transport team members but also fire, police, 911 operators, admissions clerks and emergency department personnel. From this wide selection of personnel, leaders will seldom have to debrief people with whom they work. Depending on the community, some leaders are paid while others volunteer. Cooperation among and financial support from the local hospitals, mental health agencies, police and fire departments is essential to the success of CISD teams in any given community, Recently, CISD teams have been provided for family members of emergency service workers in recognition of the impact of acute stress on the "significant others" of the workers.[23]

Critical incident debriefing

While many communities have established CISD teams, most have followed Mitchell's original format of seven formal debriefing steps. These steps are outlined briefly below.

1. Introductory Phase: The first phase involves establishing "ground rules" of confidentiality, making clear the goals of stress reduction and relief, and impressing upon the participants that the debriefing is not a critique of the event or the individuals and agencies involved. Holding thoughts and emotions in is established as self-injurious and personal expression of those thoughts and feelings are advocated to reduce one's sense of isolation and feeling of abnormality.
2. Fact Phase: Each individual participant in the debriefing is urged to recall their personal involvement in the emergency. They are asked to relate what happened from their standpoint, including what they saw, heard, and smelled. Most participants find this phase easy to comply with.
3. Thought Phase: Participants from this point forward in the debriefing process speak voluntarily. In this phase, personal thoughts, such as "the first thing I thought when I arrived on the scene," are encouraged to help personalize the experience of the workers.
4. Reaction Phase: The emotional responses of the workers are focused on during this phase. Typical questions to stimulate the

discussion of these feelings include such questions as "What was the worst part of the emergency for you?" and "How did you find yourself feeling just after the crisis was over?" Participants experience the ventilation of constrained affect associated with the event in a protected environment. Often, individuals discover similar responses among other group members and begin to feel less weak or impaired.
5. Symptom Phase: Common psychological and physical symptoms are enumerated and discussed. Professional leaders are vigilant for extreme symptoms among the participants that may warrant additional intervention. This phase signals a return to a more objective and less emotional level of discussion.
6. Teaching Phase: Leaders offer educational and information perspectives regarding stress and general stress management strategies. Participants discuss personally effective techniques for stress reduction. Leaders emphasize that the stress responses of the individuals to intense or highly personally meaningful crises are normal. The events themselves are abnormal.
7. Reentry Phase: The leaders summarize the event and the group meeting. Individuals ask any final questions or make statements to the group. Leaders provide referral information for those who would like more extended debriefing and/or counseling.

In 1991 Waters and Jaffurs[27] noted that 125 CISD teams existed in 34 states and in many foreign countries. Outcome studies therein cited suggested that CISD is effective in both reducing disability and treatment costs among emergency personnel.

Some communities have added services such as a "command consultation" of team leaders during a major emergency. This consultation is a support effort for transport team directors, police tactical commanders, and fire department officers during an actual crisis and is aimed at assisting these team leaders in utilizing emergency workers in ways that will minimize the emerging effects of stress on the workers. Additionally, Linton, Webb, and Kommor[16] added an immediate response component to the CISD concept that they called "defusing." These interventions are available to emergency teams directly upon completion of their duties in a crisis and resemble a less formal and shorter version of the full debriefing. The goal is to "defuse" intense personal responses to the event and help reduce the chance of disability among the personnel by quickly giving support.

MANAGEMENT ISSUES

Clearly, providing patient care in the emergency department, transporting victims and acutely ill patients, or working as a dispatcher, team leader, or technician in emergency service can be hazardous to one's health. Given the opportunity to experience both dependent and autonomous stress in high levels on the job, the department and team leaders have additional responsibilities to provide access to support and intervention facilities for themselves and their subordinates. Individual stress management procedures outlined above, as well as effective utilization of the concepts of critical incident debriefing, are clearly called for.

In generating support for preventive and ameliorative individual and group treatment, leaders also must recognize that in such a highly stressful job, organizational and management stressors take on increased significance. The organizational culture, with its attendant work loads, schedules, communication avenues, and relationships to its overall superstructure, also must come under scrutiny. Issues known to generate stress on an organizational level, such as under- and overwork loads, personnel shortages, shift work, and unsupportive or hostile management, must be addressed.[1] Only when these and similar organizational issues are also effectively resolved can working on an emergency response team become a position in which people can both remain healthy and remain for a long time.

DISCUSSION

To continue working as an effective caregiver in clinical transport and emergency services, individuals have three major goals to reach in order to successfully cope with the stresses of their job. First, they must maximize their opportunities for stress prevention through altering the ineffectual and counter-productive attitudes outlined above as well as developing and consistently using some form of stress reduction. Secondly, professional workers must contribute to the establishment and effective use of a stress debriefing team in their community. Simply using and encouraging others to use this mechanism of intervention can be a significant contribution to the profession. Finally, each person must help effect those changes necessary on an organizational level to insure that emergency service providers work in the most supportive and reduced-stress environments possible.

REFERENCES

1. Brown JM, Campbell EA: Stress among emergency service personnel: progress and problems, *Occupational Medicine* 41(4):149-50, 1991.
2. Cannon WB: *The wisdom of the body,* ed 2, New York, 1932, Norton.
3. Clark M, Friedman D: Pulling together: building a community debriefing team, *Journal of Psychosocial Nursing,* 30(7):27-32, 1992.
4. Clever LH, Omenn GS: Hazards for health care workers, *Annual Review of Public Health* 9: 273-303, 1988.
5. Everly RS: *A clinical guide to the treatment of the human stress response,* New York, 1989, Plenum Press.
6. Fain RM, Schreier RA: Disaster, stress, and the doctor, *Medical Education* 23:91-6, 1989.
7. Flach F: Psychological resilience. In Flach F, editor: *Stress and its management,* New York, 1989, W.W. Norton.
8. Forgione AG, Bauer FM: *Fearless flying,* New York, 1980, Houghton-Mifflin Co.
9. Freehill K: Critical incident stress debriefing in health care, *Critical care* 8(3):491-500, 1992.
10. Grossanrth-Maticek R, Eysenck HJ: Psychological factors in the prognosis, prophylaxis and treatment of coronary heart disease, *Directions in Clinical Psychology* 2:3-17, 1992.
11. Jimmerson C: Critical incident stress debriefing, *Journal of Emergency Nursing* 14(5):43a-45a, 1988.
12. Kobasa SC: Stressful life events, personality and health: an inquiry into hardiness, *Journal of Personality and Social Psychology* 37:1-11, 1979.
13. Laude J: Psychological reactions to nurses in disaster, *Nursing Research* 22:343-7, 1973.
14. Lamberg L: *American Medical Association guide to better sleep,* New York, 1984, Random House.
15. Lazarus RS, Folkman S: *Stress, appraisal, and coping,* New York, 1984, Springer.
16. Linton JC, Webb CH, Kommor MJ: Critical incident stress in prehospital emergency care, *The West Virginia Medical Journal* 88:146-7, 1988.
17. McCue JD: The effects of stress on physicians and their medical practice, *New England Journal of Medicine* 306(8):458-63, 1982.
18. Meichenbaum D, Jaremko M: *Stress reduction and prevention,* New York, 1983, Plenum Press.
19. Mitchell JT: When disaster strikes . . . the critical incident debriefing process, *Journal of Emergency Medical Services* 8:36-9, 1983.
20. Mitchell JT: Stress: the history, status, and future of critical incident stress debriefings, *Journal of Emergency Medical Services* 13:47-52, 1988.
21. Mitchell JT: Stress: development and functions of a critical stress debriefing team, *Journal of Emergency Medical Services* 13:43-6, 1988.
22. Pines AM, Arsonson E, Kafry D: *Burnout,* New York, 1981, The Free Press.
23. Rubin JG: Critical incident stress debriefing: helping the helpers, *Journal of Emergency Nursing* 14: 255-8, 1990.
24. Selye H: *The stress of life,* New York, 1956, McGraw-Hill.
25. Smith JC: *Cognitive-behavioral relaxation training,* New York, 1990, Springer.
26. Titchner JL, Kapp FT: Family and character change at Buffalo Creek, *American Journal of Psychiatry,* 133:295-9, 1976.
27. Waters J, Jaffurs W: Critical incident stress debriefing for emergency service personnel in North Carolina, *North Carolina Medical Journal* 52(12):641-3, 1991.

40

THE PSYCHOSOCIAL ASPECTS OF TRANSPORTING THE CRITICALLY ILL CHILD

JANET L. TERRY

A family experiences many stressors and crises during their lifetime. The degree of impact on the family is directly related to the severity of the event. The most traumatic event a family experiences would be the death of one of its members. The sudden and unexpected illness of a child is also highly traumatic both for the child and his family.

If the family is from a metropolitan area, they may be fortunate enough to live near a medical complex that specializes in the treatment of critically ill or injured neonates and children. This will minimize many of the stressors faced by the family, allowing them to maintain a slightly more normal life than is possible for the family whose young member must be transferred to a hospital many miles from their home.

The family suddenly finds their world turned upside down not only by the illness or injury of the child but also by the events resulting from his hospitalization and the stress exhibited by other family members. Families are rarely prepared to handle the crisis created by the illness or injury of a child. Likewise, the child is not emotionally equipped to handle such crises and tends to rely heavily on his parents as a means of support. When the child is transferred from his local or community hospital to another hospital farther from home the family frequently is taken from any existing support system, sometimes for a prolonged period of time.

It is the responsibility of the medical staff at the referring hospital as well as the Critical Care Transport Team (CCTT) to make the hospital to hospital transfer as non traumatic for the child and family as possible. This is easier if the medical personnel are accustomed to working with children, however, as the majority of the hospitals are primarily adult facilities, this is not an area where most medical staff feels comfortable. A general knowledge of some of the tasks of child development and how that development influences the child's behavior will make a difficult task much easier. While there are many tasks in each age group, only a few will be focused on. For a more comprehensive view there are numerous resources available.

CHILD DEVELOPMENT: A BRIEF OVERVIEW

A child's ability to cope with the challenges of hospitalization is directly related to his or her stage of development. Younger children have less well developed coping skills, since they lack life experiences and maturity. Each level of development the child achieves is dependent on the mastery of previous levels as a foundation. It is essential that medical personnel be familiar with the child's progression through the developmental stages. Unrealistic expectations of children and treating them as if they were younger or older will result in frustration and, frequently, in failure to achieve the desired results.

NEONATAL AND NEWBORN DEVELOPMENT

The needs of the neonate are the most basic: food, warmth, nurturing, safety and security, etc. If the neonate is born with a congenital anomaly or develops a post birth complication, it is highly possible that one or more of these needs will be left unmet in order to meet the most basic life sustaining needs. For example, a baby with a myelomeningocele will not be able to eat awaiting the surgical correction of the defect and will need to remain on his or her stomach until their back heals, even when they want to be fed, held, and cuddled. Likewise, a baby with meconium aspiration will require rapid and extensive medical interventions, including intravenous fluids, medications, supplemental oxygen and possibly intubation with ventilatory support, etc. These are but two extreme examples of medical problems the neonate may experience which would prevent the baby's normal physical needs from being met. A less extreme example would be transient tachypnea of the newborn, which might delay the baby being fed for a short time.

The premature baby has many of the same developmental needs as the term baby. The younger the baby is gestationally at the time of birth, the more attention must initially be focused on meeting physical needs, while less attention is devoted to the developmental needs of the child. Likewise, the more premature the baby the less attention initially given to the parents simply because the baby's condition is so critical and the medical staff is focused on saving the child's life. Once the premature baby has passed the initial crisis of birth and the struggle to survive, emphasis can become more evenly divided between meeting survival needs and other developmental needs, and more attention can be given to the parents.

Whether their baby is premature or suffering from a congential anomaly or birth complication, parents of the critically ill neonate face unique problems. Unlike most parents of newborn babies, these parents may wait hours before being allowed to see their child for the first time and months before being able to hold the baby they had so eagerly anticipated; some parents never touch or hold their baby while he or she is living. Before these parents can begin to face the critical illness of their newborn, they must first grieve for the loss of the perfect baby they did not have. The event becomes even more stressful when the condition of the baby requires that the child be transferred to a different hospital to receive more sophisticated medical care.

The members of the CCTT have an obligation not only to meet the medical needs of the neonate but also to help meet the needs of the family. This is accomplished in several ways, the most important being to allow the parents, if at all possible, to have contact with the baby prior to leaving for the receiving hospital. The parents should be encouraged to touch the baby and helped to understand that their touch will not be in any way detrimental to the baby. The role of all medical equipment should be explained, especially with regard to how it helps to care for the baby. If at all possible, a picture of the baby should be left with the parents to help them remember how the child looks. Ultimately this may be their only picture of the child. The picture also helps fill the void created by the baby being moved to another hospital in another city. It is important to provide the family with accurate medical information without being too technical; they need to know that everything possible is being done for their child so they can maintain hope while at the same time maintaining realistic expectations of the child's potential for recovery.

The infant: term birth to 12 months

A baby's development progresses very rapidly from birth to one year of age. Early behavior is primarily reflexive, including rooting, sucking, swallowing, crying, etc., with little if any tolerance for the delay of gratification. For the critically ill infant and the CCTT this becomes problematic when, for example, the baby becomes hungry but cannot be fed secondary to a medical problem. The child may be quieted by the use of a pacifier or by attempting to meet other needs, such as the need for security, by swaddling the baby in a blanket.

At approximately 6 months of age the baby begins to exhibit stranger anxiety, consequently it becomes important for medical staff to include the parents in the care of the child to the extent the child's medical condition allows. This might include anything from the parents simply being in the room as the child is prepared for the transport to the parents actually holding the child for less invasive procedures such as the placement of the cardiorespiratory monitor. It is important to remember that, although the parents may want to help with the care of their child, many of the procedures may be too traumatic for them to watch. It is always a good idea to give them the option of leaving the room for the procedure and returning to provide comfort once it is complete. Likewise, many procedures, such as intubation or the placement of a central line or chest tube are complicated enough that the CCTT may prefer family members wait in another room.

It is not uncommon for the child to need further stabilization prior to departing for the receiving hospital. In the event that the child is extremely critically ill, it may be necessary for the parents to wait in the waiting room while the child is prepared for the transport. This should be explained to the parents and any family, and they should be given frequent updates if possible. In this case it becomes even more important to allow the family to see the child before departure for the receiving hospital, as a child this ill may not survive until his or her parents arrive at the receiving hospital.

Between 6 and 9 months of age babies begin to experience distress when separated from their parents. This can at times be more stressful for the parents than for the baby. The baby usually calms rapidly once totally out of sight and hearing of any family members. This is frequently hard for the child's parents to comprehend because the separation is equally as hard for them. The more ill the child, the more traumatic for the family. It may help the parents to know that the majority of the children, both young and old, fall asleep within a few minutes of leaving the referring hospital. It may also be helpful for both parent and child to allow the child to carry a favorite toy or blanket on the trip. This is true even for the comatose child whom the parents may feel could awaken en route and need a reminder of them in order to feel more secure. Although a few minutes extra with the family may seem medically unnecessary, this may be the last contact the family ever has with their child and would allow their memory to be a more positive one.

Helping the infant adjust. There are several ways the CCTT and the referring medical staff can help make the transport experience easier for the infant. Perhaps the most simple is for the medical personnel, who are usually total strangers, to interact with the parents briefly before approaching the child. This allows the older infant time to adjust to the presence of strangers before they actually invade the child's space. A second way to ease the adjustment of the infant is to remember that at a very young age a child discovers their hands and begins to use them to interact with and explore the environment. Placing an IV or pulse oximeter probe on an infant's hand interferes with this ability to explore; therefore, if possible, place these, and any other medical devices such as the blood pressure cuff, on the infant's feet or lower extremities. If the infant has already begun to walk, it may not be practical to place the IV in the child's foot, so remember to be as nonrestrictive as possible with securing it. For example, try to use the child's non-dominant hand and avoid the antecubital area as it restricts movement and use of the entire arm. Finally, as previously mentioned, allow the child to hold his or her favorite stuffed animal or blanket during the transport. This provides not only the security of something familiar but also an item that may carry the parent's scent and thereby be comforting.

The toddler: 12 months to 3 years

The toddler's development continues to progress as rapidly as that of the infant. Included among the developmental behaviors and crises the toddler experiences and masters are sibling rivalry, regression, autonomy, separation anxiety, toilet training, and temper tantrums. As in the case of any hospitalized child, some developmental crises are influenced more during the illness than others. The child who is being toilet trained will use the importance of this to try to delay painful procedures. They have learned that whenever they tell their parents of their need to potty everything else is placed on hold until they have used the toilet. This training may be jeopardized during hospitalization. It is not at all uncommon for a child in the pediatric intensive care unit to be routinely placed in a diaper. Likewise, it is not uncommon for medical staff to tell the child to go ahead and potty when the child expresses his or her need during a procedure. It is important that medical staff recognize this and make provisions to meet the child's need if at all possible.

Children of any age who are placed in stressful situations may demonstrate regression to previous stages of development. This is much more common in younger children because they have not mastered present developmental tasks. This may be manifested through temper tantrums, increased dependency on parents, regression to a previous stage, and loss of recently acquired physical skills. Each of these demonstrates the child's attempt to cope with the stress but is very frightening to both the child and parents. Medical staff can be the most helpful by treating the behavioral changes as normal and reinforcing the desired behavior. It is also important that parents understand that these changes are usually temporary and that children will rapidly regain their present level of development once the crisis is past.

As children continue to develop, they learn to perform more tasks for themselves. This budding autonomy is frequently manifested through the assertion of "no" or "me do." It is important that medical staff encourage independence and allow the child to do as much as possible for themself. Autonomy is frequently inhibited by something as simple as an intravenous infusion being placed in the child's dominant hand, keeping the child from wanting to use the hand. Likewise an IV in the foot of an ambulatory child may prevent the child from ambulating, possibly prohibiting interaction with other children and the immediate environment. This emphasizes just one reason the medical team needs to be aware of child development and how the knowledge is used to minimize the trauma of illness and hospitalization.

Helping the toddler adjust. The toddlers' parents play a very important role in helping to maintain control throughout painful and invasive procedures. It is important that the medical staff be patient with the toddler but also be firm. When tested beyond the limits of a child's emotional maturity, the toddler easily loses control, and the medical staff and the child's parents must provide a substitute form of control. They also provide protection from physical harm resulting from the child struggling to avoid necessary procedures.

Children of all ages should receive liberal praise both from their parents and the medical staff, directed at even the smallest effort the child makes to cooperate and phrased to encourage the child who is out of control. Praise used in conjunction with limit setting communicates that the child is not bad but that the child's behavior is not acceptable. This prevents harm of the child's self-esteem while demonstrating that misbehavior will not be tolerated. It is important for both the staff and parents to realize that the child is not angry at them but at the situation.

When the time comes to leave the referring hospital, the toddler will usually protest more vigorously than a child of any other age. Even the child who has thus far been cooperative may become very anxious and fretful. At this point the CCTT may need to focus as much on the parents as on the child, reassuring them that once en route the child will probably sleep throughout the transport. Then the team should have the parents place the child on the transport stretcher and, after securing the child, the team should encourage the family to kiss the child and tell him or her good-bye as the team leaves. The toddler will probably cry and protest until the parents are out of sight, in an attempt to make the parents stay with them. Team members should be aware that the child may try to get off the stretcher. They should also make every effort to calm the child and make him or her feel secure.

The preschooler: 3 years to 5 years

Preschool aged children are much more verbal than their younger counterparts. Their vocabulary is growing at a seemingly exponential rate, and they seem to talk incessantly. Unfortunately, the preschooler is very egocentric, thinking everyone else thinks as they do. They are capable of carrying on a conversation, but frequently the child is the only one who really understands what is being said. Because of this it may be necessary to further explore what they are saying through other means such as interactive play. Preschool children have a very active imagination and are able to create hours of play from a few simple toys. More can be understood about the way children think in a few moments of watching them play and talk with their toys than in several hours of talking to them.

Because they can communicate better, preschoolers are slightly less prone to temper tantrums than when they were toddlers. They are becoming better able to express their emotions verbally and thus experience less frustration at the inability to express themselves. This is a relief not only to the child but also to the parents who must cope with and attempt to hide their anxieties and fears about the child's recovery while attempting to comfort their child.

Preschoolers are also able to understand more of what is said to them and are better able to follow instructions. This can become a problem for the medical staff as the child may very practically interpret what he or she is told, so for example, if the nurse says she is going to take his blood pressure the child believes she is going to take something away and not give it back.

Preschoolers also have difficulty separating thoughts and dreams from reality and tend to experience very vivid fantasies and fears. The preschoolers' most common fear is that if they are bad or have done something naughty, their parents will abandon them. This can be even more devastating for the hospitalized preschooler who needs to be transferred to another hospital but who cannot be accompanied by his or her parents. The parents and the CCTT must take special care in informing the child of the transfer to assure them that their parents will see them again at the new hospital.

Helping the preschooler adjust. The preschooler is much better able to cope with unexpected events than the toddler. Because they can communicate better, it is easier to get them to cooperate. They are much less anxious with strangers and may even be tolerant of separations from their parents, especially if given an adequate explanation for the reason for the separation and if assured that they will see their parents again at the new hospital.

At this age the child may benefit from the presence of a surrogate attachment object such as one of the members of the transport team or a favorite toy. If this is the case, it may be important for someone to be available who has not been involved in painful procedures if at all possible. In some cases the child is attached to a toy or blanket that may serve adequately for security in the absence of his or her parents.

It is much more important for the CCTT to explain procedures to the preschooler than it was with the toddler, especially if pain will be involved. It is sometimes possible to elicit their help and cooperation, although not all children will be able to cooperate at this age. As already mentioned, the preschooler has a very vivid imagination, consequently it may be advisable to limit the details of the procedure to whether it will hurt and how bad and that someone will help them hold still until it is over. If possible, explain in terminology the child will understand such as calling a shot or an IV an "ouchy" or saying that it may feel like a bee sting. This is a good age to begin helping children understand that not all things doctors and nurses do to them will hurt. If children have a doll or stuffed animal with them it may help to perform the procedure with the toy first so they can see what to expect. Another option is to first practice on a parent or older sibling, for example, before checking the vital signs of the preschooler, check them on the parent. This allows children to see that what is being done does not hurt while also letting them see that the child's parents support the intervention as a way to help the child get well. This also reinforces the concept of good touching, which many parents may have begun to teach at this age.

Although preschoolers are more tolerant of separation from their parents, they may still become upset when the time comes to leave for the receiving hospital. It will help to have parents involved in preparing children to leave by placing them on the stretcher and helping to secure the seatbelt restraints.

Then, when the time comes for the child to leave, the CCTT can become the primary caretakers, telling the child that his or her parents need to drive down in their car so they will have a way to bring the child home when he or she is feeling better and that they will see the child as soon as they get to the new hospital. Both the parents and the team members can make the trip seem like something of a game by helping children see that they will arrive before their parents thus making it seem as if the child has beaten them at a game.

The school age child: 6 years to 12 years

As children continue to grow and develop physically, they also continue to change and develop both intellectually and emotionally. School age children remain dependent on their parents and other adults to meet many of their needs, while at the same time, seeking autonomy from them and a greater involvement with their peers. They face the desire to be a part of the group of their friends while at the same time continuing to meet with parental approval. The younger school age child is more cooperative in yielding to his parents, while the older child is more independent and is more likely to follow his peers.

School age children are also becoming intellectually capable of understanding that they are sick and, as they continue to develop, they learn that sometimes people who are sick die. Younger school age children might not yet comprehend that death is permanent, but will understand that something is wrong with them and will be very sensitive about and alert to comments made by both parents and the medical staff. Even without being told of the potential terminal nature of the illness, the child may rapidly sense what is not being verbalized. This may be even more significant when the child's condition requires transfer to another hospital, because the need for the transfer may communicate to the child much more than they are being told. Children find the concept of death to be very frightening but may have difficulty expressing their feelings. They are usually more fearful of leaving their friends and family than of the process of dying, although it is not uncommon for them to express a fear of the act of dying also.

Children who have had a terminal illness for any length of time may have had thoughts of the possibility of their own death. They may have discussed these with their parents; however, if these thoughts are relatively new, they may hesitate to mention them for fear of upsetting their parents. In this case, they may find it easier to talk to the medical staff. The staff should encourage the child to express his or her fears and gently explore what has prompted the thoughts of death. It may be that they have heard someone talking about them specifically or that another child he or she knows has recently died. It is important to be supportive and allow them to express themselves while not giving false information. It may help the child to understand that at some point everyone is going to die and that while the child's medical problem is one that sometimes is fatal, everything possible is being done to help them get well. It is also appropriate to help open the communication lines between the child and parents so they can discuss his or her fears and so the child will no longer fear upsetting them by expressing his or her feelings.

The school age child's most common fear is related to the procedures they must endure, especially such things as being hurt by a needle or cut by a knife. This is exacerbated by the inability to understand the need for painful procedures, such as lumbar punctures and renal or bone marrow biopsies. All the child realizes is that the procedure hurts and that you (the nurse or doctor) will not stop. It is very difficult for them to be cooperative when they hurt and do not understand. It becomes extremely important to give the child every opportunity to exercise even a small degree of control over the situation by helping them understand what to expect during the procedure. Because the child sees things differently than an adult, the explanation must be appropriate to their level of development. For example, the pain from the placement of an IV may be related to the discomfort of a bee sting. It is also very important to explain that even though some procedures result in something being left in the child's body, such as an IV catheter, the pain will go away shortly, and they will receive a benefit such as medicines via the IV rather than a separate shot for every medicine.

As previously mentioned, school age children experience varying degrees of dependence on or independence from their parents. This may be difficult for children for several reasons. For the first time in their life, the child sees that his or her parents are not in control and may appear helpless when compared to the professionals caring for the child. This is more common when the child is in an intensive care unit connected to multiple IVs, monitors, etc. The child may have difficulty adjusting to the need to have even the most routine daily activities performed by a nurse rather than by family members. This is compounded by the fact that much of the child's time is being spent in the presence of strangers. As the length and frequency of hospitalizations increase, the child will become more familiar with the routine and will find it easier to adjust to the need for hospitalization; however the entire process is easier if the child's parents are present to provide the support.

Helping the school age child adjust. As with any age child, it is extremely important to be honest with the school age child. They are old enough to understand that they are sick and need to know what is wrong with them, what kind of treatment they need, whether the procedures will hurt, etc. They will sense whether their parents and the staff are being honest, and will learn of their condition either by being told or by listening to people talk around them.

Honesty becomes even more important when the child's condition requires medical attention not available at the home hospital, necessitating the child's transfer to another hospital. School age children have very vivid imaginations and, if not provided with honest accurate information, will create details to support the scenario they have imagined. This can be very frightening to the child and can cause both the child and parents emotional conflict, lead to a lack of cooperation by the child, and cause the exacerbation of the child's medical condition, all of which might have been prevented by more accurate information.

School age children also need to have boundaries provided for them but, at the same time, need some control over their situation. For example, the nurse might allow the child to choose which hand an IV will be placed in. This allows some control while limiting choices so they can not procrastinate. It encourages the child's cooperation and demonstrates that their needs and feelings are important. It is also good to briefly explain the procedure immediately before beginning. This informs the child but does not allow him or her the time to become unnecessarily apprehensive. It is also a good opportunity to explain how they can be the most helpful in the completion of the procedure.

In the medical transport of the potentially critically ill child, it is not uncommon for the CCTT to encounter the need to perform minor procedures in preparation for transport that were unnecessary while the child was in the referring hospital. Some of these, such as the placement of a cardiorespiratory monitor, blood pressure cuff, pulse oximeter, etc., are noninvasive and not painful but may be frightening, especially to the younger school age child who tends to be phobic and may view any new device as potentially injurious or painful. In this case the parents may participate in the child's care and demonstrate their agreement with and lack of fear of the equipment. However, as with the preschool age child, if the procedure is painful the parents should not participate but should provide support and comfort once it is complete.

Once the necessary interventions are complete at the referring hospital, it is time to leave the parents; this may or may not be difficult. The CCTT and the parents should work together in getting the child on the transport stretcher and secured in the safety restraints. These may be referred to as seatbelts "like the pilots wear," if the transport involves flying. As the CCTT and child leave the unit, the parents may also want to leave the child and begin their own journey to the new hospital. Children should be prepared ahead of time for the departure and should already know that their parents will not be traveling with them. They will probably need to be reminded of this as they leave, and as with the younger child, may find it easier if told that their parents need their car to bring the child back home when they are discharged from the new hospital. School age children are usually interested enough in the travel itself that they protest very little, if any, when their parents leave. They may be very inquisitive about the trip, asking many questions if they feel well enough, or they may simply observe their surroundings. In either case, the transport team should talk with the child providing support and information throughout the trip.

The adolescents: 13 years to 19 years

It is sometimes difficult to remember that adolescents are still in many ways children. Adolescents are in a time of rapid physical development and may already physically resemble adults, causing the medical staff and the parents to have unrealistic expectations of their behavior. They want and need to be treated like adults. The parents, however, tend to treat them like younger children, especially if the illness is newly diagnosed or has a poor prognosis. This can lead to family conflict at a time when they can least cope with it. With adolescents it is also important to remember that being critically ill does not necessarily mean being comatose or unable to perform activities of daily living.

This time of rapid physical development is very challenging even for otherwise healthy adolescents, resulting in their having many concerns about their bodies. For example, healthy adolescents may wonder if they are not developing normally, why they are developing at a different pace than their friends, why their body reacts in certain new ways, why they feel the new and strange ways they feel, etc. They may not feel free to express their concerns or curiosity about their bodies. This is further complicated for adolescents who are ill and hospitalized, with an illness that they may interpret as a betrayal by their body, over which they have no control.

As their bodies develop, adolescents become extremely self-conscious. For ill adolescents this may make activities of daily living difficult. Their medical condition may make it impossible for them to perform activities, such as bathing or using the bathroom without assistance, during a time when body changes cause them to value their privacy more than ever. It is important to encourage them by allowing them to do what they can for themselves and offering privacy and discretion in meeting the needs they are incapable of performing for themselves.

Adolescence is also a time of heightened emotions and emotional lability. Adolescents may be calm and rational one minute and depressed, angry, or irrational the next. Anger or emotional pain may be expressed through name calling, overt hostility, and verbal outbursts, or they may withdraw and refuse to communicate. Hospitalized adolescents may withdraw or expect to receive special privileges simply because they are hospitalized. This becomes more difficult because adolescents are not willing to communicate with their parents and because the parents may not yet be willing to allow their child to become independent. When this is compounded by illness, both sides must be willing to adjust their expectations. Adolescents must grow up and become more responsible, and the parents must let go of their child and allow them to make decisions about the course of their life, with parental advice and support, rather than the parents making the decisions for adolescents. This may be a source of conflict within the family and may lead to withdrawal on the part of the adolescent. Both parents and medical personnel should be alert for any expression of the adolescent's sense of loss of his or her normal adolescence through withdrawal and should encourage them to talk about how they feel. They may be more open with the medical staff as they attempt to assert their independence from their parents. Whatever the case, the adolescent should be encouraged to talk openly, and the parents should be encouraged to be open to any anger expressed and to be supportive of their child.

As with the younger child it is important for the staff and family to set limits for the adolescent who is emotionally and/or physically out-of-control. Otherwise healthy adolescents may find the mood swings and hormonal changes they are experiencing difficult enough to confront without the added burden of an illness. Although most of the time they will not acknowledge it, they appreciate having someone to help them regain and maintain control when so many areas of their life are beyond control.

It is extremely important, as with any other age group, to explain procedures and treatments to the adolescent prior to beginning them. Likewise it is important to answer their questions honestly and openly, using language they will understand but without talking down to them. The more fully they understand their illness and the necessary treatments the better they can cooperate with the staff. This is even more important when the adolescent is acutely ill and their illness necessitates transfer to another hospital for evaluation or treatment not available at the local hospital. They are old enough to understand that the condition is serious enough to require more advanced technology but lack the knowledge base to know what to expect from the trip and the other hospital. If a specialized pediatric transport team is involved in the transfer, they will be able to answer many of the questions which the patient and his or her family have and discuss their fears and feelings.

Finally, it is very important to respect the adolescent's need for privacy. In the hospital and transport setting it may not be uncommon for the medical caregiver to be of the opposite sex. For younger age children this is less of a problem, but to the adolescent it can be a major barrier and very embarrassing. It therefore becomes even more important for adolescents to be encouraged to perform as much self care as their medical condition permits, and for the staff to be cautious but matter-of-fact in administering any treatments or providing any care that might invade their privacy.

The comatose child

The CCTT is frequently involved in the transport of the comatose child. The coma may be a result of the illness, such as a diabetic coma, or secondary to closed head trauma or it may be chemically induced through the use of paralytic and sedative medications given by the medical staff in an effort to provide optimal medical care for the child. Whatever the source of the coma, it is important to remember that the child may continue to experience many of the same feelings and sensations as his alert age-equivalent counterpart. Medical personnel also need to remember that these are people who have family who care about them and expect the medical staff to provide them with the highest level of care possible.

The medical staff should interact with the child as if they were awake and alert and able to respond to them. It is important to remember things such as comfort, e.g., maintaining the child's body in proper alignment and support for optimal comfort. This communicates to the family that even though the child cannot move or respond, the medical team cares about their child. A parent who is unable to do anything to help their child feels helpless, and seeing the medical team demonstrate concern for little details such as comfort offers the assurance that their child will be properly cared for.

It is also very important to remember to talk with the child even though he or she cannot respond and does not appear to be able to hear. The patient's hearing is the last sense to fail, and the child and their family benefit from being informed about what to expect during what to them are strange and painful events and procedures. Parents of the child usually want to be as involved in their child's care as possible and will receive comfort as well as vital information about their child simply by being allowed to observe and listen to the medical staff as they care for the child. This is even more important for the critically ill child who requires medical transfer to a pediatric specialty facility.

Frequently the child's medical condition requires the undivided attention of the transport team, making them unavailable to talk with the parents prior to stabilization of the child. By allowing the parents to remain in the room and by talking with the child as if they were awake, the parents see that the child is receiving the best possible care while receiving simple information about what is being done for him or her without feeling as if they are being talked down to. In the event that their child's condition precludes the parents' presence at the bedside, the child still needs to be told which procedures will and will not be painful. Later the team can talk with the parents and explain what has been done for their child.

It is frequently medically necessary for the medical team to sedate and paralyze the child. In this case it is extremely important to administer both a sedative and a paralytic. Unfortunately, all too frequently, medical personnel forget to sedate the child before they administer the paralytic agent. One of the side effects of paralytic agents is that they cause heightened auditory and tactile senses, which, even for the ill adult is very frightening. The use of the combination of a sedative with the paralytic leads to a reduced heart rate and blood pressure, improved ventilatory capability, and produces an amnesia for the painful and frightening events. It also again demonstrates to the family a concern for the child's comfort as well as his or her medical stability, which makes it easier for them to allow strangers to take their child.

The parents and other family members

When a child becomes ill or is injured, he or she is not the only patient. Optimal patient care also involves the parents and other family members. Often this is difficult because their concern overrides their common sense at the moment and may lead to difficulty in communication. This is exacerbated when the child must be transferred to another medical facility in another city.

It is critical that health care professionals be sensitive to the parents needs as well as those of the child. Parents of a critically ill child face specific crises, including the need to develop a sense of trust in the neonatal or pediatric health care team, the need to have the opportunity to interact with and bond to their child in his or her present state of health, and the need to be able to provide at least a small degree of care for their child.

The greatest need of parents and family is the need to be informed of their child's condition. Initially following birth and/or diagnosis of the illness, parents need emotional support as well as accurate information regarding their child's condition. It is frequently necessary to repeat information multiple times in varying ways to help the parents comprehend the information, due to their impaired ability to concentrate. In the case of the critically ill child with a poor prognosis, it is not uncommon for the parents to ask the same questions of multiple people in hopes of gaining the desired information that their child will recover.

Allowing the parents to remain in the room as their child is being prepared to be transferred does much to educate the parents and help alleviate their fears while also meeting their need to be with their child and be as involved in his care as his condition permits. Team members should talk with the parents about the child's condition, answer questions, and explain necessary procedures and equipment. In all situations it is important that parents believe that they did all they could for the child and that their child received the best possible care prior to the arrival of the CCTT. This is particularly true when the referring hospital lacked the resources to provide further intervention and did all they could for the child.

The illness of their child is a time of very high stress for the parents. Their coping mechanisms are inadequate, and their support systems frequently nonexistent. This may be compounded by their child's appearance which may alter dramatically after the CCTT arrives and attaches monitors, inserts IVs, intubates, places them on a ventilator (if necessary), and administers medications.

Parents of the extremely critically ill child may also have unrealistic expectations regarding the anticipated outcome of their child once he or she has been transferred to a pediatric hospital or specialist. It is not uncommon for parents to experience a feeling of hopelessness when they are told of the transfer. They may feel that the transfer must mean their child is going to die. Conversely, parents may perceive the transfer as their child's opportunity for a miracle cure. Both areas should be addressed by the CCTT to accurately portray the child's condition and to prevent this if possible.

In addition to being concerned about their child, the parents may also be concerned about what to expect at the receiving hospital. The transport team can help alleviate many of their concerns by providing them with information about the new facility and about resources available. Information might include visiting hours for their child's unit, availability of no- or low-cost housing close to the hospital, whether or not meals are available at a reduced cost, etc. It is best to provide any important information, such as directions to the hospital and the phone number, in writing for the parents, since they have already received a vast amount of information. If the transport occurs late in the evening or at night, the parents should be prepared to stay in a hotel the first night; further resources can be explored the next day. Frequently in the case of the late evening transport, the parents need to remain in their home town throughout the night and travel to the receiving hospital the next day. Many hospitals have staff, such as social workers or chaplains, specifically for such circumstances.

SUMMARY

Medical transport of the critically ill pediatric patient involves not only specialized medical management but also particular attention to the developmental needs of the child and their family. Children respond differently to stimuli based on their age and the achievement of prior developmental tasks, and thus, have different needs based on their age. The medical staff at the referring hospital as well as the members of the CCTT need to be familiar with the developmental stages of childhood to optimally care for the critically ill child.

For the hospital who usually cares for adults, the critically ill child can be a very uncomfortable experience both medically and emotionally. This becomes less traumatic when the staff knows what to expect from the child and how to talk to the child and his or her parents. For example, many hospitals are uncomfortable allowing the parents to remain with the child especially during procedures. It is not uncommon for the referring staff to learn from the transport team, while the parents are being taught about their child's condition. Consequently, members of the transport team must be both highly skilled medically as well as willing to perform in the role of an educator. Consistent demonstration of how to best manage the critically ill child by the transport team helps prepare the referring hospital for future critically ill children and optimizes the care of all children seen by that facility.

SUGGESTED READINGS

Affonso DD and others: Stressors reported by mothers of hospitalized premature infants, *Neonatal Network* 11(6)63-70, 1992.

Cole M, Cole S: *The development of children,* ed 2, New York, 1993, Scientific American Books.

Cullen, DL: Working with children: understanding a child's developmental stages, *AARC Times* 13(11)70-2, 1989.

Dunn N: Nursing practices in neonatal transports, *Neonatal Network* 16-28, April 1983.

Epperson MM: Families in sudden crisis: process and intervention in a critical care center, *Social Work in Health Care* 2(3)265-73, 1977.

Farrell MF, Frost C: The most important needs of parents of critically ill children: parents' perceptions, *Intensive and Critical Care Nursing* 8(3)130-9, 1992.

Gohsman B, Yunck M: Dealing with the threats of hospitalization, *Journal of Pediatric Nursing* 5(5)32-5, 1979.

Gray E: The emotional and play needs of the dying child, *Issues in Comprehensive Nursing* 12(2/3):207-24, 1989.

Horner MM, Rawlins P, Giles H: How parents of children with chronic conditions perceive their own needs, *MCN* 12(1)40-3, 1987.

Kristjansdottir G: A study of the needs of parents of hospitalized 2- to 6-year-old children, *Issues in Comprehensive Nursing* 14(1)49-64, 1991.

Kruger S: Parents in crisis: helping them cope with a seriously ill child, *Journal of Pediatric Nursing* 7(2)133-40, 1992.

Kuenzi SH, Fenton MV: Crisis intervention in acute care areas, *American Journal of Nursing* 75(5)830-4, 1975.

Miron J: What children think about hospitals, *The Canadian Nurse* 86(3)23-5, 1990.

Montgomery LV: Crisis periods and developmental tasks of the premature infants' family, *Neonatal Network* 2(3)26-31, 1983.

Parkman SE: Helping families say good-bye, *MCN* 17(1)14-7, 1992.

Payne RH: Anxiety and the human family unit: a perspective, *Journal South Carolina Medical Association* 86(9)507-10, 1990.

Rutter M: Separation experiences: a new look at an old topic, *The Journal of Pediatrics* 95(1)147-54, 1979.

Sherwen LN: Separation: the forgotten phenomenon of child development, *Topics in Clinical Nursing* 5(1)1-11, 1983.

Sorensen ES: Children's coping responses, *Journal of Pediatric Nursing* 5(4)259-67, 1990.

Stewart DA and others: Psychosocial adjustments in siblings of children with chronic life-threatening illness: a research note, *Journal of Child Psychologists and Psychiatrists* 33(4)779-84, 1992.

Whaley LF, Wong DL: *Nursing care of infants and children,* ed 2, St. Louis, 1983, CV Mosby.

41

PREHOSPITAL TRANSPORT—GROUND

GEORGE L. FOLTIN
ARTHUR COOPER

The subspecialty of pediatric transport medicine has developed both from the need of pediatric critical care specialists to transport patients swiftly and safely from hospitals with limited pediatric capabilities to pediatric referral centers and the need of pediatric emergency physicians to begin resuscitation of patients with respiratory failure, shock, or trauma in the field prior to arrival at the emergency department. For the most part, patients in the former category are already known to require tertiary-level pediatric intensive care, and it is for this reason that most critical pediatric interhospital transports are staffed by hospital-based teams (physicians, nurses, and respiratory therapists) with a working knowledge of and the equipment to provide this level of care. By contrast, patients in the latter category have not been evaluated by a physician and may or may not require critical life support, but seldom have been evaluated or resuscitated to a point beyond primary and secondary assessment and intervention prior to their arrival at the hospital. Hence, they may not require providers with tertiary-level knowledge and skills. The modern discipline of pediatric transport medicine thus comprises two distinct subdisciplines, critical interhospital medicine and prehospital emergency medicine, each of which is also a subspecialty of the respective parent disciplines of pediatric critical care medicine and pediatric emergency medicine.

It is the aim of this chapter to focus upon prehospital emergency medicine: emergency medical care which is rendered in the field, either at the scene or during primary transport to the initial receiving hospital. In contrast to critical interhospital medicine, critical medical treatment that begins in the emergency department of the initial receiving hospital and continues during secondary transport to the pediatric referral center, prehospital emergency care is rendered chiefly by providers with educational backgrounds in emergency medical technology and paramedicine, acting under the overall aegis of a regional emergency medical services (EMS) system and the ultimate direction of a regional medical control physician or authority. Although the subject of prehospital emergency medicine has been discussed extensively elsewhere,[20] the fundamentals of pediatric prehospital transport, nearly all of which is ground transport, are described herein. However, the reader should always keep in mind that pediatric prehospital treatment and transport are but one aspect of emergency medical services for children (EMSC), which begins with prevention and access, continues through the prehospital emergency department, critical care, acute care, and convalescent phases of treatment, and ends with rehabilitation and recovery, all conducted within the construct of the child's medical home.[91]

PRINCIPLES OF PEDIATRIC PREHOSPITAL GROUND TRANSPORT

Pediatric prehospital emergency medicine can be distinguished in many important respects from the adult version of the specialty. Perhaps the key difference is the relative infrequency of bona fide pediatric emergencies: most reports indicate that about six percent of total ambulance runs are for children under 10 years of age, although this figure increases to ten percent if the definition of a pediatric patient includes the adolescent under eighteen years of age.* Clearly, exposure to pediatric prehospital care will be limited in low-volume emergency medical services. For example, in New York State, the average prehospital provider transports about 100 patients per year, only five to ten of whom are children (less than about one child per month).[36] By contrast, a high-volume emergency medical service, such as the New York City Emergency Medical Service, which employs some 1,500 field providers, mounts nearly 500 tours each day and responds to about 1,000,000 calls each year, may provide the prehospital emergency care professional with a rich exposure to the prehospital care of infants and children, perhaps as many as one pediatric ambulance run every third or fourth day.[35]

A second important difference is the spectrum of disease to which children are susceptible. More than half of all pediatric ambulance runs, and in some regions as many as two thirds,[36,40] are for trauma, while of the remainder the greatest single category have respiratory diseases, all of which are conditions that can theoretically be managed with basic life support (BLS) alone. By contrast, two thirds of ambulance runs in adults are for medical illnesses, many of which potentially involve cardiopulmonary diseases for which the availability of advanced life support (ALS) is crucial. Thus, a third important difference in pediatric prehospital care is the level of care required.

Unfortunately, this third difference sometimes leads to the erroneous assumption that pediatric illnesses are somehow less "acute" than adult illnesses and are therefore less deserving of critical resources,[2] when in fact, the potential for salvage, and years of productive life are actually far greater. No doubt, truly life-threatening illness and injury are rare in childhood and are typically associated not with sudden cardiac collapse but with progressive cardiopulmonary failure due to respiratory failure or shock. In each situation the child responds differently than does the adult. The child's body is capable of better preserving vital functions through various compensatory mechanisms. However, these mechanisms can only be sustained for short periods of time, and when they wear out suddenly, the child will rapidly and unexpectedly deteriorate much more quickly than an adult with the same condition. The "deceptive" presentation of respiratory failure and shock in the child represent that brief time period in which the child's compensatory mechanisms make the patient appear much less seriously ill than is actually the case. If this situation is not recognized and treated immediately, the child will often suffer an "unexpected" and frequently irreversible rapid decline. Yet, the fact that ALS interventions may therefore be required far less often in children than adults, particularly in the early phases of disease which are more likely to be encountered in pediatric patients in the field, does not mean that they are never needed or that BLS providers possess the knowledge and skills necessary to determine when these interventions should actually be performed. Nevertheless, since ALS interventions are strictly indicated probably in no more than about five percent of all pediatric ambulance runs,[2,102] delivery of prehospital care to infants and children primarily emphasizes BLS skills.

The final major difference relates to the practical aspects of pediatric prehospital care. Children are not small adults and cannot be treated and resuscitated using adult-sized tools and techniques. Unfortunately, the larger range of equipment and training which is required to care for this far smaller population often seems prohibitive to emergency medical service agencies in terms of cost-benefit analysis, let alone up-front expense. Yet, an ambulance can be fully outfitted for

* References 2, 40, 74, 84, 102, 106.

pediatric resuscitation for less than about $2,000,[17] while the cost to society of a single childhood injury death that could have been prevented through appropriate prehospital provider intervention is approximately $250,000.[76] The cost of caring for a child with neurological devastation due to inappropriate resuscitation can be even greater.

An ideal model for field treatment of pediatric patients should be based on the epidemiology of childhood illness and injury, using outcome data to support the interventions performed. Since cardiac arrest is rarely a primary event in pediatric patients,[7] the appropriate benchmark of success in prehospital care of critically ill and injured children is intervention in prearrest situations of respiratory failure and shock.[27] Cardiopulmonary resusucitation and airway interventions have been shown to be effective in pediatric near drowning and foreign body aspiration,[54,73] but evidence does not yet exist to demonstrate the improved outcome that would justify the delay inherent in providing ALS to children in the field, except for major trauma,[79] major trauma in the child is more frequently associated with respiratory failure than with shock.[16] This is not to suggest that children should be categorically denied ALS in the prehospital environment for other conditions, merely that priorities must be established.

The capabilities of BLS and ALS providers with respect to pediatric prehospital transport are shown in Box 41-1. Since pediatric prehospital care is strongly BLS-oriented, a high priority should be placed upon mastery of pediatric BLS by BLS and ALS providers alike to achieve optimal patient outcomes. EMS systems that are in the process of developing their pediatric capabilities, however, should not expect prehospital providers to feel suddenly comfortable with the care of pediatric patients, as opportunities to gain experience in treating such patients are limited. Instead, it should be understood that EMS systems will evolve gradually in their pediatric capabilities, as prehospital providers gain experience with children over time. This can be expedited by creative attempts to enhance pediatric experience for prehospital providers through emergency department, intensive care unit, and animal laboratory rotations, in addition to informal discussions and lectures.

BOX 41-1 PREHOSPITAL PROVIDER CAPABILITIES

Basic life support (BLS) interventions
- Cardiopulmonary resuscitation
- Airway opening and positioning
- Oxygen and assisted ventilation
- Extrication techniques
- Splinting and immobilization
- Emergency transport
- First aid
- Application of MAST*

Advanced life support (ALS) interventions
- All of the above, plus . . .
- Endotracheal intubation
- Nasogastric intubation
- Intravenous access
- Intraosseous access*
- Drug and fluid administration
- Electrical defibrillation
- Needle thoracostomy*
- Needle cricothyroidostomy*

* MAST: Military Anti-Shock Trousers. In regions where permitted.

PRACTICE OF PREHOSPITAL PEDIATRIC GROUND TRANSPORT

Limited data are available concerning the operation and outcome of pediatric prehospital ground transport. However, it is known that prehospital providers incompletely assess and treat pediatric emergencies in a substantial number of cases,[34,82] while circumstantial evidence suggests that there are higher death rates among children than adults with similar illnesses.[84] These findings are likely related to demonstrated shortcomings in the training and equipping of prehospital providers for pediatric emergencies,[21,86] particularly in rural areas.[83] This has led numerous emergency medical services (EMS) sys-

* References 22, 30, 49-51, 53, 66, 67, 77, 100, 101, 107.

tems nationwide to develop fully integrated systems for emergency medical services for children (EMSC), based upon the successful experience of Seidel and associates in Southern California.[85]

The outcome of asystolic cardiopulmonary arrest in children, the leading fatal dysrhythmic event in the pediatric population, is dismal, as it is in adults.* It is therefore not surprising that the salvage rate of pediatric patients following unwitnessed arrest by prehospital providers is also poor, except when cardiopulmonary resuscitation (CPR) is begun by a bystander who witnesses the arrest.[22,30] The only exception to these other wise discouraging results is for cardiopulmonary arrest associated with near-drowning, from which one third of victims may be resuscitated if prehospital ALS is promptly available.[73] Anecdotal reports also attest to the efficacy of prehospital ALS in respiratory arrest due to foreign body aspiration.[54]

Respiratory arrest

Given the propensity of the child to develop cardiopulmonary arrest as a result of progressive respiratory failure and the more favorable outcome associated with pure respiratory arrest in the pediatric age group,[49,50,100,107] prehospital providers are likely to have the greatest potential impact in the prevention of respiratory arrest through timely application of appropriate BLS and ALS interventions in the child with respiratory insufficiency. Although data on prehospital outcome of such patients is not yet available, it is known that choice of face mask and resuscitation bag both may influence the success of resuscitation: poorly fitting masks with large dead space are inadequate for infant ventilation,[98] while self-inflating bags will deliver high concentrations of oxygen only when a reservoir is attached, the pop-off valve is disabled, and a compression forceful enough to result in adequate bilateral chest rise is applied.[26,41,45] Moreover, although properly trained prehospital providers initially achieve satisfactory bag-valve-mask ventilation in simulations,[43,98,99] these skills tend to deteriorate markedly over time, especially among BLS providers.[28] However, such skill degradation may be overcome through the use of educational methodologies which reinforce the proper hand position required to achieve optimal head position, airway opening, and mask fit, hence effective ventilation.[15]

Properly taught, endotracheal intubation of pediatric patients by prehospital ALS providers will overcome the inherent limitations of bag-valve-mask ventilation of children. Indeed, success rates approaching 90% can be achieved when paramedics learn to intubate in a pediatric operating room.[52,70] Success rates, unfortunately, are significantly lower among paramedics who have not had this level of training, while complication rates are higher.[1,64] However, the success rate of pediatric prehospital endotracheal intubation can be substantially improved through experience with endotracheal intubation in live felines, conducted either in an approved animal laboratory or a veterinary teaching facility under the personal supervision of a veterinary practitioner,[81,103] as the anatomy and reactivity of the larynx in the adult feline closely mimics those of the human infant.

Major trauma

Experience with prehospital interventions for circulatory support is also increasing. Medical antishock trousers (MAST) appear detrimental to hypotensive victims of major pediatric trauma,[11] while preliminary evidence suggests that prehospital volume resuscitation may also be detrimental in such children.[13] Vascular access, which may be difficult for paramedics to achieve in patients less than one year of age,[82] may therefore prove to be more useful for management of nontraumatic conditions requiring infusion of fluids or medications, such as severe dehydration or nontraumatic cardiac arrest. Intraosseous access may be employed successfully by paramedics in young children when venous access is impossible to obtain[31,62,88,94,97] and appears cost-effective despite the relative infrequency of its use,[32,108] but IO access also may ultimately prove to have a limited role in the management of young children with life-threatening injuries.[10]

---

* References 2, 40, 74, 84, 102, 106.

Prehospital care of pediatric patients with major trauma assumes great importance not only because it is the most frequent critical pediatric emergency encountered in the field,* but also because 80% of children who die as a result of injury will not survive long enough to reach the hospital,[14] some 90% of whom will be attended by prehospital providers.[33] Most such children ultimately succumb as a result of traumatic brain injury, which induces coma, thus predisposing to soft tissue obstruction of the upper airway.[89] It is therefore not surprising that mortality rates among victims of major pediatric blunt trauma should be lower in regions where EMS systems are capable of definitive management of the airway in the field by means of endotracheal intubation.[79] Other ALS maneuvers are infrequently required in trauma, but when needed, will not delay transport if they are performed en route rather than on-scene.[48] On the other hand, the use of ALS in managing pediatric trauma victims in the field becomes difficult to justify when scene time exceeds transport time to a trauma center with pediatric capabilities, and there has been no extrication problem or traffic congestion to explain the transport delay.[74]

Problems with prehospital emergency care

Pediatric prehospital emergency care is barely a decade old in most areas of the nation, even in regions with well-organized EMS systems. Perhaps more than any other, this fact accounts for the paucity of scientific evidence documenting the efficacy of pediatric prehospital emergency care. The lack of such data in adult prehospital care has led some experts to argue that certain prehospital interventions are unproven and should be withheld, pending the availability of properly controlled scientific investigations confirming their utility.[39,90] However, it must be remembered that prehospital emergency care merely begins treatment in the field that would have been started in the emergency department, and represents commonly accepted standards of care in pediatric emergency medical practice. Thus, in the opinion of the authors, critical life support modalities should not be denied to pediatric patients in the field simply for lack of data confirming their utility in the prehospital venue. Research should focus upon the utility of particular therapies across the entire continuum of emergency care, which includes both the out-of-hospital and in-hospital phases of such care.

The overall response of the EMS system to pediatric emergencies, however, is an appropriate subject for pure prehospital research. Legitimate questions have already been raised with respect to the appropriateness of primary transport of pediatric patients by prehospital providers more accustomed to the longer scene times that are typical of adult prehospital care, particularly in short-transport urban and suburban systems: total time to definitive treatment is often shorter when patients are transported by police vehicles,[80] suggesting that police officers might have a legitimate role in pediatric transport, assuming they were appropriately trained as first responders.[92] This approach has particular appeal, given that operational logistics may result in assignment of BLS ambulances to ALS patients, and vice versa, based upon ambulance availability at the time the call requesting emergency care is made.[72] Such problems are compounded in the face of mass casualty incidents, in which the needs of pediatric patients may frequently be overlooked.[104]

Yet, the most vexing problem in pediatric prehospital emergency care is the issue of regionalization. There is now good evidence that regionalized tertiary level pediatric intensive care[71] and regionalized pediatric trauma care,[12,37,63] both result in improved mortality outcomes for children with critical illnesses and injuries of moderately great severity. However, there are no data currently available to guide prehospital providers with respect to pediatric field triage decisions. For example, while it is known that regionalized pediatric trauma care saves more children's lives, there is also evidence to suggest that adult trauma centers and surgeons achieve results which are comparable to those obtained by pediatric trauma centers and surgeons, provided that comprehensive pediatric subspecialty support is readily available.[3,29,47,75] Thus, it still remains for prehospital EMS researchers to find an answer to the key question in pediatric primary transport: under what circumstances should the prehospital provider transporting a critically ill or injured child bypass a hospital without special pediatric capabilities?

EDUCATION FOR PEDIATRIC PREHOSPITAL TRANSPORT

As stated, the ideal prehospital training system emphasizes pediatric BLS for all personnel. This entails specific BLS training of BLS and ALS providers in the care of infants and children before it undertakes the far costlier per capita training of ALS providers in more invasive modalities of care. Because response time to any emergency is a direct function of ambulance density, pediatric training of prehospital providers should not be limited to a single small segment of the prehospital provider community. Moreover, as with any critical skill that is seldom used, the frequency and intensity of this training should far exceed the actual volume of pediatric calls, for those who have limited experience in the prehospital care of children will require more practice to keep their skills sharp.

BLS certification

BLS certification at the emergency medical technician (EMT) level requires 110 hours of training at a minimum, although in some regions training may be extended by an additional 90 to 100 hours, particularly if certain ALS modalities, such as defibrillation, are determined by the region to be so essential to the public health that they are taught to BLS providers. Unfortunately, the original 110 hour emergency medical technician-ambulance (EMT-A) course,[65] which is still being taught to most emergency medical technicians nationwide, contains only 2 hours which are devoted exclusively to the prehospital care of infants and children; the only subjects covered are normal pediatric vital signs, fever, poisoning, croup, and epiglottis. Theoretically, additional time is made available in "core" sessions dealing with management of the airway, breathing, and circulation, although there is rarely ample time to cover the pediatric part of this material adequately, if indeed it is covered at all. The revised 110 hour emergency medical technician-basic (EMT-B) course recently developed under contract to the National Highway Traffic Safety Administration (NHTSA), which has been the lead agency for EMS education and training within the Federal government since 1966, devotes more than 6 hours to pediatric prehospital care and appropriately focuses upon assessment and management of respiratory failure, shock, and trauma in the child.[95]

ALS certification

ALS certification at the emergency medical technician-paramedic (EMT-P) level requires some 450 hours of training at a minimum. Although this has been extended in some areas to more than 1,000 hours, clinical exposure to the problems of infants and children, both in the hospital and in the field, varies considerably from course to course and region to region. For ALS providers at the emergency medical technician-intermediate (EMT-I) level, education in pediatrics, which obviously requires integration of new knowledge as well as mastery of new skills, is even more limited. Unfortunately, few ALS providers, even at the paramedic level, receive more than 6 to 10 hours of training in pediatrics, much of which is technically oriented.[21,83]

This is not to diminish the importance of pediatric skill training for ALS providers. Certain psychomotor skills, such as bag-valve-mask ventilation, are of such vital importance in the management of critically ill and injured children that they require constant reinforcement, stressing differences both in hands-on technique and equipment selection with respect to adults. Intubation is also essential, and, while there are many similarities between pediatric and adult intubation, there are enough differences that special training is needed for the former, although it should be based upon a strong foundation of experience with the latter. Finally, intraosseous cannulation is being used with increasing frequency to obtain venous access in infants and small children in the prehospital environment. Yet for most ALS providers, it represents a entirely new skill which will require appropriate instruction before it is introduced.

Most current ALS training courses adequately emphasize the differences between infants, children, and adults insofar as invasive techniques are concerned. This emphasis is in contrast to BLS training courses in which technical skills are seldom fully mastered for any patient group. Yet, as indispensible as skill training may be, ALS provider training must stress pediatric assessment, as this is the key to the proper application of invasive techniques in infants and children. Without such training, ALS providers are left to assume that the principal differences between pediatric and adult prehospital care are related to technique and equipment, rather than spectrum of disease and response to illness. However, although ALS providers must be aware that the diagnoses typically encountered in the pediatric age groups are different from those commonly observed in older patients, their training should focus not upon anatomic diagnosis, such as epiglottitis, but upon physiologic assessment, such as respiratory insufficiency, since the aim of pediatric prehospital care is not so much to provide definitive treatment in the field as to prevent further deterioration in ventilation, oxygenation, and perfusion during primary transport to a facility capable of providing definitive care for pediatric emergencies.

Developing and maintaining the knowledge, skills, and attitudes necessary for pediatric resuscitation requires no realignment of the basic approach to prehospital management, but does require reassurance that previously-mastered, adult-oriented knowledge and skills can be readily transferred to infants and children, so long as 1) differences in anatomy, physiology, disease spectrum, and patient assessment are well enough understood to allow a meaningful evaluation of a sick child to be obtained, and 2) special techniques, once learned, are constantly reinforced. Keen appreciation of psychological and developmental differences is also fundamental, since the interdependence between children and their parents mandates a family-centered approach to pediatric emergency care which charges the emergency provider with responsibility for the distraught parents as well as their distressed child. Still, there are additional concerns: 1) prehospital providers generally regard critical pediatric calls as the most stressful events they must face in the line of duty; 2) pediatric skills which are used infrequently are not well retained by the average prehospital provider, BLS or ALS; and 3) in times of high stress, even a well-trained prehospital provider may revert to use of adult protocols and equipment with which he or she is more familiar, even if this use is inappropriate, unless both training and retraining of field personnel are ongoing.

The current status of education and training for prehospital providers is summarized in Table 41-1. It is self evident that, for most prehospital providers, the goals and objectives of education and training for pediatric prehospital emergency care cannot be met within the framework of the basic 110-hour course in emergency medical technology, even the revised version which is currently

TABLE 41-1 TYPES OF PREHOSPITAL PROVIDERS

Provider type	*Care provided*	*Total hours required for certification*	*Total hours in pediatrics*
First responder	CPR First Aid	25	1
EMT*	All BLS	110	2
Intermediate levels†	All BLS Limited ALS	200-300	Variable
Paramedic‡	All ALS	450-1,100	6-12

* Emergency medical technician-basic (EMT, EMT-A, EMT-B, EMT-1)
† Emergency medical technician-intermediate (EMT-I, AEMT-2)
Emergency medical technician-critical care (EMT-CC, AEMT-3)
‡ Emergency medical technician-paramedic (EMT-P, AEMT-4)

BOX 41-2 MINIMUM STANDARDS FOR PEDIATRIC TRAINING OF PREHOSPITAL PROVIDERS

Basic Life Support (BLS) providers
- Knowledge
  - Anatomic and physiological differences
  - Psychological and developmental issues
  - Pediatric physical assessment
  - Pediatric vital signs
  - Spectrum of pediatric illness/injury requiring emergency care
  - Principles of neonatal/pediatric resuscitation
  - Recognition/management of pediatric respiratory distress/failure
  - Recognition/management of pediatric shock/trauma
  - Treatment of pediatric medical/surgical emergencies
    - Burns
    - Near drowning
    - Seizures
    - Poisoning
  - Recognition/reporting of child abuse
  - Recognition/management of SIDS
  - Critical incident stress debriefing
- Skills
  - Infant/child cardiopulmonary resuscitation
  - Infant/child obstructed airway clearing maneuvers
  - Infant/child airway/ventilatory management
  - Pediatric vital signs determination
  - Pediatric medical anti-shock trouser (MAST) use
  - Pediatric extrication and spine immobilization

Advanced Life Support (ALS) providers
- Review/reinforcement of all of the above, plus . . .
- Knowledge
  - Need for endotracheal/nasogastric intubation in pediatrics
  - Need for intravenous/intraosseous access in pediatrics
  - Dosage/administration of drugs in pediatric emergencies
  - Dosage/administration of fluid in pediatric emergencies
- Skills
  - Pediatric endotracheal/nasogastric intubation
  - Pediatric intravenous/intraosseous access
  - Pediatric defibrillation/cardioversion
  - Pediatric needle thoracostomy/cricothyroidostomy

being field tested. For the forseeable future, therefore, EMS systems will need to rely upon continuing education to prepare prehospital providers for the care of critically ill and injured children. However, the time investment required for most such courses is no more than about 15 hours, and all of these hours may be credited toward annual continuing education requirements already mandated for recertification. If EMS teachers impart a positive mindset toward the care of critically ill and injured children, prehospital providers will respond with an attitudinal change that may persist even when technical skills do not.

Other educational packages

Opportunities for prehospital providers to receive specific training in pediatric emergency care had been limited[83] prior to the introduction of the Pediatric Emergency Medical Services Training Program (PEMSTP) in 1985.[21] Numerous educational packages, designed for both the BLS and ALS levels of care, have appeared in recent years. Most have been developed under the auspices of the Federal EMSC Grant Program and are available through its national resource centers.[5] Many localities are also adapting the American Heart Association/American Academy of Pediatrics *Pediatric Advanced Life Support* (PALS) Course[7] for their paramedics, and this has been received enthusiastically by these providers. Minimum standards for education and training of prehospital providers, as defined by a consensus Task Force on Education and Training from the Federal EMSC projects, are shown in Box 41-2.[9]

Courses that can be self-taught or are separable into modules allow for wide dispersion of teaching materials. This approach has been successfully adopted by the Pediatric Prehospital Care Course developed jointly by the New York State Department of Health and the New York State and New York City EMSC projects.[36] Greater use of modern telecommunications technologies has also been advocated to permit the large number of rural providers in this nation to have access to training that traditionally has been centered at major teaching institutions. Such telecommunications can be used for dissemination via broadcast or mobile teaching stations, such as the interactional laser disc system developed by the Idaho EMSC project.

Properly controlled scientific studies evaluating pediatric skill retention in BLS and ALS providers and field performance have not yet been performed. However, some inferences can be drawn from pilot studies.[18,19,43,64] First, retention of basic airway skills appears somewhat better among ALS providers than among BLS providers, although in neither group is it optimal. Secondly, pediatric intubation training using the feline model serves not only to teach an important new skill but, presumably because of increased familiarity with the pediatric airway, also increases the ALS provider's overall sense of confidence in managing the critical pediatric airway. Next, intraosseus cannulation training, using the "chicken leg" model, appears no less easily mastered by prehospital ALS providers than by their physician colleagues and often has been more easily mastered. Finally, there is no objective evidence from written and oral test scores on certification or recertification examinations to suggest that pediatric ALS protocols are not understood, and there are no indication from evaluations of field performance that they have not been followed or that pediatric skills are improperly performed or applied. Indeed, prehospital providers who have successfully applied their pediatric training are among its most vocal proponents.

The relevance of these observations for ALS provider training is self-evident. However, several inferences can also be drawn with respect to BLS provider training.[23,25] Since BLS providers usually have more direct experience in the field with pediatric patients than ALS providers, the observed difference between BLS and ALS providers insofar as pediatric airway skill retention is concerned appears to be due chiefly to length of training. There is reason to believe that extended pediatric training would have the same salutary effect on pediatric airway skill retention on BLS providers as it does on ALS providers. Such extended training, for the most part, is enthusiastically received by BLS providers, among whom the perception that their pediatric training has been less than adequate is widespread. The degree of confidence in handling pediatric emergencies expressed by BLS providers who have undergone training similar in length to that which is normally offered to ALS providers in most regions appears no different from that seen in ALS providers who have undergone this training.

EQUIPMENT FOR PEDIATRIC PREHOSPITAL TRANSPORT

The Task Force on Education and Training of the Federal EMSC Grant Program has identified the minimum equipment needs for pediatric prehospital emergency care at both the BLS and ALS levels, as shown in Box 41-3.[24] The American College of Emergency Physicians (ACEP) has published a similar document.[69] While medications required by children differ little from those needed by adults, drug dosages are determined, for the most part, on the basis of size. The use of color-coded resuscitation tapes that key drug doses[55] and equipment selection[56] to body length has proved effective in the field. These color-coded tapes are now a standard item of equipment in many EMS agencies, particularly for ALS providers.

As stated, the actual cost of equipping EMS systems for pediatric resuscitation is remarkably low. Since many services already have some of the necessary equipment, meeting the currently recommended standards is relatively inexpensive. For those which do not, comparing the actual costs of obtaining this equipment with other fixed expenses may be illuminating.[17] For example, a single vehicle can be fully outfitted for considerably less than the price of a single semiautomatic defibrillator.[8]

BOX 41-3 MINIMUM STANDARDS FOR PEDIATRIC EQUIPMENT IN PREHOSPITAL VEHICLES

Basic Life Support (BLS) vehicles

- Pediatric stethoscope, infant/child attachments
- Pediatric blood pressure cuffs, infant/child sizes
- Disposable humidifier(s)
- Pediatric simple/nonrebreathing oxygen masks, all sizes
- Pediatric face masks, all sizes
- Pediatric bag-valve devices, infant/child sizes
- Pediatric airway adjuncts, all sizes
- Pediatric suction catheters, all sizes
- Pediatric Yankauer device
- Pediatric extrication collars, all sizes
- Pediatric extrication equipment (including infant car seat)
- Pediatric limb splints, all sizes
- Pediatric traction splint
- Pediatric medical anti-shock trousers (MAST)

Advanced Life Support (ALS) vehicles

All of the above, plus . . .

- Pediatric endotracheal tubes, all sizes
- Pediatric stylets, all sizes
- Pediatric laryngoscope blades, all sizes
- Pediatric Magill (Rovenstein) forceps
- Pediatric intravenous catheters, all sizes
- Pediatric intraosseous needles, all sizes
- Pediatric nasogastric tubes, all sizes
- Pediatric ECG electrodes
- Pediatric defibrillator paddles, infant/child sizes
- Pediatric dosage-packed medications/fluids
- Pediatric dosage/volume wall chart
- Mini-drip intravenous infusion sets

ROLE OF PREHOSPITAL PROVIDERS IN PREHOSPITAL TRANSPORT

As stated, prehospital care is emergency medical treatment begun prior to arrival in the emergency department that would have been started in the emergency department by an emergency physician, had the patient first sought treatment there, instead of calling for an ambulance. Hence, prehospital care should be viewed not as a separate part of emergency care, but as an extension of the emergency department into the patient environment. In some nations, mostly in Europe, critical prehospital emergency treatment is provided directly by emergency physicians on ambulances outfitted as mobile critical care units. In this nation prehospital care is rendered by emergency medical technicians or paramedics acting under the direction of a specially trained emergency physician, known as a prehospital Medical Control physician. The principles and practice of prehospital emergency medical treatment, as practiced by prehospital paraprofessionals, are embodied and delineated in a series of detailed treatment instructions termed "protocols," that constitute, in effect, a standing set of "doctor's orders" from prehospital medical control physicians to the prehospital providers practicing under their supervision. BLS protocols typically consist solely of standing orders, which are routinely executed without the need for direct physician involvement. ALS protocols, however, may also contain one or more "Medical Control physician options" that are more complex or critical in nature, and therefore require voice contact with the responsible medical control physician before they can be initiated.

As the responsible physician supervisors of paraprofessional medical personnel, prehospital medical control physicians have special obligations to critically ill and injured children who require emergency care. Pediatric patients cannot be properly evaluated or appropriately treated using protocols and procedures designed for adults. However, the special needs of infants and children may not be appreciated by professionals with limited experience in the care of pediatric medical and traumatic emergencies. Thus, it is vital that prehospital Medical Control physicians involve regional experts in pediatric emergency medicine, trauma surgery, and critical care in all phases of EMS system planning, development, oversight, and quality management. It is particularly important that Medical Control physicians involve education and training, medical control, and quality assurance as they relate to the needs of pediatric patients.

ROLE OF PREHOSPITAL PROVIDERS IN INTERHOSPITAL TRANSPORT

The focus of this chapter, thus far, has been on primary (prehospital emergency) pediatric transport. Ideally, children in need of secondary (critical interhospital) transport (onward transport from an EDAP, or emergency department approved for pediatrics,[87] to a PCCC, or pediatric critical care center[6]) are attended by a referral center-based, physician-led or nurse-led critical transport team dispatched from the PCCC to the EDAP by ground or air for this specific purpose. Realistically, relatively few regions of the nation possess this capability and must therefore rely upon health professionals (including paraprofessionals with backgrounds in emergency medical technology and paramedicine) whose training, as currently defined, does not include specific education in critical interhospital transport. Clearly, such individuals possess the basic knowledge and skills required to conduct secondary transport, provided they receive special additional training in the fundamentals of critical interhospital medicine.

Nevertheless, the severity of illness and injury in pediatric patients requiring transport,[46,58] and the stabilization time required for such patients prior to commencement of transport,[105] both suggest that critical pediatric interhospital transports should be conducted by properly qualified physicians and nurses whenever they are available. While it is clear that decisions or interventions requiring immediate physician involvement are made or performed during transport in fewer than half of all cases,[61,96] which can usually be anticipated in advance,[60] it is equally clear that it is difficult to predict with certainty which transports will actually require direct physician participation and those which will not.[68,78] The presence of an endotracheal tube and physiologic instability appear to have greater positive predictive value than other indicators of the need for physician participation in pediatric critical interhospital transport,[59] although under proper medical direction, well-trained nonphysician providers can transport intubated patients with minimal risk.[4] Yet, adverse events which do occur during pediatric critical interhospital transport and result in physiologic deterioration are due chiefly to complications associated with endotracheal intubation,[44] and happen more often during transport than they do in the pediatric critical care unit,[42] underscoring both the inherent danger of critical pediatric interhospital transport and the conventional wisdom of staffing such transports with pediatric critical care-capable physicians and nurses whenever possible.

The goal of pediatric critical interhospital transport is to mimic as closely as possible the care the patient would receive in a pediatric critical care unit, subject to the limitations of space and equipment available in the patient compartment of a moving ambulance.[93] As such, transport providers, at a minimum, must be capable of critical pediatric assessment and monitoring and must be highly skilled in the techniques of endotracheal intubation and assisted ventilation, vascular access and circulatory support, as well as fluid and drug administration in critically ill and injured children.[57,93] Ideally, such providers will perform these functions as regular members of dedicated, organized pediatric transport services in accordance with established policies and procedures that are subject to ongoing review. However, experience has also shown that transport providers must receive specific education in the actual conduct of critical pediatric interhospital transport if optimal results are to be obtained.[38,93]

Most physicians and nurses who are based in emergency departments and critical care units already possess the technical knowledge and skills required for secondary transport but may lack a clear understanding of the legal requirements imposed upon secondary transport by Federal law (see Chapter 36), or may not possess an understanding of the roles and responsibilities of prehospital paraprofessionals who may be called upon to assist them. By contrast, prehospital paraprofessionals called upon to assist during interhospital transport may possess a clear understanding of their roles, but typically lack the knowledge and skills necessary to assist hospital-based providers in conducting safe transport. Because this knowledge and skill base can be acquired in a relatively short time, and can be easily delineated in additional protocols that define and limit the scope of practice of interhospital transport-capable EMTs and paramedics, such paraprofessionals are well-suited to assist hospital-based physicians and nurses with interhospital critical transport. The general thrust of such protocols, as is also the case in the critical care unit, is maintenance and monitoring of ventilation, oxygenation, and perfusion, with reversion to prehospital standing orders for resuscitation in the case of a clinical emergency. However, they should also provide special additional instructions with respect to critical life support devices such as transport ventilators, infusion pumps, chest tubes, Gardner-Wells tongs, and the like, as well as medications not commonly utilized during prehospital emergency transport.

There are, at present, no standardized criteria or curricula available to assist ambulance service medical directors in providing this additional training to EMTs and paramedics practicing under their licenses. Clearly, however, it is the responsibility of the medical control physician to ensure that such providers are properly trained. At a minimum, such training must include instruction in the differences between prehospital emergency care and critical interhospital care, legal issues involved in transport, use of the various critical life support devices noted above, and pediatric advanced life support (using scenarios specifically developed to mimic commonly encountered problems in pediatric interhospital transport). Such training must be acceptable both to the ambulance service medical director and regional experts in pediatric emergency medicine, trauma surgery, and critical care. Ideally, this training should become a required component of basic education for prehospital personnel expected to participate in interhospital transport, and ultimately, part of a local or regional credentialing process in critical interhospital transport medicine.

Unfortunately, more often than not, local circumstances will dictate both the need for critical pediatric interhospital transport and the composition of the team available to conduct such transport. Under no circumstances, however, should transport ever be conducted by a team incapable of definitively managing the pediatric airway or performing age-appropriate vascular access, whether intravenous or intraosseous. If an endotracheal tube or physiologic instability is present or anticipated before or during transport and a critical pediatric transport team is available, it should be summoned to conduct the transport. Otherwise, a pediatrician, surgeon, or emergency physician trained in pediatric advanced life support and skilled in its application may conduct the transport, assisted as necessary by available nonphysician providers within the limits of their experience and defined scope of practice.

REFERENCES

1. Aijian P and others: Endotracheal intubation of pediatric patients by paramedics, *Ann Emerg Med* 18:489-94, 1989.
2. Applebaum D: Advanced prehospital care for pediatric emergencies, *Ann Emerg Med* 14:656-9, 1985.
3. Bensard DD and others: A critical analysis of acutely injured children managed in a adult level I trauma center, *J Pediatr Surg* 29:11-8, 1994.
4. Beyer AJ, Land G, Zaritsky A: Nonphysician transport of intubated pediatric patients: a system evaluation, *Crit Care Med* 20:961-6, 1992.
5. Brownstein D: Educational resources. In Luten R, Foltin G, editors: *Pediatric resources for prehospital care,* ed 3, Arlington, 1993, National Center for Education in Maternal and Child Health.
6. California Pediatric Critical Care Coalition: Systems approach, Appendix D. In Seidel JS, Henderson DP, editors: *Emergency medical services for children: a report to the nation,* Washington, 1991, National Center for Education in Maternal and Child Health.
7. Chameides L, editor: *Textbook of pediatric advanced life support,* Dallas and Elk Grove Village, 1988. American Heart Association and American Academy of Pediatrics.
8. Cooper A and others: Costs of equipping and training emergency personnel for pediatric resuscitation, *Ped Emerg Care* 7:385, 1991 (abstract).
9. Cooper A and others: Education and training of professionals and the public. In Seidel JS, Henderson DP, editors: *Emergency medical services for children: a report to the nation,* Washington, 1991, National Center for Education in Maternal and Child Health.
10. Cooper A and others: Efficacy of intraosseous infusions in children who present in hypotensive shock following major trauma, *J Pediatr Surg* (submitted for publication).

11. Cooper A and others: Efficacy of MAST use in children who present in hypotensive shock, *J Trauma* 33:151, 1992 (abstract).
12. Cooper A and others: Efficacy of pediatric trauma care: results of a population-based study, *J Pediatr Surg* 28:299-305, 1993.
13. Cooper A and others: Efficacy of prehospital volume resuscitation in children who present in hypotensive shock, *J Trauma* 35:160, 1993 (abstract).
14. Cooper A and others: Epidemiology of pediatric trauma: importance of population-based statistics, *J Pediatr Surg* 27:149-54, 1992.
15. Cooper A and others: Teaching paramedics to ventilate infants: preliminary results of a new method, *Ped Emerg Care* (submitted for publication).
16. Cooper A, Barlow B, DiScala C: Mortality and physiologic instability: the pediatric perspective, *J Pediatr Surg* (submitted for publication).
17. Cooper A: Systems approach, Appendix B. In Seidel JS, Henderson DP, editors: *Emergency medical services for children: a report to the nation*, Washington, 1991, National Center for Education in Maternal and Child Health.
18. Cooper A, Welborn C: Unpublished data.
19. DePrima J, Giordano L, Ross Y: *Minutes of the training and testing subcommittee, medical advisory committee, New York City Emergency Medical Services*, New York, 1988-1990, New York City Emergency Medical Services.
20. Dieckmann RA, editor: *Pediatric emergency care systems: planning and management*, Baltimore, 1992, Williams and Wilkins.
21. Eichelberger MR, Stossel-Pratsch G, Mangubat EA: A pediatric emergencies program for emergency medical services, *Pediatr Emerg Care* 1:177-9, 1985.
22. Eisenberg M, Bergner L, Hallstrom A: Epidemiology of cardiac arrest and resuscitation in children, *Ann Emerg Med* 12:672-4, 1983.
23. Elling R: Personal communication, November 10, 1990.
24. Emergency Medical Services Education & Training Taskforce, Emergency Medical Services for Children Grant Program, Bureau of Maternal and Child Health Resources Development: *pediatric ambulance equipment recommendations*, Rockville, 1988, U.S. Department of Health and Human Services.
25. Emergency Medical Services Education & Training Taskforce, Emergency Medical Services for Children Grant Program, Bureau of Maternal and Child Health Resources Development, *Summary of education & training issues survey responses*, Rockville, 1988, U.S. Department of Health and Human Services.
26. Finer NN and others: Limitations of self-inflating resuscitators, *Pediatrics* 77:417-20, 1986.
27. Foltin G and others: Developing pediatric prehospital advanced life support: the New York City experience, *Ped Emerg Care* 6:141-4, 1990.
28. Foltin G and others: EMT ventilation of infant mannequins: a comparison of mouth-to-mouth and bag-valve-mask techniques, *Pediatr Emerg Care* 4:295, 1988 (abstract).
29. Fortune JM and others: A pediatric trauma center without a pediatric surgeon: a four year outcome analysis, *J Trauma* 33:130-9, 1992.
30. Freisen RM and others: Appraisal of pediatric cardiopulmonary resuscitation, *Can Med Assoc J* 126:1055-8, 1982.
31. Fuchs S and others: A prehospital model of intraosseous infusion, *Ann Emerg Med* 20:371-4, 1991.
32. Garrison HG and others: A cost-effectiveness analysis of pediatric intraosseous infusion as a prehospital skill, *Prehosp Disast Med* 7:221-7, 1992.
33. Gausche M and others: Pediatric deaths and emergency medical services (EMS) in urban and rural areas, *Pediatr Emerg Care* 5:158-62, 1989.
34. Gausche M, Henderson DP, Seidel JS: Vital signs as part of the prehospital assessment of the pediatric patient: a survey of paramedics, *Ann Emerg Med* 19:173-8, 1990.
35. Giordano LM: Personal communication, December 31, 1993.
36. Guerin R and others: *Pediatric pre-hospital care course student manual*, Albany, 1991, New York State Department of Health Emergency Medical Services Program.
37. Hall KR and others: Traumatic death in urban children, revisited, *AJDC* 147:102-7, 1993.
38. Henning R, McNamara V: Difficulties encountered in transport of the critically ill child, *Ped Emerg Care* 7:133-7, 1991.
39. Johnson JC: Prehospital care: the future of emergency medical services, *Ann Emerg Med* 20:426-30, 1991.
40. Johnston C, King WD: Pediatric prehospital care in a southern regional emergency medical service system, *South Med J* 81:1473-6, 1988.
41. Kain ZK and others: Performance of pediatric resuscitation bags assessed with an infant lung simulator, *Anesth Analg* 77:261-4, 1993.
42. Kanter RK and others: Excess mortality associated with interhospital transport, *Pediatrics* 90:893-8, 1992.
43. Kanter RK: Evaluation of mask-bag ventilation in resuscitation of infants, *AJDC* 141:761-3, 1987.
44. Kanter RK, Tompkins JM: Adverse events during interhospital transport: physiologic deterioration associated with pretransport severity of illness, *Pediatrics* 84:43-8, 1989.
45. Kissoon N and others: An evaluation of the physical and functional characteristics of resuscitators for use in pediatrics, *Crit Care Med* 20:292-6, 1992.
46. Kissoon N and others: The child requiring transport: lessons and implications for the pediatric emergency physician, *Ped Emerg Care* 4:1-4, 1988.

47. Knudson MM, Shagoury C, Lewis FR: Can adult trauma surgeons care for injured children? *J Trauma* 32:729-39, 1992.
48. Lavery RF, Tortella BJ, Griffin CG: The prehospital management of pediatric trauma, *Ped Emerg Care* 8:9-12, 1992.
49. Lewis JK and others: Outcome of pediatric resuscitation, *Ann Emerg Med* 12:297-9, 1983.
50. Losek JD and others: Prehospital care of the pulseless, nonbreathing pediatric patient, *Am J Emerg Med* 5:370-5, 1987.
51. Losek JD and others: Prehospital countershock treatment of pediatric asystole, *Am J Emerg Med* 7:571-5, 1989.
52. Losek JD and others: Prehospital pediatric endotracheal intubation performance review, *Ped Emerg Care* 5:1-4, 1989.
53. Ludwig S, Kettrick RG, Parker M: Pediatric cardiopulmonary resuscitation: a review of 130 cases, *Clin Pediatr* 23:71-5, 1984.
54. Luten R, Foltin G, Pons P: Access to optimal care for children in the EMS system. In Luten R, Foltin G, editors: *Pediatric resources for prehospital care,* ed 2, Elk Grove Village, 1990, American Academy of Pediatrics, Committee of the Section on Emergency Medicine.
55. Luten RC and others: A rapid method for estimating resuscitation drug doses from length in the pediatric age group, *Ann Emerg Med* 17:576-81, 1988.
56. Luten RC and others: Length-based endotracheal tube and emergency equipment in pediatrics, *Ann Emerg Med* 21:900-4, 1992.
57. MacNab AJ: Optimal escort for interhospital transport of pediatric emergencies, *J Trauma* 31:205-9, 1991.
58. Mayer TA: Severity of illness and injury in pediatric air transport, *Ann Emerg Med* 13:108-11, 1984.
59. McCloskey KA and others: Variables predicting the need for a pediatric critical care transport team, *Ped Emerg Care* 8:1-3, 1992.
60. McCloskey KA, Johnston C: Critical care interhospital transports: predictability of the need for a pediatrician, *Ped Emerg Care* 6:89-92, 1990.
61. McCloskey KA, King WD, Byron L: Pediatric critical care transport: is a physician always needed on the team? *Ann Emerg Med* 18:247-9, 1989.
62. Miner WF and others: Prehospital use of intraosseous infusion by paramedics, *Ped Emerg Care* 5:5-7, 1989.
63. Nakayama DK, Copes WS, Sacco W: Differences in trauma care among pediatric and nonpediatric trauma centers, *J Pediatr Surg* 27:427-31, 1992.
64. Nakayama DK, Gardner MJ, Rowe MI: Emergency endotracheal intubation in pediatric trauma, *Ann Surg* 211218-23, 1990.
65. National Highway Traffic Safety Administration, U.S. Department of Transportation: *Emergency medical technician national standard curriculum,* ed 3, Washington, 1984, Department of Transportation.
66. Nichols DG and others: Factors influencing outcome of cardiopulmonary resuscitation in children, *Ped Emerg Care* 2:1-5, 1986.
67. O'Rourke PP: Outcome of children who are apneic and pulseless in the emergency room, *Crit Care Med* 14:466-8, 1986.
68. Orr RA, Venkataraman T, Singleton CA: Pediatric risk of mortality (PRISM) score: a poor predictor in triage of patients for pediatric transport, *Ann Emerg Med* 18:450, 1989 (abstract).
69. Pediatric Emergency Medicine Committee and Emergency Medical Services Committee, American College of Emergency Physicians: *Minimum pediatric pre-hospital equipment guidelines,* Dallas, 1991, American College of Emergency Physicians.
70. Pointer JE: Clinical characteristics of paramedics' performance of pediatric endotracheal intubation, *Am J Emerg Med* 7:364-6, 1989.
71. Pollack MM and others: Improved outcomes from tertiary center pediatric intensive care: a statewide comparison of tertiary and nontertiary care factilities, *Crit Care Med* 19:150-9, 1991.
72. Pon S and others: Utilization of pre-hospital care by pediatric patients in New York City, *Ped Emerg Care* 5:286, 1989 (abstract).
73. Quan L and others: Outcome and predictors of outcome in pediatric submersion victims receiving prehospital care in King County, Washington, *Pediatrics* 86:586-93, 1990.
74. Ramenofsky ML and others: EMS for pediatrics: optimum treatment or unnecessary delay? *J Pediatr Surg* 18:498-504, 1983.
75. Rhodes M, Smith S, Boorse D: Pediatric trauma patients in an 'adult' trauma center, *J Trauma* 35:384-93, 1993.
76. Rice DP and others: *Cost of injury in the United States: a report to congress,* Atlanta, 1989, Centers for Disease Control.
77. Rosenberg NM: Pediatric cardiopulmonary arrest in the emergency department, *Am J Emerg Med* 2:497-9, 1984.
78. Rubenstein JS and others: Can the need for a physician as part of the pediatric transport team be predicted? *Crit Care Med* 20:1657-61, 1992.
79. Rutledge R, Smith CY, Azizkhan RG: A population-based multivariate analysis of the association of county demographic and medical system factors with per capita pediatric trauma death rates in North Carolina, *Ann Surg* 219:205-10, 1994.
80. Sachetti A, Carraccio C, Feder M: Pediatric EMS transport: are we treating children in a system designed for adults only? *Ped Emerg Care* 8:4-8, 1992.
81. Sankaran K, Yadlapalli J, Zakhary G: Evaluation of a teaching method for endotracheal intubation in neonates, *Ann RCPSC* 18:135-6, 1985.
82. Schonfeld NA and others: Paramedic physical assessment and intervention in children, *Ann Emerg Med* 18:437, 1989 (abstract).
83. Seidel JS: A needs assessment of advanced life support and emergency medical services in the pediatric patient: state of the art, *Circulation* 74 (Suppl IV) :IV-129-IV-133, 1986.
84. Seidel JS and others: Emergency medical services and the pediatric patient: are the needs being met? *Pediatrics* 73:769-72, 1984.

85. Seidel JS and others: Pediatric prehospital care in urban and rural areas, *Pediatrics* 88:681-90, 1991.
86. Seidel JS: Emergency medical services and the pediatric patient: are the needs being met? II. Training and equipping emergency medical services providers for pediatric emergencies, *Pediatrics* 78:808-12, 1986.
87. Seidel JS, Henderson DP: Systems approach, Appendix C. In Seidel JS, Henderson DP, editors: *Emergency medical services for children: a report to the nation*, Washington, 1991, National Center for Education in Maternal and Child Health.
88. Seigler RS, Tecklenburg FW, Shealy R: Prehospital intraosseous infusion by emergency service personel: a prospective study, *Pediatrics* 84:173-7, 1989.
89. Sharples PM and others: Avoidable factors contributing to death of children with head trauma, *BMJ* 300:87-91, 1990.
90. Shuster M, Chong J: Pharmacologic intervention in prehospital care: a critical appraisal, *Ann Emerg Med* 18:192-6, 1989.
91. Sia CJ, Peters MI: Physician involvement strategies to promote the medical home, *Pediatrics* 85:128-30, 1990.
92. Sinclair LM, Baker MD: Police involvement in pediatric prehospital care, *Pediatrics* 87:636-41, 1991.
93. Smith DF, Hackel A: Selection criteria for pediatric critical care transport teams, *Crit Care Med* 11:10-12, 1983.
94. Smith RJ and others: Intraosseous infusion by prehospital personnel in critically ill pediatric patients, *Ann Emerg Med* 17:491-5, 1988.
95. Stoy WA: Personal communication, December 31, 1993.
96. Strauss RH, Rooney B: Critical care pediatrician-led aeromedical transports: physician interventions and predictiveness of outcome, *Ped Emerg Care* 9:270-4, 1993.
97. Stroup CA: Intraosseous infusion: prehospital use in the critically ill pediatric patient, *JEMS* 12:38-9, 1987.
98. Terndrup TE, Kanter RD, Cherry RA: A comparison of infant ventilation methods performed by prehospital personnel, *Ann Emerg Med* 18:607-11, 1989.
99. Terndrup TE, Warner DA: Infant ventilation and oxygenation by basic life support providers: comparison of methods, *Prehosp Disast Med* 7:35-40, 1992.
100. Thompson JE, Bonner B, Lower GM: Pediatric cardiopulmonary arrests in rural populations, *Pediatrics* 86:302-6, 1990.
101. Torphy DE, Minter MG, Thompson BM: Cardiopulmonary arrest and resuscitation of children, *AJDC* 138:1099-1102, 1984.
102. Tsai A, Kallsen G: Epidemiology of pediatric prehospital care, *Ann Emerg Med* 16:284-92, 1987.
103. Tunik M and others: Teaching paramedics to intubate infants, *Pediatr Emerg Care* 4:298, 1988 (abstract).
104. van Amerongen RH and others: The Avianca plane crash: an emergency medical system's response to pediatric survivors of the disaster, *Pediatrics* 92:105-10, 1993.
105. Whitfield JM, Buser MK: Transport stabilization times for neonatal and pediatric patients prior to interfacility transfer, *Ped Emerg Care* 9:69-71, 1993.
106. Yamamoto LG and others: A one-year series of pediatric prehospital care: I. Ambulance runs; II. Prehospital communication; III. Interhospital transport services, *Ped Emerg Care* 7:206-14, 1991.
107. Zaritsky A and others: CPR in children, *Ann Emerg Med* 16:1107-11, 1987.
108. Zimmerman JJ, Coyne M, Logsdon M: Implementation of intraosseous infusion technique by aeromedical transport programs, *J Trauma* 29:687-9, 1989.

42

PREHOSPITAL TRANSPORT—AIR MEDICAL

DAVID TELLEZ
KENDRA BALAZS
LINDA YOUNG

Each year nearly 25,000 children die from injuries, 100,000 children are permanently disabled, and 2.5 million children are temporarily disabled from trauma alone.[54] These statistics have led to a nation-wide effort to address the needs of critically injured children.[54] Efforts from the Academy of Pediatrics and American Heart Association have led to the development of the Pediatric Advanced Life Support (PALS) and the Advanced Pediatric Life Support (APLS) courses which are being taught to pediatric caregivers throughout the country. An EMS program (EMS-C) has been developed for children. The purpose of EMS-C is to educate EMS personnel and physicians in the care of children in the prehospital environment as well as identify qualified caregivers and institutions for injured children. Pediatric transport programs have developed as a logical extension of the neonatal and adult transport programs. Recently, the American Academy of Pediatrics developed a section on Transport Medicine as a forum for discussion of educational issues, research, development of standards, evaluation of current practice, and improvement of quality of care during transport.

Many studies have been published about interfacility transports which address the above concerns,* but little information has been produced about pediatric prehospital transports. It would be an understatement to say that the most critical phases of a child's illness/injury are prehospital assessment, stabilization, and transport. Scene transport can occur by ground or rotor wing aircraft depending upon the existing circumstances. This chapter will deal with the logistics of the rotor wing prehospital transport of the child.

* References 26, 32, 37, 43, 50, 66, 68, 80.

DEMOGRAPHICS

Before discussing issues concerning a rotorwing prehospital transport team, it is best to identify the patient population that will be encountered. Retrospective reviews of pediatric EMS ground ambulance runs have shown that approximately 55% of these children will be trauma victims, whereas 45% will present with medical problems.[5,53,62,73,78] Blunt injuries, falls, and motor vehicle accidents (MVA) were the predominate causes of traumatic injuries with the central nervous system (CNS) as the most commonly injured organ system. Respiratory distress, seizures, and ingestion were the cause of most medical transports. Younger children were more likely to be transported for medical reasons, whereas in older children the cause was most often trauma.

Though there are no published demographic data on rotorwing pediatric prehospital transports, unpublished data on 1,349 transports by Samaritan AirEvac (Phoenix, AZ) from 1989-92 was consistent with the above findings with an average age of 60 months for trauma and 33 months for medical. Further evaluation revealed that 75% of the patients were trauma related and 25% involved medical problems. The increase in the percentage of trauma transports by helicopter versus ground suggests helicopters are more likely to be used for pediatric trauma scenes because of the urgency to transport the patient to definitive care.

SCENE TRANSPORT PHILOSOPHY

Rapid response and aggressive resuscitation are hallmarks for managing the critically injured child. Because of their relatively small blood volumes, a predisposition to respiratory embarrassment, increased susceptibility to hypoxemia, and the potential for CNS deterioration after serious head trauma, children must receive expedient resuscitative care. The adult "golden hour" may be 30 minutes or less for children which has contributed to the development of the controversial "swoop and scoop" scene transport philosophy.[24,49,78] In fact, what probably affects outcome is the quality of resuscitation that occurs well before a helicopter or transport team reaches the patient. This is in contrast to the approach of bringing ICU expertise to the patient used for interhospital transports. Due to the paucity of pediatric literature in this field, it is difficult to determine what procedures are necessary and what an appropriate scene time should be. There are no established standards; this may be because no one philosophy holds true in all situations. Adult studies suggest that very little time should be spent in the field with trauma victims that are only a few minutes from a Level I Trauma Center.* There is debate regarding what procedures other than intubation should be performed on children prior to arrival at the trauma center. Any procedure of questionable benefit that delays arrival to the operating room (definitive care) could be deleterious. On the other hand, medical emergencies where definitive care (airway stabilization and medications) can be administered at the scene and rural trauma (longer transport times) may require a different approach. More time may be spent at the scene stabilizing these patients prior to transport if ALS is necessary.[38,53,57] Because of the importance of minimizing the time spent in an uncontrolled environment, all efforts should be made to effectively stabilize and transport the patient as quickly as possible.

The scene transport team must be able to immediately recognize a critically ill or injured child and be skilled at advanced life support for children. Their assessment must be accurate and promptly relayed to medical control so that decisions regarding the patient's destination and management can be made in a timely fashion. Procedures should be kept to a minimum. The basic principles of airway, breathing, and circulation as well as transport stabilization are all that need be applied during this phase of the child's illness.

GROUND VERSUS AIR TRANSPORT

Appropriate transport of ill or injured patients by air versus ground, particularly from a scene location, has been a subject of study since the beginning of the air medical transport profession. Research projects conducted by various flight programs have attempted to define specific triage criteria for appropriate use of a rotor wing aircraft based on patient outcomes.[28,56,74,75] Other retrospective research papers have been able to show improved predicted outcomes in patients transported by air.[9,11,40,46] Although most of the research projects were centered around adult patients, the implications can be transferred to the pediatric population. Limitations of these studies revolve around multiple confounding variables that exist when comparing trauma patients transported by air rather than by ground. Patient outcomes in the two groups could have been due to differences in injuries, transport personnel skills, the time from injury to arrival at the trauma center, and treatment given at the receiving facility. Defining the types of injuries that justify the additional cost of transporting patients by air has been difficult because of these variables. However, air transport can reduce the time from injury to definitive care which has been shown to make a difference in survival of trauma patients.[61,72]

In 1990 the Association of Air Medical Services (AAMS) published a document entitled "Position Paper on the Appropriate Use of

* References 7, 22, 23, 33, 63, 64.

BOX 42-1 AAMS CRITERIA FOR THE APPROPRIATE USE OF AIR MEDICAL TRANSPORT

General Criteria

1. The patient requires critical care life support (monitoring, personnel, medications, or specific equipment) during transport that is not available from the local ground ambulance service.
2. The patient's clinical condition requires that the time spent out of the hospital environment (in transport mode) be as short as possible.
3. The potential for delays which may be associated with ground transport, including road obstacles and traffic, is likely to worsen the patient's clinical status.
4. The patient is located in an area which is inaccessible to regular ground traffic.
5. The patient requires specific or timely treatment, not available at the referring hospital or facility.
6. The patient's clinical condition requires that care be given by physician(s) at the receiving hospital who are intimately familiar with the patient's history, including previously begun chemotherapy regimens and extensive prior invasive procedures.
7. The use of a local ground transport team would leave the local area without adequate EMS coverage.

Trauma Patients

1. Lengthy extrication of the patient from the accident site, and the severity of the patient's injury requires delivery of a critical care team to the accident site.
2. One or more of the following mechanisms of injury with a motor vehicle accident is present:
   - There had been structural intrusion into the patient's space in the vehicle;
   - The patient was ejected from the vehicle;
   - Another person in the same vehicle died;
   - The patient was a pedestrian struck by a vehicle traveling more than 20 mph;
   - The patient was not wearing a seat belt in a car which overturned;
   - The patient was thrown from a motorcycle traveling more than 20 mph;
   - The front bumper of the vehicle was displaced to the rear by more than 30 inches, or the front axle was displaced to the rear;
3. The patient fell from a height of greater than 20 feet.
4. The patient experienced a penetrating injury anywhere on the body between the mid-thigh and the head.
5. The patient experienced an amputation or near-amputation and required timely evaluation for possible reimplantation.
6. The patient experienced a scalping or degloving injury.
7. The patient experienced a severe hemorrhage. Included are those patients with a systolic blood pressure of less than 90 mmHg after initial volume resuscitation and those requiring ongoing blood transfusions to maintain a stable blood pressure.
8. The patient experienced burns of the skin greater than 15% of the body surface, or major burns of the face, hands, feet or perineum, or associated with an airway or inhalation injury.
9. The patient experienced, or had great potential to experience, injury to the spinal cord, spinal column, or neurologic deficit.
10. The patient suffered injuries to the face or neck which might result in an unstable or potentially unstable airway and may have required invasive procedures (such as endotracheal or nasotracheal intubation, tracheotomy, or cricothyroidotomy) to stabilize the airway.
11. The patient had a score from an objective ranking system for trauma at the scene of the accident or at the referring hospital's emergency department which indicated a severe injury.
12. The patient is a child less than 5 years of age with multiple traumatic injuries.
13. The patient is greater than 55 years of age and has multiple traumatic injuries, whether with or without preexistent illness, such as diabetes mellitus, coronary artery disease, chronic obstructive lung disease, or chronic renal failure.
14. The patient is an adult with a respiratory rate of less than 10 or greater than 30 breaths per minute or a heart rate of less than 60 or greater than 120 beats per minute.

BOX 42-1 AAMS CRITERIA FOR THE APPROPRIATE USE OF AIR MEDICAL TRANSPORT—cont'd

Adult Medical/Surgical Patients

1. The patient experienced a respiratory or cardiac arrest within the past 12 hours or is experiencing acute respiratory failure not responsive to initial therapy.
2. The patient requires continuous intravenous vasoactive medications or mechanical ventricular assist to maintain a stable cardiac output.
3. The patient requires continuous, intravenous anti-dysrhythmia medications or a cardiac pacemaker to maintain a stable cardiac rhythm.
4. The patient requires mechanical ventilator support or is at risk of having an unstable airway.
5. The patient experiences an acute deterioration in mental status.
6. The patient requires immediate invasive therapy for hypothermia.
7. The patient has an indwelling pulmonary artery catheter, intra-aortic balloon pump, arterial line or intracranial pressure monitor.
8. The patient has a respiratory rate of less than 10 or greater than 30, or a heart rate of less than 50 or greater than 150, or a systolic blood pressure of less than 90 mmHg or greater than 200 mmHg.
9. The patient has evidence of significant acidosis (such as arterial pH <7.2) not responsive to initial therapy.
10. The patient requires immediate transport in a critical care environment to a medical center that can perform organ transplantation or procurement.
11. The patient is experiencing an acute myocardial infarction, a dissecting or leaking aneurysm, or an acute cerebrovascular accident in evolution and requires therapy of diagnostic procedures not available at the referring institution.
12. The patient is experiencing seizures which cannot be controlled at the referring institution.
13. The patient is pregnant with a high-risk obstetrical condition (including placenta previa, abruptio placenta, eclampsia, preeclampsia, or premature labor with or without rupture of the membranes) and requires urgent transport to a perinatal center.

Pediatric Patients

1. The patient is experiencing or has a high risk of developing cardiac dysrhythmia or cardiac pump failure that requires interventions not available at the referring hospital.
2. The patient is experiencing or has a high risk of developing acute respiratory failure or respiratory arrest and is not responsive to initial therapy.
3. The patient requires invasive airway procedures (including endotracheal or nasotracheal intubation, tracheotomy, or cricothyroidotomy) and assisted ventilation.
4. The patient is experiencing any of the following unstable vital signs:
   - Respiratory rate < than 10 or > 60 breaths per minute;
   - Systolic blood pressure < 60 mmHg in a neonate;
   - Systolic blood pressure < 65 mmHg in an infant < 2 years of age;
   - Systolic blood pressure < 70 mmHg in a child 2-5 years old or systolic blood pressure < 80 mmHg in a child 6-12 years.
5. The patient is experiencing any of the following clinical conditions:
   - Near-drowning with signs of hypoxia or altered mental status
   - Status epilepticus
   - Acute bacterial meningitis
   - Acute renal failure
   - Unstable toxicologic syndrome
   - Reye's syndrome
   - Hypothermia
   - Multiple trauma

Modified from the *Journal of Air Medical Transport.* Copyright Sept 1990. JEMS Communications.

Emergency Air Medical Services"[8] (see Box 42-1). Included in the document are criteria for air transport of trauma, pediatric and adult medical/surgical patients for both scene and interfacility transports. This document was based on evaluation of published research and the experiences of the air medical directors nationwide who participated on the AAMS Medical Advisory Committee. Many air medical transport programs use this position paper criteria when conducting prospective or retrospective reviews of appropriate utilization of air transport.

In early 1992 the National Association of Emergency Medical Services Physicians (NAEMSP) developed a position paper for scene response entitled "Air Medical Dispatch: Guidelines for Trauma Scene Response"[48] (see Box 42-2). Guidelines for helicopter utilization were based on consensus of

BOX 42-2 NAEMSP GUIDELINES FOR HELICOPTER SCENE RESPONSE

Clinical
- General
  - Trauma victims need to be delivered as soon as possible to a regional trauma center.
  - Stable patients who are accessible to ground vehicles probably are best transported by ground.
- Specific: Patients with critical injuries resulting in unstable vital signs require the fastest most direct route of transport to a regional trauma center in a vehicle staffed with a team capable of offering critical care en route. Often this is the case in the following situations:
  - Trauma Score <12;
  - Glasgow Coma Scale score <10;
  - Penetrating trauma to the abdomen, pelvis, chest, neck, or head;
  - Spinal cord or spinal column injury, or any lateralizing signs;
  - Partial or total amputation of an extremity (excluding digits);
  - Two or more long bone fractures or a major pelvic fracture;
  - Crushing injuries to the abdomen, chest or head;
  - Major burns of the body surface area, or burns involving the face, hands, feet or perineum, or burns with significant respiratory involvement or major electrical or chemical burns;
  - Patients involved in a serious traumatic event who are less than 12 or more than 55 years of age;
  - Patients with near-drowning injuries, with or without existing hypothermia, and/or
  - Adult patients with any of the following vital sign abnormalities:
    - systolic blood pressure <90 mmHg;
    - respiratory rate <10 or >35 per min;
    - heart rate <60 or >120 per min; or
    - unresponsive to verbal stimuli.

Operational situations in which helicopter use should be considered:
- Mechanism of injury:
  - Vehicle roll-over with unbelted passengers;
  - Vehicle striking pedestrian at >10 miles per hr;
  - Falls from >15 feet;
  - Motorcycle victim ejected at >20 miles per hr;
  - Multiple victims.
- Difficult access situations:
  - Wilderness rescue;
  - Ambulance egress or access impeded at the scene by road conditions, weather, or traffic;
- Time/distance factors:
  - Transportation time to the trauma center greater than fifteen minutes by ground ambulance;
  - Transport time to local hospital by ground greater than transport time to trauma center by helicopter;
  - Patient extrication time >20 minutes; or
  - Utilization of local ground ambulance leaves local community without ground ambulance coverage.

BOX 42-3 CONSIDERATION FACTORS WHEN DETERMINING MODE OF TRANSPORT FROM A SCENE

- Patient condition
- Entrapped patient
- Distance and duration of transport to an appropriate receiving facility
- Traffic patterns and time of day
- Availability of landing site for the rotor-wing
- Geographic location of the patient
- Weather
- Expertise of the air medical transport team versus the first responder
- Community EMS services

physicians involved in day to day EMS activities. The recommendations incorporated the clinical and operational aspects of a scene which influence mode of transport.

When deciding mode of transport it is important to identify the advantages of air versus ground. Since every EMS community is different, transport decisions may be based on one or more factors, (Box 42-3) thus it is difficult to set rigid guidelines. AAMS and NAEMSP include specific descriptions of these factors in their documents.

Patient condition, time, and distance

After assessing the patient's condition, the prehospital provider must evaluate the time critical nature of the patient's illness or injury. If the patient requires rapid transport, it is necessary to determine whether a rotor wing transport will take less time than the time involved in transporting by ground. Ground transport time is contingent on distance to the receiving facility, type of roads (freeway versus city streets), time of day, and rush hour traffic patterns. When estimating the time involved in air transport, consideration must be given to aircraft response time to the scene, setting up a landing zone, preparing the patient for transport, and the time required for flying the patient to the receiving facility. Patient entrapment may add to the total prehospital time which can be minimized by using air transport. If air transport will save even minutes in moving the patient to definitive care, it should be used when warranted by the patient's condition.

Prehospital expertise

Prehospital providers usually do not receive extensive training in child care.[38,43,57,79] They may not be comfortable with their ability to assess and treat injured or seriously ill children. Opportunities to maintain their skills in intubation and insertion of IVs may be limited. These limitations may influence the decision to call on the expertise of the air medical transport team trained in pediatric care.

Geography and weather

Transport by air may be in the patient's best interest if the scene is located in an area difficult to reach by ground ambulances. Dirt roads, mountainous terrain, or other geographic deterrents may delay transport or make it impossible to reach the patient by ground transport. A long rough ride in an ambulance may also aggravate injuries. Weather must be taken into consideration as well. Generally, air medical rotor wing aircraft are limited by ice, snow, fog, low visibility, and thunderstorm activity. Ground ambulances may be delayed in weather but they can usually get to the patient and deliver them to the receiving facility.

Rural setting

If the patient is in a rural setting with personnel and equipment unable to meet the needs of the patient, then air transport may be used to bring the needed skills and equipment to the patient. The scene ambulance may be the only ambulance available to cover that community, in which case taking it out of service for a long ground transport would leave the area without EMS coverage. Air transport would also be appropriate in this situation.

EMS protocols

Another factor to consider in ground versus air transport are the EMS protocols developed by the county and/or state in which the local EMS system functions. First responders should be aware of those protocols which guide their transport decisions, since they are different from county to county and state to state.

LOGISTICS OF A SCENE TRANSPORT

The logistics of smooth orchestration of an air medical transport scene call includes appropriate communication, preparing a safe landing zone and ensuring safety on the scene. Other components to consider are treating and stabilizing the patient and triaging to an appropriate facility.

Communication

There are four communication elements of an air medical scene call. These are as follows:

- Notifying the flight team,
- Identifying a safe landing zone,
- Flight following, and
- Medical control.

Notification for helicopter response to scene calls is usually incorporated into the existing EMS network established by state or county protocols. Generally, the flow of communication consists of the prehospital personnel notifying their dispatch center who then contacts the air medical transport communication center with a brief patient report, location of the scene and radio frequency of ground personnel.

Identification of a safe landing zone requires communication between the pilot and ground personnel. Ground personnel should relay information regarding landing zone area location, possible obstructions (power lines, light poles, trees, etc.), and wind direction to the pilot. During landing, the pilot should remain in radio contact with both the flight program communication center and the ground personnel to ensure that all lines of communication remain open. Once on the scene, the pilot should remain in radio contact with the air medical personnel.

Flight following refers to the ongoing communication between the pilot and the communication center during all phases of flight. The purpose of flight following is to be able to locate the aircraft at any time should an emergency occur.

Medical control may be established by ground and/or air personnel. Each county and/or state has their own EMS base station medical control system for ground agencies and fire departments. The flight program in that area may use the existing system for medical control, or they may have their own parallel medical control physicians. Usually, first responders establish medical control for the scene with their base station. If the air medical personnel require additional medical direction they would patch with their medical control physician enroute to the receiving facility. Ideally, the best base station medical control system for pediatric scene calls would be that all ground and air personnel have access to a pediatric ED physician or PICU specialist.

Landing zone and scene safety

Landing a helicopter in the street requires coordination between the pilot and the ground personnel to ensure the safety of the aircraft, the people on board, and those on the ground. Prehospital personnel should be given rotor wing safety orientation education by the flight programs who serve their areas. Orientation to the helicopter, appropriate needs for a safe landing zone, and safety rules on how to approach the helicopter should be components of a continuing education program provided to new prehospital providers. All prehospital providers should receive recurrent training on a regular basis.

Orientation to the helicopter includes providing prehospital personnel the opportunity to sit in the aircraft, review the medical equipment, and discuss patient loading procedures (i.e., opening and closing aircraft doors, loading the stretcher, exiting the aircraft, zone of safety).

Each aircraft, as well as the rotor wing operator, have specific requirements for a safe landing zone depending on the size of the aircraft and the policies and procedures of the rotor wing operator. However, there are some general guidelines used by all flight programs for designating an appropriate landing zone (see Box 42-4). Since prehospital and law enforcement personnel are responsible for choosing and setting up a landing zone, they should know what the landing zone needs are for the flight program in their area.

The importance of educating the prehospital providers to safety in and around a rotor wing aircraft on a scene cannot be overemphasized. General safety rules should

BOX 42-4 LANDING ZONE REQUIREMENTS

- Minimum landing zone (LZ) area (can be anywhere between 60 by 60 feet and 100 by 100 feet).
- Free from overhead obstacles (i.e., wires, trees, light poles, etc.).
- Free from debris.
- Relatively level.
- Two approaches marked with secured flares, beacon, or emergency overhead lights.
- Direct illumination toward landing spot not at approaching aircraft.
- Wet down the area if dusty.
- Plan possible alternative landing site.
- Secure LZ—one tail rotor guard at 15 feet behind aircraft entire time the aircraft is on the scene.
- No vehicles or nonaircraft or nonprehospital personnel within anywhere between 60 and 200 feet of the aircraft depending on the vendor policies.

BOX 42-5 HELICOPTER SAFETY

- Keep your back toward the landing area until the dirt has settled to protect your eyes.
- Never approach the aircraft until signaled to do so by the pilot.
- Approach the aircraft from the front in view of the pilot.
- Secure any small pieces of clothing or equipment that can potentially be blown by the rotor wash.
- Wear ear protection.
- Do not raise your arms or equipment above the level of your head while under the rotor blades.
- Do not smoke or run within 50 feet of the aircraft.
- Exit the aircraft toward the front in view of the pilot.

always be followed when working around a helicopter (see Box 42-5). First responders and air medical personnel must work together in a coordinated effort for the protection of everyone on the scene.

Besides following the rules described in Box 42-5, there are two other safety aspects that must be addressed. The first is securing the tail rotor. It is vital that the flight team ensure that a tail rotor guard has been designated. This is particularly important to prevent bystanders from inadvertently walking into the tail rotor when the aircraft remains "hot" with the rotor blades turning.

The second safety aspect involves hazards at the scene. All safety rules regarding fire and electrical danger as well as hazardous materials on a scene apply to air medical personnel when approaching a motor vehicle accident or any other situation. Flight personnel should always evaluate the situation for potential hazards before proceeding to the patient.

Patient stabilization on the scene

The purpose of air medical transport is to reduce the time it takes for a patient to receive definitive care. This is especially important in the pediatric population. Lavery reported on 458 pediatric ALS responses in an urban setting over a two year period.[38] His review concluded that the two most needed interventions on scene prior to transport were intubation and IV access.

The cornerstone of pediatric medical care is stabilization of the airway. This must be done in conjunction with C-spine stabilization, since it is more likely that a prehospital rotor wing transport will be trauma related.[5,53,62,73,78] All airway procedures should be done by two caregivers with one using the jaw thrust or a similar C-spine stabilizing technique. If the patient is unable to maintain an adequate airway with assistance, then intubation or a cricothyrotomy is required. In addition, if the Glasgow Coma Score is less than 8 or the child is in a clinical state of respiratory failure, bag valve mask and preferably intubation must be performed.

Specific to the endotracheal intubation procedure, studies have noted that scene airway management in children is a difficult task.[1,34,43,48] For children less than 3 years old, one study indicated only a 50 to 55% prehospital intubation success rate though this rate increased with older children.[1] Typically, scene intubation attempts required multiple tries as compared to in hospital attempts. This was attributed to less experienced care-givers, environmental conditions, and distractions.[47] If intubation is unsuccessful, bag-valve-mask ventilation should be performed with meticulous technique until intubation can be attained. Once the airway has been established with the appropriate sized tube taped in good position at the lip (approximately 10 cm + age in yrs.), continual attention must be paid to maintaining the patency and correct placement of the tube. Breath sounds must be continually reassessed at the bases of the lung fields. Successful intubation does not automatically preclude major airway complications from occurring. These complications include a dislodged tube, a mucous plugged tube, right mainstem intubation, failure to adequately oxygenate, aspiration, anoxia secondary to repeated attempts, and a pneumothorax.[34,47] If a tension pneumothorax is suspected after reevaluating the endotracheal tube placement (i.e., difficulty bagging, unequal chest movement, unstable hemodynamics, and/or signs of chest injury), the chest should be needled with a 20 to 22 gauge catheter, usually in the second intercostal space at the mid-clavicular line. Placement of a one-way valve is recommended if the catheter is left in place.

After airway stabilization, the patient should be prepared for transport. This entails securing the patient on a backboard when indicated, applying splints and bandages if warranted, and placing basic monitoring devices on the patient (i.e., ECG monitor, pulse oximeter).

Difficulty in obtaining venous access has been a rate-limiting step in pediatric resuscitation. The importance of establishing a line prior to transport is dependant on the patient's condition and the transport time. In most cases, especially with short transport times, venous access should not delay transport. This decision can be made with medical control in difficult situations. Fortunately, with the intraosseous needle (IO) technique, time delay for venous access can be reduced. The procedure is simple to perform and can be easily taught to prehospital personnel.[65] Intraosseous access can be used for the infusion of crystalloids, colloids, and blood products as well as resuscitative medications, antibiotics, and anticonvulsants.[67,76,77] In a survey of air medical transport teams,[81] this under used technique had over an 80% success rate with few minor complications.

Ultimately, the priorities on scene are to 1) stabilize the airway and cervical spine, 2) establish IV access the best way possible without delaying transport, 3) prepare the patient for transport, and 4) transport rapidly to the nearest facility capable of providing care.

Scene triage

Scene triage in an EMS system is an important component of determining patient destination and mode of transport. The basis of triage is the determination of severity of injury or illness followed by a decision regarding destination of the patient. Though a scene triage method may have been derived from mortality statistics, it should be used as a tool for decision-making and not as a predictor of mortality. As a tool, it should be simple enough for a prehospital provider to use in a reproducible fashion within a stressful environment. Triage criteria for children are only in their infancy and have not been extensively implemented. Classically, triage has been handled from one physician or paramedic to another according to certain predetermined referral patterns. In 1984 the Pediatric Trauma Score (PTS) was developed as a protocol for rapid assessment and triage for the injured child (Table 42-1).[70] An injury receiving a PTS of 8 or less would require transport to an institution providing the highest care for children in the region.[72] Several studies have documented the relationship between the PTS and injury severity and have confirmed the validity of its use as an effective triage tool.[35,52] However, the PTS is not without error when studying overtriage and is not universally accepted as a triage tool by all EMS providers.[12,36,58] In addition, there are no established field triage mechanisms for medical illness emergencies other than those based on the common sense of the caregiver.

At present, no triage mechanism is simple to use yet accurate enough to prevent unacceptable under- or overtriage of patients.[12] Triage decisions, especially for medical patients, must be individualized with regards to

TABLE 42-1 PEDIATRIC TRAUMA SCORE

Component	*+2*	*+1*	*−1*
Size	>20 kg	10-20 kg	<10 kg
Airway	normal	maintainable	unmaintainable
Neurologic	awake	obtunded	comatose
Systolic BP	>90 mmHg	90–50 mmHg	<50 mmHg
(or pulses)	(2+ at wrist)	(1+ at groin)	(no pulse)
Open wounds	none	minor	major/penetrating
Skeletal	none	closed fx.	open/multiple fxs

availability of resources, weather, distance, geography, and cost. It is also important to note that not all trauma centers have the expertise of pediatric trauma teams and pediatric intensive care units. The ability of the trauma center to provide ongoing pediatric nursing and respiratory expertise should be considered when deciding on the child's destination, particularly when the time and distance difference is minimal by air.

AIR MEDICAL TRANSPORT TEAM

Team composition for air medical helicopters who respond to scene calls will vary with personnel availability and training. There is no specific team composition which will cover every transport in every location for every patient. Physicians may be part of the team, however, for most helicopter scene calls, the team will consist of a flight nurse and a flight paramedic.* Because transport times for scene response are critical, in most programs these team members are completely dedicated to transports.

The debate on whether pediatric transport teams should be broad-based (i.e., adult patient experienced) or dedicated specialized pediatric teams continues to be reviewed within the air medical profession.[2,18,43,60] Not only is accessibility and response time of team members a valid concern, but the issues of training and ongoing skills competency verification are also issues for concern.

In general, for prehospital scene calls, a broad-based team is capable of safely handling a wide variety of pediatric emergencies.[15,25,41] The broad-based team frequently has a quicker response to scene call requests. This is likely due to multiple, strategically based aircraft and air medical personnel (AMP) that are immediately available because they are not responsible for in hospital, primary patient care while on duty. Whichever team approach is used, broad-based or dedicated, the challenge for the air medical transport service is to ensure that the flight team provides the same or better quality care than the patient had prior to transport.[37]

The selection of potential air medical personnel is very important. Members of the flight team should have substantial medical experience and be recognized as among the best in their field before being selected. The team members must be adaptable and possess critical decision making and interpersonal communication skills. They must also be able to tolerate the stressors of flight and be able to work within the air transport environment.

Air medical control physician

The role of the Air Medical Control Physician (AMCP) is to provide physician backup for the air medical transport team after they accept transfer of care. In most cases, the flight team will not be assisted by a physician and in that regard must operate as physician extenders in the prehospital setting. The nature of this relationship is crucial because it conveys significant responsibilities to both participants. The transport team serves as the information source and treatment provider; the physician provides additional medical expertise. Trust and knowledge from both sides must be maintained or the system will not function effectively.

The qualifications of the AMCP should be similar to that of the medical director of the

* References 2, 4, 10, 13, 19, 20, 24, 27, 28, 31, 42, 44, 55, 59.

flight team. In some programs the AMCP may be the air medical director, and in others, the AMCP may be designated by the director. The AMCP should have pediatric emergency medicine or pediatric critical care expertise with transport medicine training. This physician must be thoroughly famildiar with the local EMS triage system and medical control protocols. Knowledge of the flight program's patient care guidelines, procedures, and protocols is also essential in order to provide appropriate medical direction.

Medical direction can be provided by two methods. On-line medical direction is provided by direct radio communication between the AMCP and the flight team. Off-line medical direction is provided through established guidelines, procedures, and protocols approved by the air medical director. In most instances, flight teams operate under off-line medical control unless they are first responders to the scene.

Transport physician

The transport physician must be specifically certified for pediatric transport by the Air Medical Director using the defined criteria established for the individual transport program. This physician should have skills appropriate for the treatment of seriously ill children and acts as team leader in coordinating patient stabilization management and monitoring during the transport.

The role of the physician led transport team is controversial.* Nearly all of the pediatric data is derived from interhospital transports, not scene transports where the philosophy is different. Scoring systems used to predict the need for physician staffed teams have not been validated for predicting transport morbidity. As such, patients who would benefit from a physician's presence have not been identified. Adult studies using physician-staffed prehospital transport teams are no less ambiguous.† Review of these data suggests that a physician's skills or judgement are beneficial in a small percentage of patients, but the conclusions were based on subjective analysis. Baxt and others[10] looked objectively at this issue and found a decrease in the number of predicted deaths in patients transported by physician led prehospital transport teams compared with nurse led teams. Cautious interpretation is necessary because this difference was in a very small subpopulation (N = 5) and the authors acknowledged that further training and on-line medical control would likely correct any deficiencies identified with the nurse led team. Thus, the role of a pediatric transport physician remains undefined, especially in the prehospital setting. The cost effectiveness as well as the impact on health care of a physician based transport team is unproven. With a highly skilled nonphysician flight team and appropriate medical control, most problems surrounding the stabilization of an injured child at the scene can be managed until the patient arrives at the hospital for more definitive care.

Flight nurse

The flight nurse should be a registered nurse with extensive critical care and/or emergency department experience. In addition, pediatric experience is preferred. Once hired, the nurse must complete the flight training program approved and overseen by the medical director. In most cases, the transport nurse will be the highest level of skilled caregiver at the scene and should be responsible for coordinating patient stabilization management and monitoring during transport.

Flight paramedic

The flight paramedic should have at least two years of prehospital experience. Once hired, the flight paramedic will receive additional training and clinical experience in child management overseen by the medical director. The paramedic's role is to provide prehospital expertise and assist the team leader with stabilization and management of the patient during transport.

Other team members

The majority of transport teams are composed of nurses and physicians or paramedics. However, some transport programs use respiratory therapists (RTs) or emergency medi-

* References 2, 4, 10, 13, 19, 20, 24, 27, 32, 42, 44, 57, 59.

† References 4, 19, 20, 27, 31, 55, 59.

cal technicians (EMTs) as the second team member.

TRAINING

Whatever the team composition, thorough training should be provided initially as well as on a continued basis to adequately prepare the medical flight team to care for children in a safe, consistent, and quality manner.

There are several essential components that should be included in any air medical transport organization's training program. These components include patient care management, formal orientation to aircraft flight principles and FAA regulations, aircraft safety, the proper use of aircraft radios, and communication etiquette. In addition, there should be specific training on the transport service's state and local requirements for prehospital scene control and medical direction. OSHA's bloodborne and airborne pathogen regulations and the FDA's regulations on safe medical devices should also be reviewed.

Continuous quality improvement (CQI) process information should be included with emphasis on system improvement.[18,25] Charting and documentation requirements should be reviewed with regard to the flight program's policies, procedures, and standards of care guidelines. Feedback mechanisms should be in place for the medical director to review case scenarios with the general staff as well as individual counseling with AMP about patient management issues. CQI files should be kept on all medical personnel separate from their personnel file, which documents specific patient management issues, conference discussions with the medical director, or CQI Coordinator and follow-up plans of action.

Finally, all programs should cover stress management issues to help the staff identify internal and external stressors that will be affecting their lives. These training programs should be on-going, and resources should be provided to assist the employee when indicated.

Patient management training components

Trauma related injuries are likely to be the most common reason for helicopter scene call requests. Therefore, training must focus on all aspects of trauma assessment, stabilization, and in-flight management.* Other common medical prehospital scene situations should also be covered such as submersion accidents, hypo/hyperthermia management, envenomations, and seizures. Training components for the rotor wing scene environment should emphasize rapid recognition and assessment of critical injuries, respiratory distress, and circulatory failure. General classroom training should cover all aspects of pediatric assessment with attention to the anatomical and physiological differences between children and adults.

Paramount to both the classroom and skills training are the principles and procedures for performing basic and advanced life-saving skills. Airway management of the child must be emphasized with in-depth review of anatomical differences, recognition of airway compromise, and options for controlling the airway. Options to be reviewed should include basic head positioning, bag-valve-mask and oropharyngeal airway devices, endotracheal tubes, and needle and surgical cricothyrotomies.

Finally, basic stabilization and packaging should be part of every flight training program. Proper techniques and equipment for cervical-spine, extremity immobilization, use of safety straps, and transport equipment should be covered.

Clinical lab training

Hands-on clinical experiences are vital for all air medical personnel. These experiences should be obtained through the pediatric intensive care unit, emergency department, operating room and preceptored transports for new trainees.

Specific goals for the new trainees should be in written form and signed off by the preceptor when proficiency is attained. Whenever possible, small animal labs should be included to provide the added experience and confidence in performing invasive procedures. IVs, arterial punctures, needle and surgical cricothyrotomies, intubations, chest tubes, and central and intraosseous line insertions should be reviewed.[68]

* References 5, 37, 53, 62, 73, 78.

BOX 42-6 AMP THOUGHT PROCESSES AND PLANNING

WHEN REQUESTED ON A SCENE:

- Mentally preparing themselves for the type of scene call (i.e., motor vehicle accident, drowning, medical condition, cardiac arrest, etc. and the age of the child).
- Preparing appropriate equipment/drugs for the child being transported.
- Assisting the pilot to find the location of the scene.
- Observing for obstructions and safety hazards while landing at the scene.
- Securing the landing zone.
- Receiving report from the first responders.
- Evaluating, treating, and preparing the patient for transport.
- Establishing medical control.
- Identifying the receiving facility.
- Performing patient assessment, intervention and evaluation during transport.
- Giving report to the receiving facility nurse and physician.

WHEN REQUESTED ON AN INTERFACILITY TRANSPORT:

- Mentally preparing themselves for the type of patient being transported (i.e., respiratory distress, meningitis, sepsis, seizures, trauma etc. and age of the child).
- Preparing specialized equipment such as a ventilator.
- Calling the communication center prior to lift off for more detailed report as indicated.
- Landing at the designated helipad at the referring facility and responding to the patient's unit.
- Receiving report from the patient's nurse and/or physician.
- Evaluating, treating and preparing the patient for transport.
- Patching to the pediatric medical control physician when indicated.
- Discussing the patient condition and transport with the parents when they are present.
- Performing patient assessment, intervention and evaluation during transport.
- Giving report to the receiving facility nurse and physician.

Aircraft and scene safety training

Air medical personnel (AMP) mentally prepare themselves differently for a scene transport versus an interfacility transport (see Box 42-6), consequently thought process and planning and aircraft and scene safety are crucial components of the training program. The major differences between scene and interfacility transports center around time and landing zone safety. Scene calls require immediate response of the team and aircraft to the child. This is coupled with rapid assessment, stabilization, and transport from an uncontrolled situation to an appropriate facility. Interfacility transports allow more time for preparation for the transport. The landing zone for the scene call demands the attention of the pilot, air medical personnel and ground personnel for the safety of all persons on board and at the scene. Hospital helipads are inherently safer because they are usually a secured and familiar landing site for the pilot.

COMPETENCY VERIFICATION

Competency verification validates the AMP's ability to demonstrate good clinical judgement and perform procedures. It is one of the most important continuing educational programs that can be offered in any flight program. Not only does competency verification ensure quality patient care but it also provides the staff with a sense of accomplishment and enhanced confidence. Records should be kept on a monthly and annual basis which documents the flight personnels' skills performed, including attempts and successes. Clinical judgement can be evaluated through chart review and discussion with the medical director.

Competency verification should be an integral part of the flight program, especially for broad-based teams who may not have specialty training and continual clinical experience in pediatrics. Annual procedure minimal requirements should be set by the program's medical director with provisions for additional clinical experience when identified.

PEDIATRIC EQUIPMENT AND MEDICATIONS

Equipment needed for scene pediatric transports should be geared towards its intended use and type of transport mission. This equipment must be durable and field tested to withstand vibration and extreme temperature changes. It should also be compact, portable, and easily cleaned.

A designated staff member or committee should be responsible for evaluating each piece of equipment intended for air medical transports. The items should be evaluated based on cost, safety, performance, weight, and compactness. When possible, the evaluator should contact current and past users of the equipment to determine the pros and cons of its use in the air medical environment.

Equipment that requires battery power should ideally have auxiliary power packs for use in aircraft with an invertor. Nicad batteries should be routinely deep cycled, and smaller, disposable batteries should be tested daily with back up supplies available on the aircraft.

A preventive maintenance program should be established, and all electrical equipment must be tested for performance and safety on a routine basis. Equipment failures during patient mission should be reported to the flight program administrative personnel. Policies should be established to direct the air medical personnel in the event of equipment failure, especially if it causes actual harm to the patient. Reporting forms must be available to comply with the Safe Medical Device Act.

Standardized transport bags should be designed with function and accessibility in mind. Airway adjuncts, IV supplies, and first line ACLS drugs should be positioned for immediate access. Depending on the types of missions performed, equipment used less often can be stored in the aircraft in order to

BOX 42-7 MINIMUM EQUIPMENT NEEDED FOR PEDIATRIC AIR TRANSPORT

Airway/Breathing Supplies:
- Oxygen—portable and inline aircraft
- Suction—portable and inline aircraft
- Suction catheters (6-14F)
- Bulb syringe
- Oropharyngeal airways (0-4)
- Oxygen devices (NRB, simple mask, nasal cannula)
- Bag-valve-mask (pediatric and adult) with multi-sized masks
- Laryngoscope handle and blades (sizes 0–3)
- Endotracheal tubes (2.5-5.5 uncuffed and 5.5-6.5 cuffed)
- Adjuncts—BAAM and ETCO2 detector
- Cricothyrotomy kit—surgical and needle
- Needle thoracostomy set
- Chest tube set (size 10-32)
- SVN set up
- Pulse oximeter with peds probes

Circulation Equipment:
- Cardiac Monitor/Pacer/Defibrillator
- IV Infusion pumps
- Automatic BP machine with multiple size cuffs
- IV fluids (LR and NS) and tubing (60 and 10 gtt)
- Buretrol
- IV catheters/butterfly needles (16-22 gauge)
- Central line catheters
- Intraosseous needles
- Mast pants—pediatric and adult size

Trauma Stabilization Equipment:
- Spine board
- Head immobilizer multiple sizes
- Cervical collars
- Ladder or pneumatic splints
- Arm boards
- Straps
- Keds board
- Femur traction splint

Supplemental Equipment:
- Syringes—multiple sizes
- 4 × 4 gauze pads
- Portawarms
- Cool packs
- Nasogastric tubes (10-14F)
- Tomey syringe
- Thermometer
- Dextrosticks
- Pressure bags
- Trauma pads
- Kling/Kerlix
- Delivery kit

BOX 42-8 MINIMUM PEDIATRIC MEDICATION SUPPLIES

First Line ACLS:
- Adrenaline 1:1000
- Adrenaline 1:10,000
- Atropine
- D10 and D25
- Lidocaine
- Naloxone

Other Drugs:
- Adenosine
- Albuterol
- Aminophylline
- Anectine
- Bretylium
- Calcium Chloride
- Diazepam
- Diphenhydramine
- Dobutamine
- Dopamine
- Flumarzenil
- Furosemide
- Isoproterenol
- Meperidine
- Midazolam
- Morphine
- Phenobarbital
- Promethazine
- Racemic Epinephrine
- Sodium Bicarbonate
- Terbutaline
- Vecuronium
- Verapamil (contraindicated for infants)

lighten the load of the equipment bag. Recommendations for equipment to be carried on the rotor wing aircraft for use during pediatric scene transports is found in Box 42-7. The list of medications in Box 42-8 is a minimum recommended stock for rotor wing scene transport of children. The par levels of each drug as well as additional drugs may vary from flight program to flight program depending on patient population and treatment protocols.

Proper therapy and stabilization depend on the availability of appropriate monitoring devices, respiratory care equipment, supplies and drugs. Irrespective of the length of transport or whether the flight team does primarily scene or interfacility transports, supplies and equipment should be accessible and in safe working condition. To ensure proper working condition of a full complement of supplies, the flight team should check equipment and supplies on the aircraft at the beginning of their shift.

DISCUSSION

Unlike interfacility pediatric transports, the emphasis on prehospital air transport should be on rapid patient stabilization and transport. Each EMS system should have a coordinated plan in place that specifically addresses pediatric prehospital care. The plan should include the following:

- Criteria for appropriate use of air versus ground transport,
- Designation of receiving facilities which specialize in pediatric trauma and critical care,
- Triage guidelines for transport to the closest most appropriate pediatric facility,
- Education and clinical experience in child management for prehospital providers, and
- Appropriate equipment and drugs for prehospital personnels' use during pediatric prehospital care. The challenge for the 1990s is for EMS systems to integrate pediatric emergency care into their existing programs. Sick and injured children should no longer be managed according to adult standards, but instead, definitive protocols and programs must be implemented for this specialty population.

REFERENCES

1. Aijian P and others: Endotracheal intubation of pediatric patients by paramedics [see comments], *Ann Emerg Med* 18(12):1376, 1989; *Ann Emerg Med* 18(5):489-94, 1989.
2. American Academy of Pediatrics: Guidelines for air and ground transportation of pediatric patients, *Pediatrics* 78(5):943-950, 1986.
3. American Academy of Pediatrics, Guidelines for air and ground transport of neonatal and pediatric patients, 1:27-32, 1993.
4. Anderson TE and others: Physician-staffed helicopter scene response from a rural trauma center, *Ann Emerg Med* 16(1):58-61, 1987.
5. Applebaum D: Advanced prehospital care for pediatric emergencies, *Ann Emerg Med* 14:656-9, 1985.
6. Applebaum D, Slater PE: Should the mobile intensive care unit respond to pediatric emergencies? *Clin Pediatr* 25(12):620-3, 1986.

7. Aprahamian C and others: Traumatic cardiac arrest: scope of paramedic services, *Ann Emerg Med* 14(6):583-6, 1985.
8. Association of Air Medical Services: Position paper on the appropriate use of emergency air medical services, *J Air Med Trans* 29, September 1990.
9. Baxt WG, Moody P: The impact of a rotorcraft aeromedical emergency care service on trauma mortality, *JAMA* 249(22):3047-51, 1983.
10. Baxt WG, Moody P: The impact of a physician as part of the aeromedical prehospital team in patients with blunt trauma, *JAMA* 257(23):3246-50, 1987.
11. Baxt WG and others: Hospital-based rotorcraft aeromedical emergency care services and trauma mortality: a multicenter study, *Ann Emerg Med* 14(9):859, 1985.
12. Baxt WG and others: The failure of prehospital trauma prediction rules to classify trauma patients accurately, *Ann Emerg Med* 18(1):1-8, 1989.
13. Beyer AJ and others: Nonphysician transport of intubated pediatric patients: a system evaluation, *Crit Care Med* 20(7):961-6, 1992.
14. Blumen IJ, Bunne MJ: Altitude and Flight Physiology. *Emerg* 24(7):36-43, 1992.
15. Blumen IJ, Tressa J: Transporting the critical care child, *Emerg* 22(12):36-9, 1990.
16. Bolte R, Whitfield J: Proceedings of the section on critical care/transport medicine joint session, American Academy of Pediatrics Annual Meeting, *Ped Emerg Care* 8(6):371-2, 1993.
17. Boyle MF and others: Surgical cricothyrotomy performed by air ambulance flight nurses: a 5-year experience [see comments], *J Emerg Med* 11(1):41-5, 91-2, 1993.
18. Brink LW and others: Air transport, *Pediatrics Clin N A* 40(2):439-55, 1993.
19. Burney RE, Fischer RP: Ground versus air transport of trauma victims: medical and logistical considerations, *Ann Emerg Med* 15(12):164-8, 1986.
20. Carraway RP and others: Life saver: a complete team approach incorporated into a hospital-based program, *Ann Surg* 50:173-82, 1984.
21. Controversies in pediatric emergency medicine: prehospital intravenous access in pediatric trauma, *Ped Emerg Care Care* 7(2):117-9, 1991.
22. Copass MK and others: Prehospital cardiopulmonary resuscitation of the critically injured patient, *Am J Surg* 148:20-6, 1984.
23. Cwinn AA and others: Prehospital advanced trauma life support for critical blunt trauma victims, *Ann Emerg Med* 16(4):399-403, 1987.
24. Dalton AM and others: Helicopter doctors? *Injury: Brit J Accid Surg* 23(4):249-50, 1992.
25. Day S and others: Pediatric interhospital critical care transport: consensus of a national leadership conference, *Pediatrics* 88(4):696-706, 1991.
26. Dobrin RS and others: The development of a pediatric emergency transport system, *Ped Clin N A* 27(3):633-46, 1980.
27. Duke JH, Clarke WP: A university-staffed private hospital-based air transport service, *Arch of Surg* 116:703-8, 1981.
28. Fischer RP and others: Urban helicopter response to the scene of injury, *J Trauma* 24(11):946-51, 1984.
29. Fleisher GR: Controversies in pediatric emergency medicine: prehospital intravenous access in pediatric trauma, *Ped Emerg Care* 7(2):117-9, 1991.
30. Graneto JW, Soglin DF: Transport and stabilization of pediatric trauma patient, *Ped Clin N A* 40(2):365-79, 1993.
31. Hamman BL and others: Helicopter transport of trauma victims: does a physician make a difference? *J Trauma* 31(4):490-4, 1991.
32. Harris BH and others: Aeromedical transportation for infants and children, *J Ped Surg* 10(5):719-24, 1975.
33. Ivatury RR: Penetrating thoracic injuries: in-field stabilization vs. prompt transport, *J Trauma* 27(9):1066-73, 1987.
34. Jacobs LM and others: Endotracheal intubation in the prehospital phase of emergency medical care, *JAMA* 250(16):2175-7, 1983.
35. Jubelirer RA and others: Pediatric trauma triage: review of 1,307 cases, *J Trauma* 30(12):1544-7, 1990.
36. Kaufmann CR and others: Evaluation of the Pediatric Trauma Score [see comments]. *JAMA* 263(1):69-72, 1990; Comment in *JAMA* 263(18):2447, 1990.
37. Kissoon N: Triage and transport of the critically ill child, *Prog Ped C C* 8(1):37-57, 1992.
38. Levery RF and others: The prehospital treatment of pediatric trauma, *Ped Emerg Care Care* 8(1):9-12, 1992.
39. Losek JD and others: Prehospital pediatric endotracheal intubation performance review, *Ped Emerg Care* 5(1):1-4, 1989.
40. Mackenzie CF and others: Two-year mortality in 760 patients transported by helicopter direct from the road accident scene, *Ann Surg* 101-108, September 1979.
41. Mayer TA, Walker ML: Severity of illness and injury in pediatric air transport, *Ann Emerg Med* 13(2):108-11, 1984.
42. McCloskey KA: Aeromedical transport services and AAP guideline: a commentary, *Ped Emerg Care* 8(6):318-20, 1992.
43. McCloskey KA, Orr RA: Pediatric transport issues in emergency medicine, *Ped Emerg Care* 9(3):475-89, 1991.
44. McCloskey KA and others: Pediatric critical care transport: is a physician always needed on the team? *Ann Emerg Med* 18(3):247-9, 1989.
45. Morse TS: Transportation of critically ill or injured children, *Ped Clin N A* 16(3):565-71, 1969.
46. Moylan JA and others: Factors improving survival in multisystem trauma patients, *Ann Surg* 207(6):679-85, 1988.
47. Nakayama DK and others: Emergency endotracheal intubation in pediatric trauma, *Ann Surg* 211(2): 218-23, 1990.
48. National Association of Emergency Medical Services Physicians: Air medical dispatch: Guidelines for trauma scene response, *Prehos & Dis Med* 7(1):75, 1992.
49. Panel: Prehospital trauma care—stabilize or scoop and run, *J Trauma* 23(8):708-11, 1983.

50. Pon S, Notterman DA: The organization of a pediatric critical care transport program, *Ped Clin N A* 40(2):241-61, 1993.
51. Ramenofsky ML: Emergency medical services for children and pediatric trauma system components, *J Ped Surg* 24(2):153-5, 1989.
52. Ramenofsky ML and others: The predictive validity of the Pediatric Trauma Score, *J Trauma* 28(7): 1038-42, 1983.
53. Ramenofsky ML and others: EMS for pediatrics: optimum treatment or unnecessary delay? *J Ped Surg* 18(4):498-504, 1983.
54. Report of the 97th Ross Conference on Pediatric Research: Emergency Medical Services for Children, 1989, Ross Laboratories.
55. Rhee KJ and others: Is the flight physician needed for helicopter emergency medical services? *Ann Emerg Med* 15(2):174-7, 1986.
56. Rhodes M and others: Field triage for on-scene helicopter transport, *J Trauma* 26(11):963-9, 1986.
57. Sacchetti A and others: Pediatric EMS transport: are we treating children in a system designed for adults only? *Ped Emerg Care* 8(1):4-8, 1992.
58. Sagy M: Scoring systems in emergency pediatrics: "One cannot see the forest for the trees." *Ped Emerg Care* 5(2):142-4, 1989.
59. Schmidt U and others: On-scene helicopter transport of patients with multiple injuries—comparison of a German and an American system, *J Trauma* 33(4):548-55, 1992.
60. Schneider C and others: Evaluation of ground ambulance, rotor-wing, and fixed-wing aircraft services, *Trans C Ill* 8(3):533-64, 1992.
61. Schwartz RJ and others: Impact of pre-trauma center care on length of stay and hospital charges, *J Trauma* 29(12):1611-15, 1989.
62. Seidel JS and others: Emergency medical services and the pediatric patient: III Resources of ambulatory care centers, *Pediatrics* 88(2):230-5, 1991.
63. Sloan EP and others: The effect of urban trauma system hospital bypass on prehospital transport times and Level 1 trauma patient survival, *Ann Emerg Med* 18(11):1146-50, 1989.
64. Smith JP and others: Prehospital stabilization of critically injured patients: a failed concept, *J Trauma* 25(1):65-70, 1985.
65. Smith RJ and others: Intraosseous infusions by prehospital personnel in critically ill pediatric patients, *Ann Emerg Med* 17(5):491-5, 1988.
66. Special Report: Air transport of pediatric emergency cases, *N Engl J Med* 307(23):1465-8, 1982.
67. Spivey WH: Intraosseous infusion, *J Pediatr* 111: 639, 1987.
68. Strauss RH: Aeromedical transport services accepting pediatric patients and their abidance by published guidelines, *Ped Emerg Care* 8(6):318-20, 1992.
69. Swan TH: The politics of air transportation, *Emerg* 24(7):48-50, 1992.
70. Tepas JJ and others: The pediatric trauma score as a predictor of injury severity in the injured child, *J Ped Surg* 22:14, 1987.
71. Tepas JJ and others: The pediatric trauma score as a predictor of injury severity: an objective assessment, *J Trauma* 28:425, 1988.
72. Trunkey DD: The value of trauma centers, *Am Coll Surg* 5-7, October 1982.
73. Tsai A and others: Epidemiology of pediatric prehospital care, *Ann Emerg Med* 16(3):284-92, 1987.
74. Urdaneta LF and others: Evaluation of an emergency air transport service as a component of a rural EMS system, *Am Surg* 50(4):183-8, 1984.
75. Urdaneta LF and others: Role of an emergency helicopter transport service in rural trauma, *Arch Surg* 122:992-6, 1987.
76. Warren DW and others: Intraosseous infusion rates: comparison of various intraosseous sites versus peripheral intravenous in nomovolemic and hypovolemic pigs, *Clin Invest Med* 13(4):644, 1990.
77. Warren DW and others: Pharmokinetics of radioactive tracers from multiple intraosseous sites in a pig model, *Clin Invest Med* 13(4):589, 1990.
78. Weinberg JA: Trauma and severe illness in children: how are they alike and different? Report of the 97th Ross Conference on Ped Research, 1989 May.
79. Yamamoto LG and others: A one-year series of pediatric prehospital care: I. Ambulance runs; II. Prehospital communication; III. Interhospital transport services, *Ped Emerg Care Care* 7(4):206-14, 1991.
80. Yurt RW: Triage, initial assessment, and early treatment of the pediatric trauma patient, *Ped Emerg Care* 39(5):1083-91, 1992.
81. Zimmerman JJ and others: Implementation of intraosseous infusion technique by aeromedical transport programs, *J Trauma* 29(5):687-9, 1989.

43

THE RURAL PEDIATRICIAN'S PERSPECTIVE

LORI G. BYRON

THE RURAL PEDIATRICIAN'S PERSPECTIVE

Editors' Note. This textbook is written by authors with expertise in every aspect of the transport process. One individual who is extremely important, yet frequently misunderstood, criticized, or simply not appropriately recognized, is the rural physician who refers patients to teritary care. These 'unsung heroes' may have the greatest potential impact on a critically ill child's eventual outcome, yet they often work with fewer resources (equipment and personnel) and less access to continuing medical education than other physicians, and they are geographically farthest from tertiary care (necessitating stabilization for longer duration transports). Some of these physicians have little experience with critically ill children, but put additional time and emotion into "pulling out all the stops" to provide the best possible care with all available resources. Others, who may be years out of residency training, have the instincts and experience that is invaluable in recognizing the potentially seriously ill child early enough to intervene before the situation progresses. "Rural physicians" caring for children include family practitioners, emergency medicine physicians, obstetricians, and pediatricians. This chapter is written by a pediatrician who has worked in rural Montana for the several years since her residency. She has dealt with all the potential crises in a rural setting, including multiple simultaneous trauma victims, multiple simultaneous "codes," difficulty in being able to give thorough transport reports during a crisis, blizzards precluding *any* transport out, and limited prehospital care resources. This chapter presents her view of responsibilities of the rural physician as well as her perspective on what are reasonable expectations of the referring facility.

PREVENTION STRATEGIES

Before addressing crisis intervention for a critically ill child, a discussion is needed of one of the most critical roles of the rural physician. Primary care physicians should be actively involved in injury prevention education. It is well known that trauma is the number one cause of pediatric deaths, with 50% of trauma deaths occurring within the first hour, and another 30% occurring between 1-3 hours after trauma.[12] Preliminary data from Montana show that the majority of trauma fatalities in a rural state occur before contact with prehospital emergency services. It may be hours before a victim of a motor vehicle accident (MVA) or other trauma is discovered;[10] the only real hope for these patients is injury prevention and control. Anticipatory guidance at well child visits including the American Academy of Pediatrics' The Injury Prevention Program (TIPP) sheets, car seat policies for newborn discharges, and contact with legislators on pediatric/safety issues are important components of a complex overall prevention strategy. It has been shown that after a child receives emergency department care for bicycle-related injuries, parents are no more likely to acquire helmets in the following year;[2] if major trauma does not result in behavior changes, advice from the primary physician as well as legal mandates are also needed. Continued research on effective injury prevention education is crucial, some of which is best done from private practitioner's offices.

Anticipatory guidance should address whom the parent can call for advice. Phone numbers for local ambulance services should be provided. Parents should be told which ambulance services and which hospitals are preferred for pediatrics, if there is a choice. Parents should be instructed on when to call the office versus going directly to the local emergency department. Private offices should advertise "Ask-A-Nurse" type services available by 1-800 numbers, if such a program exists locally and if the information is consistent with local standards of care.

Primary care physicians can ensure that parents are taught cardiopulmonary resuscitation (CPR) during the postpartum period in the hospital. CPR, Pediatric Basic Life Support (PBLS), and first aid courses should be made available in all communities, and primary care providers should encourage parents and patients to take the courses. High schools that offer such courses usually find an enthusiastic group of students enrolled. "Babysaver" classes for young baby-sitters also disseminate safety information in the local community.

ADVANCE PREPARATION FOR INTERHOSPITAL TRANSPORT

Emergency medical service preparation

Rural hospital personnel need intimate contact with local ambulance services. Rural physicians and local transport systems should lobby for legislation of EMS delivery and enhanced 911 systems. Rural pediatricians should consider assisting in on-line medical control or at least be willing to back-up non-ER or nonpediatric trained medical control officers. Rural pediatricians should review off-line standing orders for their prehospital providers and offer to rewrite any that seem inappropriate. They can offer to teach the pediatric/newborn sections of paramedic/EMT/First Responder courses and can offer to participate in post-run evaluations of pediatric emergencies with the prehospital providers and the medical control officer. Rural pediatricians can review the local ambulance's equipment lists and attempt to modify them as needed. (Such lists are easily available in several resource texts.[3]) If funding is limited, consider a dropbag technique for pediatric equipment in the local emergency room or with the local ambulance system that would allow a physician accompanying an ambulance on a pediatric transfer to have additional equipment and supplies available.

If a state has an organized EMS data collection system in which participation is voluntary, local physicians should encourage involvement by community hospitals and the local ambulance system. The rural hospital should ensure that the receiving hospital and the transport services used also collect data. This, combined with patient outcome statistics, must be analyzed in order to improve the EMS system. Local physicians should insist that their hospitals utilize ICD-E Codes (which classify the external cause of injury) in their business and computer department. Identified local trends can then be used to guide local injury prevention efforts.

Depending on the distances involved and availability of EMS personnel, hospitals at both referring and receiving ends should consider consolidating pediatrics at one facility.[11] Of course, this is generally not an option at the referring end. Protocols for bypass of the local facility by EMS personnel should be established and agreed upon by all parties involved. This may only be practical when prehospital personnel respond in an area relatively equidistant between their base facility and secondary/tertiary facilities. Availability of backup prehospital services must first be ensured or a county/region could be left without EMS services while the local team was out-of-county. All personnel involved need to work towards improved survival of children as their goal.

Helicopter transport teams should be capable of landing "in the field" where geographically appropriate and when police/fire/EMS personnel determine that need. These prehospital providers should have written guidelines which have been agreed upon by the medical control for the local ambulance system as well as the transport system, for these situations. Interhospital transport protocols should also address this issue.

Emergency department preparation

Crash carts should be clearly labeled with the contents periodically reviewed by the medical staff, in addition to routine nursing checks of location, quantity, and expiration dates of supplies. Pediatric equipment can be included or, preferably, located in a separate crash cart, dropbag, or tacklebox. The equipment in size gradations, such as endotracheal tubes, gastric tubes, and intravenous equipment, should be organized in a readily accessible fashion. One useful adjunct is a "respiratory roll," which rolls up compactly and unrolls to reveal progressively larger sizes of endotracheal tubes plus all other equipment required for intubation. A pediatric resuscitation measuring tape,[7] as developed by James Brosolow, M.D., should be included. Equipment can also be organized by colors using the Brosolow® tape color which corresponds to patient size; this method puts all respiratory and cardiovascular access equipment for a given sized patient in one package. Besides routine crash cart contents in pediatric sizes, intraosseous needles should also be included. Pedia-trake/Nu-trake® devices are invaluable for physicians not routinely performing tracheostomies. A high-flow oxygen setup for needle cricothyroidotomies should also be available. Laminated lists of age/weight-appropriate vital signs, code sheets, vasoactive infusion rates, and the Pediatric Glasgow Coma Scale are essential. A list of items not on the crash cart but potentially necessary in a pediatric emergency, such as umbilical artery trays, chest tube trays, warming lights, and pediatric blood pressure cuffs, should also be included.[8]

It is critical that rural hospital staff prepare for emergencies. JCAHO mandates that "a hospital is capable of instituting essential lifesaving measures and implementing emergency procedures that will minimize further compromise of the condition of any infant, child, or adult being transported."[6] A written disaster plan should be readily accessible. A phone list of all potentially available local medical personal should be immediately available and the contents known by all hospital employees. Also, numbers of all available ambulance and transport systems and numbers for subspecialty consultants should be available. Primary physicians must have linkage to secondary and tertiary centers as well as specialized centers (i.e., burn, pediatric cardiovascular, ECMO, etc.)[1] Mock case scenarios can be presented to staff in order to better prepare for actual pediatric crises.

A written disaster plan should be readily accessible. Routine disaster drills can be realistically done and aid in determining needed resources for emergencies, besides meeting JCAHO requirements. They can be arranged as a multifacility and even multicounty event, involving police and fire personnel as well as hospital and prehospital personnel. Often, helicopter transport services will participate as part of their training. Local artisans usually enjoy moulaging patients, typically hospital staff's family members and friends. Usually, the county disaster personnel or EMS services director or a hospital's environmental engineer organizes the drill; some element of surprise is ideal to truly test local resources. The drill provides a valuable learning opportunity in prehospital and hospital triage. A prearranged notification network should be used with responsible parties calling vital off-duty staff members. Utilization of hospital space and manpower in a drill frequently results in improvements in the disaster plan. A critical step in these drills is a postdrill, multidepartmental review/critique of the event.

Pediatricians should encourage personnel covering local emergency rooms to be PALS and ATLS certified. Intraosseous techniques should also be well known (and regularly practiced on chicken legs) in rural settings. Rural pediatricians should consider becoming PALS instructors to help maintain their own skills and to facilitate local course offerings. If pediatricians do not routinely cover ER shifts in small towns, they should be available for pediatric emergencies. Joint conferences are useful between ER physicians and pediatricians to periodically review pediatric emergencies. In areas where no pediatricians are located, transport services can promote access of PALS courses to rural hospital personnel, preferably by offering courses in the rural region, but at least by advertising and increasing awareness of courses already planned.)

Helicopter/fixed wing landing sites should be appropriately maintained and lighted at the local hospitals. Arrangements with police or hospital security should be made beforehand to clear and protect the landing sites during an emergency.

INDICATIONS FOR PATIENT TRANSFER

Pediatric patients are transferred to tertiary care for a variety of reasons, not all of which are related to the inability of the referring physicians to take care of the child. Transfer is indicated when the need arises for certain regionalized equipment, such as computerized tomography scanners or dialysis units. Specialized services, such as pediatric surgery or psychiatric facilities, will only be available at larger medical centers. Lack of hospital beds and nursing staff will occur more frequently in a rural area, since the numbers of each are small. In addition, staff qualified to care for seriously ill children may not be available on all shifts. A family may insist on transfer. Or, finally, a physician may be uncomfortable with managing a patient's illness.

On occasion, patient death is better accepted when in a secondary or tertiary care facility. Families may then perceive that all available resources were used for their loved one. (This reason for transport may be more closely scrutinized as health care reform progresses.) Organ donation can occur more completely and efficiently in a large medical center.

INITIAL CONTACT WITH THE TRANSPORT TEAM

Ease of access to Medical Control is critical. A single phone call should put a referring physician in touch with some member of the team, even if the Medical Control physician has to then be paged. A list of questions, preferably condensed enough to fit near key telephones, usually asked by the dispatcher should be provided to the local hospitals by the transport team (the hospital may have to request this). Referring facilities should attempt to have all the anticipated information handy prior to initiating the call.

By OBRA regulations, there must be physician to physician transfer of a patient.[15] If possible, the referring doctor needs to make the initial contact with the transport team. However, not infrequently, major trauma, multiple victim trauma, or concurrent medical emergencies occur at a small hospital and overwhelm available resources. When there is only one physician and limited ancillary staff, time is at a premium. The physician may be the only person capable of making assessments and performing procedures. Transport coordinators should be cognizant that a ward clerk or aide may be the only person available to make a call. A patient's name, age, vital signs, and a "lay" description of the situation may be all the information that they can provide. Waiting until a physician or nurse is available may take another 20 to 30 minutes. The physician will usually have a moment to speak with a transport coordinator after a unit clerk has initiated the call, the need for someone else to place the call is especially important if the transport system is one that has to page a Medical Control physician.

In some emergencies, when the referring facility's resources are overwhelmed, the physician may know that at least one patient needs transporting, yet may not know which one is most critical until the transport team is en route. The local hospital should inform the dispatcher of this and describe what is currently known about the "candidates" for transfer, so that the appropriate team and equipment are sent. If transport teams are capable of taking more than one patient at once, they should inform the referring hospital.

It is helpful to be given an approximate mobilization time during the initial phone call, and the transport coordinator should also contact the referring hospital when the team actually departs from the receiving facility. This can help the local physician prioritize what needs to be accomplished in the time remaining until the team arrives. She/he must decide, for example, if the postintubation chest x-ray is more important than the blood work if there is only one lab technician. If two large bore IVs are not in place when the transport team arrives, it may be because a chest tube or other procedure took precedence.

When unexpected delays occur, the referring physician may need to arrange for a different mode of transport. This may involve an appropriately trained physician riding in an appropriately equipped local ambulance. The Medical Control officer at the receiving facility should concur with this, if appropriate, or advise otherwise (including disclaiming liability) it if seems that the patient's safety would be compromised.

Transport frequently is required because the facility cannot handle the needs of the patient, not because the physician cannot handle the medical condition. Consequently, advice from the medical control physician may not be needed. A rural pediatrician may actually be more qualified in pediatric stabilization than a nonpediatric Medical Control physician. In other situations, especially those frequently encountered by emergency physicians (such as management of an unknown toxic ingestion), advice may be appreciated. The best situation diplomatically is for the receiving physician to ask if the referring physician would like any help with patient management.

When a tertiary care center has an emergency physician as on-line medical control, the pediatrics department should be notified of the transport. If the pediatrician is then to assume medical control, the outlying hospital should be made aware so appropriate physician to physician contact can be made as time allows.

PATIENT CARE TRANSFER

It is important for the local hospital to understand what a transport team expects from them. Some teams prefer that the medical staff remain to help, and others prefer to act independently immediately upon arrival. Generally, if a staff member is available, someone should remain with the team to answer questions, order labs, find supplies, etc. Otherwise, a contact person for the transport team to call upon should be clearly indicated when the local staff leaves the transport team alone. It may not be possible for the physician or nurse to remain with the team if other critical patients are demanding their attention. Prior on-site visits by the transport team help each side understand the needs of the other.

The legality of turning over patient care from a physician to a nonphysician (i.e., a nurse-led team) should be addressed before that situation arises. A prior visit and a written statement on this issue is appreciated by most referring hospital's administration and physician staff. The Medical Control physician is assuming a tremendous responsibility by becoming the patient's physician of record without the opportunity to examine the patient. The referring staff should understand that this situation may necessitate some additional telephone time between the team and medical control.

IMPORTANT ASPECTS OF THE TRANSPORT TEAM

Quality of pediatric training and experience of the personnel on a transport team is important, yet is frequently not a matter of choice when only one transport service is available. Literature on the transport team should include a description of the qualifications of the members. Members should be chosen for their medical skills as well as for their ability to deal sensitively with the patient, with the personnel at the referring hospital, with parents, and with each other.[3] Since the referring hospital is responsible for ensuring that the level of care during transport is appropriate under OBRA regulations, they should be informed of the specific pediatric training and experience required of team members.[4] When a dedicated pediatric team is not available, a rural pediatrician may be more likely to ride with a patient in an ambulance or to accompany the transport team if allowed.

To the local hospital, speed of arrival is frequently the most important aspect for a transport team, especially in trauma situations. In multiple victim trauma, local manpower will be stretched, and quick transport of even one of the patients allows the limited local resources to be stretched between the remaining patients. Also, speed may be critical to the survival of a patient with a surgical emergency and to other patients for whom the local hospital cannot provide definitive care.

The respect that the team gives the local facility provides strong incentive to continue to employ that particular team. The referring physician usually finds it difficult to "give up" a patient. Families and patients lacking medical expertise can easily assume that their facility and their physician are inferior, regardless of the reason for transfer. Many tertiary care centers, especially those with housestaff programs, reinforce this concept. This is difficult for the competent rural physician. Transport personnel can help families understand reasons for transfer while maintaining their trust in their local resources. The AAP Ad Hoc Task Force on Definition of the Medical Home says: "The AAP believes that the medical care of infants, children, and adolescents ideally should be accessible, continuous, comprehensive, family-centered, coordinated, and compassionate. It should be delivered or directed by well-trained physicians who are able to manage or facilitate essentially all aspects of pediatric care. The physician should be known to the child and family and should be able to develop a relationship of mutual responsibility and trust with them."[3] In order for this type of medical care to be given, the rural physician must be given credit. The patient should be returned to his/her care upon discharge from the tertiary center. The primary care physician should receive a detailed report on the patient's care, follow-up needs, and discharge medications.

SITE VISITS

It is helpful for a transport service to be informed about the facilities and the physicians with whom they deal. Offering an on-site visit to see what resources are available in a community is helpful to both the referring and receiving facilities. The frequency of on-site visits should be based on staff turnover on the transport team, in the receiving facility, and at the referring facility. An on-site community outreach program offered by the transport team is an ideal vehicle to accomplish these goals. Regional courses/symposiums sponsored by transport systems are also good for education and public relations. Details of comprehensive community outreach programs are available in the chapter on that topic.

During a visit by the transport team, members can record a checklist of available equipment and personnel, as well as the pediatric training and experience of staff. Suggestions can be offered to prompt rural facilities to update equipment, training, or protocols.

The transport team should be aware of the prehospital capabilities for any given county or otherwise defined area. Since there may be large variances in the prehospital systems from county to county, Medical Control's approval of mode of transport may differ dramatically for different referring facilities.

Written information from the transport team should include a formal transport agreement to facilitate transfers. This document should address what is required of the referring hospital, medical liability, assumption of costs, and phone numbers to activate transport. This agreement should be renewed on an annual basis. Examples of such documents are contained elsewhere.[9] The list of questions routinely asked when transport is initiated should be provided. A transfer sheet also helps the local facility to organize data and prepare for the team's arrival. Since, according to JCAHO, a referring hospital is also responsible for care given at a receiving facility, it is helpful to know that quality assurance is being addressed within the transport team and at the receiving facility.[5]

All hospitals need policies and procedure in place for interfacility transport. Issues of uninsured patients, crossing state lines, and payment for transport should be addressed. The legal responsibilities of the parties involved should be well delineated.

There should be a clear policy on whether a local physician can travel with the transport team in specific cases. Again, a local pediatrician may be more competent in some pediatric emergencies than the adult-trained nurse on the transport team. Since it often requires flying one less team member, the local physician may have to make the decision to accompany the team prior to their departure from the receiving facility.

Transfer packets are helpful to provide the patient's family. Families can sign consent forms if they must leave prior to arrival of the team. Information such as city maps, a floor plan of the receiving hospital, facilities for eating, local hotels, and phone numbers assist families during a stressful time. A form listing what is requested by the receiving facility will also help the outlying hospital prepare better for the transport (for example, sending maternal blood with the newborn on a neonatal transport).

Transport teams should not assume that an outlying hospital has infrequently used drugs such as prostaglandin E_1 or tolazoline, so these should be carried by the team if potentially needed. Smaller facilities may not stock digibind, snakebite antivenom, or dantrolene. Formularies are frequently limited, so the corticosteroid preparation used by medical control may not be available. Outlying hospitals usually have a spectrum of antibiotics to cover all critical situations, yet may not have the particular combination preferred by Medical Control. Copies of hospital formularies and equipment in rural hospitals may be worth having in the dispatch office or at least perusing during an on-site visit.

FOLLOW-UP

Brief written follow-up on the status of a referred patient is a wonderful public relations effort by the transport team. The follow-up is ideally written by someone involved in the particular transport. This note should also specify the final attending physician since patients are frequently accepted by the Emergency Department physicians. If state or facility regulations limit this note due to patient confidentiality issues, the community hospitals should be made aware of this policy.

A contact person for problems or complaints is needed. Complaints or compliments by a referring facility should be considered as feedback courteously. Written follow-up that an issue was addressed is then helpful to the local facility/physician.

DISCUSSION

The chief concern of all medical personnel involved with children should be the patient's life and safety. Politics, economics, "turf wars," and prejudice have no place. Interhospital transport fills a gap in our medical systems. Such transports can be enhanced by improved communication and understanding between rural and secondary/tertiary facilities; effort is needed at both ends to optimize pediatric health care.

REFERENCES

1. Conn A: Organization and components of combined rural and urban EMS systems. In *Report of the 97th Ross conference on pediatric research: Emergency medical services for children,* Columbus, OH, 1989, Ross Labs.
2. Cushman R and others: Helmet promotion in the emergency room following a bicycle injury: a randomized trial, *Pediatrics* 88(1):43, 1991.
3. *Emergency medical services for children: the role of the primary care provider,* Elk Grove Village, IL, 1992, American Academy of Pediatrics.
4. Frew SA and others: COBRA: implications for emergency medicine, *Ann Emerg Med* 11: 835-7, 1988.
5. Joint Commission for the Accreditation of Healthcare Organizations: *Accreditation manual for hospitals,* Chicago, 1989, JCAH.
6. Joint Commission for the Accreditation of Healthcare Organizations: *Accreditation manual for hospitals,* Chicago, IL, 1989, JCAH.
7. Lubitz DS and others: A rapid method for estimating weight and resuscitation drug dosages from length in the pediatric age group, *Ann Emerg Med* 17:576-81, 1988.
8. Ludwig S, Selbst S: A child-oriented emergency medical services system, *Curr Probl Pediatr* 141-2, March 1990.
9. McIntyre MS: *Injury control for children and youth,* Elk Grove Village, IL, 1987, American Academy of Pediatrics.
10. Espasito TE and others: *Rural preventable mortality study,* US DOT Report #DTNH22-90-C-05016, Washington, DC, 1993.
11. Simon JE: Current problems in the emergency management of severe pediatric illness. In *Report of the 97th Ross conference on pediatric research: Emergency medical services for children,* Columbus, OH, 1989, Ross Labs.
12. Trunkey DD: Trauma, *SciAm* 249:28, 1983.
13. Aoki B, McCloskey A: Medicolegal issues in interhospital transport. In *Evaluation, stabilization, and transport of the critically ill child,* St. Louis, 1992, Mosby-Year Book, Inc.

44

INTRAHOSPITAL TRANSPORT

ELIZABETH WALLEN
SHEKHAR T. VENKATARAMAN
RICHARD A. ORR

Tremendous strides been made in the past two decades in the care of the critically ill pediatric patient. An increased understanding of critical illnesses and advances in technology have improved the ability to maintain life-support in critically ill infants and children. Transport of a critically ill pediatric patient, defined as the movement of a critically ill infant or child from one site to another, is now possible because critical care can be provided outside the Intensive Care Unit (ICU) for extended periods of time. There are three categories of patient transports: prehospital, interhospital and intrahospital transports. **Prehospital transport** refers to the transport of patients from a nonhospital site of injury or illness to a local hospital. **Interhospital transport** refers to the transport of patients from one hospital to another, usually from a community hospital to a tertiary care hospital. **Intrahospital transport** refers to the transport of patients within the hospital from one patient care area to another. Studies on prehospital and interhospital transport of critically ill infants and children show that: 1) adverse events occur during transport, 2) the incidence of adverse events is related to the severity of the underlying illness, 3) physiologic deterioration may occur despite providing optimal intensive care, and 4) the transport team must optimally be composed of personnel best equipped to recognize and treat problems during transport.[16,21-25,28,29,36] Much attention has been focused on prehospital and interhospital transports, but scant attention has been paid to intrahospital transport of critically ill infants and children. Intrahospital transports occur as frequently, if not more frequently, than prehospital and interhospital transports and should be considered a part of the critical care continuum. Adverse events during intrahospital transport can be as life-threatening as during prehospital or interhospital transport.

TYPES OF INTRAHOSPITAL TRANSPORT

There are essentially two types of intrahospital transports: two-way transports from one location to another and back, or one-way transports from one location to another (Figure 44-1). Two-way intrahospital transports usually involve moving the patient from the ICU or a general ward to a noncritical care area for a diagnostic or therapeutic procedure, and after completion of the procedure, the patient is returned back to the ICU or the general ward. One-way transports usually involve: 1) transport to the ICU from the operating room (OR), the emergency department (ED), or the general ward, 2) transport to the OR from the ICU, ED, or the general ward, or 3) transport to the general ward from the ICU, the ED, or the OR. The severity of illness of patients transported and the risks associated with each type of transport differ considerably. The transport time, defined as the time taken from the initiation to the comple-

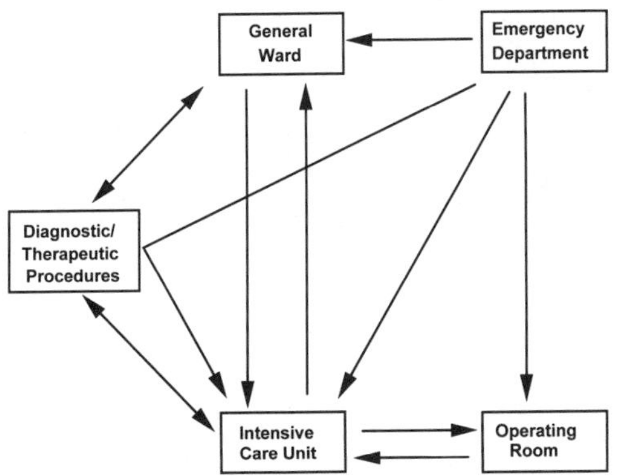

Fig. 44-1. Types of intrahospital transports. One-way transports are shown by one-way arrows, and two-way transports are shown by two-way arrows.

tion of the transport, includes the time taken for preparation, the actual transfer of the patient, and the posttransfer stabilization. In two-way transports, the transport time includes the time spent in the non-ICU area for a diagnostic or therapeutic procedure, which may vary from minutes to several hours.

TWO-WAY TRANSPORTS

Transports from the ICU for diagnostic/therapeutic studies

Nonportable diagnostic tests such as gastrointestinal radiologic studies, computerized tomography (CT), magnetic resonance imaging (MRI), cardiac catheterization, or angiography are sometimes needed in the critically ill patient to follow the course of disease and therapy. These tests take time and require the patient to be out of the ICU for a prolonged period of time. Such transports are risky because the patient is being moved from the safe environment of the ICU to a location where advanced monitoring and care are not readily available. Patients who are taken from the ED for diagnostic studies before being admitted to the ICU should also be included in this category. Adult patients who were admitted to the ICU with severe trauma experienced serious physiologic changes in heart rate, blood pressure, respiratory rate, intracranial pressure, or oxygen saturation when they were transported out of the ICU for diagnostic studies.[1,19,33,45] Indeck and others[14] have reported that one-fourth of these patients had their clinical treatment changed within 48 hours of the transport. The incidence of adverse events during such transports out of the ICU correlated with the severity of injury.[1,19] Mechanically ventilated patients transported out of the ICU experienced cardiovascular changes related to altered ventilation, or changes in intracranial pressures.[1,2,10,34,46]

In children, Venkataraman and others[41] reported that there was a significant change in heart rate, blood pressure, respiratory rate, temperature, or oxygen saturation in 72% of intrahospital transports. Half of the patients transported had at least one major event, and in 15.5% of the transported children, at least one major therapeutic intervention, defined as a fluid bolus >20ml/kg, initiation or increasing vasopressor infusion for hypotension, a change in ventilator settings in response to desaturation or hypercarbia, or treatment for increased intracranial hypertension (mannitol or hyperventilation), was performed.[41] Venkataraman and others also showed that 11% of children who were mechanically ventilated during transport required changes in their ventilator settings either during the transport or soon after arrival in the ICU. The incidence of adverse events and the requirement for at least one major intervention was related to both the severity of illness as judged by the TISS score[47] and the transport time.[41]

Transport from the general ward for diagnostic or therapeutic procedures

This type of transport involves patients from the general ward who require a diagnostic or a therapeutic procedure. Such patients often require sedation. Sedatives may depress the respiratory drive and result in hypoxia and hypercarbia. Several studies have shown that sedation in children can result in arterial oxygen desaturation.[6,11,30,35,42] These have been attributed to hypoventilation due to decreased respiratory drive and/or obstructed breathing due to floppiness of the airway.

ONE-WAY TRANSPORTS

Transports between critical care areas

A patient may require transport between the OR and the ICU, between the ICU and the OR, or between the ED and the ICU or the

OR. Insel and others[15] have shown that patients transferred from the OR to the ICU had significant increases in systolic blood pressure and heart rate. Venkataraman and others[41] showed that 59.1% of patients transferred from the OR to the ICU had at least one adverse event, 36.4% had at least one major event, 8% had at least one equipment-related mishap, and 11.4% received at least one major intervention. Even though the transport times between the OR and the ICU were quite short in both these studies, these transports were associated with clinically significant perturbations of the cardiorespiratory systems. There is potential for similar adverse events during transport of a patient from the ICU to the OR. After initial resuscitation and stabilization in the ED, some patients need to be transferred to the ICU for ongoing care. Secondary insults may occur during the transport process, and must be anticipated.[10-12] Hypoxia was seen in 15 to 22% of unconscious victims with head-trauma transferred from the ED to a neurosurgical unit.[1,9,33] An inadequately managed airway was the major reason for hypoxia in these patients.[9,33] About one-third of these patients with a compromised airway in the ED had hypoxia.[9] Other adverse events seen in these patients includes arterial hypertension or hypotension and intracranial hypertension.[1] Some of the adverse events such as inadequately managed airways are avoidable. Pretransport severity of illness correlated with the incidence of mishaps during transport.[9,33]

Transports from a critical care area

When a patient no longer requires intensive care, they are usually transferred to a non-ICU area. Such transports include postoperative patients who are transferred out of the OR to either the recovery room or the ward and patients transferred out of the ICU to the ward. These transports involve patients who are recovering and no longer require intensive care. The level of care required is less than that is provided in the critical care area from where they are transported. The anticipation in these instances is for the patient to improve progressively over time. Patients emerging from anesthesia have decreased ventilatory drive and a decreased ability to protect their airway. A decreased ventilatory drive may result in hypoxia, and an unprotected airway may result in airway obstruction from pooled secretions or floppiness of the upper airway.

McConachie and others[26] reported that nearly all children recovering from anesthesia showed a decrease in systemic blood pressure, with more than 50% having a change in blood pressure of 20% or more from preoperative values. McConachie and associates[26] also reported that 28 of 16,700 children suffered respiratory complications requiring intubation and mechanical ventilation. Cohen and others[7] reported that the risk of adverse events, both major and minor, was 35% in the perioperative period. Infants younger than 1 month of age had the highest incidence of adverse events in the recovery room.[7] Postoperative hypoxia is well recognized in patients breathing room air after surgery.[17,27,38]

Transports to a critical care area

This type of transport involves patients who require intensive care. Patients initially admitted to the ward may become more severely ill and require a level of care that cannot be provided in the general ward. In this case, patients need to be moved from an area where advanced monitoring and care are either not feasible or not available to an area where such monitoring and care are available. Secondary insults may occur during the transport process and must be anticipated.

DEFINITIONS OF POTENTIAL COMPLICATIONS OR ADVERSE EVENTS

Adverse events during intrahospital transport can be classified into changes in physiologic variables and equipment-related mishaps (Box 44-1). Physiologic variables include temperature, heart rate, breathing rate, blood pressure, and other vascular pressures, intracranial pressure, and measures of gas exchange. Hypothermia is defined as a core temperature $<36\,^{\circ}C$. A clinically significant change in heart rate, breathing rate, or vascular pressure may be defined in many ways. If the pretransport value is within normal limits for age, then a significant change can be defined as a $>20\%$ change from pre-

BOX 44-1 ADVERSE EVENTS DURING INTRAHOSPITAL TRANSPORT OF PATIENTS

Physiologic deterioration
- Significant change in vital signs (HR, BP, Temp, RR)
  - >20% change from baseline
  - Change in vital signs outside the range of normal
- Cyanosis or arterial oxygen saturation <90%
- An increase in $PaCO_2$ with an arterial pH < 7.3 in the absence of metabolic acidosis
- Altered mental status
- Intracranial hypertension (ICP > 20 cm H_2O)

Equipment-related events
- Airway and breathing related events
  - Endotracheal tube mishap (dislodgement, obstruction by secretions, etc.)
  - Loss of oxygen supply
  - Lack of suction equipment
  - Disconnection of ventilator circuit
- Equipment malfunction (power failure, non-function, etc.)
- Infiltration of IV fluids
- Dislodgement or disconnection of tubes and catheters
  - Central venous catheters
  - Tubes in the gastrointestinal tract
  - Pleural, pericardial, mediastinal, or abdominal drainage tube

transport values, or a change that falls outside the normal range for that age.[13,39] If the pretransport value is outside the normal range, then a significant change can be defined as a change that requires a therapeutic intervention. Intracranial hypertension is defined as an intracranial pressure greater than 20 cm H_2O. In infants, even an intracranial pressure of 15 cm H_2O may be considered significant enough to warrant an intervention. A significant change in oxygen saturation is defined as a reduction in oxygen saturation of greater than or equal to 5% lasting 5 minutes or longer. Hypercarbia, is defined as an increase in arterial carbon dioxide tension greater than 60 torr with a pH less than 7.35 in the absence of metabolic acidosis. Changes in vital signs may be further classified into **minor,** those not requiring immediate therapy, and **major,** those that require immediate therapy.

Equipment-related events include dislodgement of tubes or catheters, loss of oxygen supply, malfunction of equipment, and errors in medication (Box 44-1). Smith and others[37] reported that 34% of the adults who were transported out of the ICU for diagnostic studies had an equipment-related mishap. In transports involving children, Venkataraman and associates[41] showed that during intrahospital transport, there was at least one equipment-related adverse event in 10% of intrahospital transports. Equipment-related mishaps may be those that do not result in major physiologic deterioration, further classified as **minor,** and **major** mishaps may be classified as those that do result in major physiologic deterioration (Box 44-1).

PRETRANSPORT STABILIZATION AND PREPARATION

A team approach is essential for the safe transport of critically ill patients. The approach should take measures that prevent adverse events during transport and prepare to deal with problems during transport. Link and others[19] showed that major adverse events were encountered when adequate monitoring was not available but were eliminated when a dedicated transport team was involved. This phase includes assessment of: 1) severity of illness, 2) monitoring requirements, 3) equipment to be taken on transport, and 4) care plans during transport. It also includes the physical preparation of the patient and equipment for transport.

Assessment of severity of illness

Before every transport, the patient's severity of illness must be evaluated because pretransport severity of illness is associated with adverse events during transport. The level of physiologic stability, monitoring, and ongoing therapies should be assessed. Scoring systems such as the **PRISM** that reflect physiologic instability can be used to classify patients, but **PRISM** has been validated only to predict in-hospital mortality.[31] The disadvantage of the **PRISM** score is that while a high score defines a high risk group, a low score does not preclude the requirement for intensive care.[28] Venkataraman and others[41] have shown that severity of illness as assessed by a pretransport Therapeutic Intervention Scoring System (TISS),[48] a score that reflects the cumulative therapies received by the patient prior to transport, predicted the need for major interventions during intrahospital transport. The level of monitoring and the type of ongoing treatments will dictate the amount of equipment required during transport. This evaluation should include not only the monitoring and therapy the patient currently requires, but also what may be needed during transport.

"Know thy destination"

The second issue during pretransport preparation is to "know thy destination."[40] Many transports involve moving the patient to different corners of an institution and may involve delays, such as waiting for an elevator or waiting for a previous patient to finish the diagnostic procedure. Arrangements must be made to ensure no delay in transport. The transport time must be estimated before the transport because in addition to the pretransport severity of illness, the incidence of adverse events correlates with the transport time.[41] A thorough knowledge of the level of monitoring possible in these locations is also essential, so that the team can prepare to take the appropriate equipment.

Selection of personnel and equipment

The third step is the selection of personnel. In addition to the primary nurse accompanying the patient, additional personnel may be required depending on the severity of illness and the equipment required. This may include additional nurses, a respiratory therapist, a physician, and others. Generally, physicians are more readily available to escort patients on transport in teaching hospitals than in community hospitals. The team must be familiar with the patient's illness. It would be preferable for the team to consist of the same personnel who were caring for the patient before transport. The disadvantage of personnel leaving a unit is the reduction in coverage in that unit. Since the availability of personnel is different depending upon the particular unit or hospital, guidelines for intrahospital transports have to be individualized for each unit and institution.

Equipment required for monitoring and emergency management must be portable and accompany each transport. Portable equipment should be light, small, compact, easy, and safe to operate, reliable, and rugged.[32] In addition, it should have a rechargeable battery capable of providing power continuously for at least 2 hours on a single charge. Box 44-2 describes a suggested list of supplies to be carried by the transport team for transports from the ICU to the diagnostic suite. The list may be modified for other types of transport. A transport pack is a convenient way to carry all these supplies. Care must be taken to keep the transport pack manageable so that the team members can carry it without difficulty. Heart rate and respirations can be monitored by a portable display. Respirations should also be monitored clinically by examining the adequacy of chest rise, the breathing rate, the difficulty in breathing, and the color of the nailbeds and mucosa. Blood pressure can be monitored invasively or noninvasively. An ideal portable cardiorespiratory monitor should be capable of displaying the ECG and breathing efforts continuously and at least two pressure tracings, have a display that is clearly readable at a distance of 15 to 20 feet, and have built-in alarms for low and high readings.

Volumetric infusion pumps capable of infusing fluids and drugs continuously are commonplace in the intensive care unit. An ideal volumetric pump would be light, portable, capable of operating on built-in battery power, capable of delivering fractional rate of infusion at 0.1 ml/hr increments, and deliver a constant and accurate flow of fluid with a less than 5% variability. It is preferable to use the same volumetric pump in the ICU and during transport because changing pumps may result in greater variability in fluid delivery. The pump must have an occlusion alarm to alert the team members. During transport, only the most essential fluids should be administered. This includes all vasoactive drug infusions and maintenance IV fluids. Narcotic and sedative infusions can be switched over to bolus administration for the transport. It would be preferable not to infuse blood prod-

BOX 44-2 PICU TRANSPORT BAG CONTENTS

Intubation kit
Laryngoscope handles
Laryngoscope blades
Miller blades (sizes 0-3)
Wis-Hipple blade (size 11/2)
Foregger blade (size 2)
Curved MacIntosh (sizes 3 and 4)
Endotracheal tubes (2.0 through 8.5)
Oral airways (4 sizes)
Nasal airways (14 through 34)
Yankauer suction
Intubation drugs
Atropine 400 mcg/ml (1ml)
Vecuronium 10 mg vial
Large Magill forceps
Stylets
NG tubes

IV administration kit
Fluids
5% albumin
500 ml bag .9NS
Syringes (1 through 60 ml)
Needles (24 through 18 G)

Infusion drugs
150 mg nitroprusside
130 ml 1:1000 epinephrine
15 ml 40 mg/ml dopamine
120 ml 250 mg/20 ml dobutamine

Emergency drugs
5 ml 2% lidocaine abboject
10 ml 1:10,000 epinephrine
50 ml 50% dextrose
50 ml NaHCO3
10 cc vial CaCl (100 mg/ml)
2 ml narcan (0.02 mg/ml)
1 ml narcan (0.4 mg/ml)
250 ml 25% mannitol
2 ml dilantin (50 mg/ml)

Miscellaneous
Stopcock
10 cc normal saline vials
10 cc sterile water vials
Betadine ointment
Heparin (1 ml) 1:1000
Tapes
Dressing materials
T-connectors
Tourniquet
Alcohol wipes
Nonsterile gloves
Surgilube
Benzoin
ECG electrodes (small and large sizes)
Flash light
Suture removal kit
Suction machine
Suction catheters: 6Fr, 8Fr, 10Fr, 16Fr size.
250 ml .9NS irrigation solution
Normal saline bullets

ucts and routine drug infusions during transport. These steps would minimize the number of pumps to be carried on transport.

An E-size oxygen cylinder with the appropriate high-pressure regulator and flowmeter should accompany all transports and be secured safely to the stretcher or the mobile bed. The pressure in the E-cylinder should be checked before the transport to ensure that there will be sufficient gas supply during the transport. Oxygen supply tubing should be of sufficient length to provide supplemental oxygen during transport. An appropriate sized self-inflating resuscitation bag, equipped with a manometer and a PEEP valve, and a resuscitation mask should also accompany the patient for emergency manual ventilation. A pulse oximeter should be used to monitor patients on supplemental oxygen. A portable ventilator may be useful in mechanically ventilated patients in order to ensure that a preset tidal volume is reliably delivered in spite of changes in resistance and compliance of the respiratory system.[8,43] An ideal portable ventilator should be able to generate a peak inspiratory pressure (PIP) that is adequate for the pediatric population, function as a constant inspiratory flow generator, have a PIP-limiting valve that is adjustable, have minimal gas compression volume in the circuit, and have less than 10% variability in the delivered tidal volume regardless of PIP.[5] In addition, the ventilator's gas consumption should be as little as possible. Table 44-1 describes the

TABLE 44-1 CHARACTERISTICS OF PORTABLE VENTILATORS

Characteristics	*Omni-Vent Stein-Gates Medical Equipment Inc*	*Univent Impact Medical Corp*	*PLV-102 LifeCare Products*	*LP-10 Aequitron Medical*	*IC-2A Biomed Devices*	*MVP-10 Biomed Devices*
Operating modes	IMV/SIMV Assist-Control CPAP	IMV/SIMV Assist-Control CPAP	IMV/SIMV Assist-Control CPAP	IMV/SIMV Assist-Control CPAP	IMV/SIMV CPAP	IMV/SIMV CPAP1
Drive mechanism	Pneumatic	Pneumatic	Piston-driven	Piston-driven	Pneumatic	Pneumatic
Controls	Electronic	Electronic	Electronic	Electronic	Pneumatic	Electronic
Cycling mechanism	Time	Time	Time	Time	Time	Time
Inspiratory valve	Yes	Yes	Yes	Yes	Yes	No
Inspiratory flow @ 50 PSI	0-150 lpm	0-100 lpm	10-120 lpm	0.1-264 lpm	0-75 lpm	0.6-10 lpm
TV range	30-3000 ml	0-5000 ml	50-3000 ml	100-2200 ml	0-3000 ml	0-600 ml
RR range	1-150 bpm	1-150 bpm	2-40 bpm	1-38 bpm	1.3-66 bpm	0-120 bpm
Pressure relief valve (max)	100 cm H_2O	100 cm H_2O	100 cm H_2O	80 cm H_2O	100 cm H_2O	100 cm H_2O
PEEP	0-20 cm H_2O	0-20 cm H_2O	Not built-in External PEEP valves needed	0-20 cm H_2O	0-20 cm H_2O	0-20 cm H_2O
Manual trigger	No	Yes	No	No	Yes	No
Size/Wt	2 kg	<5 kg	13.6 kg	15.5 kg	3.86 kg	2.3 kg

features of some of the portable ventilators that can be used in the pediatric population. The addition of capnography may offer additional control over minute ventilation.

Preparation of the patient for transport

The airway and breathing must be secure. If a patient requires mechanical ventilation, arrangements must be made to provide mechanical ventilation during transport. If the patient is intubated, the endotracheal tube must be securely taped and well anchored. The endotracheal tube should be suctioned prior to transport to ensure its patency. Under certain circumstances, such as a newborn infant with complex congenital heart disease undergoing cardiac catheterization, it may be prudent to intubate and institute mechanical ventilation before transport. In our experience, this approach has considerably reduced the incidence of adverse events in these patients. Adequate intravenous access is essential. If immobilization of the patient is required, then arrangements need to be made prior to transport. Fever, pain, anxiety, or unnecessary movement of the patient increases oxygen consumption and may cause tachycardia and intracranial and systemic hypertension. Sedation may be required to reduce anxiety. Narcotic analgesics may be required to control pain. Neuromuscular blockade may be required in mechanically ventilated patients to control minute ventilation. If neuromuscular relaxants are used in intubated patients on mechanical ventilation, one must remember to sedate and adjust minute ventilation appropriately. The patient must be stabilized as much as possible prior to transport. The transport itself should involve the least amount of therapeutic interventions.

TRANSPORT PHASE

The transport phase involves several steps:

1. Movement of the patient from the bed to the transport stretcher,
2. Movement of the equipment and supplies to the transport stretcher,
3. Continuation of critical care,
4. Monitoring during the transport,
5. Transport to the destination,
6. Movement of the patient from the transport stretcher to the bed at the destination, and
7. Stabilization of patient.

For two-way transports, the transport phase also includes the following steps:

1. Monitoring during the test,
2. Movement of the patient from the diagnostic suite to the transport stretcher,
3. Continuation of critical care and monitoring during transport,
4. Transport back to the ICU, and
5. Movement of the patient from the transport stretcher back to the patient's bed.

The goals during the transport phase are three-fold:

1. Maintain patient stability.
2. Continue present level of management.
3. Prevent or avoid mishaps.

Patients and equipment must be moved from the bed to the transport stretcher with the utmost care. Dislodgement of tubes and catheters, disconnection of intravenous infusions, and accidental extubations are potential adverse events during this process. Several personnel may be required to coordinate the movement of both the patient and all the equipment to the stretcher. A better approach may be to use mobile beds which can be moved to the transport location for all patients on admission. This would ensure that the patient is moved only at the transport location. Decreasing the number of times the patient is moved reduces the chances of equipment-related mishaps. Due to the amount of equipment required during transport, some have suggested the use of a specially designed transport cart or mounting bracket to carry the portable devices.[18,20,44] A transport cart must be strong enough to carry the weight of the portable devices but light enough for the transport team to easily move. The advantage of such a system is convenience during transport. For patients on mechanical ventilation, the respiratory therapist should accompany the team, connect the patient to a mechanical ventilator upon arrival at the transport site (preferably the ventilator used or to be used by the patient in the ICU), and ensure that the portable oxygen cylinder is shut off.

POST-TRANSPORT STABILIZATION

This phase involves moving the patient from the transport stretcher to the bed, moving all necessary equipment back to the bedspace, and posttransport stabilization. A critically ill patient may require about 30 minutes to an hour for stabilization after an intrahospital transport. This stabilization time must be considered as an extension of the transport process. Andrews and associates[1] showed that significant cardiorespiratory changes occur posttransport in severely head-injured patients. The care provided again must reflect the severity of the underlying illness. Upon return, the team should assess the patient's clinical status, put away any extra equipment used in transport, and document the transport. The documentation should include any adverse event noted and interventions performed to correct it.

MONITORING AND APPROACH TO PROBLEMS DURING TRANSPORT

Critical care must continue to be provided at the same level as before transport. Monitoring should be appropriate for the severity of illness. In critically ill children, heart rate should be monitored continuously. In patients who have an intraarterial catheter, the blood pressure should be monitored continuously. Patients requiring supplemental oxygen would certainly benefit from pulse oximetry. Patients undergoing cardiac catheterization or diagnostic tests in radiology are prone to hypothermia, due to exposure to a cold environment. Care must be taken to clothe the patient appropriately, monitor the temperature, and if the body temperature falls below 36°C, the ambient temperature should be increased.

Hemodynamic changes that may occur during transport are bradycardia, tachycardia, hypotension, hypertension, or a dysrhythmia. Tachycardia may result from anxiety, pain, fever, untreated hypovolemia, hypotension, infusion of vasoactive drugs, or hypoxia. Bradycardia may result from hypothermia, hypoxia, or intracranial hypertension. Systemic hypertension may result from anxiety, pain, intracranial hypertension, or excessive delivery of vasoactive drugs. If a significant hemodynamic change is observed, the team must evaluate the patient to determine the cause and treat it.

Hypoxia and hypercarbia may result from hypoventilation. In spontaneously breathing patients, hypoventilation may result from excessive sedation. This is usually due to depressed breathing efforts, reduced airway muscle tone, or airway obstruction from a "floppy" airway. A patent airway can be maintained by repositioning the airway or by providing an oral or a nasopharyngeal airway. Pulse oximetry is useful in detecting desaturations in patients who are sedated in the diagnostic suites. Supplemental oxygen can prevent some of these desaturations and must be available. In spontaneously breathing patients, supplemental oxygen can be provided by a face mask or a nasal cannula. In mechanically ventilated patients, hypoventilation may result from delivery of an inadequate tidal volume or ventilator rate. Inadequate tidal volume may be the result of a disconnection of the ventilator circuit, accidental extubation, excessive leak of gas in the circuit, inadequate preset tidal volume, occlusion of the endotracheal tube, or as a result of sudden changes in the total respiratory system compliance or resistance.

Hypoxia in mechanically ventilated patients may result from hypoventilation, inadequate maintenance of positive end-expiratory pressure or mean airway pressure, or variations in inspired oxygen concentration. Pulse oximetry is useful to detect hypoxemia. Hypercarbia can be detected using either a capnograph or transcutaneous carbon dioxide electrode. If hypoxia or hypercarbia is detected, then the team must determine that the airway is secure and then manually bag the patient with 100% oxygen and ensure adequate ventilation and oxygenation. The ventilator circuit must be examined to ascertain that there is no disconnection or leak. Hypocarbia and respiratory alkalosis may result from excessive ventilation. Respiratory alkalosis may result in hypokalemia, cardiac ectopy, and leftward shift of the oxyhemoglobin dissociation curve with decreased oxygen delivery to the tissues. Excessive hypocarbia may potentially cause cerebral ischemia in patients with intracranial hypertension. If hypocarbia and respiratory alkalosis is detected, then the minute ventilation should be decreased either by decreasing the tidal volume or the ventilator rate. In mechanically ventilated adults, strict control of tidal volumes delivered during transport reduced the incidence of adverse cardiopulmonary changes.[10,46] This is achieved either by using manual ventilation with a pneumotachometer to assess delivered volumes or by the use of a portable ventilator that delivers a preset tidal volume.[10]

Intracranial hypertension is a common complication associated with head trauma, liver failure, and various encephalopathies. During intrahospital transport, clinically significant intracranial hypertension may develop spontaneously, or due to agitation, pain, hypercarbia, or hypoxia. These patients are prone to develop life-threatening brain herniation due to intracranial hypertension. Signs of brain herniation include an acute change in mental status, pupillary changes, and changes in the type and depth of respirations and systemic hypertension. Care must be taken to prevent any increase in intracranial pressure. Intracranial hypertension can be treated by hyperventilation, mannitol, or by draining the cerebrospinal fluid through an indwelling intraventricular catheter.

The endotracheal tube can become obstructed due to secretions or dislodged during movement. This may result in hypoxia and hypercarbia and can be life-threatening if it is not recognized immediately. An obstructed endotracheal tube would result in an increase in peak inspiratory pressure for patients who are receiving volume-controlled ventilation and a decrease in the delivered tidal volume. A dislodged endotracheal tube can be diagnosed by performing a direct laryngoscopy and visualizing the position of the endotracheal tube. If a direct laryngoscopy cannot be performed, then capnography can aid in the detection of a dislodged endotracheal tube. A portable colorimetric carbon dioxide detector has been recently used to verify the location of an endotracheal tube.[3,4] Loss of oxygen supply may be due to disconnection of the oxygen tubing or due to an empty oxygen cylinder. Dislodgement of intravenous catheters may be serious if vasopressor agents are being infused through those catheters. Battery powered devices may fail due to low power, and therefore require constant maintenance to ensure that they are fully charged at all times.

DISCUSSION

Intrahospital transports of critically ill patients must be considered as part of the critical care continuum. These transports are intensive in terms of utilization of personnel and resources. Advance preparation and optimal coordination of the transport process are critical toward safe transport of the critically ill infant and child. The transport team must anticipate, prevent, and treat adverse events during transport. The level of care provided should be commensurate with the severity of the underlying illness. The benefit of undertaking intrahospital transport needs to be weighed against the potential morbidity associated with it.

REFERENCES

1. Andrews PJ and others: Secondary insults during intrahospital transport of head-injured patients, *Lancet* 335:327, 1990.
2. Braman SS and others: Complications of intrahospital transport in critically ill patients, *Ann Intern Med* 107:469-73, 1987.
3. Bhende MS, Thompson AE, Cook DR, Saville AL: Validity of a disposable end-tidal CO_2 detector in verifying endotracheal tube placement in infants and children, *Ann Emerg Med* 21:142-5, 1992.
4. Bhende MS, Thompson AE, Orr RA: Utility of an end-tidal carbon dioxide detector during stabilization and transport of critically ill children, *Pediatrics* 89:1042-4, 1992.
5. Branson RD: Intrahospital transport of mechanically ventilated patients, *Respir Care* 37:775-95, 1992.
6. Casteel HB, Fiedorek SC, Kiel EA: Arterial blood oxygen desaturation in infants and children during upper gastrointestinal endoscopy, *Gastrointest Endosc* 36:489-93, 1990.
7. Cohen MM, Cameron CB, Duncan PG: Pediatric anesthesia morbidity and mortality in the perioperative period, *Anesth Analg* 70:160-7, 1990.
8. Dahlgren BE, Johnson A, Lofstrom JB: Portable emergency ventilators: a lung model study, *Acta Anaesthesiol Scand* 27:39-43, 1985.
9. Gentleman D, Jennett B: Audit of transport of unconscious head-injured patients to a neurosurgical unit, *Lancet* 335:330-4, 1990.
10. Gervais HW and others: Comparison of blood gases of ventilated patients during transport, *Crit Care Med* 15:761-3, 1987.

11. Gilger MA and others: Oxygen desaturation and cardiac arrhythmias in children during esophagogastroduodenoscopy using conscious sedation, *Gastrointest Endosc* 39:392-5, 1993.
12. Heinrichs W, Mertzlufft F, Dick W: Accuracy of delivered versus preset minute ventilation of portable emergency ventilators, *Crit Care Med* 17:682, 1989.
13. Iliff A, Lee VA: *Child development* 23:240-5, 1952.
14. Indeck M and others: Risk, cost, and benefit of transporting ICU patients for special studies, *J Trauma* 28:1020-5, 1988.
15. Insel J and others: Cardiovascular changes during transport of critically ill and postoperative patients, *Crit Care Med* 14:539-42, 1986.
16. Kanter RK, Tompkins JM: Adverse events during interhospital transport: physiologic deterioration associated with pretransport severity of illness, *Pediatrics* 84:43-8, 1989.
17. Kataria BK and others: Postoperative arterial oxygen saturation in the pediatric population during transportation, *Anesth Analg* 67:280-2, 1988.
18. Kondo K and others: Transport system for critically ill patients, *Crit Care Med* 13:1081-2, 1985.
19. Link J and others: Intrahospital transport of critically ill patients, *Crit Care Med* 18:1427-9, 1990.
20. Lippmann, Reisner LS, Mayer A: A portable mounting bracket for automatic ventilation in transport, *Anesth Analg* 52:864, 1973.
21. MacNab AJ: Optimal escort for interhospital transport of pediatric emergencies, *J Trauma* 31:205-9, 1991.
22. Mayer TA, Walker ML: Severity of illness and injury in pediatric air transport, *Ann Emerg Med* 13:108-11, 1984.
23. McCloskey KA and others: Variables predicting the need for major interventions during pediatric critical care transport, *Pediatr Emerg Med*, 1991 (in press).
24. McCloskey KA, Johnston C: Critical care interhospital transports: predictability of the need for a pediatrician, *Pediatr Emerg Care* 6:89-92, 1990.
25. McCloskey KA, Orr RA: Pediatric transport issues in emergency medicine, *Emerg Med Clin North Am* 9:475-89, 1991.
26. McConachie IW, Day A: Recovery from anaesthesia in children, *Anaesthesia* 44:986-90, 1989.
27. Motoyama E, Glazener CH: Hypoxemia after general anesthesia in children, *Anesth Analg* 65:267-72, 1986.
28. Orr RA and others: Pretransport pediatric risk of mortality (PRISM) score underestimates the requirements for intensive care or major interventions during interhospital transport, *Crit Care Med* 22:101-7, 1994.
29. Owen H, Duncan AW: Towards safer transport of sick and injured children, *Anaesth Intens Care* 11:113-7, 1983.
30. Pereira JK and others: Comparison of sedation regimens for pediatric outpatient CT, *Pediatr Radiol* 23:341-4, 1993.
31. Pollock MM, Ruttimann UE, Getson PR: Pediatric risk of mortality (PRISM) score, *Crit Care Med* 16:1110-6, 1988.
32. Roberts KD, Edwards M: *Paediatric intensive care*, Blackwell Scientific Publications.
33. Rose J, Valtonen S, Jennett B: Avoidable factors contributing to death after head injury, *Br Med J* ii:615, 1977.
34. Roth F: Der spitalinterne transport im grossen spital, *Scweiz Med Wochenschr* 120:164-9, 1990.
35. Sievers TD and others: Midazolam for conscious sedation during pediatric oncology procedures: safety and recovery parameters, *Pediatrics* 88:1172-9, 1991.
36. Smith DF, Hackel A: Selection criteria for pediatric critical care transport teams, *Crit Care Med* 11:10-12, 1983.
37. Smith I, Fleming S, Cernaianu A: Mishaps during transport from the ICU, *Crit Care Med* 18:278-81, 1990.
38. Soliman IE and others: Recovery scores do not correlate with postoperative hypoxemia in children, *Anesth Analg* 67:53-6, 1988.
39. Task Force on Blood Pressure Control in Children, National Heart, Lung, and Blood Institute. Report of the Second Task Force on Blood Pressure Control in Children—1987. *Pediatrics* 79:1-25, 1987.
40. Tompkins JM: Intrahospital transport of critically ill or injured children, *Pediatr Nurs* 16:51-3, 1990.
41. Venkataraman ST and others: Adverse events during intrahospital transport in critically ill pediatric patients, *Crit Care Med* 19:S79, 1991.
42. Verwest TM, Primosch RE, Courts FJ: Variables influencing hemoglobin oxygen desaturation in children during routine restorative dentistry, *Pediatr Dent* 15:25-9, 1993.
43. Viegas OJ, Cummings DF, Schumacker CA: Portable ventilation systems for transport of critically ill patients, *Anesth Analg* 60:760-1, 1981.
44. Vincent JL, Dufaye P, Kahn RJ: A complete system for transportation of critically ill patients with acute cardiorespiratory failure, *Acute Care* 10:33-5, 1984.
45. Waddell G: Movement of critically ill patients within the hospital, *Br Med J* ii:417-9, 1975.
46. Weg JG, Haas CF: Safe intrahospital transport of critically ill ventilator-dependent patients, *Chest* 96:631-5, 1989.
47. Weil MH, Planta MV, Rackow EC: Critical care medicine: introduction and historical perspective. In Shoemaker MC and others, editors: the textbook of critical care, Philadelphia, 1989, WB Saunders Company.
48. Yeh TS and others: Assessment of pediatric intensive care—application of the Therapeutic Intervention Scoring System, *Crit Care Med* 10:497-500, 1982.

45

INTERNATIONAL AIR MEDICAL TRANSPORT

PAUL DAVIS
KAREN N. (BATES) HAMILTON

The art and science of air medical transfer have progressed rapidly to the point that seriously ill neonatal patients, children and adults can be transported safely over long distances. Most medical conditions that can be transferred by air over relatively short distances should also be able to be transported internationally. However, certain additional issues arise when borders are crossed. These include but are not limited to differences in local air transport regulations, language barriers, lengthy crew duty times and the need for increased quantities of supplies. The keys to success are the use of a trained and experienced medical flight crew, a more detailed assessment and stabilization of the patient's condition, and an advance understanding and investigation of regional regulations.

INDICATIONS FOR TRANSPORT

International medical evacuations are usually undertaken for one or more of the following indications: 1) medical, 2) financial, 3) personal preference.

The primary medical indication for international transport is the lack of a certain type or level of care available in the country in which the patient becomes ill or injured. This circumstance may arise when a visitor from a highly developed country is hospitalized with a condition for which an underdeveloped country does not have facilities. The patient's financial condition and expectations for level of care may permit evacuation (not necessarily repatriation, i.e., not necessarily to the patient's home country) for care not expected by or available to local residents. Or a patient may undergo international transport for experimental, rare, or newly developed therapies only available in another country (i.e., certain types of organ transplantation). Another medical indication for transport is the patient's recovery from a critical condition to the point where repatriation can be accomplished safely. An example is the extremely premature neonatal patient unexpectedly born during an international vacation. The family may have the desire and resources to return home for an anticipated hospitalization of two to three months. However, if the patient's medical condition is critical and rapidly changing, and the 'birth country' has sophisticated neonatal intensive care, repatriation may be delayed until the patient is stable on a ventilator or is off the ventilator and feeding and growing. International medical transport may also be performed for patients living near a border for whom the closest site for critical care is actually across the border rather than within the home country.

Financial reasons for repatriation include insufficient or exhausted insurance benefits/personal guarantees, which may prohibit continuing treatment in the host country, and health insurance benefits that only apply in the country of domicile.

Countries which have a national health care system may find it less expensive to treat a patient in their home medical environment. Costs saved in such a situation are not just direct health care expenses. Family members may be able to return to work and child care, and the added living costs (hotel rooms, restaurant meals) for the family are eliminated.

The third indication for repatriation or at least transport to another country is patient or family request. When the patient is medically stable, it is quite reasonable to want treatment or convalescence in the home environment or in a country which uses their language, even if local facilities are adequate. Terminally ill patients may want to return home, where they feel more comfortable and have access to more of their family and friends.

Airport terminals and passenger aid facilities differ from one country to another. Hoists, steps, ramps or ground ambulances are not always available. Because the greatest risk to the patient occurs during transfer between, into, and out of vehicles, particular care to investigate the loading and off-loading facilities at each stage is imperative. Contingency plans and additional equipment to deal with the potential loading or offloading problem must be attended to before the outset of the trip.

Border post requirements, immigration and custom formalities, visas, any special local applications, and permission to comply with health regulations have to be obtained and prepared for (Table 45-1). Inadequate preparations and failure to notify authorities in advance will increase delays.

Ground transportation must be assessed and service procedures confirmed before any transfers are undertaken from one terminal or one airport to another. Full and detailed confirmations from airport authorities are essential before embarking. Ground facilities at any designated stopover airport should be investigated, including the nearest hospital's available emergency facilities and relevant telephone and other contact numbers.

LEVEL OF CARE NEEDED DURING TRANSPORT

Patients using international medical transport fall into two functional categories. The first is those who are stable and require only limited medical or nursing attention during the transfer. These patients are usually transported most cost-effectively by commercial airlines as opposed to dedicated medical aircraft. Attention must be paid to the seating accommodation of the patient, i.e., window or aisle, near the toilets, in bulkhead seats with extra leg room, or even upgrading to business or first class. For example, it is an FAA regulation that any passenger requiring oxygen must sit in a window seat in order to avoid obstructing the emergency egress of another passenger; alternatively a patient who needs to walk regularly in order to avoid complications of venous stasis will need an aisle seat. The transferring physician and flight coordinator should arrange for adequate nursing personnel and specialty care providers (i.e. respiratory therapists for ventilator dependent patients) during the trip. They should prearrange all passenger aid requirements for embarkation, disembarkation and ground transport.

The second category of patient is those who are unstable or potentially unstable (both mentally and physically). These patients must enter a specialized transportation process that will ensure a continuous level of care throughout the duration of the transfer, with all the necessary emergency and backup equipment and facilities constantly close at hand.

Detailed and particular care needs to be exercised at the danger areas in the transfer process where the patient is most at risk. These times include the point of take over by one treating team from another, and any point during the transfer when the patient is being moved, for example, from hospital bed to a stretcher, stretcher to stretcher, and embarking and disembarking from the aircraft or ground vehicle. Transport equipment, medications and emergency bags should be with the patient at all times. The patient and equipment should not be moved in separate relays unless the patient and equipment are continuously within visual and access range. On private aircraft, appropriate suction sources, oxygen tanks, air compressors and electrical inverters should be on board and ready for use.

TABLE 45-1 INTERNATIONAL GUIDELINES CHART: COUNTRY CODES, TIME DIFFERENCES, VISAS

Country	*Codes*	*TD*	*Visa*	*Notes*
Algeria	213	+5	Yes	
Am. Somoa	684	−6	No	
Andorra	33	+6	No	
Argentina	54	+2	No	
Australia	61	+14	Yes	
Austria	43	+6	No	
Bahran	973	+8	Yes	
Bangladesh	880	+11	No	must have return ticket
Belgium	32	+6	No	
Belize	501	−1	No	return ticket/proof of funds
Bolivia	591	+1	Yes	
Brazil	55	+2	Yes	
Bulgaria	359	+8	Yes	
Cameroon	237	+6	Yes	
Chile	56	+2	No	
China	86	+13	Yes	
Columbia	57	0	Yes	return ticket/tourist card
Costa Rica	506	−1	No	
Cyprus	357	+7	No	obtain upon arrival
Czechoslovakia	42	+6	Yes	
Denmark	45	+6	No	
Ecuador	593	0	No	migratory control card
Egypt	20	+7	Yes	
El Salvador	503	−1	Yes	
Ethiopia	251	+8	Yes	
Fiji	679	+17	No	need return ticket
Finland	358	+7	No	
France	33	+6	No	
Gambia	220	+5	Yes	
Germany	49	+6	No	
Greece	30	+7	No	
Guam	671	+15	No	
Guatemala	502	−1	Yes	or tourist card
Guyana	592	+2	Yes	
Haiti	509	0	No	proof of citizenship/photo
Honduras	504	−1	Yes	
Hong Kong	852	+13	No	need return ticket
Hungary	36	+6	Yes	
Iceland	354	+5	No	
India	91	+10.5	Yes	
Indonesia	62	+12	No	need return ticket
Iran	98	+8.5	Yes	
Iraq	964	+8	Yes	
Ireland	353	+5	No	
Israel	972	+7	No	return ticket/proof of funds
Italy	39	+6	No	
Ivory Coast	225	+5	Yes	
Japan	81	+14	No	return ticket
Jordan	962	+7	Yes	
Kenya	254	+8	Yes	

Continued.

TABLE 45-1 INTERNATIONAL GUIDELINES CHART: COUNTRY CODES, TIME DIFFERENCES VISAS—cont'd.

Country	*Codes*	*TD*	*Visa*	*Notes*
Korea	82	+14	Yes	North—not recommended
Kuwait	965	+8	Yes	
Liberia	231	+5	Yes	
Libya	218	+7	Yes	
Luxemburg	352	+6	No	
Malaysia	60	+13	No	
Monaco	33	+6	No	
Morocco	212	+6	No	
Netherlands	31	+6	No	
New Zealand	64	+18	No	
Nicaragua	505	−1	No	
Nigeria	234	+6	Yes	
Norway	47	+6	No	
Pakistan	92	+10	Yes	
Panama	507	0	No	return ticket/tourist card
Paraguay	595	+2	No	
Peru	51	0	No	
Phillippines	63	+13	No	return ticket required
Poland	48	+6	Yes	
Portugal	351	+5	No	
Romania	40	+7	Yes	
Saudi Arabia	966	+8	Yes	
Senegal	221	+5	Yes	
Singapore	65	+13	No	
South Africa	27	+7	Yes	
Spain	34	+6	No	
Sri Lanka	94	+10.5	No	return ticket/proof of funds
Suriname	597	+1	Yes	
Swaziland	268	+7	No	
Sweden	46	+8	No	
Switzerland	41	+6	No	
Taiwan	886	+13	Yes	
Tanzania	255	+8	Yes	
Thailand	66	+12	No	return ticket required
Tunisia	216	+6	No	
Turkey	90	+8	Yes	
Uganda	256	+8	Yes	
Uruguay	598	+2	No	
Venezuela	58	+1	Yes	and tourist card
Yugoslavia	38	+6	Yes	
Zaire	243	+6	Yes	
Zambia	260	+7	Yes	
Ximbalswe	263	+7	No	return ticket/proof of funds

Note: All time zones are based on Eastern Standard Time.
TD = Time Difference, in hours, from EST.
This information is subject to change with changing government regulations.

GENERAL CONSIDERATIONS

Transports are usually performed to bring a patient from a lower level of care to a higher one. The advisability of transfer in the face of scanty or unreliable medical information must be carefully considered. It has to be accepted that on occasion the team will arrive to find a patient who is simply too unstable for long distance transport. The initial indication for transport (i.e., repatriation for convenience vs. inability to care for the patient's condition) will determine whether transport is canceled, delayed, or diverted to a geographically closer facility.

General medical standards and available facilities of the sending institutions may vary greatly, even if the same terminology and descriptions are used. For example, the concept of an Intensive Care Unit may be vastly different in various countries, both in quality of staff and in sophistication of equipment.

All reasonable attempts should be made to assess the situation in advance of the transport, even if transport is delayed in order to make an appropriate evaluation. The patient's best interest will not be served if the team does not have a detailed understanding of the situation to be encountered.

Language barriers may make it difficult to properly understand and evaluate the patient's diagnosis, medical condition, and current treatment. International long distance phone companies offer translators in a wide range of languages. The initial patient assessment can be made via a three-way or conference call using these services. In view of the complex nature of medical terminology, it may be necessary to take an experienced translator as part of the team. Barring that, advance preparations should be made for a trained interpreter at the referring hospital. It is not appropriate to plan to assume care of a seriously ill patient with communication only through a friend or family member who "speaks some English."

Telecommunication systems may present another barrier to information exchange. Cellular phones or radio transmitter/receivers used by the team in their home country should not be expected to interface with communications equipment used at the receiving hospital. Thus, the team may be unable to receive or send information about changes in the patient's condition. In some countries regular pay phones do not accept coins and instead require special "phone cards" for payment.

Because of the additional stops for refueling, crew changes and all of the border crossing and airport formalities, international transfers may be of longer duration than would be expected by travel distance alone. There is a far greater potential for unexpected delays enroute. Local disposable supplies may not be compatible with the team's equipment and, therefore, cannot be counted on for replacement or restocking of exhausted team resources. These issues should be considered when planning equipment and medication needs for the trip. In general, supplies should be carried to care for the patient for twice the predicted time of transport. Differences in power sources may also necessitate additional battery power and use of current adapters.

Dedicated medical transport aircraft often have a shorter range than commercial carriers before requiring refueling. This means that there will be more stops enroute. Relief aircrew and perhaps also relief transport teams need to be stationed along the way. Arrangements for additional medical equipment, extra oxygen cylinders, fluids and medications enroute need to be planned for and delivery ensured in advance if necessary.

MEDICAL LEGAL ISSUES

A license to practice medicine does not automatically apply in a foreign country. It is a general rule that only when a physician is in the 'no-man's land' in the air is it truly legal to take over responsibility for patient care. However, practically speaking, most teams take over responsibility for the patient at the referring hospital. This exposes them to the whole spectrum of legal problems that may emanate from practicing medicine without a license. With this in mind, handover procedures need to be carefully planned and complied with to the letter. The referring physician can be asked to accompany the transport team to the airport and to formally turn patient care over once through immigration control. All reasonable advance efforts should

AUTHORIZATION FOR NARCOTIC TRANSPORT

To whom it may concern:
Our aeromedical crewmembers ______________ (name) and ______________ (name)
are authorized to transport and administer according to current ATS protocols (standing orders), if necessary the following narcotics:

1. Valium oral or parenteral
2. Morphine Sulfate oral or parenteral
3. Demerol oral or parenteral
4. Phenobarbital oral or parenteral
5. Ativan oral or parenteral

Our patient, ______________ (name) is being transported

from ______________ (hospital) in ______________ (city, state, country)

to ______________ (hospital) in ______________ (city, state, country)

Your cooperation in assisting our medical staff is greatly appreciated and necessary in the best interests of providing high quality medical care to this sick or injured individual.

Sincerely yours,

SAMPLE

____
Karen N. Hamilton, RNC, CEN, CCRN, CFRN
Vice President/Chief Flight Nurse
Program Director

____
John P. Bryant, M.D.
National Medical Director
FAA Medical Examiner

Fig. 45-1. Authorization for narcotic transport.

be made to obtain appropriate insurance coverage, as local policies may not cover practice in another country. Protocols for attempting to obtain temporary hospital privileges should be developed, especially for any hospital or country which regularly uses a particular international transport system.

All medications carried, especially controlled substances, must be disclosed to customs authorities upon request. A letter of explanation of potential need from the medical director of the transport team may be helpful. The formal Authorization for Narcotics letter (Figure 45-1) should also include (for controlled substances) a calculation of reasonable quantities of medication which would be used for the particular patient and a copy of the team's policies and protocols monitoring medication distribution (i.e., locked containers, signature protocols, etc). Written prescriptions for the individual patient may also be needed. It may also be helpful to note in the letter that for narcotics, as for all other medications, a greater quantity is carried than is anticipated to be needed. This would be necessary in the event that the team was to spend more time than anticipated with the patient, if the patient were sicker than anticipated, or if an additional patient or patients were to be cared for by the team.

TRANSPORT VIA COMMERCIAL AIR CARRIER

For purposes of discussion in this chapter, the United States is considered to be the base country, with the perspective that "international" means outside the U.S. Commerical airlines are frequently used for transporting moderately ill patients because of distance and cost implications. Using commercial airlines to transfer the very ill raises additional responsibility factors and protocols. Connecting flights are often involved, including those with different airlines. No two airlines are exactly the same in terms of their standing regulations for transferring ill people, loading procedures, onboard equipment and internal layout. With this in mind every effort should be made, if the patient's condition is not compromised, to seek non-stop or at least direct (no plane change at stops) flight routing, even if departure time is delayed.

Airlines are usually ambivalent about transporting seriously ill, psychotic or contagious patients. Stable patients, in general, when accompanied by a qualified aeromedical crewmember, and who will not cause embarrassment or offend fellow passengers, will be transported without too much fuss. An example of the medical questionnaire to be filled in by the attending physician gives a good indication of the requirements for the voyage (Box 45-1). Unstable patients present a very different picture to the airline, so much so that Lufthansa has designed, and will possibly soon implement, a totally self-contained medical transport module that is separate from the passengers.

BOX 45-1 AIRLINE'S MEDICAL INFORMATION SHEET

Patient's name, initials, sex, and age.

Nature of incapacitation.

Name, age, sex, and qualification of attending physician and/or escort (business/home telephone numbers).

Medical data of patient, date of diagnosis, prognosis for the trip, and contactable or contagious disease.

Is patient in any way offensive to other passengers (smell, appearance, conduct)?

Wheelchair needed (yes/no, type, etc.)?

Ambulance required (yes/no)?

In-flight requirements or arrangements, for example, special meals, equipment, oxygen, toilet use, special seating, leg rest, etc.

Arrangements that have been made for assistance at connecting points, airport of arrival, etc.

In order to properly transport a reclining patient, six to nine coach seats, or four first or business class seats, need to be purchased, the stretcher fitted, and the area screened from the remainder of the passengers. Oxygen available from the aircraft's oxygen supply delivers only 2-4 liters per minute, so arrangements need to be specifically made for extra oxygen to be taken on board. It should be ensured that the connections are compatible with transport equipment. It is rare for a commercial airliner to supply any electrical power; if available, power points may be 220 volts, 110, 28 or 14 volts. The necessary connections should be investigated in advance and a variety of socket adapters should be carried. Additional portable lighting is imperative.

If two or more airlines are used, separate and specific arrangements need to be made with each carrier. All arrangements should be reconfirmed and names of the person(s) confirming the arrangements and contact telephone numbers should be carried in writing by the team.

Ground arrangements and transfer procedures at the airports should also be double checked. Names and telephone numbers of all contacts must be carried, along with the name and telephone numbers of the airline's medical director (if that position exists). When the patient must be transferred enroute to the final destination, ensure that the nearest hospital to the airport is alerted and the local doctor and equipment are investigated in advance. A relatively standard checklist of all the questions that need to be answered for the airline's medical director is appended (see Box 45-1).

It should also be confirmed in advance that the insurance (malpractice, life and disability) of the transport staff and administrative team covers them for commercial medical transfers.

In addition to the patient, issues involving both the flight personnel and any family members accompanying the patients must be addressed. All should have appropriate travel documents such as passports, visas, and immunization records (see Table 45-1). Any companions traveling with the patient should be asked about their own past medical histories, current medications and allergies in anticipation of the unlikely event of having their own medical emergency occur during a long flight. Family members should be told to carry on their own prescription and non-prescription medications. The medical flight crew should review information on the culture, customs and climate of the destination country and any countries in which stops will be made. Attire and behavior should be appropriate to meet reasonable expectations of the local culture. The team should also carry enough cash in local currency to cover any unanticipated expenditures. Particularly of note is the fact that in many countries the ability to obtain expected assistance may in fact depend on appropriate "tipping".

Pre-flight screening should be thorough in order to avoid arrival in another country to find a patient too unstable to transport. Specific consideration should be given to the effects of altitude on the patient's condition and to the effects of pressurizing the aircraft on travel time, fuel load and need for refueling stops. In the event that the patient's condition worsens, the team should be prepared to spend a longer time then projected in the patient's country. This would specifically include taking additional clothing and additional supplies of any medications the flight crew requires for themselves personally. Travel guides for countries of likely transport should be kept in the medical office in order that medical crews may refer to them for information about climate and culture.

Ground ambulance arrangements should be established during the preflight screening. Either the patient's physician, the family or the local American Consulate can assist with this preparation. It is useful to take two separate wallets, one for U.S. dollars and the other for local currency. It should be anticipated that costs will always be higher than expected. Major credit cards should always be taken, either in the name of flight personnel or in the form of appropriately authorized corporate cards from the transport program. Traveler's checks can add security to the amount of cash taken. However, traveler's checks will not help in the arena of "tipping".

A completed Authorization for Aeromedical Transport (Figure 45-2) must be taken to announce the teams' official status and purpose for the transport. A complete list of medications, equipment and supplies should be carried in the event that airline or immigration officials require such documentation.

Airline and hotel reservations should be arranged prior to departure from the home country. Confirmation of reservations sent via FAX should be carried with the team at all times.

Commercial airline regulations will vary with regard to what type of patients they can accept and what type of services to the patient are either provided or allowed. It would be most helpful for the team to carry a copy of a letter faxed to the appropriate airline official outlining the patients condition. A written response from that official and carried by the team can carry tremendous weight if disagreements occur enroute. Specifics addressed would include whether an IV will be required to be hung, what arrangements are made for oxygen, what sort of stretcher will be used, what suctioning equipment is needed, etc. It should be noted that it generally takes three days to arrange a stretcher transport on commercial air carriers. Commercial airline stretchers may be secured in special brackets over the seats in the first class, business class or rear coach compartment of the plane.

Modified oxygen adapters should always be carried, as each airline will have different sources. The available oxygen supply should be checked for each aircraft as well as the need for portable oxygen during on-loading, off-loading or stand-by times. This oxygen, rarely available from the airline, can be provided by ground ambulance or medical oxygen services companies. Oxygen tanks should never be allowed to completely empty. If the tank is empty, condensation forms water which collects in the bottom of the tank. The tank will then be unusable for purified oxygen filling. The liter flow should be stopped at about 300psi. Ambulance crews should be reminded in advance that oxygen will have to be brought to the plane. The ambulance crew should not be released until the oxygen supply on the aircraft has been tested and found adequate for the patients needs.

A predesignated individual, for example

AUTHORIZATION FOR AEROMEDICAL TRANSPORT

To whom it may concern:

This letter is written with the intent of introducing to you our medical services. Aeromedical Transport Specialists, Inc., provides medically managed air transport services capable of making life-saving assistance accessible to anyone, anywhere in the world. Our medical personnel are specially trained in aviation physiology and critical care medicine. In order for them to properly care for our patient, certain specialized medication, equipment, and supplies will be necessary for transport. Our equipment is FAA approved and authorized to remain on board the aircraft under the direct supervision of our medical personnel. A complete detailed list is available upon your request.

Our patient, ______________________________ is being transported
(name)

from ______________________ in ______________________
(hospital) (city, state, country)

to ______________________ in ______________________
(hospital) (city, state, country)

Your cooperation in assisting our medical staff is greatly appreciated and necessary in the best interests of providing high quality medical care to this sick or injured individual.

Sincerely yours,

SAMPLE

______________________	______________________
Karen N. Hamilton, RNC, CEN, CCRN, CFRN Vice President/Chief Flight Nurse Program Director	John P. Bryant, M.D. National Medical Director FAA Medical Examiner

Fig. 45-2. Authorization for aeromedical transport. Reproduced with permission, Aeromedical Transport Specialists, Inc.

the Transport Coordinator, should be identified as the point person for all planning. That person should be informed as to all specific details of the progress of preparing for the transport. In all preparations it should be assumed that the length of the transport will be longer than actually predicted. Possible additional items needed include but are not limited to extra batteries, charging plugs and monitor chargers.

IN THE FOREIGN COUNTRY

Immediately upon the team's arrival in the foreign country, the transporting airline should be contacted to confirm arrangements. Specifically it should be determined that the stretcher and oxygen have been ordered, that security clearances are arranged, that the loading procedures are established (either through the gate at the forward entrance or via forklift for a rear entrance load), that dietary arrangements are appropriate and that wheelchair, aisle chair, and/or seating arrangements have been confirmed as appropriate.

The team should initially go to the patient's hospital to meet the patient and to review all preflight orders. The base hospital coordinator should be called to confirm arrival of the team and to provide a current report on the patients condition. The team's medical equipment should be checked for its compatibility with all adapters needed for foreign current. It should be assumed that special plugs are required and that regular battery packs for the heart monitor or suction unit should never be plugged directly into the wall in another country. The equipment charging lights should be checked after the appropriate converter system is connected. The team should remember that current in wall sockets may go off if the lights are turned off.

The team should ensure that all ground arrangements have been made and that the patient will arrive at the airport in sufficient time to board the flight. A minimum of one and a half hours at the airport should be planned prior to departure of international flights.

It is helpful if a team member or designee can arrive at the airport in advance of the patient. If that is not possible, a team member should go to the ticket counter to check on the flight and to request assistance from a special service agent. These agents can help with loading the patient, with clearing security and customs and with securing the equipment on board. They can also act as a liaison with flight attendants.

Charting should be done in the home base's time zone with local time in parentheses or written below. Maximum cabin and cruising altitudes along with their duration can be obtained from the airline crew. The names of physicians involved with the transport, ambulance personnel, customs officials, family and accompanying friends, the special service agent, the discharging nurse and the receiving nurse should all be documented. Prior to landing, the pilot should be notified to call ahead and arrange for the ambulance and for customs officials to board the aircraft to clear the patient. All paperwork including entrance cards should be in order prior to landing. When returning to the U.S., a Customs Declaration Card is required for each family. An individual should be designated to obtain baggage in the baggage claim area. Family members can help with this. At least one team member, and more if the patient is seriously ill, should remain with the patient at all times.

The team should always go with the patient to the receiving facility and should give a report directly to receiving hospital personnel. The receiving individuals should sign for all personal property, chart forms, medications, x-rays and special equipment. Unless the transport team routinely uses duplicate or triplicate forms, inflight records should be copied for the patient's new medical chart. Continuity of care dictates provision of bed to bed and physician to physician (or team to physician) transfer.

AFTER THE TRANSPORT

All transport equipment and supplies should be cleaned and restocked. Any problems encountered should be documented in writing and, if serious, communicated immediately to appropriate transport administrators. Suggestions for improvement of future international transports should also be given to appropriate personnel (i.e., Chief Flight Nurse, Medical Director, Program Director, etc.). Expense reports with receipts should be completed. Expenses should be written in U.S. dollar amounts with any foreign currency itemization clearly stated. All narcotics should be returned to the appropriate locked area and separate documentation should be made of any narcotics used during transport. Follow-up should be considered with the patient, the patient's family, the referring facility and physician, and anyone else who assisted in facilitating the transport.

MISCELLANEOUS CONSIDERATIONS

- It is useful for the team to take bendable straws if the patient is able to drink. These will be much easier to manage than a straight straw.
- If a foreign physician will be accompanying the transport team, a round trip airplane ticket will probably be necessary in order for the physician to be accepted through immigration.
- A preflight conference between team members and coordinators is useful in order to be clear that everyone has the same understanding of activities involved with the flight.
- Any equipment to be checked into the baggage compartment should be put in an appropriately secure box or suitcase.
- The patient should be visited shortly after arrival in a foreign country in order to become aware of any problems as soon as possible.
- Equipment should be kept securely locked and appropriately tagged. Pieces of tape across the opening of containers can serve to alert the team to any tampering which may have occurred.
- Suitcases and valuables should be kept secured at all times.

- Instructions for electrical converters should be reviewed prior to departure in the event that the crew has any questions about their use.
- If feasible, the patient's head should be directed toward the front of the aircraft when traveling aboard a commercial air carrier.
- The aeromedical crew members should always keep passports, airline tickets, boarding passes, etc. on their person. Friends or family members should not be allowed to be responsible for these important documents.
- Again, always take more cash than you think you will need.

SPECIAL CONDITIONS

Leg casts should be elevated with pillows and blankets for take offs and landings and with a small suitcase and pillows and blankets during flight. The best seat is in the bulkhead row, preferably at the window seat in order to prevent accidental bumping by other passengers or food service carts. The patient should be seated with their strong or unaffected side inboard.

Patients with strokes (CVA) should be seated in aisle seats with their strong or unaffected side inboard. If a posey restraint is needed, the passenger sitting behind the patient must be traveling with the patient if their food tray is obstructed and unusable.

Quadriplegic patients must be accompanied by a competent companion. Paraplegic patients are allowed to travel by themselves by most commercial airlines. Wheelchairs are not allowed on board aircraft. The passenger must be carried on board or have an aisle chair available. Currently all U.S. registered commercial jet aircraft are required to have a portable aisle chair available.

A minimum of twenty-four hours prior to departure is necessary to obtain oxygen through the airline. Oxygen may only be installed if it is four rows or ten feet ahead of or behind the smoking section. Smoking is prohibited on all U.S. commercial flights of less than six hours duration, and increasingly international carriers offer nonsmoking flights for much longer trips. As of January 1, 1995, all Delta Airlines domestic and international flights will be nonsmoking. It is usually better for the patient and the aeromedical crew to take an entirely nonsmoking flight, even if it delays the transport for a few hours. Passengers are not permitted to use their own oxygen during flight. A full oxygen tank may be checked as baggage or an empty oxygen tank may be placed in the overhead bin or under the seat in front of the patient. Most oxygen tanks provided by the airline hold twenty-two cubic feet. These "super-D" tanks are shorter and of larger diameter than an E-tank but with the carrying capacity.

There is no standard (110VAC) household current available on board commercial aircraft. A twelve volt D/C (115-400hertzAC) power source may be available on some B727's, DC10's and L-1011 aircraft. At least forty-eight hours advance notice is needed to confirm power converter availability with the airline's maintenance department.

Lead acid batteries are not allowed on board commercial aircraft. Dry cell and gel type batteries are acceptable. Batteries which are self contained in isolettes, wheelchairs, or monitors are allowed. Certain general seating arrangements should be noted. Arm rests in bulkhead seats and first class seats cannot be removed. Bulkhead seats are the best for passengers with casts and for patients with seeing eye or hearing ear dogs. Oxygen can be installed in the first class compartment of 747, DC10 and L10 aircraft as well as any aircraft in which all of first class is non-smoking. The only acceptable seats for patients to recline during takeoffs and landings are the last seat in the cabin in front of a bulkhead (first class, business class or coach) and if there are no passengers in the entire row behind the patient.

If required by the airline, medical certificates may be obtained from any ticket counter. A letter to the airline stating that the patient is "stable for commercial air transport" should be provided by an attending physician. A prescription is needed for any oxygen required for the patient and must state liters per minute/hour, whether the need is intermittent or continuous, whether or not the oxygen will be needed while on the ground or during layovers or plane changes, and the method of delivery (adult mask, pediatric mask, nasal cannula).

If the patient or another individual begins to hyperventilate, have them re-breath CO_2 into a paper bag. They can try to count to five for each inhalation and exhalation. Attempts should be made to keep the patient calm or to have him or her sing or talk as a distraction.

For middle ear pain experienced during descent, the patient should be instructed to yawn, swallow or move his or her jaw. Sucking on hard candy, chewing gum, or sucking on a pacifier can help, as can performance of the valsalva maneuver. Decongestant nasal sprays are particularly helpful in relieving this condition. Similar methods can help alleviate pain from trapped gas in sinuses.

If the patient is known to have trapped gases in the GI tract, he or she should avoid drinking large amounts of water before going to altitude. The patient should also avoid chewing gum (during ascent) and carbonated beverages and should chew food well. Assistance in relieving gases may be provided by massaging the abdomen from the right to the left.

Prevention is the key to eliminating motion sickness. Anti-emetics may be administered prior to flight. Small, easily digested meals should be eaten prior to flight. The patient or team member should rest lying down with the head low or the seat lying back. The patient should be kept in a cool, well-aired cabin environment, should avoid inflight reading or writing, should avoid sudden head movements, and should keep his or her eyes closed or fixed on a stationary object.

Patients with a pneumo or hemothorax should have their chest tubes placed to a heimlich valve for the flight. Flying for seventy-two hours after removal of a chest tube should be avoided unless a sea level cabin altitude is maintained. Chest tubes should not be clamped except in the event of an emergency, as a tension pneumothorax may develop.

Patients with gastrointestinal disorders should have tube feedings held for four hours prior to and during transport. NG tubes should be kept open to the air during transport and should not be clamped. Laxatives, stool softeners and enemas should be withheld the morning of departure. Colostomy bags should be vented at the top of the bag by making a small pin hole and covering with a bandaid after the air is released. Commercial air carriers are reluctant to accept incontinent patients. The team should make every effort to avoid odors which would be offensive to other passengers. An organic odor eliminator spray should be carried in the flight crew supply bag to help alleviate unpleasant odors.

SUMMARY

International air transport of moderately and critically ill patients, both by commercial air carriers and by dedicated air ambulances is becoming increasingly frequent. Reasons for this include increased access to international travel, disparities in medical sophistication, and technological improvements allowing safe long distance transport. Careful planning and detailed protocols can mean the difference between a complicated, frustrating and potentially dangerous transport and a safe, efficient one in which the patient is delivered in a stable or even improved condition.

46

EQUIPMENT

HARRIET HAWKINS
ZEHAVA NOAH

The provision of a high level of care during the interhospital transport of critically ill neonatal and pediatric patients demands that the equipment used meet specific requirements. It is no longer acceptable to borrow equipment from the units or the emergency department or to permit the use of poor quality equipment.

Whether the transport team is dedicated (exists only for the purpose of transport) or not, the equipment must be dedicated.[2] It should not be loaned out to other units within the hospital, regardless of how urgent the situation may be. Transport equipment must be readily available for transport and, therefore, should be reserved for use by the transport team. Although transport equipment can be easily used in the nontransport environment, the reverse is not true. Much of the equipment regularly used within the hospital setting is not adaptable for transport, either because of size, weight, or lack of battery power. Even though various units in the hospital might have equipment that will work well on transport, there is no guarantee that it will always function appropriately. If equipment has been in use in a patient care area, there may be no way of knowing how much battery life is available. The transport team must own and maintain equipment in order to be assured that it is fully charged and appropriately stocked. Although laborious, daily assessment of equipment presence and function is required to ensure availability at a moment's notice.

CHARACTERISTICS OF TRANSPORT EQUIPMENT

Weight and space limitations require that equipment be lightweight and easily portable. All necessary parts or cables must be able to be stored with the equipment, either within the piece of equipment or in a pouch attached. A two person transport team should be able to easily load all necessary equipment.

Another feature required for transport equipment is durability. Vibration, extremes of temperature, and if fixed wing transport is used, changes in barometric pressure expose transport equipment to substantial stresses not encountered in the hospital environment.[2] The external casings on equipment must be capable of withstanding occasional bumps into doors and walls and the bouncing of the vehicles.

Because the transport environment is one that is always moving, the equipment used must be easily secured during transport. This is important not only in the transport vehicle but also while moving the patient through the halls of a hospital. Equipment that does not come from the manufacturer with mechanisms for securing it must have these added prior to use on transport. The engineering and/or biomedical department of the hospital can assist in adding devices for appropriate securing.

Although the majority of vehicles used for transport will have alternating current available, all equipment used must be able to run on battery power. Battery power is needed in the transit from facility to vehicle and may be necessary in case of power failure in the transport vehicle. The suggested amount of battery life is twice the expected time of the transport.[2] In order to ascertain that all equipment is capable of working at full battery power, regular evaluations by the hospital biomedical department is mandatory. When not in use, most transport equipment must be kept charging.

Reliability is also a key factor when selecting transport equipment because there is generally no other back-up equipment available. Anytime there has been an equipment problem on a transport, regardless of how slight, the equipment should be checked as soon as possible after the termination of the transport. The equipment must be easy to troubleshoot while on transport and all staff must be well-versed in using each piece of equipment.[8]

All equipment should be cleaned after each transport. Many times, clean equipment will be needed again immediately for another transport. For this reason, the equipment must be easily cleaned using a standard hospital cleaning solution. Cloth or porous materials should be avoided whenever possible as such materials absorb the cleaning solution and, therefore, require a drying time between transports. Equipment that requires elaborate dismantling for cleaning is impractical.

The standard transport vehicles of today, whether ground or air, have sophisticated communication and navigation systems. It is important that equipment used in the vehicles have no electromagnetic interference so that patient monitoring devices and communication/navigation devices can be used simultaneously.

Transport equipment must meet all federal, state, city, and FAA codes, including hazardous material regulations if appropriate.[2] If the transport program is hospital-based, the equipment may also have to meet any codes imposed by the hospital. Dispensation of such hospital codes may be possible if the nature of the equipment use is clearly defined.

TRANSPORT EQUIPMENT AND THE BUDGET

There are multiple ways of categorizing transport equipment. From a budget standpoint, there are items that must be purchased from the capital budget and those that can be charged to the patient or come from an operating budget. Monitoring equipment, isolettes, intravenous pumps, and transport ventilators are examples of capital budget items. In beginning a new transport program, these are expensive items that must be considered in the initial budget. In addition, provisions must be made for replacing these items as they either become old and no longer function well or as they become out of date. Rapid evolution of medical technology often makes existing equipment obsolete. A transport program will have to plan to be able to keep up with current trends by purchasing new pieces of equipment as they become accepted standard of care, either in-house or for transport systems.

Disposable items needed on transport may be charged to the individual patient. These items can be restocked after each transport, using available hospital or floor stock. Mechanisms must be in place to allow for easy accessibility of these items so that the transport equipment can be restocked in a timely manner and efficiently accounted for. Medications, intravenous catheters, intravenous tubing, and gastric tubes are examples of patient charge items.

Certain items, such as alcohol swabs, syringes, and gauze pads are often hospital floor stock and are not charged to individual patients. Hospital-based transport programs may choose to restock these items from the floor stock of the receiving unit. Individual independent transport programs may have their own floor stock of these items or may choose to restock from the receiving hospital.

MONITORING EQUIPMENT

Cardiac monitors

Cardiac monitors can be divided into two types: those with a defibrillator and those without. Standard neonatal cardiac monitors do not have a built in defibrillator. These neonatal monitors and others (intended for all ages) are available in sizes very conducive to transport and generally have a long battery life. They can be equipped with modules that allow for monitoring of temperature, respiratory rate, noninvasive blood pressure, invasive blood pressure (arterial line), and oxygen saturation. A recording device is often available, allowing for continuous or intermittent recording (hard copy) of monitored data. Although frequently thought of as neonatal monitors, these monitors can be configured for use on pediatric patients and should be considered for use when transporting the critically ill pediatric patient with an arterial line in place.

Cardiac monitors with a defibrillator unit are commonly used for pediatric transports. These monitors are usually much heavier and larger in size than the monitors used for the neonatal patient. When choosing a monitor/defibrillator unit, it is important to think of the patient population for which the unit is intended. There are units available that are capable of cardioverting at the low wattage necessary for the infant or toddler. Programs that will be transporting all age groups should have such a unit available. Newer monitors are capable of external pacing, but these units tend to be quite bulky, heavy, and expensive.

Regardless of the type of monitor used, the digital display must be easily visible from a variety of angles and in various types of lighting. An audible alarm with limits that can be set to patient specific settings is desirable.

Non-invasive blood pressure monitors

As noted above, noninvasive blood pressure monitoring capability is available in combination with some cardiac monitors. In addition, separate noninvasive blood pressure monitors are available which work on battery power. These are often intended for use only on either the neonatal or pediatric patient and must be used with the correct size cuff for the individual patient. Since it may be difficult to obtain reliable manual blood pressures during transport, a noninvasive blood pressure monitor can be extremely useful when transporting the potentially hypotensive or hypertensive patient.

Pulse oximeter

Pulse oximeters for continuous oxygen saturation monitoring are available both as integral parts of cardiac monitors and as separate units. The separate units are small, lightweight, and durable and generally have a long battery life. In addition to the oxygen saturation, these monitors also display a digital heart rate, allowing for correlation between the cardiac monitor and oxygen saturation monitor.

Pulse oximeter probes may be either reusable or disposable. Reusable probes must be cleaned between each patient use. The reusable probe is efficient when continuous pulse oximetry monitoring is used as part of a transport protocol (as opposed to use only for respiratory distress), because there is generally no charge for the use of the probe. Disposable probes are commonly a patient charge item. If the transport and in-house monitors are compatible, the patient requiring oximetry after arrival at the tertiary care center can use the same probe.

The pulse oximeter only works as well as the quality of the signal that it receives. If the arterial pulsations cannot be accurately detected (as in the patient with decreased peripheral pulses from shock or during an especially bumpy ride), the arterial oxygen saturation readings will be unreliable and alternate methods of assessment must be used.

End-tidal CO_2 monitors

End-tidal CO_2 monitoring is a noninvasive method of evaluating CO_2 concentration in expired respiratory gases. For patients requiring mechanical ventilation, or patients with increased intracranial pressure this monitor can be an important adjunct for transport, especially during lengthy transports. Studies have shown that these monitors function well in the transport environment.[5]

Transcutaneous O_2 and CO_2 monitors

Combined transcutaneous O_2 and CO_2 monitors can be used in transport to monitor not only oxygenation but adequacy of ventilation. Monitors are available for use in all age groups and are small, lightweight, and have extended battery life. Such noninvasive monitors have been shown to be accurate in both ground and air transport.[6] Due to the difficulty in doing so during transport, special attention must be paid to calibrating the transcutaneous monitor and to applying the skin probe.

Doppler

The transport environment is often noisy, making the use of a standard stethoscope less than ideal. A Doppler amplifier may be used to assist in the manual evaluation of blood pressure during transport. The Doppler may also be used to facilitate the assessment of pulses, as manual assessment is difficult when the ride is bumpy. Dopplers come in a variety of small and lightweight sizes. They may also be wired with a volume control directly through the headsets used in flights. This can allow continuous or intermittent monitoring of pulse throughout a flight without necessitating removal of the headset.[4]

MECHANICAL VENTILATORS

Mechanical ventilators are extremely useful in maintaining accurate ventilatory parameters during transport. There are a variety of transport ventilators available, many of them small, lightweight, and durable. The choice of ventilator will depend on the patient population to be transported. Although patients can be ventilated manually using a bag and mask or bag and endotracheal tube a transport ventilator provides better uniformity of ventilation and also allows for the most effective use of all transport personnel.[7]

Transport ventilators are either battery powered or pneumatic. Pneumatic ventilators use a gas source (oxygen) for power. Use of this type of ventilator has the risk of depleting the oxygen supply in the transport vehicle. This must be carefully considered, especially for long distance transports. Many battery powered ventilators can run on either alternating current or battery power. Gas density decreases with increased altitude, a consideration in air medical transport as pneumatically powered ventilators will deliver a slower rate at higher altitudes.[7]

Transport ventilators should be equipped with an alarm system that alerts the team to disconnection, decrease in desired oxygen delivery, and excessively high airway pressure.[3] They must also allow for variable inspiratory/expiratory (I:E) ratios and be able to deliver positive end-expiratory pressure (PEEP) as well as a variety of rates.

Although a transport ventilator can provide consistent ventilation, in air transport the accuracy of the settings may be influenced by changes in altitude. The team must regularly assess and record the functioning of the ventilator and be prepared to make necessary changes throughout the transport.[7] In addition, the patient's oxygen requirements and tidal volume may change with altitude, and the team must be prepared to adjust the ventilator as needed.[2]

Regardless of the type or sophistication of transport ventilator, the transport team must be knowledgeable in its use and must be able to trouble-shoot when problems arise.

OXYGEN AND COMPRESSED AIR VIA BLENDER

All critically ill and injured patients will initially be placed on 100% oxygen. After initial assessment and stabilization, many patients may be weaned to a lower inspired oxygen concentration. This is of particular importance in neonatal transports. Teams transporting neonatal patients must have a blender system (for oxygen and compressed air) available. Older pediatric patients may be weaned using available mask devices, in which case oxygen alone will be adequate. For all transports, the gas source must be adequate for at least twice the anticipated duration of the transport. Portable as well as in-line gas must be available. All dedicated transport vehicles must have oxygen available as a minimum and many will also have the blender system.

INTRAVENOUS PUMPS

Maintaining patency of intravenous lines is a priority during transport. Many patients may be transported on medication drips where accuracy of rate is of utmost importance. Due to inadequate height, changes in gravity (with air transport), and small catheters in small veins (neonates and infants), intravenous fluids frequently do not infuse at the appropriate rate unless placed on a pump. Pumps used for transport are able to provide exact infusions regardless of the height of the intravenous bag, as gravity is not a factor. Intravenous controllers are not adequate, as they rely on gravity for the infusion.

Intravenous pumps need to offer a variety of rate selections. Medication infusions for a neonatal patient may need to be delivered at rates as low as 0.1 cc per hour. The older pediatric patient may need much faster flow rates.[2] The ideal pump is one that is versatile enough to provide both low and high flow rates, doing both with accuracy. Such pumps are available and can function on both battery and alternating current.

Because a critically ill patient may require multiple intravenous lines, pumps used for transport must be small and lightweight. Syringe pumps are especially useful in transport. In cold climates the syringe pump(s) can be placed in the isolette or under the covers, allowing the intravenous fluid to be warmed, thus helping to prevent hypothermia and cold stress.

SUCTION

Suction must be available throughout the transport. Most dedicated transport vehicles (ambulance, rotor craft and fixed wing aircraft) have a built in suction unit that operates off alternating current as well as battery power. An independent battery operated suction unit must also be available.[2] The appropriate sized suction catheters for each patient must be included in the transport equipment.

ISOLETTE

The word isolette generally brings to mind the neonatal or newly born patient. It should be remembered that the isolette can be used on infants less than 5 kg, regardless of age. Some brands of isolette can easily accommodate infants up to 6 kg. The isolette offers a warm environment for transport and allows constant visibility of the infant, without the necessity of bundling in blankets. Especially in cold climates, the isolette is a much safer mode of transport for small infants than a stretcher. If the isolette is to be used in air transport, FAA approval is suggested.[2]

The isolette must be able to work on alternating current as well as battery power and should be used on alternating current for as much of the transport as possible. In extremely cold temperatures there is a constant demand on the battery for a high output of heat and the battery time is greatly shortened.

All monitoring devices must be firmly secured to the isolette. Shelves and securing straps can be custom-fitted to meet the needs of each transport program. Some isolettes have shelves or drawers where equipment may be safely stored although it may not always be easily visible from such a storage shelf. It is for the safety of all involved in the transport that heavy items, such as a cardiac monitor or portable ventilator, are permanently affixed or securely tied to the isolette.

Isolettes used for critical care neonatal transports will usually be configured to include a cardiac/respiratory/temperature monitor, portable ventilator, oxygen analyzer, oxygen and compressed air tanks connected to a blender system and a pulse oximeter. Intravenous syringe pumps may be affixed to the exterior of the isolette, although this should be reconsidered when transporting in cold climates where it may be preferable to place the pumps inside of the isolette to permit warming of the fluids.

Between transports, isolettes should be kept plugged in to alternating current and charging and should be kept warm at all times. It can take as long as 30 to 40 minutes for an isolette to reach maximum temperature, especially when it is extremely cold. Keeping the isolette warmed at all times ensures that a warm environment will be readily available even when travel time is short.

During transport it is exceedingly important to minimize the exposure of the isolette to cold. Rapidly loading the isolette into the transport vehicle and avoiding long periods of standing outside in cold weather can minimize temperature fluctuations within the isolette. Covering the isolette with a blanket during the exposure to extreme cold can help in maintaining the internal temperature.

The isolette should have a restraint system to secure the infant during the actual transport. Regardless of the mode of transport, the ride can often be bumpy, causing increased stress to the infant and also potential for physical harm. Using a foam mattress inside the isolette can help cushion the ride and is especially useful for the very small premature infant.

MISCELLANEOUS PATIENT SPECIFIC EQUIPMENT

Blood pressure cuffs and manometer

Blood pressure cuffs must be available in a variety of sizes so that the appropriate size (two-thirds the length of the upper arm) can be selected for each patient being transported. A universal sphygmomanometer can be used with any size cuff.

Stethoscope

Stethoscopes are available in neonatal, infant, pediatric, and adult sizes. The appropriate size should be available and selected for each transport.

Ventilation bags

Anesthesia bags, if used, can be easily stored in a respiratory equipment bag. Self-inflating bags take up more room and may need to be selected for the individual patient, based on size. Both 450 cc or 500 cc and 1 L bags and appropriate reservoirs should be available.

Warming adjuncts

Depending on the size and condition of the patient and the climate, additional warming adjuncts may be necessary. Crushable heat packs intended for use with infants are practical for transport. They are activated by crushing the compartments within the pack and will stay warm for up to 2 hours. They can be used in an isolette or under it and bundled with a larger infant or toddler.

Mylar "space" blankets are available in a variety of sizes. These blankets help hold in the body heat and can be used along with conventional blankets to keep larger patients warm during transport. These mylar blankets are extremely lightweight, compact and can easily be carried on all transports.

MISCELLANEOUS EQUIPMENT

Camera

An instant type camera is an important piece of equipment for teams transporting neonatal patients. The new parents must be given photographs of their newly born child. When possible, these photographs should be taken prior to instituting multiple invasive procedures. It is important for the team to carry a camera in the event of transport from the rare nursery that does not have one or, more likely, for the case of the infant born precipitously in an emergency department. Unfortunately, it is possible that these may be the only pictures the parents have of their child alive.

Cellular phone

A portable cellular phone allows the transport team to contact either the referring hospital or the tertiary care center during the transport. Although many transport vehicles will have phones available, a phone belonging to the team helps ensure this contact. The usefulness of cellular phones depends largely on population density of the travel area, as very rural areas lack cellular towers. When cellular towers are not present in the local area, another means of communication (for example, through the driver's or pilot's radio) should always be available. Untested concerns exist on possible interference of the phones with aircraft navigation equipment. The pilot(s) should always be consulted before a call is placed.

Car seat

Unless the restraint system has been specially adapted, infants (too large for an isolette) and toddlers are often poorly restrained when the traditional transport vehicle stretcher is used. For this reason, when the infant or child's condition allows, a car seat should be used to safely restrain the child during transport. Although a standard infant or toddler car safety seat can be used, one made especially for use in ambulances will prove to be more versatile. This seat has a higher back with an adjustable neck support and can be used in a variety of positions. It can also be used on a large range of patient sizes and is made entirely of washable soft plastic so that it can be cleaned after each use.

ORGANIZATION OF TRANSPORT SUPPLIES

The supplies used for transport can be placed into three broad categories: respiratory, medication, and miscellaneous (everything that is not respiratory or medication). Using three separate bags for storing these supplies allows optimal organization and ease of locating particular items in an emergency.

Bags can be clearly marked as "respiratory" or "medication" so that assisting personnel can help in finding supplies in an emergency.

Each bag should have enclosed a list of all supply contents (see Appendix 46-1, pages 622-625). Each bag should also have an organizational system so that items are always placed in the same area of the bag, regardless of who is restocking after use. This ensures that each team member will be able to rapidly find each item without having to search extensively.

Supplies need to be restocked immediately after each transport so that the bags are always stored ready for use. Regular checking of the bags will ensure that all supplies are appropriately stocked and that out of date medications are replaced. Whether the bags are fully checked daily, weekly, or monthly will depend on the make-up of the team and its patient volume.

Periodic evaluation of the contents of each bag will allow the team to make changes in supplies as needed. As protocols change, some items may no longer be necessary and others may be added. Teams must always be open to changing their supplies based on the needs of the team and the patient population that is being transported as well as advances in medical practice.

There is a tendency to want to carry absolutely everything that is potentially necessary on every transport. This is not realistic as both space and weight are limited. Teams must think about what they really need in the transport vehicle to provide care. Teams that act as first responders and do scene calls will need a different quantity and type of supplies than those teams that only do interhospital transports as interhospital transport teams can use supplies at the referring hospital. There are many items that are in abundance at all hospitals in all departments, such as alcohol swabs, gauze pads, syringes, and needles. Although a few of each should be stocked in the transport bags, there is no need to carry large amounts, as they can be easily obtained. Whenever possible, necessary items should be used from the referring hospital stock, conserving team supplies for use in the transport vehicle. Items such as small endotracheal tubes, nasopharyngeal airways, and intravenous catheters or specialty gastric tubes may not be available in the referring hospital and will need to be adequately stocked by the transport team.

Teams that transport only neonatal patients can easily limit their equipment to that which is appropriate for neonates. Teams that transport pediatric patients will need to have varying sizes of equipment, as pediatric patients may range in size from a small infant to a very large teenager. Teams that transport all age groups may want to have three sets of bags: neonatal, pediatric, and adult. Additional "subspecialty" packs for trauma victims or ECMO candidates can provide extra equipment which is otherwise not necessary.

Although most pediatric transport teams will have similar equipment and supplies, each team will have their own unique needs based on patient population, mode of transport, transport personnel, terrain, and climate. In order to provide a high level of care during transport, the appropriate equipment and supplies must be readily available and in good working order.

REFERENCES

1. ASHBEAMS: *Air-medical crew national standard curriculum, advanced student manual,* ed 1, Pasadena, CA, 1988, 207-12.
2. *Guidelines for air and ground transport of neonatal and pediatric patients,* Elk Grove Village, IL, 1993, American Academy of Pediatrics.
3. Guidelines Committee of the American College of Critical Care Medicine, Society of Critical Care Medicine and American Association of Critical-Care Nurses Transfer Guidelines Task Force: Guidelines for the transfer of critically ill patients, *Crit Care Med* 21(6):931-7, 1993.
4. Mooney M: Aeromedical equipment selection: a logical planning process, *Emergency Medical Services,* 68-70, June 1987.
5. Peterson C and others: Comparative evaluation of three end-tidal CO_2 monitors used during air medical transport, *The Journal of Air Medical Transport,* 7-10, February 1992.
6. Reimer J and others: Portable transcutaneous O_2 and CO_2 monitors and pulse oximeters during transport of critically ill newborn infants, *The Journal of Air Medical Transport,* 9-13, August 1992.
7. Rouse, M: Mechanical ventilation during air medical transport: techniques and devices, *The Journal of Air Medical Transport,* 5-8, April 1992.
8. Schneider C and others: Evaluation of ground ambulance, rotor-wing, and fixed-wing aircraft services, *Crit Care Clin,* 8(3):546, 1992.

APPENDIX 46-1. SAMPLE LISTINGS OF CONTENTS

PEDIATRIC MISCELLANEOUS TRANSPORT BAG

IV and blood drawing supplies

4 T-connectors
Butterfly catheters 23 G × 2 and 25 G × 2
Angiocaths 2 16 G, 2 18 G, 4 20 G, 6 22 G, 8 24 G
Tourniquets
Needles—18 G, 20 G, 22 G (5 each)
Armboards—1 small, 1 large
4 Intraosseous needles
Syringes
  10 1 cc
  10 6 cc with needle
  10 12 cc
  1 20 cc
  3 60 cc
  2 blood gas syringes
  10 3 cc with needle
10 alcohol swabs
10 betadine swabs
2 benzoin swabs
3 2 × 2's
2 Occlusive dressings
1 razor
Bedside glucose kit (alcohol, small adherent bandages, 2 × 2's, lancets, reagent strips)
1 urine cup cut in half and taped ('house for IV')
1 medicine cup cut in half and taped ('house for IV')
1000 cc D5/.2 NS
1000 cc 0.9 NS
250 cc 5% Albumin
5 100 cc bags of D5W (for mixing medicated drips)
IV pump tubing appropriate for team pumps
2 4-way stopcocks
5 IV extension tubings
1 blood filter with adapter coupler
1 500 cc pressure bag
2 dispensing pins

MISCELLANEOUS SUPPLIES (SAME BAG AS IV SUPPLIES)

Adhesive remover
4 NS droppers (sodium chloride for inhalation)
1 penlight
1 pair scissors
Rescue blanket
Bulb syringe
1 5-in-1 connector
1 large 'Y' connector
Suction catheters
  4 5-6 FR
  3 8 FR
  1 10 FR
  1 14 FR
1 10 F Anderson gastric tube
4 Heimlich valves
3 10 FR chest tubes
2 12 FR chest tubes
10 FR oxygen catheters
Tape (silk and waterproof)
Urinary catheters (1 each)
  5 FR
  8 FR

10 FR
14 FR
Urimeter

PEDIATRIC RESPIRATORY TRANSPORT BAG

Airway adjuncts and oxygen delivery supplies

Oropharyngeal airways (sizes 00, 0, 1, 2, 3, 4, 5)
Nasopharyngeal airways
Non-rebreather masks (adult, pediatric)
Infant partial rebreather mask
Pediatric venturi mask
Aerosol masks (pediatric, infant)
Medication nebulizer and medications (Albuterol, Racemic Epinephrine)
Oxygen flowmeter
Nasal cannula—pediatric, adult
CFM—pediatric, adult
Oxygen and compressed air adaptors for transport vehicle(s)

Intubation supplies

Laryngoscope handle
Extra set of batteries for handle
Laryngoscope blades (straight 0, 1, 2, 3 and curved 2 & 3)
Magill forceps
Extra light bulbs for blades
2 stylets
1″ waterproof tape and skin prep or tincture of benzoin (to secure tube)
Endotracheal tubes (3 each)—2.5, 3.0, 3.5, 4.0, 4.5, 5.0, 5.5, 6.0 cuffed, 7.0 cuffed, 7.7 cuffed, 8.0 cuffed

Ventilation supplies

Resuscitation masks (1 each)—premature, newborn, infant, child, small adult, medium adult, large adult
Anesthesia bags (only if team is skilled in use) (1 each)—0.5 L, 1 L, 2 L
Manometer
Oxygen tubing—3 foot length and 12 foot length
Anca adapter
Appropriate size self-inflating bag with reservoir (450cc/500cc or IL)

Pediatric medication bag

The contents of this bag may vary depending on regional and hospital protocols and the types of patients to be transported. Resuscitation medications should be placed in proximity, and controlled substances must be kept in a locked container. (Antibiotics tend to be especially variable and are not included in this list. In general, 2 penicillins, an aminoglycoside, and 2 cephalosporins will cover most needs.)

Adenosine 6 mg	4 vials
Albumin 5% 50 cc	3 vials
Albumin 25% 50 cc	2 vials
Albuterol 20 cc	1 vial
Aminophylline 500 mg	3 vials
Atropine 1 mg	4 vials
Calcium Gluconate 10%	2 vials
Dexamethasone 4 mg	1 vial
Dextrose 50% (500 mg/cc)	2 vials
Diazepam 10 mg	2 vials
Digoxin 0.5 mg	2 ampules
Diphenhydramine 50 mg	2 vials
Dobutamine 250 mg	2 vials
Dopamine 200 mg	2 vials
Epinephrine 1:1000 30 cc vial	1 vial
Epinephrine 1:10,000	4 vials
Fentanyl 100 mg	2 ampules
Furosemide 20 mg	2 vials
Heparin 1000 U 1 cc vial	1 vial
Hydralazine 20 mg	2 vials
Hydrocortisone 1 gm	1 mix a vial
Isoproterenol 1 mg	2 vials
Lidocaine 1%	2 vials
Lidocaine 20% 10 cc syringe	1 syringe
Mannitol 25% (12.5 GM)	6 vials
Midazolam 10 mg	2 vials
Morphine 10 mg	1 vial
NaCl injectable 10 cc	10 vials
Naloxone 0.4 mg	6 vials
Phenobarbital 65 mg	20 vials
Phentolamine (Regitine) 5 mg	2 vials
Phenytoin 100 mg	8 vials
Procainamide 100 mg	1 vial
Sodium bicarbonate 10 mEq	4 vials
Sterile water 10 cc	6 vials
Vecuronium 10 mg vial	1 vial

Refrigerated drugs

Insulin regular or Humulin	1 vial
Lorazepam 4 mg	4 vials
Pancuronium Bromide 1 mg/cc	10 cc vial
Succinylcholine 20 mg/cc	1 vial

NEONATAL MISCELLANEOUS TRANSPORT BAG

IV and blood drawing supplies

2 blood gas syringes
Syringes
- 3 3 cc
- 3 6 cc
- 3 12 cc
- 3 20 cc
- 10 TB with needle
- 10 3 cc with needle

Butterfly catheters, 23 G × 3, 25 G × 3
Angiocaths—8 24 G, 6 22 G, 2 20 G
Needles—18 G, 20 G (5 each)
10 alcohol swabs
10 betadine swabs
2 benzoin swabs
neonatal armboard
1 medicine cup cut in half and taped ('house for IV')
1 razor
5 2 × 2's
1 tourniquet
4 rubber bands
500 cc D10W
500 cc D5W
500 cc 0.9 NS
5% Albumin (5 50 cc bottles)
IV pump tubing appropriate for team pumps
5 100 cc—empty IV bags (viaflex) for mixing drips
2 4-way stopcocks
5 IV extension tubings
4 T-connectors with injection port
1 blood filter with adaptor coupler
Bedside glucose kit (alcohol swabs, small adherent bandages, 2 × 2's, lancets, reagent strips)
Blood tubes—variety of each
Armboards—infant sized

Miscellaneous supplies (same bag as IV supplies)

Adhesive remover
Doppler
Tapemeasure
Cord clamp
Lubricant
Penlight
4 NS droppers (sodium chloride for inhalation)
Rescue blanket
1 5-in-1 connector
1 large 'Y' connector
Suction catheters
- 5 5-6 FR
- 5 8 FR
- 1 10 FR

Gastric tubes
- 1 Anderson 10 FR
- 1 8 FR
- 3 5 FR

4 Heimlich valves
4 10 FR chest tubes
1 8 FR oxygen catheter
Tape (silk and waterproof)
Rolled gauze bandages
1 Petroleum jelly gauze
1 Telfa gauze
Sterile procedure tray (for UA line insertion or chest tube insertion)
- Scalpel and blades
- Small hemostats (6)
- Iris forceps
- Catheter introducer
- 4.0 silk suture with needle × 2
- Umbilical tape
- 4 × 4's
- Betadine solution
- Scissors

Umbilical catheters—3.5 and 5.0—2 each

NEONATAL RESPIRATORY TRANSPORT BAG

Airway adjuncts and oxygen delivery supplies

Bulb Syringe
Oropharyngeal airways (sizes 00 and 0)
Partial rebreather mask (infant size)
Infant simple face mask
Infant head hood (that will fit in isolette) with baffle and white nipple adapter
Neonatal nasal cannula
Oxygen flowmeter
Oxygen and compressed air adaptors for transport vehicle(s)

Intubation supplies

Laryngoscope handle
Extra set of batteries for handle
Laryngoscope blades (straight 0 & 1)
Extra light bulbs for blades
1 Magill forceps
2 small stylets

Endotracheal tubes (4 each) 2.0, 2.5, 3.0, 3.5, 4.0
1″ waterproof tape and skin prep or tincture of benzoin (to secure tube)

Ventilation supplies

Resuscitation masks (1 each)—premature, newborn, infant
Anesthesia bags—2 500 cc bags (should be used only by personnel experienced in their use)
1 450 or 500 cc self-inflating bag with reservoir
Anca adapter
Manometer
Oxygen tubing—3 foot length and 12 foot length
Oxygen flowmeter

NEONATAL MEDICATION BAG

The contents of this bag may vary depending on hospital protocols. (Antibiotics tend to be especially variable and are not included in this list.)

Adenosine 6 mg	1 vial
Aminophylline 500 mg	1 vial
Ampicillin 2 GM	1 vial
Ampicillin 500 mg	1 vial
Atropine 1 mg	1 vial
Ceftriaxone 500 mg	1 vial
Dextrose 25%	1 10 cc vial
Dilantin 100 mg	1 vial
Dobutamine 250 mg	1 vial
Dopamine 20 mg	1 vial
Epinephrine 1 : 10,000 10 cc	1 vial
Epinephrine 1 : 1000 30 cc vial	1 vial
Fentanyl 250 mcg/5 cc	1 ampule
Gentamicin 20 mg	1 vial
Heparin 1000 u	1 vial
Midazolam 10 mg/2 cc	2 vials
Narceine 1 mg/cc	4 1 cc ampules
NaCl injectable 10 cc	8 vials
Phenobarbital 65 mg	4 vials
Phentolamine 5 mg/vial	1 vial
Prostaglandin E, 500 mg/cc	2 ampules
Sodium bicarbonate 5 mEq	4 ampules (0.5 mEq/cc)
Sterile water injectable 10 cc	4 vials
Tolazoline 100 mg/4 cc	2 ampules
Vecuronium 10 mg/vial	1 vial

47

INVASIVE PROCEDURES

JEFFREY S. RUBENSTEIN

The safe and efficient transport of critically ill infants and children often requires the completion of one or more invasive procedures. Stabilization of these critically ill children can demand any combination of advanced airway management (see Chapter 18), placement of central venous or intraosseous catheters for vascular access, arterial catheters for intravascular monitoring, thoracentesis or pericardiocentesis, or placement of thoracostomy and pericardial catheters. The health care personnel responsible for the transport of these children must be proficient with these techniques and their indications.

The indications for procedures performed immediately before or during transport differ from those in the pediatric intensive care unit (PICU). The decision to perform a procedure before or during transport should be based primarily on its ability to promote a safe and uneventful transport rather than on its need to provide the patient with definitive critical care.

Management of the airway, achievement of stable vascular access appropriate to the length of the transport and the condition of the child, and evacuation of significant air or fluid collections in the thorax are absolutely necessary for safe transport of any child. Placement of arterial catheters for blood pressure monitoring, while ideal for the hemodynamically unstable patient, is probably only indicated for longer duration transports and will not be discussed in detail. Finally, adjunctive diagnostic procedures, such as lumbar puncture or paracentesis are rarely necessary, will only delay transport, and may result in additional risk to the patient. These latter two procedures should almost always be deferred until transport is completed. A suggested classification of procedures for transport is outlined in Box 47-1.

VASCULAR ACCESS FOR TRANSPORT

The initial resuscitation and stabilization of the unstable infant or child who requires transport should be identical to that required for any critically ill patient. *After* appropriate steps have been taken to ensure the patency of the airway, and the ability to provide the patient adequate oxygenation and ventilation is ensured, vascular access must be obtained. A protocolized approach to this has been suggested by Kanter,[3] and adopted with modifications by the American Heart Association/American Academy of Pediatrics for their Pediatric Advanced Life Support (PALS) course.[2] The PALS recommendations for achieving vascular access in hemodynamically unstable infants and children are that there are to be no more than 3 to 5 minutes of attempts at peripheral intravenous cannulation, followed by an immediate change to intraosseous needle placement and infusion in children less than 6 years of age or central venous cannulation/saphenous venous cutdown in older children. Though technically more difficult, intraosseous infusion is possi-

BOX 47-1 CLASSIFICATION OF NEED FOR PROCEDURES DURING TRANSPORT

Absolutely necessary
- Venous access
- Thoracostomy for pneumothorax
- Pericardiocentesis for tamponade

Ideal
- Arterial access
- Thoracostomy for pleural effusion

Not necessary
- Lumbar puncture
- Paracentesis

ble in the older child as well. In older children, the choice between attempting central venous cannulation or saphenous cutdown should be based on the expertise of the transport personnel. The femoral vein is most commonly chosen, though the external and internal jugular and subclavian veins may also be used.

The ability to maintain the patency and integrity of venous catheters once they are placed is crucial during transport; this becomes increasingly important as the projected length of the transport increases. Central venous catheters, especially when sutured in place, are more stable than peripheral IVs and intraosseous needles, which can be dislodged when bumped. All peripheral and central IVs placed before the arrival of the transport team at the referring facility must be evaluated for patency and placement, usually by direct inspection of the site after a rapid infusion of 3 to 10 cc of fluid and/or a check for blood return.

Peripheral venous access

The technique of catheterizing peripheral veins is well known and, when possible, is the safest and easiest means of achieving intravenous access.[2] Commonly used sites are the antecubital veins (cephalic and basilic), saphenous veins, and veins located on the feet, forearm, dorsal aspect of the hands, and in children under a year of age, the scalp. In children undergoing transport, the use of indwelling plastic or Teflon catheters is preferable because of the increased stability of the placement. It is possible (but not desirable) to place metal "butterfly" needles to achieve venous access in difficult situations, although these catheters are less stable and more prone to infiltration.

Saphenous vein cutdown

The technique of saphenous vein cutdown has been well described[2] and is a reliable means of achieving peripheral venous access in experienced hands. However, with the increasing acceptance of intraosseous line placement and increasing familiarity with achieving percutaneous central access in critically ill children, saphenous cutdown is much less frequently used. The saphenous vein traverses the medial surface of the ankle approximately 0.5 cm to 1 cm anterior and superior to the medial malleolus (Figure 47-1). A tourniquet is applied to the lower leg, and the skin is prepped. Using sterile technique (and local anesthesia, if indicated) an incision is made in the location of the vein. The vein is identified using a hemostat, dissected out, and cannulated usually with a 20 or 22 gauge catheter. The skin is sutured at the conclusion of the procedure. Because of the location of the vein (distally and distinct from vital structures), there are few complications associated with saphenous cutdown except infection. In less experienced hands, the procedure is more time consuming than other means of achieving access; this has led to its decreasing role in resuscitation and transport.

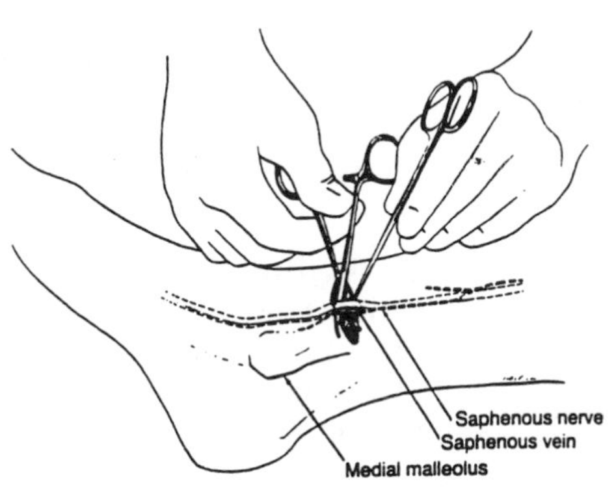

Fig. 47-1. Technique of saphenous vein cutdown. (From McIntosh BB, Dulchavsky SA: Peripheral vascular cutdown, *Crit Care Clin*, October 1992.

Intraosseous access

Placement of intraosseous needles has become a popular alternative means of vascular access in children within the last decade, although it was first described more than 50 years ago. It is particularly useful in infants and small children with hemodynamic instability or circulatory collapse in whom placement of a peripheral IV is nearly impossible. Intraosseous catheters are placed most commonly in the proximal tibia, although they can be placed in other marrow-containing bones, such as the distal femur, distal tibia, anterior and posterior iliac spines, and sternum. Although commercially available intraosseous needles are available, it is possible to use any 16 or 18 gauge needle (e.g., spinal, bone marrow) in an emergency. Needles with stylets are preferable in this situation because placement of needles without stylets may force a core of bone and marrow into the needle resulting in obstruction to fluid flow.

The technique for intraosseous placement in the proximal tibia has been well described.[4] The anterior surface of the proximal tibia is prepped in a sterile fashion after the equipment is collected (Box 47-2). The tibial tuberosity is identified and the intraosseous needle is inserted into the tibia about 2 centimeters distally (Figure 47-2). The needle is advanced with a screwing motion either perpendicularly or slightly inferiorly in order to avoid hitting the growth plate. Placement occurs when a sudden loss of resistance is felt. Confirmation of placement is assured when the needle remains upright without support, and the infusion of 5 to 10 cc of fluid does not result in noticeable soft tissue swelling. Some authors have advocated aspirating the needle to obtain marrow after placement to ensure proper location. This recommendation is controversial because of the possibility of clogging the needle, which would make it nonfunctional.

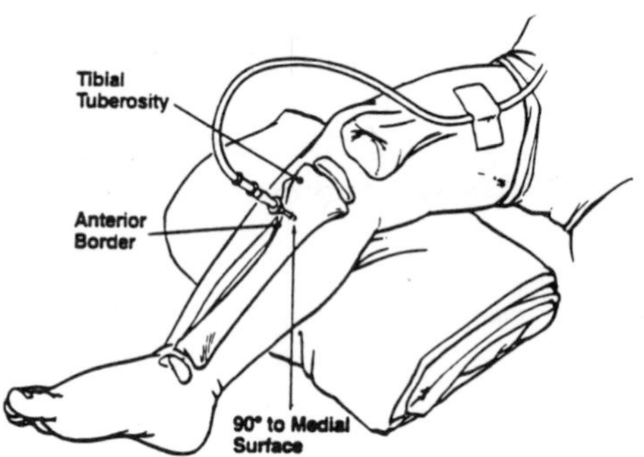

Fig. 47-2. Technique of anterior tibia intraosseous needle placement. (From McIntosh BB, Dulchavsky SA: Peripheral vascular cutdown, *Crit Care Clin,* October 1992.)

BOX 47-2 EQUIPMENT FOR INTRAOSSEOUS NEEDLE PLACEMENT

- Sterile gloves
- Antiseptic solution
- Intraosseous needle OR 16 or 18 gauge spinal needle with stylet OR bone marrow needle
- 5 or 10 cc syringe

Central venous access

Catheters placed into central veins and sutured into position are the most stable vascular access for transport. The advantages of this route for consistent access is immediately evident, especially when potent vasoconstrictor agents (e.g., dopamine, epinephrine, norepinephrine) are infused. The risk of infiltration of these substances alone may be an indication for central access.

Although central catheters are commonly placed in the femoral vein in children, the external and internal jugular and the subclavian veins can also be used. A long catheter can also be threaded up the cephalic vein into the superior vena cava, though this is rarely done in the acutely ill child requiring stabilization. All central catheters used on transport should be sutured in place.

Excepting the rare circumstance where a catheter is threaded centrally from the cephalic or other peripheral vein, central veins in infants and children are almost always catheterized using modifications of the Seldinger technique.[1] A brief summary of this technique follows. This procedure involves locating the vessel with a thin walled needle (attached to a syringe that is aspirated as attempts are made to puncture the vessel). Once the vessel is properly entered (*easy* free-flow of blood into the syringe), the syringe is then disconnected, and a flexible guidewire that is at least 1.5 times the length of the catheter (with either a "J" shaped tip or a soft end) is advanced through the needle. The needle is then removed, leaving the wire in place in the vessel, and the catheter is advanced over the wire. The guidewire is then removed, and the catheter is aspirated to ensure blood return. The procedure can be modified to include the use of a dilating catheter(s) that is advanced over the guidewire and removed (again, leaving the guidewire in place). A portion of the guidewire must always remain visible outside the patient throughout the procedure. The final position of the catheter is usually checked radiographically, though there may be instances where the expenditure of time that this check would entail is not justified. Complications of this procedure include the induction of atrial and/or ventricular arrhythmias by the catheter or guidewire, laceration of a central vessel or the heart by the guidewire or catheter, hematoma formation, inadvertent arterial puncture, and loss of the guidewire. The equipment necessary for central venous catheterization using the Seldinger technique in children is listed in Box 47-3.

BOX 47-3 EQUIPMENT FOR CENTRAL VENOUS CATHETERIZATION

Sterile gloves
Antiseptic solution
Sterile drapes
Local anesthetic/syringe/needle
3 or 5 cc syringe (preferably without Luer tip)
Infusion fluids
"Seldinger kit" consisting of:
- Hollow needle
- Catheter (single or multilumen; 3 to 7 French diameter; sufficient length)
- Guidewire (fits through needle and catheter; at least 1.5 times length of catheter)

Suture
Sterile dressing materials

Femoral vein catheterization. The femoral vein is often preferred because of easy access. During resuscitative efforts attempts can be made to catheterize it simultaneously with management of the airway. It is located in the femoral triangle, just medial to the femoral artery. To puncture the femoral vein, the patient is positioned as in Figure 47-3 with the hip externally rotated and abducted and the knee slightly flexed. After suitable skin preparation and using sterile technique, the femoral artery is palpated and the skin punctured 2 to 3 cm below the inguinal ligament just medial to the femoral arterial pulsation. The needle is advanced at a 30° to 45° angle until a free flow of blood is obtained. The catheter is then placed using the modified Seldinger technique. Should the femoral artery be accidentally punctured, a rapid assessment should be made of the advisability of catheterizing it to provide monitoring capability. If the needle is removed, pressure should be held for at least 5 minutes to prevent hematoma formation. Complications unique to catheterization of this vessel are femoral artery puncture, hematoma formation, infection, and thrombosis of the femoral vein or inferior vena cava.

Internal jugular vein catheterization. The internal jugular veins can also be catheterized. In general, the right side is preferred

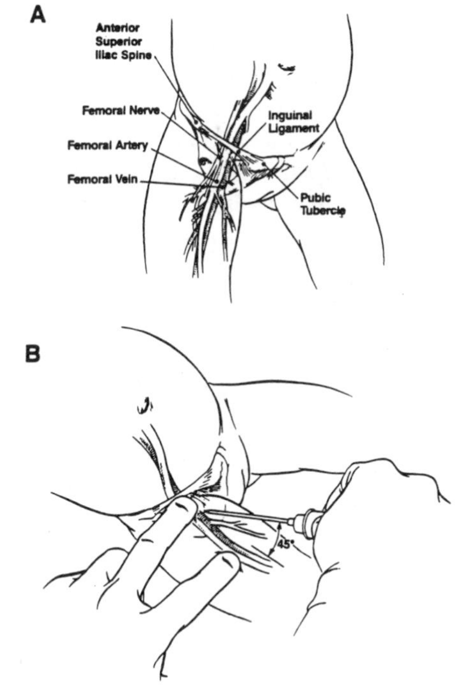

Fig. 47-3. A and B, Technique of femoral vein catheterization. (From Chameides L, editor: *Textbook of pediatric advanced life support*, Dallas, 1988, American Heart Association.)

because the right internal jugular vein has a straight course to the right atrium, the apex of the lung is lower on the right side (reducing the risk of a pneumothorax), and the thoracic duct is located on the left side in most patients. There are three approaches to catheterizing the internal jugular vein: central, anterior, and posterior. The central approach will be described; the other approaches are similarly described elsewhere.[2] The patient is prepped and placed in 20° to 30° Trendelenburg position with the neck extended and the head turned away from the site of puncture. The child is positioned in an identical position to that used for internal jugular catheterization (Figure 47-4). The needle is inserted at the apex of the triangle formed by the sternal and clavicular heads of the sternocleidomastoid muscle and the clavicle and directed at a 30° angle towards the ipsilateral nipple. During this phase, the free hand can be used to locate and retract the carotid artery, minimizing the risk of carotid puncture. Following puncture of the vein, the Seldinger technique is used to place the indwelling catheter. Immediate complications of internal jugular placement include carotid arterial puncture, hematoma formation, pneumothorax, and laceration of the thoracic duct.

Subclavian vein catheterization. Although the subclavian vein is more commonly used in adults than in infants and children, its catheterization is a safe and effective means of achieving stable vascular access.[5] The child is placed with the head turned to the side opposite the puncture, either flat or more optimally in a 20° to 30° Trendelenburg position. A roll is placed under the child along the vertebral column. After the site is prepped, the skin is punctured at the inferior edge of the clavicle, at a distance of one-third its length measured from the medial edge (Figure 47-5). The needle is aimed toward the suprasternal notch and should pass beneath the clavicle at its junction with the first rib. When freely flowing blood is obtained, the catheter is placed using sterile Seldinger technique, taking particular care to prevent aspiration of air into the vein by a forceful inspiratory effort. Immediate complications of placement usually occur because of the proximity of the subclavian vein to other vital structures. Potential complications include pneumothorax, subclavian artery puncture, and laceration of the thoracic duct (usually left-sided). Subclavian vein catheterization should not be attempted in a patient with a coagulopathy.

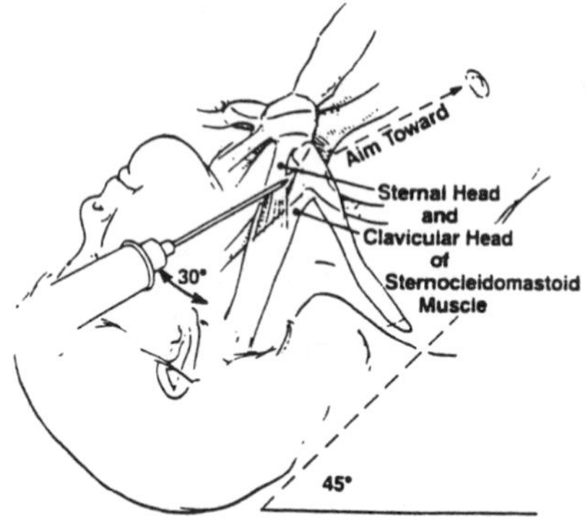

Fig. 47-4. Central technique of internal jugular vein catheterization. (From Chameides L, editor: *Textbook of pediatric advanced life support,* Dallas, 1988, American Heart Association.)

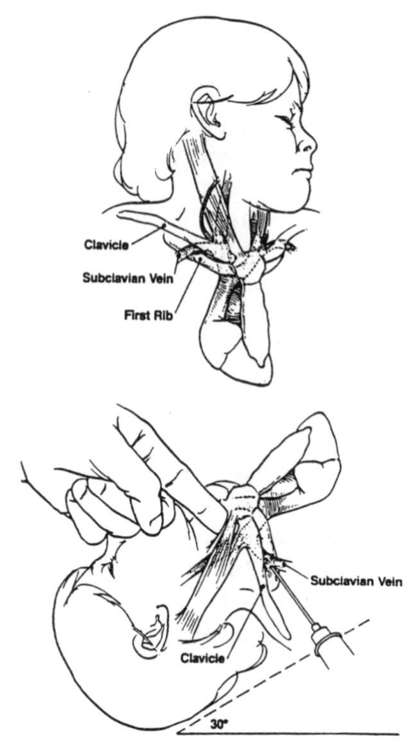

Fig. 47-5. Technique of subclavian vein catheterization. (From Chameides L, editor: *Textbook of pediatric advanced life support,* Dallas, 1988, American Heart Association.)

External jugular vein catheterization. Placement of a catheter in the external jugular vein is another means of achieving stable vascular access. Although the superficial location of this vein would seem to make it an ideal candidate for cannulation, it is often collapsed during times of hemodynamic compromise and it may be difficult to access in patients who have unstable airways or who are undergoing cardiopulmonary resuscitation. The skin is prepped, and the vein is punctured using sterile technique. The vein may be cannulated using either a standard IV catheter (catheter-over-needle) or by using Seldinger technique to place a central catheter. Because of the superficial location of this vessel, the major complication of attempts to cannulate it is hematoma formation at the site of puncture.

Umbilical vein catheterization. In newborns and neonates the umbilical vein can also be used to gain access to the central circulation. It must be stressed, though, that the likelihood of successful cannulation of the umbilical vein decreases as the neonate ages. The umbilical vein is the single, thin-walled vessel found in the umbilical stump. Equipment is collected (see Box 47-4) and the infant is placed supine with the legs and arms gently restrained. After the cord and surrounding area is prepped and draped, the cord is sectioned and the vein is identified. The catheter

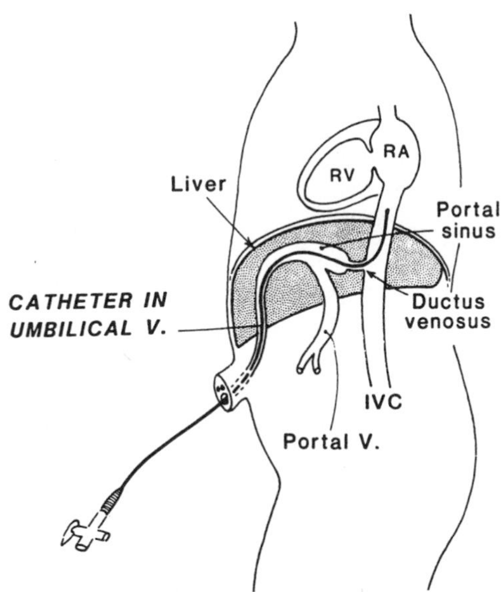

Fig. 47-6. Technique of umbilical vein catheterization. (From Ryan and others: *Practice of anesthesia for infants and children*, Philadelphia, 1986, WB Saunders.)

is placed into the vein (Figure 47-6) and advanced to one of two locations: either to the level of the right atrium (central), or just far enough that there is good blood return (peripheral). It is important that the catheter be placed in either one of these locations; intermediate placement can lead to hepatic damage from infusions being delivered directly into the liver. Complications of umbilical venous catheterization include infection, thrombosis, and the development of cirrhosis should the catheter be misplaced.

BOX 47-4 EQUIPMENT FOR UMBILICAL VEIN CATHETERIZATION

Sterile gloves
Antiseptic solution
Sterile drapes
3, 5, or 10 cc syringe
Infusion solution
Scalpel/blade
Fine, smooth tipped, curved forceps
Mosquito hemostats
Umbilical catheters (3.5 mm and 5 mm diameter; varying lengths)
Suture
Tape

THORACOSTOMY

Changes in barometric pressure that accompany changes in altitude make it necessary to remove intrathoracic air collections before initiation of air transport because these collections will expand as barometric pressure decreases during flight (see Chapter 16). Expansion of a pneumothorax or pneumopericardium can cause respiratory and/or hemodynamic compromise. Following drainage of intrapleural or intrapericardial air, a tube should be left in place for at least the duration of the transport to guard against the risk of reaccumulation. While an intrathoracic fluid collection does not carry the same risk of rapid expansion as does a pneumothorax, it should similarly be drained if it is believed to present any risk of cardiorespiratory decompensation.

Thoracostomy tubes are most commonly placed above the second rib in the midclavicular line or in the fifth, sixth, or seventh intercostal space in the mid-to-anterior axillary line (Figure 47-7). After the appropriate equipment is prepared (see Box 47-5), the skin overlying the incision area is prepped, and the area is infiltrated with a local anesthetic. A skin incision large enough to accommodate the chest tube is made. The tip of a closed, curved hemostat is then passed over the superior surface of the rib to avoid laceration of an intercostal blood vessel and through the intercostal muscles. The pleura is then punctured, and the hemostat is spread to enlarge the tract. The hemostat is withdrawn, and a finger is inserted through the tract to ensure that the lung is not adherent to the chest wall. The tube is then inserted; the hemostat may be used as a guide for the tube by grasping the tip of the tube and repassing the hemostat. The tube must be advanced until all of the side holes in the tube are intrapleural. All chest tubes should be sutured in place and taped with an occlusive dressing. The tube should be connected to a water seal and 10 to 20 cc of water of negative pressure constantly applied whenever possible. Alternatively, the tube can be connected to a flutter-valve device that does not allow air to enter the tube from outside the patient during inspiration. The tube must never be clamped, especially when patients are receiving positive pressure ventilation since the pneumothorax may reaccumulate rapidly. A chest x-ray should be taken to assess tube position and resolution of the process if the facility has the capability.

Alternatively, commercially available kits that use Seldinger-like techniques of placement may be used. After preparation of the skin with antimicrobial solutions and local anesthesia, a needle is attached to a syringe and is aspirated as the needle is introduced into the usual locations described above. When air or pleural fluid is aspirated, the syringe is disconnected and a curved tip guidewire is introduced through the needle into the pleural space. The needle is removed, leaving the guidewire in position. Care must be taken to cover the hub of the needle during this portion of the procedure so as not to permit the entry of air into the pleural space. A small skin incision is made at the site of the wire, and a dilator is introduced into the pleural space and removed. The chest tube is passed over the wire and the wire is withdrawn. The tube

BOX 47-5 EQUIPMENT FOR THORACOSTOMY

- Sterile gloves
- Sterile drapes
- Local anesthetic/syringe/needle
- Scalpel/blade
- Large curved hemostat or Kelly clamp
- Thoracostomy tubes (8 French to 20 French—dependent on size of child)
- Suture
- Occlusive dressing materials
- Pleural drainage system

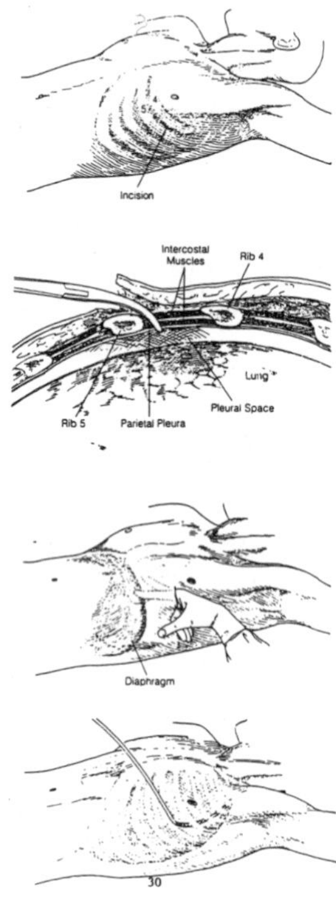

Fig. 47-7. Technique of lateral thoracostomy placement. (From *Care of the surgical patient,* Sci Amer Med 1989, section I.)

is then sutured in place and handled as described above.

Finally, in emergent situations (most commonly a tension pneumothorax), a large bore IV catheter (usually an 18 or 20 gauge) can be placed directly into the pleural space with immediate clinical improvement. Similar landmarks to those used for thoracostomy placement are used and a large syringe attached to catheter and aspirated as the needle is introduced. A rush of air or pleural fluid indicates pleural puncture, after which the catheter is slowly advanced over the needle a short distance. The catheter can then be connected to a water seal device, or in patients who are receiving continuous positive pressure breathing, the catheter can even be left open to atmosphere.

Complications of thoracostomy placement include hemothorax (from laceration of an intercostal blood vessel), pneumothorax, inadvertent puncture of the abdominal organs, infection of the pleural space, and reexpansion pulmonary edema.

THORACENTESIS

Therapeutic thoracentesis can also be performed before transport, although placement of a thoracostomy tube will usually offer a greater stability over the duration of the transport. While thoracostomy tube placement is the overwhelmingly preferable treatment of pneumothorax prior to air transport, some pleural effusions can be treated with thoracentesis alone before air transport, although in this case a chest x-ray following the procedure must show no evidence of pneumothorax. Purely diagnostic thoracentesis should be deferred until after the transport is completed. Thoracentesis can be performed in the fifth, sixth, or seventh intercostal space in the mid-to-anterior axillary line or posteriorly at the level of the inferior border of the scapula. After preparation of the skin and infiltration with local anesthetic, an 18 or 20 gauge angiocath is attached to a syringe and is inserted through the skin. The syringe is aspirated and the needle advanced until the pleura is punctured (pleural fluid or air is obtained). The fluid or air is aspirated, and the catheter and needle are removed. The complications associated with thoracentesis are similar to those associated with thoracostomy placement.

PERICARDIOCENTESIS

Pericardiocentesis (with or without placement of an indwelling pericardial drain) is indicated whenever a pericardial effusion or pneumopericardium is causing or may imminently cause hemodynamic compromise (tamponade). The echocardiogram remains the single most important diagnostic test for the diagnosis of pericardial fluid and/or tamponade, but is often not available at the time of transport. The physical signs and symptoms associated with tamponade are tachycardia, narrow pulse pressure with a large pulsus paradoxus, hypotension, muffled heart tones, and elevated central venous pressure (or associated signs such as jugular venous distention and hepatomegaly). Chest x-ray demonstrates an enlarged cardiac silhouette.

Pericardiocentesis is best performed under echocardiographic or fluoroscopic guidance. When this is not available, electrocardiographic (ECG) guidance should be used. In the absence of ECG support the following procedure can similarly be followed. A subxiphoid approach minimizes the chances of cardiac or coronary puncture. Equipment is collected (see Box 47-6), and the patient lies supine. The skin overlying and inferior to the

BOX 47-6 EQUIPMENT FOR PERICARDIOCENTESIS WITH CATHETER PLACEMENT

Sterile gloves
Antiseptic solution
Sterile drapes
Local anesthetic/syringe/needle
Entry needle
ECG machine with precordial lead attached to hub of entry needle
10 cc syringes
Pericardial catheter (typically soft material in "pigtail" shape)
Flexible J-tipped guidewire (fits through entry needle and pericardial catheter)
Suture material
Sterile dressing materials

xiphoid is prepped and anesthetized. A 14 to 20 gauge IV or spinal catheter is attached to the precordial ECG lead at the hub and to a syringe. As the syringe is aspirated the needle is placed just inferior to the xiphoid and advanced slowly at a 30 degree angle towards the left shoulder (Figures 47-8 and 47-9). Aspiration of fluid (or air in the case of a pneumopericardium) indicates pericardial puncture. A change in the ECG (altered QRS complex, or PR or ST segments) indicates contact with the heart; withdrawal of frank blood indicates cardiac puncture. In both cases, the needle should be withdrawn. Following pericardial puncture a tube may be placed using Seldinger-like techniques. A soft-tipped J-wire can be introduced through the needle, the needle removed, and a multiholed "pigtail" catheter left in place. The patency of pericardial tubes must be assured frequently throughout the transport by periodic aspiration.

Complications associated with pericardiocentesis (with or without catheter placement) include myocardial puncture, coronary artery laceration, cardiac arrhythmias, pneumothorax, and infection of the pericardial space.

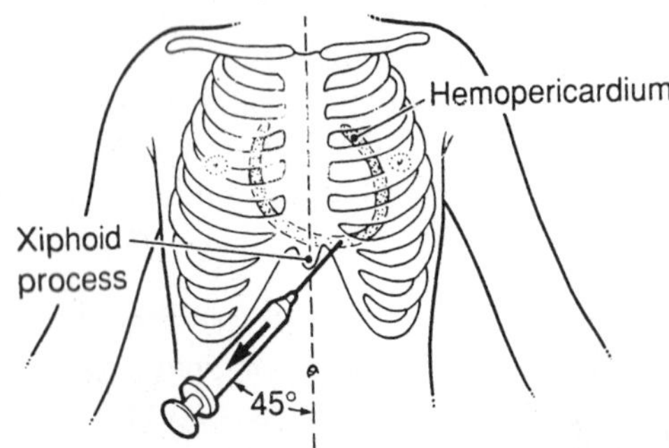

Fig. 47-8. Technique of pericardiocentesis. (From Kirkland L, Taylor RW: Pericardiocentesis, *Crit Care Clin*, October 1992.

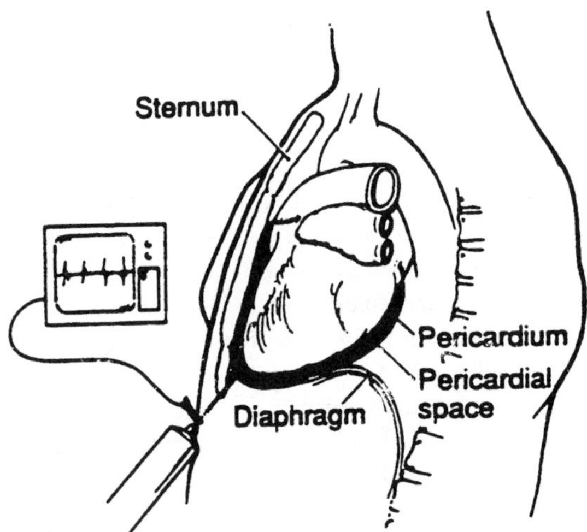

Fig. 47-9. Technique of pericardiocentesis. Schematic depicts the equipment and anatomic landmarks utilized in the subxyphoid approach to pericardiocentesis. (From Rasch D, Webster D: *Clinical manual of pediatric anesthesia*, New York, 1993, McGraw Hill.)

REFERENCES

1. Agee KR, Balk RA: Central venous catheterization in the critically ill patient, *Crit Care Clinics* 8:677-86, 1992.
2. Chameides L, editor: *Textbook of pediatric advanced life support*, Dallas, 1988, American Heart Association.
3. Kanter RK and others: Pediatric emergency intravenous access: evaluation of a protocol, *Am J Dis Child* 140:132, 1986.
4. Spivey WH: Intraosseous infusions, *J Pediatr* 111: 639-43, 1987.
5. Venkataraman ST, Orr RA, Thompson AE: Percutaneous infraclavicular subclavian catheterization in critically ill infants and children—A prospective study. *J Pediatr* 113:480-85, 1988.

48

THE TRANSPORT DATA BASE

ROBERT S. ROTH

With the arrival and spread of the microcomputer revolution, the rapid collection and analysis of data is within the reach of almost anyone with a personal computer. Those who have access to reliable data are positioned to make rapid decisions based on sound precepts and are able to have the competitive edge.

The nature of transport medicine has altered dramatically in the last decade. Directors of transport programs no longer have the luxury of worrying only about the medical aspects of transport and ignoring the business aspects. With the ratcheting down of payment to institutions, transport programs are vulnerable to limited budgets. Data is needed to support positions taken when trying to maintain a high quality transport program in a cost-effective manner.

Personnel involved in transport programs are under pressure to have available answers to questions posed by administrators of hospitals, directors of transport programs, pediatric and neonatal intensive care units, quality assurance committees, and regulators. Operating transport programs efficiently requires good transport data.

The goal is to develop a useful and meaningful transport database and to avoid the efforts that are often made which result in systems that do not meet the needs of the users. To do this it is necessary to examine and understand the types of questions that are likely to be asked, the reasons that data systems fail, the approach to system development, and the construction of the database. With an understanding of these factors, the chance of having a successful and useful transport data system will be greatly enhanced.

TYPES OF QUESTIONS

The types of questions that will be asked of a transport data base fall into several categories, demographic, financial and administrative, quality of care, and marketing.

Demographic

Most transport programs are very interested in understanding the demographic characteristics of the population that they serve, i.e., where do their patients come from? Defining the adolescent, pediatric, and neonatal mix of patients, the distances traveled, the ratio between scene work and interfacility transport, and the types of diseases and conditions treated, will all help to determine the structure of the transport program. A good understanding of these factors will help to decide what kinds of vehicles are necessary, the composition of the transport team, and the varieties of equipment needed.

Financial and administrative

How many hours are the nurses out on transport versus the total nursing hours on-call? It is very important to have good, well-presented data when making a case for additional needs to institutional administrators. A hard data understanding of personnel time requirements can be helpful for both figuring out ways to reduce cost and for obtaining the extra help needed for the program. When attempts are made to trim the budget of what appears to be a money losing transport program, good data such as ancillary charge generation, patient length of stays, and numbers of admissions that result from the availability of the transport program can be used to demonstrate the value of the program.

Quality of care

Are particular individuals having difficulty doing intubations on transport? It is imperative that transport programs maintain good quality management programs. There are many important quality issues that can be examined with the use of a transport database. Among these are team composition, carrier problems, equipment failures, monitoring of team skills and experience, response times, issues for outreach education, and patient condition during transport. The careful planning of a transport data base can automate the time-consuming parts of quality assurance. It can also move the quality assurance process closer to a concurrent monitoring system. This will allow problems to be identified and acted on quickly. In a transport environment, rapid problem solving is obviously very important.

An additional benefit is that the data can be used when the program is being reviewed by regulatory agencies such as JCAHO. With increasing frequency, regulatory agencies and insurance carriers are reviewing transport program activities and quality assurance programs.

Marketing

Who are the top ten referring physicians? Transport programs serve an important role in presenting the institution to referring hospitals. Consequently, the transport program has a role in the marketing of the institution's medical services. By using the data gathered ᐧto the transport database, the institution develop marketing strategies. As an ex-, often the transport program will be to notice changes in the referral pat- cting on this information work can begin on rectifying any problems that may have led to a loss of referrals.

PATHWAYS TO PROBLEMS OR WHY SYSTEMS FAIL

The development of a database for transport is a time consuming and expensive task. By examining the reasons systems fail, the developer can shorten the process, reduce the cost, and enhance the chances of success.

The objectives are not clearly defined

The push to rapidly develop an operating transport data system overshadows taking the time and effort that are required to understand clearly what the users of the system expect the system to do. Failure to understand the objectives can result in the installation of a system that may be used to collect data for a significant period before it is realized that it is inadequate to answer important questions posed by the users. Another mistake is sometimes made by buying hardware or software before the objectives of the program are delineated. This can result in being limited by a system incapable of meeting the needs of the users. Time must be devoted to outlining what is expected of the data system.

Users are not given primary consideration in the design

Unless the needs of the users, the working patterns, and the resources available to the users are considered in the design, the data will end up not being collected and/or the inaccuracy rate will be very high. If the program itself is not user friendly, frustration with its use will lead to the same consequences. Ultimately the users will find ways to avoid using the system.

The data system is too complicated

To succeed, the data system should be kept simple, particularly in the initial phase of development. Starting out with plans to have a data collection system that does everything that anyone in the program can imagine is a mistake. In the desire to have the best and most comprehensive transport data system, often sight is lost of what most of the requests for data will be.

While some people involved in the design

would like every physiological parameter, ventilator setting, medication dose, etc., to be recorded on every transport patient, this will bog down the data collection system until it becomes unworkable.

The result of too complex a system can be that, after a significant period has elapsed, it will be realized that the system developed still cannot generate the reports wanted or meet the program requirements. Because so much energy has gone into the development, there then develops a resistance to making needed major changes or to scrapping the system and starting over.

The data system cannot deliver data in a timely fashion

Data needed which is delivered after decisions are made is of little use. Providing data rapidly, before it is needed to make decisions, will result in the nurturing of support for the system. Users of the system will ask for more data, realize the system's value, and support the resources that the data system will need for further development.

The system is too inflexible

Medical care, transport, and computer technology are all changing very rapidly. As the data system is used frequently, it will become evident which changes are necessary to make the data system more useful or easier to work with. If a system is too rigidly developed or uses obscure program languages or operating systems, it will not be easy to keep up with the changes necessary for a modern data collection system. As time goes on the system will become more irrelevant. It is important when picking hardware and software to keep the future in mind.

Inadequate resources are committed

Dambro and others report a good case study of a failed computerized data system at an academic medical center.[2] Cost ultimately led to the system's demise, but several important issues regarding resource planning, equipment, and system design mistakes are also highlighted. For a system to survive, adequate dollars and manpower must be allocated to the project. To develop a whole data system and then realize that there is no one available to do the collection of the data or no money for ongoing support is a major mistake.

HOW TO GO ABOUT SYSTEM DEVELOPMENT

There are two major aspects to the development of a working transport data system. One is the design of the system of data collection, and the other is the construction of the database itself.

The system

Choose the developer. The first step in the development of a transport data system is to define who has the interest, expertise, time, and is willing to take the responsibility for the development and maintenance of the data system. Unless a committed individual is identified before embarking on the project, chances of success are small. Often equipment has been purchased and then languished because no one took the responsibility for the system. The person chosen may come from many different roles: physician, nurse, administrator, etc. The role of the person chosen is not as important as their interest in the system. By choosing carefully before starting any development, much wasted time and frustration will be avoided. It is very important to make sure that the developer has a vested interest in the data. If a programmer is used who will not be involved in the data, then a second person with a strong interest in the data should work side by side with the programmer during development.

Keep it simple. The single most important point in system usage is that very effective data collection systems can be developed by keeping them simple. This point cannot be overemphasized. "How can I keep it simple?" must be asked repeatedly at each step in the process. If even one variable is collected successfully, then there is a system of sorts. From this nidus, a larger and more useful transport data system can be built. It is far more important to have a limited number of useful variables then a great number with many little used or irrelevant ones.

Consider the system usage. An idea of how the system will be used should be considered. Will the system involve one microcomputer with a single person responsible for data entry, database maintenance, and report generation? Or, will there be a network of microcomputers in different locations with different individuals sharing a common database? The system concept will guide the rest of the thinking as development progresses.

Choose the data collection methods. A decision has to be made regarding what methods of data collection will be used. The first step is to examine the process by which a transport takes place at each institution. One technique used to do this is data modeling.[1,4] A diagram should be made which delineates at which point and by whom the various pieces of transport data will be collected (see Figure 48-1). Once the flow of information is understood the methods can be chosen. Whether transport data will be collected and abstracted from the written notes done on transport, on special manually or optically read forms, via radio transmitting data pads, or directly into laptop microcomputers used on transport, will be a function of how each program operates and the resources available.

By careful planning, it may be possible to eliminate duplicate efforts in data collection such as when the communication specialist, the unit physician, and transport team all collecting and recording the patient's weight in different parts of the record.

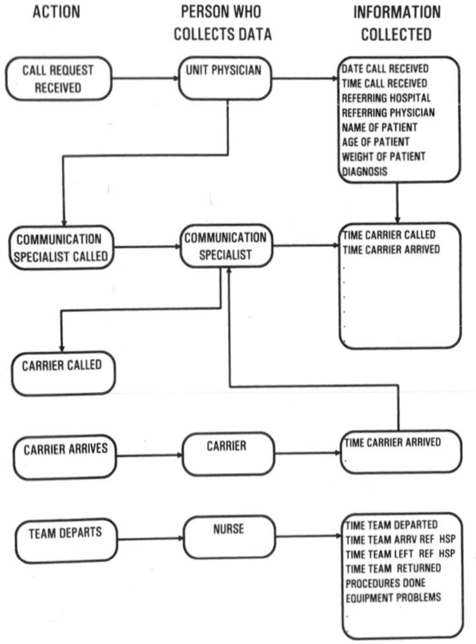

Fig. 48-1. Flow chart delineating the collection of transport data.

Plan built-in incentives. Planning for user incentives is an important part of data system development. The question must be continually asked: why would the users want to spend the time collecting and contributing to the data base? Negative incentives, such as "Do it! It's your job," result in poor compliance and lack of caring about accuracy in the data.

One type of incentive that can be built into the system to enlist cooperation is by taking the "two carrot theory" approach. In this method, the developer provides a long and short term reason for the collectors of data to want to enter data into the system.

As an example, the nurses on transport are asked to collect and record some data, including transport times, in the nursing notes. The computerized data system could provide the nurse with a list of patients, type of transports, and time spent on each for nursing certification purposes. Simultaneously, the organization would get, from the use of the transport times, budget, and planning, information regarding nursing hours spent on transport. Both parties receive something back from the data system. The nurse has an incentive to collect the data accurately because, in addition to professional responsibility, there is a personal importance to the data.

Examine the workload. It is important to make every effort to attempt to lighten the workload or decrease the stress on the collectors of the data. Major hospital-based systems have failed because the introduction of data collection by computer caused an increase in the work necessary to keep track of the same amount of data that was collected manually before the introduction of the computerized data collection system. There is a great incentive to use a system that makes an individual's job easier.

Keep in mind the issues that affect reliability of the data. The reliability of information collected in a transport database depends on the following issues:

Distance of the vested party from the data entry. If the person entering the data is far removed from the person who has a vested interest in the data, the accuracy rate will go down. The ideal situation occurs when the party most interested in the variable enters it. If the data entry is done by a clerk who does not understand the significance of the variable and is forced to make judgments about the data, then the accuracy will be less.

Inherent nature of the question being asked. In a regional transport database in Northern California, one variable asked for is whether the mother of an infant or neonate has had a positive toxicology screen. Because many institutions filling out this variable are worried about the sensitive nature of this information, the variable is seldom filled out on the collection form. A report generated using this variable would be very inaccurate.

Ease of collectibility. Some information is very difficult to collect depending on the institution and the information asked for. As an example, the type of primary payor for insurance purposes is often difficult for a clinical service to collect accurately. It is particularly hard to collect at the time of transport. To increase the accuracy of this information, ideally the information would be collected from the financial services office at the time of discharge. This may be difficult to do, and so the information is often taken from the admitting face sheet causing less accuracy in the data.

Number of passes that the data goes through. A classic example is the following scenario involving Apgar scores. Initially, a 5 minute Apgar score is assigned by the referring hospital and recorded on the labor and delivery record. The referring pediatrician arrives, asks the score, and is told verbally an incorrect number that he then records in his admitting note. The transport team arrives at the referring institution, takes a history, and records the Apgar score from the referring physician's note. When the team returns, they give an oral history to the receiving housestaff who may then mutate the score once more before an admitting note is written several hours later. Effort should be made to reduce the number of steps in data collection.

Form design. There are several ways to record data on data collection forms. When recording diagnoses, one way is to provide a check off box, which when checked indicates a diagnosis was present or not. Another method leaves a blank box in which the diagnosis can be recorded by handwriting it in. In an actual example, a nonmedical data clerk entered a diagnosis in a free form text variable as "monocrotiz embrocoli" because of unreadable handwriting. The actual diagnosis was necrotizing enterocolitis. A check off box would have prevented this type of error. In one failed hospital system, a majority of a 15% error rate was attributable to handwriting errors.[2] In another study, reporting of birth certificate information improved dramatically with redesign of the reporting form.[3]

If all of the above issues in system development are not addressed, an elegant data collection system in a technical sense may be created, but it may not be well used or may ultimately end up being discarded.

Development of a transport data base (see Figure 48-2)

Often the approach taken when developing a database is to begin by listing all of the possible variables. This will result in a database that stores many more variables then will ever be used. Further, a great deal of effort will go into the collection of data that will never be accessed. It can also result in the opposite effect of leaving out important variables because a haphazard approach was used in the

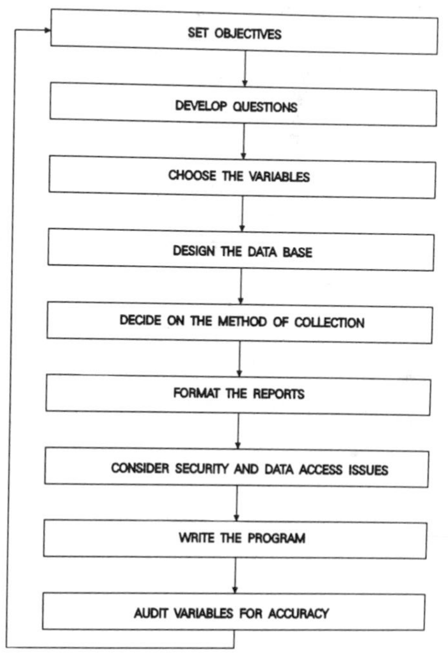

Fig. 48-2. Flow chart outlining the development of a transport database.

development. To avoid these problems, a systematic method should be used to decide which variables are necessary for each transport program.

Set objectives. The first step is to take the time to decide what kind of information is needed and for what purposes the transport database will be used. All the objectives will not be known at the start. It has been the experience of many people that, as the word spreads that a source for transport data is available, other questions that were not originally contemplated are posed to the system. Users sometimes do not know what they want until the time that they need the information. Start by defining the objectives as accurately as possible.

To understand this process, a simple example will be used. The problem in General Hospital (GH) pediatric intensive care unit is that there is too long a delay before the team leaves in response to a transport call. Besides the quality of care issue from a delayed response, New General, another nearby PICU has slowly been wooing away referrals from GH by responding to emergency transport calls more rapidly. It is very difficult to figure out where the delay is occurring. GH decides to set as an objective that 95% of the time, the team will be out the door in 30 minutes or less.

Develop questions. Pose questions that can help to decide if the objectives are being met. By doing this the next step of selecting which variables to store in the database will become evident. Asking multiple questions of each objective will make it easier to identify the precise cause of any problem if the objective is not being met.

In this example, three questions that might be asked are: (1) How long is it from the time of the request for transport until the transport team departs? (2) How long is it from the time that the carrier is called until they are prepared to depart? (3) How long does it take the team members to arrive from home? The answer to these questions will help the transport program pinpoint the source of the problem if the objective is not being met. By storing data that answers these questions, the program will know if the transport time limit of 30 minutes is being achieved and whether the problem lies with the carrier or the transport team members.

The process of designing reports that the users would like to see will sometimes help to figure out what kinds of questions to ask. Reports are really the answers to requests for data. Asking the users what reports would be helpful will generate the questions that will lead to variable selection. Interviewing the potential users about their problems and data needs will provide another avenue for question development.

Choose the variables. Select the variables needed to answer the questions. This process includes choosing the variables, applying validity tests to the variables, defining the variables, and watching for variable traps.

In this example for the first question regarding transport team departure the two variables that answer the question are the time the call was received and the time that the team departed. For the second question, the variables are the time that the carrier was called and the time that the carrier was ready for departure. The time the team was called and the time they arrived for transport are the variables that are needed for the answer to the third question. From this example, six variables have been created. Patient identification such as name, medical record number, and transport date will also be wanted to analyze individual situations where there were transport delays. This will add three more variables (see Table 48-1).

Apply several tests to each variable. These tests are (1) Does the variable help to answer the question? (2) Is it possible to collect the variable easily? (3) What is the likelihood that the collected variable will be accurate? If the variable does not meet these tests, the chance of having a useful piece of data is small. The process should be repeated until all the variables are selected, useful, collectable, and have the potential for accuracy.

The nine variables in this example would meet these tests in most transport programs.

Define the variables. When collecting data in a computer database, each variable has four major characteristics that need to be defined: name, units, type, and length.

Assign a name to each variable. The length of the name may be limited by the choice of the software used.

TABLE 48-1 VARIABLES GENERATED FROM THE GH EXAMPLE

Definition	*Name*	*Units*	*Type*	*Length*
Patient last name	LASTNAME		TEXT	16
Medical record number	RECNUM		TEXT	8
Transport date	TRANDATE		DATE	8
Time call received	TMCALLRV	24 HOUR CLOCK	TIME	5
Time team departed	TMTEAMDP	24 HOUR CLOCK	TIME	5
Time carrier called	TMCRCALL	24 HOUR CLOCK	TIME	5
Time carrier ready for departure	TMCRDEP	24 HOUR CLOCK	TIME	5
Time team called	TMTMCALL	24 HOUR CLOCK	TIME	5
Time team arrived	TMTMARR	24 HOUR CLOCK	TIME	5

Using the variables in the example, names are arbitrarily assigned within the restraints of the chosen software (see Table 48-1).

Decide on the type of units. Since many people may be involved in collection, a decision must be made as to the type of units in order to standardize the data.

In this example it must be decided for the time variables whether to use A.M./P.M. or to use the military 24 hour clock.

In other situations the choices might be between grams or kilograms for weight, numeric codes or actual names for referring physicians, or procedure codes or free form text for procedures performed on transport.

Most commercial databases demand that each variable be assigned a type. It will depend on which software that is used what the variable type will be. Types of variables include text or character, numeric, integer, date, time, or logical, i.e., true or false.

Definition of type becomes important later when reports are demanded from the system. For example, if the weight of a transported neonate has been stored as a text variable, it will probably serve for most purposes. The weight will print out on the screen and in reports with no difficulty. Should someone, however, decide they would like to look at the mean weight of a group of transported neonates, it will not be possible for the computer to do the calculation with the weights in a text format. The computer does not see a text variable as a number. It would be the same as if an attempt was made to average the last name of the patients. If the weights had originally been stored as a number this problem would not have occurred.

In the GH example, the patient's last name and medical record number will be assigned the type, text; the transport date type, date; and the six time variables will all be assigned the type, time (see Table 48-1). By assigning the medical record number as type text and not the type number, medical records that start with zero will be stored that way. Storage as a number variable would delete the leading zero.

Decide the length of each variable. For instance, if the last name of the patient is one of the variables in the database, the computer will need to know how much space to allocate for this variable. If the length is too short, the person doing the data entry will be unable to enter the entire last name. On the other hand, if the variable is too long, excess disk space will be consumed, and eventually a decrease in system speed will occur during searches. In the case of numbers, provision must be made for how many decimal spaces will be allowed.

For the sample database lengths, see Table 48-1.

Watch out for variable traps. As the variables are designed there are several traps that the designer of a transport database can fall into if planning is not done carefully.

Same variable—double meaning trap. A variable may legitimately have more than one meaning. Before the transport of a maternal high risk patient, the obstetrician may feel that the infant is 26 weeks by size. After birth the neonatologist may feel that the infant is 30 weeks by exam. Both parties make decisions based on what they believe the infant gestation to be at the time the decision is made. When trying to retrospectively examine these decisions, it is important to know what perspective and information was used. If only the gestational age by exam is stored in the data base, then conclusions about obstetrical management will not always be valid. The solution to this particular trap is to store two separate variables—the gestational age by exam and the obstetrical gestational age.

Same variable—double data trap. Multiple recordings of the same piece of data in various parts of the chart can result in inconsistency and confusion about which information to store. Often an abstracter is faced with multiple recordings of Apgar scores in the same chart: the labor room record, OB note, pediatric admitting note, transport note, etc. It is not uncommon for the scores to vary from source to source. The solution to this problem is to define which set of scores is to be consistently used, i.e., the labor room record.

A second approach is to have the person who is closest to the source of the data, the assigner of the Apgar scores, be the one who enters the data. This method, however, requires a sophisticated and complex data system.

Unknown—not available trap. This is the situation that arises when it is not clear why a piece of data is missing from the database. Two possible reasons are as follows: (1) the variable was looked for in the chart at the time of entry into the database and could not be found (not available), or (2) the data entry person did not have the chart available at the time of entry and, therefore, did not enter the variable (unknown). The consequences are that 3 years later, when someone asks a question of the data, it will not be clear to the individual asking the question whether they must go back to the chart to look for the missing data or whether this effort can be saved. If not available had been entered, they would know that the piece of information was already looked for and was not present in the patient record. A solution for this problem is to always make provision to allow the selection of either "not available" or "unknown" as possible choices during data entry.

Zero trap. Commercially available database programs handle the failure to enter a numerical value in the database in different ways. In some databases, when no entry is made, the program assumes a zero value. Other systems insert what is known as a null value, a place holder which is not equal to zero. A significant problem can occur when a user asks for a list of all transport infants with a 5 minute Apgar score of less then three, only to find that there seems to be too many infants with 5 minute Apgar scores of zero. It may then be impossible to figure out who actually had an Apgar of zero and who had no entry made at all for which the computer inserted a zero. To solve this problem, a nonsense number such as 99 can be assigned to the 5 minute Apgar score when this data is not available. This will allow future users to easily pick out the true zeros from the infant with no information. If the database program used inserts a null, this will not be a problem.

In the six time variables in the GH example, whether the database program inserts a null value or not, if the time is not entered, is very important. Many programs which do not use null values will record the time as 00 : 00 when no time is entered. This value also represents midnight. It would be very confusing to study a time problem only to find many events which seem to have occurred at midnight but in fact did not.

Turn of the century trap. This is a very unusual situation. Some programs demand that a valid date be entered when a date is called for. When the date is not known, attempts to enter nonsense dates such as 00/00/00 will be rejected by the system. To overcome this problem, some people have used remote but valid dates such as 01/01/01 when the date information is not available. In a pediatric transport program, not many patients will be near one hundred years old.

As the turn of the century approaches, caution must be used, since the year 01 will appear again soon. Either enter the full year, such as 1901, or pick a date such as 01/01/50, too old for pediatric patients and too far away to be of immediate concern. A database that allows a null value for dates would be the best solution.

Design the database. This part of the process will be greatly facilitated by using the resources of an individual familiar with how databases are constructed. In designing a database, it must be decided how the data will be grouped and used. This step is important because the speed with which the program operates, the storage space needed, and the complexity of the program will be affected significantly by the design. Proper design may also allow easier use of specialized files such as physician names and addresses in other applications.

Databases are constructed of variables (see Figure 48-3). The variables are grouped into a record or row for each entry, for example, transport patient. The records are grouped into files. The database consists of a single or several files. In a database's simplest form, one file is used. All the variables stored, regarding a single transport, are kept in the individual record. The advantage to this approach is that the creator of the database does not have to worry about the relationships between the files. All information can be found and manipulated in one file. The disadvantage is that certain pieces of information may have to be repeated unnecessarily in each patient's record. This leads to a waste of disc space and a slowing down of the ability to find information.

For instance, in a single file, if the receiving hospital stores the name and address of the referring physician for each transport, each patient record would have to contain variables for the physician name and office address. If the office address of the referring physician changed, then all the records containing that address would be inaccurate when called up later.

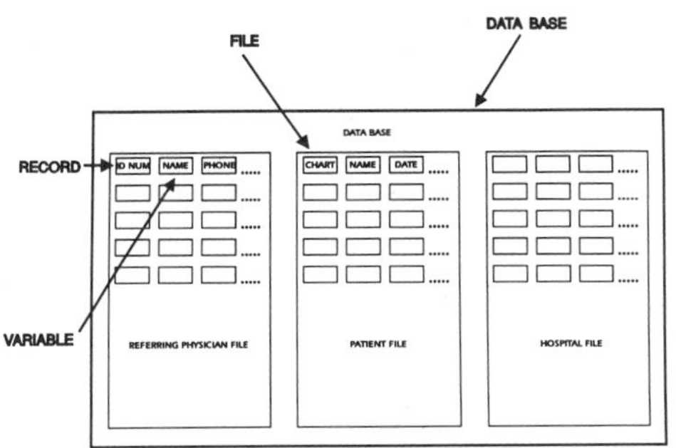

Fig. 48-3. Databases are constructed of variables grouped into records and rows.

A solution to this problem is to store a coded number representing the referring physician in the patient record and to store all information about the referring physician such as name, address, specialty, phone number, fax number, etc. along with the code number in a separate file. If information changes about the physician, by updating the record for that physician, all records of the patients containing that physician's code number are automatically updated. A second advantage is that, by having a separate physician file, this file could be copied and used for other applications.

A simple but effective structure for a transport database consists of three files, one for the patient information, the second for physician information, and the third for referring hospital data (see Figure 48-3). The files are then linked by the use of codes. By using appropriate programming techniques it will not be necessary to memorize codes or the physicians or hospitals for data entry. The amount of disc space saved when thousands of patients are stored will be considerable. The ease of updating the patient records will be greatly simplified.

Many other variations are possible. A user doing a research project may want some very specific data that is not normally collected in the patient database record. A separate file could be set up and linked to the patient records. This file would contain only the variables that the researcher called for along with an identifier for the patient. Since the study will most likely be limited in time, it would not be necessary to reserve room in every patient record in the database for these special variables. Only the patients under study would have these variables saved. Each transport program's needs will define the appropriate file structure for that program.

Decide on the method of collection. The method of collection of data will vary from institution to institution depending on who collects data and where the collection occurs. One transport program may gather the birth date from the referring hospital chart accompanying the transport patient, while another may obtain it from the nursing notes written by the transport team on transport. In order for a computerized data collection system to cause the minimum amount of disruption, and to enlist the maximum amount of cooperation, the data collection techniques should parallel as closely as possible the current working methods of the users. By using good programming techniques the computer can be set to do the work of sorting which variable goes to which file. This means that the collector of data or the data entry person will not be forced to accommodate the computer, but vice-versa. The entry screens on the computer should parallel the data collection forms.

Most transport programs will use manual forms as an intermediate step before data entry. The forms for data collection should be simple and clear. When possible, definitions for variables that might be ambiguous should be located on the forms. For example, if there is a box on a neonatal transport form that is to be checked for adequate maternal prenatal care, then a definition about what constitutes adequate care should be present on the form for the person filling out the form.

In the GH example, it would be important to write on the form that 24 hour military time is to be used so that 8:00 does not get written when 20:00 is the expected time.

Another approach is to develop a manual of definitions. This method, however, is not as useful because often the manual is not available at the time the data is being recorded on the form.

Other more exotic methods of collection such as taking a notebook computer on transport should be considered. Direct entry reduces the number of times that the data changes hands and, therefore, the error rate.

Format the reports. All the reports that the system will eventually generate do not need to be known at the time the program is written. At this stage the developers will have a very good idea of what kind of data output they would like to see. Decisions should be made regarding what type of reports are needed, who will receive the reports, and the frequency with which the reports will be distributed. Another decision must be made about whether on-line access to information needs to be available or whether printed reports delivered to the recipients will be adequate.

The process of discussing and developing which reports are needed is very important in helping the developers understand which variables will be needed for each report. This sometimes leads to discovering the need for a variable that was not considered at an earlier stage in development.

Mention should be made of the use of graphics in developing reports. Graphics are a powerful tool. Pleasing design, incorporating the use of graphics into the reports developed will help communicate the information contained in the report (see Figure 48-4). It will help to promote the value of the database.

Consider security and data access issues. With one microcomputer and one person en-

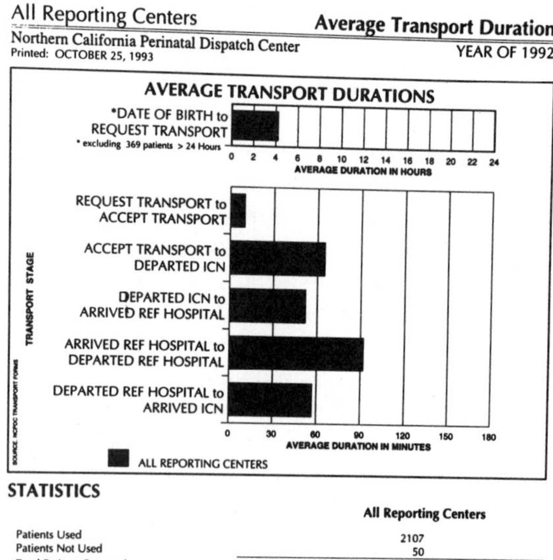

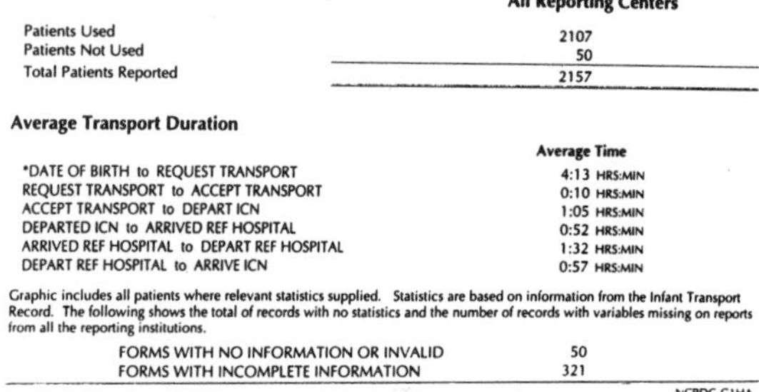

STATISTICS

	All Reporting Centers
Patients Used	2107
Patients Not Used	50
Total Patients Reported	2157

Average Transport Duration

	Average Time
*DATE OF BIRTH to REQUEST TRANSPORT	4:13 HRS:MIN
REQUEST TRANSPORT to ACCEPT TRANSPORT	0:10 HRS:MIN
ACCEPT TRANSPORT to DEPART ICN	1:05 HRS:MIN
DEPARTED ICN to ARRIVED REF HOSPITAL	0:52 HRS:MIN
ARRIVED REF HOSPITAL to DEPART REF HOSPITAL	1:32 HRS:MIN
DEPART REF HOSPITAL to ARRIVE ICN	0:57 HRS:MIN

Graphic includes all patients where relevant statistics supplied. Statistics are based on information from the Infant Transport Record. The following shows the total of records with no statistics and the number of records with variables missing on reports from all the reporting institutions.

FORMS WITH NO INFORMATION OR INVALID	50
FORMS WITH INCOMPLETE INFORMATION	321

NCPDC-G1HA

Fig. 48-4. Graphics used in reports, such as bar graphs, help to promote the value of the database.

tering and retrieving data, security and access are not a major problem. If many people will have access to the database either on one computer or on a network, further steps will have to be taken. The use of individual passwords that are changed with regularity will offer some security protection. In the design of a database with multiple users, it may become important to know who entered data and at what time. By leaving variables for the date, time, and entry person it will be possible to go back and see when the data was last entered or changed.

A decision should be made as to who will have ownership of the data. If this is not done, several people could change data one after the other with uncertainty developing as to the validity of the data.

A transport took place at GHA, and the time the carrier arrived for transport was recorded on the dispatcher form. The time showed that the carrier was late. It was subsequently discovered by the dispatcher that the time was a mistake. The form had already been sent for data entry. The dispatcher entered the database and corrected the time. Later, a data entry clerk noticed that the time on the dispatcher form differed from the time in the data base and changed the time back to the incorrect one found on the form.

It must be decided who will be allowed read access, who will be allowed write access, and who will have the right to change data.

Write the program. Once the database structure, forms, and reports are decided upon, the program can be written. Several different approaches can be taken to developing the software for a transport database. A commercially available transport database can be purchased, a standard database program can be used, or a proprietary program can be written from scratch.

The purchase of a commercial package has the advantage that no time needs to be spent in writing the software for the database. If the program is well supported by the company offering it for sale, the users will have someone to turn to for program support or problems. There are major problems with this approach. These packages are very difficult to locate. They will usually be quite expensive because of the small customer base. The companies writing the software may be small and could go out of business. When this occurs the users of the system will be stranded. If this approach is taken, upon purchase, a copy of the computer source code should be demanded.

A much preferred method is to use a commercially available database package. While this will require either the user or a programmer to write the program, many of these database programs are relatively easy to learn and to use. A rudimentary database can be ready to run in only a few days when used by someone familiar with this type of package. The cost of using a commercial database package is substantially lower than the other methods. This method will serve most transport programs needs.

If a transport program has highly complex requirements for data entry, then a computer program written specifically for the institution may have to be written. This will usually be a very expensive and time-consuming affair. It has the advantage that the users will have complete flexibility in design, and the program will do exactly what they want. When this mode is used, changes will generally require the services of a programmer.

Audit variables for accuracy. Once the database is in operation it is important to continually assess its validity. It is important to periodically audit the accuracy of the variables and ask the following questions: 1) Is the variable being collected? 2) Is the variable accurate? 3) Is the definition confusing? 4) Has the variable become outdated?

Decide what new data can or should be added. Decide which variables are no longer necessary or are not very accurate. Make adjustments in the variables used.

It is important to keep the database open to change. Do not set an arbitrary date beyond which records are closed to change. As reports are asked for over time, errors in prior data will be uncovered. By keeping the database dynamic rather than static there will be an opportunity to correct the errors and improve the accuracy of the database with time.

A well thought out transport data base is a major asset for a transport program. To summarize the major points:

1. Decide before starting who will have responsibility for the system and how it will be paid for.
2. Spend most of your development time in planning, not programming.
3. Consider what answers are expected from the system right at the start and throughout the development.
4. Never forget the user.
5. Keep it simple.
6. Remember that any data system is constantly evolving over time and needs to be examined and modified on an ongoing basis.

REFERENCES

1. Chen, P: The entity—relationship model—toward a unified view of data, *ACM Transactions on Database Systems*, 1(1), 9-36, 1976.
2. Dambro MR and others: An unsuccessful experience with computerized medical records in an academic center, *J Med Educ*, 63, 671-3, 1988.
3. Frost F and others: Birth complication reporting: the effect of birth certificate design, *Amer J Public Health*, 74(5), 505-6, 1984.
4. Kay S: Towards relevant medical information systems, *Med Inform*, 15(4), 327-31, 1990.

49
TRANSPORT SAFETY

KAREN KLEIN
DEBRA M. BILLS

In the transport environment, safety relates to accident prevention and the avoidance or minimization of personal injury and property damage. The relative security of the hospital environment is frequently taken for granted by health professionals and administrators. This attitude transfers into the transport environment in which clinical experts must function. The health profession has dedicated its most expert clinicians to extend tertiary care capabilities to patients who require extensive and highly sophisticated care. In so doing, policies, personnel, and property have been lost due to underestimating the cruel realities of mother nature and the transport environment of the ground and air. Neither of these entities is very forgiving when policies and people fail to take them into account.

The focus on safety has been a priority for the air medical profession. This is the result of the total number of aviation accidents rising to its all time high of thirteen reported in 1986. With a high patient transport volume the accident rate was 15 per 100,000 patient transports (or approximately 105,000 flight hours). The concern of the government, public, and air medical profession was heightened when the accident rate for commercial Emergency Medical Services (EMS) helicopters was found to be slightly less than twice the accident rate of 14 CFR Part 135 unscheduled air taxi helicopter operators. EMS helicopters and personnel had a greater risk of a fatal accident (approximately 3.5 times more) than those flying 14 CFR Part 135 unscheduled helicopter air taxis and all turbine helicopters. The primary causes of these accidents were related to weather conditions resulting in reduced visibility and spatial disorientation, engine failures, and obstacle strikes.[52]

Fortunately with the air medical transport profession's attention on safety enhancement, 1990 was accident free. Unfortunately, the most recent two years have again experienced accidents which were related to weather and reduced visibility.[51] Self-improvement of the profession must continue to be a priority by focusing on safety performance analyses, enhancing equipment and technology, and providing personnel protection gear and supplemental training.[56] Although costly, these measures will hopefully eliminate complacency or overconfidence in what has already been accomplished and minimize accident occurrence. The cost of prevention in the air medical environment is only a fraction of the financial and human cost of an aviation accident.

In comparison the national safety record of ambulances is difficult to ascertain. One source estimated that 12,000 emergency medical vehicle accidents occur in the United States and Canada each year as a direct result of using red lights and sirens. This does not include the accidents that do not directly involve the emergency vehicle itself. There may be five times this number secondary to the "wake effect." Emergency vehicles disrupt, startle, and confuse other drivers and result in related accidents.[19] When reviewing New York state statistics from January 1984 to December 1987, reportable accidents amounted to 1,412 occurrences, resulting in six fatalities and 1,894 injuries to ambulance occupants. These accidents are those with damage exceeding $600 or which involve personal injury.[26] One source extrapolated these statistics to the country. They estimated 5,400 injuries and 17 deaths annually as a consequence of emergency medical vehicle accidents. In addition, the majority of the New York crashes occurred on clear days with good visibility during daylight hours. They occurred on dry roads at intersections with traffic lights when ambulances were making turns or passing through the intersection. Similar characteristics were also found in emergency medical vehicle accidents that occurred in Arizona during 1983.[70] Therefore, human error again becomes the primary factor in ambulance accidents if the ambulance is adequately maintained.

To maintain safe operations in the transport environment, it is vital to initiate programs at all levels. In 1983 Roy G. Fox described the three levels of aviation safety. These levels consisted of prevention of emergency occurrence, minimization of the emergency effect, and minimization of the injuries.[37] For this discussion, these levels will be extended to the concept of transport safety. Instead of focusing on crash survivability, the focus of this chapter will be expanded to transport accidents, their prevention and impact minimization. It is important to note that the safety levels are nonexclusive. In other words, what may be beneficial for prevention may also be considered a major factor in the minimization of the effect of the emergency.

PREVENTION

Prevention is not a foreign concept to health professionals. Although frequently an idea that is difficult to quantify because its results are difficult to substantiate, it is commonly accepted that "an ounce of prevention is worth a pound of cure." Unfortunately, programs influencing these areas are frequently modified or eliminated if budgetary savings are required.

Operations in and around vehicles

In general, operations in and around ground and air vehicles share several common features. First and foremost, planning for the specific patient transport requires the evaluation of weather and road conditions. A determination of the most appropriate mode of transport and the most direct route must also be made. Weather will influence the planning and completion of either type of transport.

For air medical transports, rotorcraft using visual flight rules (VFR) may need to be abandoned for helicopters or fixed wing using instrument flight rules (IFR). The FAA has published controversial weather minimums in Advisory Circular 135-14A for air ambulance operations that must be followed as a standard (see Table 49-1). Entering inadvertent IFR or instrument meteorologic conditions (IMC) without the appropriate instruments or pilot proficiency has led to the primary cause of fatal accidents in the air medical transport profession. Resorting to an IFR aircraft, whether helicopter or fixed wing, enables the transport program to continue service in conditions that would prohibit VFR aircraft from continuing the mission. Planning is also important with these transports since a flight plan must be filed prior to departure. In addition, weather must be continuously monitored because airfields may be closed for departures and landings if their ceiling and visibility minimums are exceeded. These weather minimums are more conservative (FAR Part 135) when an actual patient is on board the aircraft than when the transport leg consists of only the flight crew and air medical personnel (FAR Part 91). Generally, if there

TABLE 49-1 AIR AMBULANCE WEATHER MINIMUMS UNCONTROLLED AIRSPACE[35]

Conditions	*Ceiling*	*Visibility*
Day local	500 feet	1 mile
Day cross country	1000 feet	1 mile
Night local	500 feet	2 miles
Night cross country	1000 feet	3 miles

is zero miles visibility and the ceiling height is zero, air medical and ground transports will be unable to be completed until there are clearer skies and roads.

Besides planning, shared operational procedures include the need and, in certain instances, the requirement to have all personnel, passengers, and patients restrained during the transport. The FAA requires by regulation that all individuals be restrained on lift off and landing.[1] It is preferred that they are also secured during the flight in case of turbulence, but this judgment may be left to the discretion of the pilot. In a review of the air medical transport accidents that occurred from 1972 to 1987, it was concluded that eight of the 82 fatalities would have been prevented with three point shoulder restraints. Eleven other fatalities and fourteen cases of severe injury may have been prevented with their use.[61] State laws should be also evaluated for seat belt requirements in ambulances. Caring for unrestrained victims of motor vehicle accidents only reinforces the need for medical personnel to keep seatbelts on during ground transports if laws are not available to mandate their use. In reviewing New York's emergency medical vehicle accidents, most of all the serious injuries occurred in those not wearing any type of restraint.[31]

Not only will restraints help limit injury in the event of an accident, but they will also limit the access of the patient to the controls of the vehicle and the pilot or driver. The need to separate the pilot and controls from the patient is further emphasized since the air medical profession[22] and FAA standards have called for solid barriers between the pilot and the patient. This keeps the patient isolated in the event they would become violent and uncontrolled by physical restraints.

Transport personnel must orient to vehicle capabilities and equipment handling. Although not their primary responsibility, they must know how to open and close doors and access emergency exits. Basic operation of each vehicles' electrical system must be understood to use and problem-solve the lighting, suction, environmental control, and radio systems. All stretchers, isolettes, equipment, and supplies should be secured to prevent projectile objects during turbulence, rough roads, and accidents. Patient loading and unloading must be completed with care to avoid damage to the vehicle and injury to personnel and patient. Although these are general procedures shared by all transport modes, they may become very specific and different for the method, make, and interior configuration of the vehicle. As a result, transport personnel must be familiar with these procedures and the idiosyncrasies of each mode of transport to operate safely.

Ambulances. Similar to the air medical profession, the evolution of the ground transport system started with old methods of transportation and developed into more sophisticated means. Horse drawn litters transitioned into horse and buggies and finally resulted in the current large, powerful ambulances. The United States Department of Transportation (DOT) has developed specifications regulating the manufacture and design of vehicles used as ambulances. The federal regulation that governs vehicles deemed ambulances is KKK-A-1822-C. It has minimum requirements in order for a vehicle to be called an ambulance.[59] Refer to Box 49-1 for specific requirements.

They also mandate the specifications of the three basic types of ground units. The Type 1 commercial cab has a conventional cab chassis that originally had no passageway between

BOX 49-1 KKK MINIMUM AMBULANCE REQUIREMENTS

- Used for emergency medical care;
- Designed to provide a driver and patient compartment;
- Carry equipment and supplies for emergency medical care;
- Safeguard patients and others from hazardous conditions;
- Carry extrication equipment;
- Provide two-way radio communication between ambulance, dispatcher, hospital, and authorities;
- Provide portable radio communication between emergency personnel when separated; and
- Designed and constructed to provide maximum safety and comfort to the patient(s).[59]

the cab and patient compartment. Special orders may be requested to connect the two compartments. Type 2 ambulances are customized, commercial vans. Type 3 specialty vans have cabs with a walk-through to the patient area in the larger, modular type body.[58] Each type of ambulance has their respective advantages and disadvantages. When selecting an ambulance for a transport system, length of transport, size of transport team, type and size of carried medical equipment, and types of roads traveled are only a few of the criteria that need to be assessed. As an example, if most of the transports will consist of short distances on crowded urban streets with a two to three man team, the large Type 3 modular ambulance should be avoided. It may consume excessive amounts of gas and be unable to fit through congested streets. Besides regulating their construction, each ambulance is also classified as either a Class 1, two-wheel drive vehicle, or a Class 2, four-wheel drive vehicle. The KKK-A-1822-C specifications are necessary to prevent modification of residential vehicles to be used as ambulances.[58]

Clinically, ambulances are rated as either Basic Life Support (BLS) or Advanced Life Support (ALS). Capabilities of EMS staff and available equipment will be different in each of these categories. Specific differences are defined by state regulation and transport teams should be knowledgeable about the resources made available by each category. Refer to Box 49-2 for examples of equipment carried by each type of service.[58] A complete summary of BLS and ALS equipment may be found in the cited reference.

Each emergency medical vehicle must also be equipped with an emergency light, sirens, air horn, and PA system.[59] These warning devices are to be used to inform pedestrians and other vehicles of an emergency. While an ambulance is responding to a request for help, the emergency medical vehicle operator must appropriately use lights and sirens. Most states have regulations governing their use. They will only allow lights and sirens for life-threatening or potentially life-threatening illnesses or injuries.[23] Examples of these may include airway obstruction or respiratory failure, cardiac arrest, uncontrolled bleeding or excessive blood loss, complicated childbirth, and trauma resulting from serious mechanisms of injury.

When traveling with lights and sirens, the operator must continue to obey traffic laws, but some areas may exempt emergency vehicles from certain traffic laws. Examples of exceptions to traffic laws for emergency medical vehicles include proceeding through a red traffic signal or stop sign after slowing and giving other motorists adequate warning; exceeding the posted speed limit if other lives are not in danger; and moving in the opposite direction of posted flow of traffic if the road is clear and adequate warning is given.[59] Although exceptions may exist, one must exercise caution at all times. Special care should be taken when approaching an intersection since this location presents the greatest risk of collision for an emergency vehicle. Other precautions include not exceeding the posted speed limit by more than ten miles per hour and maintaining the posted speed limit at intersections with green traffic lights. If a red traffic light, stop sign, or railroad crossing is

BOX 49-2 BASIC AND ADVANCED LIFE SUPPORT EQUIPMENT

BLS EQUIPMENT[58]

Airways	Pen light
Bite sticks	BP cuffs
Nasal cannula	MAST (Adult & Peds)
Cervical collars	O_2 Masks
Cold packs	Portable O_2
Eye pads	BVM resuscitators
Restraints	Splints
Gauze pads	Stretcher—patient folding scoop
OB kit	
Sandbags/head immobilizer	Suction—portable wall mounted
Tape	
Trauma dressings	Suction catheters
Backboards—long & short	Infection control kit
	Stethoscope

ALS EQUIPMENT

Monitor & defibrillator
Laryngoscopes
Endotracheal tubes
ACLS medications & miscellaneous others
Intravenous fluids & catheters
Syringes & needles

approached, the ambulance should come to a complete stop before continuing with the transport. The maximum speed of the emergency vehicle should only be 20 mph if traveling in the lane of oncoming traffic. Local considerations may influence each transport program's operations. Specific policies may need to be developed to prevent any panic on the part of other motorists. Some areas of concern include traveling through a tunnel that prohibits lane changing or across a long bridge.

A critically ill or injured patient does not justify recklessness, particularly when strobe lights, sirens, and painting ambulances with bright colors have been shown not to provide enough warning to other motorists. Many studies have been done to determine the appropriate frequency range for the human ear to hear an emergency vehicle's approach.[26] The best placement of the siren speakers has also been evaluated. Currently speakers are being placed on the front grill instead of the cabin roof to provide a better signal in the front of the ambulance.

Federal specifications provide minimum standards for visual warning devices. There has been an ongoing debate to decide the best color for these lights. Flashing lights are generally accepted to be far superior to catch bystanders' and other motorists' attention. Red, a commonly used emergency color, blends in with tail lights. One suggestion is to use a combination of colored strobe lights to provide high visibility. This could be accomplished with green or blue combined with red as an identifiable signal of danger.[27]

In addition to lights and sirens, the color of the emergency vehicle may also reduce the chance of an ambulance being involved in an accident. Although most ambulances are white with orange striping, evidence shows that lime yellow is more visible than these traditional colors. The goal is to provide the motorist with quick identification of an emergency vehicle. With this in mind, use of lime yellow as the universal color for an ambulance has been recommended to federal and state agencies.[27]

Commercial airlines. An alternate method of transportation is the use of commercial airlines. This method of travel may be considered if the patient is stable and transport time is not critical. When making these special flight arrangements, one should speak to a reservation supervisor to simplify the process. This individual will provide information regarding check in procedures, medical equipment permitted on board the aircraft, and additional costs involved.

Some airlines will arrange to accommodate a stretcher and provide oxygen. These special provisions may take up to 72 hours to arrange. Established guidelines by each airline for use of oxygen will need to be determined before the day of travel. Use of the airline's oxygen may be limited to on board the aircraft only. Arrangements may be needed for other oxygen sources while in the airport.

Fixed wing

Hazard areas. Recognizing the hazard areas of airplanes and jets is an important first step in preventing injury and damage. Generally, these aircraft are able to shut their engines down quickly, so they should not be approached until this is completed. Accidental contact with rotating propellers will cause major penetrating trauma to personnel. The exhaust temperatures of a jet engine will reach temperatures of 550 to 600°C. Even so, engines will continue to be hot and must be avoided to prevent burns. In addition, loose clothing, hats, rags, etc. must not be worn around aircraft when engines are on. If these guidelines are not followed, they may be drawn into the air intake and cause engine failure.

Airport ramp entry must be done cautiously. Ambulances waiting for the arrival and shut down of aircraft must avoid other aircraft and equipment on the field. Depending on the size of the airport, continued exposure to the experienced noise levels may lead to impaired hearing if adequate protection is not taken. There is also the danger of fire, since aircraft engines vent fuel after shut down. As a result, smoking should not occur within 50 feet of the aircraft.

Pilot responsibilities. The pilot is responsible for all aspects of the aircraft. Transport decisions regarding weather conditions and aircraft status rest with the pilot. This includes opening and closing doors and ensuring that all equipment and persons are appropriately secured in the right location. According to FAA regulations, the pilot is responsible for briefing all passengers on board the aircraft.

Briefings consist of the following information:

- Smoking is prohibited if oxygen is in use;
- Use of seat belts during take-offs and landings;
- Position of seat backs for departures and landings;
- Location and means to open doors and emergency exits;
- Location of survival equipment;
- Ditching procedures for over water operations;
- Location and use of emergency oxygen if flights exceed 12,000 feet MSL; and
- Location and operation of fire extinguishers.[47]

Rotorcraft

Normal operations. Medical personnel have special operational responsibilities during a patient transport. Communications must be maintained with the pilot in order to assist in locating air traffic and identifying obstructions on lift-offs and landings despite patient condition. The pilot should also be informed when distracting medical equipment will be used and if the patient has any special transport needs. Nonessential intercom conversation must be maintained at a minimum during the critical flight phases of lift-offs, landings, and emergencies. Proper radio terminology should be used at all times. While caring for the patient, a "hot" mike should be used only when absolutely necessary. In addition, the use of red or amber lights is preferred during night flights, since white lights may interfere with the pilot's night vision. To further avoid this complication, lights may need to be dimmed or turned off during landings at night.

Hazard areas. The main and tail rotor systems are a source of multiple hazards when working around helicopters. Almost invisible at full revolutions per minute (RPM), the main rotor tips may spin as fast as 400 mph or about 300 rpm. The smaller tail rotor may travel as fast as 2,000 rpm. Contact with either rotor would result in major trauma and death. Because of these dangers, helicopters should be approached only after making eye contact with the pilot and then being directed to advance. To stay in direct view of the pilot, the helicopter should be approached from the front, directly towards the nose of the aircraft or at 45 degree angles of the nose. The aircraft should never be approached from the rear, and personnel should generally not walk behind the tail rotor or under the tail boom. Two exceptions to this rule are the MBB BO-105 and BK-117 aircraft which have rear clam shell doors for patient loading and unloading. In these instances, personnel should never step back beyond the horizontal stabilizer. See Figure 49-1 for the safe approach and working areas around helicopters. If it is necessary to approach the aircraft while the rotors are turning, one should do so from the down slope side if the helicopter is resting on an uneven surface or slope (Figure 49-2). Tall equipment should be carried to and from the aircraft below head level. One should also avoid doing CPR and always maintain a crouched position under the revolving blades. During warm-up or cool-down stages when the rotor velocity is slower, gusts of wind may cause the main rotor blade to dip 4 to 5 feet from the ground. Despite the type and operational status of the helicopter, no one should advance towards the aircraft without the pilot and medical crew's direction.

An additional concern with rotor systems is the rotor wash that it produces. The wind produced by a helicopter may range from approximately 25 mph during warm-up or cool-down to 50 mph when the aircraft hovers over the ground or is at maximum revolutions while on the ground. Rotor wash effects increase when the aircraft is located downwind. The wind will send loose items such as dust,

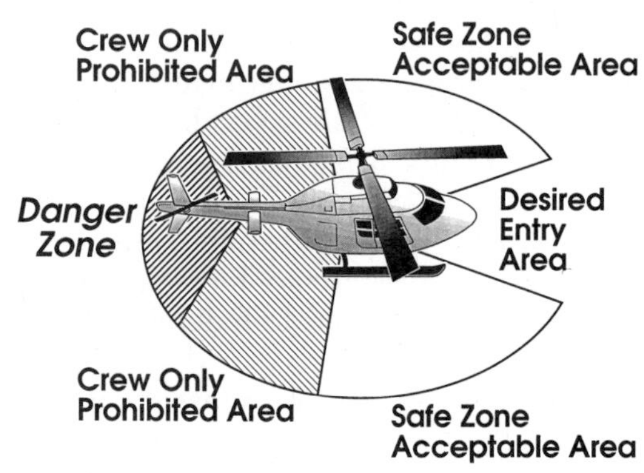

Fig. 49-1. Rotorcraft approach areas.

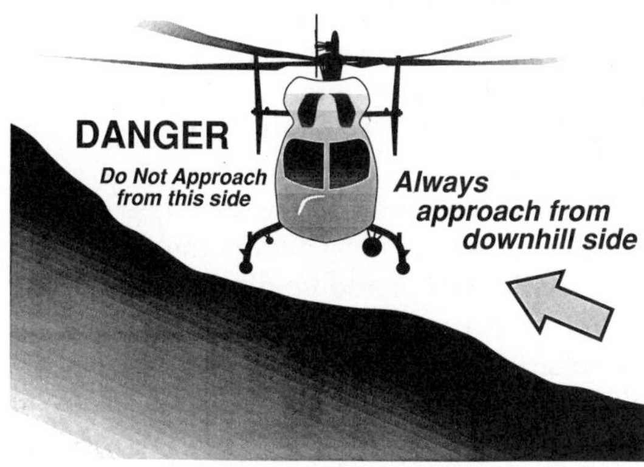
DANGER
Do Not Approach from this side
Always approach from downhill side

Fig. 49-2. Rotorcraft Approach on Slopes

snow, litter, loose clothing, and unsecured stretcher mattresses and linen flying to collide with unsuspecting victims. Eye protection should be available for ground personnel coordinating the landing of helicopters. Dry landing areas may be hosed down with water to prevent dust storms on landing. Landing areas with hard, packed snow should be selected or snow removal on helipads completed before landing. Otherwise a "white out" situation may occur and result in the pilot losing all reference to the ground. Emergency ground personnel should stay at least 100 feet away from the landing site with the patient. Not only may flying objects injure bystanders, but the possibility exists for debris to be drawn into the air intake of the engine. This could damage the engine and cause it to fail.

Rotor wash may also increase the wind chill factor under the rotating blades and damage exposed skin of personnel and patients. In an air temperature of 10°F, a wind chill factor of −30°F is created when the rotor wash is 25 mph. Skin may be damaged at these temperatures in minutes.

The engines are an added source of hazards. Depending on the helicopter make, they emit a loud, high frequency noise that may range between 90 and 100+ decibels during operation. In comparison, normal speech is 40 to 65 decibels. Constant and repeated exposure to this level of noise may create a permanent, high-frequency hearing loss if adequate protection is not taken with earplugs and/or headsets.

As previously mentioned, entry of flying debris into the engines' air intake could result in damage and failure. Also, the exhaust from the engine should be avoided because it is approximately 400°C. On shut-down, the engines may vent some fuel, therefore smoking is prohibited within 50 feet of the helicopter. When the weather is very dry, open flames, such as flares used to mark landing sites, should not be used within 150 feet of the landing area. Personnel should take special care when walking around the aircraft after venting because fuel will make cement and asphalt surfaces very slippery.

Landing sites. When establishing landing sites for helicopters, several qualities should be sought. Whether landing at a helipad or the scene of an accident, the landing area must be large enough to hold the aircraft and free of obstructions such as wires, trees, telephone poles, and towers. The National Association of EMS Pilots recommends the following dimensions for landing sites.[53]

	Day	*Night*
Large helicopter (e.g., Bell 412 or Bell 212)	120 × 120 feet	200 × 200 feet
Medium helicopter (e.g., BK-117, Dauphin, Bell 222)	75 × 75 feet	125 × 125 feet
Small helicopter (e.g., Jet Ranger)	60 × 60 feet	100 × 100 feet

It is just not sufficient to have a landing zone which is large enough. It must also have a landing and departure path into the wind which is free of obstructions. Low lying obstructions to be avoided include stumps, bushes, posts, and large rocks. Taller obstructions such as trees, towers, and electrical wires should not encompass the landing zone. The elevator shaft type of approach and departure may be necessary for landing areas with obstructions around the periphery. This requires maximum engine power to lift and land and leaves no reserve power for emergency maneuvers. In addition, as a result of the surrounding obstructions, there is nowhere to glide the aircraft to a safe landing in the event of engine failure. Pathway clearance for landings and lift-off into the wind must be allowed for obstacles of varying heights (see Figure 49-3 for Approach/Departure Path and Clearances). Ground

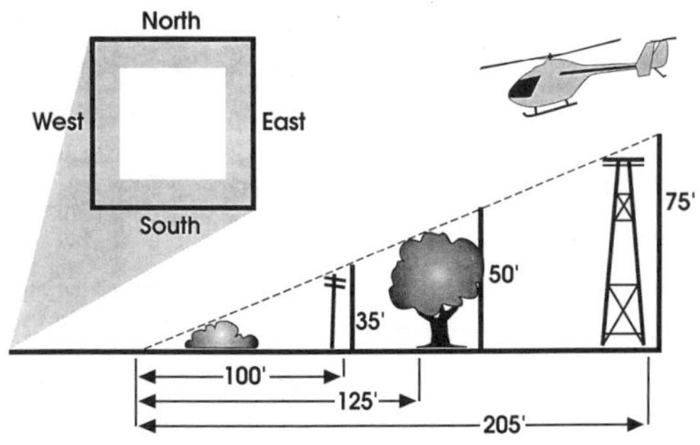

Fig. 49-3. Landing Zone Approach and Departure Path

personnel must keep the flight crew and air medical personnel informed of all obstacles. The pilot will usually complete a high and low level reconnaissance of the site prior to touchdown to ensure that all obstacles are accounted for. An alternative site is always a reasonable option if obstacles were visualized from the air which were not appreciated from the ground.

In addition to size and obstructions, other criteria for landing site selection must be maintained. The landing site should not exceed a slope angle of 8 to 10 degrees. Special considerations must be taken if hazardous materials are involved. The helicopter landing zone should be selected at least one mile upwind from incidents involving explosives, poisonous gases/vapors, radioactive gases, or chemicals at risk for exploding and burning. If the incident involves radioactive materials which are not vapors, the landing zone need only be one quarter mile upwind. Regardless of the hazardous material, low lying areas should be avoided because the toxic gases or vapors may gather in these areas.[53]

The touch-down area may be targeted by placing a well identified marker at each corner of the site. A separate marker should be placed at the point adjacent to the landing site where the wind is originating. Options for markers include beacons, vehicle headlights, flashlights, colored smoke for daytime operations, and flares. Once again, extreme caution should be exercised following the previous guidelines if flares are to be used. They must be closely managed. Sources of white light, such as headlights, searchlights, spotlights, and camera lights, should never be directed toward the helicopter. This light will ruin the pilot's night vision rendering him blind and potentially unable to control the descent of the aircraft.[29]

Fortunately, landing sites do not need to be established each time a patient must be transported. Predesignated landing zones may be established in areas where sites are limited. In these situations, the size of the area and its obstruction limitations have been evaluated prior to its use during an emergency evacuation. Flight crew and ground personnel are comfortable with the safety of the locations. They may be identified by number or descriptive characteristic for that particular locality. It is advised that the high and low level surveys be continued, since things may have changed unnoticed since the last inspection.

Predesignated landing zones may also be specially designed helipads at hospitals or other agencies. These too must adhere to the guidelines for landing site establishment. According to the Commission on the Accreditation of Air Medical Services (CAAMS), helipads must be a limited distance from the helipad to enable continuous monitoring of the patient and performance of emergent patient interventions if necessary. They are to be marked with an "H" or similar landing designation and identified by a strobe light or beacon. A device for wind direction must be available. Lights must be on hand for night operations.[22] An excellent resource to review when planning a helipad is the FAA's Heliport Design, Advisory Circular 150/5390-2. In addition, specifications must be in compliance with local, state, and other federal regulations.

Environmental factors

Leaving the protective confines of a hospital exposes medical personnel to the potential hazards of the environment. Understanding and heeding the limitations of these factors further promotes prevention of accidents. The factors that must be understood to meet this outcome are altitude, terrain, and weather.

Altitude and terrain. Altitude and terrain impact air medical transport more so than ground transport. Circumstances in which this may be otherwise would include accessing patients in areas where roads are inaccessible to ambulances or rescue vehicles (e.g., flooding, mud, etc.) or when search and rescue is part of the ground response team's mission profile. In these instances, special training may be required for handling mine, cave, wilderness, or other environmentally exposed emergencies.

For helicopters and fixed wing aircraft the impact is more straightforward and operationally oriented. Actual selection of aircraft depends on the designated geographical service area. Aircraft are rated for specific service ceilings, which is the altitude that its flight characteristics have been safely demonstrated. As altitude increases, aircraft performance is adversely affected, and the total allowable gross weight (operational weight + payload) may have to be decreased to land in high altitudes.

The terrain which is encompassed in the identified service area may limit whether a flight is accomplished and, if so, with or without special modifications. Landing sites with slopes of angles greater than 8 to 10 degrees are not recommended but may be attempted depending on the aircraft, aviation management firm or transport program policy, pilot experience, surface condition, and wind direction and velocity. As previously mentioned, landing area requirements depend on the aircraft model. Confined areas for landing zones which may have been established at preexisting helipads or at temporary sites present their own set of special problems.

Frequently, surrounding obstacles such as trees, electrical lines, or towers prevent safe angles of approach and departure and require vertical entry or exit. This places extra power demands on the aircraft when entering these phases of flight and it also leaves very little room for human or mechanical error. If a problem arises during this scenario, there is virtually no place to go to avoid obstacles and to land safely. Surface conditions which consist of snow, dust, or other granular substances (i.e., sand or coal) will impair visibility and possibly result in spatial disorientation. On the other hand, rocky or uneven landing sites result in unstable surfaces for landing and alternative sites must be found. Mountainous regions complicate the situation further because higher altitudes decrease aircraft performance during a time when slopes, confined spaces, and/or poor surface conditions demand more power. Examples of special modifications to meet the demands of some of these scenarios include snow skids for snow operations and flotation devices for over-water operations.[9]

In addition, fixed wing aircraft, which include airplanes and jets, are limited to specific runway lengths which have been established by the manufacturer. In accessing patients from distant localities, fixed wing transport may be the most cost effective and time conscious choice of transport. The major limiting factor in optimizing portal to portal transfer of care is that they must land at airports which may be of varying distances from the patient's location. If the runway of the local airport is not long enough for the aircraft being used, an alternative airport may be required. This may result in longer ground turn around times for both patient and transport team. Commercial airlines are obviously limited to major airports and their related air traffic control time constraints.

Weather. The most significant element which impacts medical transports is the weather. As weather conditions change throughout the year, the mode of transport selected, air or ground, may be influenced. For example, if skies are clear, but all roads have been blocked by a recent blizzard, it is more feasible to resort to rotorcraft transport than to an ambulance. On the other hand, if visibility is obscured by fog, then the only immediate option is to transport by ambulance unless waiting for the fog to "burn off" is a reasonable alternative.

Weather related to air and ground transport is not an easy phenomenon to understand. This is especially true when appropriately treating and transporting acutely ill or injured patients as quickly as possible is the mission of most transport programs. It is very difficult to explain to the anxious individual on the other end of the telephone line that the helicopter's lift-off is delayed because of poor visibility when they are caring for an acutely ill child in a location with clear skies. Health care providers, both those transferring and receiving patients, frequently lose sight of the fact that *safe transport* is paramount in any mission statement. They must not risk becoming part of the problem in the event of an accident which was preceded by a poor decision to depart in less than acceptable weather conditions. In addition, there is the ethical principle of nonmaleficence ("above all, do no harm") which obligates that patients NOT be exposed to any unnecessary risk.[66] As a result of these obligations, health professionals must understand the weather limitations of their transport vehicles, so informed decisions may be made regarding their selection and use. In addition, unwarranted pressure must not be placed on the individuals making these decisions.

Aircraft are affected by weather conditions which impair visibility, decrease ceiling levels (altitude of the cloud layer), diminish performance, and hamper aircraft control. These conditions include temperature, humidity, and icing; fog and precipitation in the forms of snow, rain, hail, or sleet; and turbulence, wind shear, and thunderstorms.

Temperature, humidity, and icing. Operational limits for ambient temperature exist for every aircraft and will ultimately influence which aircraft is used for a specific region.[12] When evaluating regional humidity experiences, areas with high humidity will find that the performance of selected aircraft will also be impacted. As humidity increases, the air becomes "thicker" with water molecules producing more resistance for rotors. As a result, more engine power is required to lift the aircraft and to safely land. Frequently, the challenges of increased humidity are responded to by decreasing the available payload of the aircraft (equipment and/or personnel). Decreasing the fuel load for short flights or refueling at distant airports for longer distanced flights are options. These adjustments must be completed in order to ensure the availability of engine power without exceeding the aircraft's operational limits in the event of an emergency.

On the colder side of the spectrum, icing conditions at altitude may be expected when flying in visible precipitation, such as rain or cloud droplets, and the temperature is at or below freezing. Air temperature decreases 1°C for every 330 feet gain in altitude.[47] If the aircraft is not equipped with functional deicing equipment, which is the case with the rotor blades of IFR and VFR helicopters, ice will rapidly accumulate. This effect produces increased aircraft weight and drag and reduced thrust and lift which results in the rapid deterioration of aircraft performance. Pilots must remove the ice by using available deicing equipment, leave the area of precipitation, or go to an altitude with temperatures above freezing. Icing conditions are reported as follows:

Trace—perceptible and not hazardous without the use of deicing/anti-icing equipment unless encountered for over one hour;

Light—more rapid rate of accumulation which is nonproblematic if deicing/anti-icing equipment is used, but potentially hazardous if the flight is extended over one hour;

Moderate—increased rate of accumulation which may be hazardous for short encounters and requires the use of deicing/anti-icing equipment or flight diversion; or

Severe—rate of accumulation unaffected by deicing/anti-icing equipment and requires immediate diversion.[32]

Even commercial airlines have had to divert from Pittsburgh to warmer climates when deicing equipment failed to function. In general, reported icing conditions prohibit rotorcraft flights, and this is one of those conditions which may not be totally appreciated by air medical transport users. If icing conditions are experienced on the ground, transport by ambulance may be impacted as well.

Fog, haze, and precipitation. Anything which interferes with the pilot's ability to identify objects in front of him or her impacts his/her visibility. Fog, haze, and precipitation may interfere with the completion of an air medical transport at any point in time. If severe enough, they could even interfere with safe, expeditious ground transports as well.

Fog is frequently encountered as vapor forms with temperature changes. Moisture condenses as temperatures decrease and may hang in river valleys, around the ground, or entirely engulf the area. Monitoring the spread between the dew point and temperature will assist in determining the likelihood of fog. As air cools, its capacity to hold water vapor decreases and relative humidity increases. The dew point is the temperature in which water vapor condenses into water droplets or frost.[12] The closer the temperature is to the dew point, the increased chance of fog formation.

Haze, not generally known as a weather condition, may be compounded by slow or no air movement which results in the accumulation of industrial smoke and pollution. Major forest fires have resulted in an excessive smokey atmosphere which has diminished reported visibility for air transport by VFR aircraft until the area has been cleared by winds.

Precipitation comes in the forms of rain, sleet, hail, and snow. The intensity of precipitation is measured by the rate in which the substance falls. Light precipitation falls up to 0.10 inches per hour (0.01 inch per 6 minutes). Moderate precipitation ranges from 0.11 to 0.30 inches per hour or greater than 0.01 to 0.03 inch per 6 minutes. If precipitation exceeds 0.30 inch per hour (0.03 inch per 6 minutes), then it is considered heavy.[32]

Snow will also be evaluated based on its impact on visibility. Light snow is associated with a visibility of 5/8 statute mile or more. Moderate snow intensity will result in a visibility ranging between 5/16 and 5/8 statute miles. And finally, heavy snow will impact the visibility such that it is less than 5/16 statute mile.[32] Frequently, in these situations a "white out" condition may be encountered. The pilot loses sight of all references on the ground, may become spatially disoriented, and inadvertently collide with the ground if unable to resort to his/her instruments.

Depending on the accompanying precipitation, sleet and hail will also diminish visibility for the pilot. Hail is produced when ice crystals remain at altitude in a cloud of super cooled water droplets long enough to increase in size thousands of times larger than normal. Sleet is made of ice pellets which were formed when raindrops passed through a layer of cold air close to the ground and froze.[17] In addition, sleet may be associated with additional icing problems, while hail, depending on the size and force of the stones, could damage the airframe of the aircraft on impact. Hail is frequently encountered in thunderstorms.

Turbulence, wind shear, and thunderstorms. Wind is produced when warmer air is replaced by cooler air. Its velocity must be considered when evaluating weather conditions. Aircraft have limits set for speed. Exceeding those limits will place structural strains on the airframe and rotor system. Gusting of wind may also complicate a very straightforward landing or lift-off making it more difficult to control the aircraft.

Turbulence is usually an irregular motion or swirling of air which results in rapid changes in the speed and direction of the wind. It may vary in its degree of intensity and is most commonly experienced with irregular terrains when combined with strong surface winds, gradient winds, temperature inversions, or thermal convection movements which may be associated with snow covered or glacier slopes.[50] Its intensity is reported as being light, moderate, severe, or extreme. When evaluating the weather forecast for flight acceptance, the extent of reported turbulence may impact the ability of air medical personnel to care for patients safely. Not only are they likely to experience injury if unrestrained as turbulence intensity increases, but the critically ill or injured patient may not be able to receive the necessary care during the flight. Clinical procedures such as airway maintenance for the vomiting, back boarded patient or CPR for anyone in cardiopulmonary arrest will most likely be impossible to perform if turbulence is greater than moderate intensity. Table 49-2 reflects aircraft and occupant reactions during turbulence and should be considered when evaluating acceptance of an air medical transport.

The most dangerous circumstances which involve rapid wind velocity and direction changes are frequently experienced with warm and cold front passages, thunderstorms, and clouds which produce rain but not at the intensity of thunderstorms. Wind shear may precede the passage of a warm front by up to 6 hours or follow a cold front by up to an hour or more. In arid regions, severe downdrafts may occur with the following conditions:

Rain from high-based clouds evaporates prior to reaching the ground,
Temperatures above 80°F,
Light surface winds, and
Dew point and temperature spreads exceeding 35°F.

Wind shear is particularly threatening to aircraft flying within 1,000 feet of the ground, since downward air movement velocities of 1,000 feet per minute may be encountered. This vertical movement may exceed 2,000 to 3,000 feet per minute within 200 feet of the terrain. Wind shear of this strength could force aircraft into the ground, especially on lift-off or landing. In addition, horizontal wind shear may exceed 30 knots, which would cause the aircraft to surpass its placarded "red-line" speed and again impose structural strains on the airframe and rotor system.[50]

Thunderstorms are formed when large amounts of evaporated water condense into clouds and release heavy rain. An unstable atmosphere must exist in order to develop thunderstorms. This occurs when the temperatures in the upper troposphere drop more rapidly than normal (greater than 5.5°F per 1,000 feet). Rapidly moving cold fronts overtaking warm air will frequently produce these conditions and result in brief, violent storms accompanied by strong, gusty winds and a short period of heavy rain.[17] Usually found in late spring and summer, they manifest all of the previously mentioned conditions with their inherent risks: turbulence, hail, rain, snow, icing conditions, sustained updrafts and downdrafts, and lightning.

TABLE 49-2 TURBULENCE REPORTING CRITERIA[22]

Intensity	*Aircraft reaction*	*Internal reaction*	*Reporting terms*
Light	**Light Turbulence** momentarily causes slight, erratic changes in altitude &/or attitude. OR **Light Chop** causes slight, rapid, & somewhat rhythmic bumpiness without appreciable changes in altitude or attitude.	Slight strain against seat belts or shoulder straps felt by occupants. Unsecured objects may be displaced slightly. Little or no discomfort experienced with walking.	**Occasional**—Less than $\frac{1}{3}$ of the time. **Intermittent**—$\frac{1}{3}$ to $\frac{2}{3}$ of the time.
Moderate	**Moderate Turbulence** changes altitude &/or attitude, but aircraft remains in control. It usually causes variations in indicated airspeed. Similar to light, but more intense. OR **Moderate Chop** causes rapid bumps or jolts without appreciable changes in aircraft altitude or attitude. Similar to light, but more intense.	Occupants feel definite strains against seat belts, or shoulder straps. Unsecured objects are dislodged. Walking is difficult.	**Continuous**—More than $\frac{2}{3}$ of the time.
Severe	Turbulence that causes large, abrupt changes in altitude &/or attitude. It usually causes large variation in indicated airspeed. The aircraft may be momentarily out of control.	Occupants are forced violently against seat belts or shoulder straps. Unsecured objects are tossed about. Walking is impossible.	
Extreme	Turbulence in which the aircraft is violently tossed about and is practically impossible to control. It may cause structural damage.		

Correlations between the visual appearance of thunderstorms and the severity or amount of turbulence or hail have not been made. Air or ground-based weather radar will reflect the areas of moderate to heavy precipitation. Areas of highest liquid water content of the storm result in increased radar reflectivity. Generally, the intensity and frequency of turbulence increases in these areas. In addition, severe turbulence may be expected within 20 miles of a severe thunderstorm and 10 miles in less severe storms. Avoiding thunderstorms entirely is the best policy. If a thunderstorm is approaching, sudden gusts of low-level turbulence may cause loss of aircraft control, therefore landing and take-offs should be postponed. Vivid and frequent lightning indicates the probability of a severe thunderstorm and should be circumvented using the previously mentioned distance precautions.[50]

Weather information systems. Readily accessible, current, and accurate weather information is an absolute necessity in enhancing weather decisions impacting medical transports. A number of systems are available at varying costs. The most basic mechanism is the weather channel on cable television. Not generally in an aviation format, it broadcasts movement of fronts and associated weather graphics 24 hours a day. Flight Service Stations (FSS) located throughout the country may also provide weather information which is updated hourly. A phone call may be placed into these offices to receive weather information from the FSS briefer for the areas encompassed by the flight path. Unfortunately, these services are becoming fewer in number due to budgetary cuts.

The next option would be computer access by phone modem. Sponsored by the FAA, DUATS (Direct User Access Terminal Service) provides the same weather information that is obtained from the Flight Service Station. Services may include hourly observations, terminal forecasts, notice to airmen, significant meteorological information, upper air information, radar data briefs, severe weather bulletins, satellite and radar graphics, current and forecast maps, and custom flight plan services. In the private sector, Kavouras, WSI Corporation, and Jeppesen Sanderson are a few companies which supply similar products. Other options with large price tags would include satellite and radar accessing systems to obtain concurrent weather information.[11]

Maintenance

Aircraft. In the aviation industry, maintenance of helicopters and fixed wing aircraft is scheduled and required for all U.S. registered aircraft. The scheduling routine is preventive in nature and coordinated on a daily, hourly (i.e., 25 hr, 50 hr, 100 hr, etc. flight time), predetermined lift-off and landing cycles, and/or annual basis. Aircraft components have established flight time limits or cycles before they must be inspected. In addition, unscheduled maintenance may occur for inoperable or failed components. It may also be required for FAA advisory directives (ADs) or manufacturer's service bulletins (SB). These notifications identify a problem that has been identified by either of those services which are considered potentially hazardous and require evaluation immediately or within a specified time-frame. All inspections must be signed off in the aircraft logbook to verify completion.[12]

Regardless of the type of maintenance, it must be completed by law by a certified airframe and power plant (A & P) mechanic who has been FAR 135 qualified. With the focus on accident prevention, position statements, recommended guidelines, and standards have been published by professional organizations such as Helicopter Association International (HAI), the Association of Air Medical Services (AAMS), and CAAMS regarding access to maintenance facilities and qualified personnel. The most specific set of standards which enhanced the recommendations of the other organizations was established by CAAMS, the newly established organization to accredit the air medical profession. Within these standards, A & P mechanics are required to have 2 years of rotorcraft experience with factory schooling, or an approved equivalent, in the assigned aircraft. Special training for service and maintenance of oxygen systems and the installation, inspection, and maintenance of special medical equipment were identified criteria. In addition, a procedure for advising flight and air medical personnel when aircraft were not airworthy was required. Most of these standards also apply to the mechanics servicing fixed wing aircraft as well.[22]

Even with the progress which these organizations have made, the AAMS Safety Congress II (May, 1992) charged the leaders of AAMS to investigate and address such unanswered questions as how many mechanics are necessary to adequately maintain one, if not more than one, aircraft functioning 24 hours a day; what is appropriate rest and duty time for mechanics; and what type of recurrent training standards should be established.[9] It is time to focus on some of these concerns, since safety has been questioned when pilots exceeded their duty times in busy transport programs. At this time, however, it is still acceptable, by regulation, to allow mechanics to maintain aircraft while on-duty or on-call 24 hours a day without relief until 7 consecutive days have passed. Fatigue has been an issue for pilots flying 8 out of 24 hours, but not for mechanics working extensive periods of time to get the aircraft "back in service."

Ambulances. For ambulances, the maintenance requirements are less regulatory and consist more of recommendations made by manufacturers and the auto industry for general service maintenance. Regular servicing of an emergency medical vehicle is critical to the safety of those travelling in and around the vehicle. Over time, just as with any piece of machinery, natural wear and tear will cause damage which may lead to break-down. With preventive maintenance, time and money may be saved. Routine servicing and replacement may be less costly than paying for the break-down which will occur later. Also, the time the vehicle is out of service may result in lost revenue due to the inability to respond to a call. Examples of preventive maintenance schedules recommended by owner's manuals are provided in Table 49-3. In addition, the majority of states require safety and emissions inspections on all vehicles. Safety checks evaluate the functioning of all lights, brakes, warning devices, tires, mirrors, and windshield wipers. Where they are not required, for the safety of all those involved, these suggested inspections should still be completed.[59]

Medical equipment. As many persons involved with the transport of the critically ill and injured are aware, the first known accounts of air transport dates back to the siege of Paris in 1870 with the use of balloons. Next came World War II where fixed wing aircraft transported the wounded. Air medical transport continued to evolve through the Korean

TABLE 49-3 AMBULANCE PREVENTIVE MAINTENANCE[59]

Every 3 months or 4,000 miles	*Every 6 months or 12,000 miles*
Change oil and filter	Major tuneup—Check, adjust, or replace PRN:
Grease chassis	Compression
Lubricate all moving parts	Spark plugs
Inspect tires for air pressure, damage, wear	Wiring
Check—Cooling system	Points and condenser
Exhaust system	Carburetor and choke adjustment
Battery conditon	Timing
Lights, sirens, and horn	P.C.V. valve
Condition of wipers	Fuel filter
Condition and tension of belts	Air cleaner
All fluid levels	Front wheel bearings
	Front end alignment
	Shocks and springs
	Tires balanced and rotated
	Steering system
	All services noted with three month check

and Vietnam Wars where helicopters played an important role.[60] As transportation became more sophisticated, so did the equipment used to treat these patients. Initially, no equipment was carried. First aid kits were ultimately replaced with modern pieces of electronic equipment such as IV pumps, monitors, pacemakers, ventilators, intraaortic balloon pumps, and incubators to name a few. As a result of the progress in medical technology, in 1967 the Association for the Advancement of Medical Instrumentation (AAMI) was founded in an effort to increase the understanding and beneficial use of medical devices and instrumentation.[8]

Biomedical considerations are a very important aspect to being able to safely transport a patient. The standard maintenance procedures recommended by AAMI may be modified for transport equipment focusing on preventive maintenance as a key issue. In the transport environment, regardless if the transportation is by ground, fixed wing, or rotorcraft, equipment needs to be durable and able to withstand temperature changes, vibration, mobility, moist environments, and humidity changes.[60] This environment will require more frequent biomedical checks of the equipment than a piece of equipment which will remain stationary.

Daily checks of used equipment should be routine to avoid potentially dangerous situations with malfunctioning equipment in an environment which has few, if any, spares available. One must ensure that the equipment will not interfere with the vehicle's electrical or radio communications systems prior to purchasing and also keep track of each repair required on each piece of equipment to aid in pinpointing recurrent problems. The United States Air Force Aeromedical Research Group has tested many medical products for their use in air transports. Further information on these products may be purchased from the US Government.[8]

Selection and health maintenance of personnel

The selection of transport personnel and their continued health maintenance is a broad topic which, if given enough attention, will enhance the safety of overall operations as well as individual performance. Transport personnel are exposed to unusual mobile environments, physically straining and fatiguing conditions, and health risks which they may not be normally exposed to in the hospital environment. The enclosed space of ambulances and aircraft does not enable personnel to use proper body mechanics when lifting or moving patients. Rotating and extended shift coverage promotes fatigue development which is further escalated by the unusual stresses placed on staff during air or ground transports. Throughout the medical profession, it is assumed that an experienced individual who is current in their specialty will be able to practice safer than one who is not. Extending this thought to include personal physical fitness should also enhance safe performance in this mobile environment.

Physical exams and fitness criteria. As mentioned, the interiors of ambulances and aircraft have limited work spaces which do not support the use of good body mechanics. In addition, aircraft, helicopters in particular, have a maximum gross weight limitation. Maximum gross weight is determined by the sum of the empty weight (aircraft and mounted equipment) and useful load (fuel, passengers, and carry-on equipment). As a result, all transport personnel may have to be limited to height and weight restrictions. Strength and agility may be particularly important to evaluate, since personnel are working in confined areas. Unlike pilots who must have a FAA Class II medical certificate to maintain their commercial pilot certificate, the issue of physical standards for flight personnel has been long standing and there have been no guidelines offered to assist in transport program policy development.

In an attempt to address the physical wellbeing of staff, guidelines for preemployment physicals have been developed to include physical exams encompassing head-to-toe assessment, vital signs, visual acuity with and without correction, and auditory acuity; immunization assessment for rubella, tuberculosis, and hepatitis B; and screening tests for complete blood count, chemistries, urinalysis, PPD or Mantoux test, hepatitis B antibody and antigen, ECG if older than 35, and chest x-ray as needed.[12] AAMS continues to support the standard of periodic physical and hearing examinations. Mechanisms that define physical fitness criteria had not been attempted until UCDMC Life Flight in Sacramento compiled a survey of proposed minimum physical fitness policy items. Of the 134 air medical programs surveyed, 84.3% classified how the items were being addressed in their program. Responses classified fitness items as being more strict or similarly stated in the respondent's program or acceptable as presented, too strict, or not applicable. As a result of these responses, the following minimum, uniform physical fitness guidelines were developed for consideration for air medical transport policy development:

1. Meet provisions of the FAA Class III physical exam. (See Box 49-3 for requirements.)
2. Obtain annual audiograms.
3. Report for flight duty in a mentally alert state, ready for the stress of the different working conditions and circumstances that may be encountered.
4. Be able to wear installed seat belts.

BOX 49-3 SUMMARY OF FAA CLASS III PHYSICAL REQUIREMENTS[36,71]

A. Eye
   1. Visual acuity correctable to 20/30.
   2. No serious pathology of the eye.

B. Ear, nose, throat, and equilibrium
   1. Ability to hear the whispered voice at 3 feet.
   2. No acute or chronic disease of the internal ear.
   3. No disease or malformation of the nose or throat that might interfere with, or be aggravated by flying.
   4. No disturbance in equilibrium.

C. Mental and neurologic
   1. No established medical history or clinical diagnosis of any of the following:
      a. A personality disorder that is severe enough to have repeatedly manifested itself by overt acts.
      b. A psychosis.
      c. Alcoholism, unless there is established clinical evidence, satisfactory to the Federal Air Surgeon, of recovery, including sustained total abstinence from alcohol for not less than the preceding 2 years. As used in this section, "alcoholism" means a condition in which a person's intake of alcohol is great enough to damage physical health or personal or social functioning, or when alcohol has become a prerequisite to normal functioning.
   2. No other personality disorder, neurosis, or mental condition that makes the applicant unable to safely perform the duties of air medical personnel.
   3. No established medical history or clinical diagnosis of:
      a. Epilepsy.
      b. A disturbance of consciousness without satisfactory medical explanation of the cause.
   4. No other convulsive disorder, or disturbance of consciousness that makes the applicant unable to safely perform the duties as air medical personnel.

D. Cardiovascular
   1. No established medical history or clinical diagnosis of:
      a. Myocardial infarction.
      b. Angina pectoris.
      c. Coronary heart disease that has required treatment or, if untreated, that has been symptomatic or clinically significant.

E. General medical condition
   1. No established medical history or clinical diagnosis of diabetes mellitus that requires insulin or any other hypoglycemic drug for control.
   2. No other organic, functional, or structural disease, defect, or limitation that makes the applicant unable to safely perform the duties of air medical personnel.

5. Carry a stretcher loaded with 100 lb assisted by one partner and load the same stretcher into the helicopter with one partner's assistance.
6. Do chest compressions for 5 continuous minutes in the aircraft.
7. In the event of pregnancy, the flight nurse will be expected to comply with the above standards and, within 4 weeks of diagnosis, provide written medical clearance to continue as a crew member. This clearance will include indication that the obstetrician is aware of the above activities. After the 20th week of pregnancy, written medical clearance is required every 2 weeks until removal from flight duty is recommended by the obstetrician. Upon written recommendation from the physician that the nurse shall not continue on flight duty, the flight nurse will be reassigned to the nursing float pool until the end of parental or maternity leave.[71]

These guidelines were based on a consensus by 75% or more respondents and not developed as a standard. They were presented as a working draft by which transport programs could develop their own mission-specific policies. Medical conditions which are considered a disability should be evaluated by the medical director to determine whether the risk of injury in the transport environment is increased for the applicant and others. Examples of these conditions include asthma; hearing loss greater than 25 decibels in the 500, 1000, 2000, and 3000 Hz frequencies, as measured by an audiometer; heart murmurs; history of back pain; migraines or chronic headaches; seizure disorders; thyroid and endocrine disorders, to name a few.[12]

Reporting to work in a mentally alert state is a subjective criterion but may be further expanded by addressing the use of antihistamines, prescription drugs, and/or alcohol consumption prior to duty. It is generally accepted that medication which may impair judgment or create drowsiness is not consumed within 8 hours of starting duty. This time criteria includes alcohol consumption. Personnel donating blood should not work within a 72 hour period after the donation, since physical performance may be impacted.[12]

Other areas that may need to be addressed in policy development may include carrying of special equipment (e.g., isolettes), ability to complete special procedures such as rappelling or hot off loading from a hover if search and rescue is included in the program's mission profile, weight and height ratio limits as defined by standard charts and aircraft limits, and requirements for ground transport. Endurance, muscle tone, and agility are areas that require further evaluation regarding their impact on transport personnel. A weight reduction, muscle toning, and endurance enhancing physical maintenance program may serve the system well if it helps prevent injuries and paid time off for those who are not "in shape."

Scheduling practices. In order to optimize transport personnel's performance and reinforce safe operations, personnel must be alert and well-rested. Scheduling of 24 hour shift coverage for health care providers has been controversial for a long time. Impaired performance has been related to interruptions in circadian rhythms, duration of shifts, and cumulative sleep loss. Not only have shifts been demonstrated to affect performance, but they also affect transport personnel's quality of life and relationships with family and friends. Chronobiologists who study the effect of time on living organisms have shown that fixed, rapidly rotating, and weekly rotating shift schedules impact negatively on an individual's performance. They have also shown that, in order to maximize performance, shifts should be changed infrequently in a forward rotating direction (i.e., day to evening to night for 8 hour shifts) with days off scheduled to maximize transition between shifts.[54] In addition, the total number of phase shifts, days to nights or nights to days, should be kept to a minimum. Each phase shift results in transient internal desynchronization (TID). Metabolic processes and energy levels are decreased and produce feelings of fatigue, decreased reaction times, and time disorientation. The effects of a phase shift may be diminished if personnel are permitted to sleep during the night shift.[18]

Helicopter Hospital Emergency Medical Evacuation Service (HEMES) pilots by regulation are required to have 10 consecutive hours of rest before reporting to duty. FAR 135.271 also limits the total flight time to 8 hours in a 24 hour period. If a pilot is on duty for 24 hours, he/she is also required to have 8 previously declared consecutive hours of rest during that period. This means that a pilot, by law, may turn a flight down if he/she is not going to be able to obtain an 8 hour rest period in that stretch of 24 hours. A busy shift may require a change in personnel to continue operations legally. In addition, the maximum on-duty assignment may not exceed 72 hours. To emphasize the importance of safe operations and rested pilots, the FAA recommends that no less than four pilots be assigned to each aircraft in programs providing 24 hour consecutive EMS/H coverage.[35,68]

As previously mentioned, these restrictions exist for those who fly the aircraft, but not for those who fix them. Mechanics are required to have at least 24 consecutive hours off during any seven consecutive days, or the equivalent of that, within one calendar month.[35] There are no restrictions for the number of hours in a day that a mechanic may work. If alternative aircraft are not available, this could result in abuse if the flight program "must get back into service for the good of mankind."

In the 1993 Air Medical Program Survey, air medical crews consisted of nurses, doctors, paramedics, and other personnel. Their duty shifts were described as 8 hours (3%), 12 hours (63%), 24 hours (10%), 12 and 24 hours (19%), and other (5%). Twelve hour shift utilization was down by 19% from the previous year. This ended a steady trend of increased utilization since 1988. On the other hand, 12 and 24 hour shifts were up 19%, while other undefined alternatives had increased by 4%.[14]

Developing parameters for scheduling which optimizes personnel performance and safety is a vital key to prevention. Although 24 hour shift coverage is an unavoidable practice in health care, it is a particularly risky procedure in the transport environment because requests for patient transfers may take personnel far from their base prior to oncoming relief. This leads to extended shifts, inadequate rest, and a return to duty the next day to begin the vicious cycle over again. Compounded by several transports in the day or night, rotating shifts, and not enough time off to recover from the previous duty shifts, the individual and program are potentially headed for disaster. As a result of this dilemma, the National Flight Nurse Association (NFNA) published its position as ". . . performance, alertness, and decision making would be improved if: . . . Provisions are made by all HEMS programs to assure that flight nurses receive a minimum of 10 hours of uninterrupted rest in any twenty-four hour period with back-up personnel identified to assume relief from duty if an air-medical crew member is excessively fatigued at any time."[54] They also cited the scheduling guidelines recommended by chronobiologists to maximize rest and performance. These positions were based on published research which demonstrated that alertness, fine motor skills, and judgment deteriorated when rest was not obtained.

Stress management. Stress is the condition in which the body responds to demands placed upon it. Stress results from a perceived imbalance between a demand and the individual's ability to meet the demand. Demands may be physical and involve environmental factors such as temperature and humidity extremes, noise, vibration, and/or lack of oxygen.[42] These stressors are frequently seen within the transport environment and particularly with flight. The eight stresses of flight include barometric pressure changes and hypoxia as altitude increases, thermal changes, gravitational forces, decreased humidity, noise, and vibration, all of which compound to produce fatigue.[47] In like manner, it is not unusual to find extreme changes in temperature, possibly changes in altitude, loud noises with sirens, and ambulance compartments encompassed with vibrations during ground transports. As a result, the general transport environment is fraught with physical stressors.

The second class of stressors are physiologic. They include fatigue, lack of physical fitness, sleep loss, missed meals which lead to hypoglycemia, discomfort associated with a full bladder or bowel, and any disease, chronic or acute, which the body may be battling. In addition, there are psychological stressors such as financial commitments, job pressures, family responsibilities, or the mental workload related to certain tasks or projects.[42] Life stressors, both good and bad, have been studied and rated to determine their impact on an individual's stress response. It was found that if the stress is severe enough that disease will result. Individual's with life change units (LCU) totaling between 150 and 199 points experienced health changes within a two year period (37%). For those experiencing LCUs between 200 and 299, 51% reported health changes. 79% had injuries or illnesses if their LCUs totaled over 300. Usually, health changes followed life crises by approximately one year.[43] See Table 49-4 for the Social Readjustment Rating Scale.

All of these factors combine to create stress and the body responds in three stages. The first stage is the alarm reaction in which the body recognizes the stressor and prepares for flight or fight. Fear produces a huge burst of energy, increases muscle strength, and enhances hearing and vision. Short-term, adrenalin produces an increased level of alertness and a greater capability to find the solution to the stressor. On the other hand, anger (fight) increases the blood pressure and does not enhance decision making.[42]

After the body recognizes and responds to the stressor, the resistance stage enables it to repair any damages or adapt to the stressor. The first two stages are frequently gone through, since individuals must cope with

TABLE 49-4 SOCIAL READJUSTMENT RATING SCALE[113]

Life event	*Value*	*Life event*	*Value*
Death of spouse	100	In-law troubles	29
Divorce	73	Outstanding personal achievement	28
Marital separation from mate	65	Wife beginning or ending work outside of home	26
Detention in jail or other institution	63	Beginning or ending formal education	26
Death of close family member	63	Major change in living conditions (i.e., new home, remodeling, deterioration in home or neighborhood)	25
Major personal injury/illness	53	Revision of personal habits	24
Marriage	50	Troubles with the boss or instructor	23
Being fired at work	47	Major change in working hours or conditions	20
Marital reconciliation with mate	45	Change in residence	20
Retirement from work	45	Changing to a new school	20
Major change in health or behavior of family member	44	Major change in type/amount of recreation	19
Pregnancy	40	Major change in quantity of church activities	19
Sexual difficulties	39	Major change in social activities	18
Changing a new family member	39	Taking out a minor purchase loan	17
Major business readjustment (i.e. merger, reorganization, bankruptcy, etc.)	39	Major change in sleeping habits—quantity or time of day	16
Major change in financial state	38	Major change in number of family get-togethers	15
Death of close friend	37	Major change in eating habits—quantity, time of day, or setting	15
Changing to different work line	36	Vacation	13
Major change in number of arguments with spouse	35	Christmas	12
Taking out mortgage or loan for major purchase	31	Minor violations of law	11
Foreclosure on mortgage or loan	30	12 MONTH TOTAL	____
Major change in work responsibilities (i.e. promotion, demotion, transfer)	29		
Son or daughter leaving home	29		

Reprinted with permission from The Social Readjustment Rating Scale, Oxford.

physical and emotional stressors daily. However, if the stress continues, the body will remain in the state of readiness for fight or flight until it is no longer able to keep up with the demand. This leads to the final stage of exhaustion.[42] Generally, stress may cause fatigue which is characterized by a decrease in work capacity and performance, a feeling of tiredness, and a desire to rest.

As previously mentioned, the demands of the transport environment are encumbered with stressors that include the physical environment of the aircraft or ambulance, the mental and physical challenges of caring for and transporting critically ill or injured patients in mobile surroundings, the unknown timetable of transport scheduling, and poor scheduling methodology. In addition, self-imposed stressors may compound the effects of stress and result in fatigue within the work place. Self-imposed stressors encompass:

Drugs
Exhaustion
Alcohol
Tobacco
Hypoglycemia.[45]

As a result, individual recognition and stress management programs are needed to support the well-being of transport personnel.

Reducing stress starts with recognizing its existence and working towards individual control of self. This is vital to avoid anxiety, deteriorating performance, and panic. Every attempt must be made to reduce fatigue by maintaining good general physical fitness, limiting self-imposed stressors, maintaining good living conditions, and improving working conditions to the best possible level. High workload conditions, a source of acute situational stress, may produce uncertainty, tunnel vision, errors, and erratic performance which does not usually adhere to normal performance standards. These situations must be managed by delegating, prioritizing, and preplanning actions to expand available emergency response time in order to avoid unsafe performance.[45] If transport personnel are unable to manage the day to day stressors placed upon them, stress management programs may need to be sought from clergy, social services, critical incident specialists, or psychologists.

Pregnancy. When evaluating the need for a pregnancy policy, each transport program will need to evaluate the maternal and fetal risks for the transport team member and the operational priorities of the program. A high level of performance must be maintained for the program so that safe operations and patient care are not jeopardized. Since no universal policy exists for pregnant air medical personnel at this point in time, the decision will need to be collaborative among the medical director, director of operations, department head or chief flight nurse, the individual, and their obstetrician. Recently, many flight programs were polled to determine what type of policies were in existence. The responses ranged from no policy at all to requiring a date when the medical crew member would terminate flight status. There is no consistency among flight programs as to when flying should cease.[24]

Many factors relating to the pregnancy must be constantly evaluated by the individual to be maintained on active flight status. How severe is the nausea and vomiting? What degree of fatigue is she experiencing? In the third trimester, will she be able to perform all her duties without deterioration in care and safety? Will she be able to safely enter and exit the aircraft and be able to be securely strapped?

The most obvious question in addressing this issue is the effect of fetal oxygenation at varying altitudes. A recent study was conducted to determine if there were any fetal changes as altitude increased. The pregnant women were on a commercial airline with cabin pressures of 2,395 m (7,855 ft). Despite a maternal drop of 25% in oxygen tension, there was no significant fetal distress detected.[44]

A few minor performance alterations may be made in order to assist the pregnant transport team member to continue active flight status. She may need assistance with lifting and a change in scheduling patterns (i.e., 12 hr shifts to 8 hour shifts). To combat nausea and vomiting, she may try crackers, eating smaller more frequent meals, or sitting in a forward facing seat.[24]

With so many different responses to pregnancy, a rigid policy is not feasible. There will need to be areas for deviation. When developing a pregnancy policy, one should incorporate options for alternative duties, overtime and scheduling, replacement during maternity leave, and multiple pregnancies within the transport team at any given time. In addition, the individual's obstetrician must be made aware of the physical requirements of transport duty. Encompassed in knowing what the job entails, continuation of transport duty must be confirmed by that individual with each obstetrical visit.

This is a very delicate issue. Policies need to be adopted so as not to discriminate against a pregnant employee while ensuring optimum operations within the transport program.

OSHA. In order to make the workplace safe, the Occupational Safety and Health Administration (OSHA) has developed extensive regulations for which employers and employees must adhere to or become subject to legal proceedings and fines. For the medical transport profession, operational procedures and clinical practice will be impacted by the regulations which address hearing protection, chemical exposure, and bloodborne pathogens. There are a lot of changes occurring with the interpretation of these regulations for the transport environment, and it is vital to stay current with any modifications.

Hearing protection. In the United States approximately 15 million workers are exposed to excessive noise levels. More than 8 million of these workers have been left with some degree of noise induced hearing loss.[41] With these staggering statistics, the transport profession must try to prevent any further casualties of hearing dysfunction.

From a recent hearing protection policy survey mailed to 121 air medical transport programs, only 44% of the 77 respondents had a written policy regarding auditory testing. All aircraft have varying degrees of noise levels internally and externally. For example, the noise levels of a BK-117 reach almost 110 decibels depending on the location of the reading (Figure 49-4).[62] As a result, it is very important not to forget about hearing conservation for all flight crew, air medical personnel and individuals interfacing with the aircraft.

Not only are flight crew members at risk for hearing impairment, but studies have shown that ambulance personnel may be exposed to noise levels exceeding occupational standards. Hearing loss in EMS drivers has been associated with the sirens located on the cabin roof and with opened windows.[27]

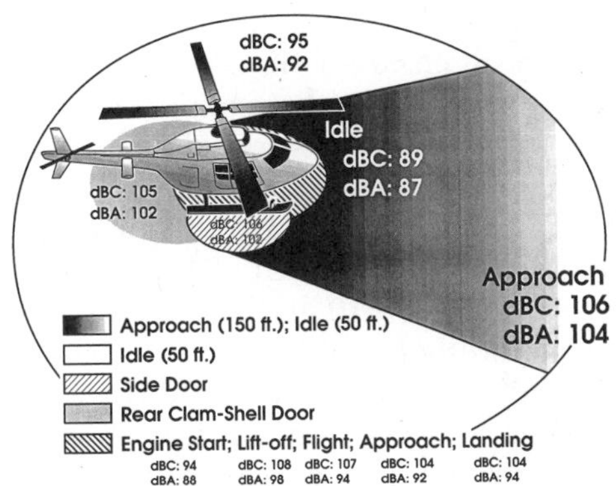

Fig. 49-4. Noise Levels Surrounding a BK-117

OSHA has devised a standard in order to protect workers from excessive sound levels. Permissible noise exposures are shown in Table 49-5. When any worker is subjected to levels greater than those in the standard, personal protective equipment must be provided by the employer at no cost to the employee. The employer must also develop a hearing conservation plan which includes exposure monitoring, employee notification, observation of monitoring, audiometric testing, and the evaluation of audiogram follow-up procedures for deviations found during the audiogram.[20]

All employees will be provided with the levels of noise exposure. It is also the responsibility of the employer to provide audiomet-

TABLE 49-5 PERMISSIBLE OCCUPATIONAL NOISE EXPOSURES[20]

Duration per day (hours)	*Sound level dBA slow response*
6	90
6	92
4	96
3	97
2	100
1.5	102
1	105
0.5	110

ric testing performed by licensed or certified personnel at no cost to the employee. A baseline audiogram must be completed prior to being exposed to the work related noise. At least annually, follow-up audiograms will be performed and compared to previous tests for Standard Threshold Shift (STS). STS is an average change of 10 decibels or more in the hearing threshold relative to the baseline audiogram at 2000, 3000 and 4000 Hz in either ear. Each test will be conducted at least 14 hours after the final work noise exposure or nonoccupational noise.[20]

OSHA also requires that records be maintained on individual audiogram results, calibration of audiometric equipment, and workplace noise level exposures. Specific criteria may be obtained from the Code of Federal Regulations, Labor 29, Hearing Standards and Amendments. OSHA requires all noise exposure records be retained for a period of 2 years and audiometric test records for the duration of employment. An employee may have access to any of these records upon request.[20]

Once the employer provides hearing protection, it is also their responsibility to provide proper training for the use and care of the devices. They are responsible for ensuring that personnel adhere to the hearing protection policy. The employer must also confirm that the specific protector used provides the adequate noise reduction for the environment in which the employee is exposed.[20]

Instituting a hearing conservation policy is the first step to ensure that each transport team member preserves their valuable gift of hearing. Failure to comply to any of these regulations may result in a substantial monetary fine.

Right to Know Act. In the transport environment the OSHA regulations and the Right to Know Act impact all involved. Transport personnel must be advised of any hazardous substances they may come in contact with while working. These hazardous materials include infectious secretions, radioactive matter, chemicals, cytotoxic materials, and gaseous substances. The act requires that personnel be provided with an annual updated list of any hazardous substance used in the workplace. They must be oriented to and trained for the safe use, proper handling, storage, emergency exposure procedures, and disposal methods for each hazardous substance. Appropriate safety equipment must be made available for the substance being handled. Transport team members must also be informed of the location and use of this equipment. Safe handling procedures are to be monitored. Policies and procedures must be in place and revised as needed to address these requirements.[57]

OSHA has developed the hazardous communication standard, HAZCOM, for keeping employees informed. The transport team's HAZCOM program should include the development and implementation of a written HAZCOM program, mechanisms to identify and track chemical hazards with Material Safety Data Sheets, chemical warning labels and warning devices, employee training, and accidental exposure procedures. All hazardous materials must have warning labels indicating the degree of health hazard, the degree of fire hazard or flash point, the degree of reactivity, and if the substance has special hazard precautions (i.e., water reactive, oxidizer, radioactive, or corrosive). It is the responsibility of each employee, as outlined by OSHA, to be familiar with the policies and procedures and to safely use all available personal safety equipment. Each team member is also responsible for reporting any adverse occurrences associated with the listed hazardous substances.[57]

Bloodborne pathogens. With the increasing public awareness of diseases being spread through blood contamination, OSHA developed standards for exposure to bloodborne pathogens which were instituted March 6, 1992. OSHA's standards were instituted to protect the more than 5 million health care providers in the United States who are at risk for occupational exposure to bloodborne pathogens. Two viruses have been specifically targeted by these standards, the human immunodeficiency virus (HIV) and the hepatitis B virus (HBV). Even though the chances of contracting either of these diseases is relatively low, health care workers may further minimize and potentially eliminate the spread of these diseases in the work environment through prevention.

Any employee at risk for occupational exposure to bloodborne pathogens is covered by the OSHA regulations. As defined by OSHA, an exposure is any "reasonably anticipated skin, eye, mucous membrane, or parenteral (i.e., needlestick) contact with blood or other potentially infectious material that results from the performance of an employee's duties."[21] In the transport environment, others will be subject to these regulations and include police, fire fighters, EMS personnel, and pilots.

OSHA has defined other types of potentially infectious material besides blood. They include all human body fluids, any unfixed human tissue or organ, blood or organs from infected experimental animals, and cultures of solutions containing HIV or HBV. Universal precautions must be used when handling any of these substances since "all blood and potentially infectious materials other than blood must be handled as if infected because it is impossible to determine if a patient or blood specimen is infected."[21] Practicing universal precautions is a vital step in complying with the OSHA standards and protecting oneself.

Under these same guidelines, any employee who is at risk for exposure to HBV may elect to be vaccinated against HBV within ten working days of starting employment. The vaccine is provided as a series of three intramuscular injections. The most common side effect is soreness at the injection site. Exemptions from this regulation include those previously vaccinated, those with HBV immunity, and when the vaccine is medically contraindicated. An employee may decline the vaccination but is mandated to sign a declaration that the vaccine is being refused. The employee may change their mind at any time and still receive the vaccine free of charge. If an employee has a positive HBV exposure, postexposure preventive treatment must also be made available. The intramuscular injection of immunoglobulin will be given to provide passive immunity to HBV after the exposure.[4,21]

Every employer is required to have a written exposure control plan. The simple goal of the plan is to eliminate or minimize exposures to infectious materials. It must include a list of job classifications in which employees are at risk for occupational exposure, a schedule for implementing the requirements on how employees will be protected and trained, a contact person if an exposure incident occurs, and a procedure to evaluate any exposure incident. Engineering controls, work practice controls, and personal protective equipment go hand in hand to eliminate or minimize exposure incidents. The use of all three control measures is mandated by OSHA.[21]

Engineering controls are items or areas which are used to isolate infectious materials away from patients and staff. They must be well maintained, pass a regularly scheduled inspection, and be repaired or replaced as needed. Examples of engineering controls include handwashing facilities which must be readily accessible. The use of antiseptic hand cleanser or towelettes may be used on a short-term basis, but hands must be washed with soap and water as soon as possible after the exposure. Containers for used sharps must be puncture resistant, leak proof, easily accessible, and labelled or color-coded for easy identification. Reusable containers must be designed so they may be emptied without risk to the person emptying them. Specimen containers used for transporting any type of specimen or contaminated object (i.e., gloves) must be kept in leak proof containers and properly labelled as regulated waste containers.[4,21]

Personal protective equipment protects employees from direct contact with blood or other potentially infectious material. It includes gloves; gowns or lab coats; face shields or masks; eye protection; and mouthpieces, resuscitation bags, and pocket masks. Personal protective equipment must be easily accessible in appropriate sizes and provided to each employee free of charge. Cleaning, disposal, repair, and replacement of personal protective equipment is also the responsibility of the employer. Selecting the appropriate protective equipment is vital.[4,21] If in doubt, use it.

Work practice controls are standards that will assist employees to perform their job in the safest manner possible. Work practice standards which must be employed include the following:

- Handwashing is the first line of defense in personal protection against bloodborne pathogens. OSHA requires that handwashing be completed immediately after removing gloves or other protective equipment. Removing devices (e.g., contaminated gloves or masks) may lead to unexpected exposures.
- Needles and sharps are to be placed in appropriate containers for disposal. OSHA standards prohibit sharps from being recapped unless there is no other alternative. If recapping is necessary, it must be completed by using a recapping device or a one handed scoop method to replace the cap.
- Handling of contaminated materials must be with techniques to prevent or minimize splashing or spraying. OSHA standards specifically prohibit pipetting or suctioning materials by mouth. If these procedures are required, mechanical means must be used.
- Food and drink must not be stored where other potentially infectious materials are kept. No eating or drinking is to occur in the work environment if any risk exists. This also includes smoking, applying cosmetics, and handling or adjusting contact lenses.
- Transported specimens must be packed in leak proof containers.
- Contaminated equipment must be cleaned appropriately prior to being repaired or shipped. If decontamination is not possible, appropriate labelling must be used to identify the source(s) of contamination.
- Routine cleaning is addressed in general housekeeping practices. A written schedule for cleaning and decontamination is required.
- Broken glass must be handled carefully if contaminated. NEVER pick up broken glass by hand. Use a brush and dust pan, tongs, or forceps. If the glass held any infectious material, the devices used to clean up the spill will be considered contaminated and must be handled and cleaned accordingly.
- Sharps containers must be puncture and leak proof. If moving a sharps container, care must be taken to prevent spillage.
- Contaminated laundry should be handled as little as possible. Ideally the laundry should be bagged at the site where it was used.[21]

In the transport environment, there has been extensive speculation regarding the application of these regulations. National organizations are working closely with OSHA to refine the interpretation of these standards for the transport of critically ill and injured patients.

If an accidental exposure occurs, three immediate actions are recommended.

1. Cleanse the exposed area to minimize the chance of infection,
2. Notify the designated contact person to begin documentation of the incident, then
3. Seek medical attention for treatment and evaluation.[21]

Confidential medical evaluation and follow-up are available at no charge to the employee. All lab testing will be done free of charge to the employee. The evaluation process consists of testing for HIV and HBV from the source unless it is already known that the source is positive for either disease. Identification of the source individual and disclosure of their results may vary according to state and local laws. Written documentation of the evaluation process and medical follow-up must be maintained. This includes the employee's HIV and HBV results, but the employee has the right to refuse blood collection and/or testing. If blood has been collected but no consent for HIV testing was given, the blood sample will be kept for 90 days. At any time, the employee may change their mind and consent to testing. Postexposure prophylaxis will be offered and consists of immune globulin for hepatitis B and the current recommendations from the Centers for Disease Control for HIV. Counseling and evaluation of any reported illnesses must also be provided to the employee at no cost.[4,21]

Confidential medical records will be maintained for all employees with occupational exposures. The employee has the right to view these records once the request is submitted in writing.[21]

In the mobile transport environment, the concern for bloodborne pathogen exposure may increase, secondary to continuous movement and limited disposal resources. Prevention is a priority and the exposure control plan should not be overlooked.

Training

In order to optimize the safe practices of transport personnel, standards of performance are established through operational policies and procedures. If not previously exposed to this ever changing environment, personnel need to be oriented to the demands of safe transport. Mechanisms for the maintenance of operational competency must also be established and employed. Currently, standards are being developed for competency performance by both voluntary and regulatory agencies. The ultimate goal is to prevent accidents in the transport environment, but if unexpected circumstances prevail, currency in responding to operational emergencies may minimize the extent of the emergency and associated injuries.

Pilots. Air medical professional guidelines which are reinforced in the CAAMS standards, require pilots to have a commercial rotorcraft-helicopter airman's certificate and experience levels of at least 2,000 hours of flight time as the pilot in command prior to assignment with an air medical service. Fixed wing pilots must have the same flight time experience and possess a commercial multiengine certificate. Also, fixed wing pilots must possess at least 500 hours multiengine time as pilot in command and 100 hours of night flight time within the 2,000 hours.

In addition to these minimum qualifications, CAAMS has established training and recurrency standards. Minimum helicopter training should consist of ground and flight training at a factory school for the specific helicopter model being used by the transport program. This may be substituted with an equivalent program. Between 5 and 10 flight hours as pilot in command is required prior to assuming independent functioning for EMS missions. Five hours is necessary if transitioning from a single to a single, a twin to a single, or a twin to a twin engine aircraft. If one is transitioning from a single to a twin engine aircraft, then 10 hours of flight time are required. In addition to these time requirements, at least 5 flight hours must be dedicated to orientation to the service area. This includes 2 hours which must be night flying as pilot in command. Fixed wing pilots should have 25 hours in the specific make and model of aircraft before flying as the pilot in command on patient missions.[22]

Minimum training standards have also been developed addressing the special nature of air medical transport. For helicopter pilots, they involve orientation to the following:

- Terrain and weather specific to the service area;
- Hospital or health care system sponsoring the transport program;
- Installed medical systems on the helicopter;
- Patient handling procedures which include loading, unloading, and infection control;
- EMS and public service agencies unique to the service area; and
- Inadvertent instrument meteorologic conditions (IMC) recovery procedures by instrument reference.[22]

Annual recurrency training should minimally consist of FAR Part 135 training requirements, IMC recovery procedures, flight by instrument reference, local routine operating procedures, hazards in the area's terrain, review of existing and changed referring and receiving hospital landing areas, and scene operational procedures.[22,56] Fixed wing pilots need to be oriented to and complete annual reviews in infection control, operational aspects of the installed medical systems, and procedures for loading and unloading patients.

Since air medical transport helicopters may be dispatched in less than ideal weather conditions to remote areas and the majority of all EMS accidents have been associated with weather and pilot error, the FAA has emphasized the need for training in two specific areas in Advisory Circular 135-14A. The first area is in instrument recovery from inadvertent instrument meteorologic conditions (IMC). The importance of this training has also been identified by CAAMS. To legally maintain instrument currency, a pilot must have six instrument approaches and 6 hours in actual IMC or under "the hood" for simulated conditions within the preceding 6 months. This does not necessarily make the pilot proficient or highly skilled. Obtaining this training will enhance the pilot's ability to control the aircraft by instruments without depending on the ground as reference in order to operate the aircraft safely.

The other program highly recommended by the FAA is training in Crew Resource Management (CRM). When evaluating problems encountered by flight crews, the emphasis in the past has been to improve technology. As the quality and dependability of the machinery has improved, investigations started identifying that 60 to 80 percent of all air carrier incidents and accidents were the result of human factors. Problems were associated with poor group decision-making, ineffective communication, inadequate leadership, and poor task or resource management. In all civil helicopter accidents, pilot error has been assigned as the causative factor 64% of the time. This statistic increases to 90% for accidents occurring during EMS missions.[34] As a result Crew (originally Cockpit) Resource Management programs were developed in the aviation profession to optimize the use of all available human, hardware, and information resources. Human resources encompass all those individuals working with the cockpit personnel, such as dispatchers, cabin crew members, maintenance personnel, and air traffic controllers. The goal is to prevent aviation accidents by optimizing the human/machine interface and accompanying interpersonal activities. Critical decision-making requires appropriate problem and resource identification, prioritization of responses, delegation of responsibilities, and planning to expand available response time. With the focus on safety in the air medical profession, CRM training programs are being developed for single pilot EMS helicopter operations.

Aircraft mechanics. To facilitate the safe flying experience of the pilots, mechanics have also been recommended to be factory schooled or its equivalency in an approved program and FAR 135 qualified to maintain the aircraft used by the air medical service. In addition, lead mechanics of these programs must be certified airframe and power plant (A & P) mechanics. These individuals require training specific to the interior modifications of the aircraft. Inspection of the installed medical equipment, its removal, and reinstallation is particularly vital. In addition, they need supplemental training on servicing and maintenance of the medical oxygen systems.[22]

Medical personnel. Education specific to the transport environment consists of patient assessment, treatment, preparation, and handling and equipment operation. EMS communications with radios and familiarization with the EMS system is necessary to operate safely. These areas pertain to both air and ground transport. In addition, air medical transport requires special understanding of day and night flying protocols, survival training pertinent to the geographic service area of the transport program, aircraft safety reviews, and ground operations. Aircraft safety reviews should consist of at least the following:

- Aircraft evacuation procedures;
- Emergency communications and frequency use;
- In-flight and on the ground fire suppression;
- In-flight emergency and emergency landing procedures (i.e., crash positions, oxygen shut off, equipment securing, and emergency fuel shut off);
- Use of the emergency locator transmitter (ELT); and
- Specific capabilities, limitations, and safety measures used for each aircraft.

Requirements for landing site establishment on scenes of accidents and notification of landing zone changes at hospitals should be understood. Patient loading and unloading during normal and "hot" situations must be practiced, as well as refueling during normal and emergency situations. These operational topics should be incorporated into the orientation and at least an annual safety review.[22] The frequency of reviews may need to be increased if flight personnel are not exposed to the air medical transport environment daily.

Ambulance drivers. The operator and the ambulance are the most basic aspects to be considered for safe ground transports. The driver's attitude is a good tool to use when determining a candidate for operating the vehicle. Qualities to look for in candidates include courtesy, patience, dependability, and consideration for others. Driving an emergency vehicle can be stressful. This stress may be intensified when transporting a pediatric patient. Not only does the driver have the lives of the patient and the crew as his or her responsibility, but the driver must be constantly aware of the persons and environment around the ambulance which may impact completion of the transport. For this reason good mental and physical health is imperative when choosing an emergency medical vehicle operator.[59]

Driving an emergency vehicle should not be compared with driving a car. Simple tasks like braking, steering, backing up, and parking become more difficult maneuvers in a larger, heavier, more powerful vehicle.[65] Being a safe emergency medical vehicle operator means having the proper attitude, sufficient knowledge, specialized training, and the skills to drive a vehicle which may exceed 11,000 pounds. There are few formal driver training courses offered for emergency vehicle operators. Most learn from on-the-job training. For those who are fortunate to be offered a training course, EVADE (Emergency Vehicle Advanced Driver Education) and the Failsafe Driving System are two examples of formal programs.

EVADE combines classroom instruction along with driving exercises in a modified ambulance named MERV (Multiple Emergency Response Vehicle). Using MERV allows students to experience power steering and brake failures and tire blow outs at 35 mph. This enables the driver to practice reacting to the unexpected in a controlled environment. Even the experienced driver will be surprised at what may be learned in this type of program.[70]

The Failsafe Driving System focuses on two types of driving strategies, high forces and low forces. The goal to practicing high force driving is to escape a dangerous situation, such as rapid lane changes, skid recovery, or off road control, once they have been introduced. On the other hand, low force driving focuses on awareness of surroundings in order to prevent the need to perform any high risk maneuver.[65]

Communications personnel. Little has been said to this point about the importance of communications personnel in regards to safety, but as the "hub" of coordination for all aspects of the transport program, these individuals play a vital role. Whether it is obtaining the initial transport information from the requesting parting or tracking the location of all the program's vehicles, communicators are a major link in the safety program's chain. Toward this end, they must be trained in ground to ground and air telecommunications for dispatching and following the progress of transports in accordance with the FCC. They must be oriented to the geographical service area with instructions in local map reading and aeronautical chart interpretation. This knowledge requires further expansion by providing training in basic navigation, weather terminology, and procedures for flight service weather advisories. The communications personnel will be the first to identify or be notified that an incident or accident has occurred. As a result, they need initial and ongoing training in incident response coordination and public relations techniques.[7]

Ground personnel. Inherent to safe operations is the coordinated interface with personnel who use the transport system for critically ill and injured patients. In order to appropriately use the system, they must be educated regarding the available transport vehicles, their advantages and limitations, and methods for requesting services. When accessing air medical transport resources, these individuals must also know how to operate safely around aircraft. Safety programs should be developed for hospital, industrial, public safety, law enforcement, and EMS personnel. These presentations provide instructions on safe operations for landings, departures, and loading/unloading of patients. Programs should include the following areas:

- Landing zone designation and preparation;
- Safety in and around the helicopter;
- Loading and unloading of the aircraft with rotors running and after shut-down;
- Procedures for day and night operations into and out of unprepared landing zones;
- Communications and coordination procedures with ground personnel;
- Emergency procedures and responses for emergency landing, fuel leaks, aircraft evacuation, and fire suppression; and
- Handling of oxygen and other equipment around aircraft.[22,35]

Without properly trained ground personnel, unexpected incidents may end in catastrophic results because someone did not know how to operate around an aircraft. Catastrophic does not always imply immediate loss of life, limb, or property. It may mean that the aircraft is rendered inoperable because a stretcher was not properly prepared for transferring a patient and linen was drawn into the engine's air intake. Delays in transport may result in irreversible repercussions in the patient's clinical progress.

Patient safety-special scenarios

Epiglottitis and upper airway obstruction. When a transport team receives a call for a child with the possible diagnosis of epiglottitis, all team members must realize the role that safety plays in the outcome of this potential fatal disease. The standard of care for epiglottitis is for the child to be taken to the operating room before transfer for emergent artificial airway placement in a controlled environment, that is, in an operating room with an anesthesiologist. Many facilities are not equipped to handle this type of medical emergency and will request that the child be transported to a pediatric tertiary care facility.

When the transport team arrives, the major concern will be to keep the child calm. If after the initial assessment the team decides the child can be safely transported to the pediatric center without endotracheal intubation, special arrangements should be made to have the parent or guardian accompany the child. This will usually prevent the child from becoming emotionally upset with the separation.[10,63,69] Securing both the parent and the child on the stretcher together while allowing the child to maintain a position of comfort works best. The parent may administer the oxygen by whatever method the child will tolerate. It will be the responsibility of the team members to monitor the child for any signs or symptoms of worsening airway obstruction. Once at the receiving facility, it may be necessary to take the child directly to the operating room for immediate airway intervention.

If the child has an endotracheal tube before transport, extreme caution will be needed to prevent accidental dislodgement. Elbow restraints and limb restraints may be beneficial, but the child will usually require substantial intravenous sedation. If intravenous sedation is not adequate, the team may need to also use a muscle relaxant to protect the airway. Adequate ventilatory support should be used to maintain a normal oxygen saturation and good chest rise on inspiration.[6] This protocol may be used not only for the child with epiglottitis but for any child with upper airway obstruction.

Car seats. When called upon to safely transport pediatric patients, securing these small bodies to large, adult-sized stretchers may be a problem. One should be knowledgeable about the national public awareness and how all 50 states require children under the age of 4 years to be secured in a child safety seat while riding in a car.[3] These patients should be secured to a stretcher, secured to a stretcher with the parent, or in a child safety seat secured either to the stretcher or to the jump seat. One should not allow parents or a team member to hold the child during transport. It is common for a child to cry when separated from the parent or guardian.[6] Fortunately, they will usually stop crying once out of site of the parent or they will fall asleep once surrounded by the constant hum of the engine.

The two methods of securing an infant or child to a stretcher are using the straps or a safety seat. When using straps, at least two should cross the patient either in a crisscross fashion across the chest or one across the chest and one just above the knees (Figure 49-5A). This may require repositioning the adult arrangement of straps or by adding another set. For the older child, an alternative method would be to use a shoulder harness in addition to a thigh strap. The shoulder harness will provide better stability over the chest and shoulders (Figure 49-5B). These restraint methods would be the most appropriate if the patient is in any way unstable.

If transport personnel believe that the infant or child is stable enough to be transported safely in a safety seat, then this is an acceptable option (Figure 49-6). Several examples of clinical conditions in which safety seats may be used include pharyngitis, failure to thrive, mild electrolyte imbalances, and a foreign body in the esophagus or stomach. For interfacility transports, the parent may volunteer the use of their own car seat. Be aware of the differences among these seats. An infant seat is made for infants from birth to 20 pounds (9 kg) only.[2] Infants without good head control, regardless of age, should be placed rear facing in the vehicle.[38] This may be done by securing the car seat to the stretcher. A convertible seat is one in which a

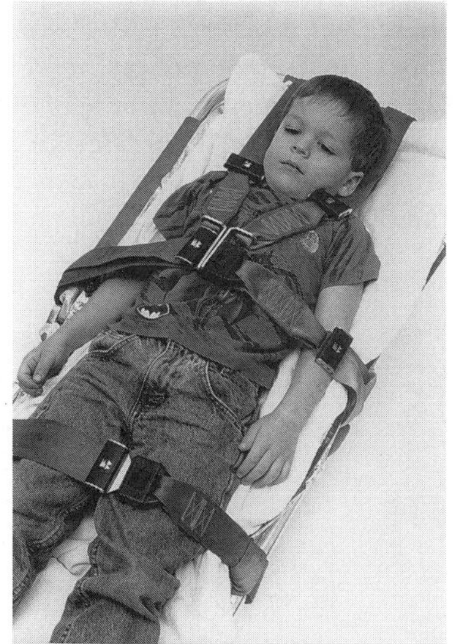

A

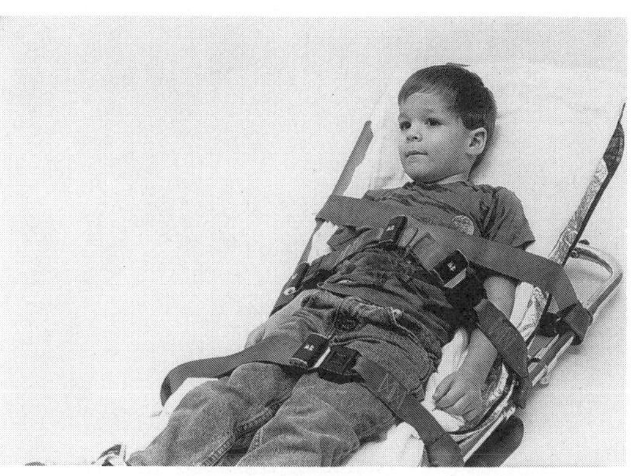

B

Fig. 49-5A,B. (A) Stretcher Restraint with Shoulder Straps (B) Stretcher Restraint with Head Elevated (Courtesy Children's Hospital, Medical Media, Pittsburgh, Pa.)

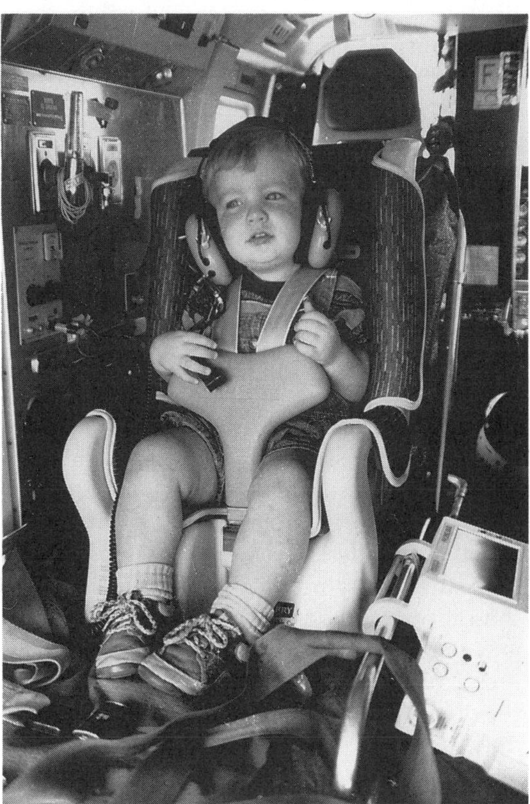

Fig. 49-6. Safety Seat Secured on Stretcher (Courtesy Children's Hospital, Medical Media, Pittsburgh, Pa.)

child from birth to 40 pounds (18 kg) may be safely restrained.[2] Frequently a cushioned insert is used for the smaller infant to provide a better fit. All child safety seats manufactured after 1985 must also comply with FAA Regulations to be an approved safety seat for use in commercial aircraft.[33]

Child safety seats may also be used when transporting children from the scene of an accident. Good assessment skills are needed prior to determining if this may be done without causing further harm to the child. The assessment should reveal a child not in shock, without hidden sources of bleeding, and with external bleeding only on exposed areas. If all these criteria are met then a decision may be made to safely transport the child in the seat. The head may be taped directly to the car seat for cervical immobilization.[15]

Restraints. As previously mentioned, all patients being transported will be required to be restrained with the appropriate safety straps. If these straps fail to protect the patient or the entire crew, then further measures must be taken. These may include the use of limb restraints, leather restraints, or the use of pharmacological agents. Patients which may require additional restraining measures include those with psychiatric problems, head injuries, and known seizure disorders; those who are intoxicated, under the influence of psychotropic agents, or suicidal; or any patient who the pilot/driver feels represents a danger.[54] If the use of physical restraints is required, these restraints may only be attached to the stretcher. In an emergency situation, the patient may still be removed on the stretcher without further removing the restraints.

Although the incidence is low, if the patient is in the custody of a law enforcement officer, the patient may need to be restrained using the officer's handcuffs. Again, the handcuffs may only be attached to the stretcher. In this case, arrangements may need to be made for the officer to accompany the patient. A policy that addresses transporting the officer's firearm will need to be developed.

Isolettes. The use of an isolette will be required when transporting an ill neonate. The isolette must be capable of providing temperature regulation, oxygen, and humidity while allowing for visibility and emergency access to the infant.[1] Methods for securing this isolette in all vehicles will need to be evaluated prior to purchasing the unit for the transport system's use. Stretcher mounts vary in transport vehicles. The isolette may need to be secured in an ambulance by using straps. A special mounting system is required in rotor or fixed wing aircraft (Figure 49-7). The use of this equipment must be inspected and approved by the FAA prior to use with a patient. In aircraft the isolette must be able to withstand 9.0 G forward, 6.6 G downward, 3.0 G upward, and 1.5 G lateral impact forces. Tie downs or mounts which secure equipment must be able to withstand 13.5 G forward, 9.9 G downward, 4.5 G upward, and 2.25 G sideward impact forces.[35] Deceleration or impact forces are dependent on the initial velocity of the object and the amount of distance it has to stop. They are expressed in meters per second or "G." The FAA also recommends the use of a cushioned head pad in the

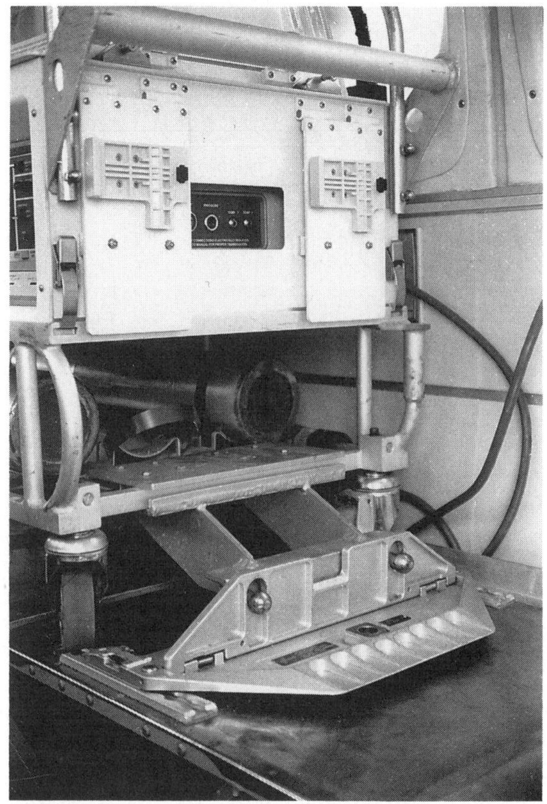

Fig. 49-7. Securing of Isolette with Bucher Mount (Courtesy Children's Hospital, Medical Media, Pittsburgh, Pa.)

isolette to protect the infants head in the event the infant would slide towards the front of the isolette. Safety restraints must be used on the infant while in the isolette to prevent sliding into the side of the isolette during normal vehicle operations.

Parent briefings. The decision to allow a parent or guardian to accompany the child during transport is a controversial issue, and in general, is not a recommended practice. Ground transports may have the room to be able to carry a parent, but there are still many things to be considered. What is the severity of the child's illness or injury? Will invasive procedures or resuscitation be required during transport? Are additional passengers insured while on the vehicle? What is the parent's or guardian's emotional state? Is there a benefit of having the parent at the tertiary care center for consent or language interpretation?[30]

In addition to these questions, there are separate issues when transporting family members in an aircraft. When considering whether to allow a parent to travel with the transport team, the pilot needs to be the first person consulted. The pilot will need to evaluate weight, balance, and aircraft performance issues. The medical crew needs to evaluate the clinical needs of the child before making the final decision. If invasive or resuscitation procedures are anticipated, the parent may not be able to emotionally handle observing what needs to be done and may inadvertently cause harm to the entire crew. The decision must be collaborative between the pilot and medical crew to justify taking the extra passenger.

Obtain a brief history from the passenger concerning motion sickness, fear of heights, claustrophobia, drug or alcohol ingestion, and inner ear problems and assess their general emotional state. Time factors may be of concern with a critically ill child who requires interventions during the trip. The parent will obviously want to know what and why these procedures are required. The crew may be distracted from the care, jeopardizing optimal care for the patient. Any one of these reasons may be cause for refusal to transport the parent or guardian.

If the decision is made to transport the parent, a thorough safety briefing must be provided by the air medical team or the pilot. This briefing includes seating arrangements, application and removal of seatbelts, use of headsets and radio etiquette, and the explanation of normal operational items such as warm-up and cool down times, aircraft vibrations, radio noise, travel time, and location of "sic-sacs" if needed. If the parent is brought in anticipation of clinical deterioration resulting from separation anxiety, this will require securing the parent on the stretcher with the child. An example of this may be seen in the case of the child with epiglottitis.

Several air medical transport programs do not allow family members to accompany the patient. Some programs require final approval from an administrator. Others may require a signed waiver for release of any liability in the event the passenger would be injured during the transport.[30] Many factors need to be considered, therefore a uniform policy may not be practical. A transport program should establish guidelines for parents or guardians accompanying children that allow some flexibility.

MINIMIZE EMERGENCY EFFECT

In the previous sections, extensive information was presented supporting accident and injury prevention. A number of these areas will also affect the extent of the emergency. Ensuring that all transport team members, patients, passengers, and equipment are secured increases the likelihood of survival in an accident. In aircraft, all installed equipment must be able to endure 9.0 G forward, 6.6 G downward, 3.0 G upward, and 1.5 G sideward impact forces.[35] The limits for tie downs and mounts are also as cited in the isolette section. Securing equipment is not enough; they must withstand the forces which would be encountered if an accident would occur. In addition, securing smaller pieces of equipment and supplies (e.g., response bags) prevents projectile objects.

The selection of a large enough landing zone without obstructions in the approach and departure paths enables the pilot to maneuver a disabled aircraft with minimal power to a hard landing, resulting in an aircraft that is damaged rather than destroyed.

The on-going emergency procedure training that pilots, medical crew members, and ambulance drivers are exposed to supports the appropriate reactions when an actual emergency occurs. The ultimate goal is to keep everyone current regarding their responsibilities during such situations and to keep the emergency in control as much as possible.

Other opportunities to minimize an emergency may be obtained through vehicle enhancements. Avionic equipment which supports safe operations during deteriorating meteorological conditions includes glide slope receivers and autopilot/stabilization capabilities. Short of being an IFR certified aircraft, these enhancements may enable the pilot to safely exit inadvertent instrument meteorologic conditions (IMC). Hopefully, the whole situation would have been avoided by using weather radar or a stormscope, although not all changing weather conditions will be detected by these instruments (e.g., fog). For those flying a single engine aircraft, transitioning to a twin engine aircraft changes an engine failure which requires autorotation to a landing with single engine power and more control. Having certified wire strike protection on the helicopter may prevent the aircraft from being incapacitated by telephone or electrical wires if inadvertently encountered during lift-off or landing.

Interior design should also be considered for both ambulances and aircraft. When studying the EMS helicopter crashes that occurred since 1972, evidence showed that occupants in the main cabin were approximately 4.5 times more at risk for experiencing an injury in survivable crashes than those individuals involved in non-EMS helicopter accidents. In addition, the EMS main cabin occupants were more likely to experience more severe injuries. This increased risk was attributed to the many changes made by the medical interior of the aircraft. This conclusion was further substantiated by 40% of all EMS respondents answering a questionnaire regarding their accident. They attributed their injuries to the on-board medical equipment.[28]

Sharp cornered designs of storage compartments should be eliminated or well padded. If the compartments are enclosed with doors, one should be sure they will not be forced open resulting in stored supplies becoming projectile objects. Equipment, such as monitors, which may protrude from the wall should be on retractable mounts. One should avoid hanging blunt, potentially penetrating (e.g., IV mounts), objects or other compartments from the ceiling. Even without an emergency, these items may become a source of injury for the distracted medical crew person who is intent on caring for the critically ill or injured patient.

MINIMIZE ACCIDENT INJURIES

Once an emergency has occurred and everything has hopefully been performed to limit its effects, the third tier of the transport program's safety plan will be launched. This is the part of the plan which was developed to minimize the amount of injuries that may occur from an accident. Addressed in this part of the plan are additional vehicle crash worthiness enhancements, post incident and accident plans, emergency procedures and crash survival techniques, personnel protective clothing, survival techniques, and emotional support.

Crash worthiness equipment enhancements

In order to make a crash survivable, the livable volume of the cabin space of the aircraft (or vehicle) must not be crushed. Enhancing crash worthiness of the vehicle enables it to withstand crash forces with minimal structural damage. Energy absorbent techniques are used to engineer a progressive structural collapse to decrease the loads on occupants. The body may endure the following impact forces:

Spineward (chest to back)	45 G for 0.044 seconds or 25 G for 0.200 seconds,
Sternumward (back to chest)	45-83 G for 0.100 seconds,
Headward	15 G for 0.150 seconds,
Tailward	15 G for 0.100 seconds, and
Lateral	20 G for 0.100 seconds.[28]

This tolerance to impact forces must be enhanced through several mechanisms.

First, as previously emphasized, restraints must be worn. Lap belts will enable the body to tolerate 15 G forward and 4 G vertical forces. Add the mandatory use of shoulder harnesses and the body will then be able to tolerate a 45 G forward and 25 G vertical force. The harness aligns the spine in an upright position to endure higher impact forces. They help prevent head injuries to enable the occupant to maintain consciousness and coherency to better deal with the emergency. Shoulder harnesses also double the injury tolerance of the body to lateral forces.[37]

Energy attenuation may then be further increased to more tolerant levels through two other enhancements. Use of energy absorbing seats with high backs enables the force of the impact to be applied to the occupant at a slower rate. With a standard seat, the occupant free-falls to the cabin floor and attempts to deform it unsuccessfully. If the seat is able to stroke or move vertically 4 inches, it will reduce the vertical loading forces from an average of 300 G to 18.6 G.[28,37] This clearly reduces the impact to a more endurable level. This advantage is only experienced if shoulder harnesses are used and if the occupant's back is snug against the seat back. Addition of energy absorbing skids further enhances these properties. This enables the skids to spread until the fuselage belly comes in contact with the ground. On the other hand, a rigid fuselage will not tolerate a high load impact.[37]

Finally, modifying aircraft with Crash Resistant Fuel Systems (CRFS) prevents massive post impact fires. This enables occupants the additional time to recover and exit the aircraft.

Emergency planning

Planning for the response to emergencies is a frequently neglected component of air medical transport programs. Although no one likes to think about an operational emergency, in actuality, a post accident and incident plan needs to be developed and practiced to increase the chances of survival for those involved. All crew members must be familiar with emergency procedures, so they become as automatic as any clinical protocol. Mock emergencies should be practiced biannually to ensure that all participants are familiar with their responsibilities.

Beginning with the communications personnel who are following the aircraft every 15 minutes, a time limit must be established for the emergency plan to be initiated if the aircraft fails to respond to the communications center. Attempts to contact the aircraft by radio for 10 minutes should be completed. Telephone inquiries to the destination site should then be made to confirm that the aircraft is overdue. The emergency plan may be initiated for medical emergencies, precautionary landings, overdue aircraft or lost communications, "MAYDAYs," and rescue and recovery for confirmed accidents. Although emergencies in aircraft may have more devastating and far reaching results, they may be used as a blueprint for similar circumstances for ground transport services.

The emergency plan may be kept in a separate binder from the rest of the operational procedures to provide easier access during these stressful events. The plan may be made in a step-by-step checklist format to ensure that all appropriate personnel and services are notified. Once the initial telephone calls are made, predesignated administrative and support personnel should arrive at the communications center. Only a limited number of individuals with specific responsibilities should be admitted to prevent chaos during communications coordination and monitoring of the radio for any distress signal from the missing aircraft. Continuation of normal operations may need to be delegated to a second communicator or an external communications center. The persons designated to respond to the communications center depends on the type of emergency and may include, but not be limited to, the medical director, director of operations, chief flight nurse or clinical supervisor, communication's supervisor, and/or a representative from the aviation or ground management firm. An alternative location should be established to allow any personnel involved in the transport program to gather for support as needed.

Since many media sources monitor EMS and fire frequencies, a flood of calls may come into the communications center. One person should be designated to handle all of the media calls to be consistent in all responses until an official, confirmed report is available. The selected individual may be the public relations spokesperson, medical director, or the aviation representative.

In the event of a confirmed emergency, the communications personnel should plot the aircraft's projected flight plan using the last known coordinates in order to mobilize assistance or initiate a search and rescue. Authorization may need to be obtained from administration to launch a second aircraft from within the program or a neighboring flight program, weather permitting, to begin the air search for the missing aircraft. Alternative air search and rescue resources may include law enforcement, military, civil air patrol, national guard, and coast guard rotorcraft or a local fixed wing aircraft. Ground search resources may be initiated by contacting local law enforcement agencies, fire and EMS, search and rescue groups, and forest rangers and park service agencies in the aircraft's anticipated flight path. Key resources for corridors and sectors within the service area should have been previously identified in the post accident/incident plan so that precious time is not lost in identifying and contacting them during the crisis. Vital information to be furnished to any search and rescue group includes:

Type and model of aircraft,
Color of the aircraft,
Number of persons on board,
Radio frequency used for transmissions, and
If an emergency locator transmitter (ELT) is on board.

Since the route of an ambulance is usually on more highly traveled roads, confirmation of a ground incident may originate from the transport team or law enforcement/EMS services which have already responded to the accident.

Once the aircraft or ambulance has been located and the nature of the emergency confirmed, arrangements for maintenance support, patient and medical crew transport completion, or emergency medical transportation of any injured must be coordinated. If the incident resulted in injuries, it is important not to transmit names of those involved over the radio.

All transport program personnel should be notified of the incident to avoid hearing about it from the media. This should be completed as early in the process as possible. Clergy and social services may be made available as needed and access of these individuals should be incorporated into the plan. Next of kin of all the transport team members involved in the incident must be notified. Another meeting place with access to clergy and social services should be set up for family members wishing to wait together. The receiving facility must be notified of the patient's delay and circumstances surrounding the delay. The patient's family may then be contacted, if needed.

Critical incident stress debriefing teams should be accessed within 24 hours of the incident in order to provide emotional support. It may be necessary to make this service available to all personnel. Many crew and family members may need long-term counseling following an emergency. All should be encouraged to seek counseling to work through the stress of the events.[46,52]

Emergency procedures

On-board emergency procedures. Prior training for any on-board emergency is the key to coping with the real situation. It is next to impossible to prepare for an ambulance accident, and only 25% of aircraft emergency landings allow time for planning.[48] For this reason, all personnel, patients, and equipment should remain securely fastened at all times.

If time allows for preparation, special attention must be directed towards removing eyeglasses, eliminating sharp objects from pockets, fastening the restraint system snugly, securing loose equipment[47] and the patient, and positioning the head of the stretcher flat. The visor of helmets should be lowered for added protection of the eyes. In addition, all sources of oxygen, on board and portable, should be turned off.

There are two types of "crash" positions which may be used. Selection of the appropriate option depends on the type of safety restraint being worn. For lap belts with shoulder harnesses, one should sit straight with feet flat on the floor, press the back firmly against the seat, and cross the arms over the chest while gripping the harness with each hand[13] (Figure 49-8). The second position will be

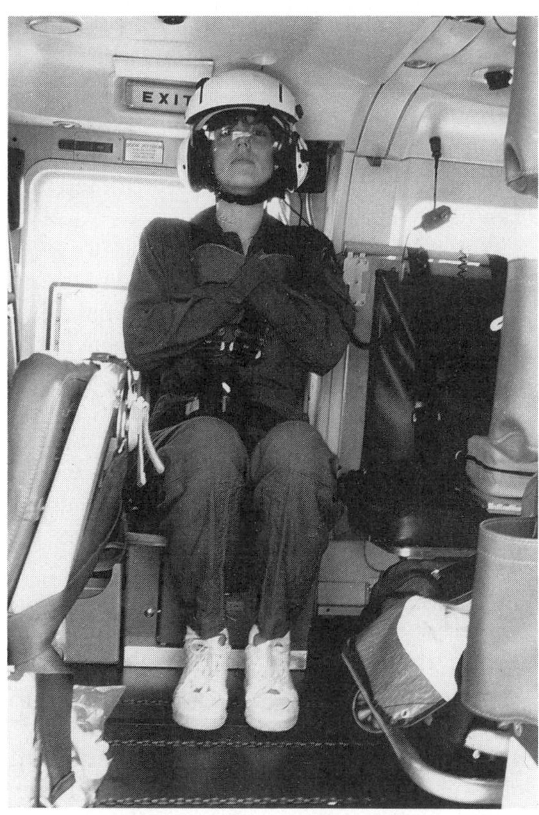

Fig. 49-8. Crash Position with Shoulder Restraints (Courtesy Children's Hospital, Medical Media, Pittsburgh, Pa.)

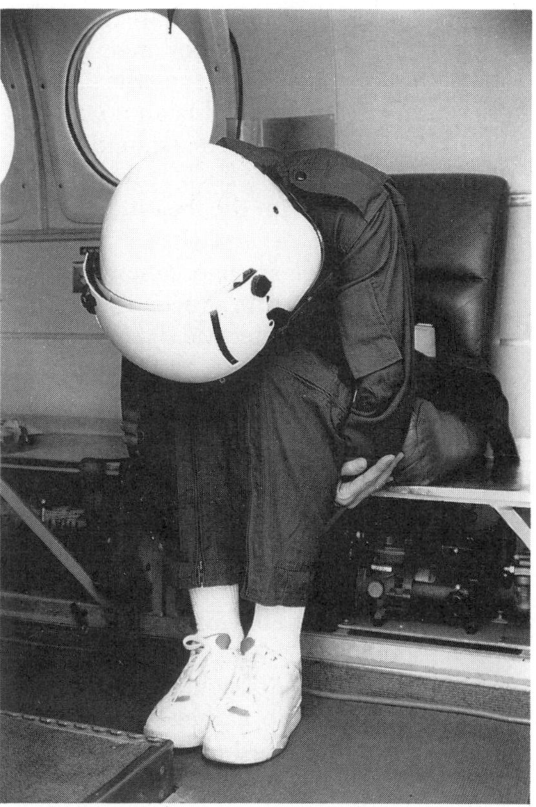

Fig. 49-9. Crash Position without Shoulder Restraints (Courtesy Children's Hospital, Medical Media, Pittsburgh, Pa.)

used if only a lap belt restraint is used. This position consists of sitting with the back pressed against the seat back, bending forward with the chest on the knees, and wrapping the arms around the thighs[13] or grasping the ankles with the hands[48] (Figure 49-9).

Other emergencies which require special training include engine failure, smoke or fire inside the aircraft, and rapid decompression. Engine failure in a twin engine aircraft may require landing at the closest airport by a helicopter or fixed wing aircraft, but the pilot's judgement to continue on with the flight is an alternative option. A single engine aircraft, on the other hand, will require the initiation of immediate emergency landing measures.[47]

Any smoke or fire must be reported to the pilot immediately. The pilot will turn off all electrical sources. Oxygen must also be turned off as soon as possible. All crew members must know the location and function of on-board fire extinguishers. It will be at the pilot's discretion whether the extinguisher will be used while still airborne.[47] Premature ignition of the fire extinguisher may obscure the pilot's vision and create a more serious emergency.

Smoke or fire in an ambulance also requires immediate action. The ambulance should be pulled off to the side of the road. The operator will turn off the electrical system and oxygen while the crew is evacuating the vehicle. Extinguish the fire with the on-board extinguisher. Alternate travel arrangements will then need to be arranged.

Rapid decompression is associated with pressurized aircraft flying at altitudes greater than 10,000 feet and occurs with a broken window or an opened exit. If this situation is encountered, the emergency oxygen system will be activated. One should place on their own oxygen mask first and then assist the other crew members and patient.[47]

Immediately after the emergency landing,

the main priority is to eliminate potential sources of fire. The pilot or crew member will need to turn off the fuel and then the battery, in that order.[47] If there had been no time to turn off all oxygen sources, this should also be attended to at this time. Each crew member should be familiar with the location of these switches.

Evacuation. After an emergency landing, the first logical step is to evacuate from the wreckage to optimize survival. Panic and disorientation among the transport team members must be minimized for the best chance of survival. The two physiological senses most involved during reorientation will be sight and touch. It is particularly important to enhance the use of touch, since many emergencies may occur at night in an aircraft without electrical power and potentially filled with smoke or water.[48] Tactile orientation may be accomplished with the hand-over-hand method. This consists of holding onto an old reference point while finding a new point with the other hand.[13] After reorientation to surroundings is accomplished, an assessment of crew member injuries must be initiated. This may be done visually or verbally.

The pilot will be in charge of the evacuation procedure and will shut off the fuel, engine, and battery. If the pilot is unable to perform these vital tasks, another crew member must take charge to see they are performed in the proper order. No one should try to leave until the aircraft's rotors have come to a complete stop. To evacuate while the rotors are still in motion may further extend the individual's degree of disorientation and potentially lead to a serious injury.[13]

Evacuation should be through the easiest, most accessible exit. Evacuation of the patient and crew may be through a jettisoned door or through a broken window if normal procedures fail to open either of them. If imminent danger of fire or aircraft instability is feared, further securing of the area may be accomplished prior to extricating the patient.[13]

Once safely out of the wreckage, all transport team members should meet at a predesignated area. Initially, 100 feet from the nose of the aircraft is the beginning point to seek. If this twelve o'clock position is unsafe, one should move around the aircraft in a clockwise direction to three o'clock, then six o'clock, etc. until a safe location is found. A safe meeting point is away from the main and tail rotors and away from smoke, fire, and fumes. It is imperative not to return to the aircraft until the pilot has determined the area to be hazard free.[13]

Water landings. Many programs fly over large bodies of water during day to day operations. The FAA requires that personal flotation devices be made available in the event of an unexpected water landing. When flying over water, special attention should be directed towards the different aspects of a water landing as part of the safety-survival program. The following guidelines should be included in the emergency procedures for these scenarios.

Bracing for impact with the water means that crew members must press their backs against the seat back while holding their heads firmly against the head rest and grasping their seat with their arms by their sides.[64] Since the helicopter is top-heavy, the aircraft may rotate as much as 160 degrees in any direction after it is submerged in the water.[64] This is important to remember so that evacuation does not occur until the aircraft has come to a complete stop. Mentally counting 8 to 10 seconds should ensure that settling is completed. As with any hard landing, find a reference point to established orientation. A point may be found with one hand while holding onto the release mechanism of the seat belt and shoulder harness.

Once counting is complete, release the seat belt system while holding onto the reference point in order to locate the nearest exit. The crew member closest to the door will need to emergency jettison it, since water pressure may prevent normal opening procedures. If you are unsure as to your position in the water, one should remember that air bubbles will always float in the direction of the surface. Once location of the water surface is realized, crew members should gently push out of the aircraft remembering that kicking feet may injure any crew members exiting behind.[64] Swim horizontally for approximately ten seconds before surfacing in order to avoid floating debris.[47] While on the surface of the water, one should move away from any additional debris and then inflate the personal flotation device.[13] Any type of flotation device should not be inflated while still inside the aircraft.

Knowing how to react during an unexpected landing may be helpful during an emergency, but special training involving emergency preparation and practice should be made available to transport team members. Practicing these survival techniques may greatly increase the chances of survival. To simulate emergencies without light, personnel should perform emergency techniques such as maintaining a patent airway, removing a patient/team member's headset, turning off the oxygen supply, and getting emergency and survival equipment while blindfolded.[13] If a water landing simulator is available, this is a very realistic way to show personnel how difficult it is to tread water while clothed in a Nomex jump suit and boots.[64] Practicing emergency procedures will assist transport team members to have a sense of what needs to be done and to react without panic, even though they may be frightened.[40] These types of exercises may help each individual in realizing what will occur during this type of landing and, in effect, increase survivability.

Wilderness survival

After surviving an air medical incident, many emotions will be encountered. Anger, panic, fear, denial, grief, and bereavement are only a few. Air medical transport personnel who have been accustomed to providing emergency care to others for years suddenly find themselves requiring these same services. A positive mental attitude will be key to surviving an emergency landing. This may be best accomplished through self confidence, setting realistic goals, and making positive decisions.[47] On the other hand, this may be very difficult to achieve if one is faced with being the sole survivor or watching as fellow crew members perish.

If an accident occurs with the ambulance, chances of survival are enhanced by staying with the vehicle on the road if risks of fire and instability have been eliminated. Survival principles will be the same.

Each region and terrain will dictate what is carried in the survival kit. Many programs will only be 24 hours away from search and rescue in poor weather conditions, while others will be longer in better conditions. The major principles when developing training programs and collecting survival equipment are to provide the necessities of survival. These include water, food, warmth, shelter, and clothing.[5] After addressing these requirements, resources and training must focus on ways to enhance the crew's rescue. Since survival begins with being prepared, daily checks of the survival kit should be as routine as inspecting any other piece of equipment or response bag that is carried for the clinical mission.[47]

Water. A healthy person may only be able to survive one week without water.[5] Depending on the extent of the sustained injuries, some may need more water than others to replace any fluids that have been lost. Maintaining adequate hydration may be difficult in this setting. If any intravenous fluids endured the landing, these may be used to orally replace fluid, electrolytes, and glucose.[47] Rationing available water may be imperative, since all water found in the wilderness should be considered contaminated and may further complicate dehydration with vomiting and diarrhea.

Appropriate measures must be taken to ensure all water will be safe to drink. The most effective way to destroy harmful organisms is to boil it for a full five minutes. There are several chemical purification processes available in sporting goods stores. Some of these systems include halazone tablets, chloride of lime, tincture of iodine, and iodine water purification tablets. These tablets will need to be stored in a cool, dry place and be replaced on a regular basis to ensure freshness. If snow is readily available, it should be melted prior to drinking to prevent any further heat loss.[5,47]

If water is at a dangerously low level, the following tips may be used to locate water sources. Areas surrounding water will be lush with plant growth. Water tends to lie near the base of hills. From a distance vegetation will be seen. In high country, water may be found near the tops of mountains. While in flat country, long winding areas of shrubs and brush will indicate that water is nearby. Following game trails will usually lead to water.[5]

In the desert, some water holes may be poisonous. Any water hole which has skeletons of animals surrounding it or does not have thriving vegetation should be avoided. When searching for water in the desert, one may need to look underground. A dry riverbed or lake may be disappointing at first, but digging down a short distance may prove productive. If a palm tree or reed grass is found, this is a sign that moisture is not far away. Cacti are able to survive due to their ability to store large quantities of water. The fluid may be retrieved by cutting the cactus into small sections, smashing each one, and then drinking the juice which is removed.[5]

Every effort should be made to avoid drinking salt water due to its cathartic property. Placing a button or a pebble in the mouth will help decrease the sensation of thirst if necessary.[5]

Food. For many transport programs rescue will be within 48 hours of landing, so food will not be a necessity. The main priority in this situation will be to maintain adequate hydration. If the aircraft has gone down in a remote area and rescue will be delayed for any reason, food then becomes more important. Food is vital to keep energy stores high and to keep the mind as sharp as possible. If any type of food is carried in a survival kit on board the aircraft, rationing for the entire crew must be initiated. When these rations are nearing the end, one should turn to the surroundings for further nourishment. One should be familiar with the particular part of the country serviced by the transport program in terms of local edible plants, berries, animals, etc.

Areas surrounded by water are good places to find different edible delicacies. No reasonable nourishment should be overlooked. All seaweed is safe to eat, whether raw or cooked. Other meals from the sea may include sea cucumbers, abalone, turtles, and fish. When in this type of survival situation, fishing or trapping small animals may become necessary. The only thing that should be totally excluded from the wilderness diet is mushrooms which have very little food value.[5]

Warmth. Being able to start a fire not only provides warmth and a means of cooking, but it will also provide light and a sense of security in the dark.[47] Matches should be an essential part of the emergency survival kit and should be kept in a watertight case or be waterproof. There are many ways to start a fire without matches. Steel striking flint, two rocks striking each other, a magnifying glass, and a bow and drill are a few examples. Birch bark is a resourceful kindling wood. Even snow covered or wet bark will still produce a flame. Once the flame has been established, larger, dry pieces of dead wood should be added. One should avoid moist wood which will not maintain a flame. It may be necessary to add wood to the fire a few times at night to prevent it from extinguishing.[5]

Shelter. Finding shelter from environmental elements is an important aspect of survival training. It will be able to keep personnel warm or cool and dry.[5] A simple resource to use would be the fuselage of the aircraft if it is deemed safe from rolling and there is no chance of any future damage from flooding or avalanches. Holes should be covered with any available material such as sheets and blankets.[47] If the wreckage is not functional, then other accommodations will need to be made.

Ingenuity is the key to survival. A cave near the site would make an excellent alternative refuge. If in snow, life-saving shelters may be built to prevent hypothermia. Houses of snow may be formed to protect against the elements. Packing a mound of snow and letting it harden for 20 to 30 minutes will provide suitable sanctuary after digging into it at right angles (Figure 49-10). Heating this small area

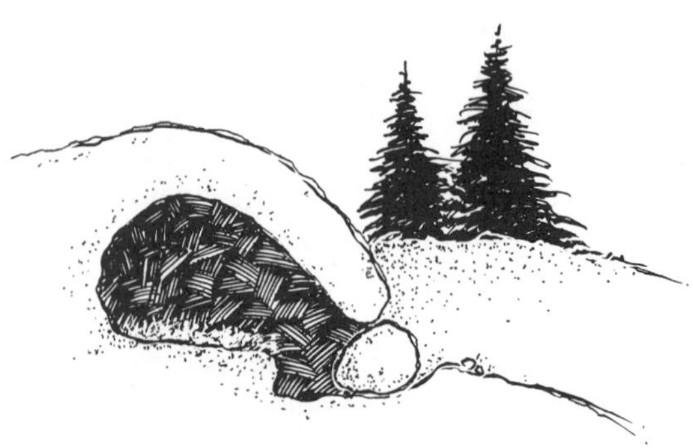

Fig. 49-10. A snow house will provide suitable shelter from the elements.

may be quite simple with the combination of body heat and a small fire.[5] If a fire is built, provide adequate ventilation to prevent the threat of carbon monoxide poisoning.

Carbon monoxide poisoning may be a hazard in any enclosed space, whether it is a tent, cave, or the aircraft's fuselage. As external temperatures decrease, the tendency is to close off any area where cold air may enter which reduces ventilation and increases the risk of carbon monoxide poisoning. Symptoms suggestive of this condition include headache, nausea, dizziness, malaise, and cardiac arrhythmias with progression into coma. If carbon monoxide poisoning occurs in these types of settings, the first thing to do is to move into fresh air and keep warm. Drink some sort of warm stimulant such as coffee, tea, or hot chocolate, if available. Lie still while keeping warm, and take deep breaths of the fresh air.[5] As soon as possible and without any further risk, eliminate the source of the carbon monoxide.

If your program travels over deserts, desert survival training must be further explored. Shelter in the desert may be found by digging two to three feet into the sand to get away from the day's blazing sun.[5]

In wooded areas a primitive lean-to may be made if no other options are available (Figure 49-11). Coverings may include a sheet, other large material that is salvaged from the aircraft, or branches from trees or shrubs.[5] Getting into thick brush will also provide protection from the weather.

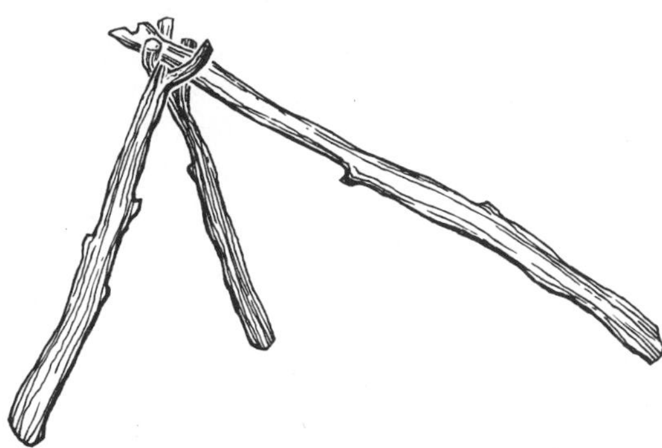

Fig. 49-11. A lean-to is fairly easy to construct and can provide adequate protection if no other options are available.

Clothing. Crew members should always dress for the season while still being functional. Tight fitting clothes should be avoided to prevent constriction. Dressing in layers will enable the body to ventilate perspiration and conserve heat. Plan to protect all parts of the body. A 2 hour fixed wing flight may pass over several different climates. Preparation for all of these climates is recommended. In addition, the team must anticipate what needs to be worn at the referring destination. In the extremes of the desert, long sleeved shirts, pants, and head and eye covers will protect against the sun.[5,47] Individualized training should be developed based on the service area of the transport program.

Signalling. If the aircraft has experienced an unscheduled landing, one should remember that it is much easier to see a downed aircraft from the air than by a person walking through the forest or desert. Keep the aircraft free of debris, snow, and frost to increase an air search party's chances of locating the wreckage and crew.[5,47] After tending to the initial needs of all involved, the next logical step is to increase the chances of being found. When the aircraft is deemed safe to return, check to see if the radio is still functioning. If the radio can transmit signals, the location of the accident should be announced to anyone who may be listening. One should initiate the transmission with "MAYDAY" which identifies the need for immediate attention. If an emergency locator transmitter (ELT) is part of the aircraft, one should check to see if it was activated on impact. If not, the ELT should be activated by hand to aide in rescue efforts.

Signal fires, mirrors, flares, and distress signals may expedite being found. The fire which may already have been started for warmth is an excellent way to be spotted either by air or ground search parties. Adding green foliage, oil, or rubber to a fire will make it smokey and easier to visualize during the day. Mirrors reflect light and may attract the attention of searchers. Any shiny object such as a piece of metal or wet glistening wood will also reflect light.[47] Flares, if available, will be seen at any time of the day, and flashlights may be used at night.[5,47]

The universal distress signal is based on the number three.[5] Placing three Xs made of sheets or debris in view of air search and rescue parties will increase the chances of being seen. One should place them against a contrasting background, such as the tops of trees or bushes to enhance visibility.[39] In addition, whistles assist nearby rescue parties to pinpoint the location of crew members. They may be used in the day or night.[5,47]

Survival equipment. As previously mentioned, the survival pack should be part of the daily transport bag checks. In addition to aircraft survival equipment, each crew member should also carry a personal survival pack. Being prepared for an unexpected landing will only enhance survival. See Box 49-4 for suggested survival equipment. Alterations may need to be made for specific cold weather and desert conditions.

Personal protective clothing

Reviewing the analysis of the increased incidence of air medical transport accidents in the late 1980s, recommendations and position papers were developed to address this crisis.[54,56] An independent review of 50 nonmilitary helicopter accidents resulting in 82 deaths from 1972 to 1987 by accident investigators, physicians, and safety experts, resulted in a prominent city newspaper publishing that eleven cases of lethal head injury would have been prevented by wearing flight helmets.[61] In 1988 the National Transportation Safety Board, which is responsible for analyzing causes of aviation accidents, recommended that "helmets, flame- and heat-resistant uniforms, and protective footwear can help reduce or prevent injury or death of pilots and medical personnel in survivable accidents."[55] Additional studies added credence to these positions.

BOX 49-4 SURVIVAL EQUIPMENT[41]

PERSONAL	
Mirror	Compass
Whistle	Extra pair of prescription glasses
Pocket knife	Contact lens case
Candy bars	Emergency foods
Sunglasses	
AIRCRAFT	
Waterproof matches	Rope
Discos lighter	Knife
Ax	Compass
Insect repellent	Mirror
Flashlight	Flares
Whistle	Sunglasses
Sunscreen	Seasonal clothing
Toilet paper	Sleeping bags (prn)
Water purification tablets	

Helmets. A 1985 DOT/FAA review of civilian helicopter crash dynamics reported that 18% of fatal and major injuries involved the head, and 9% were attributed to the face and neck.[54] In 1991 the U.S. Army evaluated severe, but potentially survivable, helicopter crashes between 1972 and 1988. Occupants wearing the SPH-4 helmet were compared to those who did not wear helmets. They concluded that individuals not wearing helmets were 6.3 times more likely to suffer a fatal head injury. Unhelmeted crew members were also 7.5 times more likely of experiencing injury if they were riding in the rear of the aircraft. Since most air medical personnel fly in the aft compartment of the helicopter, this finding is particularly important in supporting the mandatory use of helmets for transport teams.[25] One might question the validity of transferring findings from military studies to civilian air medical transport programs. The incidence of military accidents is greater due to the number of transports encountered and, at times, the mission profile, but impact with the ground of aircraft and occupants is just as devastating.

The purpose of wearing helmets for rotorcraft personnel is to enable them to "ride out" the entire accident sequence, since they are unable to eject from the aircraft. Deceleration forces are dependent on the object's initial velocity and the amount of distance it must stop. The goal of the helmet is to enable the head to tolerate more diffuse impact forces ranging from 300 to 400 G without skull fracture or concussion and to insulate it from penetrating trauma. The bone break strength of the head ranges from 30 G at the nose to 100 to 200 G for one square inch of frontal bone. On the other hand, fixed wing helmets are designed to protect the head from the ejection sequence.[25]

Understanding the purposes for helmet designs is important when selecting a helmet. Motorcycle, racing, and military fixed wing helmets will not provide the necessary impact protection in rotorcraft accidents. Other qualities to evaluate when selecting a helmet are weight, sound attenuation, interface with aircraft radio/communication system, breadth of visual field, and ability to function in the helmet.[12] All normal and emergency procedures should be practiced in the helicopter prior to its actual use on a patient mission. Visors should be used, since they protect the face from projectile objects.

Uniforms and outer wear. The potential of post crash fires in survivable air medical accidents is approximately 25%.[54] This as a result of fuel spillage from ruptured fuel tanks or lines being ignited from electrical sparks or heated surfaces. One source of ignition would be the helicopter's engine with a temperature of approximately 400°C. If a fire would occur, occupants would need to exit, possibly through the flaming fuel. For a reasonable chance of survival for crew members wearing a military issue summer weight cotton flight uniform, the individual must exit the fireball within 10 seconds of ignition. Within 20 seconds, the temperatures of the thermal environment will range from 927 to 1,260°C. The only barrier to these excessive temperatures for the crew member will be his or her clothing.

NOMEX® has been shown to provide greater protection against thermal injuries than cotton or cotton/polyester. The protection of fire-retardant material may be further enhanced by introducing a $\frac{1}{4}$ inch air gap between the material and skin in conjunction with cotton undergarments. This double layering technique offers more than three times the thermal protection of single layers. Adding more expensive NOMEX® undergarments has shown no advantage in experiments.[54]

Garments such as jackets, shoes or boots, socks, gloves, and sweaters should be made of fire-retardant or natural fabrics. These fabrics include leather, cotton, and wool which will not melt as synthetic fabrics such as polyester and nylon. In addition, any zippers in the garment or boot should be insulated with underlying material to prevent heat transfer to the skin. High top boots have been found beneficial in the prevention of ankle injuries when working in rough terrain.

Critical Incident Stress Debriefing

Critical Incident Stress Debriefing (CISD) is a program which was developed by Dr. Jeffery Mitchell to assist with the psychological intervention and recovery of individuals following a stressful event. These events need not be natural or manmade disasters which result in great loss of human life. They include such critical events as the following:

- Serious injury or death of a coworker while on duty;
- Serious injury or death to a patient as a result of equipment failure (e.g., defibrillator failed to fire, MVA with patient on board, etc.);
- Sudden death of an infant or child, particularly if associated with a criminal act by an adult;
- Any loss of life associated with prolonged expenditures of physical and emotional energy (e.g., prolonged extrications, hazardous working conditions, etc.);
- Any incident that has the potential of causing severe injury or death (e.g., MVA, hard landing, near misses with wires or obstructions, etc.); and
- Any unusual circumstance which may result in immediate or delayed, overwhelming emotional responses (e.g., repetitive transports where resources were continuously taxed, and there was no time to rest).[67]

What is overwhelming to one individual may be only momentarily disconcerting to another. Each individual reacts to life's stressful events differently. How someone responds to a stressful incident may depend on how he/she was emotionally prior to the event. Cumulative stress responses from daily stressors may make an individual more susceptible to developing symptoms associated with stress. A stressful event will result in a response in 90% of individuals. Of this group,

80% will develop stress related symptoms within 24 hours. Half will have a delayed stress reaction which will last up to 3 or 4 weeks. The other half may experience stress from 6 months to a year. Of the group who was experiencing stress, ten percent may suffer extreme effects and require professional counselling. The remaining ten percent who did not experience any stress will include approximately 7% who are in denial and 3% who will not develop any negative effects.[49]

Responses to incident-specific stressors may be categorized as physical, cognitive, emotional, and delayed. Nausea, vomiting, muscle tremors, profuse sweating, chills, and dizziness are common examples of physical responses. Common cognitive signs and symptoms include memory loss, difficulty in problem solving and decision-making, decreased attention span, and an inability to concentrate or do routine tasks. Emotional responses vary with the individual's character and include anxiety, fear, grief, depression, feelings of hopelessness, irritability, anger, and sympathy for the victims. All of these acute responses may impact personal and professional relationships. Delayed responses may be characterized by intrusive images, such as nightmares or flashbacks, or fear that the event or circumstances may recur. This fear may lead to frequent absenteeism. As stress accumulates, a constant state of fatigue, exhaustion, or frustration may lead to burnout. Personnel become apathetic, work less, and become physically and mentally exhausted.[67]

CISD assists the involved individual(s) in understanding their response to stress by accurately identifying the events, dispelling any rumors, and communicating any feelings or thoughts surrounding the event. Debriefings should occur within 24 to 72 hours. They should be facilitated by a group consisting of individuals with common interests and at the same skill level. The goal is to enhance the individual's well being and facilitate their performance in a supportive environment. Critiquing the event and individual's performance must be avoided.

Since the opening pages of this chapter, an abundant amount of information has been presented supporting the development of a comprehensive transport system safety plan. The plan should focus on the areas of prevention, emergency minimization, and injury limitation. It was not the intent to be all encompassing because many of the topics introduced here have, in themselves, volumes written. The goal was to highlight the importance of these pieces so further understanding and clarification may be obtained as individual transport program safety plans are developed. With that understanding comes rationale to prevent their exclusion when it is time to trim the budget.

It is difficult to ascertain the exact cost of safety, but can any program or institution afford not to address it? Actual financial costs of accidents include insurance policy deductibles, lost revenue as a result of the damaged vehicle, on-going lease or loan payments, loss of business secondary to lost customer confidence, cost of money while waiting for the claim to be paid, search and rescue costs, executive and staff time dedicated to the accidents investigation and any potential litigation, and the cost of increased insurance premiums. The other cost that is more difficult to quantify is that of human pain and suffering. Medical expenses, lost time and productivity, and emotional trauma are only a few sources of concern. Money will not be saved through cutting corners, reducing maintenance and training, or identifying other false economies.[16]

As a result, safety must be made a priority throughout the transport program's philosophy. It must be continuously emphasized and supported from administration to staff members.

REFERENCES

1. American Academy of Pediatrics: *Guidelines for air and ground transport of neonatal and pediatric patients,* Elk Grove Village, Illinois, 1993, The Association.
2. American Academy of Pediatrics: *1990 Family shopping guide to car seats,* Elk Grove Village, Illinois, 1990, The Association.
3. American Academy of Pediatrics: *Pennsylvania child passenger safety project,* Elk Grove Village, Illinois, 1989, The Association.

re E, Scanga J, Rocklage C: *STAT MedEvac ccident/incident plan,* Pittsburgh, 1992, for Emergency Medicine.

editor: *Flight nursing—principles and prac-* Louis, 1991, Mosby-Year Book.

gton D: Getting out while the getting's *Business and Commercial Aviation,* 5:81-6,

n E: *Critical incident stress debriefing team g handout,* Pittsburgh, 7:12-28, 1990.

an J: Helicopters and turbulence, *Hospital n,* 7:34-5, 1989.

A: Air medical safety, paying the price, *The of Air Medical Transport,* 10:26-30, 1992.

ek P, Sorenson P: Missing aircraft—if disaster , is your program prepared?, *The Journal of dical Transport,* 12:17-9, 1989.

al EMS Pilot Association: *Preparing a landing* pamphlet), Pasadena, August 1992.

al Flight Nurse's Association Safety Position Task Force: NFNA position paper—ving flight nurse safety in the air medical heli-environment, *Hospital Aviation,* 9:43-48,

al Transportation Safety Board, Bureau of Programs: *Safety study commercial emergency l service helicopter operations, NTSB/ss-88/* ashington, D.C., January 28, 1988.

al Transportation Safety Board: NTSB recom-tions for EMS industry, *Air Medical Safety rly,* 1st Quarter:26-28, 1988.

ational Safety and Health Administration: *d communication guidelines for compliance,* Department of Labor, Washington, D.C., Re-d 1990.

PE, Almaguer DR: Emergency medical ser-personnel and ground transport vehicles, *Prob-n Critical Care,* 4:470-6, 1990.

59. Peto G, Medve WJ: *EMS driving the safe way,* Englewood, New Jersey, 1992, Brady.
60. Riha CD: Biomedical equipment considerations for aeromedical transports, *Biomedical Instrumentation and Technology,* 2:22-30, 1993.
61. Schneider A: Medevac crews want changes to increase survival, *Pittsburgh Press,* November 1, 1987.
62. Schreiber V and others: Noise exposure to flight crew from the MBB BO-105 and MBB BK-117 (abstract), *The Journal of Air Medical Transport,* 9:76, 1990.
63. Smith JB: *Pediatric critical care,* New York, 1983, John Wiley and Sons Inc.
64. Stinson WF: Forced Water Landing—A Practice in Survival, *The Journal of Air Medical Transport,* 1:23-25, 1990.
65. Stout J: Emergency vehicle driver training; two schools of thought, *Journal of Emergency Medical Services,* 11:80-82, 1987.
66. Thomas F, Jacobson J: Applying ethical principles to air medical transport, *Emergency Care Quarterly,* 1:1-6, 1991.
67. Troiani TA, Boland RT: Critical incident stress debriefing—keeping your flight crew healthy, *The Journal of Air Medical Transport,* 10:21-4, 1992.
68. Walker VB, Fromm RE: Aircraft, airmen, and aviation aspects of aeromedical transport, *Problems in Critical Care,* 4:508-27, 1990.
69. Whaley LF, Wong DL: *Nursing care of infants and children,* ed 4, St. Louis, 1991, Mosby-Year Book.
70. Wood F: Evade—training for tire blow outs, *Journal of Emergency Medical Services,* 3:56-60, 1987.
71. Wraa CE, O'Malley RJ: Flight nurse physical requirements, *The Journal of Air Medical Transport,* 10:17-20, 1992.

4. American Medical Association, *For your protection: the OSHA regulations on bloodborne pathogens,* Chicago, 1992, The Association.
5. Angier A: *How to stay alive in the woods,* New York, 1984, Macmillian Publishing Company.
6. Aoki BY, McCloskey K: *Evaluation, stabilization, and transport of the critically ill child,* St. Louis, 1992, Mosby.
7. Association for Air Medical Services: *AAMS Standards,* Pasadena, 1992, The Association.
8. Association for the Advancement of Medical Instrumentation: *AAMI Standards and recommended practices,* Arlington, Virginia, 1986, The Association.
9. Association of Air Medical Services: *Air medical safety congress proceedings and recommendations* (unpublished), Pittsburgh, May 1992.
10. Barkin RM, Rosen P: *Emergency pediatrics—a guide to ambulatory care,* St. Louis, 1990, CV Mosby Company.
11. Berg KL: Is it time to upgrade your weather system, *The Journal of Air Medical Transport,* 3:11-13, 1992.
12. Bock H and others: *Air medical crew national curriculum,* Pasadena, 1988, ASHBEAMS.
13. Bush C: Emergency egress scenarios, *The Journal of Air Medical Transport,* 10:35-8, 1991.
14. Cady G: 1993 Program survey, *Air Medical Journal,* 9:306-12, 1993.
15. Campbell JE: *Basic trauma life support—advanced prehospital care,* ed 2, Englewood Cliffs, New Jersey, 1988, Brady.
16. Carnie RJ: Safety saves money, *Hospital Aviation,* 3:18, 1986.
17. Carrith G, editor: *The volume library,* Nashville, 1992, The Southwestern Company.
18. Cauthorne CV, Fedorowicz RJ: Work/rest schedules and their potential impact on flight crew performance, *Hospital Aviation,* 3:5-7, 1985.
19. Clawson JJ: Running "hot" and the case of Sharron Rose, *Journal of Emergency Medical Services,* 7:11-13, 1991.
20. Code of Federal Regulations, Labor 29, Hearing standard and amendments. (29CFR) 1910.95, Article 95 and final regulation.
21. Code of Federal Regulations, Labor 29, Occupational exposure to bloodborne pathogens, (29CFR) 1910.1030, 1991.
22. Commission on Accreditation of Air Medical Services: *Accreditation standards of the commission on accreditation of air medical services,* Anderson, South Carolina, 1991.
23. Commonwealth of Pennsylvania, Legislative Reference Bureau: *Pennsylvania Bulletin,* Vol. 19, No. 26, July 1, 1989, Harrisburg, Pennsylvania.
24. Cook RT, Flint N, Whitten DL: Programs and pregnancy—a survey of policies, *The Journal of Air Medical Transport,* 5:7-12, 1992.
25. Crowley JS, Licina JR, Bruchart JE: Flight helmets—how they work and why you should wear one, *The Journal of Air Medical Transport,* 8:19-26, 1992.
26. DeLorenzo RA: Bright l
tive are vehicle warnin
gency Medical Services,
27. Delorenzo RA, Eilers M
view of emergency vehi
of Emergency Medicine,
28. Dodd RS: *Factors relate
in emergency medical s*
tion), Baltimore, 1992.
29. Edington B: Where ea
tions at helicopter sce
Medical Services, 10:36-
30. Edington BH: Transpo
concerned parties aboa
Journal of Air Medical T
31. Elling R: Dispelling myt
Journal of Emergency Me
32. Federal Aviation Admin
tion manual, U.S. Dep
Washington, D.C., Febr
33. Federal Aviation Admin
seats recommended for
U.S. Department of T
D.C.
34. Federal Aviation Adm
management advisory
partment of Transportat
ruary 10, 1992.
35. Federal Aviation Admin
cal services/helicopter
U.S. Department of T
D.C., June 20, 1991.
36. Federal Aviation Admin
Regulations, Part 67.17
portation, Washington D
37. Fox RG: Crash surviv
Quarterly, 1st Quarter:
38. Fuchs S and others: C
tained by young childre
Pediatrics, 2:348-54, 19
39. Goshco A, Ruel R: Cold
Aeromedical Healthcare
40. Green B: Egress simula
30, 1989.
41. Harrison RK: Heari
menting and evaluating
4:107-11, 1989.
42. Helicopter Association
decision making workbo
Medical Safety Congre
ture, Pittsburgh, May, 1
43. Holmes MD, Rahe RH
rating scale, *Journal o*
11:213-18, 1967.
44. Huch R and others: Phy
nant women and their f
American Journal of Ob
1000, 1986.
45. Huswit J, Lambrose P,
management for single
tions workbook, Pittsburg
46.
47.
48.
49.
50.
51.
52.
53.
54.
55.
56.
57.
58.

50

RESPIRATORY CARE

CATHERINE PETERSON
PAUL WRIGHT
KENDRA BALAZS
LINDA YOUNG

HISTORY OF RESPIRATORY CARE PRACTITIONERS

The inception of Respiratory Care Practitioners (RCP) dates back to the 1940s and 1950s. Originally named oxygen orderlies, inhalation therapists, or respiratory therapists, they are now known as respiratory care practitioners. In the beginning, formal education was minimal and most training occurred on the job with an emphasis on technical skills.[11] As the demand for skilled personnel increased, formal education programs and credentialing exams were developed. Today, on the job training has been replaced by one year technician programs and two year respiratory therapist programs. The accrediting bodies for both types of education programs are the Joint Review Committee on Respiratory Therapy Education (JRCRTE) and the American Medical Association (AMA) Committee on Allied Health Education and Accreditation.

The National Board of Respiratory Care (NBRC) is the recognized credentialing body for RCPs. The NBRC administers and oversees the requirements for both the Certified Respiratory Therapy Technician (CRTT) and Registered Respiratory Therapist (RRT) exams. The RRT is the higher of the two credentials. The minimum requirement for the CRTT credential is graduation from a one year accredited program. The minimum requirement for the RRT credential is CRTT certification along with completion of a two year accredited program and clinical experience or a CRTT certification and combination of years of clinical experience and college credits to include specific science subjects.

The American Association of Respiratory Care (AARC) is the only professional national and international organization representing RCPs. The AARC is involved in various aspects of respiratory care which include the following:

- Promoting RCP professionalism.
- Developing clinical practice guidelines.
- Providing educational opportunities.
- Working with the NBRC on credentialing issues.
- Influencing health care policy and legislation related to health care reform.
- Lobbying for licensure in states not currently licensing RCPs.
- Supporting research and documentation of the therapeutic and cost-effectiveness of respiratory services.

The AARC is working on several projects which promote educational change and expansion of the RCP's scope of practice to meet the challenges of today and the future health care environment. Historically, physicians played a major role in promoting the profession of RCPs and continue to work closely with the NBRC and the AARC.

Since the AARC began lobbying for state licensure of RCPs, thirty five states currently have licensure requirements. Criteria may vary from state to state, however, CRTT or RRT credentials are uniform requirements.

The level of education and certification of RCPs varies, therefore, each transport program should define the specific criteria and the scope of practice for RCPs based on the mission of the program.

QUALIFICATIONS OF THE PEDIATRIC TRANSPORT RCP

Because RCPs in the transport environment must work with team members in an autonomous role, they should have a sound knowledge base and experience in the care of the critically ill and injured patients. Although no nationally recognized standard for minimum qualifications exists for pediatric transport RCPs, transport programs usually require a minimum number of years of experience (typically 2 to 3 years of critical care experience) prior to hiring air or ground medical transport personnel.[5] Flight programs should establish their own minimum qualifications. RCPs should hold at least a CRTT and/or RRT certification. Course completion of Advanced Cardiac Life Support (ACLS), Pediatric Advanced Life Support (PALS), and the Neonatal Resuscitation Program (NRP) may be required as appropriate. There is a perinatal/pediatric specialty exam that NBRC administers which transport programs may also require of RCPs.

THE ROLE OF THE RESPIRATORY THERAPIST IN PEDIATRIC TRANSPORT

Pediatric transport programs have evolved from the need to transport critically ill and injured children from rural or suburban communities to tertiary centers for intensive care services.[21] Transport programs have expanded to include specialized pediatric services to meet these needs. RCPs have become an integral part of many transport programs, particularly neonatal and pediatric transport programs, because of their education and clinical experience.

RCPs who have completed a two year program have a sound understanding of the anatomy and physiology of the cardiopulmonary system and a thorough knowledge of the gas laws that pertain to the cardiopulmonary system. Pathophysiology of various respiratory disease processes as well as their effect on the cardiac system is also emphasized in the two year program. Clinical skills encompass not only cardiopulmonary system assessment abilities, but also include oxygen and aerosol therapies, airway stabilization techniques, pulse oximetry, end-tidal CO_2 monitoring, and ventilator setup and management.

Pediatric transports frequently involve children with a variety of adverse medical conditions, many of which require respiratory support. The RCP is a vital team member because of clinical adeptness in airway stabilization, ventilation, and respiratory management. As part of the pediatric transport team, the RCP helps formulate a plan of care in the most acute and critical care settings. First, the RCP assists other team members in the collection of pertinent medical history from the family and other health care providers. Next, the team assesses and formulates a plan of treatment appropriate for the patient and implements the interventions required for stabilization and transport. Continual assessment of the patient's condition and emotional reassurance for the patient and family members are essential during transport. Other responsibilities of the transport RCP include assembling, checking and stocking respiratory transport equipment, monitoring and maintaining oxygen systems, and helping team members when necessary.

Depending on the scope of practice, the policies of the pediatric transport program and the medical director, the RCPs scope of practice may be expanded. This expansion in scope of practice may include IV insertion and IV pump setup, dysrhythmia recognition and defibrillation, intubation, ACLS drug administration, hemodynamic monitoring, and the use of immobilization devices. For patients who need unconventional therapies, the transport RCP may be required to be familiar with different types of high frequency ventilation (HFV) and extracorporeal membrane oxygenation (ECMO).

Dual credentialing of RCPs as Emergency Medical Technicians (EMT) or Emergency Medical Technician Paramedics (EMT-P) is another option for transport programs to consider. By cross training RCPs as EMTs or EMT-Ps, the RCP's knowledge base is broadened, and consequently, they become a more diverse transport team member.

EDUCATION

RCPs are responsible for providing advanced respiratory and emergency care to pediatric patients within the framework of the policies, procedures, and patient care guidelines of the pediatric transport program. Because the transport RCP role differs from the hospital role, additional education is necessary to prepare the RCP for an autonomous role. Didactic components should include, but are not limited to, the subjects listed in Boxes 50-1 and 50-2. Each program will need to make adjustments in the length of the education program and the curriculum depending on the background and experience of the RCP.

These components are only recommendations for the RCP curriculum in a transport education program. The scope of care and the mission statement of the pediatric transport program should be kept in mind when developing an educational program. The content of the curriculum for an RCP transport education program has not been standardized at this time.[21]

BOX 50-1 DIDACTIC COMPONENTS OF EDUCATION PROGRAM

Transport environment
- Aerodynamics of aircraft
- Flight physiology
- Stressors of flight
- Introduction to aircraft (fixed wing and/or rotor wing)
- Map reading and navigation
- Survival training

Equipment
- Immobilization devices
- Transport ventilators
- Cardiac monitors
- $ETCO_2$ monitoring devices
- IV pumps
- Hemodynamic monitors

BOX 50-2 DIDACTIC COMPONENTS OF EDUCATION PROGRAM

Patient management
- Neonatal and pediatric assessment
- Pediatric developmental assessment
- Neonatal/pediatric stabilization and transport
- Management of neonatal emergencies
- Management of pediatric medical emergencies
- Interpretation of pediatric and neonatal chest x-ray
- ACLS and PALS patient management and pharmacology
- Management of multisystem trauma of the pediatric patient
- Management of pediatric fluids and shock
- Intubation and airway management
- Acid base homeostasis
- Oxygen system calculations

Miscellaneous
- Introduction to the EMS system
- CQI and documentation in transport
- Legal aspects of air medical transport
- Transport program policies
- Infection control

MONITORING DEVICES USED IN TRANSPORT

Monitoring devices currently available for the evaluation of cardiopulmonary status are the pulse oximeter, end-tidal carbon dioxide ($ETCO_2$) monitor, and the transcutaneous gas tension monitor. A transport program should attempt to maintain or advance the patient's care during transport whenever possible and practical. A goal for the pediatric transport program should be to provide the same standard of care during transport that a tertiary medical center provides. There are some equipment constraints in the transport environment such as limitations on technical development and/or the laws of physics that reduce the availability of useful monitoring equipment for transport teams. Recent advances in technology have produced small, compact, durable, and more reliable monitoring devices which allow the transport team to provide continuity of care.

Although these monitoring devices provide data on oxygen saturation, $ETCO_2$, and oxygen and carbon dioxide levels, the correlation between the data obtained and the arterial blood gas (ABG) is not 100% accurate. ABG analysis will continue to be the "gold standard" against which all other monitoring technologies will be compared and may one day find practical application in the transport environment. However, the challenge for obtaining ABGs in transport is to maintain precise and repeatable gas tension measurements against a background of changing barometric pressures.

The RCP should be involved not only in the selection of the equipment to be used but must be intimately familiar with the information it provides, as well as its limitations.

Pulse oximetry

The technology of pulse oximetry grew out of the observation that arterial blood differs from venous blood in color. A substance is perceived as being a different color when it absorbs or reflects light of certain wavelengths. The breakthrough in pulse oximetry was the ability to synchronize the readings of spectral absorption with the arrival of the arterial waveform so that the readings represented an arterialized sample of hemoglobin in the tissue bed. The pulse oximeter does this by observing the overall reduction in light transmission that occurs as the tissue bed is engorged with arterial blood. From this information it obtains a calculated pulse rate that is displayed along with the saturation value, and with some monitors, an arterial waveform is displayed as well.

Limitations of pulse oximetry are related to the spectral characteristics of the various forms of hemoglobin and the total amount of hemoglobin available. A normal pulse oximetry reading implies normal oxygen content only in the presence of a normal level of functional hemoglobin.

The most obvious example of this limitation is the patient with significant anemia. In a patient with a hemoglobin level of 6.5 g/100 ml (normal hemoglobin for a child is 11.2 to 13.4 g/100 ml), a 100% saturation reading by pulse oximetry is still associated with an arterial oxygen content of slightly over half the normal value and does not mean or indicate normal oxygen delivery to the tissues.

Other less obvious examples include patients with a significant degree of methemoglobinemia, carbon monoxide, or cyanide poisoning. In these patients the pulse oximetry reading will indicate the percent of functional hemoglobin that is saturated. Without cooximetry to establish an absolute level of functional hemoglobin, it is not possible to correlate the reading by pulse oximetry with oxygen delivery to the tissues. However, trends can still be monitored to some degree even in the absence of such supporting data.

End-tidal carbon dioxide monitors ($ETCO_2$)

End-tidal carbon dioxide monitoring is relatively new to the transport environment. It relies on the physiologic principle that end-tidal carbon dioxide concentrations correlate with alveolar concentrations. Due to the rapid diffusion rate of carbon dioxide across the alveolar-capillary membrane, it should correlate with the arterial values. The development of the technology for $ETCO_2$ resembles the development of pulse oximetry in that the key obstacle was the synchronization of physical readings with some physiological event.

The typical end-tidal carbon dioxide monitor can obtain a gas sample from the exhaled air either from a ventilator adapter of a ventilated patient or from a cannula of a patient who is breathing spontaneously. After filtration and dehydration of the gas sample, the carbon dioxide concentration is measured by infrared sensors and real-time values are displayed.

End-tidal carbon dioxide monitoring is most useful if the values obtained can be initially correlated with an arterial blood gas analysis. Once the differential between $PaCO_2$ and $ETCO_2$ has been established, it will theoretically remain relatively fixed and the $ETCO_2$ values can be used to adjust ventilatory parameters. An RCP can have a high degree of confidence that the resulting arterial values will correlate. Trending $ETCO_2$ is of key importance in transport.

End-tidal carbon dioxide monitoring also has limitations in patients with changes in the pulmonary circulation (vascular) or mechani-

Normal Waveforms

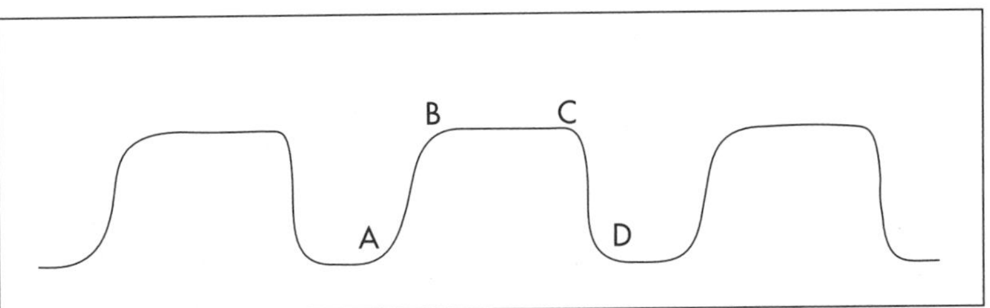

Waveform Evaluation:

* A-B: Ascending limb, expiratory portion, mixed deadspace and alveolar air with increasing concentration of CO_2. Normally starts at a baseline of zero.

* B-C: Alveolar plateau contains mixed alveolar gas with End Tidal measured at C.

* C-D: Descending limb, inspiratory portion, with decreasing concentration of CO_2. Normally returns to a baseline of zero.

Hyperventilation

A decrease in the level of the End Tidal CO_2 from previous levels.

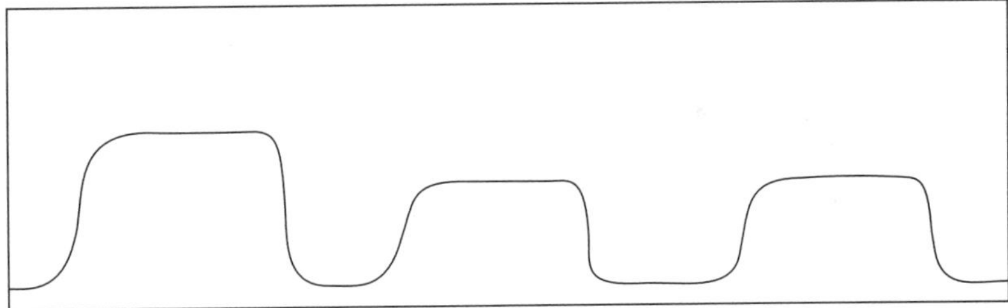

Possible Cause:

* Increase in respiratory rate
* Increase in tidal volume
* Decrease in metabolic rate
* Fall in body temperature

Fig. 50-1. Examples of normal capnogram waveforms. (Waveforms provided by Novametrix Medical System, Inc.)

cal properties (resistance and compliance) of the lungs. In the presence of significant lung disease the values obtained will be less reliable due to air trapping and other disturbances of alveolar emptying. There will be evidence of these disturbances in the morphology of the waveform on end-tidal CO_2 monitors. The differential between simultaneous arterial and end-tidal values is likely to be large (Figures 50-1 and 50-2).

Transcutaneous gas tension monitors

Transcutaneous gas tension monitors measure oxygen and carbon dioxide levels ($PtcO_2$ and $PtcCO_2$). In theory, transcutaneous monitoring most closely approximates arterial blood gas tension and measures the gas tension values in a manner similar to an arterial blood gas analyzer. Unfortunately, it suffers from the inherent inability of the air medical transport environment to provide a barometric pressure against which to reference its measurement at altitude.

In order to allow the transcutaneous gas tension to approximate those in the arteries, the transcutaneous gas tension monitors use a heat sensor. The heat from the element in the sensor causes vasodilation of the peripheral vasculature in the area under the sensor and arterialize the sample to some degree. Among the problems associated with these sensors are a need to rotate sites due to a potential of causing thermal burns under the sensor. A second potential problem is a need to secure the sensor against entry of air which can cause false values that may mask a deteriorating situation.

All of these monitoring devices are currently available in small, self-contained packages appropriate for the transport environment. Selection of specific devices should involve both transport personnel and biomedical engineering. A transport program must consider the types of the patients to be transported, availability of space, weight, power limitations, and the local standard of care.

MECHANICAL VENTILATION

A growing trend for specific diagnostic tests and/or special therapeutic interventions for critically ill patients who are mechanically ventilated increases the need for patient transfer to centers with specialized intervention and diagnostic capabilities.[22] The need to maintain sufficient oxygenation and ventilation during transport of a mechanically ventilated pediatric patient is of the utmost importance.[7,19,26]

The requirements for portable transport ventilators are growing because of the need to deliver the same continuity of care of the receiving pediatric critical care center during transport. There are a variety of commercially manufactured and designed transport ventilators available.[26] Table 50-1 shows a more in-depth description of commercially

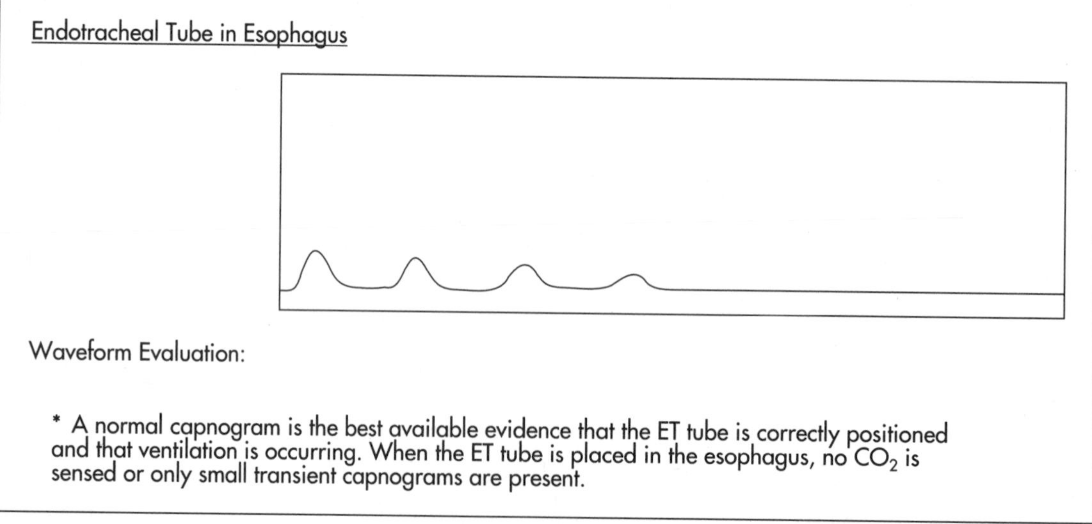

Fig. 50-2. A normal capnogram is the best available evidence that the endotracheal tube is correctly positioned and that ventilation is occurring. When the endotracheal tube is placed in the esophagus, no carbon monoxide is sensed, or only small transient capnograms are present. (Waveforms provided by Novametrix Medical System, Inc.)

available units. This table is not inclusive of every transport ventilator on the market, therefore, each program must further investigate the type of ventilator that meets their needs. This chapter is not intended to be a technical manual of portable transport ventilators but rather a discussion of what is available and some criteria that might be useful in the selection of a transport ventilator.

The ventilator must meet the needs of patients transported and be equipped with a variety of different modes such as pressure cycled, volume cycled, time cycled, or flow cycled (see Box 50-3). Transport ventilators are either electrically or pneumatically powered. Criteria such as size, weight, O_2 consumption, cost, durability, and training for personnel must be considered. Some of the new transport ventilators have built in alarms, but not to the extent of the modern ICU ventilators. Therefore, consideration of the type of monitors that the program uses for the transport ventilators is also important. To help with these decisions, there are published studies that have evaluated transport ventilators.[7-18] All criteria discussed above must be considered before purchasing a transport ventilator.

The RCP may initiate mechanical ventilatory support or continue ventilatory support of the patient. Previous studies have demonstrated superiority and increased safety of ventilatory support with a portable ventilator when compared to manual ventilation with a self-inflating bag.[16] The RCP must ensure proper ventilatory function and modify ventilator settings based on individual patient response.[20] At times, mechanical ventilation in transport requires fine tuning and can be a demanding skill. The transport team must be alert to any changes in patient ventilatory requirements.

Other considerations when using transport ventilators in-flight are possible changes in inspiratory and expiratory times as well as flow rates in pneumatically powered ventilators due to changes in barometric pressure at

TABLE 50-1 TRANSPORT VENTILATORS

Ventilators	*Power source*	*Weight (kg)*	*Size (inches)*	*Gas consumption (LPM)*	*Modes*	*Rate*
Bird AVIAN	Electronic	5	10 × 12 × 5	2	A/C SIMV CPAP	0-150
Autovent 3000	Pneumatic	.68	15 × 9 × 4.5	0.5	IMV CMV	P 9-27 A 8-20
Bio-Med IC-2A	Pneumatic	4.1	8.6 × 15.6 × 26	12	SIMV CPAP	1-66
Bio-Med MVP-10	Pneumatic	2.3	8 × 9 × 3	3	IMV CPAP	0-120
Hamilton max	Pneumatic	5.4	30 × 8 × 16.5	0.5	IMV CMV	2-30
Uni-Vent 750	Electronic	4.5	9.25 × 11.5 × 4.9	0	A/C SIMV	1-150
Newport E 100i	Pneumatic	5.9	10.5 × 9.5 × 6.5	Need to calculate	A/C IMV CPAP	1-120
Omni-Vent	Pneumatic	2	4 × 5 × 7	0	IMV CPAP PEEP	1-150

Terms: A/C—Assist Control; SIMV—Synchronize Intermediate Mandatory Ventilation; CPAP—Continuous Positive Airway Pressure; IMV—Intermediate Mandatory Ventilation; CMV—Continuous Mandatory Ventilation; PEEP—Positive End Expiratory Pressure.

different altitudes.[1] The set rate and tidal volume may change in flight and reassessment of the patient and the ventilator must be done throughout transport. The manufacturers instruction manual usually discusses the effect of altitude expected in a particular ventilator.

Patients requiring life support equipment should be under the constant surveillance of competent medical practitioners who are adept in using and troubleshooting the equipment. The possibility of machine and alarm failure that will require immediate and appropriate corrective action is always present.

BLENDERS

The use of blenders in transport can serve two purposes. The first is to supply the precise oxygen needs of the patient (constant FIO^2). The second purpose is to help conserve the oxygen supply on the aircraft by blending oxygen with compressed air, as needed, to maintain adequate flow. There have not been any documented difficulties with using the blender during transport or at altitude.

OXYGEN

Transport personnel must check oxygen levels in the transport vehicle by noting the oxygen pressure gauges at the beginning of each shift and prior to transport. The aircraft or ambulance must carry enough oxygen to complete a medical mission in the worst case scenario. Depending on the transport vehicle, two times the amount of oxygen needed for the transport would be an acceptable amount. The type of oxygen system used depends on the aircraft and which systems are available in the service area. Whether the program carries liquid oxygen or compressed gas cylinders, the transport team must be able to calculate the amount of time that the oxygen supply will last. To determine the amount of time a compressed gas cylinder will last the following formula can be used:

$$\frac{\text{cylinder size in ft}^3 \times 28.3}{\text{full tank}} = \frac{\text{Constant}}{(1/\text{psi})}$$

$$\frac{\text{Observe pressure gauge} \times \text{Constant}}{\text{gas flow in L/Min.}}$$

$$= \text{Duration of content in minutes}$$

Example: An E cylinder = 22ft^3 at 2200 psi,

$$\frac{22 \times 28.3}{2200} = 0.28 \text{ liters/psi}$$

$$\frac{700 \times .28}{5 \text{ LPM}} = 39.2 \text{ minutes}$$

FAA approved liquid oxygen systems are also available for transport and have the major advantage of allowing the transport vehicle to carry more oxygen in less space. As with compressed gas, one must be able to determine the duration of oxygen availability. For this

BOX 50-3 DIFFERENT MODES OF VENTILATION

Pressure cycled:	A pressured cycled ventilator will terminate gas delivery during the inspiratory phase when a predetermined pressure is realized.
Volume cycled:	A volume cycled ventilator requires selection of a desired volume to be delivered and will stop the gas flow when that volume of gas has been delivered.
Time cycled:	A time cycled ventilator will stop gas flow and change to the expiratory phase when a preset period of time has elapsed after the start of inspiration.
Flow cycled:	A flow cycled ventilator will stop inspiration when gas flow falls below a critical level that is independent of airway pressure, tidal volume, or duration of inspiration.

TABLE 50-2 PRESSURE AND VOLUMES OF COMMONLY USED CYLINDER

Gas	*Full cylinder pressure*	*D*	*E*	*H*
Oxygen	2200	12.7	22	244
Compressed air	2200		22	244

calculation, it is necessary to refer to the manufacturer's specifications on the size of the system used.

For aircraft operating with various oxygen systems, the program may need to look into the Federal Aviation Regulations (FARs) under which the aircraft operates to determine who can fill or replace the oxygen in the aircraft (Table 50-2).

Oxygen requirements

Critically ill and injured pediatric patients may suffer adverse effects at high altitudes from unrecognized hypoxia. To make adjustments for maintaining a constant alveolar oxygen tension, the following formula can be used:

$$\frac{\text{Current barometric pressure} \times \text{current FiO}_2}{\text{Barometric pressure at current altitude}} = \text{New FiO}_2$$

Example: A pediatric patient is being transported from sea level (760 mmhg) to 3000 feet (681 mmhg). Prior to transport the patient requires 40% FiO_2. To calculate the FiO_2 required for transport, the following example is used:

$$\frac{760 \times .4}{681} = 0.45 \text{ FiO}_2$$

The patient will require 45% oxygen to maintain the same PAO_2 at the change of altitude during the transport.

SUMMARY

It is critical that skilled personnel are part of the pediatric transport team. The risk of complication during transport can be minimized by using the most advanced equipment to monitor patients and the most beneficial team composition. It is also very important that the proper monitoring equipment is available and the transport team has the experience to use and troubleshoot the equipment.[6] Careful evaluation and management of the patient is crucial during transport. The RCP is a very important part of the pediatric transport team because of their education, knowledge base and experience. The pediatric patient in particular benefits from the RCPs expertise in respiratory care.

REFERENCES

1. ASHBEAMS and Samaritan AirEvac: Air medical crew national standard curriculum: instructor manual, Pasadena, 1988, ASHBEAMS.
2. Barnes TA: Emergency ventilation techniques and related equipment, *Respiratory Care* 37(7):673-94, 1992.
3. Bio-Med Devices IC2A adult ventilator instructors manual, Madison, Connecticut, 1984, Bio-Med Devices.
4. Bio-Med Devices MVP-10 ventilators instructors manual, Madison, Connecticut, 1992, Bio-Med Devices.
5. Brink LW and others: Air transport: transport medicine, *Pediatric Clinics of North America,* 40(2):439-63, 1993.
6. Brink LW and others: Transport of the critically ill patient with upper airway obstruction, *Critical Care Clinics* 40(3):633-47, 1992.
7. Campbell RS and others: Laboratory and clinical evaluation of the impact uni-vent 750 portable ventilator, *Respiratory Care* 37(1):29-36, 1992.
8. Day SE: Intra-transport stabilization and management of the pediatric patients, *Transport Medicine* 40(2):263-73, 1993.
9. Dayle E and others: Transport of the critically ill child, *British Journal of Hospital Medicine* 48(6): 314-19, 1992.
10. Downs JB, Marston AW: A new transport ventilator: an evaluation, *Critical Care Medicine* 5(2):112-4, 1977.
11. Eiserman JE: The expanding role of the respiratory care practitioner, *Respiratory Care* 35(12):1189-91, 1990.
12. Egan DF: Fundamental of respiratory therapy, ed 3, St. Louis, 1977, Mosby-Year Book, Inc.
13. Fluck RR, Sorbello JG: Comparison of tidal volumes, minute ventilation, and respiratory frequencies delivered by paramedic and respiratory care student with pocket mask versus demand valve, *Respiratory Care* 36(10):1105-12, 1991.
14. Gibbons M: Dual-credentialed staff, Advance for Managers of Respiratory Care, 17-23, May/June 1993.
15. Hendrik W and others: Comparison of blood gases of ventilated patients during transport, *Critical Care Med* 15(8):761-3, 1987.

16. Hurst JM and others: Comparison of blood gases during transport using two methods of ventilatory support, *The Journal of Trauma* 29(12):1637-40, 1989.
17. Jeffs M: Air medical transport in 1991, *Respiratory Care* 37(7):796-806, 1992.
18. Johannigman JA and others: Laboratory and clinical evaluation of the max transport ventilator, *Respiratory Care* 35(10):952-9, 1990.
19. Johannigman JA and others: Techniques of emergency ventilation: a model to evaluate tidal volume, airway pressure and gastric insufflation, *The Journal of Trauma* 31(1):93-8, 1991.
20. Kacmarek RM: The role of the respiratory therapist in emergency care, *Respiratory Care* 37(6):523-32, 1992.
21. Kissoon N: Triage and transport of the critically ill child, *Progress in Pediatric Critical Care* 8(1):37-57, 1992.
22. McGough EK, Banner MJ, Melker RJ: Variation in tidal volume with portable transport ventilators, *Respiratory Care* 37(3):223-39, 1992.
23. Nehrenz G: Aeromedical physiology, Unpublished manuscript, 1987.
24. Omni-Vent series D ventilator service manual, Topeka, Kansas, 1992, Omni-Tech Medical, Inc.
25. Operator's manual max, Reno, Nevada, 1989, Hamilton Medical.
26. Rouse MJ, Branson R, Semonn-Holleran R: Mechanical ventilation during air medical transport: techniques and devices, *The Journal of Air Medical Transport* 11(4):5-8, 1992.

INDEX

Page numbers in italics indicate illustrations; *t* indicates tables.

D

F

J

K

L

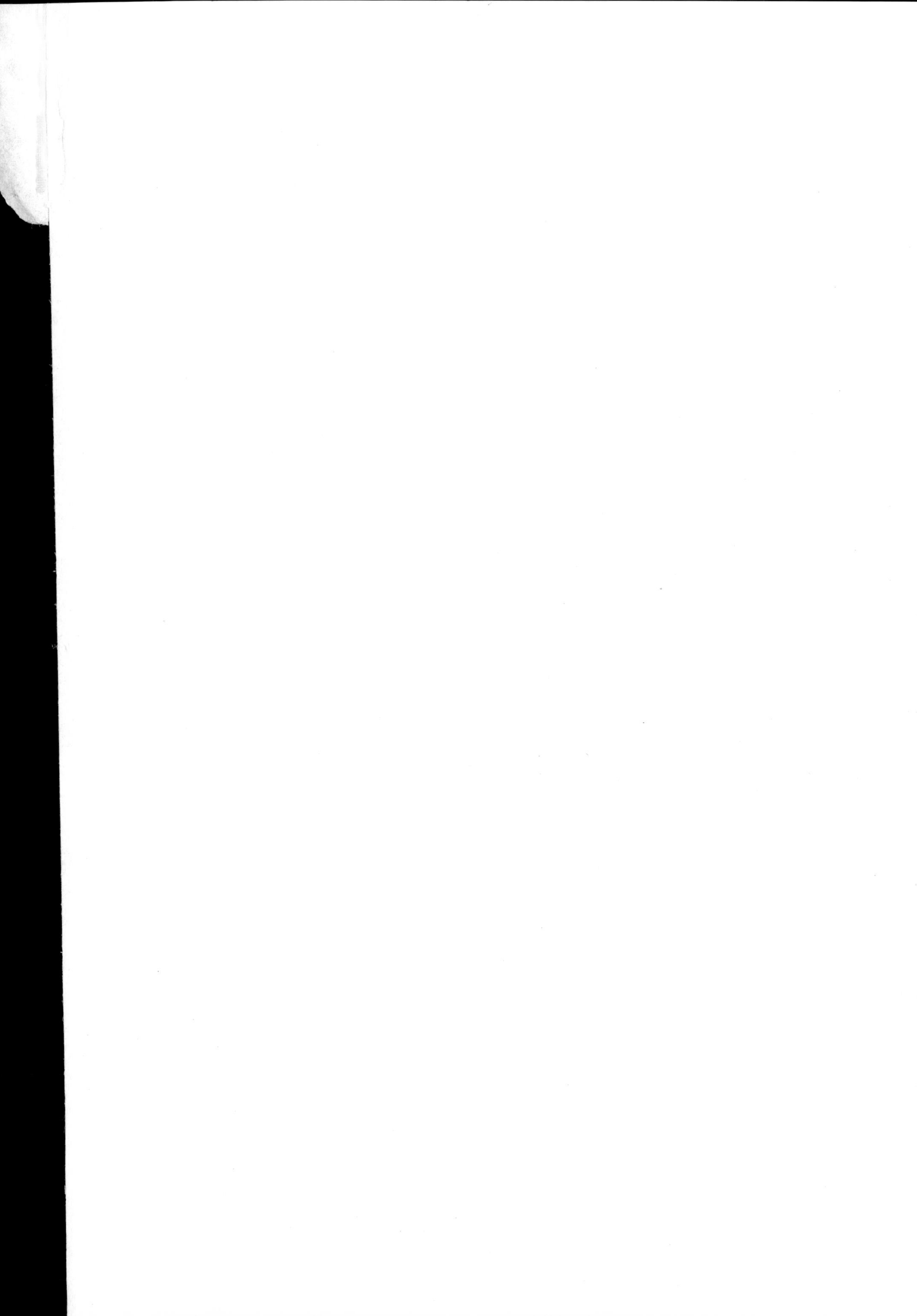